Health Promotion
Throughout the Life Span

Health Promotion
Throughout the Life Span

Eighth Edition

CAROLE LIUM EDELMAN, GCNS-BC, CMC
Private Practice
Professional Geriatric Care Management
Westport, Connecticut

ELIZABETH CONNELLY KUDZMA, DNSC, MPH, RNC
Professor; Director of MSN Program
Curry College, Division of Nursing
Milton, Massachusetts

CAROL LYNN MANDLE, PhD, CNS, FNP†
Former Associate Professor
Connell School of Nursing
Boston College
Chestnut Hill, Massachusetts;
Massachusetts General Hospital
Boston, Massachusetts

†Deceased.

ELSEVIER
MOSBY

3251 Riverport Lane
St. Louis, Missouri 63043

HEALTH PROMOTION THROUGHOUT THE LIFE SPAN, EIGHTH EDITION   ISBN: 978-0-323-09141-1
Copyright © 2014, by Mosby, an imprint of Elsevier Inc.

Previous editions copyright © 2010, 2006, 2002, 1998, 1994, 1986

Notices

Knowledge and best practice in this field are constantly changing. As new research and experience broaden our understanding, changes in research methods, professional practices, or medical treatment may become necessary.

Practitioners and researchers must always rely on their own experience and knowledge in evaluating and using any information, methods, compounds, or experiments described herein. In using such information or methods they should be mindful of their own safety and the safety of others, including parties for whom they have a professional responsibility.

With respect to any drug or pharmaceutical products identified, readers are advised to check the most current information provided (i) on procedures featured or (ii) by the manufacturer of each product to be administered, to verify the recommended dose or formula, the method and duration of administration, and contraindications. It is the responsibility of practitioners, relying on their own experience and knowledge of their patients, to make diagnoses, to determine dosages and the best treatment for each individual patient, and to take all appropriate safety precautions.

To the fullest extent of the law, neither the Publisher nor the authors, contributors, or editors, assume any liability for any injury and/or damage to persons or property as a matter of products liability, negligence or otherwise, or from any use or operation of any methods, products, instructions, or ideas contained in the material herein.

Library of Congress Cataloging-in-Publication Data
Health promotion throughout the life span / [edited by] Carole Lium Edelman,
Carol Lynn Mandle, Elizabeth C. Kudzma. -- Eighth edition.
     p. ; cm.
  Includes bibliographical references and index.
  ISBN 978-0-323-09141-1 (pbk. : alk. paper)
  I. Edelman, Carole, editor. II. Mandle, Carol Lynn, editor. III. Kudzma,
Elizabeth C., editor.
  [DNLM: 1. Nursing Care. 2. Health Promotion. 3. Nurse's Role. WY 100.1]
  RT90.3
  613--dc23   2013024901

Content Strategist: Nancy O'Brien
Senior Content Development Specialist: Maria Broeker
Publishing Services Manager: Jeff Patterson
Designer: Amy Buxton

Printed in China

Last digit is the print number: 9   8   7   6   5   4   3   2   1

In memory of our dear friend and colleague
Carol Lynn Mandle,
co-editor of *Health Promotion Throughout the Life Span* since 1986.
Carol Lynn passed away in April 2013.
She was one of those very special persons who gave the world something unique.
She will be remembered for her love, commitment, and dedication
to family, friends, colleagues, and students. We love and respect you deeply.
Rest in Peace.

CONTRIBUTORS

Gary P. Austin, PT, PhD, OCS, FAAOMPT
Associate Professor
Director, Orthopaedic Physical Therapy
   Residency Program
Doctoral Program in Physical Therapy
   Sacred Heart University
Fairfield, Connecticut
Chapter 12, Exercise

Kathleen Blais, EdD, RN
Professor Emerita
College of Nursing and Health Sciences
Florida International University
Miami, Florida
Chapter 24, Older Adult

Jennifer Elizabeth Brunton, PhD
Professor of Ethics, Bioethics and
   Philosophy
Community College of Vermont,
   Brattleboro
Brattleboro, Vermont
*Chapter 14, Complementary and Alternative
   Strategies*

Kevin K. Chui, PT, DPT, PhD, GCS, OCS
Associate Professor
University Department of Physical Therapy
   and Program in Geriatric Health &
   Wellness
College of Health Professions
Sacred Heart University
Fairfield, Connecticut
Chapter 12, Exercise

Tawna Cooksey-James, PhD, RN, CNE
Assistant Professor
School of Nursing
Ohio University
Athens, Ohio
*Chapter 2, Emerging Populations and Health
Chapter 15, Overview of Growth
   and Development Framework
Chapter 18, Toddler
Chapter 21, Adolescent*

Dee Coover, PhD, RN
Cardiac Disease Management Program
   Manager
Visiting Nurse Service in Westchester &
   Putnam
White Plains, New York
Chapter 23, Middle-Age Adult

Michael Fortin, PT, DPT
Clinician
Proaxis Physical Therapy
Spartanburg, South Carolina
Chapter 12, Exercise

Philip A. Greiner, DNSc, RN
Professor and Director
School of Nursing
College of Health & Human Services
San Diego State University
San Diego, California
*Chapter 1, Health Defined: Objectives for
   Promotion and Prevention*

Suzy Harrington, DNP, RN, MCHES
Director, Department for Health, Safety, and
   Wellness
American Nurses Association
Silver Spring, Maryland
*Chapter 9, Screening
Chapter 14, Complementary and Alternative
   Strategies*

Susan A. Heady, PhD, RN
Professor, Nursing Department
Webster University
St. Louis, Missouri
Chapter 10, Health Education

**June Andrews Horowitz, PhD, RN, PMh,
CNS-BC, FASAN**
Professor
William F. Connell School of Nursing
   Boston College
Chesnut Hill, Massachusetts
*Chapter 4, The Therapeutic Relationship
Chapter 13, Stress Management*

**Debora Elizabeth Kirsch, RN, MS,
CNS, PhDc**
Director of Undergraduate Nursing Studies
Clinical Assistant Professor
SUNY Upstate Medical University College
   of Nursing
Syracuse, New York
*Chapter 3, Health Policy and the Delivery
   System*

Yi-Hui Lee, PhD, MBA, MSN, BSN
Associate Professor
College of Nursing and Health
Wright State University
Dayton, Ohio
*Chapter 2, Emerging Populations and Health
Chapter 21, Adolescent*

Brian Pecchia, PT, DPT, ATC
Clinician
Millbrook Physical Therapy
Millbrook, New York
Chapter 12, Exercise

Roseanne M. Prunty, DPT
Physical Therapist
Acute Care and Acute Rehab
Bridgeport Hospital/Yale New Haven Health
Bridgeport, Connecticut
Chapter 12, Exercise

Anne Rath Rentfro, PhD, RN
Professor
University of Texas at Brownsville
Brownsville, Texas
Adjunct Faculty:
University of Texas Health Science Center,
   Houston
University of Texas Health Science Center,
   San Antonio
*Chapter 6, Health Promotion and the
   Individual
Chapter 7, Health Promotion and the Family
Chapter 8, Health Promotion and the
   Community
Chapter 19, Preschool Child*

Susan Scott Ricci, ARNP, MSN, MEd
Nursing Faculty
University of Central Florida College of
   Nursing
Orlando, Florida
*Chapter 16, The Prenatal Period
Chapter 17, Infant*

Jeffrey R. Ross, BFA, MA, MAT
English Teacher and ESL Tutor
Cyahoga Falt, Ohio
*Chapter 25, Health Promotion for the
   Twenty-First Century*

Ratchneewan Ross, PhD, MSc, RN
Associate Professor and Director of
   International Activities
College of Nursing
Kent State University
Kent, Ohio
*Chapter 25, Health Promotion for the Twenty-
   First Century*

Ali Salman, MD, PhD, ND
Associate Professor
Faculty of Health Studies
Brandon University
Manitoba, Canada
Chapter 2, Emerging Populations and Health
Chapter 21, Adolescent

Leslie Kennard Scott, PhD, PN-BC, CDE
College of Nursing/Pediatric Endocrinology
University of Kentucky
Lexington, Kentucky
Chapter 20, School-Age Child

Jeanne M. Sorrell, PhD, RN, FAAN
Senior Nurse Scientist, Cleveland Clinic
Professor Emerita
School of Nursing
George Mason University
Fairfax, Virginia
*Chapter 5, Ethical Issues Related to Health
    Promotion*

Toni M. Tucker, MA, RD
Woodbridge, Virginia
Chapter 11, Nutrition Counseling

Ancillary Contributors
Joanna E. Cain, BSN, RN
President and Founder
Auctorial Pursuits, Inc.
Austin, Texas
Study Questions
Case Studies

Anna K. Wehling Weepie, DNP, RN, CNE
Assistant Dean, Undergraduate Nursing
Professor, Allen College
Waterloo, Iowa
Test Bank

REVIEWERS

Janice A. Aloi, DMH, RN, CNE
Assistant Professor
Nursing Department
University of Medicine and Dentistry
Newark, New Jersey

Glenda Avery, PhD, ARNP
Associate Professor
Nursing Department
Troy University
Phenix City, Alabama

Margaret E. Barnes, RN, MSN
Assistant Professor
School of Nursing, RNBSN Post-Licensure
Division
Indiana Wesleyan University
Marion, Indiana

**Angeline Bushy, PhD, RN, FAAN,
PHCNS-BC**
College of Nursing
University of Central Florida
Orlando, Florida

Pamela N. Clarke, RN, MPH, PhD, FAAN
Professor and Director of the Center for
Community Health and Economic
Development
Fay W. Whitney School of Nursing
University of Wyoming
Laramie, Wyoming

Kim Clevenger, EdD, MSN, RN, BC
Associate Professor of Nursing
Department of Nursing
Morehead State University
Morehead, Kentucky

Nancy J. Cooley, MSN, RN, FNP-BC
Associate Professor of Nursing
University of Maine at Augusta
Augusta, Maine

Janice A. Edelstein, EdD, PHCNS-BC
Adjunct Community Health Nursing
Instructor
Nursing Department
Wisconsin Lutheran College
Milwaukee, Wisconsin

Dr. Mara Eisch
Clinical Assistant Professor Nursing
Department
University of Wisconsin—Madison
Madison, Wisconsin

Nanci Feltner, MSN/ED, RN
Assistant Professor
College of Health and Human Services
Concordia University—Portland
Portland, Oregon

Jessica Gonzales, RN, MSN
Nursing Department
North Seattle Community College
Seattle, Washington

Rosanna Henry, MSN
RN Instructor and Director, Clinical Lab
School of Nursing
Duquesne University
Pittsburgh, Pennsylvania

Carolyn Hulsen, MSN, RN
Professor of Nursing
Department of Nursing
Black Hawk College
Moline, Illinois

Vicki L. Imerman, MSN, RN
Professor
Nursing Department
Des Moines Area Community College
Boone, Iowa

**Scharmaine M. Lawson-Baker, DNP,
FNP-BC, FAANP**
CEO
Advanced Clinical Consultants
New Orleans, Louisiana

Margaret Ochab-Ohryn, CRNA, MBA
Associate Professor
Oakland Community College
Southfield, Michigan

Charlene M. Romer, RN, PhD
Associate Professor
Nursing Department
Clayton State University
Morrow, Georgia

Melissa L. Weir, MS, RN, CEN, CPEN
College of Nursing & Allied Health Sciences
Howard University
Washington, DC

Ann M. York, PhD
Associate Professor
Master of Health Care Administration
Program
Des Moines University
Des Moines, Iowa

Mary E. Abrums, RN, MN

Marinda Allender, RN, MSN, CPN

Douglas Bloomquist, PhD

Philip Boyle, PhD

Carolyn Spence Cagle, PhD, RNC

Lenny Chiang-Hanisko, PhD, RN

Jacqueline Clinton, PhD, RN, FAAN

Joni Cohen, RN, MN

Rebecca Cohen, RN, EdD

Katherine Smith Detherage, PhD, RN, CNAA

Helene Dixon, CNM, MSN

Martha Driessnack, PhD, APRN

Lea Edwards, BSN, MEd

James A. Fain, PhD, RN, RAAN

Gail Park Fast, MN

Marilyn Frank-Stromberg, EdD, NP

Carol Scheel Gavan, EdD, RN

Heather O'Brien Gillespie, MSPT

Pamela J. Grace, APRN, PhD

Qalvy Grainzvolt, BS

Sheila Grossman, PhD, APRN-BC

Krishan Gupta, MD

Lois Hancock, MSN, ARNP

Carolyn Hayes, PhD, RN

Janice Hooper, PhD, RN, CS

James S. Huddleston, MS, PT

Kathleen Huttlinger, PhD, FNP

Dennis T. Jaffe, PhD

Sally Stark Johnson, RN, MSN

Jeanette Lancaster, RN, PhD, FAAN

Gina C. Lowry, PhD, RN

Margaret K. Macali, MS, RN, CS

William Martimucci, MD

Ann Marie McCarthy, RN

Nancy Curro McCarthy, RN, EdD

Nancy Milio, PhD, FAAN, FAPHA

Katherine E. Murphy, MN, FNP

Lisa Newton, PhD

Jean M. O'Connor, MS, MPH, RNC, FNP

Reverend James O'Donahue, SJ, PhD

Ellen F. Olshansky, DNSc, RNC

Johanne Quinn, PhD, RN

Gurpal K. Sandhu, PhD

Jan Schurman, MN, FNP

Linda Snetselaar, PhD, RD

Arlene Spark, EdD, RD

Marie Truglio-Londrigan, PhD, RN, GNPC

Geraldine Valencia-Go, PhD, MA, RN, CS

Carol L. Wells-Federman, MS, MEd, RN, CS

PURPOSE OF THE BOOK

The case for promoting and protecting health, and preventing disease and injury was established by many accomplishments in the twentieth century. Americans are taking better care of themselves, and public concern about physical fitness, good nutrition, and avoidance of health hazards such as smoking has become ingrained in the lifestyles of many Americans.

Encouraging positive health changes has been a major effort of individuals, the government, health professionals, and society in general. In the United States, public and private attempts to improve the health status of individuals and groups traditionally have focused on reducing communicable diseases and health hazards. Now growing concerns exist to improve access to and reduce costs of health services and to improve the overall quality of life for all people. Americans increasingly recognized that the health of each individual is influenced by the health environments of all individuals worldwide.

Health-promotion advances require a better understanding of the environment, health risks, behaviors, and intervention measures. *Healthy People 2010* has identified important determinants of health status, which include the following:

- Individual behavior
- Biology and genetics
- Physical environment
- Social environment
- Health services

Outcome measures designed to assist individual efforts to change and improve behavior in these areas can lead to decreases in morbidity and mortality.

Professionals who undertake health-promotion strategies also need to understand the basics of health protection and disease and injury prevention. Health protection is directed at population groups of all ages and involves adherence to standards, infectious disease control, and governmental regulation and enforcement. The focus of these activities is on reducing exposure to various sources of hazards, including those related to air, water, foods, drugs, motor vehicles, and other physical agents.

Health care providers present individuals, families, and communities with disease- and injury-prevention services, which include immunizations, screenings, health education, and counseling. To implement prevention strategies effectively, it is essential to develop activities targeted to and tailored for all age groups in various settings, including schools, industries, the home, the health care delivery system, and the community.

Throughout the history of the United States, the public health community has assessed the health of Americans. In 1789, the Reverend Edward Wigglesworth developed the first American mortality tables through his study in New England. The *Report of a General Plan for the Promotion of Public and Personal Health* was completed by Lemuel Shattuck in 1880. *Healthy People, The Surgeon General's Report on Health Promotion and Disease Prevention,* was first published in 1979, and was followed by *Healthy People 2000: National Health Promotion and Disease Prevention Objectives,* which listed three goals to be achieved by the year 2000:

1. Increase the span of healthy life for Americans.
2. Reduce health disparities among Americans.
3. Achieve access to preventive services for all Americans.

Healthy People 2010 addressed these health problems by establishing goals and objectives for the first decade of the new millennium. The vision for *Healthy People 2010* was "Healthy People in Healthy Communities" because, as nursing has long recognized, the health of each individual is inseparable from the health of families, communities, the nation, and the world. Health is significantly affected by the environments in which each individual lives, works, travels, and plays. Dimensions of the environment are not only physical but also psychosocial and spiritual, including the behaviors, attitudes, and beliefs of each individual. Specific objectives in 28 focus areas supported 2 major goals:

1. Increase quality and years of healthy life.
2. Eliminate health disparities.

Released in 2010, *Healthy People 2020* reflects these assessments of major risks to health, changing public health priorities, and emerging issues related to our nation's health preparedness and prevention. The following vision was established: A society in which all people live long healthy lives.

The mission within this vision is improving health through strengthening policy. *Healthy People 2020* will:

- Identify nationwide health improvement priorities.
- Increase public awareness and understanding of the determinants of health, disease, and disability and the opportunities for progress.
- Provide measurable objectives and goals that can be used at the national, state, and local levels.
- Engage multiple sectors to take action that are driven by the best available evidence and knowledge.
- Identify critical research and data collection needs.

The overarching goals for *Healthy People 2020* continue the tradition of earlier *Healthy People* initiatives of advocating for improvements in the health of every person in our country. They address the environmental factors and place particular emphasis on the determinants of health:

- Eliminate preventable disease, disability, injury, and premature death.
- Achieve health equity, eliminate disparities, and improve the health of all groups.
- Create social and physical environments that promote good health for all.
- Promote healthy development and healthy behaviors across every stage of life.

These databases continue to provide assessments of health status and risk for evaluations and future planning, not only for health policymakers and health care providers but also for individuals, families, and communities at the local, regional, national, and global levels. (Subscribe to the *Healthy People* listserv for the latest information and to receive e-mail notices of related news, events, and publications at http://healthypeople.gov/hp2020.)

The information in this edition of *Health Promotion Throughout the Life Span* includes these and other data and recommendations for health promotion, health protection, preventive services, and surveillance data systems, including those to the U.S. Preventive Services Task Force (www.ahrq.gov/clinic/cps) and the Guide to Community Preventive Services (www.thecommunityguide.org).

APPROACH AND ORGANIZATION

This edition presents health data and related theories and skills that are needed to understand and practice when providing care. This book focuses on primary prevention intervention, based on the Leavell and Clark model; its three main components are: (1) health promotion, (2) specific health protection, and (3) prevention of specific diseases. Health promotion is the intervention designed to improve health, such as providing adequate nutrition, a healthy environment, and ongoing health education. Specific protection and prevention strategies, such as massive immunizations, periodic examinations, and safety features in the workplace, are the interventions used to protect against illness.

In addition to primary prevention, this book discusses secondary prevention intervention, focusing specifically on screening. Such programs include blood pressure, glaucoma, and diabetes screening and referral (the acute component of secondary prevention is not addressed in this book).

This text is presented in five parts, each forming the basis for the next.

Unit 1, *Foundations for Health Promotion,* describes the foundational concepts of promoting and protecting health, and preventing diseases and injuries, including diagnostic, therapeutic, and ethical decision-making based on the nursing emphasis of health patterns as described by Margaret Newman.

Unit 2, *Assessment for Health Promotion,* focuses on individuals, families, and communities and the factors affecting their health. The functional health pattern assessments developed by Gordon serve as the organizing framework for assessing the health of individuals, families, and communities.

Unit 3, *Interventions for Health Promotion,* discusses theories, methodologies, and case studies of nursing interventions, including screening, health-education counseling, stress management, and crisis intervention.

Unit 4, *Application of Health Promotion,* also uses Gordon's functional health patterns, emphasizing developmental, cultural, ethnic, and environmental variables in assessing the developing person. The intent is to address the health concerns of all Americans regardless of gender, race, age, or sexual orientation. Although the human development theories discussed are primarily based on the research of male subjects, emerging theories based on female subjects have been included. The hope is to describe human development that more accurately reflects the complexity of human experiences throughout the life span.

Unit 5, *Challenges in the Twenty-First Century,* presents a single chapter that discusses changing population groups and their health needs as well as related implications for research and practice in the twenty-first century. Throughout the text, research abstracts have been added to highlight the science of nursing practice and to demonstrate to the reader the relationship among research, practice, and outcomes.

Throughout these units, the evolving health care professions and the changing health care systems, including future challenges and initiatives for health promotion, are described. Emphasis is placed on the current concerns of reducing health care costs while increasing life expectancy and improving the quality of life for all Americans. This promotes the reader's immediate interest in thoughts about the content of the chapters.

Key Features

- A **full-color design,** including color photos, has been implemented throughout for better accessibility of content and visual enhancement.
- Each chapter starts with a list of **objectives** to help focus the reader and emphasize the content the reader should acquire through reading the book. **Key Terms** including quality and safety terms are listed at the front to acquaint readers with the important terminology of the chapter.
- Each chapter's narrative begins with **Think About It,** the presentation of a clinical issue or scenario that relates to the topic of the chapter, followed by critical thinking questions. This promotes the reader's immediate interest in and thought about the chapter.
- **Research for Evidence-Based Practice** boxes provide brief synopses on current health-promotion research studies that demonstrate the links between research, theory, and practice.
- **Diversity Awareness** boxes offer cultural perspectives on various aspects of health promotion.
- **Hot Topics** explores current ethical issues, controversies, and dilemmas with respect to health promotion, providing an opportunity for critical analysis of care issues.
- The **Case Study** highlights a real-life clinical situation relevant to the chapter topic.
- The **Care Plan** relates to the Case Study with the standardized sections of Defining Characteristics, Related Factors, Expected Outcomes, and Interventions, and details nursing diagnoses relevant to health-promotion activities and the related interventions.
- **Innovative Practice** boxes highlight inventive and resourceful projects, programs, and research studies that draw upon new ways of implementing health promotion.
- *Healthy People 2020* boxes present a list of selected objectives that are relevant to each chapter's topic.
- **Website Resources** include expanded chapter resources, such as assessment tools, developmental charts, and immunization schedules.
- **Study Questions** are located on the book's website to offer additional review and self-study practice.

New Features

1. Objectives of *Healthy People 2020* (http://healthypeople.gov) and a link to new listings of the developing data and goals for 2020 on the book's Evolve website
2. More comprehensive research to further develop evidence-based practices
3. Comprehensive emphasis on quality and safety, including information from the Quality & Safety Education for Nurses (QSEN) project
4. Updated photos and figures throughout the book
5. Specific emphasis on growth and development throughout the life span
6. Expanded content in Chapter 3 on financing and global health
7. Updated information on the *Dietary Guidelines for Americans* including the recommended content of each dinner plate

Evolve Resources

The expanded website for this book provides materials for both students and faculty, and is accessible at http://evolve.elsevier.com/Edelman/.

For Students

- **Website Resources:** Resources that supplement the chapter discussion
- **Study Questions:** Multiple choice and in NCLEX® format
- **Glossary:** Comprehensive list of all Key Terms and their definitions; search capability allows searching by term, definition, or chapter

For Instructors

- **TEACH for Nurses,** including Nursing Curriculum Standards, Teaching Activities, and Case Studies
- **Research Evaluation and Critique**
- **Image Collection,** with all images from the book
- **Lecture Slides,** in PowerPoint
- **Test Bank,** 700 questions in NCLEX format, including the new innovative item format

The current trend to emphasize the developing health of people mandates that health care professionals understand the many issues that surround individuals, families, and communities in social, work, and family settings, including biological, inherited, cognitive, psychological, environmental, and sociocultural factors that can put their health at risk. Most important is that they develop interventions to promote health by understanding the diverse roles these factors play in the person's beliefs and health practices, particularly in the areas of disease and injury prevention, protection, and health promotion. Achieving such effectiveness requires collaboration with other health care providers and the integration of practice and policy while developing interventions and considering the ethical issues within individual, family, and community responsibilities for health.

Carole Lium Edelman
Elizabeth C. Kudzma
Carol Lynn Mandle

ACKNOWLEDGMENTS

We had the good fortune of receiving much assistance and support from many friends, relatives, and associates. Our colleagues read chapters, gave valuable advice and criticism, helped clarify concepts, and provided case examples.

We also acknowledge the contributions of all the authors. In developing this text, they gave the project their total commitment and support. Their professional competence aided greatly in the development of the final draft of the manuscript. Special thanks go to Diana Seib for assistance with the manuscript.

The editors worked and learned from each other during the planning and development of this book; throughout the entire process, close contact prevailed. Elizabeth Kudzma, a long-standing contributor, is now part of the text's editorial team. She has added much knowledge and perspective to the eighth edition.

Many thanks to the Elsevier editorial team: Nancy O'Brien, Maria Broeker, Jeanne Genz, and Jacqueline Kiley. We appreciate and thank them for their ongoing help and support. It was a true pleasure working with them.

I am fortunate to have faith in the Lord, who gives courage and strength to face life's difficulties in a positive manner. My children, John and Megan Gillespie, Tom and Heather Gillespie, and Deirdre O'Brien, and my grandchildren, Ryan, Caroline, Meredith, and Colleen, bring joy to me as a grandmother and mother. Their patience and love are truly appreciated.

Rachel Pennacchia provides much encouragement and support. Fredric Edelman gives continued joy and happiness in our marriage.

Carole Lium Edelman

In the continued development of health, I acknowledge our faith in God and the joy of friends; the love of marriage and family with Robert, Elizabeth, Jonathan, Stephanie, David, Fiona, and Adeline; the commitments of nurses to social justice in the care of all people; and the knowledge we are continually becoming...

Carol Lynn Mandle

As a contributor from the first edition to the present, I thank Carole Edelman and Carol Mandle for inviting me to assist with this eighth edition. The insights and clinical experiences of Curry College faculty colleagues and students are continuing sources of enrichment. Thanks also to my family, including my sister and brother (Mark and Mary), daughter Katherine, and especially to my husband Daniel, who provided support, discussion, and insight throughout this project.

Elizabeth Connelly Kudzma

To our wonderful families, friends, students, and colleagues—
that they promote health in themselves and others.

CONTENTS

UNIT 2   ASSESSMENT FOR HEALTH PROMOTION

UNIT 5   EMERGING GLOBAL HEALTH ISSUES

Health Promotion
Throughout the Life Span

UNIT 1

Foundations for Health Promotion

Health Defined: Objectives for Promotion and Prevention

Philip A. Greiner

 WEBSITE

http://evolve.elsevier.com/Edelman/
- Study Questions
- Glossary

OBJECTIVES

After completing this chapter, the reader will be able to:
- Analyze concepts and models of *health* as used historically and as used in this textbook.
- Evaluate the consistency of *Healthy People 2020* goals with various concepts of health.
- Analyze the progress made in this nation from the original *Healthy People* document to the foci in *Healthy People 2020.*
- Differentiate between health, illness, disease, disability, and premature death.

- Compare the three levels of prevention (primary, secondary, and tertiary) with the levels of service provision available across the life span.
- Critique the role of research and evidence as well as the nurse's role in health education and research for the promotion of health for individuals and populations.

KEY TERMS

Adaptive model of health
Applied research
Asset planning
Clinical model of health
Community-based care
Cultural competence
Disease
Ecological model of health
Empathy
Epidemiology
Ethnocentrism
Eudaimonistic

Eudaimonistic model of health
Evidence-based practice
Functional health
Health
Health disparities
Health promotion
Health-related quality of life (HRQoL)
Healthy People 2020
High-level wellness
Illness
Interprofessional practice
Levels of prevention

Person-centered care
Qualitative studies
Quality of life
Quantitative studies
Racism
Role performance model of health
Social determinants of health
Specific protection
Well-being
Wellness
Wellness-illness continuum

Use of Complementary and Alternative Therapies

One of the biggest challenges to health care providers is the blending of Western medicine and health practices with the health practices from other cultures and ethnic groups. The federal government formed the National Center for Complementary and Alternative Medicine (NCCAM) [http://nccam.nih .gov/] to conduct and support basic and applied research and training and to disseminate information on complementary and alternative medicine to practitioners and the public. As demographics of the United States shift, more people use a combination of therapies in self-care and for the treatment of specific illnesses.

- What questions should the student ask to obtain information from people about their use of nontraditional therapies?
- What information should the student know about the benefits or limitations of using complementary therapies, such as acupuncture, spiritual healing, herbal remedies, or chiropractic?
- What resources should the student trust for information on the efficacy and use of herbal remedies relative to prescription medications?
- Which ideas of health would be most compatible with the use of alternative therapies?
- How can alternative therapies be integrated into *Healthy People 2020* objectives, given that the emphasis of these objectives is the use of available community resources and the development of partnerships?

Health is a core concept in society. This concept is modified with qualifiers such as *excellent, good, fair,* or *poor,* based on a variety of factors. These factors may include age, gender, race or ethnic heritage, comparison group, current health or physical condition, past conditions, social or economic situation, geographic location, or the demands of various roles in society. In addition, there is growing evidence that larger societal and environmental concerns determine health outcomes. This chapter will discuss health as a concept and related concepts such as wellness, illness, disease, disability, and functioning. These concepts are frequently embedded in theories, such as theories of health behavior (Pender et al., 2010) or health planning (Issel, 2009). Some motivating factors behind the move to disease prevention and health promotion in society will be examined with an introduction to *Healthy People 2020,* the federal government's health objectives for the nation. The implementation of these concepts as nursing actions will also be addressed from ideal and pragmatic standpoints. Research and evidence supporting these concepts, and recommendations for further research, will be presented.

Nurses understand the pivotal role they play in promoting health and preventing disease, the important role of research in the knowledge of what is "healthy," and the central role of epidemiology (the study of health and disease in society) and public health theories in the everyday practice of nursing.

EXPLORING CONCEPTS OF HEALTH

Dr. Margaret Newman (2003), a nursing theorist, states that definitions of health in the nursing literature can be classified broadly within two major paradigms. The first paradigm is the wellness-illness continuum, a dichotomized portrayal of health and illness ranging from high-level wellness at the positive end to depletion of health at the negative end. High-level wellness is further conceptualized as a sense of well-being, life satisfaction, and quality of life. Movement toward the negative end of the continuum includes adaptation to disease and disability through various levels of functional ability. The wellness-illness conceptualization was the focus of early research and is consistent with some of the categories Dr. Judith Baigis Smith (1983) identified in her philosophical analysis of health. Research based on this paradigm conforms primarily to scientific methods that seek to control contextual effects, provide the basis for causal explanations, and predict future outcomes (for example, see Kaplow and Reed [2008]).

The second paradigm characterizes health as a perspective developmental phenomenon of unitary patterning of the person-environment. The developmental perspective of health has been present in the nursing literature since 1970, but it was not identified clearly with health until the late 1970s and early 1980s. It has been conceptualized as expanding consciousness, pattern or meaning recognition, personal transformation, and, tentatively, self-actualization. This shift toward a developmental perspective has had clear implications for the way in which health is conceptualized (Newman, 2003). Although not endorsing the developmental perspective to the extent of Rogers (1970) and Reed (1983), Pender and colleagues (2010) and Allen and Warner (2002) state that health is an outcome of ongoing patterns of person and environment interactions throughout the life span. Research within this paradigm seeks to address the dynamic whole of the health experience through behavioral and social mechanisms over time. Health can be better understood if each person is seen as a part of a complex, interconnected biological and social system.

A more recent and comprehensive developmental approach is the ecological model of health (Institute of Medicine [IOM], 2003), which is useful for promoting health at individual, family, community, and societal levels. This model was updated in 2008 (and the 2010 report adding quality of life) with an emphasis on the social determinants of health—those factors in society that have an influence on health and the options available to people to improve or maintain their health. (These models are also reviewed in Richard, Gauvin, and Raine [2011].) In this way, the ecological model of health is more compatible with Smith's descriptions of health as adaptation and eudemonia (self-actualization). The social determinants of health also form the basis for *Healthy People 2020* (U.S. Department of Health and Human Services [USDHHS], 2011). Each of these ideas will be examined in more detail throughout this chapter.

People involved in health promotion must consider the meaning of health for themselves and for others. Recognizing differences in the meaning of health can clarify outcomes and expectations in health promotion and enhance the quality of health care. Because health is used to describe a number of entities, including a philosophy of care (health promotion and health maintenance), a system (health care delivery system), practices (evidence-based health practices), behaviors (personal health behaviors), costs (health care costs), and insurance (uninsured health care), the reason that confusion continues regarding the use of the term "health" becomes clear. People's use of the term "health," and its incorporation into these various entities, has also changed over time.

Americans born before 1940 experienced the greatest changes in how health is defined. Because infectious diseases claimed the lives of many children and young adults at that time, health was viewed as the absence of disease. The physician in independent practice was the primary provider of health care services, with services provided in the private office. The federal government was only beginning to establish its role in working with states to address public health and welfare issues (Barr et al., 2003).

As the national economy expanded during and after World War II in the 1940s and 1950s, the idea of role performance became a focus in industrial research and entered the health care lexicon. Health became linked to a person's ability to fulfill a role in society. Increasingly, the physician was asked to complete physical examination forms for school, work, military, and insurance purposes while physician practice became linked more directly to hospital-based services. The federal government expanded its role through funding for hospital expansion and establishment of a new Department of Health, Education, and Welfare (DHEW), currently the Department of Health and Human Services (DHHS) (Barr et al., 2003). It was recognized that a person might recover from a disease yet be unable to fulfill family or work roles because of residual changes from the illness episode. Concepts of disability and rehabilitation entered the health care arena. The work or school environment was viewed as a possible contributor to health, illness, disability, and death.

From the 1960s to the present, there have been incredible changes in the health care delivery system while federal and state governments attempted to control spending and health care costs escalated (Barr et al., 2003). Primary care providers, including nurse practitioners and other advanced practice nurses, now attempt to involve individuals and their families in the delivery of person-centered care, and teaching individuals about individual responsibilities and lifestyle choices has become an important part of their job. Health care became an interdisciplinary endeavor even while managed care companies limited the health promotion options available under insurance plans. During this time, the idea of adaptation had an important influence on the way Americans view health. Increasingly health became linked to individuals' reactions to the environment rather than being viewed as a fixed state. Adaptation fit well with the self-help movement during the 1970s and with the progressive growth in knowledge from research about disease prevention and health promotion at the individual level.

Emphasis is being placed on the quality of a person's life as a component of health (USDHHS, 2000; USDHHS, 2011). Research on self-rated health (Cano et al., 2003; Idler & Benyamini, 1997) and self-rated function (Greiner et al., 1999) indicates that there are multiple factors contributing to a person's perception of his or her health, sometimes referred to as functional health (Gordon, 2010) or health-related quality of life (HRQoL) (Andresen et al., 2003; DHHS, 2011). There are multiple tools available for measuring quality of life, including a general measure established by the World Health Organization (WHO, 2004) (The World Health Organization Quality of Life, WHOQOL-BREF) and the McGill Quality of Life Questionnaire (Cohen et al., 1997) for use at the end of life (Box 1-1: Quality and Safety Scenario).

Models of Health

Throughout history, society has entertained a variety of concepts of health (David, 2000). Smith (1983) describes four distinct models of health in her classic work:

Clinical Model

In the clinical model, health is defined by the absence and illness by the conspicuous presence of signs and symptoms of disease. People who use this model may not seek preventive health services or they may wait until they are very ill to seek care. The clinical model is the conventional model of the discipline of medicine.

Role Performance Model

The role performance model of health defines health in terms of individuals' ability to perform social roles. Role performance includes work, family, and social roles, with performance based on societal expectations. Illness would be the failure to perform roles at the level of others in society. This model is the basis for occupational health evaluations, school physical examinations, and physician-excused absences. The idea of the "sick role," which excuses people from performing their social functions, is a vital component of the role performance model. It is argued that the sick role is still relevant in health care today (Davis et al., 2011; Shilling, 2002).

Adaptive Model

In the adaptive model of health, people's ability to adjust positively to social, mental, and physiological change is the measure of their health. Illness occurs when the person fails to adapt or becomes maladaptive to these changes. As the concept of adaptation has entered other aspects of American culture, this model of health has become more accepted. For example, spirituality can be useful in adapting to a decreased level of functioning in older adults (Haley et al., 2001).

Eudaimonistic Model

In the eudaimonistic model exuberant well-being indicates optimal health. This model emphasizes the interactions between physical, social, psychological, and spiritual aspects of life and the environment that contribute to goal attainment and create meaning. Illness is reflected by a denervation or languishing, a lack of involvement with life. Although these ideas may appear to be new when compared with the clinical model of health, aspects of the eudaimonistic model predate the clinical model of health. This model is also more congruent with integrative modes of therapy (National Institutes of Health, National Center for Complementary and Alternative Medicine [NIH/NCCAM], 2011), which are used increasingly by people of all ages in the United States and the world. In this eudaimonistic model, a person dying of cancer may still be healthy if that person is finding meaning in life at this stage of development.

Fall Prevention in the Home

Falls in the home are a common yet preventable source of both fatal and nonfatal injuries. In 2012, the Centers for Disease Control and Prevention reported in their *Morbidity and Mortality Weekly Report, QuickStats* section that older adults ages 75 and older had the most nonfatal injury falls in which health care providers were consulted because of the injury. These data, from a 2010 *National Health Interview Survey*, indicate that 12% of this older adult population experience a fall significant enough to seek health care.

There are specific factors that contribute to fall risk, including changes to the person attributable to age, medication use, and environmental hazards. Nurses are in key roles to work with older adults to assess fall risks and help them gain control over this aspect of their health. The National Center for Injury Prevention and Control at CDC provides guidelines for fall prevention in older adults at www.cdc.gov/ncipc/pub-res/toolkit/checklistforsafety.htm.

Risk factors attributable to the aging process include visual, hearing, and functional limitations. Although pets have proven to be a benefit for older adults by providing companionship and comfort, they can also scamper underfoot or the older adult may trip over the pet because the pet is not seen or heard. Loss of night vision and depth perception also can contribute to falls when lighting is poor or when moving from room to room. Older adults should be encouraged to always wear prescribed vision and hearing aids when moving about the house or apartment. Loss of upper and lower body strength can also contribute to fall risk. Lower body strength is needed to lift legs and feet high enough to navigate stairs and changes in texture of flooring. Upper body strength allows the use of supports when moving about. Watch the person maneuver about the living space and note the use of furniture, walls, and other objects for support.

Medications can contribute to disequilibrium. A careful review of currently used medications, both prescribed and over-the-counter, can help identify possible medications that could contribute to fall risks. Environmental risks include clutter, too much furniture for the room, placement of items in typical walkways, lighting problems, needed repairs to flooring and walls, and the need for supports such as grab bars and railings. Again, watching the person navigate through the home is helpful in recognizing potential trip hazards and areas where additional supports are needed. Adequate hydration is another consideration, especially if the person is taking medications that contribute to dehydration without regular fluid replacement or if the temperature of the home and environment is too high.

Health outcomes for the person can be significant. Falls can cause minor injury and embarrassment, but they can also cause life-threatening injuries such as fractures and head injuries. If a fall has occurred, it is helpful to do a root cause analysis to determine those factors that contributed to the fall. Ask permission before attempting to make any alteration to the home, because items and their placement may have sentimental importance to the person. Address medication changes with the person, pharmacist, and/or primary care provider. Some medication habits may be hard for the person to change.

The nursing implications of fall risk are many and varied. Assessment skills must be practiced in a variety of settings so that the nurse is vigilant for potential hazards and individual factors that might precipitate a fall. Older adults should be routinely observed performing their daily routines to identify visual, hearing, and functional decline. Also, if a person reports a fall, that report should trigger a more extensive evaluation of that individual because falls may be indicative of future fall risk.

Falls are a frequent but preventable occurrence, especially for older adults. Falls also contribute millions of dollars each year to the cost of health care as a result of personal injury and disability. That is why fall prevention is a key feature of quality and safety education for nurses.

Questions
- Can you identify at least four items in your own environment that may contribute to your fall risk?
- How would you structure an interview with an older adult to determine the presence of fall risks in that person's home?
- What evidence and arguments would you use to encourage an older adult to modify the home environment to decrease the risk of a fall?

Sources: Adams, P. F., Martinez, M. E., Vickerie, J. L., & Kirzinger, W. K. (2010). Summary health statistics for the U.S. population: National Health Interview Survey, 2010. *Vital Health Statistics 2011*, 10, 251; CDC. (2012). QuickStats: Rate of nonfatal, medically consulted fall injury episodes, by age group. *Morbidity Mortality Weekly Report, 61(04),* 81.

These ideas of health provide a basis for how people view health and disease and how they view the roles of nurses, physicians, and other health care providers. For example, in the clinical model of health, a person may expect to see a health care provider only when there are obvious signs of illness. Personal responsibility for health may not be a motivating factor for this individual because the provider is responsible for dealing with the health problem and returning the person to health. Therefore attempts to teach health promoting activities may not be effective with this person. On the other hand, those who adopt a eudaimonistic model of health may find that practitioners working under a clinical model do not address their more comprehensive health needs. They may instead seek out a practitioner of alternative medicine or the council of a priest, rabbi, or minister to complement the services of the more traditional health provider.

Wellness-Illness Continuum

The wellness-illness continuum, as stated earlier, is a dichotomous depiction of the relationship between the concepts of health and illness. In this paradigm, wellness is a positive state in which incremental increases in health can be made beyond the midpoint (Figure 1-1). These increases involve improved physical and mental health states. The opposite end of the continuum is illness, with the possibility of incremental decreases in health beyond the midpoint. This depiction of the relationship of wellness and illness fits well with the clinical model of health.

High-Level Wellness

From a dichotomous representation of health and illness as opposites, Dunn (1961) developed a health-illness continuum that assessed a person not only in terms of his or her relative health compared with that of others but also in terms of the favorability of the person's environment for health and wellness (see Figure 1-1). Adding this second dimension to the health-illness continuum created a matrix in which a favorable environment allows high-level wellness to occur and an unfavorable environment allows low-level wellness to exist.

With this addition, it became possible to combine the clinical model of health with models based on social and environmental parameters. The concept demonstrates that a person can have a

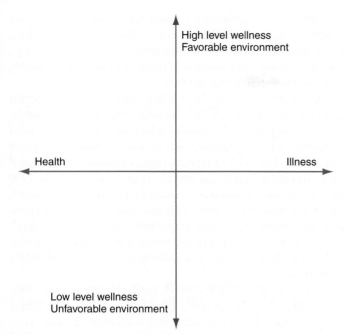

FIGURE 1-1 Wellness-illness continuum with high-level wellness added. Moving from the center to the right demonstrates movement toward illness. Moving from the center to the left demonstrates movement toward health. Moving above the line demonstrates movement toward increasing wellness. Moving below the line demonstrates movement toward decreasing wellness. (Adapted from U.S. Department of Health and Human Services, Public Health Service, 1982.)

terminal disease and be emotionally prepared for death, while acting as a support for other people and achieving high-level wellness. High-level wellness involves progression toward a higher level of functioning, an open-ended and ever-expanding future with its challenge of fuller potential and the integration of the whole being (Ardell, 2007). This definition of high-level wellness contains ideas similar to those in the eudaimonistic model of health. Additionally, high-level wellness emphasizes the interrelationship between the environment and the ability to achieve health on both a personal and a societal level.

Health Ecology

An evolving view of health recognizes the interconnection between people and their physical and social environments. Newman (2003) expressed this interconnection within a developmental framework, and the work of Gordon (2010) applies this interconnection to functional health patterns as presented in subsequent chapters. Health from an ecological perspective is multidimensional, extending from the individual into the surrounding community, and including the context within which the person functions. It incorporates a systems approach within which the actions of one portion of the system affect the functioning of the system as a whole (IOM, 2003, 2010). This view of health expands on high-level wellness by recognizing that there are social and environmental factors that can enhance or limit health and healthy behaviors. For example, most people can benefit from physical activity such as walking, and people are more likely to walk in areas where there are sidewalks or

walking paths and where they feel safe. Nurses can encourage people to walk, but may also need to advocate for safe areas for people to walk and work with others to plan for people-friendly community development.

Functioning

One of the defining characteristics of life is the ability to function. Functional health can be characterized as being present or absent, having high-level or low-level wellness, and being influenced by neighborhood and society. Functioning is integral to health. There are physical, mental, and social levels of function and these are reflected in terms of performance and social expectations. Function can also be viewed from an ecological perspective, as in the example of walking used previously. Loss of function may be a sign or symptom of a disease. For example, sudden loss of the ability to move an arm or leg may indicate a stroke. The inability to leave the house may indicate overwhelming fear. In both cases, the loss of function is a sign of disease, a state of ill health. Loss of function is a good indicator that the person may need nursing intervention. Research in older adults indicates that decline in physical function is a sentinel event and may indicate the future loss of physical function and death (Boltz et al., 2012; Greiner et al., 1996).

HEALTH

Health, as defined in this text, is a state of physical, mental, spiritual, and social functioning that realizes a person's potential and is experienced within a developmental context. Although health is, in part, an individual's responsibility, health also requires collective action to ensure a society and an environment in which people can act responsibly to support health. The culture and beliefs of people can also influence health action. This definition is consistent with the World Health Organization (WHO) definition of health as the state of complete physical, mental, and social well-being and not merely the absence of disease and infirmity (WHO, 2004), but moves beyond this definition to encompass spiritual, developmental, and environmental aspects over time. The physical aspect includes one's genetic makeup, which when combined with the other aspects influences one's longevity. This broader definition is applicable across the life span, as well as in situations where illness may be a chronic state. For example, in this broader definition of health, a person with diabetes may be considered healthy if she is able to adapt to her illness and live a meaningful, spiritually satisfying life. Health is considered to be part of the metaparadigm for nursing (Fawcett, 1984), which includes the four components of person, health, environment, and nursing. As can be seen in the discussion thus far, health can be viewed in a variety of ways.

ILLNESS, DISEASE, AND HEALTH

It is easy to think of health or wellness as the lack of disease and to consider illness and disease as interchangeable terms. However, health and disease are not simply antonyms and disease and illness are not synonyms. Disease literally means "without ease." **Disease** may be defined as the failure of a person's adaptive mechanisms to counteract stimuli and stresses adequately, resulting in functional or structural disturbances. This definition is an ecological concept of disease, which uses multiple factors to determine the cause of disease rather than describing a single cause. This multifactorial approach increases the chances of discovering multiple points of intervention to improve health.

Illness is composed of the subjective experience of the individual and the physical manifestation of disease (Hollingsworth & Didelot, 2005). Both are social constructs in which people are in an imbalanced, unsustainable relationship with their environment and are failing in their ability to survive and create a higher quality of life. Illness can be described as a response characterized by a mismatch between a person's needs and the resources available to meet those needs. Additionally, illness signals to individuals and populations that the present balance is not working. Within this definition, illness has psychological, spiritual, and social components. A person can have a disease without feeling ill (e.g., asymptomatic hypertension). A person can also feel ill without having a diagnosable disease (e.g., as a result of stress). Our understanding of disease and illness within society, overlaid with our understanding of the natural history of each disease, creates a basis for promoting health.

PLANNING FOR HEALTH

Public health has always had the prevention of disease in society as its focus. However, over the past 30 years, the promotion of health and individual responsibility moved to the forefront within public health, become a driving force in health care reform.

A key milestone in promoting health was the advent of *Healthy People* (U.S. Department of Health, Education, and Welfare [USDHEW], Public Health Service, 1979), the first Surgeon General's report on health promotion and disease prevention issued in the later years of President Carter's administration. This document identified five national health goals addressing the reduction of death in adults and children and the reduction of sick days in older adults.

- To continue to improve infant health, and, by 1990, to reduce infant mortality by at least 35%, to fewer than 9 deaths per 1000 live births
- To improve child health, foster optimal childhood development, and, by 1990, reduce deaths among children ages 1 to 14 years by at least 20%, to fewer than 34 per 100,000
- To improve the health and health habits of adolescents and young adults, and, by 1990, to reduce deaths among people ages 15 to 24 by at least 20%, to fewer than 93 per 100,000
- To improve the health of adults, and, by 1990, to reduce deaths among people ages 25 to 64 by at least 25%, to fewer than 400 per 100,000
- To improve the health and quality of life for older adults, and, by 1990, to reduce the average annual number of days of restricted activity attributable to acute and chronic conditions by 20%, to fewer than 30 days per year for people 65 and older

Further, the document identified three causes of the major health issues in the United States as allowing careless habits, environmental pollution, and harmful social conditions (e.g., hunger, poverty, and ignorance) to persist that destroy health, especially for infants and children.

Healthy People was a call to action and an attempt to set health goals for the United States for the next 10 years. Unfortunately, a change in political leadership, a lack of political and social willpower, and the spiraling costs of hospital-based health care intervened. The need to report progress toward these national objectives led a larger, renewed effort in the form of *The 1990 Health Objectives for the Nation: A Midcourse Review* (USDHHS, Public Health Service, 1986). This midcourse review noted that, although many goals were achievable, the unachieved goals were hindered by current health status, limited progress on risk reduction, difficulties in data collection, and a lack of public awareness.

Healthy People 2000 (USDHHS, Public Health Service, 1990) and its *Midcourse Review and 1995 Revisions* (USDHHS, Public Health Service, 1996) were landmark documents in that a consortium of people representing national organizations worked with U.S. Public Health Service officials to create a more global approach to health. Additionally, a management-by-objectives approach was used to address each problem area. These two documents became the blueprints for each state as funding for federal programs became linked to meeting these national health objectives. While the objectives became more widely implemented, methods for collecting data became formalized and the data flowed back into the system to form the revisions set in 1995. The core of these health objectives remained: that is, prevention of illness and disease was the foundation for health. *Healthy People 2000* established three broad goals:

- Increase the span of healthy life.
- Reduce health disparities.
- Create access to preventive services for all.

Additionally, the work included 22 specific areas for achievement, with objectives in each area based on age, health disparities, and health needs. By 1995, progress was made on 70% of the objectives. However, for 30% of the objectives, movement toward goals was in the wrong direction, had experienced no change, or could not be determined because of a lack of data.

Healthy People 2010 (USDHHS, Public Health Service, 2000), introduced two overarching goals:

- Increase quality and years of healthy life.
- Eliminate health disparities.

The first goal addressed the issues of longevity and quality of life. Both longevity and quality of life address the concern that people are living longer but frequently with numerous chronic health problems that interfere with the quality of their lives. However, quality of life is also an issue for people who are unable to achieve a long life. Combining these two ideas placed an emphasis on both longevity and quality of life as areas that need improvement.

The second goal, eliminating health disparities, addressed the continuing problems of access to care; differences in treatment based on race, gender, and ability to pay; and related issues such as urban versus rural health, insurance coverage, Medicare and

Medicaid reimbursement for care, and satisfaction with service delivery.

From these goals, the *Final Report* (CSDH, 2008) was completed using the 733 objectives (of the original 969 objectives) for which tracking data were available. A total of 23% of these objectives were met, with another 48% moving toward their targets, representing positive responses on 71% of the objectives. However, 5% of the objectives demonstrated no change from baseline and 24% of the objectives moved in a negative direction from target. For example, look at Focus Area 19: Nutrition and Overweight. Of 22 objectives, none were met, 2 moved toward the target, 3 demonstrated no change, and 15 moved away from the target. These findings are consistent with the epidemic of overweight and obesity in the United States and reflect the continuing influence of factors in our society that contribute to inactivity and weight gain (Ogden et al., 2006).

HEALTHY PEOPLE 2020

Goals

For *Healthy People 2020* (U.S. Department of Health and Human Services, 2011), there are four overarching goals:

- Attain high quality, longer lives free of preventable disease, disability, injury, and premature death.
- Achieve health equity, eliminate disparities, and improve the health of all groups.
- Create social and physical environments that promote good health for all.
- Promote quality of life, healthy development, and healthy behaviors across all life stages.

These four goals established the territory in which health promotion and disease prevention efforts take place. Research in a variety of areas has clearly indicated that health disparities are directly and indirectly linked to longevity and quality of life issues (Williams & Mohammed, 2009). For example, the American Cancer Society reports that African American men die from prostate cancer more than any other racial or ethnic group, with their death rate almost 2.4 times higher than that in White men (American Cancer Society, 2005) (Box 1-2: Diversity Awareness).

The *Healthy People 2020* focus areas include Adolescent Health; Blood Disorders and Blood Safety; Dementias, Including Alzheimer's Disease; Early and Middle Childhood; Genomics; Global Health; Healthcare-Associated Infections; Health-Related Quality of Life and Well-Being; Lesbian, Gay, Bisexual, and Transgender Health; Older Adults; Preparedness; Sleep Health; and Social Determinants of Health. These focus areas are an expansion on previous areas and incorporate recent evidence more directly in each area.

The detailed objectives can be found at www.healthypeople.gov/2020/topicsobjectives2020/pdfs/HP2020objectives.pdf. These focus areas span age categories from conception to death and incorporate prevention, access, treatment, and follow-up at the individual, family, provider, work site, and community levels. The 42 topical areas lead to specific objectives for each topical area. One example is used here for illustration.

BOX 1-2　DIVERSITY AWARENESS

Influence of Personal Cultural Values on Health Care Delivery

Culture influences every aspect of human life, including beliefs, values, and customs regarding lifestyle and health care. As health care providers, nurses need to be aware of their own beliefs, values, and customs and how these ideas translate into behavior. It is easy to assume that an individual's own perspective is correct and shared by others. This is especially true when working with other health care providers who share the same culture. This concept is referred to as **ethnocentrism** and can lead to a devaluing of the beliefs, values, and customs of others, known as **racism**. Although it is impossible for any person to ignore the cultural influences on their lives, nurses and other health care providers have a special obligation to be aware of their own social and cultural biases. Our focus as nurses must be on the cultural influences in the daily lives of individuals through the development of **cultural competence** and cultural humility. The ability to view other persons' situations from their perspective is known as **empathy.** Diversity awareness will continue to challenge providers to lifelong learning about the persons for whom they provide care as the racial and ethnic mix in society changes.

Objective PA-2.1. Increase the proportion of adults who engage in aerobic physical activity of at least moderate intensity for at least 150 minutes/week, or 75 minutes/week of vigorous intensity, or an equivalent combination. This objective directly addresses each of the overarching goals, either directly or indirectly. Physical activity can contribute to the maintenance or improvement in mobility, which improves the quality of life and prevents disability. It is something in which most people can participate. It enhances positive mental health through stress reduction and physical fitness, which contribute to the development of healthy behaviors. However, it takes social action and awareness to address the need for social and physical environments that support physical activity across the life span.

Access to health care to obtain a complete physical examination before starting to exercise and the quality of the work or neighborhood environment available for exercise can contribute to success or failure of this objective. This objective is related to other objectives such as nutrition, obesity, and stroke prevention.

Additionally, current knowledge about physical activity and specific populations was considered when creating the *Healthy People 2020* objectives. Women, low-income populations, Black and Hispanic people, people with disabilities, and those older than age 75 exercise less than do White men with moderate-to-high incomes (U.S. Department of Health and Human Services, 2012). These health disparities can influence the number of people in these groups who develop high cholesterol or high blood pressure measurements, which further increases their risk of heart disease and stroke. Although this objective addresses adults, other objectives address the need for beginning exercise activities at an early age and encouraging young adults to be actively engaged in exercise. How might this objective be adjusted to the needs of an older adult population?

The target for this objective is that 47.9% of adults engage in aerobic physical activity of at least moderate intensity for at least 150 minutes/week, or 75 minutes/week of vigorous intensity, or an equivalent combination. This target represents a 10% increase over the 2008 baseline. This approach emphasizes personal responsibility but now includes society's role in addressing the social and physical environments within which those choices are made (U.S. Department of Health and Human Services, 2012).

Health care providers need to be responsible for offering health promotion, providing preventive health services, and monitoring behaviors. Unfortunately, many of the financial incentives for providers are to perform tasks and procedures rather than to counsel and help individuals choose between various behaviors. The Patient Protection and Affordable Care Act (U.S. Congress, 2010) now requires primary care providers to provide free wellness services to older adults and others, and to provide person-centered care. Providers need to take the time to discuss behaviors that may improve the quality of life and extend years of life. For example, the addictive nature of tobacco and its effect on the development and course of a variety of chronic health conditions are now well recognized. Providers should be asking every person if they use tobacco and should be providing them with ways to quit smoking, including economic and social incentives.

Providers also need to look for partnership in the community through which they can better serve the needs of individuals. *Healthy People 2020* emphasizes that person-centered care is essential to health promotion. One approach to person-centered care to build partnerships is the use of community nursing centers as a partnering organization (www.nncc.us/site/). The Health Promotion Center (HPC) operated by Fairfield University School of Nursing in Fairfield, Connecticut, was one example. The nurses and nursing students who provided health education, screening, and referral services at the HPC worked with existing community organizations to better meet the health care needs of underserved people. The HPC worked with senior housing and senior centers to provide comprehensive

cardiovascular screenings and medication review. As an extension of this work, funding was secured for a program called *Step Up to Health*, a project to increase physical activity in this population through interactive planning and consumer ownership of the activities. The project was part of the National Blueprint Project supported by the Robert Wood Johnson Foundation (www.agingblueprint.org). The project engaged older adults in walking programs, line dancing, gardening, and low-impact exercise programs, including programs from the National Arthritis Foundation (www.arthritis.org/). Another approach to partnerships is to have providers serve as active participants on community boards and advisory committees, which allows providers to become aware of the service needs in the community and the resources available to meet those needs.

Work sites and communities need to become partners in providing opportunities for people to lead healthy lives through flexible work schedules, work site wellness programs, accessibility of safe parks, and availability of exercise facilities. Converting empty lots into community gardens provides beautification of the area, an opportunity for exercise in caring for the garden, and a source of fresh vegetables. The availability of bike paths encourages physical activity (Box 1-3: Innovative Practice).

Churches, temples, and mosques can be vital partners in meeting *Healthy People 2020* objectives. Faith communities can break economic, social, racial, and gender barriers, making them an excellent source for sharing information on health promotion and disease prevention. Parish nurses are becoming increasingly prevalent and they incorporate *Healthy People 2020* objectives into their activities (International Parish Nurse Resource Center, 2012).

Public health officials at all levels are necessary partners in meeting *Healthy People 2020* objectives. As part of the core public health functions of assessment, policy development, and assurance, the U.S. Public Health Service and all state, county, and local health departments need to collect data, make information available to the public, create policies that support

---

✳ BOX 1-3 INNOVATIVE PRACTICE

Process for Assessing, Evaluating, and Treating Overweight and Obesity in Adults

Overweight and obesity are major concerns in public health because they contribute to other health problems such as high cholesterol, high blood pressure, diabetes mellitus, heart disease, functional limitations, and disability. As part of the National Heart, Lung and Blood Institute's (NHLBI, 2000) Obesity Education Initiative, titled *Aim for a Healthy Weight*, nurses have an important role to play in health education related to obesity prevention and control. More complete information and guidelines updated in 2012 can be retrieved from www.nhlbi.nih.gov/health/public/heart/obesity/lose_wt/index.htm.

Make the Most of the Individual's Visit and Set an Effective Tone for Communication: Nurses ask individuals about their weight history, weight-related health risks, and desire to lose weight. The approaches used need to be respectful of a person's lifestyle, habits, and cultural influences. Discussions need to be nonjudgmental and goal directed.

Assess Individual's Motivation/Readiness to Lose Weight: Nurses explain body mass index and why it is the preferred method of determining overweight and obesity in adults. Individuals need to understand the methods of data collection and measurement of height and weight, as well as waist

circumference, risk factors, and comorbidities. Nurses develop skill in determining readiness and motivation to lose weight in their patients.

Build a Partnership with an Individual: Nurses work with individuals to determine what each person is willing to do to achieve a lower weight. This approach includes knowing the best practices in weight management and weight loss. Fad diets, dietary supplements, and weight loss pills may be inappropriate for most people, and formal weight loss programs may be too expensive for low- and moderate-income families. Use recommended diets that restrict caloric intake, set activity goals with your patients, encourage the person to keep a weekly food and activity diary, and provide information on diet and activity. Be sure to record individual goals and the treatment plan, including a health education plan. Nurses are knowledgeable about current treatment options and their success. Holistic approaches are needed, since food behaviors are influenced by many factors. Listen to individuals' stories about food and its role in their lives. Therapies should fit the individual's goals and lead to lifestyle change.

Healthy People 2020 objectives, and ensure that needed services are available from a competent workforce.

CASE STUDY

Refer to the Case Study that appears at the end of this chapter along with the Care Plan. Read carefully, because some of the concepts covered in those boxes are applied in the following sections.

Problem Identification

How many problems are present in Frank's situation? The answer depends on who is asked the question and his or her position in relation to Frank. Each point of view focuses on different aspects of Frank's life. His physician, using a clinical model of health, might say that Frank has coronary heart disease with an acute myocardial infarction, hypertension, hyperlipidemia, chronic bronchitis, and obesity. But Frank's problems also represent a failure to meet several of the *Healthy People 2020* objectives on a personal level. His nurse can add that he has paid little attention to his lifestyle, even after changes were recommended. He continues to overeat, drink too much, smoke, not exercise, and live a stressful life. Frank's employer sees a man who has potential, but who is now too disabled to take on new responsibilities and perhaps unable to continue performing his previous duties. Frank's children might feel that he can no longer take them on trips or play with them. His wife, Sada, knows that their plans for educating their children, and for travel and enjoyment, might suffer. The human resource personnel who manage Frank's health insurance and pension programs would say that he has an expensive disease, and the state health planner would point out that Frank's problem is only one of a growing number of disabling illnesses that result from preventable causes. A reviewer for *Healthy People 2020* might see Frank as part of the aggregated data on heart disease, indicating a continuing increase in heart disease among Black non-Hispanic men.

To Frank, his health problems are multidimensional. His initial fear of dying, pain, dependence, and frustration decreased as he began to feel better, but Frank is haunted by his realization that he might never be able to achieve his dreams for himself and his family. Although theoretically in his prime, Frank suddenly sees himself as far older than his years, both in body and in social achievement. He believes he has reached his limit and that he will never again have the freedom to choose his future. He and his family needed to evaluate their situation and make alternative plans based on asset planning. A care plan has been developed based on the situation of Frank and his family. (See Care Plan at the end of this chapter.)

Planning Interventions

Rather than emphasizing the chronic health issues and related problems, the nurse can begin with asset planning within the family. **Asset planning** is a planning approach that, given the realities of the present, helps focus the family and their providers on the building blocks for their future. It focuses on the assets or strengths of the individual, the family, and the community, applying those assets to improve or maintain the current level of functioning.

Frank's physician and nurse can begin with the fact that Frank survived his first myocardial infarction. The coronary damage resulting from this event becomes the baseline for determining future change in the lives of Frank and his family. Earlier, Frank's physician had taken a broader time perspective when he advised Frank to reduce his cigarette smoking, which was contributing to both his bronchitis and his hypertension, and to change his high-fat diet and sedentary habits, which contributed to his weight problem and his high blood pressure. These lifestyle changes now become tools for Frank's recovery and for change within his family. His cardiac event also becomes a risk factor for heart disease in the lives of his children.

Looking at the immediate future, Frank's employer saw the effect of the event on Frank's position within the company. Frank would have a long recovery that could be successful if he adhered to his cardiac rehabilitation program. Asset planning at this level means examining how to move Frank back into his work role without further jeopardizing his health. Frank and Sada also need to examine if he could continue in this position, given its potential effect on his health.

Frank and his family used a broader perspective than the medical personnel or the corporation. They knew that to achieve the family's economic and educational goals and still spend time together, they had to make decisions that would ultimately affect Frank's health. Similar to many Americans, they had been willing to live with Frank's job pressures and stressful lifestyle caused by the economy. The family members were aware of their impoverished roots and had no wish to return to them. However, they also recognized that the strength of their family, their ability to work together to achieve goals, and their faith were assets that could be used for support.

Frank's social network of friends, relatives, and church members became an additional asset. They helped the family through the difficult initial weeks at home by delivering meals, taking care of the yard work and laundry, and providing companionship so Sada could shop and have time alone. As Frank recovered, they would provide support for the social and lifestyle changes that Frank and his family needed to make.

The nurse-led cardiovascular rehabilitation group played a vital role in Frank's recovery. As the physician continued to monitor Frank's cardiac status, the nurse began the long process of working with Frank to modify his habits. He had stopped smoking while in the hospital, but with more free time than usual, he was craving to smoke again. Using an asset planning approach and Gordon's functional health patterns (2010), the nurse identified the changes that Frank needed to make to decrease the risk of a second heart attack. A plan was developed to help Frank begin to take control of his life through behavior changes. These changes included relaxation techniques, diet modification, smoking cessation, and mild chair exercises. The support of the family was enlisted to reinforce the changes Frank was willing to make, since social support and environmental changes are shown to enhance personal decision-making. His employer was contacted and agreed to a plan enabling Frank to work from home using a computer while the workplace became smoke-free. Frank became an asset to the workplace, serving as a spokesperson for the benefits of lifestyle change. He was enlisted to talk with other employees about stress management, exercise, weight reduction, and smoking cessation based on his personal experiences.

Health planners and public health officials used the broadest perspective in asset planning by viewing Frank as an example of a person whose potential shifted as a result of a preventable, disabling illness. The planners looked to public and private community patterns and policies that increase healthful habits and living conditions. Work schedules and work load; stress and safety in work environments; affirmative action programs for jobs and wages; availability of public transportation systems, recreational facilities, and economically accessible housing; farm price subsidies for food and tobacco crops that affect buying patterns; excise taxes and regulation of health damaging drugs such as alcohol and nicotine were all taken into consideration (Grzywacz & Fuqua, 2000). The asset planning approach emphasized the positive actions that could be made at the personal, employment, community, and societal levels to minimize the effects of Frank's illness and related diseases, thereby addressing all levels of the ecological model of health.

What Was the Actual Cause of Frank's Problem?

It is not possible to separate one cause from another because heart disease is a multifactorial disease. In Frank's case, the sources of illness were found in the many interrelationships in his life. Attempting to treat or change each factor as a separate entity can have only a limited effect on the improvement of overall health. Frank's health problems were numerous. In addition to a poor diet, weight gain, lack of exercise, and smoking, his hyperlipidemia, an adaptive biological response to the pressures in his life, further debilitated him. It eventually led to clogged coronary vessels and his responses became maladaptive. His hypertension, resulting from his diet and time-constrained lifestyle, complicated by the buildup of plaque secondary to hyperlipidemia, was also a biological attempt to adjust to a situation that contributed to an imbalance between his personal resources and the demands of his family and the economic world. Frank's smoking was a psychosocial means to help him relieve some of the emotional pressures. It may have served this short-term purpose, but only at a silently rising cost to his health. Cigarette use by persons who have hypertension or high serum cholesterol levels multiplies their risk of coronary heart disease (Izzo & Black, 2003).

Evaluation of the Situation

The health status of an individual or population depends on a sustainable balance of the complex responses between physiological, psychological, and social and environmental factors. Health was initially conceived as a biological state, with genetic endowment as the starting point. However, health involves psychological and social aspects and is interpreted within the context of the immediate environment.

The interconnections between biophysical, psychological, and environmental causes and consequences did not end with Frank's heart attack. His heart attack was only the most dramatic sign that health damaging responses outweighed health promoting ones. The "tip of the iceberg" analogy is frequently used to illustrate the importance of identifying individuals with subclinical symptoms. High blood lipid levels, high blood pressure, obesity, smoking, and persistent worrying were no less important than the infarction in shaping the status of Frank's health. Repairing the damage to Frank's heart without changing his lifestyle, habits, and work environment would only buy a brief amount of time before further damage would occur.

The infarction and resulting disability also permanently reshaped Frank's environment. After a few months of working full time, Frank realized that he needed to find a less stressful job. He recognized that his sales administration skills were an asset and began interviewing in the nonprofit sector. Ultimately, he landed a job at half his previous salary, but with excellent benefits and a flexible work environment. His reduced income meant that his children's educational opportunities were more limited than they were before his heart attack, but his family responded by seeking tuition support from community organizations. Frank found that his contacts in both the corporate and the nonprofit sectors increased his value to his new employer. Frank's entire life, internal and external, had changed. He had learned to adapt to his health problems and had developed a more eudaimonistic approach to health and life.

Frank's situation illustrates how causes and effects in life and health tend to merge into constant, inseparable interconnections between individuals and their worlds. A person's health status is a reflection of a web of relationships that characterize that person's life. Health is not an achievement or a prize, but a high-quality interaction between a person's inner and outer worlds that provides the capacity to respond to the demands of the biological, psychological, and environmental systems of these worlds.

After reviewing the list of *Healthy People 2020* Focus Areas listed in Box 1-4, which of the focus areas apply to the promotion of Frank's health? Clearly, the area of heart disease and stroke is most applicable. The *Healthy People 2020* website (www.healthypeople.gov/2020/default.aspx) has a number of objectives that relate directly to the prevention of heart disease, hypertension, and hyperlipidemia, including objectives that relate to treatment options and training the public to recognize and respond to nutrition and weight (Box 1-5: *Healthy People 2020*). Referring to the information about Frank and his experience, determine what his children should be taught based on the *Healthy People 2020* objectives in this focus area.

Healthy People 2020 can form the basis for planning, service delivery, evaluation, and research in every aspect of the health care system. The nurse needs to be familiar with this document and its intent. Nurses should compare their practices with the objectives in *Healthy People 2010*. Additionally, the nurse needs to be aware of the research and practice changes that occur as a result of the work toward these objectives.

LEVELS OF PREVENTION

Prevention, in a narrow sense, means averting the development of disease in the future. In a broad sense, prevention consists of all measures that limit disease progression. Leavell

---

♥ BOX 1-4 THE 13 FOCUS AREAS IN HEALTHY PEOPLE 2020

- Adolescent Health
- Blood Disorders and Blood Safety
- Dementias, Including Alzheimer's Disease
- Early and Middle Childhood
- Genomics
- Global Health
- Healthcare-Associated Infections
- Health-Related Quality of Life and Well-Being
- Lesbian, Gay, Bisexual, and Transgender Health
- Older Adults
- Preparedness
- Sleep Health
- Social Determinants of Health

From U.S. Department of Health and Human Services, Public Health Service. (2010). *Healthy People 2020*. Retrieved February 19, 2012, from www.healthypeople.gov/2020/about/new2020.aspx.

♥ BOX 1-5 HEALTHY PEOPLE 2020

Selected National Health Promotion and Disease Prevention Objectives for Nutrition and Weight Status

- Increase the proportion of adults who are at a healthy weight.
- Reduce the proportion of adults who are obese.
- Reduce the proportion of children and adolescents who are considered obese.
- (Developmental) Prevent inappropriate weight gain in youth and adults.
- Increase the contribution of fruits to the diets of the population aged 2 years and older.
- Increase the variety and contribution of vegetables to the diets of the population aged 2 years and older.
- Increase the contribution of whole grains to the diets of the population aged 2 years and older.
- Reduce consumption of calories from solid fats and added sugars in the population aged 2 years and older.
- Reduce consumption of saturated fat in the population aged 2 years and older.
- Reduce consumption of sodium in the population aged 2 years and older.
- Increase consumption of calcium in the population aged 2 years and older.

From U.S. Department of Health and Human Services, Public Health Service. (2010). *Healthy People 2020* Objectives. Retrieved February 19, 2012, from www.healthypeople.gov/2020/topicsobjectives2020/default.aspx.

---

and Clark (1965) defined three levels of prevention: primary, secondary, and tertiary (Figure 1-2). While the levels of prevention are related to the natural history of disease, they can be used to prevent disease and provide nurses with starting points in making effective, positive changes in the health status of the persons for whom they provide care. Within the three levels of prevention, there are five steps. These steps include health promotion and specific protection (primary prevention); early diagnosis, prompt treatment, and disability limitation (secondary prevention); and restoration and rehabilitation (tertiary prevention).

Some confusion exists in the interpretation of these concepts; therefore, a consistent understanding of primary, secondary, and tertiary prevention is essential. The levels of prevention operate on a continuum, but may overlap in practice. The nurse must clearly understand the goals of each level to intervene effectively in keeping people healthy.

Primary Prevention

Primary prevention precedes disease or dysfunction. However, primary prevention is therapeutic in that it includes health as beneficial to well-being, it uses therapeutic treatments, and, as a process or behavior towards enhancing health, it involves symptom identification when teaching stress reduction techniques. Primary prevention intervention includes health promotion, such as health education about risk factors for heart disease, and specific protection, such as immunization against hepatitis B. Its purpose is to decrease the vulnerability of the individual or population to disease or dysfunction. Interventions at this level encourage individuals and groups to become more aware of the means of improving health and the actions they can take at the primary preventive health level and the optimal health level. People are also taught to use appropriate primary preventive measures. However, primary prevention can also include advocating for policies that promote the health of the community and electing public officials who will enact legislation that protects the health of the public.

Health Promotion

The definitions of **health promotion** vary. O'Donnell (1987, p. 4) has defined health promotion as "the science and art of helping people change their lifestyle to move toward a state of optimal health." Kreuter and Devore (1980) proposed a more complex definition in a paper commissioned by the U.S. Public Health Service. They stated that health promotion is "the process of advocating health in order to enhance the probability that personal (individual, family, and community), private (professional and business), and public (federal, state, and local government) support of positive health practices will become a societal norm" (Kreuter & Devore, 1980, p. 26).

The Theoretical Basis of Health Promotion. The theoretical underpinnings for health promotion have evolved since the early 1980s. Most of these theories are behaviorally based, derived from the social sciences, and extensively researched. These theories include the theory of reasoned action by Ajzen and Fishbein (1980), theories of behavior by Bandura (1976, 1999, 2004), the health belief model by Rosenstock (Janz et al., 2002), Pender's health promotion model (Pender et al., 2010), and stages of change theories by Prochaska (Prochaska et al., 2004). Internet searches on each of these theories will provide numerous sites where more detailed information is available.

The Social Nature of Health Promotion. Health promotion goes beyond providing information. It is also proactive decision-making at all levels of society as reflected in the *Healthy People 2020* objectives. Health promotion holds the best promise for lower-cost methods of limiting the constant increase in health care costs and for empowering people to be responsible for the aspects of their lives that can enhance well-being. Based

Primary Prevention

Health Promotion
• Health education
• Good standard of nutrition adjusted to
  developmental phases of life
• Attention to personality development
• Provision of adequate housing, recreation,
  and agreeable working conditions
• Marriage counseling and sex education
• Genetic screening
• Periodic selective examinations

Specific Protection
• Use of specific immunizations
• Attention to personal hygiene
• Use of environmental sanitation
• Protection against occupational hazards
• Protection from accidents
• Use of specific nutrients
• Protection from carcinogens
• Avoidance of allergens

**Leavell and Clark's
Three Levels of Prevention**

Secondary Prevention

Early Diagnosis and Prompt Treatment
• Case-finding measures: individual and mass
  screening surveys
• Selective examinations to:
  • Cure and prevent disease process
  • Prevent spread of communicable disease
  • Prevent complications and sequelae
  • Shorten period of disability

Disability Limitations
• Adequate treatment to arrest disease process and
  prevent further complications and sequelae
• Provision of facilities to limit disability and
  prevent death

Tertiary Prevention

Restoration and Rehabilitation
• Provision of hospital and community facilities for
  retraining and education to maximize use of remaining
  capacities
• Education of public and industry to use rehabilitated
  persons to fullest possible extent
• Selective placement
• Work therapy in hospitals
• Use of sheltered colony

FIGURE 1-2 The three levels of prevention developed by Leavell and Clark. (Data from Leavell, H., &
Clark, A. E. [1965]. *Preventive medicine for doctors in the community*. New York: McGraw-Hill.)

on the need for health promotion activities within the health care system, efforts must be made to identify the multiple determinants of health, determine relevant health promotion strategies, and delineate issues relevant to social justice and access to care. Individuals, families, and communities must be active participants in this process so that the actions taken are socially relevant, economically feasible, and supportive of changes at the individual level.

The Active and Passive Nature of Health Promotion. Health promotion efforts, unlike those efforts directed at specific protection from certain diseases, focus on maintaining or improving the general health of individuals, families, and communities. These activities are carried out at the public level (e.g., government programs promoting adequate housing or reducing pollutants in the air), at the community level (e.g., Habitat for Humanity or community health centers), and at the personal level (e.g., voting to offer low-income housing or to elect public officials who recognize the need for public oversight). Nursing interventions are actions directed toward developing people's resources to maintain or enhance their well-being—a form of assets-based planning.

Two strategies of health promotion that involve the individual may be either passive or active. Passive strategies involve the individual as an inactive participant or recipient. Examples of passive strategies are public health efforts to maintain clean water and sanitary sewage systems to decrease infectious diseases and improve health, and efforts to introduce vitamin D in all milk to ensure that children will not be at high risk for rickets when living in areas where sunlight is scarce. These passive strategies must be used to promote the health of the public when individual participation might be low but the benefit to society is high.

Active strategies depend on the individual becoming personally involved in adopting a proposed program of health promotion. Two examples of lifestyle change are performing daily exercise as part of a physical fitness plan and adopting a stress-management program as part of daily living. A combination of active and passive strategies is best for making an individual or society healthier. Reexamine the case study to determine when Frank could have incorporated some of these strategies to decrease his risk of heart disease.

This text is concerned almost entirely with active strategies and the nurse's role in these strategies. Some passive strategies are presented, but they are presented with the implicit belief that each individual must take responsibility for improving health. It is undeniable that passive strategies also have a valuable role, but they must be used within a context of encouraging and teaching individuals to assume more responsibility for their health.

An Application of Theory to the Practice of Health Promotion. The Transtheoretical Model (TTM) is an excellent example and can be applied to this case study. TTM incorporates Stages of Change (readiness to take action), Decisional Balance (benefits to and detractors from changing a behavior), Self-Efficacy (personal confidence in making a change), and Processes of Change (cognitive, affective, and behavioral activities facilitating change). The bases of TTM are the stages of change—six stages that people spiral through on a path toward making and sustaining a behavioral change to promote health. These stages are:

Precontemplative	Not considering change
Contemplative	Aware of but not considering change soon
Preparation	Planning to act soon
Action	Has begun to make behavioral change (recent)
Maintenance	Continued commitment to behavior (long-term)
Relapse	Reverted to old behavior

Each stage offers opportunities for the nurse to provide information and support behavioral change. Encouraging people and suggesting changes to their environment that support behavioral change can increase individuals' self-efficacy and their chances of maintaining a change. This model also recognizes that people need multiple opportunities to make behavioral change before achieving success and that relapse should be expected (Prochaska et al., 2004).

Although health promotion would seem to be a practical and effective mode of health care, the major portion of health care delivery is geared toward responding to acute and chronic disease. Preventing or delaying the onset of chronic disease and adding new dimensions to the quality of life are not as easy because they take time to implement and evaluate and require personal action. These actions are more closely associated with everyday living and the lifestyles adopted by individuals, families, communities, and nations. Habits such as eating, resting, exercising, and handling anxieties appear to be transmitted from parent to child and from social group to social group as part of a cultural, not a genetic, heritage. These activities may be taught in subtle ways, but they influence behavior and have as much of an influence on health as does genetic inheritance. Although the public may not appreciate the causal relationships between behavior and health, it should be apparent to health professionals. Arguably, the concept of risk is the most basic of all health concepts, since health promotion and disease protection are based on this concept.

Health promotion strategies have the potential of enhancing the quality of life from birth to death. For example, good nutrition is adjusted to various developmental phases in life to account for rapid growth and development in infancy and early childhood, physiological changes associated with adolescence, extra demands during pregnancy, and the many changes occurring in older adults. Good nutrition is known to enhance the immune system, enabling individuals to fight infections that could lead to disabling illnesses. Other individual activities are adapted to the person's needs for optimal personality development at all ages. As seen in Unit 4, much can be done on a personal or group basis, through counseling and properly directed parent education, to provide the environmental requirements for the proper personality development of children. Community participation is also an important factor in promoting individual, family, and group health (see Chapters 6, 7, and 8).

Personal health promotion is usually provided through health education (see Chapter 10). An important function of nurses, physicians, and allied health professionals, health education is principally concerned with eliciting useful changes in human behavior based on current research. The goal is to inculcate a sense of responsibility in individuals for their own health and a shared sense of responsibility for avoiding injury to the health of others. For example, encouraging child-rearing practices that foster normal growth and development (personal, social, and physical) addresses both the individual parent and the needs of society. Health education nurtures health promoting habits, values, and attitudes that must be learned through practice. These must be reinforced through systematic instruction in hygiene, bodily function, physical fitness, and use of leisure time. Another goal is to understand the appropriate use of health services. For example, a semiannual visit to a dentist may teach a child better oral health habits and to visit the dentist regularly, although this is not the primary purpose of the visit. Parents, teachers, and caregivers play a vital role in health education. In addition to teaching individuals, nurses need to develop skills in group teaching and in providing education within community organizations.

Available research clearly shows an increase in longevity, a decrease in mortality and morbidity, and an improvement in the quality of life for individuals who have been involved in health promotion activities such as physical activity and avoidance of smoking (Crimmins et al., 2011). It must be emphasized that health promotion requires lifestyle change. Once a lifestyle change has been adopted, vigilance is needed to ensure that the lifestyle change is maintained and modified to fit developmental and environmental changes.

Empirical data linking risk factors, health promotion activities, and outcomes are sufficient to drive the development of the *Healthy People 2020* objectives and to be incorporated into quality improvement measures in managed care. One of the challenges posed in *Healthy People 2020* is the development of measurable outcome objectives that are based on more realistic economic models.

Health promotion is an important concept for nursing because it embodies many other concepts that nursing is concerned with today. As stated earlier, much of the nursing role is involved with health teaching. Standard 5B of the *Nursing: Scope and Standards of Practice* document (American Nurses Association [ANA], 2004, p. 28) requires nurses "to promote health and a safe environment" through health teaching and evaluation of teaching effectiveness in clinical practice (Box 1-6: Hot Topics). Health education is clearly a nursing role.

Specific Protection

This aspect of primary prevention focuses on protecting people from injury and disease, for example, by providing immunizations and reducing exposure to occupational hazards, carcinogens, and other environmental health risks. These hazards and risks include not only protection of adults from work-related injuries (e.g., back injuries in nurses, dismemberment in machinists, exposure to chemicals used in boat repair or to inhaled sawdust by carpenters) but also protection of infants and children from potential carcinogens (e.g., exposure of children to diesel emissions, damage to a fetus caused by radiation).

Primary prevention interventions are considered health protection when they emphasize shielding or defending the body (or the public) from specific causes of injury or disease. Implementing nursing interventions that prevent a specific health problem may seem easier than promoting well-being among individuals, groups, or communities because the variables are delineated more clearly in prevention than in promotion and the potential influences are less diverse.

Examples. Two examples may help demonstrate these differences. Immunization for influenza is quite popular and has become a regular activity for people at risk each fall. Nurses can participate in this specific protection role by giving the influenza injections in clinics and offices. Another example is creating nut-free schools to protect hypersensitive children from life-threatening allergic reactions to peanut and other nut products. Such initiatives have largely been the result of grassroots parent organizations working with formal community

---

🔥 BOX 1-6 HOT TOPICS

Health Promotion Program Incentives

The concept of health promotion program incentives is multidimensional. Incentives are best defined relative to their purpose, type, and form for either groups or individuals.

An incentive is a reward designed to influence an individual to make a desired change where he/she might otherwise not make the behavioral change solely on the intrinsic benefit of the changed behavior. For example, a person may not choose to stop smoking because of the cost of the smoking cessation materials. If the person is given the smoking cessation materials for free and provided with a $10 incentive each week for using the materials, then that person might decide to make the change. The benefits of not smoking were not enough of an incentive to stop smoking, but the incentives helped to make the behavioral change possible.

One example of an integrated incentive program in an employee wellness program is the *HEALTH Plus Program* at Vanderbilt University (2012)

(www.vanderbilt.edu/HRS/wellness/healthplus.htm). Full-time employees and faculty can participate in an incentive program that rewards them for participation and achievement of specific health and wellness goals. Participants receive monetary incentives for completing a Health Risk Assessment on-line. They can then select a level of behavior change based on increasing levels of commitment (bronze, silver, or gold). For each level, participants choose wellness categories and actions they are willing to take within each category. They then work on those actions over the next year and complete another Health Risk Assessment at the end of the year to note specific achievement. Information is available on each category and action, and wellness staff can assist participants in reaching desired goals. The incentive for the participants is an additional $10 to $15 in each paycheck, participation in groups working on specific actions, and recognition of achievement of each level. The university benefits from healthier employees, which increases productivity, limits health care costs, and improves quality of life.

organizations to adopt policies that protect the health of these children. Nurses may be involved in the parent organizations or the school or public health boards that review the proposed policies. Additionally, nurses must be able to address the need to protect specific portions of the population at risk.

Secondary Prevention

Although primary prevention measures have decreased the hazards of chronic diseases such as cardiovascular disease, conditions that preclude a healthy quality of life are still prevalent. Secondary prevention ranges from providing screening activities and treating early stages of disease to limiting disability by averting or delaying the consequences of advanced disease.

Screening is secondary prevention because the principal goal is to identify individuals in an early, detectable stage of the disease process. However, screening provides an excellent opportunity to offer health teaching as a primary preventive measure. Screening activities now play an important role in the control of diseases such as heart disease, stroke, and colorectal cancer. Additionally, screening activities provide early diagnosis and treatment of nutritional, behavioral, and other related problems. Nurses play an important role in screening activities because they provide clinical expertise and educationally sound health information during the screening process.

Delayed recognition of disease results in the need to limit future disability in late secondary prevention. Limiting disability is a vital role for nursing since preventive measures are primarily therapeutic and are aimed at arresting the disease and preventing further complications. The paradox here is that health education and disease prevention activities seem similar to those used in primary prevention, but are applied to a person or population with an existing disease. Modifications to the teaching plan must be made based on the individual's current health status and ability to modify behavior. In the case study, Frank needed secondary prevention after his heart attack. The lifestyle changes needed to prevent a second heart attack were similar to the steps he could have taken to prevent his initial heart attack, but with a recognition that his coronary status was now compromised. As a result, exercise had to be increased gradually as part of a cardiac rehabilitation program and diet modifications had to be made with support from a registered dietitian to ensure adequate nutrition and weight loss.

Tertiary Prevention

Tertiary prevention occurs when a defect or disability is permanent and irreversible. The process involves minimizing the effects of disease and disability by surveillance and maintenance activities aimed at preventing complications and deterioration. Tertiary prevention focuses on rehabilitation to help people attain and retain an optimal level of functioning regardless of their disabling condition. The objective is to return the affected individual to a useful place in society, maximize remaining capacities, or both. The responsibility of the nurse is to ensure that persons with disabilities receive services that enable them to live and work according to the resources that are still available to them. When a person has a stroke, rehabilitating this individual to the highest level of functioning and teaching

lifestyle changes to prevent future strokes are examples of tertiary prevention.

THE NURSE'S ROLE

Evolving demands are placed on the nurse and the nursing profession as a result of changes in society. Emphasis is shifting from acute, hospital-based care to preventive, community-based care, which is provided in nontraditional health care settings in the community. This demand for community-based services, with the home as a major community setting for care, is closely related to the changing demographics of the United States. While the home and community become the existing sites for care, nurses must assume more blended roles, with a knowledge base that prepares them to practice across settings using evidence-based practice. Within these roles, nurses assume a more active involvement in the prevention of disease and the promotion of health. Nurses can be more independent in their practice and place a greater emphasis on promoting and maximizing health, and more than ever nurses are accountable morally, ethically, and legally for their professional behavior.

Nursing Roles in Health Promotion and Protection

Although nurses often work with persons on a one-to-one basis, they seldom work in isolation. Within today's health care system, nurses collaborate with other nurses, physicians, social workers, nutritionists, psychologists, therapists, individuals, and community groups. In this interprofessional practice, nurses play a variety of roles.

Advocate

As advocates nurses help individuals obtain what they are entitled to receive through the health care system, try to make the system more responsive to individual and community needs, and help persons develop the skills to advocate for themselves. In the role of advocate, the nurse strives to ensure that all persons receive high-quality, appropriate, safe, and cost-effective care. The nurse may spend a great deal of time identifying and coordinating resources for complex cases. Other examples of advocacy will be seen in subsequent chapters.

Care Manager

The nurse acts as a care manager to prevent duplication of services, maintain quality and safety, and reduce costs. Information gathered from reliable data sources enables the care manager to help individuals avoid care that is unproven, ineffective, or unsafe. Reliable sources of information on best practices, evidence-based practices, and standard protocols are available from Internet sites sponsored by the federal government (e.g., www.nih.gov; www.cdc.gov), specialty organizations (e.g., www.arthritis.org; www.nursingworld.org; www.caremanager.org), and private foundations (e.g., www.rwjf.org; www.jhart-found.org). Successful care management depends on a collaborative relationship among the care manager, other nurses and physicians, the individual and his or her family, the insurance provider, and other care providers who work with the person. The wishes of the individual and family need to be clear to the care manager as part of person-centered care provision. Facilitating communication among parties is one of the care manager's most important functions.

Consultant

Nurses may provide knowledge about health promotion and disease prevention to individuals and groups as a consultant. Some nurses have specialized areas of expertise or advanced practice, such as in gerontology, women's health, or community/public health, and they are equipped to provide information as consultants in these areas of specialization (ANA, 2004). A gerontological nurse specialist might be on a community planning board offering advice about what types of health promotion activities should be considered in planning a new senior housing development. All nurses need to develop consultation skills that can be integrated into practice and allow the individual nurse to take advantage of opportunities to provide support on an individual level or for future development at the organizational level (Norwood, 2003).

Deliverer of Services

The core role of the nurse is the delivery of direct services such as health education, flu shots, and counseling in health promotion. Visible, direct delivery of nursing care is the foundation for the public image of nursing. The public demands that nurses be knowledgeable and competent in their delivery of services. This role is clearly expressed in *Nursing's Social Policy Statement* (ANA, 2003) and in the ANA's *Code of Ethics for Nurses with Interpretive Statements* (ANA, 2008).

Educator

Health practices in the United States are derived from the theory that health components such as good nutrition, industrial and highway safety, immunization, and specific drug therapy should be within the grasp of the total population. Even with its rich resources, society falls far short of attaining the goal of maximal health for all. The problem is not a lack of knowledge, but rather the lack of application; therefore it is incumbent on nurses to be excellent health educators. To teach effectively, the nurse must know essential facts about how people learn and the teaching-learning process (see Chapter 10).

In addition to their storehouse of scientific knowledge, nurses who are committed to their teaching role know that individuals are unique in their response to efforts to change their behavior. Teaching may range from a chance remark by the nurse, based on a perception of desirable individual behavior, to structurally planned teaching according to individual needs. Selection of the methods most likely to succeed involves the establishment of teacher-learner goals. Health promotion and protection rely heavily on the individual's ability to use appropriate knowledge. Health education is one of the primary prevention techniques available to avoid the major causes of disability and death today and is a critical role for nurses.

Healer

The role of healer requires the nurse to help individuals integrate and balance the various parts of their lives (McKivergin, 2004).

Healing resides in the ability to glimpse or intuit the "interior" of an individual, to sense and identify what is important to that other person, and to incorporate the specific insight into a care plan that helps that person develop his or her own capacity to heal. It requires a mindful blending of science and subjectivity (Benner et al., 2010; Siegel, 2007). Nurses have a special ability to help people heal. The art of nursing is the extraordinary ability to manage a broad array of information to create something meaningful, sensible, and whole (see Chapter 14).

Researcher

In today's health care environment, nurses are constantly striving to understand and interpret research findings that will enhance the quality and value of individual care. To provide optimal health care, nurses need to use evidence-based findings as their foundation for clinical decision-making. When nurses or other clinicians use research findings and the best evidence possible to make decisions, the outcome is termed evidence-based practice. Evidence-based practice is defined as the conscientious, explicit, and judicious use of current best evidence in making decisions about the care of individuals. The practice of evidence-based nursing means integrating individual clinical expertise with the best available external clinical evidence from systematic research (ANA, 2004).

The National Institute of Nursing Research (NINR) serves as the focal point in developing research themes for the future of the profession. NINR supports research to establish a scientific base for the care of individuals throughout the life span—from the management of individuals during illness and recovery to the reduction of risks for disease and disability. The five "investment" themes NINR has identified are to: enhance health promotion and disease prevention; improve quality of life through symptom management; improve palliative and end-of-life care; enhance innovation in science and nurse practice; and encourage a new generation of nurse scientists (NINR Strategic Plan, 2011). Notice how the *Healthy People 2020* objectives match many of these themes.

Evidence-based practice involves searching for the best evidence with which to answer clinical research questions. Research evidence can be gathered from quantitative studies that describe situations, correlate different variables related to care, or test causal relationships between variables related to care (Levels I to IV). Such studies become incorporated into screening and treatment standards such as those from the U.S. Preventive Services Task Force (2010). Research evidence can also be gathered from qualitative studies that describe phenomena or define the historical nature, cultural relevance, or philosophical basis of aspects of nursing care (Levels V to VII). Applied research is done to directly affect clinical practice (Burns & Grove, 2003). Sackett and colleagues (1996) stressed the use of the best evidence available to answer clinical questions and explore the next best evidence when appropriate. The next best evidence may include the individual clinical judgment that nurses acquire through clinical experience and clinical practice and other qualitative approaches to research.

Nurses need to recognize that research is important as a basis for their practice and that they need to participate in the research process. For example, both home health nurses and nurses in long-term care facilities are required to collect extensive data on the cognitive and physical functioning of individuals through the OASIS and MDS assessment tools. These data are used as part of the quality improvement process to indicate areas for improvement in care, thereby contributing to nursing protocols. Nurses in hospital settings are asked to participate in research as part of the Magnet Hospital designation process.

Chapters 16 to 24 contain specific health promotion research studies. Time should be taken to review these studies and explore the relationship between behavior and disease, to identify which population groups are at risk, and to discover what types of health promotion programs work and why they work. Through knowledge of research, nurses can strengthen their confidence in making daily decisions about quality care (Box 1-7: Research for Evidence-Based Practice).

IMPROVING PROSPECTS FOR HEALTH
Population Effects

Cultural and socioeconomic changes within the population unequivocally influence lay concepts of health and health promotion. Currently there are areas of the United States where the Hispanic population is larger than any other population group. By the year 2050, it is predicted that the majority of people in the United States will not be of White European descent (U.S. Census Bureau, 2010a). Taken together as a portent for future health promotion strategies, these predictions about the population indicate that current knowledge about and approaches to health promotion may not meet the needs of the future U.S. population (see Chapter 2).

In addition to changes in the ethnic and racial distribution within the population, the projected changes in age distribution will affect health promotion practice. Considerable growth is expected in the proportion of the population that is 25 years of age and older. For example, the post–World War II baby boom will increase the number of persons in the 65-and-older age group between the years 2010 and 2030 (U.S. Census Bureau, 2010b). While there was a drop in births after 1960, this decrease has been offset by an increase in immigration, both

legal and illegal. More restrictive immigration rules related to Homeland Security have limited legal immigration since 2002 (U.S. Department of Homeland Security, 2011). Analysis of these population trends and projections helps health professionals determine changing needs. Additionally, analysis of the social and economic environment is necessary for developing social policy concerning health.

SHIFTING PROBLEMS

The provision of personal health services must be influenced by current information regarding environmental health. Environmental pollution is a complex and increasingly hazardous problem. Diseases related to industry and technology, including asthma and trauma, have become important threats to health.

The physical and psychological stresses of a rapidly changing and fast-paced society present daily problems, such as psychosocial and spiritual poor health habits. Post-traumatic stress disorder is becoming a more common diagnosis. Obesity, partly attributed to a lack of exercise and increasing food portion size, is a growing health issue. The ingestion of potentially toxic, non-nutritious, high-fat foods is another contributing factor (see Chapter 11). The abuse of tobacco, drugs, and alcohol also negatively affects health.

The emphasis on treating disease through the application of complex technology not only is costly but also contributes minimally to the improvement of health. An orientation toward illness clearly focuses on the effects rather than the causes of disease.

A substantial change in wellness patterns is occurring. Infectious and acute diseases were the major causes of death in the early part of the twentieth century, whereas chronic conditions, heart disease, cerebrovascular accident (stroke), and cancer are the major causes today. An emphasis on the diagnosis and treatment of disease, which were highly successful in the past, is not the answers for today's needs, which are closely related to and affected by the individual's biochemical functioning, genetics, environment, and personal choices. The Patient Protection and Affordable Care Act (2010) was enacted to begin the process of

BOX 1-7   RESEARCH FOR EVIDENCE-BASED PRACTICE
Preventing Functional Decline in Hospitalized Older Adults

The ability to function independently is important throughout life, but especially as one ages. While some loss of independence in physical functioning may be expected over time, hospitalization should not contribute to physical function loss. Current practice in most hospitals is to limit a person's mobility and independence in activities of daily living. At times these limitations are imposed to prevent falls or other events for the benefit of the individual. But at other times limitations are imposed for the convenience of the staff or to decrease the risk of liability.

Older adults are at risk of losing their functional abilities if the hospitalization imposed limitations interfere with their normal level of activity. A prolonged hospitalization and rehabilitation period can lead to deconditioning, where the person loses muscle mass, strength, and range of motion as a result of a decrease

in their activity. Research has demonstrated that such declines can further limit the activities of daily living for these older adults (Graf, 2006).

Evidence is now available to improve the quality of hospital and long-term care of older adults. Actions include establishing functional baseline data through geriatric assessments at time of admission and at other set times during the stay; using protocols to improve self-care, nutrition, sleep quality, and cognition; minimizing the adverse events that may further influence loss of physical function; and improving the hospital environment to better serve an older adult population (Kleinpell et al., 2008). It is still the nurse caring for the individual person who is most likely to see the need for applying this evidence to improve the care of the hospitalized older adult.

paying for health promotion by providing insurance coverage for more people and by covering preventive health services.

MOVING TOWARD SOLUTIONS

Solutions are neither simple nor easy, but they can be focused in two major directions: individual involvement and government involvement. The first direction concentrates on actions of the individual, especially actions related to lifestyle choices across the life span. The learning and the inherent changes that are involved require the adoption of a new set of skills by people who will need the assistance of nurses to make those changes. Approximately one fifth of the population in the United States is faced with the problem of getting the basic necessities of food and shelter. The other four fifths, whose basic needs are met, must overcome problems resulting from affluence (U.S. Department of Health and Human Services, 2011).

Motivational factors play a large role in influencing attitudinal change. As discussed in Chapter 10, programs for health promotion and health education are only part of the answer.

Financial incentives for prevention may be another motivating factor, and health advocacy by professionals in the health field is critical. Additionally, private and public action at all levels is needed to reduce social and environmental health hazards. Toxic agents in the environment such as particles from diesel emissions and social conditions such as school overcrowding can present health hazards that may not be detected for years; therefore, it is necessary for individuals and government to play a role.

Legislation and financing that relate to primary prevention are discussed in Chapter 3. Government activity, in the form of legislation, is currently increasing in this area. For example, increasing the activity time in schools, mandating seat belt use, and implementing taxes on gasoline use are specific areas for governmental intervention. Health ecology and planning are important areas for government involvement in the future. The redirection of the existing health care delivery system, putting more emphasis on primary prevention, is probably the most difficult and the most far-reaching goal; however, an emphasis on a wellness system is necessary to improve the health of the U.S. population.

CASE STUDY

Health Assessment: Frank Thompson And Family

Frank Thompson's large brick home is located off a sparsely traveled country road. A few yards away stands the uninhabited shack where Frank was born during World War II.

Frank was raised knowing the odds that he faced as a poor tenant farmer. He helped his father, Ben, with their small tobacco and corn crops. They were unaware that the hazardous chemicals in the pesticides they used would later affect Ben's life. As his father often reminded him, Frank had to do better than others in school so he would not be doomed to the tenant farmer's life. However, Frank's school attendance was erratic because it was interrupted by the frequent demand of tending field crops. Thin and often tired, Frank had recurrent infections. The school nurse helped the Thompson family obtain the necessary medication for Frank's initial infection, but the family was never able to afford the penicillin that was necessary to prevent recurrent infections.

Inspired by the early work of Martin Luther King, Jr., Frank was intent on helping at home and building something better for his future. Frank managed to more than compensate for his lost time at school. He passed his college entrance examinations and was awarded one of the new equal opportunity grants, which offered him a choice of attending any of the Ivy League schools in the Northeast. Instead, he chose the prestigious Southern University and eventually earned a masters of business administration (MBA) degree. He married Sada, his longtime girlfriend, and the two planned their future.

With a good job in a large local sales firm, Frank built his house and started a family. He moved from a salesman to a division head and often traveled to regional meetings, sometimes accompanied by Sada and their three children. Frank's dream of sharing his success with his family included using part of his earnings to help his brothers and sisters with their education.

This new way of life meant little time for relaxation and frequent attendance at business luncheons and career-promoting social occasions. Frank kept late hours and worked long weekends. Good food, drinks, and cigarettes helped Frank relax before and after important business and social encounters; these softened the edges of hard bargaining and were status symbols.

Not surprisingly, Frank gained weight. He had a persistent cough, which was probably a result of the smoking habit that developed during the early years of his career. Frank's physician, with whom Frank visited regularly at the corporation's

health maintenance organization (HMO), said Frank's blood pressure and serum lipid levels were both higher than normal and that he had chronic bronchitis. The physician urged Frank to take the actions that Frank already recognized: reduce smoking, drinking, and intake of saturated fats and calories; get more exercise; and find ways to relax. However, Frank's life was too busy for exercise. He had to work harder as he was promoted in his company, but he also had to appear relaxed, which was an essential characteristic for a prospective vice president. To meet these goals, Frank tended to drink and smoke more. He also refused to take medication for problems he could not see. Without the outward signs of disease, Frank believed he was out of shape, but generally healthy. Then Sada noted that his chance for promotion might actually improve if he lost some weight; therefore, Frank registered for a physical fitness program for executives that he could attend on Sunday mornings and before work during the week. At his first workout, the classic sharp pain gripped his chest and Frank had a massive heart attack.

Weeks later, Frank was convalescing at home after being released from the university's coronary care facility. He was lucky to survive the heart attack and he was also fortunate to have most of the health care services covered by his medical insurance plan; in addition, 80% of his earnings were protected by the company's disability pension. (Most people in the United States do not have this protection.)

However, Frank's dreams of promotion were shattered. For many months he could go to the office only two or three times a week at most, simply to deal with routine matters. He could not travel, for business or otherwise, for a long time. He was also skeptical about his cardiac rehabilitation program because his heart attack happened during exercise.

Reflective Questions

1. As a nurse, how would you explain to Frank that his heart attack was not caused by his exercise?
2. How might a family approach to diet and exercise work with this family, given its structure and background?
3. Are there negative behaviors in your life that you see as status symbols?

◎ CARE PLAN

Health Assessment: Frank Thompson and Family

*NURSING DIAGNOSIS: Risk for Ineffective Coping due to change in role performance and self-esteem

Defining Characteristics
- Inability to complete tasks
- Lack of focus on needs
- Feelings of inadequacy
- Inability to make decisions
- Sense of being overwhelmed
- Rest and sleep disturbance
- Frequent stress-related headaches
- Emotional fragility
- Assessment of situations does not match assessments of others

Related Factors
- Unexpected life changes
- Diagnosis of chronic disease
- Stressful life events
- Unsure of family supports
- Unrealistic expectations of self
- Unpredictable future
- Need to reassess abilities
- Insecure job status

Expected Outcomes
- The person will develop realistic expectations of capabilities based on rehabilitation potential.
- The nurse and person will set mutually agreeable milestones for resuming functions.
- The person will develop a revitalized sense of self.
- The person and family will use available resources to examine social and role shifts that affect the family.
- The person and spouse will express to each other their hopes and fears about the future.

Interventions
- Listen to the concerns of the person and spouse regarding job, social, family, and medical concerns.
- Counsel the individual and spouse about realistic goals and expectations of cardiac rehabilitation.
- Assist the individual in setting realistic and reachable short-term goals.
- Assist the individual in developing more effective problem-solving skills.
- Provide support and positive feedback as short-term goals are met.
- Explore available community services that match the goals of the family.
- Facilitate family access to needed services through advocacy and supportive guidance.
- Supervise and teach about the use of prescribed and other medications.
- Coordinate communications between providers, employers, and other organizations to meet coping needs of the individual and his or her family.

*NANDA Nursing Diagnoses—Definitions and Classification 2012-2014, Herdman T.H. (ED). Copyright © 2012, 1994-2012 NANDA International. Used by arrangement with John Wiley & Sons Limited. In order to make safe and effective judgments using the NANDA-I nursing diagnoses it is essential that nurses refer to the definitions and defining characteristics of the diagnoses listed in this work.

SUMMARY

The ways individuals define health and health problems are important because definitions influence attempts to improve health and care delivery. In the case study, Frank Thompson's health was affected by obvious, immediate, and personal factors, such as his diet and employment pressures. Nevertheless, his problems had their roots in the social and economic conditions of his parents; in his own early history of illness, education, and work; and in his and his family's hopes and aspirations. His physician defined Frank's problem in immediate biomedical terms. Public health planners, who saw Frank's problem on a longer-term population basis, sought policy solutions to the problem of preventing cardiovascular disease.

The view taken in this text is that a broad and longer-term perspective of health is the best guide to promoting health more effectively, even as nurses deal with individual problems on a daily basis. Health is a sustainable balance between internal and external forces. Health allows people to move through life free from the constraints of illness and promotes healing.

Illness represents an imbalance that human choices (intertwined social, political, spiritual, professional, and personal choices) create. In the United States, communities may still have time to reduce the onslaught of chronic disability and shift the direction, slow the pace, and humanize the scope of economic and social life.

Shifting directions in today's health care patterns may be possible only when nurses and other health professionals do what is expected of them as leaders in the care of health: to work with others through open processes; to provide leadership in finding the vision and the path; and to inform, educate, and reeducate themselves, their colleagues, the media, and the general public using research findings and evidence-based practice methods.

The responsibility of nurses as health professionals today is to see the health problem in new ways and help others to do the same. Responsibility means developing new roles and examining the problem through others' viewpoints, including those of individuals, the public, other professionals, and other nations. Responsibility also means evaluating the social and individual consequences, the long-term and short-term effects, and the public and private interests that are involved when deciding on the set of tools to use in the care of health.

REFERENCES

Ajzen, A., & Fishbein, M. (1980). *Understanding attitudes and predicting social behavior.* Upper Saddle River, NJ: Prentice Hall.

Allen, F. M., & Warner, M. (2002). A developmental model of health and nursing. *Journal of Family Nursing, 8*(2), 96–135.

American Cancer Society. (2005). *Cancer facts and figures for African Americans 2005-2006.* Atlanta, GA: Author.

American Nurses Association. (2003). *Nursing's social policy statement*. Washington, DC: ANA Publications.

American Nurses Association. (2004). *Nursing: Scope and standards of practice*. Washington, DC: ANA Publications.

American Nurses Association. (2008). *Code of ethics for nurses with interpretive statements*. Washington, DC: ANA Publications.

Andresen, E. M., Catlin, T., Wyrwich, K. W., & Jackson-Thompson, J. (2003). Retest reliability of surveillance questions on health related quality of life. *Journal of Epidemiology and Community Health*, *57*(5), 339–343.

Ardell, D. B. (2007). *What is wellness?* Retrieved February 19, 2012, from www.seekwellness.com/wellness/what_is_wellness.htm.

Bandura, A. (1976). *Social learning theory*. Upper Saddle River, NJ: Prentice Hall.

Bandura, A. (1999). *Self-efficacy: The exercise of control*. New York: W.H. Freeman.

Bandura, A. (2004). Health promotion by social cognitive means. *Health Education Behavior*, *31*(2), 143–164.

Barr, D., Lee, P., & Benjamin, A. (2003). Health care and health policy in a changing world. In H. Wallace (Ed.), *Health and welfare for families in the 21st century* (2nd ed.). Boston: Jones & Bartlett.

Benner, P., Sutphen, M., Leonard, V., & Day, L. (2010). *Educating nurses: A call for radical transformation*. San Francisco: Jossey-Bass.

Boltz, M., Resnick, B., & Galik, E. (2012). Interventions to prevent functional decline in acute care settings. In M. Boltz, E. Capezuti, T. Fulmer, & D. Zwicker (Eds.), *Evidence-based geriatric nursing protocols for best practice* (pp. 104–121). New York: Springer.

Burns, N., & Grove, S. K. (2003). *Understanding nursing research* (3rd ed.). Philadelphia: Saunders.

Cano, A., Scaturo, D., Sprafkin, R., Lantinga, L., Fiese, B., & Brand, F. (2003). Family support, self-rated health, and psychological distress. *Primary Care Companion Journal of Clinical Psychiatry*, *5*, 111–117.

Cohen, S. R., Mount, B. M., Bruera, E., Rowe, J., & Tong, K. (1997). Validity of the McGill Quality of Life Questionnaire in the palliative care setting. A multi-center Canadian study demonstrating the importance of the existential domain. *Palliative Medicine*, *11*, 3–20.

Commission on Social Determinants of Health (CSDH). (2008). *Closing the gap in a generation: Health equity through action on the social determinants of health. Final Report of the Commission on Social Determinants of Health*. Geneva: World Health Organization.

Crimmins, E. M., Preston, S. H., & Cohen, B. (2011). *Explaining divergent levels of longevity in high-income countries*, The National Research Council. Retrieved May 20, 2012, from www8.national academies.org/onpinews/newsitem.aspx?RecordID=13089.

David, R. (2000). Keynote address: Leadership for innovation in health care. In *Ford Foundation, John F. Kennedy School of Government, Summary of Proceedings, Local Innovations in Health Care Conference*, Cambridge, MA: June 28-30, 2000.

Davis, M. A., Weeks, W. B., & Coulter, I. D. (2011). A proposed conceptual model for studying the use of complementary and alternative medicine. *Alternative Therapies in Health and Medicine*, *17*(5), 32–36.

Dunn, H. (1961). *High-level wellness*. Arlington, VA: R.W. Beatty.

Fawcett, J. (1984). The metaparadigm of nursing: Present status and future refinements. *Journal of Nursing Scholarship*, *16*(3), 77–87.

Gordon, M. (2010). *Manual of nursing diagnosis* (12th ed.). Sudbury, MA: Jones & Bartlett.

Graf, C. (2006). Functional decline in hospitalized older adults. *American Journal of Nursing*, *106*, 58–67.

Greiner, P., Snowdon, D., & Greiner, L. (1996). The relationship of self-rated function and self-rated health to concurrent functional ability, functional decline, and mortality: Findings from the Nun Study. *Journal of Gerontology. Series B, Psychological Sciences and Social Sciences, S, 51B*(5), S234–S241.

Greiner, P., Snowdon, D., & Greiner, L. (1999). Self-rated function, self-rated health, and postmortem evidence of brain infarcts: Findings from the Nun Study. *Journal of Gerontology. Series B, Psychological Sciences and Social Sciences*, *54*(4), S219–S222.

Grzywacz, J., & Fuqua, J. (2000). The social ecology of health: Leverage points and linkages. *Behavioral Medicine*, *26*(3), 101–115.

Haley, K., Koenig, H., & Bruchett, B. (2001). Relationship between private religious activity and physical functioning in older adults. *Journal of Religion and Health*, *40*(2), 302–312.

Hollingsworth, L., & Didelot, M. (2005). *Illness: The redefinition of self and relationships*. Paper presented at the 4th Global Conference—Making Sense of: Health, Illness, and Disease, Mansfield College, Oxford: Great Britain.

Idler, E., & Benyamini, Y. (1997). Self-rated health and mortality: A review of twenty-seven community studies. *Journal of Health and Social Behavior*, *38*(1), 21–37.

Institute of Medicine. (2003). *The future of the public's health in the 21st century*. Washington, DC: National Academies Press.

Institute of Medicine. (2010). *The future of nursing: Leading change, advancing health*. Retrieved April 28, 2012, from http://iom.edu/Reports/2010/The future of Nursing-Leading-Change-Advancing-Health.aspx.

International Parish Nurse Resource Center. (2012). *Resource catalog*. Retrieved May 20, 2012, from www.parishnurses.org/.

Issel, L. M. (2009). *Health program planning and evaluation: A practical, systematic approach for community health* (2nd ed.). Sudbury, MA: Jones & Bartlett.

Izzo, J., & Black, H. (2003). *Hypertension primer* (3rd ed.). Philadelphia, PA: Lippincott Williams & Wilkins.

Janz, N., Champion, V., & Strecher, V. (2002). The health belief model. In K. Glanz, B. Rimer, & F. Lewis (Eds.), *Health behavior and health education: Theory, research and practice* (3rd ed.). San Francisco: Jossey-Bass.

Kaplow, R., & Reed, K. (2008). The AACN synergy model for patient care: a nursing model as a force of magnetism. *Nursing Economic$*, *26*(1), 17–25.

Kleinpell, R., Fletcher, K., & Jennings, B. (2008). Reducing functional decline in hospitalized elderly. In R. G. Hughes (Ed.), *Patient safety and quality: An evidence-based handbook for nurses*. Rockville, MD: Agency for Healthcare Research and Quality. Retrieved May 31, 2012, from www.ncbi.nlm.nih.gov/books/NBK2629/?report=printable.

Kreuter, M., & Devore, R. (1980). Update: Reinforcing the case for health promotion. *Family & Community Health*, *10*, 106.

Leavell, H., & Clark, A. E. (1965). *Preventive medicine for the doctor in his community*. New York: McGraw-Hill.

McKivergin, M. (2004). The nurse as an instrument of healing. In B. Dossey, L. Keegan, & C. Guzzetta (Eds.), *Holistic nursing: A handbook for practice* (pp. 233–254). Sudbury, MA: Jones & Bartlett.

National Heart, Lung and Blood Institute (NHLBI). (2000). *Obesity education initiative. The practical guide: Identification, evaluation, and treatment of overweight and obesity in adults*. NIH Publication No. 00-4084. Bethesda, MD: U.S. Government Printing Office.

National Institute of Nursing Research (NINR). (2011). *NINR strategic plan*. Retrieved February 19, 2012, from www.ninr.nih.gov/NR/rdonlyres/8BE21801-0C52-44C2-9EEA-142483657FB1/0/NINR_StratPlan_F2_508.pdf.

National Institutes of Health, National Center for Complementary and Alternative Medicine. (2011). *What is CAM?* Retrieved January 20, 2012, from http://nccam.nih.gov/health/whatiscam/.

Newman, M. (2003). A world of no boundaries. *Advances in Nursing Science, 26*(4), 240–245.

Norwood, S. (2003). *Nursing consultation: A framework for working with communities* (2nd ed.). Upper Saddle River, NJ: Prentice Hall.

O'Donnell, M. (1987). Definition of health promotion. *American Journal of Health Promotion, 1*(1), 4–5.

Ogden, C., Carroll, M., Curtin, L., McDowell, M., Tabak, C., & Flegal, K. (2006). Prevalence of overweight and obesity in the United States, 1999-2004. *Journal of the American Medical Association (JAMA), 295*(13), 1549–1555.

Pender, N. J., Murdaugh, C. L., & Parsons, M. A. (2010). *Health promotion in nursing practice* (6th ed.). Upper Saddle River, NJ: Pearson/Prentice Hall.

Prochaska, J., Gill, P., & Hall, S. (2004). Treatment of tobacco use in an inpatient psychiatric setting. *Psychiatric Services, 55,* 1265–1270.

Reed, P. G. (1983). Implications of the life span developmental framework for well-being in adulthood and aging. *Advances in Nursing Science, 6*(1), 18–25.

Richard, L., Gauvin, L., & Raine, K. (2011). Ecological models revisited: Their uses and evolution in health promotion over two decades. *Annual Review of Public Health, 32,* 307–326.

Rogers, M. (1970). *An introduction to the theoretical basis of nursing.* Philadelphia: F.A. Davis.

Sackett, D., Rosenberg, W., Gray, J., Haynes, R., & Richardson, W. (1996). Evidence based medicine: What it is and what it isn't. *British Medical Journal, 312,* 71–72.

Shilling, C. (2002). Culture, the "sick role" and the consumption of health. *British Journal of Sociology, 53*(4), 621–638.

Siegel, D. (2007). *The mindful brain: Reflection and attunement in the cultivation of well-being.* New York: W.W. Norton & Co.

Smith, J. A. (1983). *The idea of health: Implications for the nursing profession.* New York: Columbia University Teachers College Press.

U.S. Census Bureau. (2010a). *The Hispanic population: 2010.* C2010BR-04. Retrieved May 22, 2012, from www.census.gov/prod/cen2010/briefs/c2010br-04.pdf.

U.S. Census Bureau. (2010b). *The older population: 2010.* C2010BR-09. Retrieved May 22, 2012, from www.census.gov/prod/cen2010/briefs/c2010br-09.pdf.

U.S. Congress. (2010). *Patient Protection and Affordable Care Act ("PPACA"; Public Law 111–148).* Retrieved February 19, 2012, from www.healthcare.gov/law/full/index.html.

U.S. Department of Health, Education, and Welfare, Public Health Service. (1979). *Healthy People.* Washington, DC: U.S. Government Printing Office. U.S. Department of Health and Human Services.

U.S. Department of Health and Human Services, National Institutes of Health, National Heart, Lung and Blood Institute. (2012). *Obesity education initiative.* Retrieved February 19, 2012, from www.nhlbi.nih.gov/health/public/heart/obesity/lose_wt/index.htm.

U.S. Department of Health and Human Services, Office of Disease Prevention and Health Promotion. (2011). *Healthy People 2020* Washington, DC. Retrieved February 19, 2012, from www.healthypeople.gov/2020/.

U.S. Department of Health and Human Services, Public Health Service. (1986). *The 1990 health objectives for the nation: A midcourse review,* Washington, DC: U.S. Government Printing Office. U.S. Department of Health and Human Services.

U.S. Department of Health and Human Services, Public Health Service. (1990). *Healthy People 2000: The Surgeon General's report on health promotion and disease prevention.* U.S. Department of Health and Human Services (Publication No. 7955071), Washington, DC: U.S. Government Printing Office.

U.S. Department of Health and Human Services, Public Health Service. (1996). *Healthy People 2000 midcourse review and 1995 revisions.* Boston: Jones & Bartlett.

U.S. Department of Health and Human Services, Public Health Service. (2000). *Healthy People 2010 (conference edition, in two volumes).* U.S. Department of Health and Human Services, Washington, DC: U.S. Government Printing Office.

U.S. Department of Homeland Security. (2011). *Enforce and administer our immigration laws.* Retrieved May 22, 2012, from www.dhs.gov/xabout/gc_1240610592951.shtm.

U.S. Preventive Services Task Force. (2010). *Guide to clinical preventive services, 2010-2011.* Retrieved February 19, 2012, from www.ahrq.gov/clinic/pocketgd.htm.

Vanderbilt University. (2012). *HEALTH Plus Program.* Retrieved February 19, 2012, from http://healthandwellness.vanderbilt.edu/healthplus/.

Williams, D., & Mohammed, S. (2009). Discrimination and racial disparities in health: Evidence and needed research. *Journal of Behavioral Medicine, 32,* 20–47.

World Health Organization. (2004). *The World Health Organization Quality of Life (WHOQOL)-BREF.* Retrieved May 14, 2012, from www.who.int/substance_abuse/research_tools/en/english_whoqol.pdf.

CHAPTER

2

Emerging Populations and Health

Ali Salman, Yi-Hui Lee, and Tawna Cooksey-James

℮volve WEBSITE

http://evolve.elsevier.com/Edelman/
- Study Questions
- Glossary
- Website Resources
  2A: Cultural Values Orientation
  2B: Comparison of Folk and Professional Care Systems
  2C: Selected Models for Transcultural Nursing

OBJECTIVES

After completing this chapter, the reader will be able to:
- Differentiate among ethnicity, ethnic group, race, and minority group.
- Describe demographic data relative to emerging populations:
  - Arab Americans
  - Asian Americans/Pacific Islanders
  - Black/African Americans
  - Latino/Hispanic Americans
  - Native Americans
  - Homeless Persons

- Describe health concerns and issues of emerging populations.
- Discuss selected cultural factors that may have an impact on the health and well-being of emerging populations.
- Contrast the folk healing system with the professional care system.
- Explain strategies of the nursing profession to meet the needs of emerging populations.
- Describe initiatives to address the health care concerns of emerging populations.

KEY TERMS

Chi
Complementary and alternative medicine (CAM)
Cultural competency
Culture
Emerging populations
Ethnic group
Ethnicity
Ethnocentric perspective

Female genital mutilation
Folk healing system
Health disparities
Health equity
Homelessness
Hot and cold concept of disease
Jing
Minority group
Professional care systems

Race
Taoism
Transcultural nursing
Value orientations
Values
Yang
Yin

❓ THINK ABOUT IT

A New Brand of Outreach for Chemically Dependent Homeless People Living with HIV/AIDS

- Access to health care services is often a major barrier for people who are considered underserved by the health care system. Community outreach programs have shown some success in reaching persons with different types of health problems. However, outreach programs for certain marginalized populations have not always been successful in their efforts to reach the "hard-to-reach."
- A new approach in outreach programs for chemically dependent homeless people living with HIV/AIDS is harm reduction. This approach "acknowledges the reality that drug use is a part of life. Rather than condemn or condone, harm reduction practitioners seek to work collaboratively with the client."
- Harm reduction as a part of outreach programs:
  - Aims to build on the ability of individuals to make decisions about their own lives.
  - Views drug use along a spectrum, ranging from heavy use to abstinence.
  - Honors self-determination and individual dignity.
  - Functions as an alternative model of treatment that reinforces a hierarchical physician-client relationship.
- Practitioners who view harm reduction as an essential component of outreach:
  - See the clients as experts of their lives and their addiction.
  - Consider the structural factors that influence adoption of healthy lifestyles.
- Facilitate an egalitarian relationship between the client and the provider.
- Consider all the multiple pressures affecting client functioning in all spheres of life.

With the above premises and beliefs, an outreach program explored the service utilization of chemically dependent persons living with HIV/AIDS. The study's purpose was to investigate whether hard-to-reach participants, lodged through a harm reduction program at single-room occupancy hotels, access health services at the same level as those who report at the agency's drop-in center. Data indicate that low-threshold harm reduction outreach did increase access to health services by reducing barriers to services.

The researcher concluded that this component of outreach is a "valuable intervention for increasing utilization among this highly marginalized group" (p. 26). Will this philosophy of outreach be effective in helping persons with chronic illnesses such as diabetes, hypertension, or obesity just to name a few? Something to think about!

More comprehensive information on the harm reduction approach for chemically dependent individuals with HIV/AIDS is available online at www.aids.org/topics/harm-reduction-and-hiv/.

Source: Shepard, B. (2007). Harm reduction outreach services and engagement of chemically-dependent homeless people living with HIV/AIDS: An analysis of service utilization data to evaluate program theory. *Einstein Journal of Biology and Medicine, 23*, 26-32.

HEALTH DISPARITIES AND HEALTH EQUALITY

Many magnitudes of disparity, particularly in health, exist in the United States. There has been a growing awareness that racial and ethnic minority groups experienced poorer health compared to the general population in the United States. Various factors such as race or ethnicity, gender, age, disability, and socioeconomic status contribute to an individual's capability to attain good health. *Healthy People 2020* endeavors to improve the health of all groups (Hansen, 2011).

"Health disparities" is an umbrella term that includes disparities in health and in health care. It was defined by *Healthy People 2020* as "a particular type of health difference that is closely linked with social, economic, and/or environmental disadvantage," and "health disparities adversely affect groups of people who have systematically experienced greater obstacles to health based on their racial or ethnic group; religion; socioeconomic status; gender; age; mental health; cognitive, sensory, or physical disability; sexual orientation or gender identity; geographic location; or other characteristics historically linked to discrimination or exclusion" (U.S. Department of Health and Human Services, 2011). Health disparities represent a lack of efficiency within the health care system and account for unnecessary costs and diminish the quality of life for persons seeking care (Hansen, 2011).

"Health equity" is the accomplishment of the highest level of health for all people. Attaining health equity requires valuing everyone equally with focused and ongoing societal efforts to deal with preventable inequalities, historical and contemporary injustices, and the elimination of health and health care disparities (U.S. Department of Health and Human Services, 2011).

Although the diversity of the American population is one of the best assets for this country, one of the greatest challenges is reducing the disparity in health status of America's racial and ethnic minorities and other health disparity populations. The U.S. Department of Health and Human Services (2011) and the Institute of Medicine (IOM, 2008) have well documented that racial and ethnic minorities, compared to Whites, have less access to health care, receive lower-quality health care, and have higher rates of illness, injury, and premature death. The issue of racial and ethnic health disparities has become one of the most urgent problems to plague the U.S. health care system.

Efforts to eliminate disparities and achieve health equity have focused primarily on diseases or illnesses and on health care services. However, the absence of disease does not automatically equate to good health. An individual's ability to achieve good health could be affected because of race or ethnicity, gender, sexual identity, age, disability, socioeconomic status, and geographic location.

EMERGING POPULATIONS IN THE UNITED STATES

Currently, emerging populations include ethnic minorities and persons who are homeless. Ethnic minority populations could include Asian Americans/Pacific Islanders, Blacks/African Americans, Latinos/Hispanic Americans, Native Americans, and Arab Americans (Box 2-1: *Healthy People 2020*).

The increasing population of immigrants has been a significant contributor to the presence of increasing numbers of major ethnic groups in the United States. Between 2000 and 2010, the immigrant population in the United States increased

♥ BOX 2-1 HEALTHY PEOPLE 2020

Selected National Health Promotion and Disease Prevention Objectives for Emerging Populations

- Increase the number of persons with health insurance to 100%. (Baseline: 83.2% [lower in ethnic minorities] of persons under 65 years covered by health insurance in 2008)
- Increase the proportion of persons who have a specific source of ongoing care to 89.4%. (Baseline: 81.3% in 2008)
- Reduce the overall cancer death rate. Target: 160.6 deaths per 100,000 of the population. (Baseline: 178.4 deaths per 100,000 of the population in 2007)
- Prevent diabetes. Target: 7.2 new cases per 1000 per year, ages 18-84. (Baseline: 8 new cases in past 12 months, 2006-2008)
- Increase the proportion of persons with diabetes who receive formal diabetes education. Target: 62.5%. (Baseline: 56.8% of persons with diabetes received formal education in 2008)
- Reduce coronary heart disease deaths. Target: 100.8 deaths per 100,000. (Baseline: 126 coronary artery disease deaths per 100,000 in 2007)
- Reduce AIDS among adolescents and adults. Target: 13 new cases per 100,000. (Baseline: 14.4 cases of AIDS, aged 13 and older in 2007)

From U.S. Department of Health and Human Services. (2012). *Healthy People 2020* (Vol. 1). Washington, DC: U.S. Government Printing Office. Also see developing data and goals for the *Healthy People 2020* at www.healthypeople.gov.

by 8.8 million (Migration Policy Institute, 2012). In 2009 the U.S. immigrant population accounted for about 12.5% of the total U.S. population (Batalova & Terrazas, 2010). One in three Americans in the United States identifies himself/herself as African American, American Indian/Alaska Native, Asian, Native Hawaiian/Pacific Islander, Hispanic/Latino, or multiracial. It was estimated that this number is expected to increase to one in two Americans by 2050 (Kaiser Family Foundation, 2008). The increasing populations of ethnic groups are one of many factors producing disparities in health status and access to the health care system in the United States. The disparities in the health care system may cause increases of social costs attributable to the lost productivity or use of health care services among the ethnic minority populations.

ETHNICITY, ETHNIC GROUP, MINORITY GROUP, AND RACE

Race and ethnicity categories in the United States are defined by the Office of Management and Budget (OMB), with the latest set based on a 1997 revision of a 1977 standard (Humes et al., 2011). The minimal race categories for collecting data on race and ethnicity are Black/African American, American Indian/Alaska Native, Asian, Native Hawaiian and other Pacific Islander, and White; and the minimal ethnicity categories are Hispanic/Latino and Not Hispanic/Latino origin (Humes et al., 2011).

Race and ethnicity are different but somewhat alike. Race is associated with power and indexes the history or ongoing imposition of one group's authority above another. Ethnicity focuses on differences in meanings, values, and ways of living (practices) (Markus, 2008). Race has been defined as "a dynamic set of historically derived and institutionalized ideas and practices that: sorts people into ethnic groups according to perceived physical and behavioral human characteristics; associates differential value, power, and privilege with these characteristics and establishes a social status ranking among the different groups; and emerges (a) when groups are perceived to pose a threat (political, economic, or cultural) to each other's world view or way of life; and/or (b) to justify the denigration and exploitation (past, current, or future) of, and prejudice toward, other groups" (Markus, 2008, p. 654). A definition provided for ethnicity is that "ethnicity is a dynamic set of historically derived and institutionalized ideas and practices that allows people to identify or to be identified with groupings of people on the basis of presumed (and usually claimed) commonalities including language, history, nation or region of origin, customs, ways of being, religion, names, physical appearance, and/or genealogy or ancestry; can be a source of meaning, action, and identity; and confers a sense of belonging, pride, and motivation" (Markus, 2008, p. 654).

A minority group consists of people who are living within a society in which they are usually disadvantaged in relation to power, control of their own lives, and wealth (Hammond & Cheney, 2009). In the 2010 U.S. Census, just one third of the U.S. population reported their race and ethnicity as something other than non-Hispanic White alone, and this group was referred to as the "minority" population for the report (Humes et al., 2011). The minority population in the United States increased from 86.9 million to 111.9 million between 2000 and 2010, and this represented a growth of 29% during the decade (Humes et al., 2011).

CULTURE, VALUES, AND VALUE ORIENTATION

Ethnicity is evidenced in customs that reflect the socialization and cultural patterns of the group. Culture, as an element of ethnicity, refers to integrated patterns of human behavior that include the language, thoughts, communications, actions, customs, beliefs, values, and institutions of racial, ethnic, religious, or social groups (The Office of Minority Health, 2005). It is "shaped by values, beliefs, norms, and practices that are shared by members of the same cultural group" (Giger & Davidhizar, 2008, p. 2).

Values are beliefs about the worth of something and serve as standards that influence behavior and thinking. Cultural values "are unique, individual expressions of a particular culture that have been accepted as appropriate over time. They guide actions and decision-making that facilitate self-worth and self-esteem" (Giger & Davidhizar, 2008, p. 2). Relative to health, cultural values "shape human behaviors and determine what individuals will do to maintain their health status, how they will care for themselves, and others who become ill, and where and from whom they will seek health care" (Boyle, 2008, p. 266).

Value orientations, learned and shared through the socialization process, reflect the personality type of a particular society. The dominant value orientations are shared by the majority of the group. Kluckhohn's model (1953) of value orientations incorporates themes regarding basic human nature, the relationship of human beings to nature, human beings' time orientation, valued personality type, and relationships between human beings. **Website Resource 2A** shows various solutions to the questions proposed by Kluckhohn.

BOX 2-2 DIVERSITY AWARENESS
Female Genital Mutilation: Taboo or Tradition

Some practices of individuals or groups are deeply rooted in beliefs connected to culture. These practices are considered unhealthy and/or unsafe in other cultures who do not share the same beliefs. This is the case for **female genital mutilation (FGM)**. What is the likelihood of health care providers having an encounter with circumcised women? It is probably high because "although the incidence of FGM in women is worldwide, rough estimates range from 114–130 million women" (Little, 2003, p. 30). The increasing migration of circumcised women to the United States and the fact that "female circumcision has been practiced in the U.S. since the 19th century" (Webber & Schonfeld, 2003, p. 65) increase the probability of these women's presence in health care settings. In countries that legally prohibit FGM, parents often feign a holiday or vacation to the native country, where they have the young daughter circumcised.

Female circumcision and female genital mutilation have unknown origins. However, it is believed that the practice can be traced "in Africa as far back as the 5th century B.C. and has taken place in ancient Egypt, ancient Rome, Arabia, and Tsarist Russia" (Little, 2003, p. 30). There are four types of FGM:

- Type 1, also known as clitoridectomy, is the excision of the clitoral prepuce and may also involve the excision of all or part of the clitoris.
- Type 2 is the excision of the clitoris and may also involve the excision of all or part of the labia minora.
- Type 3, also known as infibulation, involves excision of part or all of the external genitalia and the stitching or narrowing of the vaginal opening.
- Type 4 refers to all other genital procedures (Momoh, 2004, p. 631).

It is a myth that FGM is advocated by specific individuals in cultures or societies that advocate and support this practice. Leval and colleagues (2004) analyzed the ways Swedish midwives discussed sexuality in circumcised African women. Their encounters with spouses in maternity wards dispelled the myth that men are the power holders. They were described as "always tender, caring, power shares, or even subordinates in the relationship" (p. 753). Support for this mythbuster is seen in societies where adult women advocate and support the practice as an affirmation of their roles and high regard for their bodies (Little, 2003). Parents of young girls support the practice as an assurance of economic security for their daughters (Gruenbaum, 2005). In some societies, powerful women leaders who are feared and respected promote this practice (Little, 2003).

There are many explanations for female circumcision. Gruenbaum (2005) offers a comprehensive discussion of these. Her analysis to approaches for proposed changes in the practice or its elimination through the passage of laws is extremely enlightening and provides a deep understanding of the complexities of FGM. There are cultural reasons for this practice, including providing health benefits, preserving virginity before marriage, serving as a rite of passage, and providing economic security for women as well as for the persons performing such acts (Berg et al., 2009; Gruenbaum, 2005; Little, 2003). Cultural beliefs about sexuality and sexual responses are also a factor (Leval et al., 2004).

FGM has many complications. The immediate ones include hemorrhage, infections, abscesses, and urinary difficulties such as retention and straining. Long-term complications include difficulty voiding, urinary and reproductive tract infections, and incontinence. Other complications are infertility, painful intercourse, keloids, introital and vaginal stenosis, dermoid cysts, and pain. For the circumcised woman during labor, there is obstructed labor, fetal distress, perineal tears, perineal wound infection, and postpartum hemorrhage and sepsis. Obermeyer (2005) contends that complications or consequences of FGM are poorly documented because of many methodological issues, including the quality of data collected. Valid research on female circumcision is a fertile ground. Obermeyer's (2005) review of studies on FGM is an excellent resource for interested researchers.

What are the care implications for nurses? Midwives and nurses whose area of practice is women's health are more likely to have experiences with circumcised women. "It is essential that midwives recognize the cultural complexities of FGM and show sensitivity when caring and supporting women with FGM during pregnancy, labour, and the postnatal period" (Momoh, 2004, p. 634). Identification can start by asking questions such as the following: "Have you been closed?" "Did you have the cut or operation as a child?" Referrals to a specialist would facilitate discussion of legal issues and possible reversal of the procedure (infibulation). Procedures to reverse infibulation during labor might be performed. Other invasive procedures need to be avoided to eliminate possible sources of pain and stress.

Following delivery, before reinfibulation or restitching is done, the health care provider needs to consider the laws governing the practice of FGM. Mother and baby, if female, are cared for with a view towards the future of the baby.

The information presented is but a very small representation of the continuing interests and work of people from diverse backgrounds. One powerful statement made by these scientists and caregivers is that whatever is done to eliminate FGM, "the cultural integrity of the people" (Little, 2003) must be preserved. Readers are strongly urged to read the cited references for a fuller understanding of FGM.

Sources: Berg, R. C., Denison, E., Lewin, S., & Odgaard-Jensen, J. (2009). *International Initiative for Impact Evaluation: Interventions to reduce the prevalence of female genital mutilation/cutting in African countries.* Retrieved May 15, 2012, from www.ieimpact.org/admin/pdfs_synthetic/011%20protocol.pdf; Gruenbaum, E. (2005). Socio-cultural dynamics of female genital cutting: Research, findings, gaps, and directions. *Culture Health Sexuality, 7*(5), 420-441; Leval, A., Widmar, C., Tishelman, C., & Ahlberg, B. M. (2004). The encounters that rupture the myth: Contradictions in midwives' descriptions and explanations of circumcised women's sexuality. *Health Care for Women International, 25,* 743-760; Little, C. M. (2003). Female genital circumcision: Medical and cultural considerations. *Journal of Cultural Diversity, 10*(1), 30-34; Momoh, C. (2004). Attitudes to female genital mutilation. *British Journal of Midwifery, 12*(10), 631-638; Obermeyer, C. M. (2005). The consequences of female circumcision for health and sexuality: An update on the evidence. *Culture Health Sexuality, 7*(5), 443-461; Webber, S., & Schonfeld, T. (2003). Cutting history, cutting culture: Female circumcision in the United States. *American Journal of Bioethics, 3*(2), 65-66.

Ethnic groups have their unique beliefs and attitudes about health and health care services (Box 2-2: Diversity Awareness). Incongruent beliefs and attitudes about health and health care services among ethnic groups versus the rest of the population, particularly health care providers, are major barriers in improving the health status of ethnic group members. Health care providers need to become responsive to the cultural values of different peoples and to realize how this cultural understanding could augment effective and humanistic care delivery. Knowledge and culturally competent practices are essential for nurses to function effectively in rapidly changing multicultural societies to provide quality and safe care to all.

CULTURAL COMPETENCY

Culture may have an impact on people's health, healing, wellness belief systems, perceived causes of illness and disease, behaviors of seeking health care, and attitudes toward health care providers. Culture may also have influence on the delivery of health care services by the providers who use their own limited set of values to view the world.

Every culture has diverse illustrative models of illness and belief systems regarding health and healing. These models and wellness belief systems include views about the pathophysiology of diseases, the cause and the onset of symptoms, the natural history of illnesses, and the appropriate treatments for various health issues.

Cultural competency is one of the major elements in eliminating health disparities; it starts with an honest desire to disregard personal biases and to treat every person with respect. Although the number of racial and ethnic populations is growing in the United States, it has produced a challenge to the system of health care delivery services. Health care providers and persons seeking care bring their individual cultures and health beliefs and values to the health care experience. Hence, understanding the cultural underpinning of care is a challenging task because of the complexity and interaction between the person seeking care and the health care provider's cultural beliefs (Salman et al., 2007). In addition, providing health care services that are respectful of and responsive to diverse individuals' health beliefs, practices, and cultural needs is believed to contribute to fewer negative health outcomes (Management Sciences for Health, n.d.; The Office of Minority Health, 2005).

It is very important for health care providers to be aware of how persons interpret their health issues or illnesses and to be capable of providing culturally competent care (Box 2-3: Hot Topics). Simply recognizing and accepting cultural diversity is

insufficient to attain cultural competency in health care. Culturally competent health care professionals should be able to consistently and thoroughly recognize and understand the differences in their culture and the culture of others; to respect others' values, beliefs, and expectations; to understand the disease-specific epidemiology and treatment efficacy of different population groups; and to adjust the approach of delivering care to meet each person's needs and expectations (Management Sciences for Health, n.d.). Cultural competency is usually reflected in a health care provider's attitude and his or her communication style.

FOLK HEALING AND PROFESSIONAL CARE SYSTEMS

Within its cultural and/or ethnic customs and traditions, each group has a healing system that incorporates the beliefs and practices deemed essential in maintaining and restoring health. Three components of the healing systems of people were defined: self-care, professional care systems, and folk healing systems (Andrews, 2008). Professional care is "characterized by specialized education and knowledge, responsibility for care, and expectation of remuneration of services rendered" (Andrews, 2008, p. 71). A folk healing system embodies the beliefs, values, and treatment approaches of a particular cultural group that are products of cultural development. Folk health practices are seen in a variety of settings, including community groups, kinship groups, private homes, and healers' shrines. Unlicensed practitioners such as lay midwives, bone setters, and herbalists are part of the folk sector, as are religious practitioners such as spiritualists, Christian Scientists, and scientologists. Other areas of differences between folk and professional care systems are summarized in **Website Resource 2B.**

The choice of a health care system varies among ethnic groups and among individuals within the same group. Ethnic individuals' preference for their folk healing systems is motivated by their familiarity with the folk healer, who usually speaks the same language and is knowledgeable about the beliefs, customs, and traditions of the ethnic group. Easy access and the individual's ability to pay for the healer's services are real advantages when compared with the difficulty of getting appointments, the long waits, and the unfamiliar institutional settings in the professional care system. When folk healing practices are not effective, the individual may turn to the professional care system. Through a culturally sensitive assessment process, nurses can determine which specific folk remedies individuals are using and whether their continued use would interfere with the prescribed medical regimen. Andrews and Boyle (2008) and Giger and Davidhizar (2008) have developed transcultural assessment guides, such as *Andrews & Boyle Transcultural Nursing Assessment Guide,* that nurses and other health care providers can use when working with ethnically diverse individuals. Selected cultural models by transcultural nurses can be found in **Website Resource 2C.** Health care professionals must avoid an ethnocentric perspective when working with ethnic groups. An ethnocentric perspective, which views other ways as inferior, unnatural, or even barbaric, can serve as a major obstacle in

---

🔥 BOX 2-3   HOT TOPICS

Culturally Competent Care Among Nurses

Cultural competence is becoming an integral part of delivering quality health care services to an increasingly diverse population that includes people from all over the world immigrating to the United States. Both immigrants and individuals belonging to ethnic minority groups are more likely to experience disparities in health care and to have inadequate access to health care services as compared to non-Hispanic Whites. People from different cultural backgrounds have a divergent approach to and understanding of their health and how to utilize health care services. Culturally competent care contributes to mitigating health disparities and increases the likelihood of diagnosing diseases that would most likely affect a given culture. Given the diversity of the U.S. population and the unique impact of culture on health, preparing nurses who are able to provide culturally competent care is indispensable to improve the health status of immigrants and minorities.

Many studies have been conducted on various ethnic groups in the United States with the hope of advancing peoples' understanding and competence to provide culturally appropriate health care to all people in this multicultural society. Several studies were also done to assess the status of cultural competence among nurses and to evaluate the effects of cultural training programs. For example, Salman and colleagues (2007) assessed cultural awareness and cultural competence levels among staff nurses who participated in a continuing education program aimed at increasing knowledge of cultural competent care of the geriatric population. Staff nurses who participated in this training program had a higher cultural competence level as compared to nurses who did not join this training program.

establishing and maintaining good working relationships with consumers of health care services.

Ethnic groups will continue to use folk remedies and healing. Therefore, health care professionals need to appreciate the many positive aspects of folk systems. A caring, holistic approach that incorporates family and support systems and considers the individual's viewpoint is one of the more positive aspects of folk systems. This approach is receiving recognition by the professional care system. A blend of both systems would optimize health care for ethnic Americans.

ARAB AMERICANS

Arab Americans come from several countries; Lebanon is the home of most. Other countries include Syria, Palestine, Iraq, Egypt, Yemen, and Jordan. Arab Americans came to the United States in three immigration waves. The first wave of immigrants who came between the late 1800s and World War I were mostly from Greater Syria. The second wave came after the close of World War II and included many Muslims and refugees displaced by the 1948 Palestine War. The last wave occurred in the 1960s and consisted of many professionals, entrepreneurs, and skilled and semiskilled laborers (Abraham, 1995; Stussy, 2000).

The U.S. Census of 2000 was a milestone survey because it recognized Arab Americans for the first time as a separate ethnic group. There are at least 1.7 million Americans who reported an Arab ancestry (Arab American Institute Foundation, 2007-2009). The three largest groups are the Lebanese, Syrians, and Egyptians. Arab Americans live in all 50 states, but one third of them live in California, New York, and Michigan. About 94% of Arab Americans live in metropolitan areas. The top five metropolitan areas of Arab American concentration are Los Angeles, Detroit, New York City/New Jersey, Chicago, and Washington, DC. One of the largest groups of Arab Americans lives in Dearborn, Michigan (Arab American Institute Foundation, 2007-2009). Three major religions are represented among Arab Americans including Christianity, Judaism, and Islam (Arab American Institute Foundation, 2007-2009). More than 45% of Arab Americans have a bachelor's degree or higher, compared to 28% of Americans at large. About 18% of Arab Americans have a postgraduate degree, which is nearly twice the American average (10%). Other statistical data and information on Arab Americans can be found at the website of the Arab American Institute (www.aaiusa.org/pages/demographics/).

Health Care Issues of Arab Americans

There is limited health-related information and a scarcity of scholarship about Arab Americans. Similar to other ethnicities Arab Americans suffer from chronic health problems such as diabetes and coronary artery disease. Several factors place Arab Americans at high risk for developing adult-onset diabetes and cardiovascular disease including obesity, age, gender, and low employment rates.

Another health concern is mental health and the role of acculturation in Arab Americans. Aprahamian and colleagues (2011) looked at the concept of mental health and degree of acculturation and the implications for mental health counselors

of Arab American clients. They reported that age at migration, length of stay in the United States, religion, and discrimination experiences were significant predictors of mental health. Mental health counselors need to be aware of and consider these factors when helping Arab American clients. Many Arab Americans seek their immediate and extended family, community, and traditional values and cultural practices for help during a health crisis. Consequently, given the unique nature of mental illness, many Arab Americans do not receive professional mental health attention when needed.

A health issue on the rise among Arab American adolescents is tobacco consumption, which is considered to be a major risk factor for many health problems affecting the respiratory and cardiovascular systems. Tobacco can be consumed in many ways; however, tobacco chewing, cigarette smoking, and using a Shisha (waterpipe) are the three major methods used to consume tobacco products. Arabs, both men and women, have long traditions of using Shisha and cigarettes with their friends and families and at other social gatherings. Weglicki and colleagues (2008) reported that the percentage of Arab American youth smoking cigarettes was lower than that of non–Arab American youth. However, waterpipe smoking was seen more often in Arab American youth when compared to non–Arab American youth. Tobacco use has been linked to a higher rate of chronic health problems such as heart disease, hypertension, and diabetes among Arab Americans than among non–Middle Eastern Whites (Jamil et al., 2008). Current waterpipe use has been better predicted by being Arab and having a lower educational level.

Access to culturally suitable and current care is essential given that the Arab American population suffers from a wide spectrum of diseases. Many barriers exist that prevent Arab Americans from using professional care services. These include religious beliefs and practices, cultural norms relating to modesty, family values of upholding the family's reputation, gender issues such as preference for same-sex health provider, use of folk remedies, and stresses of assimilation and acculturation such as lack of English skills (Figure 2-1, A-B). There are also barriers related to the health providers including a lack of culturally competent services and the possession of attitudes such as stereotyping and discrimination (Williams et al., 2008).

Selected Health-Related Cultural Aspects

Arabs value the family and the ties it maintains; therefore, the extended family, a clan, and a tribe are common kinship groups. Customs center on hospitality around food, family, and friends (Andrews, 2008). Arab American families are, on average, larger than non–Arab American families and smaller than families in Arab countries. Traditionally, more children meant more pride and economic contributors for the family. The cost of having large families in the United States, however, and adaptation to American customs seem to encourage smaller families. Religion plays an important part in Arab culture and there are dietary rules and prescribed rituals for praying and washing (Kavanaugh, 2008). Arab Americans are present-oriented and view the future as uncertain (Kavanaugh, 2008).

FIGURE 2-1 (A, B) The Arab culture values prescribed rituals for praying and cultural dress.

ASIAN AMERICANS/PACIFIC ISLANDERS

Asian Americans/Pacific Islanders (AAPIs) represent people from many different countries, so their origins, cultures, lifestyles, and religions are diverse. The number of AAPIs in the United States is about 15 million, and they speak more than 100 languages and dialects (Africa & Carrasco, 2011). Beginning in 1997, the Asian or Pacific Islander racial category was separated into two categories (one being Asian and the other being Native Hawaiian and Other Pacific Islander) by the Office of Management and Budget directive (U.S. Census Bureau, 2012a). "Asian" refers to a person having origins in any of the original peoples of the Far East, Southeast Asia, or the Indian subcontinent (Humes et al., 2011). Chinese, Koreans, and Filipinos are currently the three largest groups of Asians in the United States. According to the 2010 Census, the estimated number of U.S. residents of Asian descent comprised 5.6% of the total U.S. population. Between the 2000 census and 2010 census, Asian American and Pacific Islanders are the fastest growing (46% of growth) ethnic minority in the United States. In 2009 Chinese Americans were the largest Asian group, and following Spanish, Chinese was the most widely spoken non-English language in the United States. Most AAPIs live and reside in metropolitan areas; California is the state with the largest Asian population followed by New York. In Hawaii, 57% of the total population are Asians. Texas and New Jersey also have large concentrations of AAPIs.

AAPIs are often referred to as a "model minority"; this stereotype is frequently accepted because most AAPIs are viewed as being successful, resilient, hard-working, intelligent, and healthy. Education is highly valued in the AAPI communities. According to the reports from the U.S. Census (U.S. Census Bureau, 2012a), Asian Americans have the highest percentage of college graduates of any racial or ethnic group. About 50% of Asian Americans have a bachelor's degree or higher level of education, compared with 28% of the total population in the United States. Approximately 17.2% of Asian Americans reported having no health insurance coverage in 2009. Native Hawaiians or Pacific Islanders refer to people having origins of Hawaii, Guam, Samoa, or other Pacific Islands (Humes et al.,

2011). According to the 2010 U.S. Census, Native Hawaiians and Other Pacific Islanders comprised the largest proportion (26%) of the total population in Hawaii. The poverty rate among those who identified themselves as Native Hawaiian and Other Pacific Islander was about 5.1%. Approximately 17.3% of Native Hawaiians and Other Pacific Islanders were reported without health insurance (U.S. Census Bureau, 2012a).

A look at the status of AAPIs as a group reveals that they are doing relatively well in the United States. For instance, the median family income is higher than the national median income for all households. Compared to other ethnic groups their poverty level is lower (U.S. Census Bureau, 2012a).

Health Care Issues of Asian Americans/Pacific Islanders

Health care issues of AAPIs are relative to their ethnicity, religion, and status as immigrants. Some Asian American immigrants have carried diseases from their home countries, and they may now experience new diseases because of their new lifestyle and living conditions. However, AAPIs are more likely to be healthier than Whites and other ethnic groups. Asian American women have the highest life expectancy (85.8 years) among all ethnic groups in the United States (Centers for Disease Control and Prevention, 2012). However, Asian Americans are challenged with various factors that threaten their health. Some negative causes are associated with infrequent medical visits as a result of language/cultural barriers, lack of health insurance, and fear of transportation (Centers for Disease Control and Prevention, 2012; The Office of Minority Health, 2012c).

In general, AAPIs have health problems similar to those of the U.S. population as a whole. Cancer, heart disease, stroke, unintentional injuries, and diabetes are the top five leading causes of death among AAPIs (U.S. Department of Health and Human Services, 2010a). Asian Americans also have a high prevalence and risk factors for chronic obstructive pulmonary disease, hepatitis B, human immunodeficiency virus/acquired immunodeficiency syndrome (HIV/AIDS), smoking, tuberculosis, and liver disease (U.S. Department of Health and Human Services, Office of Minority Health, 2011). In 2007 AAPI women were 30% less likely to have breast cancer compared to non-Hispanic White women (The Office of Minority Health, 2012c). AAPI women are less likely to die from breast cancer, and death rates are lower compared to the other ethnic groups. However, AAPIs are three times more likely to have stomach cancer compared with non-Hispanic Whites. Asian/Pacific Islander men are 40% less likely to have prostate cancer as White men, but they are twice as likely to have stomach cancer. In general, AAPIs have lower rates of being overweight and having hypertension and are less likely to be current cigarette users compared with White adults. By the end of 2009 AAPI cases accounted for approximately 1% of the total HIV/AIDS population in the United States (Centers for Disease Control and Prevention, 2011b). Although the numbers of infected persons are low compared to the other groups in the United States, the increased rates of HIV/AIDS infections among AAPIs from 2006 through 2009 have raised concerns about this population (Centers for Disease Control and Prevention, 2011b).

Disparities in the health status of AAPIs are primarily a result of subcultures within the larger group. There are many divergent and segregated cultures within AAPIs; however, all ethnic populations of AAPIs are currently often classified and viewed as an unvarying group. About two thirds of AAPIs were foreign-born, whereas nearly 38% of Asian Americans do not speak English fluently (Ponce et al., 2009). The classification and cultural barriers (such as language) limit public awareness and restrain effective and culturally appropriate disease prevention for subgroups of the AAPI population. However, few studies have focused on AAPIs and even fewer researchers have examined the subgroups, and this often creates a generalized and inaccurate picture of the experience and needs of AAPIs in the United States. The heterogeneity of subgroups among AAPIs and their relatively small representation in the U.S. population make it challenging to have sufficient and representative samples from the AAPIs. Information about health status among the different subgroups of AAPIs is extremely limited; more studies are needed to fully understand their health issues.

Selected Health-Related Cultural Aspects

AAPIs share many traditional values. A comprehensive description of traditional values in several Asian groups indicates commonalities and differences (Andrews & Boyle, 2008; D'Avanzo & Geissler, 2007).

The family is the most important social institution for AAPIs (Kavanagh, 2008). The extended family has significant influence on Asian Americans. Although family dynamics and structure vary in the different AAPI subgroups, family is often the major source of functional and psychological support for AAPIs. Usually, the interests and honor of the family are more important than those of individual family members. Older family members are usually respected and have authority that is often unquestioned. For instance, among Filipinos, calling older persons by their first names is a sign of disrespect. Male friends of one's parents or grandparents are addressed as "Tito" (uncle) followed by the first name. For female friends it is "Tita" (aunt). These terms, denoting respect, have been substituted for Filipino terms that do not have English translations.

In the culture of Asian Americans, the oldest male family member often is the decision maker and spokesperson. Maintaining harmony is an important value in Asian cultures, and avoiding conflict and direct confrontation is strongly emphasized. Authorities and professionals are usually respected in the Asian American communities. Mostly, physicians and their recommendations are powerful and highly respected and valued. However, as a result of respect for authorities, AAPIs may avoid showing their disagreements with the recommendations of health care professionals. The health care providers need to recognize that lack of disagreement with recommended treatments or therapies does not mean that the Asian American patient and family agree with or will abide by the treatment recommendations.

Rates of psychological distress in AAPIs are similar to those of the general U.S. population; however, AAPIs have a tendency to be the least likely to seek mental health services among all ethnicities. A variety of factors related to cultural values, such as stigma, cultural impact of shame, and language barriers, may contribute to their low utilization of mental health services (Africa & Carrasco, 2011). Asian cultures consider that the behavior of the individual reflects on the family; therefore, mental illness or any behavior that indicates lack of self-control is viewed as producing shame and guilt to the family. Consequently, Asian Americans may be reluctant to discuss symptoms of mental illness or depression. Suicide was reported as the fifth leading cause of death among Asian Americans, compared to the ninth cause of death for White Americans; Among all U.S. women older than age 65, Asian American women have the highest suicide rate (The Office of Minority Health, 2012c).

In addition to reduced access to mental health care, the culture and values of AAPIs are associated with other health problems and risk factors that threaten health and act as barriers to accessing health care. For example, sexually related issues are taboo topics and considered a private matter that should not be discussed with other persons except the spouse. Women may feel it is embarrassing to discuss sex, to visit physician clinics for sexually related health issues, or to receive some forms of physical examinations (e.g., Pap smear). Such fears may have prohibited the willingness of AAPIs to access health care services and prevented health care providers from approaching this population for interventions. For example, the taboo topic of sexual issues was identified as one of the key barriers that makes it difficult for health care providers to approach Chinese American youths for HIV/AIDS prevention (Lee et al., 2012).

Many people find the task of parenthood in a new country difficult because some of their cultural values conflict with the mainstream cultural values—for example, passivity to avoid conflict versus assertiveness. Exposure of children to different cultures in schools and in their neighborhood facilitates their adoption of other cultural beliefs and attitudes in their socialization (Vance, 2008). Additionally, the employment of immigrant women outside the home has exposed their children to other caretakers. Grandparents are often the caretakers of young grandchildren. Filipino American grandparents view their roles as part of their family responsibility (Kataoka-Yahiro et al., 2004).

Asian folk medicine and philosophies have a strong Chinese influence as a result of early Chinese migration throughout Asia. Therefore, the folk medicines of Filipinos, Japanese, Koreans, and Southeast Asians are all imbued with Chinese principles. Taoism was the philosophical and theoretical foundation of Chinese medicine. The "Tao" is rooted in the idea of balancing natural processes and forces (such as yin and yang) and is closely related to Asians' activities of daily living including traditional health practices such as acupuncture, holistic medicine, herbalism, meditation, and martial arts. According to Tao doctrine, humans are microcosms within the universe. Achieving harmony between the two is essential because the energies of both intertwine. Yin and yang are the two forces that keep innate energy, called chi, and sexual energy, called jing, in balance. Yin is feminine, negative, dark, and cold; yang is masculine, positive, light, and warm. An imbalance in energy can be caused, for instance, by yielding to strong emotions or eating an improper diet. In their interactions, humans and the universe are both susceptible to the elements of earth, fire, water, metal, and wood (Andrews, 2008; Kavanaugh, 2008).

Asian folk medicine uses a wide variety of herbs for healing purposes, including roots, leaves, seeds, tree bark, and parts of flowers. Some aspects of Asian folk medicine have gained popularity within the professional care system. In general the use or nonuse of healing traditions seems to be consistent with how closely Asians identify with their heritage (Tashiro, 2006). Of these, the best known is acupuncture (Andrews, 2008). Similar alternative treatment modalities that are slowly gaining wide acceptance are meditation, therapeutic touch, massage, imagery, relaxation, and bipolarity. Box 2-4: Research for Evidence-Based Practice discusses the use of complementary and alternative medicine (CAM) in the United States.

LATINO/HISPANIC AMERICANS

The terms Hispanic or Latino are used interchangeably because the Office of Management and Budget (OMB) demands federal agencies to use a "Hispanic or Latino" category to identify individuals from specific national origin. The OMB definition of Hispanic or Latino origin "refers to a person of Cuban, Mexican, Puerto Rican, South or Central American, or other Spanish culture or origin regardless of race." The largest Hispanic American subgroups are Mexicans, Puerto Ricans, and Cubans. Most Hispanics live in Texas, New York, Florida, and California (The Office of Minority Health, 2012d).

Data from U.S. Census 2010 showed that the 50.5 million Latino/Hispanic people of the United States accounted for 16.3% of the total U.S. population, making this population the nation's

---

BOX 2-4 RESEARCH FOR EVIDENCE-BASED PRACTICE

Use of Complementary and Alternative Medicine (CAM) in the United States

The National Center for Complementary and Alternative Medicine (NCCAM, 2011) defines complementary and alternative medicine (CAM) as a set of varied medical and health care practices, systems, and products that are not usually considered part of conventional medicine. Medicine is practiced by holders of M.D. (medical doctor) or D.O. (Doctor of Osteopathic Medicine) degrees and by their allied health professionals such as physical therapists, psychologists, and registered nurses. Conventional medicine is also called Western or allopathic medicine and is practiced by medical doctors and doctors of osteopathic medicine. Doctors of Osteopathic Medicine (DOs) are fully licensed physicians. They provide a full range of services, from prescribing drugs to performing surgery, and employ a "whole person" approach to health care. DOs focus special attention on the musculoskeletal system, a system of bones and muscles that makes up about two-thirds of the body's mass. They may use osteopathic manipulative treatment, a system of manual therapy, to treat mechanical strains affecting all aspects of the anatomy, relieve pain, and improve physiologic function.and by other related health professionals (such as psychologists, physical therapists, and registered nurses). Acupuncture, biofeedback, relaxation, music therapy, massage, art, music, and dance therapy are some examples of CAM. Western medicine, supported by improved knowledge and advances in technology, has been successful in addressing numerous illnesses. However, there remains a cadre of chronic illnesses and conditions that do not respond well to allopathic treatment. Persons who do not experience relief from chronic conditions often resort to complementary and alternative medicine. However, the boundaries between CAM and conventional medicine are not fixed, and several CAM practices (for example, acupuncture and music therapy) have been becoming more widely accepted.

A national survey found that about 38% of Americans use complementary and alternative medicine, a group of diverse medical and health care systems, practices, and products that are not presently considered to be part of conventional medicine. Complementary medicine is used together with conventional medicine, and alternative medicine is used in place of conventional medicine (NCCAM, 2011). Another study used a comparative analysis of data from the 2002 and 2007 National Health Interview Survey (NHIS) of the civilian noninstitutionalized U.S. population to investigate recent trends in complementary and alternative medicine (CAM) (Su & Li, 2011). The findings of this study suggest that CAM use has increased significantly in the United States. This increase was more obvious among non-Hispanic Whites than among racial and ethnic minorities. The non-Hispanic White Americans had the highest prevalence rate of using at least one CAM therapy in the period from 2002 to 2007, followed by Asian Americans, African Americans, and Hispanics. This study also revealed that the use of CAM becomes more probable when there is limited access to conventional care. This study also pointed out that the increasing cost of conventional medical care has resulted in increasingly limited access to medical care and is a contributing factor to the rising prevalence of CAM use.

The dynamic interplay of many factors that serve as barriers for many ethnic groups to accessing traditional health care and the person's own cultural beliefs warrant a close look at how CAM can greatly augment health care services. This study revealed a growing prevalence of CAM use in the United States; however, the growth in CAM use was not equally distributed across racial and ethnic groups in the United States. The increasing prevalence and the increasing gap in CAM use across racial and ethnic groups highlight the critical need for assessing the health consequences of CAM therapies. There is limited information about efficacy and the possible side effects associated with the use of any specific CAM therapy and its interactive effects with conventional medicine. More studies are needed to provide information about which CAM therapies can be used as an alternative or supplement to conventional medical care.

Sources: NCCAM. (2011). *What is complementary and alternative medicine?* Retrieved July 4, 2012, from http://nccam.nih.gov/health/whatiscam#definingcam; Su, D., & Li, L. (2011). Trends in the use of complementary and alternative medicine in the United States: 2002-2007. *Journal of Health Care for the Poor and Underserved, 22,* 295-309.

largest ethnic or racial minority (U.S. Census Bureau, 2012c). A 43% increase in the Hispanic population between 2000 and 2010 makes Hispanics the fastest-growing minority group in the United States. It was estimated that the Hispanic population of the United States will constitute 30% of the nation's population by 2050 (U.S. Census Bureau, 2012c). The large size of the Hispanic population makes Mexico the only country worldwide that has a larger Hispanic population than the United States, and 63% of people of Hispanic descent in the United States were from Mexico (U.S. Census Bureau, 2012c). About 76% of Hispanics age 5 years and older speak Spanish at home, and more than half of these Spanish speakers speak English "very well" (U.S. Census Bureau, 2012c). The poverty rate among Hispanics increased from 23.2% in 2008 to 25.3% in 2009, and the percentage of Hispanics who lacked health insurance also increased from 30.7% in 2008 to 32.4% in 2009. Among the Hispanic population 25 years and older, 14% of them had a bachelor's degree or higher level of education in 2010.

Health Issues of Latino/Hispanic Americans

Hispanic Americans' health is often associated with factors such as language/cultural barriers, lack of access to preventive care, and lack of health insurance. Latinos/Hispanic Americans (LHAs) have many health issues complicated by multiple cultural, economic, political, and social factors. Hispanics are the highest uninsured racial or ethnic group within the United States (U.S. Census Bureau, 2012c).

The leading causes of illness and death among Hispanics include heart disease, cancer, HIV/AIDS, stroke, and diabetes. Hispanic men and women have higher incidence and mortality rates for stomach cancer (U.S. Department of Health and Human Services, CDC, 2012a). Mexican American adults are almost 2 times more likely than non-Hispanic Whites to have diabetes and 1.5 times as likely to die from this disease (U.S. Department of Health and Human Services, CDC, 2012b). Although cardiovascular disease (U.S. Department of Health and Human Services, 2011) and cancer are the first and second causes of morbidity and mortality among LHAs, their incidence in the general population is higher (U.S. Department of Health and Human Services, CDC, 2012a). Hispanic women were less likely to have a mammogram within the past 2 years; however, they were slightly more likely to have a Pap smear during the past 3 years when compared to non-Hispanic White women (U.S. Department of Health and Human Services, CDC, 2012a). In addition, Hispanic adults age 50 and over were 34% less likely to report having colonoscopy, sigmoidoscopy, or proctoscopy as non-Hispanic Whites (Agency for Healthcare Research and Quality [AHRQ], 2011). Hispanic adults living in the United States generally have lower rates of prostate and breast cancer as compared to non-Hispanic White adults (U.S. Department of Health and Human Services, CDC, 2012a).

Some other health conditions and risk factors that significantly affect Hispanics include asthma, chronic obstructive pulmonary disease, HIV/AIDS, obesity, suicide, and liver disease. LHAs had the second-largest numbers of persons with HIV/AIDS at the close of 2005 (Centers for Disease Control and Prevention, 2011b).

The difficulties experienced by LHAs in receiving appropriate health care services are comparable to those of the poor and other ethnic minorities. Other barriers include the lack of racial and ethnic diversity in the leadership and workforce of the health care system, lack of interpreter services for Spanish-speaking people, and lack of or inadequate culturally appropriate health care resources. Many Hispanic Americans may not readily seek care because they have continued reliance on their folk system of healing. Their preference for this is logical given their lack of health insurance and perceived difficulties negotiating the health care system because of language and other sociocultural barriers.

Selected Health-Related Cultural Aspects

Each subgroup of the LHA population has distinct cultural beliefs and customs. However, a common heritage determines similar values and beliefs. For instance, the two most important aspects of all Hispanic cultures are the emphasis on family and religion. For older Hispanic Americans, the family is an important component of good health. The family is the most important source of support; therefore, the needs of the family as a whole supersede the needs of the individual. During times of illness and crisis, the family is there for the individual. Older family members and other relatives are accorded courtesy and respect and are often consulted on important matters (Andrews, 2008).

LHAs' dependence on spiritual strength to aid them in illness and dying is evident in their use of prayer. LHAs attribute the origins of disease and illness to spiritual or natural punishments, hot and cold imbalances, magic, dislocation of internal organs, natural diseases, and emotional and mental issues. The hot and cold concept of disease was derived from the Hippocratic theory of pathology. Illness occurs when there is an imbalance. This concept of hot and cold guides Hispanics when they categorize illnesses and select appropriate treatments. For example, an elevated body temperature is managed by giving the person a cool drink to lower the fever. For a person who has a cold, drinking warm fluids would be considered therapeutic (Chong, 2002).

LHAs attribute illness and disease to many supernatural and psychological causes. The evil eye or the "mal de ojo" is an example. Fright or "susto" and hysteria or "ataque de nervios" are caused by strong emotions, crises, and traumatic experiences (Chong, 2002). LHAs still resort to many home remedies and consult folk healers including the curandero, spiritualist, *yerbero,* and the *sabador. Curanderos* use a variety of folk remedies, including prayers, rituals, herbs, and the laying on of hands. Spiritualists use medals, amulets, and prayers to affect a cure. The *yerbero* is knowledgeable in the use of herbs, whereas the *sabador* is an expert in massage and manipulation of bones and muscles (Andrews, 2008). Other Hispanic Americans, such as Cubans, practice *Santeria.* Persons who are ill may seek the advice of a "godfather" who is a member of the *Santeria.* Wearing white clothes for a year, performing rituals, and following dietary restrictions are involved in bringing forth a cure to an illness (Carbonell, 2002).

Folk remedies are used in combination with professional care approaches. The individual's belief in the folk remedy can have positive effects on the person's well-being. Therefore, professional care personnel need to find ways to blend the two systems to the optimal benefit of LHAs and their families.

BLACKS/AFRICAN AMERICANS

The "Black or African American" (BAA) refers to people having origins in any of the Black racial groups of Africa (Humes et al., 2011). According to the 2010 Census, the 4.2 million people of the Black/African American population made up 13.6% of the total U.S. population, and it is estimated that this population would constitute 15% of the total population of the United States (U.S. Census Bureau, 2012b). African Americans are the second largest minority population, following the Hispanic/Latino population (U.S. Census Bureau, 2012b).

As one of the largest ethnic groups in the United States, Blacks/African Americans are considered a minority group, a label originating from their slavery roots. Therefore, they continue, in many ways, to experience extreme segregation and exclusion from mainstream society, and discrimination by the majority group.

The majority of Blacks in the United States lived in the Southern states with the largest Black population in 2010 found in New York, Florida, Texas, Georgia, California, North Carolina, Illinois, Maryland, Virginia, and Ohio (The Office of Minority Health, 2012e). BAAs that lived outside of the South have a tendency to be more concentrated in metropolitan areas. The places with the largest Black population were New York, Chicago, and Detroit, and Michigan was the state with the greatest proportion of BAAs (Rastogi et al., 2011).

BAAs have made substantial progress in many areas in the past century. However, there are still inequities in many areas such as business, education, political participation, and leadership. The reports of the 2010 U.S. Census indicated that the rate of living at the poverty level for African Americans was three times that for non-Hispanic Whites (The Office of Minority Health, 2012e). Educationally, BAAs have made substantial gains; 18% of Black/African Americans who were 25 or older had a bachelor's degree or more in 2010 (U.S. Census Bureau, 2012b).

Health Issues of Blacks/African Americans

A complex set of social, economic, and environmental factors can be identified as contributors to the current health status of Blacks/African Americans. However, poverty may be the most profound and pervasive determinant of health status. Individuals and families who are below the poverty level or lack adequate resources have limited access to health care services such as prenatal and maternal care, childhood immunizations, dental checkups, well-child care, and a wide range of other health promoting and preventive services. In 2010 the poverty rate in this population was reported as 27.4%; 20.8% of this population was reported without health insurance during all or part of 2010 (U.S. Census Bureau, 2012b).

Two indices of the effects of poverty can be seen in the high rates of infant mortality and maternal mortality. Despite changes in living conditions, advances in infection control, and improved standards in neonatal care, BAAs still experience high infant and maternal mortality rates. In 2007 the infant mortality rate for BAAs was 2.4 times higher than that of non-Hispanic Whites (The Office of Minority Health, 2011b). BAAs have the second-highest percentage of women who lack prenatal care in the first trimester of pregnancy (The Office of Minority Health, 2011b). African Americans have lower life expectancies than other races at age 65. In 2010 life expectancy for African American males was 79 years compared to 82 for all American males. For BAA females, life expectancy was 83 years compared to 85 in all female Americans (U.S. Social Security Administration, 2012).

Black American children living below the poverty level also experience numerous health problems, including malnutrition, anemia, and lead poisoning. These problems and the lack of immunizations combine to inhibit normal growth and development and affect school performance. Poverty-stricken families usually live in depressed socioeconomic areas where housing conditions are unsafe and unhygienic. Unsafe buildings and other environmental structures cause accidents and injuries among young children. Young children have fallen to their deaths from windows that were unprotected by metal railings. Older people have suffered falls and other injuries from poorly lit stairways and hallways. Other hazards include uncollected garbage and abandoned buildings that are used as dumpsites or as meeting places for a variety of illegal activities.

African Americans are affected disproportionately by the leading causes of death in the United States, including cancer, HIV/AIDS, obesity, diabetes, heart disease, and hypertension. The incidence of cancer and mortality rates for BAAs is higher than that for White Americans. In 2007 the death rate for African Americans was higher than that of Whites for heart diseases, stroke, cancer, asthma, influenza and pneumonia, diabetes, HIV/AIDS, and homicide. African American women are 36% more likely to die from breast cancer, and they are 2.2 times more likely to die from stomach cancer (The Office of Minority Health and Health Disparities, 2007). Although African Americans are only 13% of the U.S. population, they account for 48% of HIV/AIDS cases in 2008. African American males have 8 times the AIDS rate as White males. African American females have 20 times the AIDS rate as White females (The Office of Minority Health, 2011c).

Severe high blood pressure is more common for Black Americans in both men and women. African American adults are 40% more likely to have high blood pressure but 10% less likely to have blood pressure under control than their non-Hispanic White counterparts, and African Americans are 30% more likely to die from heart disease compared to non-Hispanic White men (The Office of Minority Health, 2012f). BAA adults are 60% more likely to have a stroke and males are 60% more likely to die from a stroke (The Office of Minority Health, 2012g).

Other health issues including obesity and its contributing factors are also receiving attention. BAAs are twice more likely to be diagnosed with diabetes than non-Hispanic Whites, and they are more likely to suffer complications from diabetes (The Office of Minority Health, 2012h). This higher rate of diabetes may be related to higher obesity rates among African

Americans. BAAs had the greatest prevalence of obesity compared with other races in the United States (Flegal et al., 2012; U.S. Department of Health and Human Services, 2009).

Selected Health-Related Cultural Aspects

Differences in cultural beliefs, attitudes, and practices exist between rural and urban Black Americans; however, they share some basic cultural beliefs. Black American culture is centered on the family and religion. The family, the strongest institution, provides strong extended kinship bonds with grandparents, aunts, uncles, and cousins. The family is considered the strongest source of support, especially in times of crisis and illness (Gary et al., 2003). Family members and relatives are consulted before BAAs seek care elsewhere.

Religion and religious behavior are an integral part of the BAA community. The church is a significant support system for many African Americans; it serves many purposes beyond worship and formation including: serving as a place to meet where members could pass news, take care of business, and find strength of purpose; providing direct social welfare services; acting as a stabilizing force in the community; facilitating citizenship training and community social action; serving as a transmitter of cultural history; and providing the means for coping and surviving in a hostile world (McGadney-Douglass, 2000).

Africa Americans believe in the healing power of prayer (Vaughn et al., 2009). African Americans were found to use more prayer for health reasons (Su & Li, 2011). The BAA church and spirituality play an important role in health issues. For instance, prostate education for older men is received more favorably when done within the parish nursing approach (Lambert et al., 2002).

BAAs define *health* as a feeling of well-being and the ability to fulfill role expectations. Diseases can be caused by natural or spiritual forces (Kavanaugh, 2008). Therefore, BAAs' approach to health care is guided by these beliefs. Family members, such as grandmothers and other community members, are often consulted for traditional home remedies. Traditionally, roots, herbs, potions, oils, powders, rituals, and ceremonies are still used in many Southern communities. The use of healers is also common, including the old lady, who is knowledgeable about folk remedies and child care; the spiritualist, who assists with financial, personal, spiritual, or physical problems; and the voodoo priest or priestess, who is knowledgeable about herbs, signs, and omens (Andrews, 2008).

As noted with the folk health practices of Asian and Hispanic Americans, BAAs' folk healing beliefs and practices can augment the professional care system. Black Americans often find comfort in the support that their religious leader or traditional healer can give them. Health care providers must find an appropriate place for these nontraditional modalities when caring for BAAs.

AMERICAN INDIANS/ALASKA NATIVES

"American Indian or Alaskan Native" (AIAN) refers to people who have origins of North and South America (including Central America) and who maintain tribal affiliation or community attachment (Humes et al., 2011). Native Americans lived in America for thousands of years before the arrival of Europeans. AIANs are the original people of the land now occupied mainly by the Europeans. Evidence shows that AIANs have settled in North America for more than 75,000 years (Josephy, 1991). Native Americans came to be known as Indians, a label given by Columbus when he encountered the native peoples in the West Indies that he mistook for the East Indies. This label was then extended to all the native peoples of North and South America, from the Arctic to Tierra del Fuego. Before 1492 there were an estimated 5 million Native Americans. Columbus' discovery brought colonization and settlement by various European groups (Snipp, 2000). Thus, the ancestral lands of the Native Americans were usurped, and the people were forced to labor on farms and in mines. Thousands died from disease and hard labor or were killed in attempts to escape from slavery. Other events, such as the removal of the Southeastern tribes in 1830, the Navajos' Long March to Fort Sumner in 1864, and the massacre at Wounded Knee in 1890, caused the Native American population to dwindle to 250,000 by 1890 (Fixico et al., 2001).

In 2010, 5.2 million people in the United States were identified as American Indian and Alaska Native, about 1.7% of the total U.S. population (U.S. Census Bureau, 2012d). Native Americans are concentrated in Oklahoma, California, Arizona, New Mexico, Alaska, Washington, North Carolina, Texas, New York, and Michigan. Of the total Native American population, 22% live on reservations or other trust lands and about 60% live in metropolitan areas (The Office of Minority Health, 2012a). There are 565 federally recognized AIAN tribes, and more than 100 state recognized tribes (The Office of Minority Health, 2012a). The Cherokees make up the largest tribe (Ogunwole, 2006).

Native American percentages for higher education degrees are low in proportion to their total number. Among American Indians and Alaska Natives who are 25 and older, 13% obtained a bachelor's degree or higher (U.S. Census Bureau, 2012d). Native Americans are making some progress in all levels of college education. However, low continuing educational attainment and low income levels combined with higher rates of poverty are socioeconomic issues that affect health and the quality of life of this population. Native Americans experience the many negative situations that confront poor people both on the reservations and in the larger society.

Health Care Issues of Native Americans

Many of the health problems of Native Americans can be linked directly to the social and economic conditions described here. These conditions predispose Native Americans to illnesses and health problems that afflict the poor. Some of these problems have been discussed in the section on BAAs. Although Native Americans have responded well to prevention and treatment of infectious diseases, other health problems are closely linked with poverty and harmful lifestyle practices (The Office of Minority Health, 2012a).

Cultural barriers, geographic isolation, inadequate sewage disposal, and low income are factors that prevent American Indians/Alaska Natives from receiving quality medical care.

Some of the leading diseases and causes of death among American Indians/Alaska Natives are heart disease, cancer, unintentional injuries (accidents), diabetes, and stroke. American Indians/Alaska Natives also have a high prevalence and risk factors for mental health and suicide, obesity, substance abuse, sudden infant death syndrome (SIDS), teenage pregnancy, liver disease, and hepatitis (The Office of Minority Health, 2012a).

American Indians and Alaska Natives have an infant death rate 60% higher than the rate for non-Hispanic White Americans (The Office of Minority Health, 2012a). Native American adults are 2.1 times more likely than White adults to have diabetes (The Office of Minority Health, 2012b). AI/ANs have disproportionately high death rates from unintentional injuries and suicide (The Office of Minority Health, 2012a). Many mental health problems also confront Native Americans. Difficult life situations and stresses of daily life contribute to an array of problems, including feelings of hopelessness, desperation, family dissolution, and substance abuse, specifically alcohol. Native Americans are twice as likely to have hepatic cancer and more likely to be obese than White adults. Their AIDS rates are 40% higher compared to non-Hispanic Whites (Centers for Disease Control and Prevention, 2011b). The infant mortality rate is 1.6 times that of non-Hispanic Whites (The Office of Minority Health, 2012a).

The health problems of Native Americans are complicated by difficult access to health care. Poor health and limited health care options among urban American Indian and Alaska Native populations have been well documented in many studies (The Office of Minority Health, 2012a). Since 1972, the Indian Health Service (IHS), a government agency in the U.S. Department of Health and Human Services, has stated a series of initiatives to fund health-related activities in off-reservation settings, which make health care services accessible to urban American Indians and Alaska Natives. Federally recognized tribes are provided health and educational assistance through IHS (The Office of Minority Health, 2012a). Approximately 1.9 million American Indians and Alaska Natives receive a health service delivery system operated by the IHS. About 36% of the IHS service area population resides in non-Indian areas, and 600,000 are served in urban clinics (The Office of Minority Health, 2012a). Even though the IHS attempts to provide comprehensive, high-quality health care services to AIAN people, the quality of care and access to health services need to be improved.

Selected Health-Related Cultural Aspects

Native Americans are generally present-oriented: they emphasize events that are occurring now rather than events that will happen later. They take one day at a time, and in times of illness they cope by hoping for improvements the next day (Kavanaugh, 2008). Native Americans also value cooperation rather than competition. Sharing of resources, even among the poor, is an important component of this cultural value. Family and spiritual beliefs are important for Native Americans. Native Americans place great value on their families and relatives. Three or more generations form an extended kinship system, which is enlarged by the membership of nonrelatives who are included through various religious ceremonies (Boyle, 2008).

Despite the great diversity in Native American groups in their beliefs and practices concerning health, illness, and healing, they share a common philosophical base. Native Americans believe that optimal health exists only when a person lives in a condition with balance and harmony in the inner and outer domains of life (Grandbois, 2005). The earth is seen as a living entity that should be treated with respect; failure to do so harms the body. Instead of viewing illness as changes in a person's physiological state, Native Americans view it as an imbalance between the person and natural forces (Boyle, 2008; Grandbois, 2005). Native Americans believe that a person's sickness can be traced directly to having committed a violation against natural and spiritual laws; an individual can also inherit such a violation. The violation causes the person to have an imbalance that causes illnesses mentally, physically, emotionally, and spiritually.

Many AIANs proudly express spirituality, traditional medicinal practices, and cultural ceremonies in their lives. AIAN people frequently seek traditional practitioners, who are medicine women or men known as shamans and are believed to have hypnotic powers, the gift of mind-reading, and expertise in concocting drugs, medicine, and poisons; and who carry out rituals and healing ceremonies that are believed to restore the sense of balance, harmony, and unity that the acute or traumatic event has caused (Grandbois, 2005).

THE EMERGING RURAL AND URBAN POPULATIONS: HOMELESS PERSONS

Homelessness: A Continuing Saga

Homelessness is a complex social and economic problem that continues to persist and grow. Many services and programs have been developed to address the issue, yet homelessness remains a significant problem. Homelessness could be defined as a lack of fixed, regular, and adequate nighttime residence resulting from extreme poverty and/or unsafe or unstable living environments (National Association for the Education of Homeless Children and Youth [NAEHCY], 2007-2011; National Alliance to End Homelessness, 2012; National Coalition for the Homeless, 2009). In many studies, homeless people were counted as individuals who are in shelters or on the streets (National Coalition for the Homeless, 2009). However, homelessness is considered a temporary situation, not a permanent condition. Instead of the number of "homeless people," it has been suggested that the number of "people who experience homelessness over time" is a more appropriate measure of the magnitude of homelessness (National Coalition for the Homeless, 2009). It was estimated that about 3.5 million people (1.35 million of them children) are likely to experience homelessness in a given year (National Coalition for the Homeless, 2009). It was estimated that 42% of the homeless population are African American, 39% are White, 13% are Hispanic, 4% are Native American, and 2% are Asian (National Coalition for the Homeless, 2009).

Why Families and Persons Become Homeless

Both structural and personal factors alone or in combination lead to lack of resources to secure and/or maintain housing. An increasing shortage of affordable rental housing and a simultaneous raise in poverty are two trends largely responsible for the growth of homelessness over the past 20 to 25 years (National Coalition for the Homeless, 2009a). Between 2005 and 2007, the number of repeated homeless individuals in the United States declined by 28% because of an increased number of permanent supportive housing in the country. Recently, foreclosure has been a factor closely related to the increased number of people who experience homelessness in the United States (National Coalition for the Homeless, 2009b). Factors such as poverty, eroding work opportunities, a decline in public assistance, and lack of affordable housing are also significantly contributing to homelessness (National Coalition for the Homeless, 2009b) (Figure 2-2). Within the context of poverty and the lack of affordable housing, other additional major factors, such as lack of affordable health care, domestic violence, mental illness, and addiction disorders, can also contribute to homelessness (National Coalition for the Homeless, 2009b).

Health Issues of Homeless Persons and Families

Poor health is both an effect and a cause of homelessness. Homelessness and health care are closely interlinked. A serious health problem could force a person who does not have adequate health insurance to choose between paying bills for health care or paying rent for a place to live. The National Health Care for the Homeless Council reported that half of all personal bankruptcies in the United States are caused by health problems (National Coalition for the Homeless, 2009c).

Homelessness is associated with various behavioral, social, and environmental risks that expose individuals to many diseases. People experiencing homelessness usually have complex health problems. The lives of homeless persons and families are constant battles for daily survival. Homeless persons experience exposure to extremes in temperatures, unsanitary living conditions, crowded shelters, poor nutrition, and unsafe situations, wherever they live. They experience the same situations relative to health care—poor access because of lack of health insurance and inadequate resources to travel to health facilities.

As a result of poor living conditions and limited access to health care, homeless people are at a higher risk of being exposed to disease, violence, unsanitary conditions, malnutrition, stress, and addictive substances. The rates of serious illnesses and injuries among homeless people are three to six times the rates seen among the rest of the population (National Health Care for the Homeless Council [NHCHC], 2010). This complex mixture of severe physical and/or psychiatric illness, substance abuse, and social problems is frequently found in homeless people (NHCHC, 2010). Many diseases, including heart disease, cancer, liver disease, kidney disease, skin infections, HIV/AIDS, pneumonia, and tuberculosis, are common among the homeless population (National Coalition for the Homeless, 2009c). HIV/AIDS and homelessness are intricately associated. The homeless population has a higher prevalence of HIV/AIDS infections than the general population in the United States. It was estimated that 3.4% of homeless people were HIV-positive in 2006, compared to 0.4% of adults and youths in the general population (National Coalition for the Homeless,

FIGURE 2-2 A homeless man works at a day labor job to earn some money.

2009d). The conditions of homelessness may increase an individual's risk of becoming infected with HIV. Suffering from substance abuse disorders and sharing or reusing needles to intravenously inject drugs greatly increase homeless peoples' risks of being HIV infected. The homeless environment (such as limited privacy and communal sleeping and bathing at shelters) is not conducive to stable sexual relationships and makes it more likely for the homeless person to engage in risky sexual behaviors, therefore increasing the likelihood of contracting HIV (National Coalition for the Homeless, 2009d). Psychosocial distresses are not only associated with many mental health problems in homeless people but also influence behaviors that could affect the progression of HIV/AIDS (National Coalition for the Homeless, 2009d). Limited access to medical care severely prevents homeless persons from receiving adequate HIV/AIDS treatment as well as education concerning HIV/AIDS prevention and risk reduction (National Coalition for the Homeless, 2009d). The homeless condition may also make adherence to HIV treatment regimens challenging for homeless patients and their caregivers (National Coalition for the Homeless, 2009d). To provide comprehensive services such as health education, HIV testing, case management, and mental health services, basic health care is needed for homeless persons living with HIV/AIDS.

Stress, depression, and other mental health problems are also common in homeless people. People who are homeless experience extreme stress on a daily basis. Multiple stresses of living in shelters and on the streets, physical problems, lack of resources, psychosocial issues such as shame and stigma, and feelings of hopelessness and despair often tax the homeless person's ability to cope. About half of people experiencing homelessness suffer from mental health issues. Although only 6% of the general American population are severely mentally ill, about 25% of homeless people in the United States have serious mental illness, including chronic depression, bipolar disorder, and schizophrenia (National Alliance to End Homelessness, 2012a; National Coalition for the Homeless, 2009e).

The prevalence of substance abuse among homeless people is much higher than that among the general population

(National Coalition for the Homeless, 2009f). It is estimated that more than half of all persons experiencing homelessness suffer from substance abuse disorders (United States Interagency Council on Homelessness [USICH], 2011). Substance abuse is both a leading cause and a consequence of the continuance of homelessness among individuals. Substance abuse was reported as the single major cause of homelessness for single adults and as one of the top three causes of homelessness for families, and more than half of homeless people reported that drugs and/or alcohol were major causes of their homelessness (National Coalition for the Homeless, 2009f). Substance abuse also often arises after individuals become homeless. Homeless people abuse substances in an attempt to obtain temporary relief from their problems and eventually rely on drugs and alcohol to cope with their daily struggles; however, the substance dependence only worsens their problems and makes it more difficult for them to escape their homeless status (National Coalition for the Homeless, 2009f). Substance abuse and drug abuse often co-occur with mental health problems among homeless people. It is estimated that almost half of all persons experiencing homelessness suffer from substance abuse disorders, and most of the homeless individuals with substance abuse disorders also suffer from moderate to severe mental illness (USICH, 2011).

Most homeless people do not have health insurance or the ability to pay for needed health care, and many providers refuse to treat homeless persons (NHCHC, 2010). Even though federally funded health care services provide primary care for homeless people, the homeless individuals who are able to benefit from these services are far fewer than those who desperately need care (NHCHC, 2010). Several barriers that prevent access to health care have been recognized. These barriers include lack of knowledge regarding where to receive treatment, lack of access to transportation, and lack of identification (National Coalition for the Homeless, 2009c). Widespread access to affordable, high-quality, and comprehensive health care is necessary to stop homelessness (National Coalition for the Homeless, 2009c). On March 23, 2010, President Obama signed the Affordable Care Act into law, establishing new directives to improve access to affordable health coverage for all Americans and to protect Americans from obnoxious practices of insurance companies. The new law gives all Americans access to care by choosing affordable health insurance that fits their needs; this law also attempts to control health care costs without jeopardizing quality of care (U.S. Department of Health and Human Services, 2012).

Strategies to Address Homelessness

Homelessness has long been recognized as a multidimensional problem of modern day society. The homeless situation is a problem not only of individuals, but also of families, communities, and societies. This problem needs to be addressed as a dynamic and not a static phenomenon, because as societies continue to change and evolve, there will always be those who are excluded and suffer consequences. These are the risks that must be actively anticipated so that strategic planning could forestall any devastating and long-lasting effects.

Many initiatives to address the issues of homeless people are being implemented by the National Health Care for the Homeless Council, which works with people who have experienced homelessness, health care and service providers, and policymakers; provides advocacy, research, and training; and collaborates clinical resources to break the connection between poor health and homelessness (National Health Care for the Homeless Council, 2012). For more information about services and projects initiated by the National Health Care for the Homeless Council or its partners, please visit www.nhchc.org.

Resolving health problems and resolving homelessness are dependently interrelated. Many health problems are highly prevalent in people experiencing homelessness. Health conditions such as diabetes, HIV/AIDS, addiction, and mental illness require ongoing treatment. Without a stable place to stay, treating health conditions and finding time for healing and recovery from health problems are almost impossible. Preventive care can also be difficult for homeless people to access because it is often unaffordable (National Alliance to End Homelessness, 2012a). To end homelessness, mental and physical health conditions should be considered when designing effective, efficient strategies, and permanent stable housing together with supportive services are needed (National Alliance to End Homelessness, 2012a; NHCHC, 2010). The Health Care for the Homeless Clinicians' Network has created clinical practice guidelines for the care of homeless patients. The recommended guidelines are available at www.nhchc.org/wp-content/uploads/2011/09/General-Recommendations-for-Homeless-Patients.pdf.

Research and practice have shown that permanent supportive housing works because housing is an essential part of treatment (National Coalition for the Homeless, 2009b). In addition to providing permanent supportive housing, some other strategies to assist homeless persons include helping them gain access to the health care system and benefits, working with the community to obtain services and resources, educating homeless persons about their health, and educating health care personnel about homeless persons. Communities need to continue their in-kind work with homeless persons. Many schools and houses of religious worship have worked with local governments in extending support to the homeless. Food, clothing, night shelter, and short-term socializing have been provided. Parishioners may donate their time preparing meals, preparing the shelter, and serving as chaperones during the night. Much work is still needed to reduce homelessness. The needs of the recently identified rural homeless must be addressed. Every citizen should be educated so each person can serve as an advocate, and neighborhood coalitions should be established to prevent an increase in the number of homeless persons and to support the return of the homeless person as a dignified, contributing member of society. Health care providers must continue to seek effective ways to coordinate their efforts through the creation of comprehensive resource materials. Technology must be used at its maximal capability to facilitate assessment and monitoring. Preparation for nursing and health care for the homeless in both rural and urban settings should be strengthened as an essential part of the curriculums of the health care disciplines. Finally, more research regarding health care outcomes should be supported and data should be disseminated in a timely manner.

There is a greater degree of optimism today in dealing with the problems of homelessness. Individuals and communities are showing concern through increased involvement. Homelessness is everyone's problem, and people can ultimately effect the establishment of priorities to facilitate an improved quality of life. Increasing awareness and knowledge of the current status of homeless people will aid in understanding the problem and its ramifications. This understanding will serve as an excellent guide in providing input, taking necessary action, and making the final decision regarding the changes needed to make a healthy nation.

Nurses play a significant role in helping homeless persons. It is important for nurses to be capable of meeting the complex health needs of homeless people. Creative care planning is necessary for the homeless patient because standards of care may not be suitable for an individual who experiences homelessness and does not have a home where the basic requirements for self-care and recovery are available (Billings & Kowalski, 2008). Community health nurses are also at the forefront of advocacy for the homeless as they work to effect changes and develop strategies to deal with the problems associated with the health status of homeless people.

THE NATION'S RESPONSE TO THE HEALTH CHALLENGE

The National Institutes of Health (NIH) has proclaimed health disparities as a major concern. The NIH is putting significant effort into addressing and reducing health disparities involving cancer, diabetes, infant mortality, AIDS, cardiovascular illnesses, and many other diseases (National Institute on Minority Health and Health Disparities [NIMHD], 2012). Beginning in 2008, the Centers for Disease Control and Prevention's Racial and Ethnic Health Disparities Action Institute (REHDAI) also expanded support to communities by taking action in addressing health disparities (Centers for Disease Control and Prevention, 2011a). In 2010, the U.S. Congress stressed its commitment to health equity by elevating the National Center on Minority Health and Health Disparities (NCMHD) to the National Institute on Minority Health and Health Disparities (NIMHD). In 2011 the U.S. Department of Health and Human Services released two plans (*The National Stakeholder Strategy for Achieving Health Equity* and the *HHS Action Plan to Reduce Racial and Ethnic Health Disparities)* to reduce health disparities (Hansen, 2011). For more information regarding the two plans and the National Conference of State Legislatures (NCSL), please visit the NCSL website at www.ncsl.org/.

Healthy People 2020

Healthy People 2020 outlines a comprehensive, nationwide health promotion and disease prevention agenda. This initiative is designed to serve as a roadmap for addressing and improving the health of all persons in the United States. In the past 2 decades, one of the *Healthy People's* primary goals has concentrated on disparities. In *Healthy People 2010,* the primary focus was not just as in *Healthy People 2000* to reduce health disparities among Americans, but also to eliminate health disparities. In *Healthy People 2020,* the goal has been expanded further: to achieve health equity, eliminate disparities, and improve the health of all groups (U.S. Department of Health and Human Services, 2010b). For more information about topics and objectives in *Healthy People 2020,* please visit the website at http://healthypeople.gov/2020/default.aspx.

Office of Minority Health

The Office of Minority Health (OMH) was created in 1986, and it was reauthorized by the Patient Protection and Affordable Care Act of 2010 (The Office of Minority Health, 2011a). The Office of Minority Health has been working for more than 20 years to improve and protect the health of racial and ethnic minority populations through the development of health policies and programs that concentrate on eliminating health disparities. The OMH is leading the charge to put into practice the *HHS Disparities Action Plan* at all levels of the Department of Health and Human Services and in the communities with whom it works.

In recent years, OMH started two initiatives (the National Partnership for Action to End Health Disparities [NPA] and the Strategic Framework for Improving Racial and Ethnic Minority Health and Eliminating Racial and Ethnic Health Disparities) to guide its efforts toward eliminating health disparities in the United States. Both initiatives implemented a coordinated, systems-level approach that focused on eliminating health disparities and was contingent on science and knowledge to notify and continually improve policies and programs. The goals of the National Partnership for Action to End Health Disparities (NPA) are to enhance awareness of the importance of health disparities and actions needed to improve health outcomes for racial and ethnic minority populations, strengthen and expand leadership for dealing with health disparities at all levels, improve health and health care outcomes for racial and ethnic minorities and underserved populations and communities, improve cultural and linguistic competency in delivering health services, and improve coordination and utilization of research and evaluation outcomes. The main purpose of the Strategic Framework for Improving Racial and Ethnic Minority Health and Eliminating Racial and Ethnic Health Disparities is to direct, organize, and coordinate the systematic planning, implementation, and evaluation of efforts that are targeted at improving racial and ethnic minority health and addressing racial and ethnic health disparities. For more information about *Trends in U.S. Public Awareness of Racial and Ethnic Health Disparities* please visit http://minorityhealth.hhs.gov/assets/pdf/checked/1/2010StudyBrief.pdf. Another initiative established by the Centers for Disease Control and Prevention is the Racial and Ethnic Approaches to Community Health (REACH), established in 2010. Its objective is to "eliminate disparities in health access and outcomes. These six health areas were selected for emphasis because they reflect areas of disparity that are known to affect multiple racial and ethnic minority groups at all life stages" (The Office of Minority Health and Health Disparities, 2007). These areas include infant mortality; deficits in breast and cervical health promotion and disease prevention; and child and adult immunizations.

There are also minority health research initiatives sponsored by the National Institutes of Health, Centers for Disease Control and Prevention, and the Agency for Healthcare Research and Quality. Support for these initiatives and future ones must continue at all levels.

NURSING'S RESPONSE TO EMERGING POPULATIONS AND HEALTH

The American Nurses Association's (ANA) *Code of Ethics* explicitly states the profession's commitment to provide service to people regardless of background or situation (American Nurses Association, 2010). Nurses have responsibilities to be aware of specific health needs and respond to illness in all populations (American Nurses Association, 2010). The ANA's Council on Cultural Diversity supports the work of nurses in their development of culturally competent care. The organization and its leadership, through the Ethnic-Minority Fellowship Program, have played an essential role in supporting the work and efforts of AAPIs, BAAs, LHAs, and Native Americans with graduate and doctoral work. Nurses continue to make many positive moves toward understanding culturally diverse populations. See the Case Study and Care Plan about Mr. and Mrs. Arahan, an older adult immigrant couple at the end of this chapter, which propose nursing interventions to ensure their quality of life in their later years. Nurses' awareness and understanding of transcultural issues have been facilitated by the works of leaders such as Leininger, Giger, Davidhizar, Andrews, and Boyle, just to name a few. In addition, wide dissemination of research findings has been made possible through the *Journal of Transcultural Nursing* and through annual conferences and other sponsored workshops. Additionally, nurses with advanced preparation have committed their time and energy to developing approaches and models for transcultural nursing. These models can be found in **Website Resource 2C.**

Several nursing journals focus on cultural diversity, such as the *Journal of Cultural Diversity* and the *Journal of Multicultural Nursing and Health.* These journals and a variety of other publications are constantly increasing professionals' knowledge of health-related cultural issues. In addition, the *Minority Nurse Newsletter* provides excellent summaries of research studies, legislative updates affecting ethnic minorities, and relevant topics in education and practice. Ethnic nursing organizations are having an effect on greater cultural understanding through their dissemination of important works by clinicians, educators, and researchers (Box 2-5: Innovative Practice).

Major organizations such as the ANA, the National League for Nursing (NLN), and the American Association of Colleges of Nursing (AACN) publish culturally relevant materials to guide students, clinicians, and educators. Accrediting bodies for nursing education such as the NLNAC and the Commission on Collegiate Nursing Education (CCNE) support diversity with the inclusion of standards for maximizing with diversity in the academic preparation of students pursuing baccalaureate and master's degrees (American Association of Colleges of Nursing, 2007). Additionally, there is a cadre of nurses whose research on the cultural practices and beliefs of individuals and families gives professionals a sound base for improving practice and designing cost-effective and humanistic health care strategies. The quest to deliver culturally competent care has provided the impetus for nursing faculty to require transcultural courses in the nursing curriculum to facilitate awareness and understanding of cultural diversity. Transcultural nursing is an area of nursing study and practice that focuses on discovering and explaining cultural factors that influence the health, well-being, illness, or death of individuals or groups and seeks to provide culturally based appropriate care to people of diverse cultures (Leininger, 2001). Culture Care Diversity and Universality theory (Leininger, 2002), developed by Madeleine Leininger, is a well-recognized theory used globally by many nurses, and it has significantly contributed to the establishment and advancement of transcultural nursing research knowledge and practice. It is essential for nurses to plan culturally tailored and competent care to mitigate health disparities and provide effective care in our rapidly changing multicultural societies, thereby delivering quality and safe care to all (Box 2-6: Quality and Safety Scenario).

Additionally, major textbooks focusing on specific clinical areas of practice devote material to health care issues of ethnic minorities. Other resources include a chapter or two on cultural diversity. In addition, discussion of specific health care problems and nursing care always includes cultural aspects. In the clinical setting, health care workers, through staff development and in-service programs, are provided opportunities to learn and develop culturally sensitive care approaches (see Box 2-7).

✳ BOX 2-5   INNOVATIVE PRACTICE

Spiritual Practices and Health

Spirituality and its relationship with health outcomes have been the focus of considerable interest in recent years (Como, 2007). Spirituality can be defined as an individual's sense of peace, purpose, and connection to others as well as the person's beliefs about the meaning of life. Many people believe that spirituality plays an important role in their lives (Gillum & Griffith, 2010; National Cancer Institute, 2012).

A growing amount of evidence reveals that spirituality and spiritual care play an important role in health and health care (Ehrlich, 2011). Considerable evidence has shown spiritual practices as an important and effective coping strategy and a common approach to dealing with health problems, particularly chronic diseases such as cardiovascular disease and cancer (Como, 2007; Medical University of South Carolina, 2012; National Cancer Institute, 2012). Spiritual practices are likely to improve coping skills and social support, promote feelings of optimism and hope, encourage healthy behavior, decrease feelings of depression and anxiety, and support a sense of relaxation (National Cancer Institute, 2012). Many studies have found that spiritual or religious beliefs and practices help patients with cancer as well as their caregivers to cope with the disease (National Cancer Institute, 2012). Studies also suggest that many patients would like health care providers to consider spirituality as a factor into their health care. It was reported that 94% of people admitted to the hospital agree that spiritual health is as important as physical health, and some studies show that health care providers' support of spiritual well-being helps improve patients' quality of life (National Cancer Institute, 2012).

A spiritual assessment may help health care providers understand how religious or spiritual (RS) beliefs will affect the way a patient copes with diseases and health problems. Few tools for assessing spiritual history and/or spiritual practices have been developed to help health care professionals consider patients' spiritual needs and/or plan appropriate spiritual interventions for their patients. A *Spiritual Practices Checklist* (Quinn-Griffin et al., 2008) was developed to identify the RS interventions used and the frequency of use of RS interventions. The 12 items of the checklist include most commonly used spiritual practices (e.g., prayer) and complementary and alternative medicine (CAM) interventions (e.g., meditation, yoga). Other examples of tools are the FAITH, the HOPE, and the FICA tools that help physicians assessing patients' history of spirituality (Medical University of South Carolina, 2012). More information about the HOPE tool can be found at www.aafp.org/afp/2001/0101/p81.html?printable=afp.

It has been suggested by The Joint Commission (TJC) that a spiritual assessment should be performed on every patient to identify patient's values, beliefs, and spiritual practices (Wesa & Culliton, 2004). Each person may have different spiritual needs, depending on cultural and religious traditions. For example, African Americans and Hispanic Americans were found more likely than European Americans to report prayer for health reasons (Gillum & Griffith, 2010). In order to better counsel and care for the patients, health care providers should be aware of the common ethnic patients who may have more and special spiritual and religious needs and the common spiritual practices used by patients.

Sources: Como, J. M. (2007). Spiritual practice: A literature review related to spiritual health and health outcomes. *Holistic Nursing Practice*, *21*(5), 224–236; Ehrlich, S. D. (2011). *Spirituality*. Retrieved July 16, 2012, from www.umm.edu/altmed/articles/spirituality-000360.htm; Gillum, F., & Griffith, D. M. (2010). Prayer and spiritual practices for health reasons among American adults: The role of race and ethnicity. *Journal of Religion and Health*, *49*(3), 283–295; Medical University of South Carolina. (2012). *Spirituality and cultural diversity*. Retrieved July 16, 2012, from http://academicdepartments.musc.edu/family_medicine/Spirituality_and_Health/spiritualityculturaldiversity.htm; National Cancer Institute. (2012). *Spirituality in cancer care (PDQ®)*. Retrieved July 16, 2012, from www.cancer.gov/cancertopics/pdq/supportivecare/spirituality/Health Professional; Quinn-Griffin, M., Salman, A., Lee, Y., & Fitzpatrick, J. J. (2008). A beginning look at the spiritual practices of older adults. *Journal of Christian Nursing*, *25*(2), 100–102; Wesa, K. M., & Culliton, P. (2004). Recommendations and guidelines regarding the preferred research protocol for investigating the impact of an optimal healing environment on patients with substance abuse. *Journal of Alternative and Complementary Medicine*, *10*(1), 193–199.

✓ BOX 2-6   QUALITY AND SAFETY SCENARIO

Immigrants and Health Care Providers

Mr. Jade and Madam Nora have four children: Nirman (6 months), Julia (18 months), Hady (4 years), and Jamella (6 years). Mr. Jade is an economist who immigrated to the United States from Iraq 4 years ago. The family has come to the well-baby clinic because Madam Nora has been concerned about Nirman; Nirman's skin appears paler than her siblings and she is also not gaining weight. Mr. Jade gave a brief health history of Nirman's situation because his wife cannot express herself in English. "My wife believes that Nirman is not growing like the rest of our children. She breastfeeds her every 2 hours but she is not eating." My wife is "upset that Nirman is not becoming bigger." The vital signs are as follows: pulse, 125 beats/min; respirations, 22 breaths/min; blood pressure, 100/70 mm Hg; and rectal temperature, 99.4° F. Nirman's weight is 10 lb, 0 oz, and her length is 22 inches. Nirman appears pale. Madam Nora, age 28, is wearing a headscarf covering her hair, and a long dress. When Mr. Jade and Madam Nora are left alone, nurses can hear them arguing and raising their voices in a foreign language (Arabic), and Madam Nora appeared very upset. The medical history revealed a full-term baby female born by normal vaginal delivery with a normal birth weight. No history of vomiting, diarrhea, or fever was reported. Pallor and

jaundice were noted on physical examination. The family history revealed that both Mr. Jade and Madam Nora came from the same village and are Muslim and second-degree cousins. No genetic studies have been performed for the family members. Nirman's initial diagnosis is hemolytic anemia.

Nurses should consider the unique cultural background and family dynamics and functioning while providing care to this immigrant family to ensure safe and quality care. The family has an ineffective communication pattern and an inability to navigate through the complexity of the health care system. Madam Nora needs to communicate with health care providers through her husband, who, in turn, is not familiar with medical terminology. The fact that no genetic testing was performed among family members may be due to the unfamiliarity and complexity of the health care system in the United States as compared to the health services in their native country. It is important for nurses to have culturally competent skills and to identify cultural beliefs that may impact how immigrant patients may communicate with them. Hence, effective approaches may be implemented to provide safe and quality care for this population and to mitigate health disparities.

BOX 2-7   STUDENT HEALTH PROMOTION PROJECT

When students are retaking a clinical nursing course, they have a unique opportunity to strengthen theoretical concepts introduced in their first attempt at the course. To avoid duplication of learning experiences, the faculty needs to be creative and resourceful in enhancing critical thinking and creating experiences that would support students' achievement of course objectives. In their first attempt at the course, students are often unsuccessful in course examinations that test higher levels of learning in the cognitive domain. Therefore, learning experiences must motivate students to overcome their anxiety about failing for the second time and also inspire them to do their best.

In the first attempt at the course, a community-focused health promotion project is implemented at a senior citizen center. For the second attempt at the course, students have dual roles, both teacher and learner. First, students prepare for the experience by examining the health issues and concerns of young and middle adulthood, since these are the two age stages of the group members. The course textbook and multimedia resources in the learning center provide a review of developmental tasks, prevalent health problems, cultural aspects, and appropriate health care and nursing approaches. In a seminar format, students share their information with each other including their own experiences and perspectives as young or middle adults.

Second, students then survey the professional literature for appropriate resources, including assessment instruments on specific health issues and culturally appropriate approaches. Students agree that the prevalent issues of the group members are stress, unhealthy lifestyles, and time management.

Third, students agree on one tool to be used for the assessment, and data are collected as students interview one another. The data are comprehensive, and students are very much surprised at the commonalities among them. Results of their assessment indicate that all of the students have multiple roles, each with overwhelming demands on their time. In their pursuit of a nursing degree, students confront studying for many hours, reading voluminous numbers of pages, doing many written assignments, and reviewing for challenging examinations that they all agree tax their energy reserves. Sleep is often sacrificed, and most resort to unhealthy eating as a way to cope.

Fourth, the students develop a teaching plan using the concepts on client education taught to them during the first attempt of the course. The students formulate realistic and measurable objectives for themselves as learners. They have commented that selecting and writing these objectives seemed easier because they were the learners and realized the importance of achieving these. The healthy lifestyle strategies selected are those that they could implement with their busy schedule but would be effective nevertheless.

Fifth, the presentation of the project is held in a room that has multimedia capabilities. Using current technology, students present their material on stress and strategies to address unhealthy lifestyles through nutrition, exercise, and time management. An actual demonstration of exercises that can be done while studying or working in front of the computer is well received. Each student gets an opportunity to try out the exercises. Using a similar approach, the second group of students presents strategies on time management to cope with the multiple demands on each student's time. Student presenters discuss an awareness of one's body rhythms. They inform their peers of the value of matching the demand of the task on hand and one's corresponding energy and attention level. Culturally specific food recipes that can be prepared in a short period of time are shared with the group.

Sixth, the evaluation of the learning is done later in the semester as opposed to almost immediately after students taught at a senior center. Students see each other at least twice per week after the presentation. All the students believe that they have met the learning objectives and are continuing the strategies taught by their peers. They comment that the teaching "hit home" and that they have come to realize that as future health care professionals, health promotion activities should be for the self first before they can address the health issues of others. From the faculty's perspectives, students gain a better understanding of the concepts of client education and appreciation of a comprehensive assessment as well as use of culturally appropriate and creative approaches to teaching. The students' success in their second attempt at the course gives them a much stronger foundation for subsequent courses and a deeper appreciation of staying healthy as a priority goal of every future health care professional.

CASE STUDY

An Older Immigrant Couple: Mr. and Mrs. Arahan

Mr. and Mrs. Arahan, an older couple in their seventies, have been living with their oldest daughter, her husband of 15 years, and their two children, ages 12 and 14. They all live in a middle-income neighborhood in a suburb of a metropolitan city. Mr. and Mrs. Arahan are both college educated and worked full-time while they were in their native country. In addition, Mr. Arahan, the only offspring of wealthy parents, inherited a substantial amount of money and real estate. Their daughter came to the United States as a registered nurse and met her husband, a drug company representative. The older couple moved to the United States when their daughter became a U.S. citizen and petitioned them as immigrants. Since the couple was facing retirement, they welcomed the opportunity to come to the United States.

The Arahans found life in the United States different from that in their home country, but their adjustment was not as difficult because both were healthy and spoke English fluently. Most of their time was spent taking care of their two grandchildren and the house. As the grandchildren grew older, the older couple found that they had more spare time. The daughter and her husband advanced in their careers and spent a great deal more time at their jobs. There were few family dinners during the week. On weekends, the daughter, her husband, and their children socialized with their own friends. The couple began to feel isolated and longed for a more active life.

Mr. and Mrs. Arahan began to think that perhaps they should return to the home country, where they still had relatives and friends. However, political and economic issues would have made it difficult for them to live there. Besides, they had become accustomed to the way of life in the United States with all the

modern conveniences and abundance of goods that were difficult to obtain in their country. However, they also became concerned that they might not be able to tolerate the winter months and that minor health problems might worsen as they aged. They wondered who would take care of them if they became very frail and where they would live, knowing that their daughter had only saved money for their grandchildren's college education. They expressed their sentiments to their daughter, who became very concerned about how her parents were feeling.

This older couple had been attending church on a regular basis, but had never been active in other church-related activities. The church bulletin announced the establishment of parish nursing with two retired registered nurses as volunteers. The couple attended the first opening of the parish clinic. Here, they met one of the registered nurses, who had a short discussion with them about the services offered. The registered nurse had spent a great deal of her working years as a community health nurse. She informed Mr. and Mrs. Arahan of her availability to help them resolve any health-related issues.

Reflective Questions

1. What strategies could be suggested for this older adult couple to enhance their quality of life?
2. What community resources can they utilize?
3. What can the daughter and her family do to address the feelings of isolation of the older couple?
4. What health promotion activities can ensure a healthy lifestyle for them?

An Older Immigrant Couple: Mr. and Mrs. Arahan

NURSING DIAGNOSIS: Risk for continued feelings of isolation

Defining Characteristics
- Couple no longer has a great deal of caretaking responsibilities.
- Daughter and husband spend a great deal of time on their careers.
- Family dinners during the week are seldom.
- Daughter and her family socialize with their own friends.
- Older adult couple is thinking of returning to native country.
- Couple is concerned about life in the United States with harsh winters and their minor health problems.
- Couple is concerned about advancing years and future living arrangements.

Related Factors
- Transition from native country to the U.S.
- Differing religious, ethnic, and cultural backgrounds between native country and U.S. influence care decisions
- Differing roles in family structures between the native country and the U.S.
- Conflicting roles between the two generations
- Limited opportunities for social support and assimilation for older immigrants to the U.S.
- Health and health care needs, multiple and complex, for elder population in the U.S.

Expected Outcomes
The Arahans will:
- Join a senior citizen center for socialization and other activities.

- Volunteer at a nearby hospital or school several mornings or afternoons per week.
- Work with daughter and her family to plan at least one family meal per week.
- Pursue some neglected hobbies.
- Get involved in a church group or in a civic organization.
- Begin a discussion on future alternate living arrangements.
- Make periodic visits to the native country to see relatives and friends.

Interventions
- Encourage the couple to have open discussions about their concerns with their daughter and her family.
- Support them in their choice of meaningful activities such as joining the senior center and volunteering.
- Provide information on resources for future living arrangements in the United States.
- Develop a plan for health monitoring on a regular basis.
- Provide a list of organizations that address issues and concerns of older adults such as the American Association of Retired Persons (AARP).
- Utilize their experience and expertise (if any) in managing the parish nursing clinic.
- Initiate an older support group in the parish with the Arahans as the first members.

The Arahans' situation is a very common one in most immigrant groups. The interventions outlined above would need to consider the cultural traditions, personal preferences, health status, motivation level, physical ability, and resources of the couple to ensure positive outcomes and goal achievement.

SUMMARY

This century will continue to be a time of great challenges as the population of the United States continues to be a nation of diverse peoples. The nation and its people have repeatedly overcome devastations by both nature and humankind itself. As citizens, emerging populations share similar concerns about life, including health, an acceptable standard of living, and quality of life. An array of cultural, economic, educational, social, and political barriers are being eroded at the local, national, and global levels to ensure the health and well-being of the people of the United States. The government, public and private industries, health care professions, and all individuals can work together to reduce health disparities and ensure a healthy nation for future generations.

REFERENCES

Abraham, N. (1995). Arab Americans. In R. J. Vecoli, J. Galens, A. Sheets, & R. V. Young (Eds.), *Gale encyclopedia of multicultural America* (Vol. 1, pp. 84–98). New York: Gale Research.

Africa, J., & Carrasco, M. (2011). *Asian-American and Pacific Islander mental health*. Retrieved July 3, 2012, from www.nami.org/Template.cfm?Section=Multicultural_Support1&Template=/ContentManagement/ContentDisplay.cfm&ContentID=115281.

Agency for Healthcare Research and Quality. (2011). *National healthcare disparities report*. Retrieved July 6, 2012, from www.ahrq.gov/qual/qrdr11/index.html.

American Association of Colleges of Nursing. (2007). *Draft: Revision of the essentials of baccalaureate nursing education*. Retrieved December 18, 2007, from www.aacn.nche.

American Nurses Association. (2010). *Code of ethics for nurses with interpretive statements*. Retrieved June 20, 2012, from http://ana.nursingworld.org/MainMenuCategories/EthicsStandards/CodeofEthicsforNurses/Code-of-Ethics.aspx.

Andrews, M. M. (2008). The influence of cultural health belief systems on health care practices. In M. M. Andrews, & J. S. Boyle (Eds.), *Transcultural concepts in nursing care* (5th ed., pp. 66–81). Philadelphia: Wolters Kluwer Health: Lippincott Williams & Wilkins.

Andrews, M. M., & Boyle, J. S. (2008). Andrews/Boyle transcultural nursing assessment guide for individuals and families. In M. M. Andrews, & J. S. Boyle (Eds.), *Transcultural concepts in nursing care* (5th ed., pp. 453–457). Philadelphia: Wolters Kluwer Health: Lippincott Williams & Wilkins.

Aprahamian, M., Kaplan, D. M., Windham, A. M., Sutter, J. A., & Visser, J. (2011). The relationship between acculturation and mental health of Arab Americans. *Journal of Mental Health Counseling*, 33(1), 80–92.

Arab American Institute Foundation. (2007-2009). *Quick facts about Arab Americans*. Retrieved January 21, 2012, from www.aaiusa.org/pages/demographics/.

Batalova, J., & Terrazas, A. (2010). *US in focus: Frequently requested statistics on immigrants and immigration in the United States*. Retrieved June 29, 2012, from www.migrationinformation.org/USFocus/display.cfm?ID=818#1.

Billings, D. M., & Kowalski, K. (2008). Teaching tips. Increasing competency in the care of homeless patients. *Journal of Continuing Education in Nursing*, 39(4), 153–154.

Boyle, J. S. (2008). Culture, family, and community. In M. M. Andrews, & J. S. Boyle (Eds.), *Transcultural concepts in nursing care* (5th ed., pp. 261–296). Philadelphia: Wolters Kluwer Health: Lippincott Williams & Wilkins.

Carbonell, A. A. (2002). Cuba. In C. E. D'Avanzo, & E. M. Geissler (Eds.), *Mosby's pocket guide to cultural health assessment* (3rd ed., pp. 218–233). St Louis: Mosby.

Centers for Disease Control and Prevention. (2011a). *Racial and Ethnic Health Disparities Action Institute (REHDAI): Impacting health equity at state and local levels.* Retrieved January 17, 2012, from www.cdc.gov/Features/DisparitiesInstitute/.

Centers for Disease Control and Prevention. (2011b). *HIV surveillance report, 2009.* Retrieved January 20, 2012, from www.cdc.gov/hiv/topics/surveillance/resources/reports/.

Centers for Disease Control and Prevention. (2012). *CDC celebrates Asian American & Pacific Islander heritage.* Retrieved July 4, 2012, from www.cdc.gov/Features/AAPIHeritageMonth/.

Chong, N. (2002). *The Latino patient: A cultural guide for health care providers.* Yarmouth, Maine: Intercultural Press.

D'Avanzo, C. E., & Geissler, E. M. (Eds.), (2007). *Pocket guide to cultural health assessment* (4th ed.). St Louis: Mosby.

Fixico, D., Kolata, A. L., & Neely, S. (2001). American Indian. *The world book encyclopedia.* (Vol. 10). Chicago: World Books. 136–185.

Flegal, K. M., Carroll, M. D., Kit, B. K., & Ogden, C. L. (2012). Prevalence of obesity and trends in the distribution of body mass index among U.S. adults, 1999-2010. *Journal of the American Medical Association, 307*(5), 491–497.

Gary, F. A., Yarandi, H. N., & Scruggs, F. C. (2003). Suicide among African Americans: Reflections and a call to action. *Issues in Mental Health Nursing, 24*(3), 353–375.

Giger, J. N., & Davidhizar, R. E. (2008). Introduction. In J. Giger, & R. Davidhizar (Eds.), *Transcultural nursing: Assessment and interventions* (5th ed., pp. 2–19). St Louis: Mosby.

Grandbois, D. (2005). Stigma of mental illness among American Indian and Alaska Native nations: Historical and contemporary perspectives. *Issues in Mental Health Nursing, 26*, 1001–1024.

Hammond, R. J., & Cheney, P. (2009). *Intro to sociology: Glossary of terms.* Online free book. Retrieved June 29, 2012, from http://freebooks.uvu.edu/SOC1010/index.php/glossary-of-terms.html.

Hansen, M. (2011). *Strategies to eliminate health disparities.* Retrieved January 21, 2012, from www.ncsl.org/issues-research/health/strategies-to-eliminate-health-disparities.aspx.

Humes, K. R., Jones, N. A., & Ramirez, R. R. (2011). *Overview of race and Hispanic origin: 2010.* Retrieved January 20, 2012, from www.census.gov/prod/cen2010/briefs/c2010br-02.pdf.

Institute of Medicine. (2008). *Challenges and successes in reducing health disparities. Workshop summary.* Retrieved May 29, 2012, from www.iom.edu/Reports/2008/Challenges-and-Successes-in-Reducing-Health-Disparities-Workshop-Summary.aspx.

Jamil, H., Templin, T., Fakhouri, M., Rice, V. H., Khouri, R., & Fakhouri, H. (2008). Comparison of personal characteristics, tobacco use, and health states in Chaldean, Arab American, and non-Middle Eastern White adults. *Journal of Immigration and Minor Health, 11*(4), 310–317.

Josephy, A. M. (1991). *The Indian heritage of America.* Boston: Houghton Mifflin.

Kaiser Family Foundation. (2008). *Eliminating racial/ethnic disparities in health care: What are the options?* Retrieved July 3, 2012, from www.kff.org.

Kataoka-Yahiro, M., Ceria, C., & Yoder, M. (2004). Grandparent caregiving role in Filipino American families. *Journal of Cultural Diversity, 11*(3), 110–117.

Kavanaugh, R. R. (2008). Transcultural perspectiveness in mental health nursing. In M. M. Andrews, & J. S. Boyle (Eds.), *Transcultural concepts in nursing care* (5th ed., pp. 226–259). Philadelphia: Wolter Kluwer Health: Lippincott Williams & Wilkins.

Kluckhohn, C. (1953). Dominant and variant value orientations. In C. Kluckhohn, H. A. Murray, & D. A. Schneider (Eds.), *Personality in nature, society, and culture* (2nd ed.). New York: Alfred A. Knopf.

Lambert, S., Fearing, A., Bell, D., & Newton, M. (2002). A comparative study of prostate screening, health beliefs, and practices between African American men and Caucasian men. *ABNF Journal, 13*(3), 61–63.

Lee, Y. -H., Salman, A., & Wang, F. (2012). Recruiting Chinese-American adolescents to HIV/AIDS related research: A lesson learned from a cross-sectional study. *Applied Nursing Research, 25*(1), 40–46.

Leininger, M. (2001). The theory of culture care diversity and universality. In M. M. Leininger (Ed.), *Culture care diversity and universality: A theory of nursing* (2nd ed., pp. 5–68). Boston: Jones & Bartlett.

Leininger, M. (2002). Culture care theory: A major contribution to advance transcultural nursing knowledge and practices. *Journal of Transcultural Nursing, 13*(3), 189–192.

Management Sciences for Health. (n.d.). *The providers guide to quality and culture: Health disparities.* Retrieved July 4, 2012, from http://erc.msh.org/mainpage.cfm?file=7.1.0.htm&module=provider&language=English"

Markus, H. R. (2008). Pride, prejudice, and ambivalence: Toward a unified theory of race and ethnicity. *American Psychologist, 63,* 651–670.

McGadney-Douglass, B. F. (2000). The Black Church response to the mental health needs of the elderly. In S. L. Logan, & E. M. Freeman (Eds.), *Health care in the Black community: Empowerment, knowledge, skills, and collectivism* (pp. 199–214). New York: Haworth Press.

Migration Policy Institute. (2012). *2012 American community survey and Census data on the foreign born by state.* Retrieved August 27, 2012, from www.migrationinformation.org/DataHub/acscensus.cfm.

National Alliance to End Homelessness. (2012). *Federal policy brief: Changes in the HUD definition of "homeless."* Retrieved July 9, 2012, from www.endhomelessness.org/content/article/detail/3006.

National Alliance to End Homelessness. (2012a). *Mental/physical health.* Retrieved July 12, 2012, from www.endhomelessness.org/section/issues/mental_physical_health.

National Association for the Education of Homeless Children and Youth (NAEHCY). (2007-2011). *Facts about homeless education.* Retrieved July 9, 2012, from www.naehcy.org/facts.html.

National Coalition for the Homeless. (2009). *Who is homelessness?* Retrieved July 4, 2012, from www.nationalhomeless.org/factsheets/who.html.

National Coalition for the Homeless. (2009a). *Why are people homelessness?* Retrieved July 4, 2012, from www.nationalhomeless.org/factsheets/why.html.

National Coalition for the Homeless. (2009b). *Strategies of state mental health agencies to prevent and end homelessness.* Retrieved July 12, 2012, from www.endhomelessness.org/content/article/detail/2592.

National Coalition for the Homeless. (2009c). *Health care and homelessness.* Retrieved July 9, 2012, from www.nationalhomeless.org/factsheets/health.html.

National Coalition for the Homeless. (2009d). *HIV/AIDS and homelessness.* Retrieved July 9, 2012, from www.nationalhomeless.org/factsheets/hiv.html.

National Coalition for the Homeless. (2009e). *Mental illness and homelessness.* Retrieved July 9, 2012, from www.nationalhomeless.org/factsheets/Mental_Illness.html.

National Coalition for the Homeless. (2009f). *Substance abuse and homelessness.* Retrieved July 9, 2012, from www.nationalhomeless.org/factsheets/addiction.html.

National Health Care for the Homeless Council (NHCHC). (2010). *Homeless and health: What's the connection?* Retrieved June 22, 2012, from www.nhchc.org/wp-content/uploads/2011/09/Hln_health_factsheet_Jan10.pdf.

National Health Care for the Homeless Council (NHCHC). (2012). *About the council.* Retrieved July 11, 2012, from www.nhchc.org/about/mission/.

National Institute on Minority Health and Health Disparities (NIMHD). (2012). *Mission and vision.* Retrieved January 10, 2012, from www.nimhd.nih.gov/about_ncmhd/welcome.asp.

Ogunwole, S. U. (2006). *We the people: American Indians and Alaska Natives in the United States.* U.S. Department of Commerce Economics and Statistics Administration, Washington, DC: U.S. Census Bureau.

Ponce, N., Tseng, W., Ong, P., Shek, Y. L., Ortiz, S., & Gatchell, M. (2009). *The state of Asian American, Native Hawaiian and Pacific Islander health in California report.* Retrieved July 4, 2012, from www.healthpolicy.ucla.edu/pubs/Publication.aspx?pubID=32.

Rastogi, S., Johnson, T. D., Hoeffel, E. M., & Drewery, M. P., Jr. (2011). *2010 Census brief: The black population 2010.* Retrieved July 6, 2012, from www.census.gov/prod/cen2010/briefs/c2010br-06.pdf.

Salman, A., McCabe, D., Easter, T., Callahan, B., Goldstein, D., Smith, T. D., et al. (2007). Cultural competence among staff nurses who participated in a family-centered geriatric care program. *Journal of Nurses Staff Development, 23*(3), 103–111.

Snipp, C. M. (2000). Selected demographic characteristics of Indians. In E. R. Rhoades (Ed.), *American Indian health* (pp. 41–57). Baltimore: The Johns Hopkins University Press.

Stussy, S. A. (2000). Arab Americans. In C. J. Moose, & R. Wilder (Eds.), *Racial and ethnic relations in America* (Vol. 1, pp. 102–107). Pasadena, CA: Salem Press.

Su, D., & Li, L. (2011). Trends in the use of complementary and alternative medicine in the United States: 2002-2007. *Journal of Health Care for the Poor and Underserved, 22,* 295–309.

Tashiro, C. J. (2006). Identity and health in the narratives of older mixed ancestry Asian Americans. *Journal of Cultural Diversity, 13*(1), 41–49.

The Office of Minority Health. (2005). *What is cultural competency?* Retrieved January 22, 2012, from http://minorityhealth.hhs.gov/templates/browse.aspx?lvl=2&lvlID=11.

The Office of Minority Health. (2011a). *About OMH.* Retrieved January 22, 2012, from http://minorityhealth.hhs.gov/templates/browse.aspx?lvl=1&lvlID=7.

The Office of Minority Health. (2011b). *Infant mortality and African Americans.* Retrieved July 2, 2012, from http://minorityhealth.hhs.gov/templates/content.aspx?lvl=2&lvlID=51&ID=3021.

The Office of Minority Health. (2011c). *HIV/AIDS and African Americans.* Retrieved January 22, 2012, from http://minorityhealth.hhs.gov/templates/content.aspx?lvl=2&lvlID=51&ID=3019.

The Office of Minority Health. (2012a). *American Indian/Alaska Native profile.* Retrieved January 1, 2012, from www.minorityhealth.hhs.gov/templates/browse.aspx?lvl=3&lvlid=26.

The Office of Minority Health. (2012b). *Diabetes and American Indians/Alaska Natives.* Retrieved January 12, 2012, from www.minorityhealth.hhs.gov/templates/browse.aspx?lvl=3&;lvlid=26.

The Office of Minority Health. (2012c). *Asian American/Pacific Islander profile.* Retrieved January 20, 2012, from www.minorityhealth.hhs.gov/templates/browse.aspx?lvl=3&lvlid=29.

The Office of Minority Health. (2012d). *Hispanic/Latino profile.* Retrieved January 20, 2012, from www.minorityhealth.hhs.gov/templates/browse.aspx?lvl=3&;lvlid=31.

The Office of Minority Health. (2012e). *Hispanic/Latino profile.* Retrieved January 20, 2012, from http://minorityhealth.hhs.gov/templates/browse.aspx?lvl=3&lvlid=23.

The Office of Minority Health. (2012f). *Heart disease and Africa Americans.* Retrieved July 5, 2012, from http://minorityhealth.hhs.gov/templates/content.aspx?lvl=2&lvlID=51&ID=3018.

The Office of Minority Health. (2012g). *Stroke and Africa Americans.* Retrieved July 5, 2012, from http://minorityhealth.hhs.gov/templates/content.aspx?lvl=2&lvlID=51&ID=3022.

The Office of Minority Health. (2012h). *Diabetics and Africa Americans.* Retrieved July 5, 2012, from http://minorityhealth.hhs.gov/templates/content.aspx?lvl=2&lvlID=51&ID=3017.

The Office of Minority Health and Health Disparities. (2007). *About minority health.* Retrieved September 25, 2007, from www.cdc.gov/omhd/Amh/AMH.htm.

United States Interagency Council on Homelessness (USICH). (2011). *Substance abuse.* Retrieved July 12, 2012, from www.usich.gov/issue/substance_abuse.

U.S. Census Bureau. (2012a). *Asian/Pacific American heritage month: May 2011.* Retrieved January 21, 2012, from www.census.gov/newsroom/releases/archives/facts_for_features_special_editions/cb11-ff06.html.

U.S. Census Bureau. (2012b). *Black (African-American) history month: February 2012.* Retrieved January 21, 2012, from www.census.gov/newsroom/releases/archives/facts_for_features_special_editions/cb12-ff01.html.

U.S. Census Bureau. (2012c). *Hispanic heritage month 2011: Sept. 15-Oct. 15.* Retrieved January 21, 2012, from www.census.gov/newsroom/releases/archives/facts_for_features_special_editions/cb11-ff18.html.

U.S. Census Bureau. (2012d). *American Indian and Alaska Native heritage month: November 2011.* Retrieved January 21, 2012, from www.census.gov/newsroom/releases/archives/facts_for_features_special_editions/cb11-ff22.html.

U.S. Department of Health and Human Services. (2009). *Morbidity and Mortality Weekly Report (MMWR): Differences in prevalence of obesity among Black, White, and Hispanic adults—United States, 2006-2008.* Retrieved July 6, 2012, from www.cdc.gov/mmwr/preview/mmwrhtml/mm5827a2.htm.

U.S. Department of Health and Human Services. (2010a). *Health, United States, 2010: With special feature on death and dying.* Retrieved January 20, 2012, from www.cdc.gov/nchs/data/hus/hus10.pdf#026.

U.S. Department of Health and Human Services. (2010b). *About Healthy People: Disparities.* Retrieved January 17, 2012, from www.healthypeople.gov/2020/about/DisparitiesAbout.aspx.

U.S. Department of Health and Human Services. (2011). *National partnership for action: Health equality & disparities.* Retrieved January 17, 2012, from www.minorityhealth.hhs.gov/npa/templates/browse.aspx?&;lvl=2&lvlid=34.

U.S. Department of Health and Human Services. (2012). *The Affordable Care Act Becomes Law.* Retrieved July 13, 2012, from www.healthcare.gov/law/features/index.html.

U.S. Department of Health and Human Services, Office of Minority Health. (2011). *Asian American/Pacific Islander profile.* Retrieved January 22, 2012, from http://minorityhealth.hhs.gov/templates/browse.aspx?lvl=2&lvlid=53U.S.

U.S. Department of Health and Human Services, Centers for Disease Control and Prevention. (2011). *National Vital Statistics Reports.* Retrieved July 6, 2012, from www.cdc.gov/nchs/data/nvsr/nvsr59/nvsr59_10.pdf.

U.S. Department of Health and Human Services, Centers for Disease Control and Prevention. (2012a). *Health United States 2011: With special feature on socioeconomic status and health.* Retrieved July 6, 2012, from www.cdc.gov/nchs/data/hus/hus11.pdf.

U.S. Department of Health and Human Services, Centers for Disease Control and Prevention. (2012b). *Summary health statistics for U.S. adults: National health interview survey 2010.* Retrieved July 6, 2012, from www.cdc.gov/nchs/data/series/sr_10/sr10_252.pdf.

U.S. Social Security Administration. (2012). *Social security is important to African Americans.* Retrieved July 6, 2012, from www.ssa.gov/pressoffice/factsheets/africanamer.htm.

Vance, A. R. (2008). Filipino Americans. In M. M. Andrews, & J. S. Boyle (Eds.), *Transcultural concepts in nursing care* (5th ed., pp. 467–493). Philadelphia: Wolter Kluwer Health: Lippincott Williams & Wilkins.

Vaughn, L. M., Jacquez, F., & Baker, R. C. (2009). Cultural health attributions, beliefs, and practices: Effects on healthcare and medical education. *Open Medical Education Journal, 2,* 64–74.

Weglicki, L. S., Templin, T. N., Rice, V. H., Jamil, H., & Hammad, A. (2008). Comparison of cigarette and water-pipe smoking by Arab and non-Arab-American youth. *American Journal of Preventive Medicine, 35*(4), 334–339.

Williams, D. R., Neighbors, H. W., & Jackson, J. S. (2008). Racial/ethnic discrimination and health: Findings from community studies. *American Journal of Public Health, 98*(9 Suppl), S29–S37.

Health Policy and the Delivery System

Debora Elizabeth Kirsch

evolve WEBSITE

- Study Questions
- Glossary

OBJECTIVES

After completing this chapter, the reader will be able to:
- Examine key developments in the history of health care that influenced the philosophical basis of American health care and separated preventive from curative measures.
- Differentiate between private and public sector functions and responsibilities in the delivery of health care.
- Describe the mechanisms by which health care in the United States is financed in both private and public sectors.
- Analyze the influence of health legislation on health care delivery.

- Differentiate between the purposes, benefits, and limitations of Medicare, Medicaid, and other government-sponsored programs in achieving health equity.
- Compare and contrast the health care delivery systems of the United States and other countries.
- Discuss the major provisions of the Patient Protection and Affordable Care Act of 2010 and its impact on vulnerable populations.

KEY TERMS

Accountable care organizations (ACOs)
Advanced practice nurses (APNs)
Advocate
Affordable Care Act (ACA)
Capitation rate
Concierge care
Fee-for-service
Gatekeeper
Health insurance exchanges

Health maintenance organizations (HMOs)
Health savings accounts (HSAs)
High-deductible health insurance plans (HDHPs)
Hospitalist
Indemnity insurance plan
Independent practice associations (IPAs)
Insurance

Managed care
Medicaid
Medicare
Nursing centers
Point-of-service (POS)
Preferred provider organizations (PPOs)
Primary care provider (PCP)

❓ THINK ABOUT IT

The Federal Health Care Reform Law

The passage of the new health care federal reform law called the Patient Protection and Affordable Care Act has reignited the national conversation on the role of government oversight in the provision of health care. As the court systems battle the legalities of the many provisions of the law, questions remain on how best to serve the health care needs of all Americans.

- Will the provisions of the law solve the problems of rising health care costs, quality and safety issues, and access to health care?
- Should there be a federal government mandate to require all American citizens to have health insurance coverage?
- Why is the American health care system the most costly in the world?

The health care delivery system in the United States is a complex, multilayered entity that has the capacity to provide the newest technological treatments and implement the most advanced health care in the world. Research findings have sparked the development of international gold standards for practicing evidence-based medical and nursing care. The market-driven American health care system is distinct from any other health care delivery system in the world, employing more than 14.3 million health care workers in 2008, serving over 312 million people. The U.S. Bureau of Labor reports 10 of the 20 fastest growing occupations are health care related (U.S. Department of Labor, 2010). The American health care system is massive—but so is the cost. The rising cost of health care is consuming a growing percentage of the nation's gross domestic product (GDP). Preliminary figures in 2010 indicate national health expenditures consumed 17.9% of the nation's GDP (i.e., 2.59 trillion dollars), which equates to $8402 per person, the highest dollar amount per capita of all industrialized countries (Centers for Medicare & Medicaid Services, 2011).

Despite the vast resources devoted to financing the health care system, unequal access to care exists, especially among vulnerable populations. The rising cost of health insurance premiums is a growing burden to working American families, and the number of uninsured individuals and families is growing, in part because of the recent economic decline and high unemployment rates. Although the provision of health insurance is an important factor in health equity, vulnerable populations face additional obstacles leading to health disparities across the nation. Health disparities (a particular type of health difference that is closely linked with social, economic, and/or environmental disadvantage) adversely affect groups of individuals—especially vulnerable populations. Health care reform in the past consisted of incremental steps, mainly targeted at the poor and older adult populations (Medicare and Medicaid); however, with escalating health care costs and concern for improvement in the quality and safety of care, a more substantive reform effort was taken. The vision of *Healthy People 2020* is *a society in which all people live long healthy lives.* One of the overarching goals of *Healthy People 2020* is the attainment of the highest level of health for all people (U.S. Department of Health and Human Services [USHHS], 2011a). The new health care federal reform law called the Patient Protection and Affordable Care Act (ACA) was signed into law on March 23, 2010. The federal law requires the largest change in the financing of the American health care system since public Medicare and Medicaid programs were enacted in the 1960s. The implementation of the many provisions of the law began immediately and are slated to be fully enacted by 2018. The law is designed to address the issues of affordability, accessibility, and financing of health care, with focused efforts on meeting the needs of vulnerable populations. The Affordable Care Act will require substantial changes in public insurance programs, private health insurance market regulations, and other components of the health care system. Lacking bipartisan support for the original law, a change in the political landscape of the Senate or House of Representatives as well as actions filed in the federal court system challenging the constitutionality of the Affordable Care Act may result in the appeal or additional amendments to some of the current and future provisions. The Supreme Court ruled in favor of the ACA in June of 2012 (Kaiser Family Foundation [KFF], 2011a; KFF, 2012a).

The next several years will be challenging times for state governments to arrange the many provisions of the Affordable Care Act. For example, individuals who do not have employer insurance coverage will be able to purchase coverage through a public or private health insurance exchange. States will need to establish the structure for these new health insurance exchange programs and meet requirements for the required essential health benefit packages.

This chapter will analyze the health status of this nation compared to other countries; examine historical influences in the delivery of health care; and describe the structure and mechanisms to deliver public (Medicare and Medicaid) and private health care in the United States and select other countries, the financing of the health care system, and key federal legislation with emphasis on the provisions of the Patient Protection and Affordable Care Act (ACA) of 2010, which will strive to improve teamwork and communication between all these system pieces. Savings in health care expenditures could be realized if individuals engage in health promotion practices and avoid costly consequences of chronic disease. The Affordable Care Act is also hoping that some savings will be realized from decreasing unnecessary hospital readmissions. Nurses need to keep abreast of the various provisions and amendments of the law while they occur and be politically active in influencing health policy as an advocate of social justice for individuals and families.

THE HEALTH OF THE NATION

Health, United States is an annual published document prepared by the U.S. Department of Health and Human Services; it reports the health status of the nation by tracking a variety of specific, measurable health indicators. This annual report serves several key functions, but the main goal is to inform policymakers, the President, and Congress of the trends in the nation's health to guide the development of sound health policy and allocate resources to maintain and improve the health of the nation's citizens. The 2010 report indicates the health of the nation has improved in many areas as a result of substantial funding of public health programs, research, provision of health care, and initiatives to support consumer education. Emerging trends indicate success in the reduction of morbidity and mortality of many diseases, control of widespread infectious diseases through widespread vaccination programs, improvement in motor vehicle safety, and reduction of cardiovascular-related deaths. Life expectancy has increased for both men and women, and maternal and infant mortality rates on average are declining in many geographic locations. Heart disease is the number one cause of death for Americans, responsible for 25% of all deaths in 2007, followed by cancer, with 23% of all deaths in the same year. Education regarding leading a healthy lifestyle, controlling hypertension, using cholesterol-lowering medications, and participating in routine screening has contributed to better health for Americans, but concern about sedentary lifestyle, rising obesity trends, and chronic disease is noted. Recent national smoking cessation interventions did not demonstrate effectiveness because the number of individuals 18 years or older engaging in cigarette smoking in 2008 and 2009 was stagnant at 20.6% of the population. Other risk factors remain problematic with more than 33% of adults older than 20 years obese and 32.6% hypertensive. The report cites childhood obesity as a growing concern—between 2007 and 2008, 10.4% of children ages 2 to 5 years, 19.6% of children ages 6 to 11 years, and 18.1% of children ages 12 to 19 years were obese. As obesity trends often continue into adulthood, these children are at greater risk for developing diabetes, hypertension, and cardiovascular disease earlier in life and developing the sequelae of chronic disease in adulthood. Improvements in the nation's health have not been uniform, because some factors affecting health equity are an individual's income, race, gender, ethnicity, education level, and geographic location (National Center for Health Statistics [NCHS], 2011). The most effective intervention to decrease the growing cost of health care is to keep Americans healthy—preventing chronic diseases such as diabetes, heart disease, asthma, and human immunodeficiency virus (HIV)-related disease (Kovner & Knickman, 2011).

Healthy People 2020

As discussed in the opening chapter, on December 2, 2010, *Healthy People 2020* was launched, providing a 10-year agenda for improving the health of all Americans. The new overarching goals are listed in Box 3-1: *Healthy People 2020*.

One of the goals of *Healthy People 2000* was to reduce health disparities among Americans. Ten years later, *Healthy People 2010's* goal was to eliminate health disparities. The current 2020 goal is broader—to achieve health equity, eliminate disparities, and improve the health of all groups as measured by leading health indicators. Health disparities adversely affect groups of people who have systematically experienced greater obstacles to health based on their racial or ethnic group; religion; socioeconomic status; gender; age; mental health; cognitive, sensory, or physical disability; sexual orientation or gender identity; geographic location; or other characteristics historically linked to discrimination or exclusion (USHHS, 2011a). Individuals and groups at risk for health disparity are considered vulnerable populations. A more complete list of vulnerable populations can be found in Box 3-2. Public health nursing practice promotes and preserves the health of populations, looking at the community as a whole and its effect on the health of individuals, families, and groups. Community health nursing practice promotes, preserves, and maintains the health of populations through care provided to individuals, families, and groups and studies the effect of their health status on that of the community as a whole (Stanhope & Lancaster, 2012). A healthy community promotes a high quality of life and well-being, which can be measured by social networks, physical assets, economic opportunity, human development, and local institutions that sustain respect and support each of the dimensions (Community Health and Empowerment through Education and Research [CHEER], 2011). *Healthy People 2020* supports the need for an effective public health infrastructure for planning, delivering, and evaluating public health, with the key components being a capable and qualified workforce, up-to-date data and information systems, and public health agencies capable of assessing and responding to public health needs (USDHHS, 2011a).

Health Indicators of a Nation

Standard measures used to compare the health status of the population of one nation with another are actually death indicators. Although mortality-based indicators do not directly measure the health status of the living population, the data indirectly reflect the general health of a nation and are more readily available through government and world agencies. Table 3-1, International Comparisons of Core Health Indicators (estimates) for 2011, compares the average life expectancy by gender as well as infant mortality rates of populations in selected countries. According to Central Intelligence Agency statistics (CIA, 2012), the life expectancy of a U.S. male in 2011 was 76 years compared to 78.8 years in Sweden and 78.8 years in Canada, while females in America were reported to have a life expectancy of 80.9 years compared to 85 years in France and 84.1 years in Canada. Mexico was significantly lower for both males (73.65 years) and females (79.43 years). In 1950, life

---

♥ BOX 3-1   HEALTHY PEOPLE 2020

Overarching Goals for Healthy People 2020

- Attain high-quality, longer lives free of preventable disease, disability, injury, and premature death.
- Achieve health equity, eliminate disparities, and improve the health of all groups.
- Create social and physical environments that promote good health for all.
- Promote quality of life, healthy development, and healthy behaviors across all life stages.

BOX 3-2   VULNERABLE POPULATIONS

- Residents of rural areas
- Undocumented immigrants
- Low-income individuals and families
- Racial and ethnic minorities
- People with no health insurance coverage
- People with multiple chronic conditions
- People with language or cultural barriers
- The physically disabled or handicapped
- The terminally or mentally ill
- Persons with HIV/AIDS
- Alcohol or substance abusers
- Homeless individuals
- Individuals who do not speak English
- Individuals with communication difficulties
- Low education levels or illiteracy
- Anyone lacking health literacy

From Shi, L., & Stevens, G. (2010). *Vulnerable populations in the United States* (2nd ed.). San Francisco, CA: Jossey-Bass; Urban Institute: *Health policy center vulnerable populations*. Retrieved January 2, 2011, from http://urban.org/health_policy/vulnerable_populations/index.cfm.

TABLE 3-1   INTERNATIONAL COMPARISONS OF CORE HEALTH INDICATORS FOR 2011

	AFGHANISTAN	CANADA	FRANCE	GERMANY	MEXICO	SWEDEN	UNITED KINGDOM	UNITED STATES
Life expectancy at birth: males (years)	44.79	78.81	78.0	77.8	73.65	78.8	78.0	76.0
Life expectancy at birth: females (years)	45.25	84.1	85.0	82.4	79.43	83.5	82.0	80.9
Life expectancy at birth: both genders (years)	45.02	81.38	81.0	80.0	76.47	81.1	80.0	78.4
Infant mortality rate (per 1000 live births)	175.9	4.92	3.29	3.54	17.29	2.74	4.6	6.1

Data from the Central Intelligence Agency: *The world factbook.* Retrieved January 21, 2011, from www.cia.gov/library/publications/the-world-factbook/.

TABLE 3-2   INTERNATIONAL COMPARISON OF LIFE EXPECTANCY RATES (IN YEARS) OVER TIME FOR 1990, 2000, AND ESTIMATES OF 2011

LOCATION	TIME PERIOD	MALE	FEMALE	BOTH GENDERS
Afghanistan	2011	45	45	45
	2000	44	48	46
	1990	42	46	44
Australia	2011	80	84	82
	2000	77	82	80
	1990	74	80	77
Canada	2011	79	83	81
	2000	77	82	79
	1990	74	80	77
China	2011	73	77	75
	2000	70	73	71
	1990	68	69	68
Denmark	2011	76	81	79
	2000	75	79	77
	1990	72	78	75
France	2011	78	85	81
	2000	75	83	79
	1990	73	81	77
India	2011	63	66	65
	2000	60	62	61
	1990	57	58	57
Mexico	2011	73	78	76
	2000	72	77	74
	1990	68	74	71
United Kingdom	2011	78	82	80
	2000	75	80	78
	1990	73	78	76
United States of America	2011	76	81	79
	2000	74	80	77
	1990	72	79	75

Data from World Health Organization: *Global health observatory data repository.* Retrieved January 10, 2012, from http://apps.who.int/ghodata; Central Intelligence Agency: *The world factbook.* Retrieved January 21, 2011, from www.cia.gov/library/publications/the-world-factbook/.

expectancy in the United States for men was 56.2 years and for women 65.5 years (Social Security On-Line [SSOL], n.d.). Overall, life expectancy rates have risen sharply in the past 60 years in the United States and now average 78.4 years for both genders. In stark comparison are life expectancy rates in Afghanistan, a country with very low levels of health care provisions. The average male life expectancy is 44.79 years and for females it is 45.25 years. Compared to the United States, this gap is greater than 30 years. Over the preceding 2 decades, most nations have slowly improved life expectancy by 4 to 5 years (see Table 3-2 for select countries). Although India is behind in life expectancy compared to the other countries listed (average life expectancy in 2011 is 65 years for both genders), they have improved by 8 years and China by 7 years in the last 2 decades (NCHS, 2011).

Infant mortality rates (refer to Table 3-1) are one of the most important indicators of the health of a nation because they are associated with factors such as maternal health and access to health care. The U.S. mortality rate in 2011 was reported as 6.1 (number of deaths of infants in the first year of life per 1000 live births), a dramatic improvement from 29.2 reported in 1950 but higher than mortality rates in other developed nations (CIA, 2012; SSOL, n.d.). Mexico has an infant mortality rate of just greater than 17, which is similar to other poorer nations like India, which has an infant mortality rate of more than 47. An outlier for an extremely high infant mortality rate is Afghanistan, reporting more than 175 deaths of infants in their first year of life per 1000 live births. One reason the United States ranks less favorably in health indicators than other industrialized nations is attributed to the large disparities in health status by geographic areas, race, ethnicity groups, and social class (MacDorman & Matthews, 2008). For example, infant mortality rates for African American babies were more than twice those of Whites and Hispanics (Table 3-3). The infant mortality rate for non-Hispanic White infants in the United States was 5.63, which is below the overall average of 6.75 years in 2011, but Black or African American, non-Hispanic women have a disproportionately high rate of 13.31 infant deaths in the first year of life and American Indian/Alaska Natives have a rate of 9.22 deaths. There has been a persistent racial disparity in the United States, especially among Black infants (Bartfield, 2011). The U.S. infant mortality rate is higher than that of the other industrial nations presented in Table 3-1. Another indicator used to measure infant mortality (women of similar socioeconomic status) rates is by determining the years of education completed or the educational attainment of mothers. Large differences in infant death rates are readily apparent as shown in Table 3-4. The 2003 to 2005 infant mortality rate of White mothers who were 20 years of age or older with a college education was 4.2 whereas that for Asian women was even lower at 3.8. These statistics are much more congruent with those of other industrialized countries. African American women with less than a high school education have the highest infant mortality rates, reported as 15.1. For most races and ethnicities the higher a woman's educational achievement, the lower the overall infant mortality rate, as shown in Figure 3-1. In research terms, this indicates a positive correlation between educational attainment of women and infant mortality rates. To improve health indicators and reduce health disparities of a population, interventions

to promote educational attainment of women at least through high school need to occur as one strategy to decrease infant mortality rates. Geographic variations exist within the United States as well with the age at which women give birth. The highest percentage of women younger than age 20 years giving birth is in the state of Mississippi at 15.5%, compared to the national average of 9.3%. The greatest number of preterm births for all age groups (17.6% compared to the national average of 12%) and the highest number of women delivering infants with

TABLE 3-3   INFANT MORTALITY RATE IN THE UNITED STATES BY RACE/ETHNICITY, 2007

RACE/ETHNICITY	INFANT DEATHS PER 1000 BIRTHS*
Asian and Native Hawaiian/Pacific Islander	4.78
Hispanic or Latina	5.51
White, Non-Hispanic	5.63
American Indian/Alaska Native	9.22
Black or African American, Non-Hispanic	13.31
All mothers	6.75

Data from *National Vital Statistics, 59*(6), 2011, Table A. Retrieved January 21, 2011, from www.cdc.gov/nchs/data.
*Births are categorized according to race/ethnicity of mother.

TABLE 3-4   INFANT MORTALITY RATES IN 2007, BY TRIMESTER IN WHICH PREGNANCY CARE WAS STARTED, SMOKING STATUS DURING PREGNANCY, AND EDUCATION OF MOTHER

CHARACTERISTIC	RATE
Prenatal care beginning in first trimester	5.57
Prenatal care beginning in second or third trimester	6.3
No prenatal care	27.13
Smoker during pregnancy	10.41
Nonsmoker during pregnancy	6.1
Educational attainment:	
Less than high school diploma	7.78
High school diploma	7.17
Some college or technical school	5.79
Bachelor's degree or higher	3.77

Data from *National Vital Statistics, 59*(6), 2011 (Table II: 19 State Reported Area). Retrieved January 21, 2011, from www.cdc.gov/nchs/data/nvsr/nvsr59/nvsr59_06.pdf.

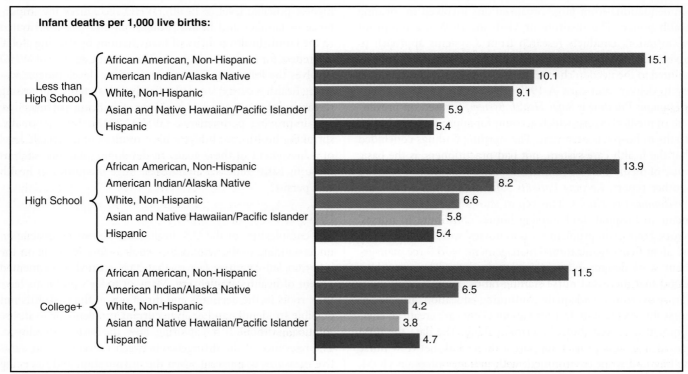

FIGURE 3-1 Infant mortality rates for mothers ages 20 years and older by race/ethnicity and education, 2003 to 2005. (Data reported from 37 states, DC, and NYC. Data from Centers for Disease Control and Prevention/National Center for Health Statistics, National Vital Statistics System, Linked Birth/Infant Death Dataset, Source, *Health,* United States, 2008, Table 19.)

low birth weights (12.1% compared to the national average of 9.3%) also occur in women giving birth in the state of Mississippi. Other states with similar correlations include Louisiana, Alabama, Arkansas, and New Mexico (Martin et al., 2011). In summary, decreasing the nations' infant mortality rates will require community interventions to decrease teen pregnancy, promote educational attainment for all women to high school level or greater, and provide targeted interventions for specific racial groups and geographic areas.

Historical Role of Women in Health Promotion

Nurses have a long tradition of involvement in health promotion, beginning with Florence Nightingale, the founder of modern nursing. While caring for wounded soldiers in the Crimean War, she fought for hospital reform by crusading for cleanliness and against overcrowding and lack of ventilation. Her careful recordings of care outcomes quantified needed reform in health promotion (Kudzma, 2006). Later, Lillian Wald, appalled by the lack of medical care, ignorance, and living conditions of the poor in 1893, developed a settlement program in New York City that trained nurses, provided care to families, and developed education programs for the community. Wald, a leader in political activism, spearheaded organized public health in the direction of health promotion for families and communities (Holder, 2004). These pioneers and others set the stage for nurses' unique role in health promotion.

A SAFER SYSTEM

The health care delivery system in the United States is experiencing significant changes sparked by health care reform, recommendations from large organizations involved in forming health policy. The Institute of Medicine (IOM), a nonprofit organization, conducts research from a systems approach to advise the nation in improving health. Several early reports pointed to the need to change the structure of health care delivery to deliver safer care. A 1999 IOM research report, *To Err is Human: Building a Safer Health System,* focused on prevention of medical errors, which account for approximately 98,000 deaths in hospitals each year. The startling findings concluded that the health care system, not bad practitioners, is the basic cause of medical errors (IOM, 1999). In 2003 the IOM released another report, *Keeping Patients Safe: Transforming the Work Environment of Nurses.* This report shows that work environments in hospitals and nursing homes contribute to nurses' errors. Four main problem areas in nurses' work environments are identified: organizational management; workforce management; work design; and organizational culture. The researchers found that increased nurse staffing ratios, fewer nurses, mandatory overtime, inadequate continuing education, and lack of nurse involvement in decisions about client care create an environment that contributes to error making. The data the IOM provided in this project support a direct link between nurse staffing and work environment with patient outcomes (IOM, 2003). Other person safety issues arise from poor workplace communication between shifts and providers. Other efforts by the IOM to improve the health of the nation include the 2006

report *Preventing Medication Errors: Quality Chasm Series,* released in July of 2006. The report found in any given week, medication errors in prescribing or taking medication were not only common but also costly to the nation and recommended a comprehensive approach to decreasing the prevalence of medication errors by making changes in the health care system (IOM, 2006). The IOM has been productive in releasing a variety of reports and workshop summaries of pressing concerns related to health and the health care system. A report released in January of 2012 discussed how standards of care can be defined as the level of health and medical care capable of being delivered when preparing for public health emergencies such as pandemic influenza, large-scale earthquake, or any major disaster scenario in which the health system may be destroyed or stressed (IOM, 2012). The IOM has made recommendations in other areas promoting safety within the health care system. In 2011, recommendations were made to improve transparency in the reporting of health information technology and promoting health literacy to encourage prevention and wellness. To provide safe, evidence-based care nurses have a responsibility to understand the system in which they practice. Although health care often is equated with medical care, which focuses on the treatment of illness, this chapter presents the evolution and ongoing development of a broader concept of health based on the definition given in Chapter 1.

GLOBAL HEALTH

The World Health Organization's (commonly referred to as WHO) overriding objective is to influence health opportunities and outcomes for all people so that they can attain the highest possible level of health. WHO recognizes the importance of families and health promotion, and has contributed to the family health policies of many nations by shaping global awareness for health promotion. The current agenda of WHO involves the following six goals: promoting development; fostering health security; strengthening health systems; harnessing research, information, and evidence; enhancing partnerships; and improving performance (WHO, 2012). Internationally, shrinking health care budgets have resulted in a variable level of achievement of these goals. In developing nations, such as those in Latin America and Africa, huge inequities in health care persist.

Historical Perspectives

The complexities of the U.S. health care system necessitate an understanding of the system as a whole before focusing on the intermingled causative factors that have created a fragmented system of health care delivery. Many of today's problems have their roots in the decisions and directions of the past. It is not possible to identify and analyze current problems or to devise solutions without first exploring how the system developed. The relevance of the divergence between preventive and curative measures is apparent when the organization and financing of the delivery system are examined. The United States has established a system that uses two basic divisions of society to provide service: the public sector and the private sector. The merger of public health and welfare policies in the public sector is rooted in the Puritan ethic inherent in the historical development of the United States. The current focus on managed care as both an organizational strategy and a financing mechanism is highlighted in a discussion of how health care is delivered and financed.

HISTORY OF HEALTH CARE

Early Influences

Historical records of early civilizations (Egyptian, Indian, Chinese, Aztec, and Greek) show that ancient peoples were concerned with disease and practiced various methods of treatment. The earliest views of health can be seen as holistic in the sense that they emerged from an integrated worldview. Primitive peoples understood illness in mystical terms: sickness and cure theories were tied to the cosmic view of life, with natural and supernatural forces often inseparable. Most religions include a person's hygiene as part of their practice. For thousands of years, epidemics were viewed as divine judgments on human wickedness, with a gradual awareness that pestilence (any epidemic disease with a high death rate) has natural causes such as climate and other aspects of the physical environment. During the Middle Ages, infectious diseases in epidemic proportions (leprosy, bubonic plague, smallpox, and tuberculosis [TB]) were the leading causes of death. Clearly, health was viewed in terms of survival and absence of disease.

Industrial Influences

The population of the Western world began to increase during the 1600s, when America was first being explored. The New World had many things to offer explorers. An adequate food supply made it possible for the population to live longer, and advances in transportation made distribution of food supplies and other goods and services possible. Manufacturing advances during the eighteenth century, through the invention of the flush toilet and cast iron pipe, made sanitary engineering possible, saving many lives by preventing diseases such as typhoid, paratyphoid, and gastroenteritis.

Socioeconomic Influences

Although the Elizabethan poor laws (1601) in England provided a system of relief for the poor, which included infants, sick and older people, and laborers in the workhouses, a new poor law was enacted in 1834 based on the harsher philosophy that regarded pauperism among able-bodied workers as a moral failing. If the worker did not earn a subsistence-level income, the attitude toward that worker was suspicious and punitive. These poor laws were the legal implementation of the Protestant work ethic that the Puritan forebears brought to the United States. According to this view, people are held directly accountable for their state in life, and health maintenance is the responsibility of the individual. The far-reaching implications of this ethic can be seen today in the organization, financing, and delivery of health services.

Public Health Influences

Edwin Chadwick (1800-1890) is known as the father of British and American public health. Chadwick established an English Board of Health, which emphasized environmental sanitation but excluded physicians outside times of crisis. Additionally, Chadwick was secretary of the Poor Law Commission, which strove to improve the health of the masses for economic reasons. Chadwick's rationale was that disease among the poor was a major factor in their inability to support themselves. Therefore governmental health and welfare policies have been joined in England since the nineteenth century.

Lemuel Shattuck, a leader of the public health movement, began the movement in the United States. He used the British system as the model, with public health services and welfare combined, despite the contradictory emphasis. Public health has focused on improving the health of the poor, whereas welfare has dictated subsistence at the minimal level. The influence of the Puritan ethic on the American health care system is apparent in the emphasis on the value of work and the attitude toward the poor. Today, health and welfare departments continue their contradictory approach to the poor.

Scientific Influences

Until the twentieth century, epidemics of infectious disease (plague, cholera, typhoid, smallpox, and influenza) were the most critical health problems and major causes of death and disability for Americans. Scientific advances during the nineteenth century by Louis Pasteur (germ theory), Robert Koch (origin of bacterial infection), Joseph Lister (antisepsis), and Paul Ehrlich (chemotherapy) expanded public health from its earlier concentration on sanitation to control of communicable diseases through a broad biological base. Public health became an important force in decreasing death rates and increasing life expectancy through the application of bacteriology. International environmental conditions were improved by developing systems that safeguard water, milk, and food supplies; promote sanitary sewage disposal; and monitor the quality of urban housing.

Between 1936 and 1954, the discovery and use of sulfonamides and other antibiotics to treat bacterial infections reduced the death rate to its lowest point in history, with deaths caused by primary infections reduced to 4%, as compared with 33% only 50 years earlier (in 1886). The death rate did not change significantly between 1954 and the mid-1960s. Another decline in the death rate began after the mid-1960s and has continued (with the exception of a slight increase in 1995) with the control of many infectious diseases (Arias & Smith, 2003). As the life expectancy of the population increases, chronic diseases such as heart disease, cancer, chronic lower respiratory tract disease, cerebrovascular disease, unintentional injury, Alzheimer's disease, diabetes, influenza and pneumonia, nephritis, and suicide in descending order are the top 10 leading cause of total death in the United States as reported by the Centers for Disease Control and Prevention (CDC, 2012a).

Despite the progress in conquering infectious diseases, in vulnerable populations infections are once again among the top leading contributors to death in the United States. For children ages 1 to 4 years, influenza and pneumonia are the sixth leading cause of death and ninth for ages 5 to 14 years. Although not in the top 10 causes of death, diseases that were thought to be under control, such as measles and TB, are resurfacing and a new group of pathogens have emerged.

The most effective strategy for eliminating TB is to monitor those infected to ensure completion of treatment is by direct observed therapy, which requires monitoring a person's medication adherence for 6 months to 2 years. Resources are needed at local public health departments to provide monitoring and follow-up in this typically elusive TB-infected population. The national TB surveillance system reports declining TB incidence cases on average with 2010 data reporting the lowest number of TB cases in the United States since national reporting began in 1953. This is significant progress since TB cases peaked in 1992. In 2010, 60% of the reported number of TB cases were foreign-born individuals (18.1 cases per 100,000) compared to U.S.-born individuals (1.6 cases per 100,000). This is an 11 times increase in foreign-born TB transmission. Rates of TB in ethnic and racial populations vary as well. Asian and Native Hawaiians and other Pacific Islanders have rates of more 20 per 100,000 persons. Interventions to eliminate TB require adequate local community resources, targeted to groups at risk (CDC, 2012c). Globally, TB is one of the world's deadliest diseases with one third of the world being infected. Interventions need to be distributed over a wide region because the risk of infection to the population is more widespread. There are an estimated 1.4 million TB-related deaths worldwide, and in 2010, 9 million people around the world became ill with TB. TB is also the leading cause of death in individuals who are HIV-infected. New strains of extremely drug-resistant TB (XDR-TB) are now emerging that are resistant not only to isoniazid and rifampin, which are the most effective first-line TB treatment drugs, but also to second-line anti-TB drugs as well. Although TB multidrug-resistant rates are low in the United States (88 cases in 2010 and 94 cases in 2009), of those cases over 80% of patients are foreign-born. TB remains an urgent public health problem with more than 75% of the cases in just 15 countries. Global interventions to reduce TB infection include targeted population- and age-specific interventions such as administering the bacille Calmette-Guérin (BCG) vaccine to children (CDC, 2012b).

An effective, comprehensive public health system is imperative to enable the United States to respond to local, national, and global concerns. As new diseases emerge, older diseases reemerge (sometimes in drug-resistant forms), and natural and man-made disasters occur, a functioning public health system is warranted. The Affordable Care Act calls for the establishment of a council within the USDHHS to be known as National Prevention, Health Promotion, and Public Health Council, required to provide coordination and leadership at the federal level among all federal departments and agencies. The council is charged with obtaining input from relative stakeholders to develop a plan to improve the health status of Americans and reduce the incidence of preventable disease, disability, and illness, which will require the integration and coordination of many of the divisions of the USDHHS (Office of the Legislative Council, 2010). The Centers for Disease Control and Prevention is the frontline agency for providing national health security and must remain vigilant in rapidly detecting and controlling disease outbreaks

in the United States and abroad. The CDC's Emergency Operations Center (EOC) is the command center for monitoring and coordinating emergency response to public health threats in the United States and worldwide, such as pandemic flu, natural disasters, and terrorist attacks. Recent global outbreaks of the Hendra virus (1994); H5N1 bird flu (1997); Nipah virus (1999); severe acute respiratory syndrome–associated coronavirus (2003); monkey pox, mad cow disease, and avian flu (2006); and H1N1 (2009), pose challenges to global public health (CDC Foundation, 2012) (see Chapter 25). According to the CDC, influenza pandemic occurs approximately three times a century, and in 1918 a severe influenza pandemic killed about 1% of those who contracted the virus. When the bird flu virus H5N1 emerged in 1997, the CDC and others began tracking the novel form of influenza, fearing a potential pandemic. Because about 60% of individuals who contracted bird flu died, concern heightened when another influenza virus, H1N1, was first recognized in Mexico in 2009. The virus was identified as influenza A, H1N1, the same virus responsible for the 1918 Spanish influenza pandemic, which was responsible for 50 million deaths. Fearing another deadly pandemic, the CDC took quick actions and developed a vaccine that was distributed to as many Americans as possible—targeting infants, young adults, and pregnant women. Although the H1N1 flu outbreak of 2009 (known also as the swine flu) killed 12,500 individuals, millions of Americans were protected against H1N1, preventing thousands of hospitalizations and deaths. The CDC remains on constant alert for new, deadly influenza viruses and other airborne diseases (CDC Foundation, 2012).

Special Population Influences

The second goal of *Healthy People 2020,* as previously stated, is to achieve health equity, eliminate disparities, and improve the health of all groups. Vulnerable populations, especially those living in poverty, are at great risk to experience health disparities (USDHHS, OMH, 2012). For many of these disadvantaged people, the issues of preventing disease and promoting good health are often secondary to the problems associated with everyday survival. Determinants of health in a population are related strongly to socioeconomic status and education level, with populations in the lower strata having worse outcomes. However, individual lifestyle behaviors including dietary choices, level of physical activity, use of alcohol and tobacco, substance abuse, and risky sexual behavior play a significant role in the health status of an individual. Access to health care for prevention, early detection, and treatment are paramount in diminishing health disparities, but programs promoting positive individual lifestyle behaviors are also needed (USDHHS, OMH, 2012) (Box 3-3: Diversity Awareness).

Political and Economic Influences

Political and economic considerations influence the health care system, and politics determines the decision makers who will negotiate a desired outcome. Economics defines the resources that are distributed and the manner in which they are distributed. The effect of economics and politics on the delivery of health care is illustrated by the situation in the United States

BOX 3-3 DIVERSITY AWARENESS

Health and Human Services Action Plan to Reduce Racial and Ethnic Health Disparities

Community-Driven Approach to Reduce Health Disparities in the United States

As a nation, health equity does not exist especially among racial and ethnic populations. Health disparities, as discussed in the report, are differences in health outcomes that are closely linked with social, economic, and environmental disadvantage, which are often driven by the social conditions in which individuals live, learn, work, and play. Marked differences in social determinants, such as poverty, low socioeconomic status (SES), and lack of access to care, exist along racial and ethnic lines, leading to poor health outcomes. The economic burden between 2003 and 2006 attributable to health disparities was estimated to be $1.24 trillion. The major dimensions of racial and ethnic health disparities outlined are the following:

- Lack of insurance negatively affects the quality of health care received by minorities. One third of the population consists of racial and ethnic minorities but constitutes more than half of the 50 million individuals without health insurance.
- Minorities are overrepresented among the 56 million people in America who have inadequate access to a primary care physician. Minority children are less likely than non-Hispanic White children to have a usual source of care.
- Racial and ethnic minorities often receive poorer quality of care and face more barriers in seeking care, including preventive care, acute treatment, or chronic disease management, than non-Hispanic Whites.
- African Americans have higher hospitalization rates from influenza than other populations and African American children are more than four times as likely to die from asthma as non-Hispanic White children. Higher obesity rates in the African American population contribute to the onset of diabetes, hypertension, and cardiovascular disease.

As the demographics of the United States continue to become more diverse, nurses need to be culturally competent as one strategy for eliminating racial and ethnic disparities. In 2004, the IOM report titled *In the Nation's Compelling Interest: Ensuring Diversity in Health Care Workforce*, diversity in the workforce was a key element of patient-centered care. Efforts to match the ethnic and racial composition of the health care workforce with the U.S. population will contribute to addressing health disparities. Providers who speak a second language will also be needed because 24 million adults have limited English proficiency. Shortages of primary care providers in underserved areas significantly affect the health of ethnic and racial minorities. The primary care nurse practitioner is ideally suited to care for underserved populations in urban and rural areas. Additional funds from the ACA are funding Communities Putting Prevention to Work (CPPW) programs, which support statewide and community-based policy and environmental changes in nutrition, physical activity, tobacco control, and other factors that harm people's health. *Healthy People 2020* provides a comprehensive set of 10-year national goals and objectives with 42 topic areas and more than 600 evolving objectives. The Leading Health Indicators outline high-priority health issues. One of the goals is to ensure that federal, state, tribal, and local health agencies have the necessary infrastructure to effectively provide essential public health services. A capable and qualified workforce, up-to-date data and information services, and public health agencies capable of assessing and responding to public health needs are three components necessary for an effective public health infrastructure (USDHHS, 2011a). Nurses can play key roles as educators and providers of care in their communities to meet the needs of vulnerable populations and close the health disparity gap.

Sources: U.S. Department of Health and Human Services, Office of Minority Health (USDHHS, OMH, 2012): *HHS action plan to reduce racial and ethnic health disparities*. Retrieved January 5, 2012, from www.minorityhealth.hhs.gov/npa/templates/content.aspx; U.S. Department of Health and Human Services (USDHHS). (2011a). *Healthy People 2020: Leading health indicators*. Retrieved December 23, 2011, from www.healthypeople.gov/2020/LHI/data/.

following the Great Depression. Roosevelt's New Deal had an effect on health care, specifically in the passage of the Social Security Act (SSA) in 1935, which authorized grants-in-aid to individual states to improve state and local public health programs. Funds were available for categorical assistance programs, with cash grants first given to needy blind and older individuals and later to disabled people. Medical care, through subsequent amendments, was an allowable budget item, but payments often were distributed for food, shelter, or other needs. Later, the SSA developed programs such as Medicaid and Medicare.

Split Between Preventive and Curative Measures

The link between environmental health and personal medical care developed when sanitarians (people who work to maintain a clean environment) realized that their efforts alone were not sufficient to prevent and cure the diseases of the population as a whole; improvement of personal health was also necessary. Early preventive services directed toward individuals originated in medical practice rather than public health but were limited to welfare medicine (caring for individuals through state programs). Community health centers that developed in America before World War I limited their scope to prevention and health education and, with the exception of some prenatal clinics, were generally located in poor neighborhoods. Delivery

of preventive services developed separately from clinical medicine and became associated with public health. Most physicians, educated in hospitals, were interested in individuals for whom prevention had failed and whose illnesses brought them to the hospital ward.

Despite the separation of preventive and treatment services, the benefits of prevention eventually were incorporated into clinical medicine for individuals. Preventive and early detection measures became a part of pediatrics and obstetrics during the early part of the twentieth century, when vaccines and vaginal cytology examinations became available and accepted. Later in the twentieth century, internal medicine incorporated early detection of diseases such as diabetes, glaucoma, obesity, and hypertension. A shift to preventive medicine for the individual occurred, but the separate educational programs for public health and medicine still divided these areas. Not until the 1960s did the emphasis begin to turn from individual to societal values (Freyman, 1980).

This new emphasis on societal values parallels another evolution in the role of health in society. Greater governmental involvement in financing the health care delivery system has improved access to health care for many populations. Technological developments include computerized medical records, which should improve access to care through better communication with labs, primary care offices, hospitals, and care delivery agencies. The recent Patient Protection and Affordable Care Act (PPACA) of 2010 reforms certain aspects of the private health insurance industry and public health programs, increases coverage for individuals with pre-existing conditions, and expands access to insurance for a projected 30 million more Americans (OLC, 2010). This sweeping mandate extends a heavy layer of federal and state oversight and will require most Americans to obtain or purchase health insurance through a public or private plan, significantly diminishing the number of individuals who are uninsured.

ORGANIZATION OF THE DELIVERY SYSTEM

The health care delivery system in the United States is a mammoth system composed of a network of public and private interrelated and in some cases overlapping components, designed to provide health care to the American people. The structure and financing of the health care delivery system is a system of multifaceted and complex interrelationship involving providers, consumers, and settings, with both private and public sectors providing services. The public sector includes voluntary and nonprofit agencies, and official or governmental agencies. The United States Department of Health and Human Services (USDHHS) is the principal federal regulatory agency charged with providing health and other essential human services so Americans can live healthier, more prosperous, and more productive lives (USDHHS, 2011b). Delivery of services is organized on three levels in both sectors: local, state, and national. Each of the three levels consists of private providers combined with official or voluntary public agencies. The nurse is often the professional who assists the health consumer to navigate throughout the complex delivery system; therefore, a basic understanding of the system's organization is essential.

Private Sector
Independent Practice
Traditionally, a person enters the health care delivery system by contracting directly with a health care provider for individual care based on fee-for-service. Free choice of provider has been the hallmark of the American free-market system. However, more recently physicians and other health care providers have been working within managed health care organizations. Although private practice traditionally has been disease oriented, the current emphasis on primary care necessitates a much broader perspective. Primary care involves continual and comprehensive care that includes efforts to keep people as healthy as possible and to prevent disease.

Private care may be delivered in numerous settings, from inpatient (hospital or extended care facility) to outpatient (ambulatory) settings. Outpatient care is defined as any health care services that are not provided on the basis of an overnight stay in which room and board costs are incurred. Ambulatory settings include two major categories: care provided by owners and providers or care provided in service settings (Box 3-4). These categories overlap, because many providers practice in their own offices and contract with one or more managed care organizations.

Nursing centers are nurse-managed health centers, often situated in medically underserved rural and urban areas, which primarily serve vulnerable populations in the provision of primary care to individuals and families. Nursing centers trace their origin to the Henry Street Settlement for the sick and poor of New York City, founded by Lillian Wald in 1893 and another visionary, Margaret Sanger, who opened the nation's first birth control clinic. The modern movement to establish nursing centers began in 1965 when the nurse practitioner (NP) role was created, which allowed nurses to provide primary care to individuals and families. Nursing centers (ambulatory care centers, family practice nursing centers, community nursing centers, and birthing centers) have provided high-quality nursing care from certified nurse midwives, nurse practitioners, and other advanced practice nurses (APNs). A number of nursing centers are academic nursing centers, established to provide nursing services to communities, learning experiences for students, and settings for faculty practice and research. The key components of a community nursing center include the following: a nurse as chief manager; a nursing staff that is accountable and responsible for care and professional practice; and nurses as the primary providers of care. Using a multidisciplinary collaboration framework, nurses have the opportunity to provide comprehensive primary care services, including a focus on wellness and health promotion, public health programs, and targeted interventions for populations with special needs. The Institute for Nursing Centers is a network of organizations whose focus is to promote and enhance the work of nursing centers by providing educational programs as well as a national repository of data for nurse-managed health centers funded by the W. K. Kellogg Foundation. Members of the Council for Nursing Centers also provide mentoring and consultation to support colleagues in developing and advancing nursing centers (Institute for Nursing Centers, n.d.). The Affordable Care Act specifically addresses nurse-managed health centers, describing them as a nurse practice arrangement managed by advanced practice nurses who provide primary or wellness services to underserved or vulnerable populations. The new law has provisions to award grants for the operation of nurse-managed health centers that meet requirements (OLC, 2010, p. 542).

Advanced practice nurses (APNs), an umbrella term for nurses who practice in the roles of nurse practitioners, clinical nurse specialists, nurse midwives, or nurse anesthetists, are well suited to provide cost-effective, quality care to individuals and families, as well as serve economically disadvantaged and vulnerable populations. APNs not only have specialized clinical knowledge and skills at the master's or doctoral level but also have pursued an advanced curriculum that includes research and theoretical foundations to determine best practices, evaluate health policy issues, and understand the intricacies of health care financial management. Nurse practitioners play a key role within the health care system and often care for vulnerable populations in rural areas and inner cities, as well as practice in primary, acute, and long-term care settings.

Move to Managed Care

Before the 1990s the traditional means for paying for health care was with indemnity insurance plans. A person would choose a physician or care provider and receive care, and the provider would either bill the individual's insurance company or be paid on a fee-for-service basis. Each separate service generated a professional fee and the provider would receive payments directly from the insurance plan; alternatively, the individual would pay the provider, file an insurance claim for each covered expense, and receive reimbursement. The provider had autonomy to treat the person without oversight from the insurance company. In a traditional fee-for-service insurance system, there are no incentives to constrain cost and care (Barr, 2008). In an effort to control costs, managed care began to regulate the utilization of health care. Physicians contracted with an insurance company for a negotiated fee-for-service, usually at a discounted rate. Today, managed care plans include a network of individual providers, and individuals who choose providers within their network usually have full coverage. Individuals who choose providers outside of the managed care network may be uncovered or covered for a lesser amount, and thus face greater out-of-pocket expenses. Within the network, a person has a primary care provider (PCP), who serves as a gatekeeper and is the foundation of the managed care concept in controlling health care costs within the organization. The primary care provider may be a physician, physician assistant, or an advanced practice nurse. Physician PCPs are usually general or family practitioners, but they may also be internists, pediatricians, or obstetrician-gynecologists. Physician assistants are educated and prepared to work under the direct supervision of physicians. Advance practice nurses who serve as primary care providers are typically nurse practitioners or certified nurse midwives.

In 2002, 95% of workers who carried employer-based health insurance were enrolled in some type of a managed care health plan. The principal force behind the growth of managed care is the belief that health care costs can be controlled by managing the way in which health care is delivered and costs can be controlled because providers of care must be careful to provide only care that is absolutely necessary (Barr, 2008).

As a "gatekeeper," the role of the primary care provider is to coordinate and oversee an individual's care. The gatekeeper concept is designed to manage the individual's use of resources, to reduce self-referral to specialists, and to protect the individual from unnecessary procedures and overtreatment (Shi & Singh, 2005). Decreasing hospital admission rates and costly procedures as well as limiting patient referrals to specialists then achieve successful cost containment of health care. An oversupply of physician specialists has occurred in some areas, and a lack of primary care providers occurs in many rural areas. Specialist salaries typically exceed those of primary care providers, and the number of specialists has increased as technology has developed. Providers of specialty care typically earn higher salaries than primary care providers, making career selection in a specialty area more attractive. Box 3-5 provides a glossary of key terms used in managed care.

Health Maintenance Organizations

Health maintenance organizations (HMOs) deliver comprehensive health maintenance and treatment services to a group of enrolled individuals who prepay a fixed fee. The health maintenance organization accepts responsibility for the organization, financing, and delivery of health care services for all enrolled members. Several HMO models have evolved. The traditional HMO structure was a group or staff model, in which the HMO owns the hospital and employs a group of physicians and some specialty services to provide care to its members. Salaried providers generally spent all of their time serving members of the HMO with no financial incentive to provide more care. An example is Kaiser Permanente Health Care System, which also has its own hospitals. A capitation method of payment is used in which a service provider receives a fixed amount per person (the capitation rate) and in turn agrees to provide all necessary care to each enrolled member. A monthly or annual rate is paid directly to the HMO either by the employer or by the employee. Staff models were described as closed panel, because employed physicians provided care only for members of the HMO. A community physician could not care for a member of the HMO without prearrangement or authorization by the HMO. In an HMO plan, individuals pay low out-of-pocket expenses, but must see a PCP first in order to be referred to a specialist. In a group-model HMO, the organization operates a health plan but contracts with groups of physicians and hospitals to provide care. The medical group receives a share of the capitation rate received by the HMO and the group agrees to provide all necessary physician services for the member. The physician can be paid by salary or fee-for-service. An independent practice association (IPA) HMO will be discussed later. For all types of HMOs, a fixed amount of money is available each year for health care, based on the capitation fee and the number of members enrolled (Barr, 2008). In 2011, 17% of workers were enrolled in an HMO (KFF, 2011c). Medicare enrollees since the 1970s have been offered the option of enrolling in fee-for-service or HMO plans. An earlier health reform law, the Medicare Modernization Act of 2003, renamed the program to include Medicare Advantage Plans. In 2009, 63% of Medicare beneficiaries enrolled in a Medicare Advantage Plan HMO (KFF, 2009).

BOX 3-5   A GLOSSARY OF MANAGED CARE TERMS

Access to health care: The degree to which individuals are inhibited or facilitated in their ability to gain entry to and to receive care and services from the health care system

Benefits: The dollar amount available for the cost of covered medical services

Beneficiary: Any person, either a subscriber or a dependent, eligible for service under a health plan

Blue Cross/Blue Shield: A combined medical plan offered through a worker's place of employment that combines both hospital and physician coverage

Capitation: A fixed amount of payment per patient, per year, regardless of the volume or cost of services each client requires

Copayments: A fixed dollar payment that is made by the patient to the provider at the time of service

Cost sharing: Provision of an insurance policy that requires the insured to pay some portion of the covered expenses (does not refer to or include cost of the premium)

Deductible: A fixed dollar amount that the patient must pay before reimbursement begins

Gatekeeper: A physician or APN who provides primary care and who makes referrals for emergency services or specialty care

Health care policy: Decisions, usually developed by government policymakers, for determining present and future objectives pertaining to the health care system

Health maintenance organization (HMO): A prepaid health plan delivering comprehensive care to members through designated providers, having a fixed monthly payment for health care services, and requiring members to be in a plan for a specified period of time

Indemnity: Monies paid by an insurer to a provider, in a predetermined amount in the event of a covered loss by a beneficiary

Independent practice association (IPA): An organization that physicians in private practice can join so that the organization can represent them in the negotiation of managed care contracts

Managed care: A health care plan that integrates the financing and delivery of health care services by using arrangements with selected health care providers to provide services for covered individuals. Plans are generally financed by capitation fees. There are significant financial incentives for members of the plan to use the health care providers associated with the plan.

Out-of-pocket expenditures: The portion of medical expenses a patient is responsible for paying

Point-of-service plan (POS): A plan that contains elements of both HMOs and PPOs. They resemble HMOs for in-network services in that they both require copayments and a primary care physician. Services received outside of the network are usually reimbursed on a fee-for-service basis

Preferred provider organization (PPO): A health plan generally consisting of hospital and physician providers. The PPO provides health care services to plan members usually at discounted rates in return for expedited claims payment

Primary care: Basic health care that emphasizes general health needs rather than specialized care

Primary care provider (PCP): A physician or APN who provides basic and routine health care services usually in an office or clinic

Reimbursement: Payment of services. Payment of providers by a third-party insurer or government health program for health care services

Self-insured plan: Plan offered by employers and other groups who directly assume the major cost of health insurance for their employees or members

Third-party payer: In health care finance, this is an insurance carrier, Medicare, and Medicaid or their government-contracted intermediary, managed-care organization, or health plan that pays for hospital or medical bills instead of the patient

Underinsured: Refers to people who have some type of health insurance, such as catastrophic care, but not enough insurance to cover all their health care costs

Uninsured: Individuals or groups with no or inadequate health insurance coverage

Utilization review: Evaluation of the necessity, appropriateness, and efficiency of the use of health care services, procedures, and facilities

From United States National Library of Medicine, National Institutes of Health: *Health economics information resources: A self-study course.* Retrieved January 20, 2012, from www.nlm.nih.gov/nichsr/edu/healthecon/glossary.html.

Medicare Advantage Plans

Medicare Advantage plans are private health plans that receive payments from Medicare for each enrollee. In 2011, 10.9 million Medicare individuals were enrolled in 1 of almost 540 plans offered. Enrollees in a Medicare Advantage plan tend to be in better health than the traditional Medicare enrollee and a number of Medicare Advantage plans fall under the category of HMOs. Because of the funding formula, those in Medicare Advantage plans often have extra benefits (vision and hearing, wellness plans) when compared to the traditional Medicare population (KFF, 2009) (Box 3-6: Hot Topics).

Independent Practice Associations

Independent practice associations (IPAs) are organizations composed of independent physicians in solo or group practices who provide health care services to members of an HMO in their private offices, eliminating the expense of the staff model HMO, which furnished and owned the facility in which care was provided. The HMO for a fee-for-service or prepaid price can purchase hospital care and specialty services not within the IPA group. Physicians in an IPA contract may be restricted to caring only for members enrolled in the IPA, but some

contracts may allow providers to care for nonmembers as well. Other variations of the staff model and IPAs exist. In a group practice model, an HMO contracts with all physicians and specialists needed by the HMO enrollees, but physicians remain independent. Some contracts are exclusive, requiring physicians to restrict care to members of an individual HMO, and other variations allow physicians to care for members outside the HMO. In a network model, HMOs contract with individual physicians and with physician groups for both primary and specialty services. The HMO maintains control over fee arrangements (Barr, 2008).

Accountable Care Organizations

Accountable care organizations (ACOs) will be a key component in the new Affordable Care Act reform law. Accountable care organizations in structure will be similar to traditional HMOs that are responsible for the quality and cost of care delivered to a defined population. An organization, either public or private, would be created that has a group of primary care physicians, providers, specialists, and hospitalists, to provide health care in a local area. Physicians would accept the responsibility for the quality of care provided and overall costs of delivering

BOX 3-6   HOT TOPICS

Medicare Advantage Plans

Derived from survey data on 53 performance measures, for a number of years the Centers for Medicare & Medicaid Services (CMS) have been rating contracts (individual Medicare Advantage plans are grouped together into contracts) with a 1 to 5 star system, with 5 stars indicating the highest level of service, 3 stars designating average performance, and 1 star signifying poor performance. The quality performance measures include keeping enrollees healthy (screenings, tests, vaccines), managing chronic long-term conditions, monitoring drug plan customer service and pricing, rating health plan responsiveness, and registering plan member complaints. Every Medicare Advantage plan covered under the same contract receives the same quality star rating. In 2012 provisions of the 2010 Affordable Care Act reform will reward Medicare Advantage plans with bonus payments based on the contract's quality star rating. Determined by geographic benchmark considerations, the amount one contract receives may be different than that received by another contract with the same star rating. Originally, the 2010 law specified a plan must achieve a star rating of 4 or more to receive a bonus payment. In 2011 not-for-profit plans achieved significantly higher quality ratings (4.09 stars) but served only 29% of Medicare Advantage enrollment while for-profit plans on average achieved only 3.22 stars yet served 71% of enrollees. To provide incentive for 3 star rated plans to improve performance, in 2012 the CMS launched a 3-year demonstration that increases the size of bonuses to highly rated plans and also provides scaled bonuses for plans that rated average. Since 59% of Medicare Advantage enrollees are in plans rated 3 to 3.5, the financial incentive is high to improve a contract's star rating. High performance plans have incentives to continue providing quality care and maintain their high star rating, and average performance plans now have incentives to rapidly improve annual performance measures. Of the 9% of contracts that are rated less than 3 stars or not yet rated, the bonus initiative to achieve a higher star rating may spur quality improvement measures to then be eligible for a bonus. The 3-year CMS demonstration initiative is expected to improve quality in all of the performance measures and thereby result in overall improvements in Medicare Advantage plans. The $3.1 billion budget in 2012 is projected to equate to a bonus payment of approximately $347 per enrollee in a not-for-profit plan versus $255 per enrollee in for-profit plans, a difference of $92 per enrollee. Kaiser Permanente has the highest average rating (4.54 stars) and is projected to receive more than $400 per enrollee in 2012, in contrast to Humana with a 3.08 rating, which is projected to receive more than $200 per enrollee. Overall, both companies will receive the same amount in total monies because Humana has about 730,000 more enrollees than Kaiser Permanente in 2011. The plans receiving bonus payments are required to use the monies to provide extra benefits to enrollees (such as eyeglasses, hearing aids, transportation to appointments, wellness plans), thus encouraging more attractive benefit packages. The overall Medicare cost per enrollee is higher if an individual is enrolled in a Medicare Advantage plan, which fuels further debate. Several other arguments have come into play regarding Medicare Advantage plans. First, some argue that plans with the same star rating should receive equal bonus monies regardless of geographic location. In some areas, there is a large difference between the bonus money awarded between contracts with the same rating and the HMOs are geographically located fairly close together. The second stronger argument is that under this bonus system, two thirds of bonus payments will be provided to 271 contracts rated at 3 or 3.5 stars in 2011, rewarding companies with only average quality large sums of bonus monies. Studies suggest few older adults are aware of the star rating system or use a plan's quality rating in selecting a plan (KFF, 2009; 2011b). Those individuals with high health literacy skills and familiarity with insurance plan options may select higher quality plans, whereas others may choose to enroll in low-quality plans because of lack of understanding of quality indicators, perpetuating health disparities among vulnerable populations.

care to a defined population of patients (Kovner & Knickman, 2011). In the new law, ACOs will become an important part of Medicare reform. An ACO that serves a person in the Medicare system will be required to be composed of physicians, specialists, and hospitals that manage the health needs of a minimum of 5000 Medicare beneficiaries for a minimum of 3 years. In October of 2011, proposed rules were released describing the manner in which ACOs were to be established. Accountable care organizations will have financial incentives in place to encourage providers to keep health care costs low by not ordering unnecessary tests and procedures, and by focusing on prevention and management of patients with chronic disease out of the hospital. Performance and savings benchmarks would be in place with a financial reward system as well as penalties. An ACO would function much like an HMO of the 1990s, but individuals would be free to see physicians of their choice outside the network without paying more (Kovner & Knickman, 2011; USDHHS, 2011c). Current HMOs, such as Kaiser Permanente, already fit the definition and have the structure required to be called an accountable care organization (Kovner & Knickman, 2011).

Concierge Medical Practices

According to a U.S. Government Accountability Office (GAO) report to Congressional Committees, concierge care is a newer model for providing primary care in a medical practice in which physicians charge individuals a membership fee averaging $1500 to $1900 per year (range reported as $60 to $15,000 per year) in return for enhanced health care services or amenities. Only a small number of physicians have established concierge care practices. Amenities most often include same-day or next-day appointments for nonurgent care, 24-hour telephone access to the physician, and routine periodic preventive examinations. Some concierge physicians do not accept insurance but 75% report billing a person's health insurance for covered services and Medicare. Individuals are encouraged to carry health care insurance for services utilized outside of the practice. Although there is wide variation in the amenities offered, no–waiting time office visits, access to physicians via cell phones and e-mail, and the option of house calls may be provided and serve as attractive incentives for individuals. Physicians who provide concierge care typically care for fewer persons (800 compared to an average load of 4000), allowing physicians more time to spend with each person and to provide expanded preventive services and practice amenities that are not available in a traditional practice. Concierge physicians benefit as well, with more time for their own families, research, and professional activities as well as an enhanced income from membership fees (GAO, 2005).

The concept of concierge medical care originated in Seattle, Washington, by an athletic team physician who realized that the level of service provided to athletes was remarkable and could be expanded to nonathletes. Physicians in this practice provide comprehensive primary care to no more than 100 persons per physician and currently charge annual membership (or retainer) fees of $13,000 per individual. This group does not bill any form of health insurance (GAO, 2005; Marquis, 2004). Described as boutique, platinum, premier, or Ritz-Carlton medical care, this level of health care caters to those who are affluent enough to pay the annual membership fees. The number of concierge medical care practices is growing, but there are those who oppose a form of care that favors the rich (country club elitism) and does not serve the needs of the poor or vulnerable populations (GAO, 2005; Marquis, 2004).

Hospitalist Movement

Responding to the same impetus that spurred managed care in outpatient settings, hospitalist programs—supported by HMOs, hospitals, and medical groups—were formed to control hospital costs without compromising quality or satisfaction with client care. Hospitalists are physicians or advanced practice nurses whose professional focus is caring for the hospitalized client. They provide direct inpatient primary, critical, and consultative care to hospitalized clients and are available 24 hours in hospitals with programs. Hospitalists engage in clinical care, teaching, research, and leadership in the field of hospital medicine. Study findings have found that hospitals with a hospitalist model program have improved both quality and safety of care with reduced lengths of stay, cost per case, readmission rates, mortality rates, and complication rates. Hospitalist practices have increased hospital efficiency and improved customer satisfaction rates (Jeter, 2007; Kuo & Goodwin, 2011). As the hospitalized persons' needs become more complex, the number of physicians and APNs functioning in a hospitalist role has grown. Another important role of the hospitalist is safe transitioning of the individual from the acute care hospital setting to post–acute-care facilities or home (Society of Hospital Medicine, n.d.).

Point-of-Service Plans

Point-of-service (POS) plans evolved in response to concern with restrictions of consumer choice in selecting providers and services. Point-of-service plans allow members, for an additional fee and higher copayment, to use providers outside of the individual HMO network. Members can choose to pay for this enhanced POS or stay within the HMO network for reduced copayments. If the individual receives care from a physician or hospital not within the list of providers or hospitals, the person pays a substantial portion of the cost of care (30% to 40% more), usually as out-of-pocket expenses (Barr, 2008). In 2011, 55% of all covered workers in employer plans were enrolled in a PPO, making PPOs the most common plan type (KFF, 2011c).

High-Deductible Health Insurance Plans

High-deductible health insurance plans (HDHPs) are structured similar to traditional managed care plans and fee-for-service plans, but have a very high annual out-of-pocket deductible of $1000 to $2000 for individual coverage. A growing number of employers are offering these types of plans, and for those individuals who are generally healthy, the low monthly premium is an attractive option compared to the cost of other types of

employer insurance plans. Plans usually have a set annual out-of-pocket limit. Attached to these plans, an employer can offer health savings accounts (HSAs) or savings options (SOs). Typically an employer will make quarterly or annual deposits into the individuals' health savings account, and the employee can elect to have additional funds withheld on a pre-tax basis to deposit into the account, up to the annual Internal Revenue Service (IRS) maximum. Individuals can withdraw money from the account at any age for health-related expenditures. The remaining money in the fund can be withdrawn at retirement without penalty. Most HDHPs are paired with in-network providers for additional savings. Some plans allow preventive services (e.g., adult physical examinations, cancer screenings, mammograms, routine gynecological visits, and well-child care) for no charge if an in-network provider is used. Office visits for sickness, laboratory tests, emergency and urgent care, and hospitalizations are covered all or in part after the deductible is met. Because out-of-pocket expenses are significant, up until the deductible is met, individuals may decide to delay or not seek health care if the deductible has not been met. Seventeen percent of workers were enrolled in HDHP plans with savings options (HDHP/SOs) in 2011, up from 13% of covered workers in 2010 (KFF, 2011c).

Preferred Provider Organizations

Preferred provider organizations (PPOs) are a type of managed care plan in the private sector that has a preselected list of providers who have agreed to provide health services for those individuals enrolled in the plan. Contracted providers in the PPO agree to deliver services to members for a fee-for-service prenegotiated rate, which is usually discounted. To control costs, members must receive care exclusively from providers within the PPO or incur additional costs if a provider is used outside of the PPO. Individuals are typically required to pay a small copay each time services are given. If an individual chooses to see a provider outside of the network, he or she will pay additional costs. To control costs, the provider must receive preauthorization from the PPO for a member to be hospitalized, and second opinions are required before major procedures or surgeries are performed. The more willing a person is to receive care from a limited choice of physicians (those within the contract), the less the person pays (Barr, 2008).

The Kaiser Family Foundation conducts an annual survey that reveals the distribution of the health plan type for individuals enrolled in employer health plans. Some employers, often those that are large, offer a variety of health plans to their employees. Distribution of health plan enrollment for covered workers (see Figure 3-2) reveals that slightly more than 50% of workers have been enrolled in employer PPO plans since 2002 (55% in 2011), with diminishing numbers of employees enrolled in HMOs (17% in 2011) and POSs (10% in 2011) and a growing segment of workers enrolled in HDHPs (17% in 2011).

Public Sector

The public sector contains official and voluntary public health agencies operating at the local, state, federal, and international levels. Before 1900, public health was concerned with problems related to environmental risks and infectious diseases. After the

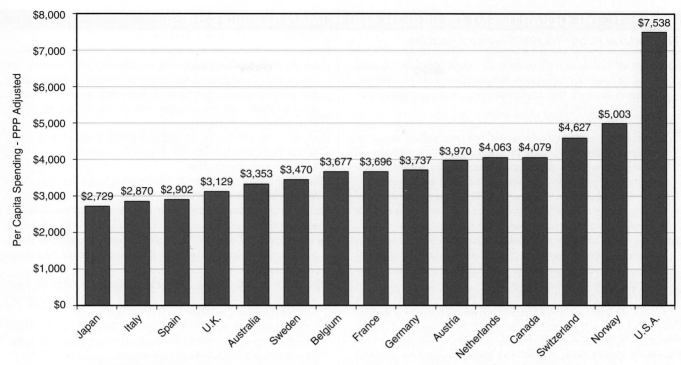

FIGURE 3-2 Total health expenditure per capita, United States and selected countries, 2008. (Source: Organisation for Economic Co-operation and Development. [2010]. *OECD health data.* OECD Health Statistics [database]. Accessed February 14, 2011, from doi:10.1787/data-00350-en.)

1900s the public health agenda expanded to address the needs of children and mothers. By midcentury, treating chronic disease had also been added to its agenda. As the century progressed, public health issues came to include substance abuse, mental illness, teen pregnancy, long-term care, epidemics of violence and/or human immunodeficiency virus/acquired immunodeficiency syndrome (HIV/AIDS), and most recently bioterrorism and disaster preparedness (Nies & McEwen, 2007).

Source of Power

The U.S. Constitution is based on the sharing of sovereign power between federal and state governments. The powers of the federal government in relation to health are not delineated specifically in the Constitution; they are derived from its authority to tax and to spend for the general welfare and from powers delegated to it by the states. The state governor or legislature usually appoints a health commissioner or secretary of health, who directs the health agency (usually the public health department) to protect citizens from communicable diseases and environmental hazards from waste, water, and food (Nies & McEwen, 2007). State health authority is based also on the Tenth Amendment, which reserves for the states, or for the people, those powers not delegated to the federal government by the Constitution. The states then use their powers to create local governments and delegate authority to them in health matters. The United States Public Health Service falls within the larger Department of Health and Human Services and Box 3-7 lists various departments and functions of the federal Public Health Service agencies that fall under the Department of Health and Human Services.

Influence of Political Philosophy

The prevailing political philosophy regarding societal health needs affects the relationship among federal, state, and local governments. Although the federal government gained power to promote health and welfare in the early twentieth century by the passage of the Sixteenth Amendment (giving it the authority to levy federal taxes), states retained sovereign power because the resources were distributed at the state and local levels. Beginning in the 1930s, however, New Deal philosophy began to displace power from the state and local governments to the federal government. Passage of the Hill-Burton Act of 1946 and establishment of what is now known as the CDC increased the federal government's power over state and local affairs. The trend toward increased federal government involvement continued during the Kennedy-Johnson era, when the government focused on societal needs and health care to an unprecedented degree. During the Nixon-Ford era, the trend began to reverse as a New Federalism movement called for less federal encroachment into states' responsibilities and greater state and local responsibility. Clearly, the federal government's role varies according to political philosophy.

During the 1980s the Reagan administration supported free-market competition among insurance plans, physicians, and hospitals to offer the best possible services with the lowest price. Reagan was adamant in his opposition to adopting national health insurance legislation for what he labeled "socialized medicine." Reagan's procompetition policies supported a decrease in federal responsibility for health care, preferring to give states power by providing block grants and control at the state level.

BOX 3-7   THE DEPARTMENT OF HEALTH AND HUMAN SERVICES (HHS)

The Federal Public Health Service Agencies

Administration for Children and Families (ACF): Federal agency funding state, territory, local, and tribal organizations to provide family assistance (welfare), child support, child care, Head Start, child welfare, and other programs relating to children and families

Administration on Aging (AoA): Federal agency responsible for the concerns and interests of older people and their caregivers. AoA works with and through the Aging Services Network to promote the development of a comprehensive and coordinated system of home- and community-based long-term care that is responsive to the needs and preferences of older people and their family caregivers

Agency for Healthcare Research and Quality (AHRQ): Federal agency whose mission is to improve the quality, safety, efficiency, and effectiveness of health care for all Americans. Supports research with grants and funding

Agency for Toxic Substances and Disease Registry (ATSDR): Federal agency that serves the public by using best science, taking responsive public health actions, and providing trusted health information to prevent harmful exposures and disease-related toxic substances

Centers for Disease Control and Prevention (CDC): Working with states, provides a system of health surveillance to monitor and prevent outbreaks of disease

Centers for Medicare & Medicaid Services (CMS): Federal agency that runs the Medicare program and works with states to run the Medicaid program

Food and Drug Administration (FDA): Federal agency responsible for protecting the public, which includes ensuring foods are safe, wholesome, sanitary, and properly labeled; guaranteeing human and veterinary drugs, vaccines, and other biological products and medical devices intended for human use are safe and effective; protecting the public from electronic product radiation; ensuring cosmetics and dietary supplements are safe and properly labeled; and regulating tobacco products

Health Resources and Services Administration (HRSA): Primary federal agency for improving access to health care services for people who are uninsured, isolated, or medically vulnerable

Indian Health Service (IHS): Responsible for providing federal health services to American Indians and Alaska Natives

National Cancer Institute (NCI): Part of NIH, principle agency for cancer research and training

National Institutes of Health (NIH): Provides leadership and direction to programs designed to improve the health of the nation by conducting and supporting research

Office of the Inspector General (OIG): Office dedicated to combating fraud, waste, and abuse and to improving the efficiency of HHS programs. Provides oversight of Medicaid and Medicare, CDC, NIH, and the FDA

Substance Abuse and Mental Health Services Administration (SAMHSA): Strengthens the nation's health care capacity to provide prevention, diagnosis, and treatment services for substance abuse and mental illness

From U.S. Department of Health and Human Services. Retrieved January 22, 2012, from www.hhs.gov/open/contracts/index.

During the Bush administration (1989 to 1993), incremental steps occurred in moving new legislation toward health care reform with a system of checks and balances in place so that no single political party controlled the White House, Senate, and House of Representatives. To avoid increasing taxes, President Bush proposed a system of tax deductions or tax credits to reduce the cost of private health insurance for families not covered by Medicaid or Medicare. Bush proposed the creation of large networks of small businesses to purchase group health insurance for their employees, voluntary measures to reduce insurance paperwork, encouragement of enrollment in HMOs, and legislation to reduce medical malpractice suits. Because of an economic recession, many workers employed by small businesses did not have employer health insurance plans and these measures would have assisted in covering working families. However, Congressional Democrats refused to support the proposed reform because it did not include an expansion of federal power with a plan for universal coverage or control over the growing cost of insurance premiums.

In 1993 the Clinton administration proposed the Health Security Act to achieve universal health care coverage in the United States by mandating that all employers provide health insurance to their employees and by giving small businesses and unemployed Americans subsidies with which to purchase insurance. The plan met severe opposition from the insurance industry and the business community. Mass media advertisements by these stakeholders questioned whether HMOs would provide choice and access to health care services. Large segments of the American public, especially the 80% who had employer-based private health insurance, began to fear being forced into HMOs, which would diminish their choice of, access to, and quality of health care. The cost of a socialized, universal health care coverage system was estimated to reach trillion-dollar levels. The act was defeated in Congress and a time of political caution followed, stalling any further movement toward universal health care. Small incremental health reform was passed such as the portability of health care coverage in 1996 (Health Insurance Portability and Accountability Act [HIPAA]), allowing persons to access health care throughout the United States, and the focus shifted to balancing the federal budget. Other incremental legislation included the passage of the Balanced Budget Act (BBA) of 1997, which made significant reforms in Medicare, as well as the formation of a new public insurance program—the State Children's Health Insurance Program (SCHIP). SCHIP is a public state insurance program supported by federal monies to provide insurance to low-income children 18 years or younger, including those who are homeless. Each state operates their own SCHIP and some states have renamed the program; for example, Georgia's program is called Peachcare and New Mexico named their program Mexikids. The federal funding of SCHIP, however, requires the program to be renewed every few years.

One group at risk for being uninsured is immigrant children. Immigrant children who have been in the country for 5 years legally and are classified low-income usually meet eligibility requirements, which vary by state for SCHIP. For this group of children, parents must supply immigrant status information and, in some states, the child's Social Security number to meet eligibility requirements (Centers for Medicare & Medicaid Services [CMS], n.d.). To facilitate the enrollment of low-income children into SCHIP, some states (44 in all) used technology

BOX 3-8 RESEARCH FOR EVIDENCE-BASED PRACTICE

Connecting Eligible Immigrant Families to Health Coverage and Care: Key Lessons from Outreach and Enrollment Workers, October 2011

The 2014 provisions of the Affordable Care Act will significantly expand insurance coverage for low- and moderate-income families through an expansion in Medicaid eligibility and by making tax credits available to help individuals and families purchase insurance coverage through new Health Care Exchanges. As of 2010, 38 million immigrants reside in the United States, which is 12.5% of the population. Seventeen million are naturalized citizens and 21 million are noncitizens. Noncitizens include both lawfully present and undocumented individuals. There are many more individuals who live in families with mixed immigration status, such as a U.S.-born child with one or both parents' noncitizens. As of 2009, it was estimated 5.6 million children were living with at least one noncitizen parent. The majority of natural citizens have employer or private insurance coverage whereas noncitizens are nearly three times as likely to be uninsured compared to U.S. citizens. Since 1996, lawfully residing noncitizens are not eligible to enroll in Medicaid and SCHIP during the first 5 years of legally residing in the United States. Some states eliminated or reduced the 5-year requirement to care for pregnant women and children. Undocumented immigrants are individuals who are not in the United States legally and are prohibited from enrolling in Medicaid or purchasing coverage through Health Exchanges. Individuals who enter any country illegally are typically not entitled to receive health care or other benefits provided to their citizens and legal residents.

In 2014, when the ACA provision takes effect to expand coverage to individuals with incomes up to 133% of the federal poverty level ($14,484 for an individual or $24,645 for a family of 3 in 2011), many more individuals will be eligible for Medicaid and individuals with incomes of up to 400% of the federal poverty level ($43,560 for individuals or $74,120 for a family of 3 in 2011) will be able to buy coverage through new Health Benefit Exchanges using tax credits to help pay for the coverage. Lawfully residing immigrant families are expected to significantly benefit from the coverage expansion. In order to realize the benefit of the health reform law, enrolling immigrant families will be key and targeted outreach efforts will need to be employed. Immigrant families face numerous challenges in accessing needed care because of limited transportation options and language barriers. Immigrant families may also experience fear and confusion in navigating the health care system and being cared for by a primary care provider who may not have the capacity to provide culturally and linguistically appropriate services.

Methodology

To gain increased insight into barriers to coverage and care facing eligible immigrants, and to develop successful strategies to overcome these barriers, Health Outreach Partners and the Kaiser Commission on Medicaid and the Uninsured hosted focus group discussions with outreach and enrollment professionals who serve immigrant communities. Thirty-five professionals participated in one of four focus groups—with one group held in Florida; one focus group held in Washington, DC; and two focus groups held in California. Using a structured interview guide, participants were asked questions concerning barriers to coverage, strategies they employ to overcome these barriers, and perceptions of the potential impact of the coverage expansion on immigrant communities. Participants gave consent to have interviews recorded and transcribed. Data were analyzed using qualitative software and supplemented with relevant research and data from a recent farmworker health outreach national needs' assessment report. Participants were individuals who provide outreach and enrollment assistance in immigrant communities.

Successful strategies to overcome barriers to coverage and care were revealed, which included:

- Utilizing trusted community organizations and individuals to provide outreach and enrollment assistance
- Providing direct one-on-one assistance from individuals with a shared background or experience
- Educating families about coverage options and the enrollment process
- Providing families with a list of required documents and identifying alternative options
- Offering both English and Spanish forms to document income
- Providing cards that families can present to request translation assistance
- Maintaining contact over time to assist families with renewal

Recommendations and Conclusions

Addressing barriers that immigrant families face will require significant changes in processes and systems as well as a cultural shift among local eligibility offices that is focused on promoting coverage. Findings support the need both to provide outreach and enrollment assistance that meets the needs of immigrant families and to offer strengthening messages to dispel fears among the immigrant community.

From Kaiser Family Foundation. (2011d). *Connecting eligible immigrant families to health coverage and care: Key lessons from outreach and enrollment workers.* Menlo Park, CA: The Henry J. Kaiser Family Foundation. Retrieved January 22, 2012, from www.kff.org. Publication #8249. October 27, 2011.

to modernize eligibility and enrollment processes, by matching electronic data with information from the Social Security Administration to more efficiently and accurately verify citizenship for children. States also made improvements in streamlining the renewal process to increase the retention of eligible children and eliminate gaps in coverage when eligibility income requirements changed (KFF, 2012b). Another major expansion in the role of the federal government occurred in 2003, when Congress passed the Medicare Prescription Drug Act Part D, and in 2007 when legislation was signed to continue funding SCHIP programs. The biggest expansion of federal oversight since Medicare and Medicaid from the 1960s came when the PPACA was signed into law in March of 2010 (Box 3-8: Research for Evidence-Based Practice).

Current Health Policy

On March 23, 2010, President Obama signed into law the Patient Protection and Affordable Care Act (PPACA) of 2010. The goals of the massive health care reform act were to dramatically reduce the number of uninsured Americans; pay for coverage without adding to the national debt; slow the rising cost of health care; and encourage a more efficient health care system (Kovner & Knickman, 2011). When first elected into office, President Obama pushed for health care reform and gained the support from a strong Democratic majority in both the House of Representatives and the Senate. Before becoming law, bitter debates between Democratic and Republican members of the House and Senate occurred. Democratic control of the Senate and House of Representatives allowed the bills to be

BOX 3-9   SECTIONS OF THE AFFORDABLE CARE ACT

TITLE I
Quality, Affordable Health Care for All Americans
TITLE II
The Role of Public Programs
TITLE III
Improving the Quality and Efficiency of Health Care
TITLE IV
Prevention of Chronic Disease and Improving Public Health
TITLE V
Health Care Workforce
TITLE VI
Transparency and Program Integrity
TITLE VII
Improving Access to Innovative Medical Therapies
TITLE VIII
Community Living Assistance Services and Supports Act (CLASS Act)
TITLE IX
Revenue Provisions
TITLE X
Reauthorization of the Indian Health Care Improvement Act

quickly voted out of committee and introduced to the floors. In December of 2009, the Senate bill passed with the partisan support of all Democrats. No Republican Senators voted in favor of the bill. In March of 2010 the bill came to a vote in the House of Representatives. This time there was bipartisan support against the bill with 178 Republicans and 34 Democrats voting against it. The bill passed by 7 votes (219 vs. 212), and 2 days later the health reform act of 2010 was signed into law and an amended version was passed in May 2010 (OLC, 2010). The 974-page document is long and complex with many provisions and a timeline for incremental sections to be enacted with the majority of the provisions taking place by 2014 (see http://healthreform.kff.org/timeline.aspx for a timeline of detailed provisions by year).

The major provisions of the law are focused on expanding health insurance coverage for the current millions of Americans who are uninsured. See Box 3-9 for a section-by-section title list of the Affordable Care Act.

Future Health Policy

Historically there has been a lack of consensus among the major political parties and stakeholders regarding health care reform. Since the Affordable Care Act became law in March of 2010, a number of states, individuals, and other organizations have filed actions in state and federal courts challenging the constitutionality of the law. The federal Supreme Court determined the constitutionality of the various provisions of this law in March 2012. Since the implementation of the law will occur over time (from 2010 to 2018), later provisions may also be met with legal opposition at the state and federal levels, which may result in amendments to the provisions. The timeline for full implementation of the many provisions will also span over two Presidential terms.

If the political landscape should change and Democrats lose control, certain provisions of the ACA could also be repealed or amended. The new health care reform law enables massive regulation by the executive branch of the federal government and requires state governments to assist with implementation of the many provisions of the law. Substantial efforts will be needed to constrain and reduce the cost of health care.

Nursing's Role in Leading Change—2010 Recommendations of the IOM

Report on the Future of Nursing. The Robert Wood Johnson Foundation (RWJF) and the Institute of Medicine (IOM) in 2008 launched a 2-year initiative to respond to the need to assess and transform the nursing profession. The IOM appointed the committee on the RWJF *Initiative on the Future of Nursing* and charged the committee with producing a report that would make recommendations for an action-oriented blueprint for nursings' future. The nursing workforce, composed of more than 3 million nurses, is the largest segment of the nation's health care workforce. The IOM recognized that nurses can play a key role in helping realize the objectives set forth in the 2010 Affordable Care Act but a number of barriers exist that prevent nurses from being able to respond effectively to rapidly changing health care settings and an evolving health care system. The committee developed the following four key messages and seven recommendations (IOM, 2010):

- Nurses should practice to the full extent of their education and training.
- Nurses should achieve higher levels of education and training through an improved education system that promotes seamless academic progression.
- Nurses should be full partners, with physicians and other health care professionals, in redesigning health care in the United States.
- Effective workforce planning and policy making require better data collection and an improved information infrastructure.

For IOM's report on the future of nursing recommendations, see Box 3-10: Innovative Practice.

Official Agencies

Official agencies are tax supported and therefore accountable to the citizens through elected or appointed officials or boards. The purpose and duties of official agencies are prescribed or mandated by law. This discussion is from the perspective of the individual gaining knowledge of or access to the health care system.

Local Level. The health department of a town, city, county, township, or district is the local health unit and is usually the first line of access and health responsibility for the population that it serves. The mayor, the board of health, or some other executive governing body appoints the chief administrator, the health officer. The local health department's role and functions usually center on providing direct services to the public and depend on the state mandate and community resources. Local governments, but usually not health departments, have the responsibility to provide general health care services for the poor.

✳ BOX 3-10   INNOVATIVE PRACTICE

IOM's October 5, 2010, Report on the Future of Nursing Recommendations

Recommendation 1: Remove scope-of-practice barriers. Advanced practice registered nurses should be able to practice to the full extent of their education and training.

Recommendation 2: Expand opportunities for nurses to lead and diffuse collaborative improvement efforts. Private and public funders, health care organizations, nursing education programs, and nursing associations should expand opportunities for nurses to lead and manage collaborative efforts with physicians and other members of the health care team to conduct research and to redesign and improve practice environments and health systems. These entities should also provide opportunities for nurses to diffuse successful practices.

Recommendation 3: Implement nurse residency programs. State boards of nursing, accrediting bodies, the federal government, and health care organizations should take actions to support nurses' completion of a transition-to-practice program (nurse residency) after they have completed a prelicensure

or advanced practice degree program or when they are transitioning into new clinical practice areas.

Recommendation 4: Increase the proportion of nurses with a baccalaureate degree to 80% by 2020. Academic nurse leaders across all schools of nursing should work together to increase the proportion of nurses with a baccalaureate degree from 50% to 80% by 2020. These leaders should partner with education accrediting bodies, private and public funders, and employers to ensure funding, monitor progress, and increase the diversity of students to create a workforce prepared to meet the demands of diverse populations across the life span.

Recommendation 5: Double the number of nurses with a doctorate by 2020.

Recommendation 6: Ensure that nurses engage in lifelong learning.

Recommendation 7: Prepare and enable nurses to lead change to advance health.

Recommendation 8: Build an infrastructure for the collection and analysis of interprofessional health care workforce data.

Data from the Institute of Medicine of the National Academies. The Future of Nursing: Leading Change, Advancing Health Report Recommendations. Retrieved January 10, 2011, from www.iom.edu/Reports/2010/The-Future-of-Nursing-Leading-Change-Advancing-Health.aspx.

State Level. Public health services are organized by each state, with wide variation from one state to another. The chief administrator is usually a state health officer or commissioner appointed by the governor. One agency, typically the state health department, carries out the primary responsibilities in policy, planning, and coordination of programs and services for local units under its jurisdiction.

Federal Level. The federal government assumes overall responsibility for the health protection of its citizens. Although all three branches of the government make health-related decisions, the major policy decisions are made by the president and his staff (executive branch) and by Congress (legislative branch). These two branches determine health policy. Once policy is determined, other government agencies are responsible for oversight to ensure implementation.

The United States Department of Health and Human Services (USDHHS), the main federal body concerned with the health of the nation, consists of a number of separate operating agencies (see Box 3-7). Under each of the federal public health service agencies listed are numerous other departments. USDHHS agencies that relate directly to nursing include the Health Resources and Services (HRSA) and the National Institutes of Health (NIH). The Bureau of Health Professions, within the Health Resources and Services Administration, contains a division of nursing, which is a source for nursing education and training grants. The National Institute of Nursing Research within the NIH funds nursing research, including health promotion and illness prevention studies.

Chief Nursing Officer. The Chief Nursing Officer (CNO) serves in the U.S. Public Health Service (USPHS) and is responsible for providing leadership and coordination of the Public Health Service (PHS) nursing professional affairs for the Office of the Surgeon General and the Department of Health and Human Services (HHS). The CNO provides guidance and advice to the Surgeon General, the Nurse Professional Advisory Committee (N-PAC), and the nation's

nursing community on matters such as prevention, primary care, health systems development, recruitment, readiness, and career development of PHS nurses. As director of the Office of Global Health Affairs, the CNO develops strategies to maximize HRSA's participation in efforts to improve health care for vulnerable populations worldwide and coordinates and advances international health policy and resource development with HRSA. The Chief Nursing Officer also serves as a consultant to the HHS Office of the Secretary's Global Health Affairs and other HHS agencies, the World Health Organization, and other international groups on a variety of health and nursing issues. The current CNO, Rear Admiral (RADM) Kerry Paige Nesseler, was appointed in November of 2009. RADM Nesseler is an advanced practice nurse who once practiced with the Indian Health Service on a reservation in Cloquet, Minnesota, as a maternal child health nurse specialist (U.S. Public Health Nursing Services, n.d.).

Federal Emergency Management Agency (FEMA). The United States Department of Homeland Security is another large branch of federal agencies with numerous offices, many of which have a connection with health care. The Federal Emergency Management Agency (FEMA) now is part of (since 2003) the U.S. Department of Homeland Security (U.S. Department of Homeland Security, 2011). FEMA was established in 1979 by an executive order merging many separate disaster-related services into a single entity to assist states when a disaster overwhelms a state's capacity to respond. A disaster, as defined by FEMA, includes a hurricane, earthquake, tornado, flood, fire, hazardous spill, act of nature, or act of terrorism. The role of FEMA is to support citizens and first responders to build, sustain, and improve capacity to prepare for, protect against, respond to, recover from, and mitigate all hazards. Assistance is provided to individuals, communities, and states that are determined to be eligible. There are 10 regional FEMA offices located throughout the country with headquarters in Washington, DC. In 2006 the Post-Katrina Emergency Management Reform Act created a "new FEMA" with an expanded mission and homeland security preparedness responsibilities in the areas of recovery, response, and logistics. The response directorate, for example, provides coordinated federal operational and logistical disaster response capability needed to save and sustain lives, minimize suffering, and protect property in a timely manner in communities overwhelmed by a disaster. FEMA also manages the National Flood Insurance Program and other programs to reduce future losses to homes, businesses, schools, public buildings, and critical facilities from floods, earthquakes, tornados, and other disasters. The U.S. Fire Administration is also an entity of FEMA and provides fire and emergency services in prevention, preparedness, and response (U.S. Department of Homeland Security, 2011).

Military Health Systems at the Federal Level. The Military Health System (MHS) is a unique partnership of medical educators, medical researchers, health care providers, and support personnel who are prepared to respond anytime or anywhere with comprehensive medical capability to military operations, natural disasters, and humanitarian crises around the world and to ensure world class health care to all Department of Defense service members, retirees, and their families. The Military Health System promotes a fit, healthy, and protected armed force by reducing noncombat losses, optimizing healthy behavior and physical performance, and providing casualty care (U.S. Department of Defense, n.d.).

The Veterans Administration (VA), an independent agency directly under the President, provides health care services for veterans through the Department of Defense, which sponsors health care for military personnel on active duty. The VA utilizes an advanced computerized information system, which allows a person's medical record to be accessed in any VA site nationally, increasing efficiency in the provision of care. For active-duty service members and retirees of the seven uniformed services, their family members, survivors, and others who are registered in the defense enrollment eligibility reporting system (DEERS), military health care is covered through the former Civilian Health and Medical Program for the Uniformed Services (CHAMPUS) insurance program, now named TRICARE. TRICARE is also available to members of the National Guard and Reserves and their families (U.S. Department of Defense, n.d.).

Wounded Warrior Care. When a soldier is severely injured, prolonged care and rehabilitation is often required before a decision can be made whether the soldier should remain on active duty. The Military Health Service (MHS) is responsible for providing clinical care to return service personnel to duty or to assist them in making the transition from MHS care to the VA health care system. Tremendous progress has been made in the rehabilitative care of injured combatants and coordination of MHS care with the VA health system (U.S. Department of Defense, n.d.). For example, Haben (2008) reports that concussion known as mild traumatic brain injury (TBI) may affect 10% to 20% of soldiers and Marines engaged in combat in Iraq and Afghanistan. More than 80% are treated with complete recovery and are redeployed. Others may need extensive rehabilitation and assistance in returning to civilian life.

Americans with Disabilities. Starting in 1992 health care providers, both as employers and as providers of public services,

were required to comply with requirements of the Americans With Disabilities Act of 1990. The act is considered the most sweeping civil rights legislation since the Civil Rights Act of 1964. The two parts that apply most directly to health care providers are the prohibitions of employment discrimination and the requirements for provision of services to people with disabilities. An example of health care provider accommodation is to install wheelchair lifts in shuttle bus systems. Despite their need for health promotion and disease prevention, individuals with disabilities face numerous problems gaining access to health promotion programs and preventive services. The barriers are financial, social, physical, and logistical.

In 1990, President George H. Bush signed the Patient Self-Determination Act, which took effect in December 1991. This law was designed to increase individual involvement in decisions about life-sustaining treatment, ensuring that advance directives for health care are available to physicians at the time that medical decisions are being made and ensuring that individuals who have not prepared such documents are aware of their legal rights. As a condition of Medicare and Medicaid payment, the Patient Self-Determination Act requires health care facilities to comply with the law. The ACA law has several provisions expanding the access requirements for services to people with disabilities.

Federal Health Information Privacy Law. Developed by the Department of Health and Human Services (HHS), as part of the Health Insurance Portability and Accountability Act of 1996 (HIPAA), federal privacy standards were enacted by Congress requiring new safeguards to protect the security and confidentiality of health information including paper, electronic, and oral communications. Health plans, pharmacies, physicians, nurses, and other health care providers must have a written privacy procedure, provide employee training on HIPAA, and designate a privacy officer to ensure procedures are followed. The privacy law permits disclosures without individual authorization to public health authorities authorized by law to collect and receive information for the purpose of preventing or controlling disease, injury, or disability (USDHHS, n.d.).

International Level. World Health Organization (WHO), the United Nations' specialized agency for health as previously discussed, was established in 1948. Comprised of membership of more than 190 countries, WHO's core functions include giving worldwide guidance in the field of health; setting global standards for health; cooperating with governments in strengthening national health programs; and developing and transferring appropriate technology, information, and standards. The following is the six-point agenda of the WHO: promoting development; fostering health security; strengthening health systems; harnessing research, information, and evidence; enhancing partnerships; and improving performance. The WHO agenda was discussed earlier. WHO also encourages and coordinates international scientific research (WHO, 2012).

Voluntary Agencies

The voluntary (not-for-profit) health movement, which began in 1882, stems from the goodwill and humanitarian concerns that are part of the nongovernmental, free enterprise heritage of the people of the United States. Nonprofit entities that maintain a tax-free status are often powerful forces in the health field, voluntary agencies, foundations, and professional associations. The tax-free status of these organizations is challenged at times based on charges that some of them serve only a limited population. Voluntary agencies are influential in promoting health affairs and research agendas at the national policy level and often have significant influence on health legislation. Their prominent role was demonstrated by the American Cancer Society's early mass media announcements about the health hazards of smoking. An example of another voluntary agency is the Alzheimer's Association, which has local chapters that provide resources for families including publications, services, respite for the caregiver, and support groups for individuals and families. In 2011 Alzheimer's disease was listed as the sixth leading cause of death for persons 65 years and older with a mortality rate in 2007 of 24.7 deaths per 100,000 people, and preliminary data for 2008 show an increase to 27.1 per 100,000. On average, people 65 years and older survive an average of 4 to 8 years after a diagnosis of Alzheimer's disease with 40% of the total number of years a person is afflicted by Alzheimer's consisting of the most severe stage of the disease. Two thirds of those with Alzheimer's die in nursing homes (Alzheimer's Association, 2011).

Philanthropic foundations provide valuable stimulation to the health field and operate under fewer constraints than do other sources in supporting research or training projects. Nurses interested in research or advanced clinical study that relates to the special interests of voluntary agencies or foundations may find grant monies available to support their work. For example, The John A. Hartford Institution is a foundation established in 1929 and supports efforts to improve health care for older Americans. Recently, the trustees of this foundation awarded a $5 million, 5-year grant to create the John A. Hartford Foundation Institute for Geriatric Nursing at New York University. The Hartford Institute promotes initiatives to improve care of older adults and training projects to prepare faculty to teach care of older adults in baccalaureate nursing programs. The institute has also raised the profile of geriatric nursing by creating nationally recognized awards for excellence in research and practice (John A. Hartford Foundation, 2012). Professional associations, organized at the national level with state and local branches, are powerful political forces. Nurses can support their professional organizations in influencing the direction of health policy through membership and active participation.

The American Red Cross. The American Red Cross is a well-known volunteer-led humanitarian organization that is officially sanctioned by the federal government as a congressional charter, meaning it is not supervised by the government because it is not a governmental agency, but is recognized officially. Founded in 1881 by Clara Barton, the International Red Cross aids victims of war and natural disasters throughout the world. There are more than 700 local American Red Cross chapters in the United States with more than 500,000 volunteers and 35,000 employees. The American Red Cross responds both to small local emergencies to help victims (such as in the case of a house fire) and to large natural disasters (such as hurricanes and earthquakes). The Red Cross is the largest supplier of blood and blood products in the United States, helps thousands of U.S. service members separated from their families maintain communication, and offers communities a range of health and safety courses. The global network of national societies relies on public donations of money, time, and blood. Local Red Cross opportunities exist including the donation of blood and assistance with blood drives and other volunteer activities (American Red Cross, 2012).

FINANCING HEALTH CARE
Costs

The health care industry is the largest service industry in the United States today and the most powerful employer in the nation, employing 14.3 million health care workers (U.S. Department of Labor, 2010). National health expenditures in the United States were greater than those in any other country, with $2.593 trillion spent in 2010, a marked increase from the $1.9 trillion spent in 2004. In 2010 health spending consumed 17.9% of the gross domestic product and is projected to be 19.3% by 2019. Hospital spending, which accounts for 31% of the national health expenditure, is expected to grow at a rate of more than 6% per year over the next decade, and the cost of prescription drugs, which accounts for 10% of national health expenditures, increased by 5.2% in 2009 to $246 billion. The trend is expected to continue on a growth path of 6.3% per year over the next decade (Centers for Medicare & Medicaid Services, 2011). In 2010 the per capita expenditure for health care (amount of money on average spent on each individual in the United States) was $8402, the highest of all countries. Figure 3-2 lists selective countries with per capita cost comparisons for the year 2008. Canada, for example, which borders the United States, is reported to spend just more than $4000 per person, which is half of what the United States spends. Many other countries spend far less per capita, yet life expectancy is greater and infant mortality rates are lower. In addition to spending more health care dollars per person than any other country, the rate of growth in per capita health expenditure in the United States is much steeper than that of other countries. The graphic representation listed as Figure 3-3 illustrates that beginning in 1970, the range of per capita expenditures between countries was narrow, but within less than a decade, the United States began to outpace all other countries and spend more per capita. Another measure of comparison is the amount of money a country devotes to health care in terms of gross domestic product (GDP). Over time, the United States again outpaces the other nations in the percent of GDP devoted to health care (Figure 3-4). In 2010, of the 305.2 million Americans, 49% had employer-based health insurance, 5% had private health insurance, 12% were enrolled in Medicare, 17% were enrolled in Medicaid, and 16% of the population were uninsured (Figure 3-5). A major focus of the Affordable Care Act law is aimed at reducing the number of uninsured Americans. These figures and expenditures, although numerous, introduce the topic of health care financing.

Health care analysts predict the accelerations in health care costs will continue, putting pressure on public and private

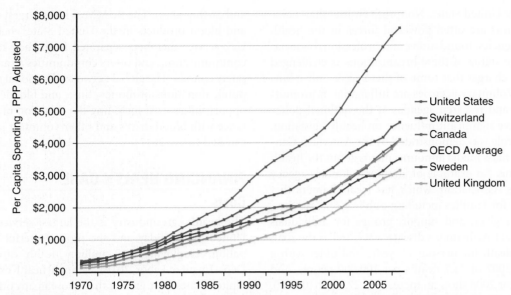

FIGURE 3-3 Growth in total health expenditure per capita, United States and selected countries, 1970 to 2008. **Notes:** Data for Canada, Norway, and Switzerland, are OECD estimates. Numbers are PPP-adjusted. Break in series: CAN (1995); SWE (1993, 2001); SWI (1995); UK (1997). Numbers are PPP-adjusted. Estimates for Canada and Switzerland in 2008. (Source: Organisation for Economic Co-operation and Development. [2010]. *OECD health data.* OECD Health Statistics [database]. Accessed February 14, 2011, from doi:10.1787/data-00350-en.)

	1970		1980	1990		2000		2008	
Australia	4.1%	*	6.1%	6.7%		8.0%		8.5%	*
Austria	5.2%		7.4%	8.3%	b	9.9%		10.5%	
Belgium	3.9%		6.3%	7.2%		9.0%	de	11.1%	de
Canada	6.9%		7.0%	8.9%		8.8%		10.4%	e
France	5.4%		7.0%	8.4%		10.1%		11.2%	
Germany	N/A		N/A	N/A		10.3%		10.5%	
Italy	N/A		N/A	7.7%		8.1%		9.1%	
Japan	4.6%		6.5%	6.0%		7.7%		8.1%	*
Netherlands	N/A		7.4%	8.0%		8.0%		9.9%	e
Norway	4.4%		7.0%	7.6%		8.4%		8.5%	e
Spain	3.5%		5.3%	6.5%		7.2%		9.0%	
Sweden	6.8%		8.9%	8.2%		8.2%		9.4%	
Switzerland	5.4%		7.3%	8.2%		10.2%		10.7%	e
U.K.	4.5%		5.6%	5.9%		7.0%		8.7%	
U.S.	7.1%		9.0%	12.2%		13.4%		16.0%	
Average	**5.2%**		**7.0%**	**7.8%**		**9.0%**		**10.1%**	

FIGURE 3-4 Total expenditure on health care as a share of GDP. **Notes:** Data from Australia and Japan are 2007 data. 2008 data from Belgium, Canada, Netherlands, Norway, and Switzerland are OECD estimates. 2000 numbers for Belgium are OECD estimates. Numbers are PPP-adjusted. Break in Series: AUS(1998); AUSTRIA(1990); BEL(2003, 2005); CAN(1995); FRA(1995); GER(1992); JAP(1995); NET(1998, 2003); NOR(1999); SPA(1999, 2003); SWE(1993, 2001); SWI(1995); UK (1997). Starting in 1993, Belgium used a different methodology. (Source: Organisation for Economic Co-operation and Development. [2010]. *OECD health data.* OECD Health Statistics [database]. Accessed February 14, 2011, from doi:10.1787/data-00350-en.)

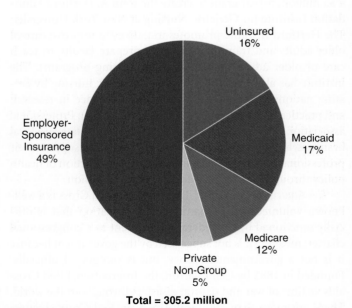

Total = 305.2 million

FIGURE 3-5 Total expenditure on health care as a share of the GDP. **Note:** Medicaid also includes other public programs: CHIP, other state programs, military-related coverage. Numbers may not add to 100% because of rounding. (Source: KCMU/Urban Institute analysis of 2011 ASEC Supplement to the CPS.)

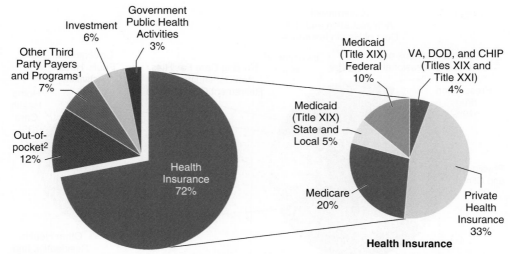

FIGURE 3-6 Nation's health dollars, calendar year 2010: where it come from. **Note:** Sum of pieces may not equal 100% because of rounding. [1]Includes worksite health care, other private revenues, Indian Health Service, workers' compensation, general assistance, maternal and child health, vocational rehabilitation, Substance Abuse and Mental Health Services. [2]Includes copayments, deductibles, and any amounts not covered by health insurance. (Source: Centers for Medicare & Medicaid Services, Office of the Actuary, National Health Statistics Group.)

payers to finance them. Factors driving costs include general inflation; health care cost inflation; application of new and more advanced technologies; growth in the proportion of older adults; government financing of health care services; growth of prescription drug usage and costs; misdistribution of health care providers and services; expansion of medical technology and specialty medicine; and the growing number of uninsured and underinsured people (KFF, 2010a, 2010b, 2010c). For example, diagnostic and therapeutic techniques—including computer-aided technology and noninvasive imaging (such as magnetic resonance imaging), cardiac surgery, organ transplantation, joint replacements (particularly hips and knees)—enhance the capabilities of medicine while increasing costs.

A combination of the following factors results in hospitals having less time to offer prevention or health promotion education to individuals—changes in hospital care and use of hospitalists, increased utilization of outpatient services, shorter inpatient stays, and increased time caring for chronic illness as opposed to acute illness. Moreover, workforce shortages, especially in nursing, increase the use of nonprofessional caregivers, and inadequate resources, reimbursement, and numbers of nurses may prevent health care professionals from offering the range of health promotion educational efforts requested in the new *Healthy People 2020* objectives.

Sources

Ultimately, the American people pay for all health care costs. Money is transferred from consumer to provider by various mechanisms. The major sources are government (federal, state, and local monies collected by taxes), third-party payment (private insurance), independent plans, and out-of-pocket support, which totaled 2.6 billion dollars in 2010. The

Centers for Medicare & Medicaid Services provide statistics on the source of the nation's health care dollars and the manner in which they are spent. In 2010 (Figure 3-6) the largest percentage of the nation's health care dollars came from private health insurance (33%), and 12% of health care costs were out-of-pocket payments made by consumers. The cost of Medicare accounted for 20% of the health care dollar and Medicaid and SCHIP 15%. In all, 72% of the nation's health care is funded by some form of health insurance. Figure 3-7 provides a similar schematic but displays where health care dollars are spent. Almost one third (31%) of health care dollars is spent on hospital care, 20% on physicians and clinics, 10% on prescription drugs, 6% on nursing home facilities, 7% on dental care, 7% on administrative costs, and 14% on non–acute care. As discussed earlier, keeping Americans healthy and out of the hospital would save a tremendous amount of money.

Employer Health Benefits

According to the 2011 employer health benefits survey conducted by the Kaiser Family Foundation, the overall inflation rate of employer-sponsored health insurance for families has risen dramatically in the past decade. In 2011 premiums rose 9%, significantly higher than the 3% increase of the previous year. The average employer-sponsored health insurance annual premium in 2011 was $5429 for individuals and $15,073 for family coverage. Since 2001, the average annual premium for family coverage has increased 113%. The worker contribution for family coverage in 2001 was $1787 per year and in 2011 grew to $4129, while the employer contribution in 2001 was $7061 and jumped to $15,073 in 2011, making it difficult for both individuals and employers to pay for higher health care premiums (Figure 3-8). Interestingly, employees in small firms (3 to 199 workers) on average paid less for premiums than

FIGURE 3-7 Nation's health dollars ($2.6 trillion), calendar year 2010: where it went. **Note:** Sum of pieces may not equal 100% because of rounding. [1]Includes research (2%) and structures and equipment (4%). [2]Includes durable (1%) and nondurable (2%) goods. [3]Includes expenditures for residential care facilities, ambulance providers, medical care delivered in nontraditional settings (such as community centers, senior citizens centers, schools, and military field stations), and expenditures for Home and Community Waiver programs under Medicaid. (Source: Centers for Medicare & Medicaid Services, Office of the Actuary, National Health Statistics Group.)

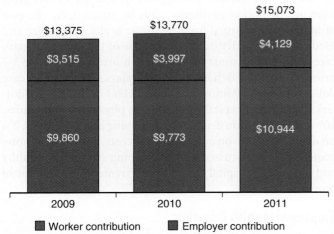

FIGURE 3-8 Average annual health insurance premiums and worker contributions for family coverage, 2009 to 2011. (Source: Kaiser/HRET Survey of Employer-Sponsored Health Benefits, 2009-2011.)

workers in large firms (200 or more workers) ($14,098 vs. $15,520) (KFF, 2011c).

As discussed previously, the majority of covered workers (55%) were enrolled in PPOs, followed by 17% in HMOs, 10% in POS plans, and 1% in conventional plans. The number of workers enrolled in high-deductible health plans with a savings option (HDHP/SO) continues to rise and accounts for 17% of covered employees. Most employees with single coverage (except 29% of those workers enrolled in HMOs) paid general

annual deductibles of $675 (copayments for office visits, laboratory testing, and prescription drugs) with 98% having prescription drug coverage plans. The survey also exposed that only 60% of employers offered health benefits in 2011 to their workers. In looking at the previous 12 years, the lowest percent of firms offering health benefits was 59% in both 2007 and 2009. The highest percent of firms offering health insurance was in 2010, with 69% followed by 68% in 2000 and 2001. Firms that employed 3 to 9 workers offered health benefits the least (47% in 2005 and 2009; high of 59% in 2010) and large firms (200 or more workers) consistently offered health benefits—97% to 99% of the time between the years 1990 and 2011 (KFF, 2011c).

Federal and state Medicaid spending showed an increasing pattern similar to that discussed earlier in this chapter, with Medicaid spending reported to be $5.3 billion in 1970, $207.0 billion in 2000, $309.0 billion in 2004, $317.7 billion in 2008, and $366.5 billion in 2009. As a cost savings mechanism, by 2000, 55.8% of Medicaid recipients were enrolled in some form of managed care plan. Although costly, the Medicaid program finances health care for low-income children, adults, seniors, and people with disabilities. Children comprise 49% of individuals in the program but account for only 20% of the spending of Medicaid dollars, whereas older adults comprise 10% of enrollment but account for 25% of the spending. The blind or disabled individuals in the program, representing only 15% of those enrolled, consumed 43% of Medicaid spending (Figure 3-9). The largest share of Medicaid monies, 61.9%, is spent on acute care and 33.3% is spent on individuals in long-term care (Figure 3-10, KFF, 2010). Medicaid is the nation's only source of significant long-term care spending, covering 6 out of 10 nursing home residents. The Affordable Care Act of 2010 will add millions of previously noneligible individuals younger than age 65 to state Medicaid plans, since expansion will allow individuals below 133% of the federal poverty level to enroll. This one measure is expected to decrease the number of uninsured by 32 million Americans (KFF, 2011a, 2012b) but significantly increase the cost of the Medicaid program.

Each state receives from the federal government a matching formula percentage of revenue to run a Medicaid program, leaving state budgets responsible for the remaining cost. Federal tax dollars must fund a minimum of 50% of a state's Medicaid cost. In 2012, 14 states—Alaska, California, Colorado,

Connecticut, Illinois, Maryland, Massachusetts, Minnesota, New Hampshire, New Jersey, New York, Virginia, Washington, and Wyoming—were funded at the minimal level of 50%, whereas other states—for example, Mississippi 74.18%, West Virginia 72.62%, Kentucky 71.18%, Utah 70.99%, Arkansas 70.17%, and Idaho 70.23%—received a much greater share of the cost of their Medicaid programs from the federal government (KFF, 2012b). The greater the percentage of federal support, the less the state has to pay with state monies. For example, when a state only receives 50% of federal funding the remaining 50% must be generated by state taxes. This is a tremendous burden on state residents. As the cost of the program increases and/or the number of persons enrolled in Medicaid increases, the taxpayers of the state must support the program often by raising state, county, and local taxes. Because Medicaid is an entitlement program, any one individual who meets Medicaid's eligibility requirements is entitled to receive benefits; therefore, there is no way to cap the Medicaid budget at the federal or state level under current law. Many states have more lenient eligibility requirements than those set by the federal government and offer more health services than are mandated. The Affordable Care Act will address some of these disparities. For example, the ACA will provide financial incentives for states that qualify, to provide enhanced services to Medicaid recipients by increasing their federal matching funds by a 1% increase. One way states have cut costs in Medicaid programs in the past is to decrease provider payment rates. This practice can jeopardize provider participation (providers willing to care for patients enrolled in a Medicaid program) and limit access to care for Medicaid

FIGURE 3-9 Medicaid enrollees and expenditures, fiscal year 2008. (Source: KCMU/Urban Institute estimates based on data from FY 2008 MSIS and CMS Form-64, 2010.)

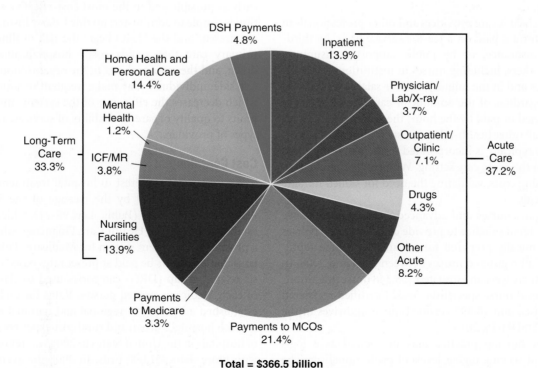

Total = $366.5 billion

FIGURE 3-10 Medicaid expenditures by service, 2009. Note: Total may not add to 100% because of rounding. Excludes administrative spending, adjustments, and payments to the territories. (Source: Urban Institute estimates based on data from CMS Form-64, prepared for the Kaiser Commission on Medicaid and the Uninsured.)

recipients. Decreasing eligibility requirements for individuals and families to qualify for Medicaid coverage is only part of the solution to reduce the number of uninsured. Since more individuals will now qualify for Medicaid, individual states need to enhance or develop efficient user-friendly systems to facilitate the enrollment process. Health care delivery systems in each state need to be formed to accommodate the increased number of Medicaid enrollees in the provision of safe and efficient quality care. The Affordable Care Act has some provisions to increase payments for primary care services provided by primary care providers (KFF, 2011a) because Medicaid provider reimbursement rates for services provided are typically much lower than other sources of payment.

The provisions in the ACA will result in the increase in the number of individuals eligible to enroll in state Medicaid programs because Medicaid will be expanded to include all individuals under age 65 with incomes up to 133% of the federal poverty rate. The overall total percent change in spending for 2014 to 2019 is projected to result in a 22.1% increase in federal spending and an average of 1.4% in state spending. The variation in both federal and state projections is great. The percent of change in federal spending from 2014 to 2019 is expected to be single digits for six states (Vermont 1.9%, New York 3.3%, Massachusetts 3.5%, Arizona 4.2%, Delaware 6.2%, and District of Columbia 8.3%) whereas all other states are projected to see double-digit increases in federal spending, the highest being Oregon 50.6%, Nevada 49.8%, and Oklahoma 48.2% (KFF, 2011a, 2012b).

Mechanisms
Payment
Although some health care providers and other professionals in the private sector are paid on a fee-for-service basis, by third-party private insurance, or by public-supported insurance, most health workers, including nurses in institutional or community agencies and in the military, receive salaries or are paid by the hour regardless of the amount of care provided. Since nurses are salaried or paid by the hour, the separation of nursing costs from all other health-related costs is difficult. The cost of nursing care typically is incorporated in the daily room and board charge in the acute care setting. Without documentation of specific nursing costs, validating the need for skilled nursing services is difficult.

In recent years, nurses and advanced practice nurses have entered independent practice to provide direct services. Nurses who are academically prepared for advanced practice represented 8.2% of all registered nurses between 2004 and 2008. In March of 2008 there were an estimated 158,348 nurse practitioners, 59,242 clinical nurse specialists, 32,523 certified registered nurse anesthetists, and 18,492 certified nurse midwives in the United States (USDHHS, 2010).

Independent nursing practice may be viewed as a logical outgrowth of seeking higher levels of professionalism. The nurse practice acts of some states encourage nurses to use their knowledge more comprehensively than many agencies sanction. Although legislation in 1997 included the reimbursement of advanced practice nurses by Medicare, not all plans and

provider groups include these nurses as primary care practitioners. Clearly, the nursing practice roles and prescriptive authority of APNs vary between states. Incremental steps have been taken to advance the APN role at both the federal and the state levels. Some states have passed laws for nurse practitioners to practice and prescribe without physician oversight. The IOM's 2010 report titled *The Future of Nursing: Leading Change, Advancing Health* supports nurses practicing to the full extent of their education and training.

Alternative forms of payment for APNs are salary and capitation. The salary system involves a set amount for services provided in a specified time frame. This system provides the employee with a fixed nursing income that is protected from changes in supply and demand, includes fringe benefits, and obviates fee collection problems. The salary system's flexibility makes it easier to fill unpopular jobs or jobs in underserved areas. Disadvantages of this system include a limit on income and constraints on schedules, vacations, and peer review. A nurse in a salaried position may not be able to earn overtime depending upon the facility. Nurses who work beyond the scheduled hours are then uncompensated for additional time under a salary arrangement, which may lead to job dissatisfaction and burnout.

In the capitation system, such as in an HMO, each provider receives a flat annual fee for each participant regardless of how often services are used. Individuals who enroll in an HMO pay a fixed amount on a monthly basis whether or not they use the services; prepayment provides an incentive to provide efficient care. The objective is to keep people healthy to prevent costly services. Cost consciousness dictates that illness be treated as early as possible and in the most cost-effective setting. Capitation is simple to administer; no third-party insurance payments are present and the HMO bears the risk of illness. Preventive primary care that avoids costly hospitalization keeps costs down, and the savings revert to the organization. On the negative side, individuals may make frequent or unnecessary visits, which decreases the efficiency of the system, and there may be limits to quality of care, availability of services, and access to all types of providers.

Cost Containment
The government's interest in hospital treatment cost containment was exemplified by the passage of the Social Security Amendments of 1983 (Public Law 98-21), which mandate the establishment by the Health Care Financing Administration of a prospective payment system for Medicare. This system stipulates that providers be paid at preset rates based on 470 diagnosis-related group (DRG) categories used to classify the illness of each Medicare-insured person. Rates for each diagnosis are established according to regional and national amounts based on each hospital's urban and rural cost experience. The number of hospitals in the United States in 2008 was reported to be 5815 with more than 951,000 beds. In 2008 the average occupancy rate in hospitals was 68.2%. Large hospitals with 500 beds or more reported higher rates of almost 75%, whereas the smallest hospitals, those with 6 to 24 beds, had 33.8% occupancy rates (Centers for Disease Control Foundation, 2010).

Another piece of legislation that targeted cost containment was the Balanced Budget Act of 1997, which also affected Medicare. This act reduced Medicare spending by limiting provider payments, increased options in the choice of managed care plans, and made medical savings accounts an option. As of 2007, medical savings accounts were linked to high-deductible Medicare Advantage plans (Medicare private health plans) and are currently available in some states. Medicare makes an annual deposit into an interest-bearing account on behalf of enrollees, who use the funds to pay for qualified health care expenses until they meet the deductible, at which point the plan will pay for all Medicare-covered services.

The Medicare Modernization Act of 2003 promotes private managed care plans to reduce the burden on the economy of Medicare entitlements. These HMO plans, called Medicare Advantage (MA) plans, discussed previously, typically have clients who are healthier than the average Medicare client. Older adults who are enrolled in these plans pay a monthly premium and are required to choose providers within the network. If care is provided outside of the network of providers, individuals usually must pay out-of-pocket costs similar to those of other HMOs discussed earlier. This can be confusing to the older person because there are many MA plans to choose from and the person may not realize how an MA plan is different from traditional Medicare coverage. Provisions have been made for enrollees to change MA plans or to be disenrolled during specific time frames. Providers have been lobbying for increased reimbursement because Medicare dictates reimbursement fees based on a predetermined formula.

Care Management. Care management began through public programs with nurses in public health departments, social workers in public welfare systems, and caseworkers in mental health departments. In care management, an experienced health care professional, such as a nurse, social worker, or gerontologist, helps determine the nursing care that is necessary, monitors that care, and arranges for individuals to receive care in the most cost-effective and most appropriate setting. Care managers are especially effective in meeting the needs of individuals recently discharged from the hospital, older adults, persons with medical conditions that are costly to treat (e.g., spinal cord injuries or persons with high-volume diseases such as chronic illnesses), persons with complex health and social needs, and other cases requiring multiple levels of care. The care manager must achieve a balance between cost and quality and must collaborate effectively with all providers involved, both inside and outside the health plan, and with the person's family to ensure appropriate quality care. Emphasis must be on health management across the continuum of health care services. As Medicaid and Medicare managed care systems continue to develop, demand for nurses to fill the care management role will continue to grow. In addition to working within organizations, care managers can have their own independent practices. Managed care organizations rely on care management to reduce inappropriate use of services, improve quality of care, and control costs (Nies & McEwen, 2007). Basic care management services are described in Box 3-11.

BOX 3-11 CARE MANAGEMENT SERVICES

- *Assessment:* Evaluating a person's physical, social, functional, psychological, financial, and spiritual needs, including the family within a specific environment
- *Care planning:* Setting goals and identifying specific services to meet individual and family needs, including how to allocate resources and refer to other resources
- *Service coordination and referral:* Facilitating and coordinating access to needed providers
- *Care monitoring and periodic reassessments:* Evaluating progress, access to and use of services, and changes in needs

---

Managed Care Issues

Managed care options will once again become more plentiful as states devise health care delivery systems to meet the Affordable Care Act mandates. Concern about the quality of care provided when the overall emphasis is cost control is an issue. Gatekeeping by the primary care provider is not seen by some individuals as a way to maintain or improve quality of care; rather, the PCP may be seen as the way managed care attempts to limit health care costs by decreasing the amount of care provided, especially by limiting referrals. Managed care has created new systems, with groups of providers delivering care in more efficient ways. The Internet has become a valuable resource for informing consumers and employers about health care issues and allowing them to search and compare information on various types of health care plans. The Internet is also a tool nurses can use for their own continuing education needs, as well as to enhance other's education within a facility, public library, or home. Nurses can steer individuals toward appropriate websites for health promotion and disease-oriented information (see Case Study at end of chapter). With the rapid expansion of scientific advances in health and medicine, it is not possible for the nurse to stay abreast of the growing body of research evidence without Internet assistance. Evidence-based practice is key in the provision of safe, quality nursing care. Registered nurses and APNs need to be able to obtain the best evidence, appraise the findings, and then apply them to practice with consideration to the culture and beliefs of the individual (Melnyk & Fineout-Overholt, 2011).

Health Insurance

Positive elements of the health care system in America include excellent clinicians, health care facilities, and equipment—all of which are available to people with good health insurance or adequate finances. The U.S. system exhibits a high degree of technological change and innovation and excellent information, quality, and cost-accounting systems. Numerous studies have found that those who do not have health insurance are at risk for poorer health outcomes. ACA 2010 will significantly decrease the number of those uninsured because Americans will be required by law to purchase or obtain health insurance. A high number of uninsured individuals are disproportionately low-income persons and measures as discussed previously will increase the number of individuals in both private and public health plans.

The plan does not address noncitizen foreign-born persons who have entered and are living in the United States illegally.

Private Health Insurance

In the private sector, the following five types of organizations provide health care insurance:

- Traditional insurance companies (including the earliest insurer, Blue Cross and Blue Shield, a nonprofit charitable organization) and for-profit commercial insurance companies
- PPOs acting as "brokers" between insurers and health care providers
- HMOs, which are independent prepayment plans
- POS plans, which combine features of classic HMOs with person choice characteristics of PPOs
- Self-insurance and self-funded plans, in which either the employer takes on the role of insurer or the enrollee sets up a trust account with tax savings

Traditionally, private insurers charged employers or individuals annual premiums and provided services on a fee-for-service basis. Organized at the state and local levels, Blue Cross and Blue Shield generally complement each other, with Blue Cross reimbursing hospitals and Blue Shield covering physicians and other providers. After World War II, insurance companies began to provide health insurance plans in competition with Blue Cross and Blue Shield. Today, more than 800 commercial, profit-making insurance companies, such as Metropolitan Life and Aetna, offer policies that cover hospitalization and in-hospital or office-based physician care, and other major medical expenses. Much of the individual insurance sold today is supplementary, such as that designed to supplement Medicare, known as Medigap. These plans reimburse only deductibles and co-insurance payments associated with Medicare.

HMOs attempt to lower health care costs by emphasizing preventive rather than curative care, decreasing the progression and severity of some illnesses. Care is provided in outpatient settings when possible. HMOs tend to use fewer services, with emphasis on the least costly means of providing a service.

POS plans enable enrollees to choose, at the point of service, whether to use the plan's provider network or seek care from non-network providers. Typically, network providers are paid on a capitated or discounted fee basis, and non-network providers are paid on a fee-for-service basis.

Another change in the structure of the insurance industry is the growth of self-insured or self-funded plans. Self-insurance means that an employer (or union) assumes the claims risk of its insured employees, whereas self-funding refers to paying insurance claims from an established fund, such as a bank account or trust fund.

Public Health Insurance and Assistance

Medicare. Medicare is a federal health insurance program that finances medical care for people older than 65, disabled individuals who are entitled to Social Security benefits, and people with end-stage renal disease requiring dialysis or a kidney transplant. The Medicare program, also known as Title XVIII of the Social Security Amendment (SSA), began in 1966 after decades of debate and is currently operated under the administrative oversight of the Centers for Medicare & Medicaid Services. Medicare is an entitlement program, meaning individuals who contributed to Medicare through taxes are 'entitled' to the benefits regardless of the amount of income and assets they have. The intent of Medicare was to protect older adults against the catastrophic financial debts often incurred in managing chronic illness and to assist in the payment of health care. In 1983 Medicare added hospice benefits for the last 6 months of life to cover services for the terminally ill. Hospice is based on a philosophy that views death as a normal part of the life cycle and emphasizes living the remainder of life as fully and comfortably as possible. Hospice care accounts for only a small amount of total Medicare expenditures. The total Medicare benefit payments in 2011 equaled $551.3 billion with 26% hospital inpatient services, 23% Medicare Advantage plans, and 5% skilled nursing, accounting for almost 50% of the total budget. There are four parts in the Medicare plan: Medicare Part A, Medicare Part B, Medicare Part C, and Medicare Part D.

Medicare Part A is financed largely through a mandatory tax of 2.9% of earnings paid by employees and their employers (1.45% each) into the Hospital Insurance Trust Fund. Part A covers inpatient care in hospitals, skilled nursing facilities (not custodial or long-term care), home health services, and hospice care. For those individuals who have contributed to or had a spouse contribute for 10 years of Medicare-covered employment, there is no monthly premium. For those individuals who have contributed 30 to 39 quarters of Medicare-covered employment, the monthly premium is $248.00; and for those who have less than 30 quarters of Medicare-covered employment and are not otherwise eligible for premium-free hospital insurance, the monthly premium is $451.00 per month for the year 2012. Medicare Part A accounted for 31% of benefit spending in 2011. The Part A benefits are subject to a deductible ($1156 in 2012) and copayments, which may be difficult for many older adults to manage as a result of fixed incomes.

Part B is supplementary voluntary medical insurance financed through a combination of general tax revenues and premiums paid by beneficiaries ($99.90 per month in 2012 with a $140 deductible); Part B covers physician visits, outpatient services, preventive services, and home health visits and accounted for 18% of benefit spending in 2011.

Part C refers to the Medicare Advantage program as previously discussed. About 25% of beneficiaries or 12 million older adults are enrolled in these private plans and account for 21% of benefit spending.

Part D is the voluntary, subsidized outpatient prescription drug benefit with additional subsidies available for low-income beneficiaries. The Part D benefit is offered through private plans that contract with Medicare. There are Medicare Advantage prescription plans and stand-alone prescription plans. Part D accounts for 12% of benefit spending and more than 29 million individuals are enrolled in this part.

The ACA includes a number of provisions that will enhance benefits and gradually eliminate the Part D prescription drug coverage gap known as the donut hole. Characteristics of the Medicare beneficiaries reveal a mixed group with half of the persons having incomes less than $22,000 per year and half of all beneficiaries with savings of less than $60,000. Approximately 29% of Medicare enrollees have cognitive impairments and 28% report poor health. Eight million Medicare beneficiaries are nonelderly individuals with disabilities and

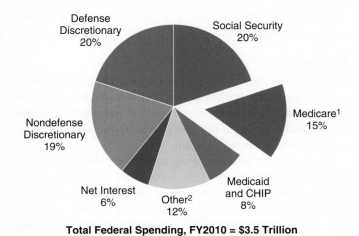

Total Federal Spending, FY2010 = $3.5 Trillion

FIGURE 3-11 Medicare spending as a percent of total federal spending, fiscal year 2010. **Notes:** FY is fiscal year.[1]Amount for Medicare includes offsetting premium receipts.[2]Other category includes disaster costs and negative outlays for Troubled Asset Relief Program. (Source: Office of Management and Budget, FY2011 Budget, Summary Tables, February 2010.)

2 million (4%) live in a long-term care facility. About 12% are over the age of 85 years. Different sections of Medicare are funded in a variety of ways, but overall 42% is funded by general revenues, 37% by payroll taxes, and 13% by beneficiary premiums. Individuals enrolled in both Medicare and Medicaid programs are considered vulnerable populations (older adults and poor) and Medicare premiums are subsidized. Medicare benefit payments accounted for 15% of the total federal budget in 2010 (Figure 3-11). Estimates predict that by 2024 Medicare's trust fund (HI Trust) will be depleted. The projected year to insolvency has varied, and the impact of the ACA has not been fully realized. Future challenges include increased costs of health care services, increased costs of technology, and increased volume and utilization of services attributable to population growth of older adults and increasing life expectancy. By 2030, 79 million people are expected to be enrolled in Medicare compared to 39 million in 2000 (Figure 3-12). Neither Part A nor Part B of Medicare offers comprehensive coverage. Inherent in the program are deductibles, set amounts that the individual must pay for each type of service before Medicare begins to pay, and co-insurance, a percentage of charges paid by the individual. There are also limitations on the amount of coverage provided.

Out-of-pocket expenses do not include premium payments for Part B or for supplemental private health insurance, which can add significantly to out-of-pocket expenses. A comprehensive booklet available online or through the Centers for Medicare & Medicaid Services details information on enrollment, costs, and covered and noncovered services. With some exceptions, noncovered services include acupuncture, chiropractic

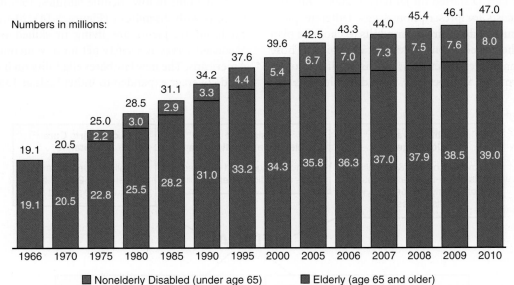

■ Nonelderly Disabled (under age 65)   ■ Elderly (age 65 and older)

FIGURE 3-12 Medicare enrollment, 1966 to 2010. **Notes:** Numbers may not sum to total because of rounding. People with disabilities under age 65 were not eligible for Medicare before 1972. (Source: Centers for Medicare & Medicaid Services, Medicare Enrollment: Hospital Insurance and/or Supplemental Medical Insurance Programs for Total, Fee-for-Service and Managed Care Enrollees as of July 1, 2008: Selected calendar years 1966-2008; 2009-2010, HHS Budget in Brief, FY 2011.)

services, custodial care (bathing and toileting), dental care and dentures, routine eye care and glasses, routine foot care, hearing aids, long-term care (if only custodial care is needed), and health care while traveling outside of the United States. Items not covered, especially custodial care, contribute significantly to out-of-pocket expenses. The main population at risk, the older adult, may have limited financial resources to seek preventive health services not covered. Some low-income enrollees may qualify for Medicaid services if income requirements are met and others may have additional benefits through private insurance (KFF, 2011e).

In the Omnibus Budget Reconciliation Act of 1989 (OBRA), Medicare revised its payment scheme for physicians, assigning relative values to services based on the time, skill, and intensity required to provide them, and a second limit was set on the amount that physicians could charge individuals above the amount that Medicare pays. This restriction was designed to limit growth of Medicare costs for physician payments.

The Balanced Budget Act (BBA) of 1997, the Balanced Budget Refinement Act of 1999, and the Benefits Improvement and Protection Act of 2000 added services to the Medicare benefits package. These services include coverage for some screening tests, diabetes monitoring and diabetes self-management, and some immunizations.

The missing Medicare benefit causing great concern was the rising cost and lack of coverage for outpatient prescription drugs. On December 9, 2003, President George W. Bush signed into law the Medicare Prescription Drug, Improvement, and Modernization Act of 2003, Public Law 108-173. This lengthy piece of legislation amended Title XVIII of the SSA to provide for a voluntary program for prescription drug coverage and to modernize the Medicare program. The Medicare prescription drug benefit Part D started on January 1, 2006, and covers some of the costs for prescription drugs. Different plans cover different drugs and require older adults to choose a plan that best meets their needs from a plethora of choices. Those with low education or literacy levels, as well as debilitated older adults in long-term care facilities, may have difficulty selecting the best plan for their individual needs. The average monthly premium cost in 2012 is projected to be about $39.00 but may be higher in some plans and for those with higher incomes. The original Part D plan required the first $250 in prescription drug costs to be paid by the older adult each year. Medicare then pays 75% of the next $2000 worth of drugs on the Plan's formulary. After that, there is a gap in coverage known as the "donut hole" where individuals pay 100% of drug costs until another $2850 has been spent out-of-pocket. At that point, Medicare will begin paying about 95% of the cost of covered drugs until the end of the calendar year. The Affordable Care Act reform law will gradually close the donut hole gap in prescription coverage.

Medicaid

Medicaid is an essential health insurance program available to certain low-income individuals and families who fit into an eligibility group that is recognized by federal and state law (Figure 3-13). Medicaid pays health care providers directly if they participate in the Medicaid program.

Medicaid is an assistance program, commonly referred to as welfare, managed jointly by the federal and state governments to provide partial or full payment of medical costs for individuals and families of any age who are too poor to pay for the care. Medicaid legislation, Title XIX of the amendments to the SSA, went into effect in 1967. The federal government provides funds to states on a cost-sharing basis, with 50% to almost 80% from the federal government and the remainder from the state, according to the per capita income of each state, to guarantee medical services to eligible Medicaid recipients (see previous discussion).

Medicaid is an integral part of the health care system providing health insurance coverage for 29 million children, 15 million adults in low-income families, 15 million elderly, and persons with disabilities (Figure 3-14). More than 1 million Medicaid recipients are living in skilled nursing facilities. Medicaid serves as a safety net for low-income and high-need Americans. The new law bases eligibility on income with Medicaid coverage expanded to individuals at 133% of the federal

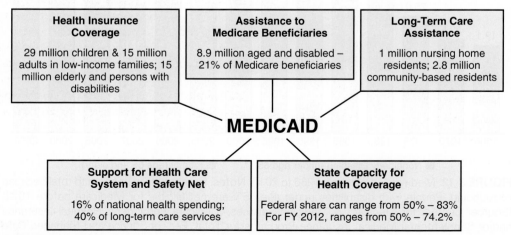

FIGURE 3-13 Medicaid has many vital roles in our health care system. (Source: Kaiser Commission on Medicaid and the Uninsured, 2011.)

poverty level ($14,404 for individuals or $29,326 for a family of 4 in 2009). The program will also support individuals and families with subsidies for insurance coverage in state-based Health Benefit Exchanges. Individuals and families with income levels 133% to 400% of poverty levels will be eligible. Previously, states established income eligibility requirements, and 47 states had income-eligibility levels for children in the Medicaid/SCHIP program at 200%. Before the current reform, states could not cover nondisabled adults without children under Medicaid.

Additionally, Medicaid pays the Medicare premiums, deductibles, and co-insurance for certain low-income Medicare recipients. Medicaid plans are open-ended, meaning a state must admit into the program at any time all individuals who meet the criteria. A state is not allowed to cap the Medicaid budget for a particular fiscal year, thus making it difficult to determine exactly how much money needs to be appropriated.

States administer Medicaid under broad federal requirements and guidelines. All states must provide federally prescribed minimal benefits to enrollees. However, many states have provided enhanced benefits. A state determines its own eligibility standards; establishes the scope, type, duration, and amount of services to be provided; sets the rate of payment; and administers its own program. Programs varied widely among states in terms of services covered. The ACA law mandates minimal essential health benefits, typically those that are offered in an employer's health plan. States will still have the option to offer a more comprehensive plan. The ACA law also invests in community health centers to allow greater access to care for enrollees. The reform law of 2010 includes a significant expansion of the Medicaid program, covering more

of the uninsured and providing subsidies to help low-income individuals buy coverage through newly established Health Benefit Exchanges.

The federal government, in the passage of the Deficit Reduction Act of 2005, made it harder for individuals to qualify for Medicaid nursing home benefits by increasing penalties on individuals who transferred assets for less than fair market value during the previous 5 years. Since long-term care is expensive, purchasing private long-term care insurance to cover nursing home care became an option in some states. Individuals who already have long-term care needs are not eligible and the cost of the premium increases with an individual's age. For older persons, the cost of the premium makes long-term care insurance unaffordable.

Passage of the welfare reform bill in 1996 (Personal Responsibility and Work Opportunity Reconciliation Act of 1996, Public Law 104-193) revealed a significant philosophical shift in federal thinking about welfare assistance in the United States. For the first time, Medicaid was not linked directly to welfare programs. Ending a 61-year guarantee of federal aid, the TANF (Temporary Assistance for Needy Families) program (formerly Aid to Families With Dependent Children) established by this legislation provides temporary financial aid with a 5-year lifetime limit. Legal immigrants who arrive in the United States after the passage of this bill must wait 5 years to become eligible for programs. The aim was to help parents become self-sufficient through welfare-to-work programs.

As part of the BBA of 1997, the State Children's Health Insurance Program (SCHIP) was enacted to provide health insurance coverage to children whose family's income is below 200% of the federal poverty level or whose family has an income 50% higher than the state's Medicaid eligibility threshold. Some states have expanded SCHIP eligibility to include family coverage. The program was approved for funding fiscal years 1998 to 2007 and was renewed in the ACA 2010 law.

Pharmaceutical Costs

The spiraling cost of prescription drugs continues to add to the complexity of providing adequate health care. Newer drugs cost more than the drugs they replace and contribute 50% of the increased cost. Increased utilization of prescription drugs adds to an increased cost per day of medications. Consumer demand sparked by drug advertisements, new indications for use, and increased consumer knowledge of available drugs has increased the demand for prescription medications. Increased drug cost is attributed to inflation, more days of therapy per user, greater number of drugs per user, cost of research and drug development, and advertising costs.

The Uninsured: Who Are They?

The United States has the highest proportion of population with no health insurance of all developed countries. The number of uninsured Americans younger than age 65 was estimated to be 46 million in 2008 and that number has risen as a result of the recent economic downturn and the growing cost of health plan premiums. The Affordable Care Act is

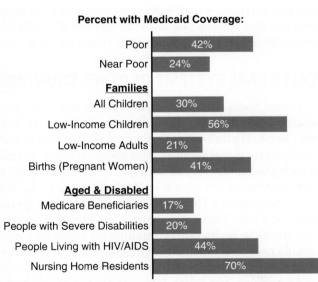

FIGURE 3-14 Medicaid's role for selected populations. (Source: Kaiser Commission on Medicaid and the Uninsured and Urban Institute analysis of 2009 ASEC Supplement to the CPS; Birth data from *Maternal and Child Health Update: States Increase Eligibility for Children's Health in 2007*, National Governors Association, 2008; Medicare data from USDHHS.

expected to reduce the number of uninsured by 60% with the expansion of Medicaid, subsidies to pay premiums in health insurance exchanges, a federal mandate requiring most legal citizens to enroll in an insurance plan or face tax penalties for noncompliance, and a provision allowing children to remain on their parents' employer family insurance until the age of 26. Previously, when children reached the age of 19 and were not full-time college students they were deleted from employer family insurance plans. The uninsured are a diverse population with greater numbers living in the South and West. By income, 41% of the uninsured are below 100% of federal poverty level (FPL), 37% are between 100% and 250% of FPL, 13% are between 251% and 399% of FPL, and 10% are above 400% of FPL. Most uninsured individuals are living in families in which there is at least one full-time worker. More men than women are uninsured (47% and 38%, respectively), and 15% are children (boys and girls). Of women who are uninsured, 28% are single parents, 39% are Latina, 38% have less than a high school education, 35% are foreign born, and 42% are below 100% of FPL. For all women in the 18 to 64 year old age group, 18% are uninsured.

The diversity of the uninsured population will require targeted outreach efforts and strategies to increase enrollment in available Medicaid and other insurance plans (KFF, 2010b, 2011b). Even with all the new options afforded by the ACA, a number of individuals will remain uninsured. Undocumented immigrants (those who are noncitizens and are living in the United States illegally) do not qualify for Medicaid or any other public insurance plan. As noncitizens they are also exempt from paying the federal tax penalty. This population is extremely vulnerable because of language and cultural barriers and fear of being discovered as an illegal immigrant; therefore, they typically do not seek health care. Provisions in current law require emergency care to be provided as well as care to pregnant women, regardless of alien status (KFF, 2010c). Another group of individuals are those who choose not to enroll and instead elect to pay the annual federal tax penalty. Once this portion of the law is enacted, it is expected that some Americans will seek legal recourse, questioning whether compulsorily insurance can be mandated as a violation of rights. Noncitizens who are legally travelling within the United States may not have health insurance coverage unless they have purchased secondary travel insurance before entering the United States.

Illegal Immigrants

The National Center for Policy Analysis reports the number of noncitizens illegally entering and living in the United States has significantly declined as a result of more effective border control and the recession resulting in fewer job opportunities. From 2000 to 2005, it was estimated that 850,000 illegal immigrants entered the United States each year for a total of about 12 million people. From 2007 to 2009, the PEW Hispanic Center and the Department of Homeland Security estimated approximately 300,000 illegal immigrants enter the United States each year. There were 7.8 million undocumented workers in the workforce in 2009, for a total of 11.1 million illegal immigrants (National Center for Policy Analysis, 2010). According to federal law, anyone entering an emergency room must be treated regardless of ability to pay or immigration status. U.S. border hospitals from Brownsville, Texas, to San Diego, California, are especially hard hit with the number of illegal immigrants crossing state lines and then seeking health care. Millions of dollars of uncompensated services are provided to undocumented immigrants across the country annually (National Center for Policy Analysis, 2010).

Another step toward addressing part of the problem for the uninsured and underinsured was the Health Insurance Portability and Accountability Act (HIPAA) (Public Law 104-191), which was passed in 1996 and took effect in 1997. The portability provision means that individuals with health insurance who lose or leave their jobs can maintain coverage even when they are sick. However, cost may be a prohibitive factor, because it does not regulate premium costs. Insurers are also prohibited from refusing coverage based on an individual's health status, although limited waiting periods may apply. Additionally, the bill allows individuals in small firms, uninsured individuals, or self-insured individuals with high-deductible plans to form a tax-exempt medical savings account (MSA) (see previous discussion). This MSA allows tax deductions for long-term care insurance premiums for those who qualify; provides support for unreimbursed home health and long-term care services; allows the terminally ill earlier access to earnings accrued in life insurance policies without tax penalties; establishes fraud and abuse guidelines; provides liability coverage for medical volunteers who provide free medical care to low-income individuals in medically underserved areas; and mandates that USHHS develop regulations and standards for the electronic transfer of medical information, confidentiality, and a unique health identifier. One of the most costly and complicated changes mandated by HIPAA is that health care companies must design interactive data systems that allow the transfer of health data while maintaining client confidentiality (USDHHS, n.d.).

HEALTH CARE SYSTEMS OF OTHER COUNTRIES

The United States spends the highest proportion of its gross domestic product (GNP) on health care of all industrialized countries (see Figure 3-4) with a reported GNP of 16% in 2008, 5.9% above the global average for the countries listed. America has the highest cost per capita (see Figure 3-2), reporting $7538 dollars were spent per person in 2008 compared to the next highest (Norway) at a little over $5000 and the lowest reported (Japan) at $2700. Figure 3-3 shows a graphic representation of the growth in health care expenditure per capita with other countries over time. Countries represented in Figures 3-2 and 3-3 all have some version of a universal health care plan and spend less money per capita. Life expectancy rates are higher and infant mortality rates are lower in these countries compared to the United States. Although each country has a different type of health plan, all share many of the same problems of the American free-market system. As mentioned earlier, rising health care costs; issues of access and affordability; workforce shortages of health care providers; increased concern over medical errors, quality of care, and safety; changing demographic population trends; and escalating health care costs are some of the inherent issues faced by all nations in providing health care.

Canadian Health Care System

The Canadian health care program, called Medicare, is a group of socialized health insurance plans that provide health coverage to all Canadian citizens regardless of medical history, personal income, or job status. The Canada Health Act, legislated at the federal level, determines what services must be provided, similar to the Medicaid program in the United States, but provinces and territories are not obligated to provide services not listed in the Act. The Act specifies basic services including primary care and hospitalizations, leaving the individual province or territory responsible for the management, organization, and delivery of health services for their residents. The Canada Health Act does not include services such as physical therapy, dental coverage, corrective lenses, home care, or prescription medicines but separate provinces can elect to provide enhancements. The five principles in the Canada Health Act are outlined in Box 3-12. Every Canadian citizen has the same basic primary health insurance that is covered by the national health care plan. Each Canadian citizen applies for a provincial health card and, once issued, the card accesses a person's medical information and is used when visiting a physician or health care provider, eliminating the need to fill out forms. Canadians pay for health care through a variety of federal and provincial taxes, just as Americans pay for Social Security and Medicare through

payroll taxes. The federal government appropriates funds to the provinces and territories through cash and tax transfers. Because the government is the primary payer of medical bills, Canada's health care system is referred to as a single-payer arrangement. Some provinces gain additional funds through sales tax, lottery proceeds, and health premiums. Additional benefits vary among the provinces, but most provide prescription drugs to older adults and low-income clients. Many services are not provided through the public health care provincial plans, so some Canadians either have supplemental private insurance obtained through their employers or have purchased insurance packages from private insurance providers to help pay for uncovered services such as dental care. In addition to public health care, private clinics offer specialized services not covered by the public health plan. Canadians covered by private health insurance typically have 80% of the costs covered at private clinics and receive specialized services not covered by the public health plan. Higher-income Canadians can pay out-of-pocket for care received at private clinics, which typically offer services with reduced wait times. For example, obtaining a magnetic resonance imaging (MRI) scan in a hospital may require a waiting period of months, whereas a private clinic could offer the scan much earlier. Canadians with private health insurance and higher incomes have access to greater health care services and more expedient health care.

At one time, the Canadian system seemed to be an ideal model that the United States should adopt; however, increasing health care costs, access issues, delays in treatment, and workforce shortages of health care providers have caused political controversy and debate in Canada. Queuing refers to a system where a person is placed on a wait list before receiving certain types of tests or surgery, allowing a person who is in need of more immediate care to receive priority. If care needs are determined to be non–life-threatening, persons may need to wait for MRIs, heart bypass surgeries, cataract removal, or hip replacement procedures for months since persons in urgent need of the procedures are higher on the list. Although all citizens receive the same level of public health care, private insurance allows a two-tiered system favoring Canadians with private health insurance or other financial resources to receive expedited care. If a person can pay out-of-pocket, they may elect to travel elsewhere (for example, to the United States) to receive expedited care. A major shortage of physicians and nurses in Canada is due in part to lower reimbursement rates by the public health system as well as lower salaries, causing some health care providers to leave Canada and practice in other countries such as the United States. Over the years, the federal government has decreased contributions to the provinces and territories because of large federal budget deficits and limited fee increases to physicians for services. Regionalization of hospitals has caused access to care issues for those outside of major cities. Expansion to offer better access to home care and community-based services is an emerging issue. A greater percentage of physicians are PCPs, not specialists like in the United States (Barr, 2008; NCHS, 2011).

BOX 3-12 FIVE PRINCIPLES OF THE CANADA HEALTH ACT

- *Universality:* All insured residents of a province or territory must be entitled to the same level of health care provided by the provincial or territorial health care insurance plan. Excluded persons are tourists, a transient visitor to the province, serving members of the Canadian Forces or Royal Canadian Mounted Police, and inmates of federal penitentiaries.
- *Portability:* A resident who moves to a different providence or territory is still entitled to coverage from his/her home province during a minimal wait period. This also applies to residents who leave the country.
- *Accessibility:* Residents of a providence or territory are entitled to have access on uniform terms and conditions to insured health services at the setting where the services are provided and as the services are available in that setting.
- *Comprehensiveness:* Provincial plans must cover all insured health services provided by hospitals, physicians, or dentists (includes only surgical-dental services that require a hospital setting).
- *Public administration:* All administration of provincial health insurance must be carried out by public authority on a nonprofit basis and must be accountable to the province or territory.

From *Canadian Health Act.* Retrieved January 22, 2012, from http://canadianhealthcare.org/page2.html.

CASE STUDY

Health Teaching: Using The Internet to Increase Health Literacy

Ella, age 34, has been married for 10 years to her husband Joe and recently moved to a new area with their 2 children, Billy, age 11 and Olivia, age 6. Joe just started a new position in a state agency and Ella plans to work 3 to 4 days a week as a home health aide. Joe completed a 2-year college degree and Ella took a few college courses but never finished her degree. The family is new to a primary care clinic and Ella asks the nurse for advice in choosing a health plan that will best meet the needs of her family. Ella and her husband would like to have a third child in the next year or so. Her husband Joe was given a folder at his new job with multiple health plans to choose from and asked Ella to "just pick one" because they are too complicated to understand. Joe considers himself healthy and active, although he has had recommendations in the past to lose 30 pounds, is borderline hypertensive, and has slightly elevated blood lipid levels. He has a strong family history of coronary artery disease and his father died from a myocardial infarction at the age of 65. Ella also struggles with a few extra pounds and often relies on fast food for quick dinners on the days she works. Their son Billy was diagnosed with attention-deficit/hyperactivity disorder (ADHD) and Olivia has asthma. Both children are above the recommended body mass index levels for their ages. The family has a home computer with Internet access and Ella states she is "getting better at using it as her 6th grade son is learning computer literacy in school and is teaching Mom."

The nurse discusses the family's general health promotion and protection needs and the special needs presented by the diseases that have been identified.

She provides some resources for Ella to learn more about the health plans available to her and consumer-friendly health information websites.

Reflective Questions

1. What additional information does the nurse need to assess this family's needs?
2. What are the priority area teaching needs for this family?
3. What community resources might be available to Ella and her family?
4. What are some appropriate websites that Ella might find useful?

Before leaving, the nurse suggests the following:

- From the Agency for Healthcare Research and Quality (AHRQ), a federal government agency with health information for consumers on guidelines in choosing a health plan: www.ahrq.gov/consumer/insuranceqa/
- From the U.S. Department of Labor, a federal agency that provides information on health plans, benefits, and has many links: www.dol.gov/
- For health care information on multiple topics:
  Health-Care Information.org: www.health-care-information.org
  *Web*MD: http://webmd.com/
  Healthfinder/: http://healthfinder.gov/
  Mayo Clinic: www.mayoclinic.com/

SUMMARY

The nursing workforce, composed of more than 3 million nurses, is the largest segment of the nation's health care workforce and nurses will be key players in moving forward the objectives set forth in the 2010 Affordable Care Act and *Healthy People 2020*. In order to move these agendas forward, nurses need to understand the complexity of the health care system— the structures (federal, state, and local) and the financing mechanisms (public and private)—so interventions can be targeted to reduce health disparities and promote health equity for all Americans. The IOM recognized a number of barriers exist that prevent nurses from being able to respond effectively to rapidly changing health care settings and an evolving health care system. Nurses need to be proactive in shaping policy that affects the health care system and need a working understanding of the complexity of the health care system to be able to educate individuals and families about health care resources, to coordinate services, and to influence health care policy at the local, state, and national levels. To accomplish this task, nurses need to become and remain well-informed citizens and health care consumer advocates.

A historical perspective and a description of the current health care delivery system in the United States provide a framework for the analysis of trends, values, and needs related to health. Awareness of global health indicators sets the stage for the nurse to then compare the health of the nation as a whole. The structure and financing of the health care system, both public and private sectors, are complicated. The influence of recent health reform, the PPACA of 2010, sparks an opportunity for nurses to be key players in engaging effectively to deliver high-quality evidence-based nursing care and move forward the agendas of *Healthy People 2020* and the IOM's *Future of Nursing*.

REFERENCES

Alzheimer's Association. (2011). *2011 Alzheimer's disease facts and figures.* Retrieved January 22, 2012, from www.alz.org/downloads/Facts_Figures_2011.pdf.

American Red Cross. (2012). *American Red Cross homepage.* Retrieved January 23, 2012, from www.redcross.org/portal/site.

Arias, E., & Smith, B. (2003). Deaths: Preliminary data for 2001 (Online). *National Vital Statistics Report, 51*(5), 1–44. Retrieved May 1, 2004, from www.cdc.gov/nchs/data/nvsr/nvsr51/nvs51r_05.pdf.

Barr, D. (2008). *Introduction to U.S. health policy: The organization, financing, and delivery of health care in America* (2nd ed.). Baltimore, MD: Johns Hopkins University Press.

Bartfield, W. (2011). *Infant mortality prevention: A community and public health approach.* Retrieved January 25, 2012, from www.ced.gov/reproductivehealth/.

Centers for Disease Control and Prevention (CDC). (2012a). *Department of Health and Human Services. Injury prevention and control: Data statistics.* Retrieved January 20, 2012, from www.cdc.gov/injury/wisqars/leadingcauses.html.

Centers for Disease Control and Prevention (CDC). (2012b). *Global TB.* Retrieved January 2, 2012, from www.cdc.gov/tb/topic/global tb/default.htm.

Centers for Disease Control and Prevention (CDC). (2012c). *Trends in tuberculosis fact sheet 2010.* Retrieved January 2, 2012, from www.cdc.gov/tb/publications/factsheets/statistics/TBTrends.htm.

Centers for Disease Control Foundation. (2010). *Hospitals, beds, and occupancy rates by type of ownership.* Retrieved January 21, 2012, from www.cdc.gov/nchs/data/hus/2010/116.pdf.

Centers for Disease Control Foundation. (2012). *How CDC saves lives by controlling REAL global disease outbreaks.* Retrieved January 20, 2012, from www.cdcfoundation.org/content/how-cdc-saves-lives-controlling-real-global-disease-outbreaks.

Centers for Medicare & Medicaid Services (CMS). (2011). *National health expenditure projections 2010-2020 forecast summary and selected tables*. Retrieved January 22, 2012, from www.cms.gov/NationalHealthExpandData/03_download.

Centers for Medicare & Medicaid Services (CMS). (n.d.). *State children's health insurance program (SCHIP) homepage*. Retrieved January 22, 2012, from www.cms.gov/apps/firststep/content/schip-qas.html.

Central Intelligence Agency. (2012). *The world fact book*. Retrieved January 25, 2012, from http://cia.gov/library/publications/the-world-factbook.

Community Health and Empowerment through Education and Research (CHEER). (2011). *What is a healthy community?* Retrieved January 25, 2012, from http://communitycheer.org/indicators/health/what-is-a-healthy-community/.

Freyman, J. G. (1980). *The American health care system: Its genesis and trajectory*. Huntington, NY: Krieger.

Government Accountability Office (GAO). (2005). *Physician services: Concierge care characteristics and considerations for Medicare*. Retrieved January 10, 2012, from http://gao.gov/new.items/d05929.

Haben, J. (2008, January 17). *Army news releases*. Retrieved from www.armymedicine.army.mil/news/releases/20080117tbitfrepart.cfm.

Holder, V. (2004). From handmaiden to right hand—The infancy of nursing. *AORN Journal, 79*(2), 374–382, 385–390.

Institute for Nursing Centers. (n.d.). *Home page*. Retrieved January 20, 2012, from www.nursingcenters.org/.

Institute of Medicine of the National Academies (IOM). (1999). *To err is human: Building a safer health system*. Retrieved January 23, 2012, from www.iom.edu/Reports/1999/To-Err-is-Human-Building-A-Safer-Health-System.aspx.

Institute of Medicine of the National Academies. (2003). *Keeping patients safe: Transforming the work environment of nurses*. Retrieved January 20, 2012, from www.iom.edu/Reports/2003/Keeping-Patients-Safe-Transforming-the-Work-Environment-of-Nurses.aspx.

Institute of Medicine of the National Academies. (2006). *Preventing medication errors: Quality chasm series*. Retrieved January 18, 2012, from www.iom.edu/Reports/2006/Preventing-Medication-Errors-Quality-Chasm-Series.aspx.

Institute of Medicine of the National Academies. (2010, October 5). *The future of nursing: Leading change, advancing health*. Retrieved January 2, 2012, from www.iom.edu/Reports/2010/The-Future-of-Nursing-Leading-Change-Advancing-Health.aspx.

Institute of Medicine of the National Academies (IOM). (2012). *Barriers to integrating crisis standards of care principles into international disaster response plans-workplace summary*. Retrieved January 25, 2012, from www.iom.edu/Reports/2012/Barriers-to-Integrating-Crisis-Standards-of-Care-Principles-into-international.*

Jeter, L. (2007, November). *Hospitalist movement gaining ground*. Medical News Papers, Inc. Retrieved from www.medicalnewsinc.com/news.php?viewStory=94.

John, A., & Hartford Foundation. (2012). *About us*. Retrieved January 22, 2012, from www.jhartfound.org/about_us.htm.

Kaiser Family Foundation (KFF). (2009). *Medicare advantage fact sheet*. Menlo Park, CA: The Henry J. Kaiser Family Foundation. Retrieved from www.kff.org, Publication #2052-12.

Kaiser Family Foundation (KFF). (2010, October). *Kaiser Commission on Medicaid facts, Medicaid and the uninsured*. Retrieved from www.kff.org, Publication #7580–07.

Kaiser Family Foundation (KFF). (2010a). *Focus on health reform: Explaining health care reform: Questions about Medicaid's role*. Menlo Park, CA: The Henry J. Kaiser Family Foundation. Retrieved January 24, 2012, from www.kff.org, Publication #7920–02, April 2010.

Kaiser Family Foundation (KFF). (2010b). *Health policy center: The uninsured*. Menlo Park, CA: The Henry J. Kaiser Family Foundation. Retrieved January 24, 2012, from www.urban.org/health_policy/uninsured/index.cfm.

Kaiser Family Foundation (KFF). (2010c). *Health policy center: Vulnerable populations*. Menlo Park, CA: The Henry J. Kaiser Family Foundation. Retrieved January 24, 2012, from www.urban.org/health_policy/vulnerable_popuations/index.cfm.

Kaiser Family Foundation (KFF). (2011a). *Focus on health reform: Summary of new health reform law*. Menlo Park, CA: The Henry J. Kaiser Family Foundation. Retrieved January 24, 2012, from www.kff.org, Publication #8061, April 15, 2011.

Kaiser Family Foundation (KFF). (2011b). *Medicare advantage plans star ratings and bonus payments*. Menlo Park, CA: The Henry J. Kaiser Family Foundation. Retrieved January 24, 2012, from www.kff,org, Publication #8257, November 2011.

Kaiser Family Foundation (KFF). (2011c). *Employer health benefits: 2011 summary of findings*. Menlo Park, CA: The Henry J. Kaiser Family Foundation. Retrieved January 24, 2012, from www.kff.org, Publication #8225, November 2011.

Kaiser Family Foundation (KFF). (2011d). *Connecting eligible immigrant families to health coverage and care: Key lessons from outreach and enrollment workers*. Menlo Park, CA: The Henry J. Kaiser Family Foundation. Retrieved January 22, 2012, from www.kff.org, Publication #8249, October 27, 2011.

Kaiser Family Foundation (KFF). (2011e). *Medicare at a glance*. Menlo Park, CA: The Henry J. Kaiser Family Foundation. Retrieved January 22, 2012, from www.kff.org, Publication #1066–14, November 2011.

Kaiser Family Foundation (KFF). (2012a). *Kaiser health tracking poll: The APA and the Supreme Court*. Menlo Park, CA: The Henry J. Kaiser Family Foundation. Retrieved January 24, 2012, from http://healthreform.kff.org/scan/2012/january.

Kaiser Family Foundation (KFF). (2012b). *Kaiser Commission on Medicaid and the uninsured*. Menlo Park, CA: The Henry J. Kaiser Family Foundation. Retrieved January 24, 2012, from http://kff.org, Publication #8272–2.pdf.

Kovner, A., & Knickman, J. (2011). *Jonas & Kovner's health care delivery in the United States* (10th ed.). New York: Springer.

Kudzma, E. (2006). Florence Nightingale's application of statistics to promote reform. *Nursing Science Quarterly, 19*(1), 61–64.

Kuo, Y., & Goodwin, J. (2011). Association of hospitalist care with medical utilization after discharge: Evidence of cost shift from a cohort study. *Annals of Internal Medicine, 155*(3), 152–159.

MacDorman, M., & Matthews, T. (2008). *Recent trends in infant mortality in the United States. NCHS Data brief #9*. Retrieved January 20, 2012, from www.cdc.gov/nchc/data/databriefs/db09.htm.

Marquis, J. (2004). *Concierge medical practice expanding across the nation*. Warner, Norcross & Judd. Retrieved from www.wnj.com/concierge_22004/.

Martin, J., Hamilton, B., Ventura, S., Osterman, M., Kirmap, S., et al. (2011, November). Births: Final data for 2009. *National Vital Statistics Report, 60*, 1–72.

Melnyk, B., & Fineout-Overholt, E. (2011). *Evidence-based practice in nursing and healthcare: A guide to best practice*. Philadelphia: Wolters Kluwer Health: Lippincott Williams & Wilkins.

National Center for Health Statistics (NCHS). (2011). *Health, United States, 2010 with special features on death and dying.* Hyattsville, MD: Author.

National Center for Policy Analysis. (2010). *Fewer illegal immigrants entering United States.* Retrieved January 20, 2012, from http://ncpa.org/sub/dpd/index.php?Article_ID=19785.

Nies, M., & McEwen, M. (2007). *Community/public health nursing: Promoting the health of populations* (4th ed.). Philadelphia: Saunders.

Office of the Legislative Council (OLC). (2010, May). *Compilation of Patient Protection and Affordable Care Act as amended through May, 1, 2010.* 111th Congress. PPACA Public Law 114–148.

Shi, L., & Singh, D. (2005). *Essentials of the US health care system.* Sudbury, MA: Jones & Bartlett.

Social Security On-Line. (n.d.). *History.* Retrieved January 10, 2012, from www.ssa.gov/history/lifeexpect.html.

Society of Hospital Medicine. (n.d.). *Definition of a hospitalist and hospital medicine.* Retrieved January 10, 2012, from www.hospitalmedicine.org/AM/Template.cfm?Section=Hospitalist_Definitions&;Template=/CM/HTMLDisplay.

Stanhope, M., & Lancaster, J. (2012). *Public health nursing: Population-Centered Health Care* (8th ed.). St Louis: Mosby.

U.S. Department of Defense (USDOD). (n.d.). *Military Health System. Frequently asked questions.* Retrieved January 20, 2012, from www.health.mil/About_MHS/FAQs.aspx.

U.S. Department of Defense (USDOD). (n.d.). *TRICARE overview.* Retrieved January 22, 2012, from www.tricare.mil/mybenefit/ProfileFilter.

U.S. Department of Homeland Security. (2011). *Federal Assistance Management Agency homepage.* Retrieved January 23, 2012, from www.fema.gov/.

U.S. Department of Health and Human Services (USDHHS). (2011a). *Healthy People 2020: Leading health indicators.* Retrieved December 23, 2011, from www.healthypeople.gov/2020/LHI/data/.

U.S. Department of Health and Human Services (USDHHS). (2011b). *Plan for retrospective review of existing rules.* Retrieved December 23, 2011, from www.hhs_final_retrospective_review_plan_8-19-11_4.pdf.

U.S. Department of Health and Human Services (USDHHS). (2011c). *Medicare fact sheet: What providers need to know-accountable care organizations.* Retrieved January 19, 2012, from http://healthreform.kff.org/Document-Finder/CMS/CMS-ACO-Fact-Sheet-for-Providers.aspx.

U.S. Department of Health and Human Services, & Office of Minority Health (USDHHS-OMH). (2012). *HHS action plan to reduce racial and ethnic health disparities.* Retrieved January 5, 2012, from www.minorityhealth.hhs.gov/npa/templates/content.aspx.

U.S. Department of Health and Human Services (USDHHS). (n.d.). *Health information privacy.* Retrieved January 12, 2012, from www.hhs.gov/ocr/privacy/hipaa/understanding/index.html.

U.S. Department of Health and Human Services (USDHHS), Health Resources and Services. (2010). *The registered nurse population: Initial findings from the 2008 national sample survey of registered nurses.* U.S. Department of Health and Human Services: HRSA Health Resources and Services Administration.

U.S. Department of Homeland Security. (n.d.). *FEMA.* Retrieved January 2, 2012, from www.fema.gov/Homepage.

U.S. Department of Labor. (2010). *Bureau of labor statistics: Career guide to industries (CGI), 2010-2011 edition.* Retrieved from www.bls.gov/oco/cg/cgs035.htm.

U.S. Public Health Nursing Services. (n.d.) *Chief nurse.* Retrieved January 22, 2012, from http://phs-nurse.org/index.php/chief-nurse.html.

World Health Organization. (2012). *The WHO agenda.* Retrieved January 20, 2012, from www.who.int/about/agenda/en/index.html/.

The Therapeutic Relationship

June Andrews Horowitz[*]

WEBSITE

http://evolve.elsevier.com/Edelman/
- Study Questions
- Glossary

OBJECTIVES

After completing this chapter, the reader will be able to:
- Evaluate values clarification as a prerequisite to effective health promotion.
- Examine the elements and process of communication.
- Analyze differences between functional and dysfunctional communication.

- Develop strategies to promote therapeutic relationships with diverse populations across clinical settings, contexts, and nursing roles.
- Synthesize knowledge of the therapeutic relationship as an essential component of health promotion.

KEY TERMS

15-minute interview
Communication process
Countertransference
Empathy
Feedback
Health literacy
Helping or therapeutic relationship
Input
Johari window
Metacommunication

Milieu
Nonverbal communication
Output
Practical reflection
Process
Proxemics
Rapport
Reciprocity
Reflection
Relationship stages

Self-concept
Self-disclosure
Self-esteem
Telehealth or mhealth
Therapeutic use of self
Transference
Values clarification
Verbal communication

*Assistance with this chapter revision was provided by Christy Tran, Undergraduate Research Fellow, Wm. F. Connell School of Nursing, Boston College.

THINK ABOUT IT

How Does a Nurse Respond When an Individual's Values Conflict with the Nurse's Value of Promoting Healthy Behaviors?

Samantha, a 17-year-old girl, comes into the health clinic at her school to ask the nurse practitioner to prescribe birth control pills for her and to check her for a vaginal discharge. The nurse begins the appointment by asking Samantha about her chief complaint of discharge. Samantha answers these questions until the nurse asks about her relationship with her boyfriend. Samantha comments, "Don't worry about me. We're in love and I just need birth control pills so I won't get pregnant." When the nurse introduces the topic of health risks associated with unprotected sex, Samantha says, "Look, I don't need a lecture. You sound like my mother. I know what I'm doing and I don't need condoms because he's not with anyone else."

As you read this chapter, think about how you could use the content to answer the questions.

- How can this nurse bridge the apparent gap between the nurse's values and Samantha's values?

- In this brief encounter, how can the nurse begin to establish a therapeutic relationship?
- What responsibilities does the nurse need to weigh in responding to Samantha's request?
- What health risks exist if the nurse accepts or refuses to grant Samantha's request?
- What does the nurse need to know about policies and care decisions for individuals who are not legal adults? What school health policies might affect the nurse's scope of practice and dialogue with Samantha? How might the nurse use this encounter to promote communication among stakeholders including elected officials (e.g., school committee members), school administrators, school nurses, parents, and students?
- What strategies could the nurse use to engage Samantha in a conversation about her sexual behaviors and related health issues?

The therapeutic relationship is the milieu in which nursing care occurs. Nursing practice is shaped by the caregiver's ability to focus on the interests, concerns, and needs of the individual (Peplau, 1991). As illustrated in the above scenario, a therapeutic relationship will be critical in problem resolution. Nurse-person interaction is an "interpersonal process in which both parties have an emotional involvement with each other, there is a degree of mutuality and reciprocity whereby needs and expectations are shared" (Carter, 2009, p. 394).

Particularly in health promotion, the nurse-person relationship is the context for care. Health promotion requires sensitivity to each person's goals and values—the individual's and the nurse's. Helping a person adopt health-promoting behaviors requires more than giving information. Health promotion also requires effective communication, which is why communication is a focus area of *Healthy People 2020* (U.S. Department of Health and Human Services, 2010) and thus a priority for nursing practice. Successful health promotion involves interpersonal skills, personal insight, accountability, mutual respect, and a supportive working milieu. Essential to this interactional process are values clarification, communication, and the helping relationship. See Box 4-1: *Healthy People 2020* for the Leading Health Indicators and Priorities for Action.

VALUES CLARIFICATION

Definition

Values are qualities, principles, attitudes, or beliefs about the inherent worth of an object, behavior, or idea that guide action by sanctioning certain behaviors and disavowing others. Values and beliefs are essential factors in design and implementation of nursing interventions. To serve the unique and diverse needs of patients, it is imperative that nurses understand the importance of cultural differences by valuing, incorporating, and examining their own health-related values and beliefs and those of their health care organizations, for only then can they support the principle of respect for persons and the ideal of transcultural care (Bjarnason et al., 2009). Cognitive values are those

BOX 4-1   HEALTHY PEOPLE 2020

Leading Health Indicators
- Access to health services
- Clinical preventive services
- Environmental quality
- Injury and violence
- Maternal, infant, and child health
- Mental health
- Nutrition, physical activity, and obesity
- Oral health
- Reproductive and sexual health
- Social determinants
- Substance abuse
- Tobacco

Priorities for Action
- Adopt the 12 *Leading Health Indicators* as personal and professional guides for choices about how to make health improvements.
- Encourage public health professionals and public officials to adopt the *Leading Health Indicators* as the basis for public health priority setting and decision-making.
- Urge public and community health systems and our community leadership to use the *Leading Health Indicators* as measures of local success for investments in health improvements.

From U.S. Department of Health and Human Services. (n.d.). *Healthy People 2010. Leading health indicators.* Retrieved January 5, 2012, from www.healthypeople.gov/2020/LHI/default.aspx#.

a person ascribes to verbally and intellectually. Active values, in contrast, are those a person physically acts out. Judging the power of a given value by its ability to influence action is important. For example, a nurse may claim to value the worth of all people equally, but may treat individuals of various races differently and provide the most time and concern for those who are racially similar to the nurse. This cognitive value has little power to shape the nurse's behavior. If the nurse treated people of all races with equal respect, the value would also be active and have great power to motivate behavior.

BOX 4-2 THE VALUING PROCESS

Choosing
1. Choosing freely
2. Choosing from alternatives
3. Choosing after careful consideration of potential outcomes of each alternative

Prizing
4. Cherishing and being happy with personal beliefs and actions
5. Affirming the choice in public, when appropriate

Acting
6. Acting out the choice
7. Repeatedly acting in some type of pattern

BOX 4-3 TECHNIQUES FOR ASSISTING INDIVIDUALS TO CLARIFY VALUES

Identify the Individual's Values
"What is important to you?"
"Which of the following statements sounds most like the way you think?"
"What do you value most in life?"

Use Reflection to Restate the Value and Make it Explicit
"In what you've just told me, I hear that it is very important to you that..."
"I understand that you value..."

Identify Value Conflicts or Conflicts Between Values and Actions
"What connection does this value have to your current health or illness and to the healthy behaviors, interventions, or treatments needed to maintain or restore your health?"
"How does this particular value affect your behavior and health?"
"What are some ways that you might put your values into action?"
"Are your actions consistent with your values? If not, then what might you change?"

Many forces shape values. Passed down from one generation to another, values color an individual's identity, goals, and sense of personal meaning. Values are embedded in the culture and taught within a family and social context, giving meaning to the life events and happenings outside the family's boundaries (Wright & Leahey, 2009). To engage in health promotion, the nurse must appreciate that values are culture-bound and explore how culture, traditions, and practices in a multiethnic and multicultural society influence health-related values. Without this understanding, the nurse is likely to relate to individuals with a limited awareness of their assumptions and inadequate sensitivity to the uniqueness and perspective of the person, family, or community.

Values evolve; they are not static. Life events and social processes can spark a reappraisal of personal values. **Values clarification** is a method for discovering one's values and the importance of these values (Raths et al., 1978). Values clarification does not tell a person how to act, but it helps people recognize what values they hold and evaluate how those values influence their actions.

Box 4-2 outlines seven steps in the valuing process. The first three steps involve a cognitive process, the next two steps involve the affective or emotional domain, and the final steps involve behavior (Raths et al., 1978; Stuart & Laraia, 2009). The nurse uses values clarification to examine personal values and their potential influence on nursing care, and to help people identify their values and reflect on their connection to health-related behaviors. Box 4-3 lists suggestions for putting values clarification into action. For a values clarification exercise, try following the steps outlined in Box 4-3 in regard to a personal value.

Values clarification becomes a clinical aim when individuals' values lead to behaviors that conflict with the nurse's value of promoting health. For example, a nurse tells a childbirth education class consisting of pregnant women and their coaches that alcohol use poses serious risks to the fetus. After the class, one woman comments, "Do you really think that having a drink once in a while is bad for the baby? I'm sick of being told that I can't do things because of the baby." In this example, an apparent conflict in values between the nurse and the individual exists. Intervention is needed to examine how this woman's wish for freedom from restrictions clashes with her desire to have a healthy child. Nurses must consider their own values related to health promotion for the individual and the fetus and must

weigh the importance of respecting individuals' rights to make decisions about their own health behaviors. Such value conflicts result in ethical dilemmas. Resolution rests on the nurse's ability to examine conflicting values and available evidence about possible outcomes when fashioning health-promotion interventions.

Values and Therapeutic Use of Self

The self, the most precious and unique of all human endowments, is a personal concept of individuality as distinct from other people and objects. **Therapeutic use of self** is the application of one's cognitions, perceptions, and behaviors to create interpersonal encounters that promote health in another person, family, group, or community. Without self-awareness and clarification of values, therapeutic use of self is impaired. **Self-concept** and **self-esteem** are interrelated components of individuals' judgments and attitudes about themselves. Self-concept is a mental picture of the self—a composite view of personal characteristics, abilities, limitations, and aspirations. Self-esteem, the affective component of self-perception, refers to how individuals feel about the way that they see themselves. Internalized appraisals from others also influence self-concept and self-esteem.

Self-concept evolves throughout life. From birth, family experiences and parental identification mold the child's sense of identity. The classic research studies of Coopersmith (1967) and Sears (1970) demonstrated positive relationships between the self-reliance, self-esteem, and self-confidence of parents and children. Self-esteem is learned from experience (Roth-Herbst et al., 2008). To cultivate children's self-esteem and enable them to have a realistic perception of their strengths and weaknesses, parents should focus on positives, give feedback on abilities and limitations, and provide the child with a sense of belonging and realistic confidence. Positive, rewarding, anxiety-free interactions contribute to security, esteem, and positive self-view. Positive but realistic appraisals from significant others, especially the parents, help the young child to develop this healthy self-view (Brown, 2008; Sullivan, 1953).

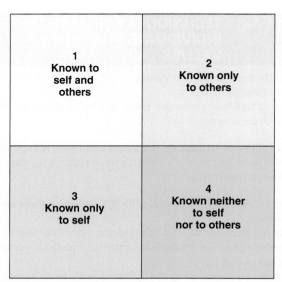

1 Known to self and others	2 Known only to others
3 Known only to self	4 Known neither to self nor to others

FIGURE 4-1 Johari window. (From Luft, J. [1984]. *Group processes: An introduction to group dynamics* [3rd ed.]. Palo Alto, CA: Mayfield. Reprinted with permission from Mayfield.)

The self does not develop solely in response to the reflected appraisals of others. Genetic endowment, experiential opportunities, and the individual's action shape self-concept. People can accept or reject the appraisals of others and modify their behavior. The ability to control actions and evaluate outcomes of interactions allows individuals to modify and alter their views of self. As such, the self is dynamic, changing through interaction with the outside world and in response to the various maturational and situational crises of life.

The ability to examine, reflect on, and evaluate the self is a uniquely human talent. Self-awareness involves interactions between the self and the external world and the symbolic connections created by the individual. The self includes an unconscious component that is only partially accessible and influences behavior. Self-awareness is influenced by the degree to which an individual has an accurate concept of all dimensions of the self. The Johari window (Luft, 1984) provides a schema for understanding the various components of the self (Figure 4-1). Box 4-4 lists these four components of the self.

Together, these windowpanes represent the total self. Three principles guide an understanding of how the self functions in this representation: change in one portion influences all other portions; the smaller the first portion, the poorer the ensuing communication; and interpersonal learning enlarges the first portion and decreases the size of one or more other portions (Luft, 1969). The goal of self-awareness is to increase the size of the first windowpane while reducing the size of the other three areas (Stuart & Laraia, 2009) (Figure 4-2).

Consider the differences between windows A and B of Figure 4-2. Window A represents an individual with little self-awareness. Windowpane number 4 is large, suggesting that a good deal of the person's experiences, thoughts, and feelings are repressed or suppressed, probably a result of associated anxiety. Additionally, window A suggests a large "not me" portion of the self. In contrast, window B represents a person who is open to the world and is comfortable with his or her self-concept.

BOX 4-4   COMPONENTS OF THE SELF

1. The *public self*, which is shown to others
2. The *semipublic self*, which is seen by others but may be outside the individual's awareness
3. The *private self*, which is known to the individual, but not revealed to others
4. The *inner self*, which is the unconscious portion not known even to the individual because it has anxiety-provoking content

The goal of high self-awareness, as illustrated in window B of Figure 4-2, is reached through three steps. The first step is listening to oneself and paying attention to emotions, thoughts, memories, reactions, and impulses. Frequently, people ignore their feelings and thoughts because they are anxious or because they are in a hurry to accomplish some other task. Without self-reflection, people act automatically and lose some of the meaning of living. To improve the ability of self-reflection, ask questions such as the following:

- What am I feeling now?
- What emotions have I experienced today and in the past day or so? What were my thoughts?
- What events led to these thoughts and feelings?
- What actions did I take? Did my behavior fit with my thoughts and feelings, or was there a lack of harmony?
- Was I aware of my reactions at the time that they took place?
- How have I responded in clinical situations lately?
- How did I react in response to a particularly happy, sad, or difficult situation? In what way might I alter my actions now? What feelings and reactions did I experience while interacting with this individual?

The second step is listening to and learning from others. Feedback from others that conflicts with self-image can produce anxiety. In response, the feedback is ignored or translated incorrectly to preserve self-image and reduce anxiety. However, this pattern of responding limits knowledge of the self and inhibits the ability to examine the appraisals of others, resulting in limited personal growth. Asking reflective questions enables the nurse to use feedback effectively. Helpful questions include "What feedback have I received today?" and "What is the other person trying to tell me now?" A person also can ask others directly for feedback. For example, a student nurse might ask another student how he or she comes across. The feedback might be used to alter aspects of behavior that are ineffective or problematic before asking a faculty member for evaluative feedback. Using clinical supervision and consultation with colleagues provides needed opportunity for reflection on practice. How the nurse comes across to the individual, family, or community is crucial to successful health promotion, making self-awareness and sensitivity to feedback essential.

The third step is self-disclosure; sharing aspects of the self enriches interpersonal life. Through self-disclosure, people come to know themselves better because they have exposed their thoughts, actions, and feelings for examination with others. Self-disclosure is an indicator of a healthy personality

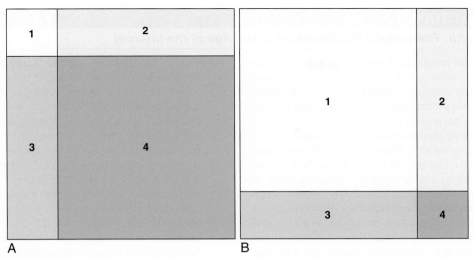

FIGURE 4-2 Johari windows illustrate varying degrees of self-awareness. **A,** Person has little self-awareness. **B,** Person has great amount of self-awareness. *1,* Public self; *2,* semipublic self; *3,* private self; *4,* inner self. (From Stuart, G. W., & Laraia, M.T. [2009]. *Principles and practice of psychiatric nursing* [9th ed.]. St Louis: Elsevier Mosby.)

and a strategy for developing one (Jourard, 1971; Stuart & Laraia, 2009). Self-disclosure by one person tends to trigger self-disclosure by another in a reciprocal pattern of interaction. Therapeutic interactions characterized by reciprocity involve a mutual exchange—a pattern of communication between the nurse and an individual, not a one-way intervention from the nurse to the other person. Traditionally, clinicians have been wary of self-disclosure because it may cross a boundary from a professional to a personal relationship. Additionally, the nurse's self-disclosure might burden the individual and shift the focus of attention from the individual to the nurse. Although these guidelines are considered in order to prevent excessive or inappropriate self-disclosure, appreciation that self-disclosure occurs within human interactions is needed. Dziopa and Ahern (2009b) found that experienced psychiatric nurses identified appropriate self-revelation as an effective component of therapeutic relationship. Nurses are not blank screens, robots, or technicians delivering care; individuals value nurses who engage in interactions as real people and who are willing to share information about themselves. Seeking consultation from a colleague is helpful whenever a concern arises regarding limits of appropriate self-disclosure.

Practical reflection involves deliberating one's own thoughts and recollections of events to understand them and to take needed corrective action. In reflection thoughts are pondered to be interpreted or analyzed. The process tends to be triggered by a seminal or meaningful event or situation and the process results in increased understanding or awareness. These insights can then be used in the future when faced with a similar event or situation (Sanders, 2009). The process of practical reflection dovetails with steps toward self-awareness previously described and offers complementary helpful tips. First, the nurse recalls an incident when something went wrong. Then the nurse experiences the incident again by remembering images and by privately retelling events, statements, outcomes, and associated emotions. Next, the nurse interprets the story of communication that failed by examining expectations, ideals, goals, influences, personal actions, and others' actions that occurred during the event. The last step involves honest inspection of the nurse's own role in the story. Insights gained may be applied to prevent repetition of the problem.

Why is it important for a nurse to clarify personal values and increase self-awareness? The nurse's values and self-understanding influence behavior. The self is the nurse's greatest tool; to use the self effectively, the nurse must be fully aware of how it functions. Thus, reflection and self-awareness guide the nurse's practice framework. In addition, sensitivity to individuals' perspectives is required to build a collaborative partnership, the cornerstone of the nurse-person relationship (Doss et al., 2011). Helping individuals to explicate their values and direct their actions accordingly toward health-related goals embodies patient-centered care as defined by QSEN (Quality and Safety Education for Nurses [QSEN], 2012): "Recognize the patient or designee as the source of control and full partner in providing compassionate and coordinated care based on respect for patient's preferences, values, and needs."

THE COMMUNICATION PROCESS

The communication process is the forum for all thought and relationships shared among people. In conjunction with the use of scientific and technological advances, communication is an essential tool for the nurse to engage in health-promotion interventions. Communication is the foundation for any professional relationship. Nurse-patient communication plays a vital role in the formation and development of the nurse-patient relationship. It is the glue that connects individuals' learning and satisfaction with care (Tejero, 2011). Communication is an information exchange between individuals through shared symbols and signs and commonly understood behavior (Ruesch &

BOX 4-5 HOT TOPICS

Telehealth/mHealth: Therapeutic Relationships in the Age of the Internet

Technological advances have produced rapid changes in communication. Automatic teller machines have replaced human tellers at banks for routine transactions. Voicemail rather than a receptionist routinely answers calls, and messages are recorded electronically. An electronic response to many calls directs the caller to a series of options that may not even include speaking to a person. E-mail, instant messaging, and "texting" are ubiquitous. Information in many areas is now available via access to a computer and an Internet connection. Wireless Internet access ("WiFi") increasingly is used as a perk to lure customers to the local coffee spot and to ease passengers' irritation during long flight delays. Nurses use electronic records and communicate updated information via hand-held devices.

Over the past decade, we have witnessed exponential increases in computer penetration (Thielst, 2010). Such technology can improve work and expand capabilities. Who would prefer to use a traditional typewriter to prepare papers and documents after mastering a word-processing program? Yet many issues deserve examination as we move into the age of telehealth.

Telehealth or mhealth (i.e., mobile health)—the use of telecommunications and data technologies to deliver health care services including diagnostic services, treatment, consultation, and health information—is now omnipresent. Rather than replacing traditional care, telehealth is best understood as a complementary approach to long-distance care delivery, and faster and easily delivered contact. Telehealth has the potential to expand access to care, particularly for individuals receiving home care and those in remote areas, and to contain costs (Luptak et al., 2010). Moreover, the concept of telehealth also encompasses remote teaching, conferencing, and consulting (Ackerman et al., 2010).

Technological advances have produced benefits; however, technology also can reduce the need for direct interpersonal contact. Barriers to use include the need for financial investment to establish networks, inadequate reimbursement mechanisms, possible risks to confidentiality with electronic transmission, and licensure issues when care is transmitted across state lines. Challenges include conducting systematic evaluation of outcomes and cost-effectiveness, and ensuring that individuals' economic status and health literacy do not constrain access.

Perhaps the most important threat is that care can become impersonal when face-to-face contact is replaced by electronic interface. Thus, preserving core nursing values as electronic care systems are created, tested, and implemented is a crucial goal. Innovative practices to safeguard core professional values in the emerging age of telehealth include:

- Avoid a "one size fits all" approach through individualized or tailored algorithms and design features specific to the system's use. Moreover, clinician behaviors that facilitate a patient-centered style of communication include using open-ended questions, building partnerships, sharing decision-making and information, providing counseling, and using statements of concern, agreement, and approval. This style more successfully addresses individual needs and is associated with greater patient satisfaction, better psychosocial adjustment, and improved health outcomes (Agha et al., 2009). Adding opportunities for on-line questions and answers or an open electronic or telephone chat with a clinician can facilitate tailoring in this delivery approach. Text and/or e-mail prompts also can facilitate adherence to care.
- Develop and maintain therapeutic relationships by inviting exchanges between the nurse and person; for example by creating a series of layered screens that first introduce the nurse (visually and with a biography) and later invite exchanges, feedback, and sharing of experiences and stories from individuals.
- Foster individual autonomy by building components that encourage decision-making, problem-solving, and knowledge development that are timely and specific to the health problem and stage of treatment or management (Agha et al., 2009).
- Create flexible technology applications that work across a variety of platforms (e.g., computer, smartphone, tablet).

Consider the following questions about telehealth:
- What effects do technological changes have on the therapeutic relationship?
- Will face-to-face interaction become a rare occurrence? In the future, might therapeutic interactions take place primarily via technology, such as voicemail, the Internet, and videorecorded transmission? What advantages and disadvantages will appear with the increasing use of technology in nursing practice?
- What creative approaches may evolve using technology in therapeutic relationships?
- How can electronic communication systems be used in disaster preparedness to alert people at risk and direct actions to increase safety when a human-caused or natural disaster is suspected, imminent, or in progress?

Sources: Ackerman, M. J., Burgess, L. P., Filart, R., Lee, I., & Poropatich, R. K. (2010). Developing next-generation telehealth tools and technologies: Patients, systems, and data perspectives. *Telemedicine and e-Health, 16*(1), 93+. Retrived from http://dx.doi.org/10.1089/tmj.2009.0153; Agha, Z., Schapira, R., Laud, P., McNutt, G., & Roter, D. (2009). Patient satisfaction with physician-patient communication during telemedicine. *Telemedicine and e-Health, 15*(9), 830-839, Retrieved from http://dx.doi.org/10.1089/tmj.2009.0030; Luptak, M., Dailey, N., Juretic, M., Rupper, R., Hill, R., Hicken, B., et al. (2010). The care coordination home telehealth (CCHT) rural demonstration project: A symptom-based approach for serving older veterans in remote geographical settings. *Rural and Remote Health, 10*(2), 1375; Thielst, C. (2010). At the crossroads: NRTRC white paper examines trends driving the convergence of telehealth, EHRs and HIE. *World Hospitals and Health Services, 46(4)*, 17-23.

Bateson, 1987). This exchange involves all the modes of behavior that an individual uses, consciously or unconsciously, to affect another person. Communication includes the spoken and written word and nonverbal communication (gestures, facial expressions, movement, body messages or signals, and artistic symbols). Furthermore, communication errors between clinical providers and individuals or their proxies as well as ineffective communication among practitioners have been identified as a major source of personal and health care delivery safety problems (Hughes, 2008). Thus promoting clear communication is a major component of promoting an individual's safety and quality care.

Increasingly, communication is electronic. Telehealth or mhealth (i.e., mobilehealth)—the use of telecommunications and data technologies to deliver health care services including diagnostic services, treatment, consultation, and health information—is rapidly growing as a communication system. Such electronic communication can encompass the spoken and written word, and nonverbal forms of communication. Yet the format and interface differ from the modes of human communication available until the latter part of the twentieth century, and changes will be exponential in the years to come. (For additional discussion, see Box 4-5: Hot Topics.)

BOX 4-6 STRATEGIES ASSOCIATED WITH PERSON-CENTERED COMMUNICATION

- Permitting people to tell their stories in their own words and chronology
- Using a conversational interviewing style
- Being friendly through humor and social conversation, and nonverbal cues such as smiling
- Eliciting people's views, perspectives, thoughts, wishes, goals, values, and expectations
- Inquiring about the nature of the person's life
- Attending to the person's needs
- Avoiding overemphasis on technical aspects of care and tasks
- Not being too busy to talk

- Responding to cues concerning emotional issues and problems
- Giving information about self-care and participation in decision-making
- Developing mutual understanding
- Creating collaborative health care plans
- Showing empathy and concern for the individual's well-being
- Connecting with individuals through humor, touch, and selective self-disclosure
- Tuning in to individuals' preferences and style
- Attending to and advocating for individuals' needs
- Maintaining confidentiality

Modified from Dziopa, F., & Ahern, K. (2009b). What makes a quality therapeutic relationship in psychiatric/mental health nursing: A review of the research literature. *Internet Journal of Advanced Nursing Practice, 10*(1), 1-19; Bolster, D. (2010). Person-centered interactions between nurses and patients during medication activities in an acute hospital setting: Qualitative observation and interview study. *International Journal of Nursing Studies, 47*(2), 154-165.

BOX 4-7 RESEARCH FOR EVIDENCE-BASED PRACTICE
The Mediating Role of Nurse-Patient Dyad Bonding in Patient Satisfaction

Study Overview

Using a correlational path analytical research design, Tejero (2011) conducted a study to examine the direct and indirect relations of nurse characteristics and patient characteristics to patient satisfaction, as mediated by nurse-patient dyad bonding. A sample of 210 nurses and 210 patients from medical-surgical, obstetrics, gynecological, otolaryngological, and ophthalmological units; the trauma ward; and medical intensive care units participated in the study. Characteristics of nurses and patients were gathered through observation, interview, and chart review. Instruments were used to measure nurse-patient bonding during observation and to measure patient satisfaction with nursing care in the interview. In addition, a checklist was used to collect information on patient complexity, vulnerability, and predictability as well as information on nurse clinical judgment and facilitation of learning.

Results

Results confirmed the importance of the nurse's role in the formation of a therapeutic dyadic relationship that results in patient satisfaction—a critical part of

quality outcomes in health care. Openness and engagement of nurses during interactions were significantly and positively correlated with patient satisfaction. Path analysis showed that nurse facilitation of learning was particularly important in mediating nurse-patient dyad bonding. Nurses' efforts to educate and provide information to patients displayed openness and engagement, which leads to openness and engagement from the patient. The manner, tone, and emotion of the nurse also were shown to affect patient satisfaction.

Implications

Formation of nurse-patient therapeutic dyadic relationships plays a major role in the quality of patients' experiences. Tejero (2011) stated that a key implication is that the nurse is the healthy individual in the dyad and clinical expert in the interaction, who is obligated to initiate and steer the dyadic relationship towards a therapeutic bond. Findings of this study showed that nurse facilitation of patient learning should be emphasized in practice and in teaching students in order to provide evidence-based practice and improve patient satisfaction.

From Tejero, L. M. S. (2011). The mediating role of the nurse-patient dyad bonding in bringing about patient satisfaction. *Journal of Advanced Nursing.* doi:10.1111/j.1365-2648.2011.05795.x.

In nursing, communication is the cornerstone of a positive nurse-person relationship. Communication refers to a set of strategies and actions to enhance reciprocity, mutual understanding, and decision-making. Focusing the clinical discussion on the person's story rather than a version reformulated by the provider is essential to person-centered communication. Box 4-6 highlights strategies associated with person-centered communication based on evidence from the research literature.

Considerable evidence supports the effectiveness of these strategies. Research study results showed that nurses communicate effectively when they use a person-centered approach or nurse-person relational approach comprised of being attentive, caring, accepting, empathetic, friendly, comfortable, calm, interested, sincere, and respectful (Carter, 2009; Doss et al., 2011; Tejero, 2011). Although these strategies sound simple and basic, such appraisals are noticeably absent in many instances and their presence is essential to quality nursing care (Box 4-7: Research for Evidence-Based Practice). Furthermore, research

findings have indicated that nurses seek communication with individuals that supports openness and engagement of both the nurse and the person to form a bonding factor between them (Tejero, 2011).

Function and Process

Ruesch and Bateson (1987) delineated the following functions of communication:

- To obtain and send messages and to retain information
- To use the information to arrive at new conclusions, to reconstruct the past, and to look forward to future events
- To begin and to modify physiological processes
- To influence others and outside events

Communication transmits information, both interpersonally and intrapersonally, and it provides the basis for action.

The process of communication consists of four components (Watzlawick et al., 1967). Nurses must be able to diagnose communication difficulties in any of these components. **Input**

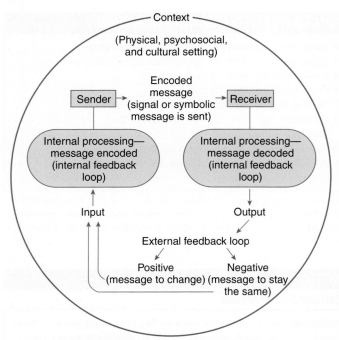

FIGURE 4-3 Communication system.

involves taking in information from outside the individual or group. Once taken in, input must be transformed in some manner to be used. For example, symbols must be translated into words to transmit ideas. The flow and transformation of processed input refers to the way information is analyzed and stored within the individual, or the way it is transmitted from person to person within a human system (group or family) before communication with the external environment occurs. The outcome of information processing, output, involves further exchange with the environment or other person. A new information exchange is triggered at this point in the cycle by the response called **feedback,** a monitoring system through which the person or group controls the internal and external responses to behavior (output) and accommodates these responses appropriately. A feedback **loop** shows the dynamic nature of communication. Each piece of communication is both a stimulus designed to elicit a response and a response to a different stimulus (Figure 4-3).

When interpersonal communication is analyzed, two types of feedback can be identified: positive (encouraging change) and negative (encouraging homeostasis or no change). Parents' commands to a young child illustrate these types of feedback: positive, "Try that again; you almost had it" and negative, "Don't touch that; it's hot." The first statement shows the parent's attempt to encourage the child to continue new behavior; the second illustrates an effort to curtail undesired behavior. Rather than meaning "good" or "bad," positive feedback and negative feedback refer to promotion of system change and stability, which is the process of balancing the direction and magnitude of change. Both types of feedback are needed, depending on the situation.

The situational context of communication is important. The context of communication is the setting's physical, psychosocial, and cultural dimensions. It includes the relationship

between sender and receiver; their previous experiences, feelings, values, cultural norms, age, and developmental stage; and the physical location (Stuart & Laraia, 2009).

Types of Communication

All human communication occurs in three forms: (1) verbal, (2) nonverbal, and (3) **metacommunication.** Each affects the meaning and influences the interpretation of the message.

Verbal Communication

Verbal communication is the transmission of messages using words, spoken or written.As symbols for ideas, words impart meaning defined by a specific language. Communicating with language is a critical ability.

People who are deaf or hard of hearing often use sign language to communicate. Signs, similar to spoken or written words, are used consistently to represent a particular meaning. Words also may be spelled out through finger spelling in a manner parallel to written communication. Braille assists blind and visually challenged people to read. Touch is used to interpret markings that represent letters and words. Sign language and braille blend aspects of verbal and nonverbal communication, but both forms of communication transmit meaning through a consistent language system.

Verbal communication with people who speak a different language poses a challenge. As societies become increasingly multicultural, assistance from specially trained interpreters is essential to providing culturally competent care. Confidentiality issues, the complexity of health information, and the need to validate understandings and reach mutual decisions make it inappropriate to use untrained personnel or relatives to interpret simply because they are available.

The importance of language development is apparent in its three functions: informing the person of others' thoughts and feelings; stimulating the receiver of a message by triggering a response; and serving a descriptive function by imparting information and sharing observations, ideas, inferences, and memories (Watzlawick et al., 1967). The ability of verbal communication to fulfill these functions is influenced by many factors, including the communicator's social class, culture, age, milieu, and ability to receive and interpret messages.

Nonverbal Communication

Nonverbal communication or language encompasses all messages that are not spoken or written. The channels of nonverbal communication are the five senses. Movement, facial and eye expressions, gestures, touch, appearance, and vocalization or paralanguage all constitute nonverbal modes of communication (Blondis & Jackson, 1982). Although all communication has the potential of being misunderstood, nonverbal communication is particularly subject to misunderstanding because it does not always reflect the sender's conscious intent. Nonverbal messages also tend to be nebulous, without specific beginnings and endings.

Body motion or kinetic behavior includes facial expression (or facies), eye movements, body movements, gestures, and posture (Blondis & Jackson, 1982). When observing facial expression, the nurse notices the affect or emotion that is communicated. Does the person appear happy or sad; alert, distracted, or sleepy; contented, agitated, or anxious? The degree of emotion expressed should also be noted. Does the person's face express what generally is considered an excessive degree of feeling for the situation, too little, or none at all? Eyes, in conjunction with the movement of other facial muscles, move in ways that convey affect. Eye contact conveys messages of interest or trust; lack of eye contact can imply lack of interest or anxiety; constant eye contact can send a message of hostility.

All of these nonverbal messages are culturally and situationally bound. Nonverbal behavior, particularly facial and eye expressions, is contextual. For example, in certain circumstances and cultures, avoidance of direct eye contact between some people can be a sign of respect. Yet, in other situations and cultures, it can be interpreted as indicative of disinterest, avoidance, or disrespect.

Sign language combines features of both nonverbal and verbal communication. Sign language involves nonverbal communication because, although it uses symbols that are communicated through specific signs, these are enhanced by facial expressions and body postures. However, sign language shares many aspects of verbal communication. It has syntax and grammar, words may be spelled out, and a standard meaning is assigned to specific signs to create symbolic language, just as words share common definitions.

Importance of Nonverbal Communication. Nonverbal communication has great power to transmit information about another's thoughts and feelings; therefore, careful observation is essential. Even silence can be very revealing. The significance of nonverbal communication is best captured by the axiom, "Actions speak louder than words." Nurses' nonverbal messages that communicate distance from the person, or signal an unfriendly or uncaring attitude, thwart development of a therapeutic relationship (Henry et al., 2011) and thereby render health-promotion efforts unproductive.

Metacommunication

Besides verbal and nonverbal communication, a phenomenon called metacommunication refers to a message about the message. Watzlawick and colleagues (1967) described metacommunication as the impossibility of not communicating: that is, "one cannot not communicate. Persons transmit a message about what is being communicated even when words are not spoken" (p. 49). Metacommunication is the relationship aspect of communication. In a sense, metacommunication involves reading between the lines or going past the surface content of the message to glean nuances of meaning. When the content and the relationship aspects, or metacommunication aspects, of a message are incongruent, interpreting the communication accurately may be difficult, leaving the receiver uncomfortable and confused.

Group Process

In group settings, a special type of metacommunication is called process. A basic principle of group theory states that all communication has content and process. Content is what is said;

process is the relationship aspect of what is communicated. Group process occurs during every group encounter. Staff meetings and clinically oriented psychoeducation, therapy, and counseling groups always involve group process. For example, consider two individuals in a smoking cessation group who always support each other by agreeing with each other and offering comments or criticism to any group member who disagrees. Although this pairing between the individuals offers them some protection from anxiety that may result from self-examination and feedback, it isolates them and curtails feedback from others. Examination of this group process is an essential task. The nurse leader and participants can transform this problematic situation into a learning opportunity by identifying the pattern by pointing out the behavior after it has occurred frequently; helping the pair and other group members consider what needs are being met through this pattern; looking at each person's role in fostering this process (e.g., why other group members have failed to confront the pair); and discussing potential outcomes of changing the behavior. These steps can be applied in clinical situations when greater self-understanding is a goal.

Effectiveness of Communication

Understanding what makes communication effective improves the nurse's ability to assess needs and to intervene successfully to promote individuals' health. Steps to functional communication include firmly stating the case; clarifying the message; seeking feedback; and being receptive to feedback when it is received. Implementing these steps to functional communication between nurses and individuals, and between nurses and other care providers, is essential to ensure patient safety and quality care (QSEN, 2012).

To state the case, the sender needs to make the content and the metacommunication congruent; when they conflict, the message is confusing. For example, a nurse is angry with a colleague for making statements to an administrator that undermined the nurse's plans for reconfiguring a health-promotion program in their agency. When the nurse had a chance to speak with this colleague, they exchanged pleasantries without mention of what the nurse thought about the colleague's statements to the administrator. When the colleague asked if something was bothering the nurse, the nurse responded that nothing was wrong. The colleague senses that the nurse's verbal and nonverbal communication did not match; in other words, the content of the message and the metacommunication were incongruent. The colleague was left feeling uneasy, and the nurse failed to express his or her thoughts or to take effective action to rectify the perceived problem with the colleague. To make the communication functional, the nurse needed to bring thoughts and feelings into awareness and reflect on the intended message. Once these steps are accomplished, the message's content and metacommunication can be adjusted to match, and the nurse's communication is likely to be effective. This example typifies ineffective communications.

To clarify the message, the sender must give a complete message. Important features should be emphasized and specifics of any request must be stated, not assumed. The message's importance also must be indicated. To illustrate, a woman mentions to her nurse that it is nearly June. The nurse responds that he has noticed how warm the weather is becoming. On the surface, this communication may seem functional until the intent of the woman's message is considered. She meant to imply that June is the 5-year anniversary of her remission from cancer, and she hoped that her nurse would somehow know that she wanted him to comment on the significance of this anniversary. To make this communication functional, the woman needed to expand the message (e.g., "My anniversary after cancer treatment is coming up") and then clarify her wish for a sensitive response from the nurse (e.g., "This anniversary marks the goal for you to be cancer-free." "What will you do to celebrate?"). Additionally, she needed to show how important the message was (e.g., "I'd really like to do something special to mark this date"). If the nurse had been attuned to the metacommunication in this exchange, he could have clarified this woman's intent and met her need for recognition and dialogue.

One technique for clarifying and qualifying messages is called the *"I" statement*. Use of "I" statements helps the sender state what he or she wants, feels, thinks, or plans (including likes and dislikes). For example, "I felt unimportant when you forgot to recognize this anniversary" is an "I" statement that the person could have used to communicate effectively. Soliciting such "I" messages is a therapeutic technique to be encouraged.

Questions can clarify and qualify, depending on the type of question asked. Open-ended questions tend to elicit descriptive responses rather than one-word answers. For example, the question, "Tell me what you did for exercise this week," is likely to yield a more elaborate description of a health behavior from a person than the question, "Did everything go okay with your exercise plan?" However, direct questions that seek a one-word answer are useful when a specific piece of information is sought. "Did you spend 15 minutes or more walking today?" may be a better approach than "What was your activity like today?" when it is important to discuss and promote minimal exercise requirements. Also, for individuals having trouble expressing more than the simplest thoughts, asking direct questions that call for brief replies can be helpful, such as, "Did you eat breakfast?" This approach is particularly useful with people who are depressed, regressed, cognitively impaired, or unable to handle complex information or communication at a particular time; or when a specific yes/no response is needed.

Seeking feedback is another element of functional communication. Consensual validation, confirming that both sender and receiver understand the same information, calls for the use of the clarification skills just described. In family communication, the parent, as the sender, should model this behavior for children by asking the child, as the receiver, to explain his or her sense of the message and how to ask the sender for further explanation. For example, "I want you to clean your room" (message from parent) can be followed by, "Tell me how you think you will do that" (validating that child and parent agree about what the task entails). This style of seeking validation can be adapted to nurse-nurse or nurse–other professional exchanges between colleagues and to therapeutic interactions, and is critical to effective clinical care (Institute of Medicine [IOM], 2010). Such confirmation in communication also is essential when

providing health-promotion interventions. Without validating that the person understands the information and its importance, and that the person has a behavior plan to follow, health-promotion efforts are likely to fail. Moreover, failure to validate is a significant risk to patient safety (QSEN, 2012).

Being open to feedback also is crucial. A "no questions" attitude blocks functional communication, whether in the home, classroom, or clinical setting. Children, students, individuals, and even other nurses may be afraid to question anyone in authority or may assume that the person should magically know what is intended or expected. For example, a person may avoid confronting a nurse who fails to explain the clinical plan and then communicates that the person should know how to follow through. Statements by the sender such as "Tell me what you think" and "What is your understanding of what I said?" are helpful.

Receiving and sending messages involves many of the same processes. Evaluation of the intent of the message, both the content and the metacommunication, is the first step. The receiver frequently needs to seek clarification and validate understanding of the message for communication to be effective. Clarification of expectations, active exchange of information, power sharing, and negotiation will enhance the quality of nurse-person communication. The outcome is a nurse-person relationship based on trust and partnership (Carter, 2009; Doss et al., 2011), critical ingredients to patient-centered care (IOM, 2010).

Factors in Effective Communication
Listening

Effective listening, an important part of communication, is more than passively taking in information. Effective listening is actively focusing attention on the message. Asking questions to explore what is meant helps the listener reach an accurate assessment of the message's meaning.

Many forms of nonverbal communication have been identified that, from a Western or European perspective, commonly convey that the person is listening. These nonverbal communications include direct gazing and eye contact, head nodding, orienting one's body to maintain interpersonal closeness, leaning forward, making facial expressions such as eyebrow animation and smiling, and using brief verbal statements that indicate interest, such as "Please go on" or "Tell me more about that…."

For behavior to communicate that the person is listening also depends on the context and intensity of the activities, and the cultural norms of each person. For example, leaning close to a person might be interpreted as intrusive. Yet, the same behavior could be seen as a sign of support, depending on the context and perspective of those involved. Sensitivity to nuances in communication and validation of meaning can be particularly helpful strategies when the nurse and person come from different cultural backgrounds.

Reciprocity, the patterning of similar activities within the same interval by two people, can help the nurse communicate a listening stance in an effective way. When the nurse matches nuances of the individual's type and style of behavior, the chances that the person will interpret the nurse's behavior as an indication of active listening are increased, and the likelihood of misinterpretation is reduced. Nurses can enhance the quality of their communication, even when encounters are brief, by attending to reciprocity in their interactions and by validating whether or not reciprocity is associated with shared interpretations of meaning.

Poor listening blocks the nurse's understanding of the person. The nurse's failure to listen may be caused by anxiety; lack of experience, which leads to excessive talking by the nurse; preoccupation with personal thoughts; or lack of practice (Stuart & Laraia, 2009). The importance of focusing on the individual's needs and concerns through effective listening is a recurrent theme in research concerning therapeutic interaction (Doss et al., 2011; Shipley, 2010) and a cornerstone of patient-centered and safe care (IOM, 2010; QSEN, 2012).

Flexibility

Flexibility is a balance between control and permissiveness. In overcontrol, every message is monitored. In exaggerated permissiveness, anything can be communicated in any way. For communication to be functional, rules are needed about what is appropriate, without rigid prescriptions that inhibit meaningful interchange. For example, the guideline that nurses will not answer questions concerning intimate details of their lives sets an appropriate limit; however, this does not mean that nurses should refuse to answer any question about themselves.

Silence

Silence between people is often uncomfortable for the nurse who is somewhat insecure about what should occur during a therapeutic encounter. However, silence can be beneficial when used carefully. When seeking a verbal response, silence can be perceived as a lack of interest. At other times, silence allows individuals to reflect on what is being discussed or experienced, lets them know that the nurse is willing to wait until they are ready to say more, or simply provides them with comfort and support. Each situation needs evaluation and sensitivity. Rather than asking a flurry of questions to break the silence, the nurse allows the person time to decide when to comment or should make brief comments that do not demand answers, such as "It can be helpful to take time to think about what we've been discussing." Also, comments such as "Try putting your thoughts or feelings into words" can help the person to share these thoughts or feelings when silence is blocking rather than improving the communication.

Humor

Humor is part of being human; it relieves tension, reduces aggression, and creates a climate of sharing. Humor can block communication when it is used to avoid subjects that might be uncomfortable or when it excludes other people. Humor can also inflict emotional pain and communicate negative views or stereotypes about particular individuals or groups through teasing and jokes concerning race, ethnicity, culture, country of origin, occupation, age, gender, sexual activity, or other traits that stand out or are devalued. A direct response to the latent content or message in this type of humor is an effective way to curtail its use and minimize its effect. For example, "That kind of joke makes me very uncomfortable. I don't find it funny to describe [the specific group in question] that way, and I would like you to

FIGURE 4-4 Touch is a powerful form of nonverbal communication. (Catherine Yeulet/Getty Images)

BOX 4-8   ZONES OF SPACE COMMON TO INTERACTION IN NORTH AMERICA

1. *Intimate space:* up to 18 inches (45.5 centimeters); used for high interpersonal sensory stimulation (see Figure 4-5, *A*)
2. *Personal space:* 18 inches to 4 feet (45.5 centimeters to 1.2 meters); appropriate for close relationships in which touching may be involved and good visualization is desired (see Figure 4-5, *B*)
3. *Social-consultative space:* 9 to 12 feet (2.7 to 3.6 meters); less intimate and personal, requiring louder verbal communication (see Figure 4-5, *C*)
4. *Public space:* 12 feet (3.6 meters) and over; appropriately used for formal gatherings, such as giving speeches (see Figure 4-5, *D*)

Source: Hall, E. (1973). *The silent language.* Garden City, NY: Doubleday/Anchor Press.

stop." To be helpful, the meaning of the humor must be understood and its purpose supportive to the individual. Clarification of the meaning should be used when there is doubt or concern.

Touch

Touch is an interesting means of nonverbal communication for nurses, who often touch individuals while administering care. The nurse's concern can be expressed by a gentle or soothing application of touch. Nevertheless, in some instances touch is inappropriate. For example, in interactions with individuals who have trauma histories or acute psychiatric disturbances, touch might be misinterpreted. A woman who has been raped might interpret touch during an examination as an attack. Evaluation of the context and meaning of touch to the individual is based on knowledge of that person and interpretation of feedback. Figure 4-4 illustrates appropriate use of touch.

Space

Space between communicators varies according to the type of communication, the setting, and the culture. Hall (1973) researched **proxemics,** the use of space between communicators, and identified four zones of space commonly used in interaction in North America that are presented in Box 4-8 and Figure 4-5.

FIGURE 4-5 **A,** Intimate distance communication. **B,** Personal distance communication. **C,** Social-consultative distance communication. **D,** Public distance communication.

Understanding the appropriate distance for a given type of interaction helps the nurse to make nonverbal and verbal communication congruent and to avoid violating spatial norms. Awareness of cultural customs concerning distance is important in shaping communication and interpreting the behavior of others. When people from different cultures or groups communicate, there may be discomfort about the acceptable distance between them when speaking. Recognition of differences helps the nurse adjust the distance and interpret the meaning of this nonverbal communication.

Many traits and components discussed in this chapter characterize functional communication. However, communication is a subtle and intricate process. Communication cannot be reduced to a set of parts and principles; its roles and nuances are far more complex and variable. Communicating by language and symbols is a special human ability. Healthy communication enables people to move from being alone to being together—clearly one of the crucial tasks of living. Effective

communication is also the foundation for the helping relationship. Moreover, effective communication is essential to providing quality care and ensuring patient safety and well-being (QSEN, 2012).

THE HELPING OR THERAPEUTIC RELATIONSHIP

A **helping or therapeutic relationship** is a process through which one person promotes the development of another person by fostering the latter's maturation, adaptation, integration, openness, and ability to find meaning in the present situation (Peplau, 1969). The therapeutic relationship emerges from purposeful encounters characterized by effective communication. In this relationship, the nurse respects the individual's values, attends to concerns, and promotes positive change by encouraging self-expression, exploring behavior patterns and outcomes, and promoting self-help (Doss et al., 2011). The therapeutic relationship is the foundation of clinical nursing

- Self-awareness and self-reflection
- Openness
- Self-confidence and strength
- Genuineness
- Concern for the individual
- Respect for the individual
- Knowledge
- Ability to empathize
- Sensitivity
- Acceptance
- Creativity
- Ability to focus and confront

practice—the essential element of quality care with every individual in every situation (Hughes, 2008; QSEN, 2012). Techniques, technology, interventions, and contexts vary, but the relational aspect of nursing practice produces a cohesive unity, allowing each nurse to see people holistically and as unique individuals. Although many components of the helping relationship are most germane to relationships that extend over time, essentials of the helping relationship apply to even brief therapeutic encounters.

No perfect profile or personality of a helping person exists. However, certain traits can be nurtured without thwarting the nurse's unique personality. These characteristics enable the nurse to be an agent of therapeutic care (Peplau, 1963; Stuart & Laraia, 2009). Box 4-9 lists characteristics associated with therapeutic effectiveness.

Characteristics of the Therapeutic Relationship

No recipe is available for a successful therapeutic relationship. Techniques and concepts serve only as tools. As a nurse develops and evaluates a helping relationship, be it long-term or brief in nature, the following guidelines may be useful.

Purposeful Communication

Purposeful communication means that the nurse focuses communication toward a particular goal. Social chitchat, communication without a goal, should not make up the bulk of therapeutic interaction. This does not mean that the nurse should never discuss a social topic; nonetheless, there should be some purpose. For example, discussing the weather with a somewhat disoriented older adult individual serves the purpose of orienting that person to the environment. Discussing the Superbowl with an avid football fan may provide valuable assessment data and engage the person in a current topic of social interest. Goals guide the nurse in focusing communication.

Rapport

Rapport is a harmony and an affinity between people in a relationship (Rogers, 1965). By using many of the traits listed for helping a person, the nurse can establish an atmosphere in which rapport can develop. To let the person know that his or

her concerns interest the nurse and that working together may alleviate some of his or her difficulties and encourage growth, it is important to be genuine, open, and concerned.

Trust

Trust is a necessary component of any helping relationship. Trust is the reliance on a person to carry out responsibilities and promises, based on a sense of safety, honesty, and reliability. Trust is an important component of partnership (Carter, 2009). The nurse promotes trust by modeling and structuring the relationship appropriately. The following strategies promote trust:

- Trusting the individual to do as promised
- Clearly defining the relationship parameters and expectations, particularly the purpose and specifics of time, place, and anticipated behavior
- Being consistent
- Examining behaviors that interfere with trust

Empathy

Empathy is the ability to understand another's feelings without losing personal identity and perspective. Empathic nurses draw on emotions and experiences that enable them to place themselves in the other person's situation. While the person senses increasing understanding and acceptancefrom the nurse, the individual's distress decreases. Outcomes from research studies are building knowledge about the role that empathic nursing care plays in outcomes. For example, Allan and Dixon (2009) conducted a phenomenological study to explore the experience of being nurtured while depressed. Interviews with hospitalized participants revealed the importance of nursing presence that included spending time listening and assisting participants to discuss problems, fears, and anxieties.

Nurses learn behavioral approaches that enhance empathic relations with people through supervised experiential learning. For example, nurses do not empathize by switching the focus of the interaction to themselves or by sympathizing (e.g., "I know exactly how you feel; that happened to me once"). Rather, they use clinical and personal experience to appreciate the individual's feelings and experiences. Using personal understanding while maintaining boundaries is the essence of empathy in the helping relationship. With empathic understanding, the nurse acknowledges the affective domain of personal experiences and uses this knowledge to appreciate the person's reactions. Empathy enables the listener to share human experiences as the basis for providing care.

Goal Direction

A helping relationship is special in its goal-directed nature. Although most human relationships focus on mutual benefit, a helping relationship exists solely to meet some need or to promote the growth of the recipient. Although the nurse may benefit from the interaction, the relationship is centered on the recipient.

Goals are formulated as desired individual behaviors. Short-term goals are likely to be achieved within 10 days to 2 weeks; all other goals are long term. All goals should be stated in measurable terms and should focus on a positive change or on the

---

BOX 4-10   GUIDELINES FOR ETHICAL INTERPERSONAL COMMUNICATION

Ethical interpersonal communication involves:
- Being aware and open to changing concepts of self and others
- Attending to role responsibilities; individual sacrifice, when it is required to make a "good" decision; and emotions, while guarding against letting emotions be the sole guide of our behavior
- Sharing personal views candidly and clearly
- Communicating information accurately, with minimal loss or distortion of intended meaning
- Communicating verbal and nonverbal messages with congruent meanings
- Sharing responsibility for the consequences among communicators
- Recognizing the multicultural context of all communication
- Respecting the dignity of every person
- Avoiding coercion and use of power in communicating
- Being sensitive to gender and cultural contexts of communication and interpretation

- Eliminating any elements of your communication that denigrate, stereotype, or devalue
- Facilitating open and accurate communication among professional groups, professionals, staff and families, clinical care unit and department staffs or administrators, and clinical care facilities

Unethical communication involves:
- Purposefully deceiving
- Intentionally blocking communication—for example, changing subjects when the other person has not finished communicating, cutting a person off, or distracting others from the subject under discussion
- Scapegoating or unnecessarily condemning others
- Lying or deceiving that causes intentional or unintentional harm
- Verbally "hitting below the belt" by taking advantage of another's vulnerability

Modified from Johannesen, R. L. (2008). *Ethics in human communication* (6th ed.). Prospect Heights, IL: Waveland Press.

decrease of problematic behavior. Ideally, a person works with the nurse to establish goals. However, some individuals, such as those who are seriously ill, depressed, psychotic, or cognitively impaired, may be unable to establish goals. When an individual is unable to negotiate appropriate goals, the nurse establishes realistic goals and shares them with the person, who is free to participate or to reject efforts to reach these goals.

Ethics in Communicating and Relating

Ethical decision-making is closely linked with the goal-directed nature of helping relationships. Ethical issues are present in human interactions whenever behavior may affect others, whenever actions involve conscious choices of methods and ends, and whenever actions can be evaluated in reference to standards of right and wrong (Johannesen, 2008). Guidelines that may be adapted as ethical standards for interpersonal communication are highlighted in Box 4-10.

Frequently the nurse may wish to set goals that the individual does not want to reach; the nurse must remember that the problem belongs to the person, as does the choice of care alternatives. The nurse assists the individual in decision-making, with the decision based on the individual's value system. However, the nurse should not take a laissez-faire approach and avoid assisting the person. The nurse's responsibility is to help the individual to examine values, identify conflicts, and prioritize goals and desired health care outcomes. Action follows from understanding values and the best available information. Both the individual and the nurse must bring interpreted facts and personally clarified values to the interaction to establish goals. Recognizing this interplay, the nurse must clarify personal values, subsequently respect the individual's rights, and act to support and protect the integrity of the person, family, group, or community.

Therapeutic Techniques

Occasionally, clinicians who are novices in establishing helping relationships assume that they are bound to "say the wrong thing" and cause terrible damage to the person, or that they will learn some magical phrases and questions to create instant rapport. No nurse or other professional is so powerful that a "wrong word" will destroy the individual's self-concept or self-esteem. Even people with physical and emotional problems are resilient and have coped, at least to some degree, with a lifetime of stresses. Alternatively, no magical saying exists that the nurse can always plug into an interaction to communicate successfully. Although some techniques are often useful, they must be applied with purpose, skill, and attention to the individuality of each person and to the context of the interaction. The following techniques therefore should be viewed as guidelines, rather than prescriptions, for effective shaping of the therapeutic relationship.

Focus on the Individual

The first step to therapeutic communication is focusing on the individual and the reason that the interaction is occurring. The nurse is not the focus; the person is. Although an overly business-like style fails to communicate concern and support (Dziopa & Ahern, 2009a), delving into one's own personal life to the extent that it diverts attention from the other person's concern also is problematic. Avoiding nurse-directed conversation can be difficult; a useful rule of thumb is to answer or respond to obvious questions and to switch the focus back to clinical concerns when other questions are asked. For example:

Individual (looks at female nurse's wedding ring): "Are you married?"
Nurse: "Yes, I am."
Individual: "What does your husband do for a living?"
Nurse: "Rather than get distracted by a discussion about me, let's get back to planning how you will manage at work."

Keeping focus on the person's concerns includes identifying the portion of the message that is clear and relevant to the purpose of the interaction, seeking validation, and helping the individual to clarify the rest of the message.

Help the Individual to Describe and Clarify Content and Meaning

Too often the nurse rushes to offer an interpretation of the nature of the problem and quickly follows up by suggesting

✔ BOX 4-11   QUALITY AND SAFETY SCENARIO

Steps in Promoting Problem-Solving

Describe the Experience or Event of Concern
Helpful Verbal Nursing Strategies
"Tell me what happened."
"Describe the experience to me."

Analyze the Parts of the Experience and See Relationships to Other Events
Helpful Verbal Nursing Strategies
"What meaning does this have for you?"
"What pattern is there?"

Formulate the Problem
Helpful Verbal Nursing Strategies
"In what way is this problematic?"
"What do you want to see changed?"

Validate the Formulation
Helpful Verbal Nursing Strategies
"Do you mean…?"
"Let me tell you what I understand you to be saying."

Use the Formulation to Identify Ways to Solve or Manage the Difficulty
Helpful Verbal Nursing Strategies
"What would you do the next time?"
"In what way has your view changed?"
"What actions are needed to solve the problem that you've identified?"

Try Out the Solutions, Judge the Outcomes, and Adjust the Plan Accordingly
Helpful Nursing Strategies
Encourage application in new situations through role playing or through practice in appropriate settings; help the individual cycle through the preceding sequence as needed to evaluate the outcome and make adjustments to the plan.

Modified from Peplau, H. E. (1963). Process and concept of learning. In S. Burd, & M. Marshall (Eds.), *Some clinical approaches to psychiatric nursing* (pp. 333-336). New York: Macmillan.

a solution. Solving problems efficiently makes the nurse feel effective, important, and powerful; however, the person's needs may not be met. A crucial step in using the therapeutic relationship effectively is to assist the individual to describe a particular experience or concern. Description is enhanced when the nurse prompts the person to clarify the description and interpret its meaning.

Use of who, what, where, and when questions helps the person to clarify and expand the content and meaning of what is communicated. Phrases such as "tell me," "go on," "describe to me," "explain it to me," and "give me an example" are also likely to elicit description of important content and to diminish distracting generalizations and abstractions. By seeking feedback, the nurse helps the individual to explain the meaning further. In clarifying, the nurse should avoid threatening, detective-like questions. Questions that begin with "why" often increase the person's anxiety because they demand reasons, conclusions, analysis, or causes (Peplau, 1964). Reformulating questions to obtain data first and then helping the individual to analyze links among events, thoughts, feelings, actions, and outcomes is generally a more helpful approach.

A problem-solving approach by the nurse assists the person to describe and clarify the content and meaning of experience. Sequential steps help the individual to explain events, to change circumstances and responses that interfere with health, and to solve problems (O'Toole & Welt, 1989; Peplau, 1963). This problem-solving approach can be adapted for use in health promotion to assist the person in problem-solving by working through the steps outlined in Box 4-11: Quality and Safety Scenario. These steps are a useful guideline for keeping the focus of concern on the individual and his or her definition of the problem. Rather than telling the person what is

wrong and how to fix it, the nurse's primary goal is helping the person to describe the problem and formulate solutions in partnership.

Use Reflection

Reflection is the restatement of what the individual has said in the same or different words. This technique can involve paraphrasing or summarizing the person's main point to indicate interest and to focus the discussion. Effective use of this approach does not include frequent, parrot-like repetition of the individual's statements. Instead, reflection is the selective paraphrasing or literal repetition of the person's words to underscore the importance of what has been said, to summarize a main concern or theme, or to elicit elaborated information. In addition, to verify understanding of health information, the nurse can ask the person to restate what has been communicated. Failure to confirm understanding interferes with desired clinical care outcomes. For example, Bolster and Manias (2010) identified failures in communication, including lack of comprehension of information from providers, as a barrier to consumers' participation in their care.

Use Constructive Confrontation

Confronting an individual means that the nurse points out a specific behavior and then helps the person to examine the meaning or consequences of the behavior. For example:

> *Nurse:* "You missed your appointment for the consultation we had scheduled."
> *Individual:* "Oh, I didn't notice the date."
> *Nurse:* "You are usually very aware of time and appointments. What do you think was going on with you that you didn't notice the date this time?"

This type of confrontation is not an angry exchange, but a purposeful way of helping the person examine personal actions and their meaning.

Use Nouns and Pronouns Correctly

Some individuals have difficulty separating themselves from others or specifying the object or subject in their language. These individuals misuse pronouns by referring to we, us, they, she, he, him, and her, without clearly identifying the referent, and by making vague statements such as "They don't like me. They told me I was useless." Others may use general nouns, such as everyone, people, doctors, and nurses, to avoid clear communication about specific persons. The nurse can clarify by asking, "Who are they?" or "To whom are you referring?" Additionally, the nurse must be careful to use separate pronouns when speaking of herself or himself and the individual, particularly when the person has disordered thinking. For example, when communicating with an individual who is confused or exhibits disordered thinking, the nurse should say you and I, rather than us or we, to promote clear thinking and communication and to assist the individual to maintain personal boundaries (Peplau, 1963).

Use Silence

Allowing a thoughtful silence at intervals helps the individual to talk at his or her own pace without pressure to perform for the nurse. Silence also permits time for reflection. Particularly helpful to the depressed or physically ill person, silence can reduce pressure and conserve energy. After several moments, the nurse can ask the person to share some thoughts. For example, "Try putting your thoughts into words," "Tell me what are you thinking or feeling now," or "I'll be here when you feel ready to talk."

Barriers to Effective Communication

Barriers to effective communication can originate with the nurse, the individual, or both. The most obvious barrier is the nurse's failure to use the types of therapeutic techniques just described. Lack of knowledge or experience can limit the nurse's ability to assess the individual's needs and repertoire of skills. Supervision and study can help the nurse apply the steps of the nursing process by using effective intervention approaches.

Communication is also ineffective when some part of the communication-feedback loop breaks down. Failure to send a clear message, receive and interpret the message correctly, or provide useful feedback can interfere with communication. Diagnosing the source of the communication breakdown, taking steps to correct it, and using knowledge of the communication process and appropriate therapeutic techniques are the nurse's responsibility.

Anxiety

When the nurse or individual is highly anxious during an interaction, perception is altered and the ability to communicate effectively is curtailed sharply. Defense mechanisms, such as denial, projection, and displacement, reduce anxiety but block understanding of the true meaning of an interaction. Severe anxiety and defense mechanisms distort reality and lead to disordered communication. To enhance interpersonal communication, the nurse identifies the feeling of anxiety and its source and uses anxiety-reducing interventions.

Attitudes

Biases and stereotypes can limit the nurse's and individual's ability to relate. When the difficulty is the individual's problem, the nurse can assist by examining those views that interfere with the person's relationships. When the problem is the nurse's, openness in the supervisory relationship to examination of personal behavior is crucial. When the nurse fails to examine his or her attitudes toward the person, negativity may be communicated and perceptions of the interaction may be distorted.

Gaps Between Nurse and Individual

Related to attitudinal barriers, differences in gender, age, socioeconomic background, ethnicity, race, religion, or language can block functional communication between the nurse and individual. These factors can cause differences in perception and block mutual understanding. Newly licensed nurses have attributed communication problems to differences in language proficiency among nurses, including English as a second language, as well as to problems in understanding non–English-speaking individuals (Smith-Miller et al., 2010). To reduce such gaps, nurses can question unclear verbal or written communications, seek clarification or assistance from translators, and explore the ways in which perceptions may differ and meanings can be clarified (Box 4-12: Diversity Awareness and Chapter 2).

Resistance

Resistance comprises all phenomena that inhibit the flow of thoughts, feelings, and memories in an interpersonal encounter and behaviors that interfere with therapeutic goals. Resistance arises from anxiety when a person feels threatened. To reduce this anxiety, the person implements resistant behavior, most often in the form of avoidance, such as being late, changing the subject, forgetting, blocking, or becoming angry.

Initially, the nurse should identify the behavior, whether it is the nurse's or the individual's behavior, and then attempt to interpret it in the context of the interaction. Exploration of possible threats in the relationship, goals, or a particular topic can lead to understanding the source of the resistance and finding the ability to handle these difficulties. Anxiety reduction is often a necessary step in dealing with resistant behavior.

Transference and Countertransference

Transference is reacting to another person in an exchange as though that person were someone from the past. Transference may involve a host of feelings that generally are classified as positive (love, affection, or regard) or negative (anger, dislike, or frustration). Typical transference reactions involve an important figure from the past such as a mother or father; however, at times transference may be more general to include all authority figures. Something about another person's characteristics, behavior, or position, in combination with individual dynamics, triggers this response. People in a therapeutic relationship

🌐 BOX 4-12 DIVERSITY AWARENESS
Multicultural Context of Communication

As health care providers, nurses might believe that they have expert knowledge about health promotion and the treatment of illness that will be beneficial to others. Therefore it seems logical that nurses would select appropriate information to share with individuals to help them maintain health and manage illness or alterations in health status. However, consider the possible influences of cultural differences between the nurse and individual.

Much of the knowledge generated from nursing-related disciplines and the sciences is rooted in a Western perspective. Particularly in the United States, knowledge is developed and interpreted from the perspective of the dominant cultural group, a White, Anglo-Saxon, Christian point of view. When this perspective remains unexamined, alternative perspectives are ignored and invisible. Nurses who are members of the dominant cultural group may be well-intentioned, but ineffective, when they attempt to engage a person of a different cultural group in a relationship without questioning how culture influences interactions, interpretations of events and information, and beliefs and values concerning health and health care practices. Preconceived ideas about people based on some characteristic or group affiliation, such as racial or ethnic identity, religion, country of origin, gender, or sexual orientation, can interfere with nurses' abilities to relate to people as individuals. At the same time, a lack of knowledge of other cultural groups hampers nurses' understanding of the individual's point of view.

Guidelines for recognizing the multicultural context of communication in therapeutic relationships include the following:
- Make ethnocultural assessment a critical component of every clinical evaluation.
- Allow other people to define themselves.
- Ask the person, and family as appropriate, about cultural health care practices and traditions.
- Respect cultural practices and traditions while providing opportunity for the person to voice preferences and make choices.
- Respect the language of others and do not assume superiority in language.
- Collaborate with trained translators and health promoters (people with the same ethnic or racial background as the individuals).
- Avoid use of racist, sexist, ageist, and other forms of denigrating language.
- Do not perpetuate stereotypes in communication.
- Adapt communication to the uniqueness of the individual.

- Reject humor that degrades members based on gender, race, ethnicity, religion, sexual orientation, country of origin, and so forth.
- Respect the rights of others to have different practices and customs.
- Do not allow injustice to continue through silence.
- Present information clearly to all people to help them make informed choices.
- Do not judge values, traditions, and practices based on their similarity or difference from personal values, traditions, and practices, but based on whether they facilitate human potential.

The following are some issues for the nurse to consider:
- When the nurse works with a person from a different cultural background, what are common barriers to establishing a therapeutic relationship?
- In learning about different cultural groups, is there a risk of creating new stereotypes that interfere with the ability to treat people as unique individuals?
- If the nurse has little or no knowledge about a person's culture, how can the nurse provide meaningful nursing care?
- Are the two previous questions contradictory? How can the nurse meet the different challenges that they imply?
- Research measurements typically are developed from the perspective of the dominant culture. If the nurse wishes to use a standardized instrument to measure clinical or research variables among members of different cultural groups, then what questions about the instrument should the nurse ask, and what problems might the nurse encounter? What would need to be done to determine whether or not an instrument truly measures the same phenomenon across different populations?
- Consider the possible influences of cultural differences between the nurse and the individual. Think of an example of two people from diverse cultural groups who developed a relationship. Examine how they got to know each other and what differences and similarities they uncovered. Did barriers to understanding each other exist? If so, how did they bridge these barriers? What did they learn about themselves? What did they learn about the ways that culture shapes perspective and interactions? Think about how a nurse can apply these insights to his or her relationships with people from cultural groups that differ from their own.
- How would a multicultural perspective change the practice?

Guidelines developed by the author based on data from Johannesen, R. L. (2008). *Ethics in human communication* (6th ed.). Prospect Heights, IL: Waveland Press; Bjarnason, D., Mick, J., Thompson, J., & Cloyd, E. (2009). Perspectives on transcultural care. *Nursing Clinics of North America, 44*(4),495-503. doi:10.1016/j.cnur.2009.07.009.

often develop strong transference feelings toward the helping professional, arising from the interaction's intensity and the care provider's authoritative or nurturing role. To work with a person's transference reactions effectively, the nurse first helps the person to examine feelings and thoughts about the nurse. Then the nurse assists the person to compare and contrast the nurse with people from the person's past to remove distortions and comprehend the present reality.

Countertransference basically is the same phenomenon, but it is experienced by the health care professional rather than the person. The nurse experiences many feelings toward the person; these feelings are not problematic, unless they remain unanalyzed and block the nurse's ability to work effectively with the individual. For example, if a nurse has strong feelings for the person and thinks that the person cannot possibly function after discharge without the nurse's aid, the nurse is likely to distort the person's abilities, encourage a childlike dependency,

and interfere with the person's progress. This nurse needs to examine such personal feelings to understand their source. Once understood, countertransference reactions generally cease to interfere with the relationship. Consultation with an advanced practice psychiatric nurse is recommended whenever transference or countertransference reactions are persistent and problematic.

Sensory Barriers

When the individual has sensory limitations, the nurse may need to use extra skill in communicating. Use of the other senses to send or receive messages should be attempted. Special help is often available from trained therapists and teachers; for example, many agencies have access to interpreters for deaf people, and visual aides may be useful. Nurses must be as creative as possible, learn from others who are skilled in alternative forms of communication, and make referrals as necessary. As technology evolves, new communication methods will continue to decrease these barriers. For example, voice recognition software programs assist persons with visual and motor challenges to communicate via text.

Failure to Address Concerns or Needs

Failure to meet the individual's needs or to recognize the individual's concerns is the most serious barrier to effective interaction. This failure can arise from inadequate assessment; lack of knowledge; inability to separate the nurse's needs from the individual's needs; and confusion between friendship and a helping relationship, including unrecognized or unresolved sexual issues. To correct this problem, the nurse should recognize that a barrier to relating with the person exists. Using the supervisory process to determine the problem's source, the nurse should then take corrective action, such as obtaining more information or knowledge, performing a self-assessment with values clarification, and examining reactions, biases, and expectations.

Setting

The setting of a therapeutic interaction can affect the goals and the nature of the communication. The most important aspect of any setting is that the nurse and individual are able to attend to each other. The nurse's attention to the person helps create this atmosphere. The nurse assesses the influence of factors such as lighting, noise, temperature, comfort, physical distance, and privacy; potentially disturbing factors can be altered or controlled within the limits of the setting. Occasionally the nurse has only minimal control over the setting, as in a busy clinic, health center, inpatient unit, or the individual's home. Although far from the ideal of a quiet, pleasant, well-lit private office, these typical clinical settings can be used effectively by creating a sense of private space. Curtains can be drawn, doors shut, and two chairs pulled to a corner to shape an environment for interaction. When possible, however, nurses seek offices or rooms to establish privacy during significant communication or when imparting important or complex health information. The nurse can also acknowledge verbally that some aspect of the environment, such as an interruption or noise, is bothersome. This strategy shows people that the nurse recognizes possible concentration difficulties and is sharing the environment with them.

Stages

Therapeutic relationships follow sequential phases, which may overlap, vary in length, or involve issues that appear over time rather than in a set sequence. Orientation (introductory), working, and termination phases have been identified by researchers and clinicians (Canabrava, 2011; Stuart & Laraia, 2009).

Originally these relationship stages were identified from clinical interactions that developed over a prolonged period of time. However, they can be observed in brief encounters that are effective; that is, interactions that meet individuals' needs rather than therapeutic interactions that have been reduced to little more than quick question-and-answer sessions. Whether the nurse is engaged in a long-term or short-term relationship with an individual, attention to the relationship stages is important. Brief therapeutic relationships will telescope the stages; therefore, it is

---

BOX 4-13   KEY TOPICS OF DISCUSSION DURING THE ORIENTATION OR INTRODUCTORY PHASE OF THE THERAPEUTIC RELATIONSHIP

- What to call each other
- Purpose of meeting
- Location, time, and length of meetings
- Termination date or time for review of progress through follow-up
- Confidentiality (with whom clinical data will be shared)
- Any other limits related to the particular setting

---

particularly important that the nurse focus on meeting the key demands of each relationship phase. It is important to note that individuals may move in and out of direct care episodes while a therapeutic relationship is maintained over a longer period. A relationship exists even when the nurse and individual do not see each other for an extended period, and each encounter takes place within the trajectory of the relationship stages.

Orientation or Introductory Phase

The orientation or introductory phase begins when the nurse and individual meet. This meeting typically involves some feeling of anxiety; neither party knows what to expect. When the therapeutic relationship is primarily a counseling type of relationship, part of the nurse's role is to help structure the interaction by discussing several topics during the initial meeting and sometimes during the first few meetings. Box 4-13 lists topics appropriate to this phase. Discussion of these issues establishes a contract or pact and involves a mutual understanding of the parameters of the relationship and an agreement to work together.

The orientation stage is a critical juncture in any therapeutic relationship. Without successful transition through the orientation phase, no working alliance will exist and treatment goals will remain unmet. Establishing a connection during the orientation phase is facilitated by consistency, sensitive pacing of communication, active listening, conveying concern and warmth, and paying attention to comfort and control. In contrast, factors that hamper relationships include inconsistency, unavailability, individual factors associated with trust, nurses' feelings about the other person, confrontation of delusions or strongly held views, and unrealistic expectations.

When the therapeutic relationship is not structured primarily as counseling with a specific number of sessions, the orientation phase may appear less distinct and the topics noted may seem irrelevant. In this case, the nurse can adapt the suggested topics to meet the specific situation. However, except in true emergencies, initial encounters should always include introductions by name, discussion of the purpose, and presentation of a plan for ongoing care or specific follow-up.

Working Phase

The working phase of the therapeutic relationship emerges when the nurse and the individual collaborate as partners in promoting the person's health. The working phase may last for an established number of sessions, as in brief psychotherapy, or it may extend over a longer period if the nurse is the primary care provider or long-term caregiver in any setting or context for an individual or family. During the working phase, the relationship is the context through which change takes place. Goals are set, and the nurse and individual work mutually toward their accomplishment. Interventions are tailored to the specific situation and health needs of the person and family. Solving problems, coping with stressors, and gaining insight are all part of the working phase. The nurse and individual recognize each other's uniqueness. Carter (2009) identified trust as the first step in establishing a working relationship. Moreover, these researchers found that the long-term involvement characteristic of successful case management requires realistic expectations and efforts to find flexible ways to persevere over time.

Resistant behaviors may be observed during this phase while the nurse and individual become closer and work on potentially anxiety-producing problems. The person may pull away through the use of defense mechanisms because change can be difficult. Overcoming the resistance becomes an important nursing task.

Termination Phase

Termination marks the end of the relationship established in the therapeutic contract or negotiated in accordance with the limits of the contract. Ending a relationship can cause anxiety for both the individual and the nurse. Termination represents a loss; therefore, it can trigger feelings of sadness, frustration, and anger. Termination in this case is the loss of a relationship and the loss of future involvement, with its attendant realistic expectations or fantasies. Termination also reawakens feelings of previously unresolved losses, such as a death or divorce.

Working through any feelings related to termination is an important part of clinical care. Some individuals require the nurse's assistance to experience the feelings of loss and to connect present reactions to past real or symbolic losses. Box 4-14 lists additional interventions for use during the termination phase.

Both the nurse and the individual can learn much during termination; the process directs both participants to examine problems and progress in the relationship, feelings, and reactions. The experience also helps the nurse and individual gain practice in ending relationships and in exploring reactions, which can be most helpful when future losses occur.

Brief Interactions

Time constraints in practice are unavoidable. Although challenging, brief therapeutic encounters can be meaningful and useful. Limited time is not a valid reason to avoid interviewing or interacting with individuals. Rather, nurses purposefully can structure brief interactions to achieve specific clinical outcomes (Wright & Leahey, 2009). Box 4-15 delineates key ingredients for a 15-minute (or shorter) interview with a family.

These guidelines for brief interactions with families can be adapted for interviews with individuals. An effective 15-minute (or shorter) interview is feasible if nurses plan to introduce themselves, state the purpose of meeting, validate understanding with the person or family, clarify such parameters as time, focus and listen, and elicit significant individual and family data. Most important, the goal of the interaction must be realistic and clearly

> **BOX 4-14 INTERVENTIONS FOR USE DURING THE TERMINATION PHASE OF THE THERAPEUTIC RELATIONSHIP**
>
> - Let the person know why the relationship is to be terminated.
> - Remind the person of the date and how many meetings or appointments are left.
> - Collaborate with other staff so that they are aware of how the person is reacting and any special needs that the person may have.
> - Help the person to identify sources of support and other people with whom a relationship is possible.
> - Review the gains and the remaining goals.
> - Discuss the pros and cons experienced during the relationship to help the person develop a realistic appraisal.
> - Make referrals for follow-up care as needed.

> **BOX 4-15 KEY INGREDIENTS FOR A 15-MINUTE (OR SHORTER) FAMILY INTERVIEW**
>
> - Use manners to engage or reengage. Make an introduction by offering your name and role. Orient family members to the purpose of a brief family interview.
> - Assess significant areas of internal and external structure and function (obtain information from genogram concerning basic family composition and external support data).
> - Ask family members three key questions.
> - Commend the family on one or two strengths.
> - Evaluate usefulness and conclude.

defined. For example, the purpose may be to elicit a family's view of the problem for which the person has sought care or to prioritize problems to be treated. Even when time is limited, the interview is structured to provide an opportunity for the person or family to engage in dialogue as an active participant in care, and the nurse's attention is completely focused on the individual.

Circumstances also can dictate the need for immediate and instructive communications that command specific actions. For example, during a crisis directive clear communication is paramount. Miller and McCurley (2011) demonstrated the importance of preparedness and communication strategies during disaster-related events. Planning in anticipation of human-caused and natural disasters is critical in order to have functional communications systems in place. Such systems increasingly will employ various methods of telecommunication. After tragic events including shootings on college campuses, efforts to communicate more effectively are paramount. Universities, for example, have responded by instituting systems to communicate rapidly with a large campus community. Widely deployed strategies feature instant text messaging and e-mailing (see Box 4-5: Hot Topics).

Health Literacy

Clear communication improves the quality of health care encounters. Health literacy, the capacity to read, comprehend, and follow through on health information, is a critical component of health promotion. Yet, nearly 9 out of 10 adults encounter problems using everyday health information to make good decisions about health (Institute of Medicine, 2011). To combat low health literacy, nurses can encourage individuals to ask three essential questions at every health visit (Ask me 3. Good questions for your good health, n.d.; Speros, 2011):

"What is my main problem?"

"What do I need to do?"

"Why is it important for me to do this?"

Nurses also promote health literacy by creating a safe and comfortable environment, sitting to establish eye contact rather than standing when communicating, using visual aids and models to illustrate conditions and procedures, and verifying understanding of care instructions by having individuals then teach the content (Speros, 2011). In the emerging age of tele-health, developing strategies for confirming understanding and individualizing methods of communicating health information are critically important (see Box 4-5: Hot Topics). The following Case Study presents a detailed scenario of a home visit and questions related to how the nurse can develop a therapeutic relationship with the person. The Care Plan presents a plan of care for the person, including communication interventions.

CASE STUDY

A Health-Promotion Visit: Maria Sanchez-Smith

As part of a health-promotion visit for Maria Sanchez-Smith and Thomas, her 2-week-old infant, Jessica Mills, a registered nurse, planned to conduct an infant assessment, provide breastfeeding support, teach about normal infant development and care activities, and assess Mrs. Sanchez-Smith's adaptation to motherhood and her postpartum recovery status. Before the visit, Ms. Mills reviewed the clinical information she obtained during Mrs. Sanchez-Smith's hospitalization. Mrs. Sanchez-Smith is a 34-year-old Hispanic, primiparous woman who delivered a 7-pound, 10-ounce healthy boy (Thomas) after a 12-hour labor. The labor had progressed well without complication. Mrs. Sanchez-Smith received epidural anesthesia at 6-cm dilation and the baby was delivered vaginally. Her husband, Mark Smith, provided labor support and was present for the delivery. After a 2-day hospital stay, Mrs. Sanchez-Smith was discharged. At discharge, the infant was breastfeeding, had normal newborn examination findings, and weighed 7 pounds, 5 ounces. Ms. Mills had been impressed by both parents' preparation for the birth. They had attended childbirth classes and read several books about infant development and parenting. Mrs. Sanchez-Smith planned to take an 8-week maternity leave from her position as a lawyer in a large practice and had arranged for a childcare provider to come to the family's home to take care of the infant beginning 2 weeks before the end of her maternity leave. Mr. Smith had not planned to take time off from his job, because he had recently been promoted to a high-level managerial position in his company that required increased travel and time at work. He was able to postpone a business trip to be present at the delivery and had sent a plane ticket to his mother-in-law so she could come and stay at their home during the first week after Mrs. Sanchez-Smith and Thomas were discharged from the hospital.

During the visit, Ms. Mills first assessed the infant. She incorporated teaching concerning normal infant development and concluded that Thomas was a healthy 2-week-old infant who was feeding well. Thomas' circumcision was healing without complication and he had regained his birth weight.

When Ms. Mills asked how Mrs. Sanchez-Smith was doing, Mrs. Sanchez-Smith hesitated and then responded, "I'm not sure. I'm very glad that Thomas is doing well…but I worry sometimes that I'm not going to be able to do everything right for him. It's funny, but I've spent so many years getting an education and establishing my law career. It was hard work, but I managed to do well. Now a little infant overwhelms me. I don't know how I'll manage this." When Ms. Mills asked Mrs. Sanchez-Smith to talk more about her concerns, Mrs. Sanchez-Smith described how incompetent she felt while her mother was staying with her. "My mother could do everything so easily. I fumbled with every diaper. It felt like she criticized how I did things. When she told me about what she did when she had children, I felt pushed to do things 'her way' and not the way that I had planned. She even wanted to give him a bottle when I was trying so hard to get breastfeeding going. At least the doctor said Thomas had gained enough weight. Thomas' weight gain made me feel like I wasn't a total failure. I couldn't wait for her to go, but I fell apart after she left. I was alone. Mark is out of town until the weekend, and I couldn't get Thomas to stop crying yesterday. I thought I would scream so I put him down in his crib and I just sat there crying. What's wrong with me? I've never felt so out of control before. I want to be a good mother, but I feel like I can't give any more right now."

In response to Ms. Mills' follow-up questions about mental status, Mrs. Sanchez-Smith described frequently feeling irritated and sad, crying a few times over the last several days, having difficulty sleeping even when the baby was asleep, feeling fatigued, and being worried about how she would be able to go back to work in only a few weeks. Ms. Mills also inquired about the family's cultural, ethnic, and religious backgrounds. Mrs. Sanchez-Smith responded, "Interesting that you should ask. That's actually another issue right now. I'm from New Mexico and my family is Hispanic and Catholic, but I'm not a practicing Catholic now. You might guess that I'm Latina from my hyphenated name. I added my maiden name to Smith when I got married to honor my family. Mark is Protestant, but not really religious. His family comes from New Jersey. They are very nice and were supportive when we got married. We were lucky that our families accepted us together. I have to admit, though, that we didn't really figure out what we would do about raising the baby. Mark thinks that we'd be hypocrites to have a Catholic christening. Plus my mother told me that I'd be selfish to go back to work so soon. Can you help me? I feel like I'm going out of my mind and I don't know what to do."

This case study raises a variety of clinical concerns. As the nurse in this encounter, Ms. Mills could begin by considering the following questions.

Reflective Questions

1. What are my feelings as I listen to her story and her distress? Am I aware of how my values and expectations affect my interaction with this person? How can I establish a therapeutic relationship to support Mrs. Sanchez-Smith during this stressful period?

2. What is the significance of the distress symptoms that Mrs. Sanchez-Smith reported? Given that the period during which many women experience postpartum blues has passed, what is the most appropriate action to obtain a thorough mental status examination for postpartum depression?

3. Who is the most appropriate health care provider to evaluate her for postpartum depression, and treat her if it is confirmed? How can I facilitate getting her the care she needs and can I remain available to her? How can I assist Mrs. Sanchez-Smith to meet the infant's developmental needs during this stressful period?

4. In what ways do family dynamics, values, and expectations related to differing cultural and religious heritages contribute to the problems described? What can I do to explore these issues further? What strengths can be harnessed? How can I engage support systems to ameliorate rather than exacerbate the difficulties? What can be done to engage both Mr. Smith and Mrs. Sanchez-Smith in a therapeutic relationship to focus on the couple and parenting concerns, and to involve both partners in treatment strategies?

CARE PLAN
Transition to Parenthood: Maria Sanchez-Smith

*NURSING DIAGNOSIS: Risk for Impaired Parenting related to stress involved in transition to parenthood

Defining Characteristics
- Feeling overwhelmed with responsibilities of new parenthood
- Insecurity about tasks of infant care
- Crying
- Sadness
- Feeling out of control
- Difficulty sleeping even when the baby is asleep
- Worry about going back to work soon

Related Factors
- Transition from high career achievement to new role as mother
- Differing religious, ethnic, and cultural backgrounds of the two parents and extended families
- Confusion and lack of decisions about religious and cultural traditions to follow for their infant
- Conflicting expectations of extended families, particularly from Mrs. Sanchez-Smith's mother
- Job pressures on Mr. Smith to travel and be away from home
- Unanticipated social isolation for Mrs. Sanchez-Smith during this postpartum period
- Limited social support (particularly from husband due to work-associated travel)

Expected Outcomes
- Competent mothering and infant care are displayed.
- Mrs. Sanchez-Smith describes her feelings, concerns, and needs.
- Indicators of postpartum depression are evaluated and referral for follow-up made for positive findings.
- Social supports are engaged.
- Mrs. Sanchez-Smith and Mr. Smith successfully negotiate immediate decisions about religious and cultural practice concerning their baby and agree to use counseling services to work out decisions concerning their child's upbringing and involvement of extended family.

Interventions
- Health information is provided about normal newborn and postpartum adjustment.
- Infant care information is provided based on Mrs. Sanchez-Smith's needs.
- Expectations about postpartum adjustment and parenthood are elicited.
- Health information about postpartum depression is provided regarding prevalence and common symptoms.
- Personal and family history is conducted, with a focus on mental health.
- Postpartum depression is evaluated using interview questions and an assessment measure, such as the Edinburgh Postnatal Depression Scale (Cox et al., 1987) or the Postpartum Depression Screening Scale (Beck & Gable, 2001).
- If symptom levels suggest postpartum depression, a referral for mental health evaluation is made. If any signs of safety risk to self or others, immediate protective action (e.g., emergency mental health evaluation) is taken.
- Sources of social support are solicited and specific plans are made to use available support, such as husband, friends, and hired infant care providers.
- Conflicts and areas of shared values, plans, goals for raising the baby are explored.
- Pros and cons of options for raising the baby are examined in relation to religious, ethnic, and cultural considerations.
- A follow-up plan is made to reassess symptoms of postpartum depression and to discuss ongoing concerns about how to raise the baby with Mrs. Sanchez-Smith and Mr. Smith.
- Referral is made to local support and psychoeducational programs for interfaith couples.

*NANDA Nursing Diagnoses—Definitions and Classification 2012-2014, Herdman T.H. (ED). Copyright © 2012, 1994-2012 NANDA International. Used by arrangement with John Wiley & Sons Limited. In order to make safe and effective judgments using the NANDA-I nursing diagnoses it is essential that nurses refer to the definitions and defining characteristics of the diagnoses listed in this work.

SUMMARY

Relating to persons offers many challenges and rewards for nurses. Although some aspects of this work are predictable, each person and family is unique and provides a chance for the nurse to learn, grow, and help in new ways. This chapter provides guidelines for developing therapeutic relationships, but these guidelines do not guarantee success or an easy job. The desire and skill of the individual nurse bring this information to life. The blend of the nurse's artistry, humanity, knowledge, skill, and ethics sparks concern and the ability to help another human being communicate effectively—essential components of the nurse-person relationship.

The therapeutic relationship is the primary arena for health promotion. Values clarification, communication, and the helping relationship are its core components. For nurses, applying this knowledge to their varied roles is essential to promoting health and providing quality care.

Rising use of technology and mounting pressures for cost-effective care are here to stay. In this climate, the importance of the therapeutic relationship is underscored (see Hot Topics box). Without a relational context, the care dimension in health care is lost, and health promotion is reduced to standardized, recipe-like prescriptions. Effective health promotion directed to the needs of individuals, families, and communities requires reflection on the value of caring, effective communication, and a helping relationship.

REFERENCES

Ackerman, M. J., Burgess, L., P., Filart, R., Lee, I., & Poropatich, R. K. (2010). Developing next-generation telehealth tools and technologies: Patients, systems, and data perspectives. *Telemedicine and e-Health, 16*(1), 93+. doi:10.1089/tmj.2009.0153.

Agha, Z., Schapira, R., Laud, P., McNutt, G., & Roter, D. (2009). Patient satisfaction with physician-patient communication during telemedicine. *Telemedicine and e-Health, 15*(9), 830–839.

Allan, J., & Dixon, A. (2009). Older women's experiences of depression: A hermeneutic phenomenological study. *Journal of Psychiatric and Mental Health Nursing, 16*(10), 865–873.

Ask me 3 good questions for your good health. (n.d.). Retrieved from www.npsf.org/askme3.

Beck, C. T., & Gable, R. K. (2001). *Postpartum depression screening scale.* Los Angeles, CA: Western Psychological Services.

Bjarnason, D., Mick, J., Thompson, J., & Cloyd, E. (2009). Perspectives on transcultural care. *Nursing Clinics of North America, 44*(4), 495–503. doi:10.1016/j.cnur.2009.07.009.

Blondis, M. N., & Jackson, B. E. (1982). *Nonverbal communication with patients: Back to the human touch* (2nd ed.). New York: John Wiley & Sons.

Bolster, D., & Manias, E. (2010). Person-centred interactions between nurses and patients during medication activities in an acute hospital setting: Qualitative observation and interview study. *International Journal of Nursing Studies, 47*(2), 154–165.

Brown, B. V. (2008). *Key indicators of child and youth well-being: Completing the picture.* New York: Lawrence Erlbaum Associates.

Canabrava, D.D.S. (2011). Nursing consultation of mental health supported by the interpersonal relations theory: Report of experience [portuguese]. *Ciência, Cuidado e Saúde, 10*(1), 150–156.

Carpenito, L. J. (2009). *Handbook of nursing diagnoses* (13th ed.). Philadelphia: Lippincott Williams and Wilkins.

Carter, M. (2009). Trust, power, and vulnerability: A discourse on helping in nursing. *Nursing Clinics of North America, 44*(4), 393–405.

Coopersmith, S. (1967). *The antecedents of self-esteem.* San Francisco: W.H. Freeman.

Cox, J. L., Holden, J. M., & Sagovsky, R. (1987). Detection of postnatal depression: Development of the 10-item Edinburgh Postnatal Depression Scale. *British Journal of Psychiatry, 150,* 782–786.

Doss, S., DePascal, P., & Hadley, K. (2011). Patient-nurse partnerships. *Nephrology Nursing Journal, 38*(2), 115–124.

Dziopa, F., & Ahern, K. (2009a). Three different ways mental health nurses develop quality therapeutic relationships. *Issues in Mental Health Nursing, 30*(1), 14–22.

Dziopa, F., & Ahern, K. (2009b). What makes a quality therapeutic relationship in psychiatric/mental health nursing: A review of the research literature. *Internet Journal of Advanced Nursing Practice, 10*(1), 1–19.

Hall, E. (1973). *The silent language.* Garden City, NY: Doubleday/Anchor Press.

Henry, S., Fuhrel Forbis, A., Rogers, M.A.M., & Eggly, S. (2011). Association between nonverbal communication during clinical interactions and outcomes: A systematic review and meta-analysis. *Patient Education and Counseling, 86*(3), 297–315.

Hughes, R. G. (2008). *Patient safety and quality: An evidence-based handbook for nurses.* Rockville, MD: Agency for Healthcare Research and Quality. (Prepared with support from the Robert Wood Johnson Foundation.) AHRQ Publication No. 08–0043.

Institute of Medicine (IOM). (2010). *The future of nursing: Leading change, advancing health.* Retrieved from www.iom.edu/Reports/2010/The-Future-of-Nursing-Leading-Change-Advancing-Health.aspx.

Institute of Medicine (IOM). (2011, March 10). *Innovations in health literacy: Workshop summary.* Retrieved from www.iom.edu/Reports/2011/Innovations-in-Health-Literacy.aspx.

Johannesen, R. L. (2008). *Ethics in human communication* (6th ed.). Prospect Heights, IL: Waveland Press.

Jourard, S. (1971). *The transparent self* (rev. ed.). New York: Van Nostrand Reinhold.

Luft, J. (1969). *Of human interaction.* Palo Alto, CA: National Press Books.

Luft, J. (1984). *Group processes: An introduction to group dynamics* (3rd ed.). Palo Alto, CA: Mayfield.

Luptak, M., Dailey, N., Juretic, M., Rupper, R., Hill, R., Hicken, B., et al. (2010). The Care Coordination Home Telehealth (CCHT) rural demonstration project: A symptom-based approach for serving older veterans in remote geographical settings. *Rural and Remote Health, 10*(2), 1375.

Melnyk, B. M., & Fineout-Overholt, E. (2011). *Evidence-based practice in nursing & health care: A guide to best practice* (2nd ed.). Philadelphia, PA: Wolters Kluwer Health: Lippincott Williams & Wilkins.

Miller, C., & McCurley, M. C. (2011). Federal interagency communication strategies for addressing radiation emergencies and other public health crises. *Health Physics, 101*(5), 559–561.

O'Toole, A., & Welt, S. R. (1989). *Interpersonal theory in nursing practice.* New York: Springer.

Peplau, H. E. (1963). Process and concept of learning. In S. Burd, & M. Marshall (Eds.), *Some clinical approaches to psychiatric nursing* (pp. 348–352). New York: Macmillan.

Peplau, H. E. (1964). *Basic principles of patient counseling* (2nd ed.). Philadelphia: Smith Kline and French Laboratories.

Peplau, H. E. (1969). Professional closeness: As a special kind of involvement with a patient, client, or family group. *Nursing Forum, 8*(4), 342–360.

Peplau, H. E. (1991). *Interpersonal relations in nursing.* New York: Springer.

Quality Safety and Education for Nurses (QSEN). (2012). *Patient centered care.* Retrieved from www.qsen.org/definition.php?id=1.

Raths, L., Harmin, M., & Simon, S. (1978). *Values and teaching.* Columbus, OH: Charles E. Merrill.

Rogers, C. (1965). *Client-centered therapy.* Boston: Houghton Mifflin.

Roth-Herbst, J., Borbely, C. J., & Brooks-Gunn, J. (2008). Developing indicators of confidence, character, and caring in adolescents. In B. V. Brown (Ed.), *Key indicators of child and youth well-being: Completing the picture* (pp. 167–196). New York: Lawrence Erlbaum Associates.

Ruesch, J., & Bateson, G. (1987). *Communication: The social matrix of psychiatry.* New York: W.W. Norton.

Sandars, J. (2009). The use of reflection in medical education: AMEE Guide No. 44. *Medical Teacher, 31*(8), 685–695.

Sears, R. R. (1970). Relation of early socialization experiences to self-concepts and gender role in middle childhood. *Child Development, 41,* 267–289.

Shipley, S. (2010). Listening: A concept analysis. *Nursing Forum, 45*(2), 125–134. doi:10.1111/j.1744-6198.2010.00174.x.

Smith-Miller, C. A., Leak, A., Harlan, C. A., Dieckmann, J., & Sherwood, G. (2010). Leaving the comfort of the familiar: Fostering workplace cultural awareness through short-term global experiences. *Nursing Forum, 45,* 18–28. doi:10.1111/j.1744-6198.2009.00163.x.

Speros, C. (2011). Promoting health literacy: A nursing imperative. *Nursing Clinics of North America, 46*(3), 321–333.

Stuart, G. W., & Laraia, M. T. (2009). *Principles and practice of psychiatric nursing* (9th ed.). St. Louis: Elsevier Mosby.

Sullivan, H. S. (1953). *The interpersonal theory of psychiatry.* New York: W.W. Norton.

Tejero, L. M.S. (2011). The mediating role of the nurse-patient dyad bonding in bringing about patient satisfaction. *Journal of Advanced Nursing.* doi:10.1111/j.1365-2648.2011.05795.x.

Thielst, C. (2010). At the crossroads: NRTRC white paper examines trends driving the convergence of telehealth, EHRs and HIE. *World Hospitals and Health Services, 46*(4), 17–23.

U.S. Department of Health and Human Services. (2010). *Healthy People 2020: Improving the health of Americans.* Washington, DC: U.S. Government Printing Office.

U.S. Department of Health and Human Services. (n.d.) *Healthy People 2010. Leading health indicators.* Retrieved from www.healthypeople.gov/2020/LHI/default.aspx#.

Watzlawick, P., Beavin, J. H., & Jackson, D. D. (1967). *Pragmatics of human communication: A study of interactional patterns, pathologies and paradoxes.* New York: W.W. Norton.

Wright, L. M., & Leahey, M. (2009). *Nurses and families: A guide to family assessment and intervention* (5th ed.). Philadelphia: F.A. Davis.

Ethical Issues Related to Health Promotion

Jeanne Sorrell

 WEBSITE

http://evolve.elsevier.com/Edelman/
- Study Questions
- Glossary

OBJECTIVES

After completing this chapter, the reader will be able to:
- Discuss health promotion as a moral endeavor.
- Describe the relationship of health care ethics to health promotion.
- Analyze the relationship of various ethical theories to the nursing role in health promotion.
- Discuss the historical development and importance to nursing of the codes of ethics.
- Describe contemporary ethical issues in health promotion (e.g., genetics, culture, end-of-life decision-making).
- Analyze problems related to health promotion using an ethical decision-making framework.

KEY TERMS

Advocacy
Applied ethics
Autonomy
Beliefs
Beneficence
Civil liberties
Codes of ethics
Confidentiality
Consequentialist
Consent
Descriptive theories
Duty-based theories

Ethical dilemmas
Ethical issues
Feminist ethics
Genetic counseling
Informed consent
Justice
Maleficence
Metaethics
Moral
Moral agency
Moral distress
Moral philosophy

Nonmaleficence
Normative theories
Paternalism
Preventive ethics
Privacy Rule
Self-determination
Social justice
Trust
Utilitarian theories
Value theories
Veracity

Assisted Suicide or Emotional Support?

A nurse in a clinic is accountable for ongoing assessments of pain management. One of the long-term clients, Ana, has required increasing amounts of narcotics for her pain management over the last year. The nurse has known for more than a year that Ana's husband, Victor, has amyotrophic lateral sclerosis, or Lou Gehrig's disease. Victor's disease adds a great deal of stress to both their lives, which has had a negative effect on Ana's physical health. The nurse assesses the emotional toll of Victor's illness as part of Ana's pain assessment. During one of these discussions, Ana asks the nurse how much of her narcotic medication her husband would need to take to end his life.

- What does it mean to provide someone with the "means" to commit suicide?
- What questions would you have for Ana at this point of the conversation?
- What would you do with the answers?
- Do you have any obligations to Victor?
- Do you collaborate with Victor's physician?
- What is in Ana's "best interests"?
- Who or what are your resources?
- What does nursing as a discipline believe about assisted suicide?
- What is the law in your state?
- What should you do?

HEALTH PROMOTION AS A MORAL ENDEAVOR

When nurses provide service to society through health-promotion interventions, their care for individuals can be seen as a moral endeavor. Moral issues are confronted in the process of attempting to enhance the well-being of a society overall, as well as promoting and protecting health for individual members of a society. Health is considered a human good because it helps people to have a desirable quality of life and achieve life goals. At the level of the individual, health promotion involves providing services that help people achieve their potential.

In order to set a higher standard of health for all people, there needs to be a change in our approach to understanding health and the development of health-promotion ethics (Murphy, 2008). Understanding the contexts of people's lives is crucial to health-promotion endeavors. This entails consideration of a variety of factors that can affect a person's health status, such as mental, physical, spiritual, environmental, cultural, social, and genetic factors. Viewing health promotion as a moral endeavor—some would even call it a moral imperative (Marks & Shive, 2007)—is consistent with the intent and goals of the U.S. government's prevention agenda for the nation as presented in *Healthy People 2020* (see www.healthypeople.gov).

The following are the four overarching goals of *Healthy People 2020*:

- Attain high-quality, longer lives free of preventable disease, disability, injury, and premature death.
- Achieve health equity, eliminate disparities, and improve the health of all groups.
- Create social and physical environments that promote good health for all.
- Promote quality of life, healthy development, and healthy behaviors across all life stages.

The purpose of health-promotion efforts, as discussed throughout this book, is to ensure that people have access to the tools and strategies to live at the highest level of well-being possible. Health-promotion efforts address environmental obstacles to human health, such as pollution, marketing of harmful products, and economic disparities. Thus health promotion is not the province of a single discipline but involves individuals, health care providers, and institutions working together to create a positive environment for health and achieve health goals (Ruger, 2008).

This chapter focuses on understanding the health professional's moral responsibilities toward individuals and society with regard to facilitating health and well-being, or the relief of suffering. Professional responsibilities are obligations incurred by disciplines that provide a service to society. For example, the *Code of Ethics for Nurses with Interpretive Statements* written by the American Nurses Association (ANA, 2001) promises that "nursing encompasses the prevention of illness, the alleviation of suffering, and the protection, promotion, and restoration of health in the care of individuals, families, groups and communities" (p. 5). This document, along with the ANA's *Nursing's Social Policy Statement* (ANA, 2010), describes the ethical responsibilities of U.S. nurses (Boxes 5-1 and 5-2). The WebLinks for this chapter on the book's Evolve site include a link to the ANA's *Code of Ethics*. The International Council of Nurses (2006) also has a *Code of Ethics*, revised in 2005, which serves as a standard for nurses worldwide and is easily accessible via the Internet.

Ethical issues focused on health promotion are best viewed as a subset of health care ethics that, in turn, has its roots in moral philosophy and value theory. This chapter discusses factors that can affect health promotion across the life span in diverse health care settings. The development, scope, and limits of ethical theories and perspectives are explored in relation to problems in health promotion. A basic assumption of this chapter is that the anticipation and prevention of ethical problems is a critical component of ethical professional action. A variety of real and hypothetical cases are presented to illustrate how ethical issues relate to health promotion. Strategies to aid the health care professional in identifying, anticipating, and addressing ethical issues are provided throughout.

The terms *ethical* and *moral* are used interchangeably throughout the chapter. Even though the two concepts are sometimes characterized differently, they have the same root meanings. The term ethics is derived from the Greek word "ethos," meaning customs, conduct, or character. The term **moral** is derived from the Latin word "mores" and originally referred to doing something from a custom or habit (Davis et al., 2010).

BOX 5-1   CODE OF ETHICS FOR NURSES

- The nurse, in all professional relationships, practices with compassion and respect for the inherent dignity, worth, and uniqueness of every individual, unrestricted by considerations of social or economic status, personal attributes, or the nature of health problems.
- The nurse's primary commitment is to the person, whether an individual or part of a family, group, or community.
- The nurse promotes, advocates for, and strives to protect the health, safety, and rights of the person.
- The nurse is responsible and accountable for individual nursing practice and determines the appropriate delegation of tasks consistent with the nurse's obligation to provide optimal person care.
- The nurse owes the same duties to self as to others, including the responsibility to preserve integrity and safety, to maintain competence, and to continue personal and professional growth.

- The nurse participates in establishing, maintaining, and improving health care environments and conditions of employment conducive to the provision of quality health care and consistent with the values of the profession through individual and collective action.
- The nurse participates in the advancement of the profession through contributions to practice, education, administration, and knowledge development.
- The nurse collaborates with other health professionals and the public in promoting community, national, and international efforts to meet health needs.
- The profession of nursing, as represented by associations and their members, is responsible for articulating nursing values, for maintaining the integrity of the profession and its practice, and for shaping social policy.

From American Nurses Association. (2001). *Code of ethics for nurses with interpretive statements*. Washington, DC: Author; American Nurses Association. (2008). *Guide to the code of ethics for nurses: Interpretation and application*. Washington, DC: Author. ©2001 American Nurses Association. Reprinted with permission. All rights reserved.

BOX 5-2   NURSING'S SOCIAL POLICY STATEMENT

Excerpt: Knowledge Base for Nursing Practice

The knowledge base for nursing practice includes nursing science, philosophy, and ethics.

Nurses partner with individuals, families, communities, and populations to address such issues as:

- Promotion of health and safety
- Care and self-care processes
- Physical, emotional, and spiritual comfort, discomfort, and pain
- Adaptation to physiological and pathophysiological processes
- Emotions related to experiences of birth, growth and development, health, illness, disease, and death

- Meanings ascribed to health and illness
- Decision-making and ability to make choices
- Relationships, role performance, and change processes within relationships
- Social policies and their effects on the health of individuals, families, and communities
- Health care systems and their relationships with access to and quality of health care
- The environment and the prevention of disease

From American Nurses Association. (2010). *Nursing's social policy statement* (3rd ed.). Silver Spring, MD: Author. ©2010 American Nurses Association. Reprinted with permission. All rights reserved.

HEALTH CARE ETHICS

Origins of Applied Ethics in Moral Philosophy

The discipline underlying practice, or applied ethics, is moral philosophy. Moral philosophy is concerned with discovering or proposing what is right or wrong, or good or bad, in human action toward other humans and other entities such as animals and the environment. Singer (1993, p. vii) described the crucial questions of moral philosophy as "What ought I to do? How ought I to live?" Among the tasks of moral philosophy is that of formulating theories or frameworks to guide action. Using a moral theory to propose and implement appropriate actions in troubling situations guides the decision maker toward good and the avoidance of harmful actions.

The theories that emerge as a result of philosophical inquiry about good action are called value theories because they are concerned with either discovering what humans seem to value (descriptive theories) or proposing what they ought to value (normative theories) to achieve predetermined goals.

Types of Ethical Theories
Descriptive Value Theories

Value theories are based on observations of human behavior over time and in a variety of settings. Descriptive theories do not tell us what actions we ought to take. They are not directive; they merely tell us how people act toward each other and their environments and what they seem to believe are good or moral actions.

Normative Value Theories

Normative theories, on the other hand, are concerned with ensuring good actions. They are reasoned explanations of the moral purpose of human interactions, or they are divinely "revealed" truths about good action (religious ethics). Actions that are in accord with the foundational principles of the theory are the type of right or good actions we should take given that we believe the principles (e.g., fairness and trust are valid). What is often called the golden rule is a classic example of a normative principle. The golden rule essentially commits us to treating other people in the manner that we, ourselves, would wish to be treated, given similar circumstances. Normative theories permit judgments about the value of actions based on the extent to which these actions are consistent with the assumptions of the theory. They are key to decision-making and relevant for health promotion, but often overlooked by policymakers (Bennett & Smith, 2007).

Consequentialism Theories. The foundational principle of John Stuart Mill's (1861) theory proposes that actions are good insofar as they are aimed at yielding the greatest amount of happiness or pleasure or causing the least amount of harm or pain to individuals and overall society. This theory is often formulated as the greatest good for the greatest number. Mill viewed pleasure as a complex concept, with qualitative as well as quantitative aspects. This perspective is consequentialist: it holds that the consequences or intended consequences of actions matter. Therefore from the consequentialist perspective, any decision about intended actions or interventions must take into account all knowable potential consequences. Among the implications of this type of theory for health care professionals is the imperative that data gathering must be thorough and complete. Additionally, the professional is accountable for possessing the appropriate skills and knowledge to undertake actions that will promote good. The professional's decision can be evaluated as bad or good to the extent that actions are in accord with the theory: in this case "right actions" would be those that are directed toward promoting the greatest good or causing the least harm. The propositions of the theory direct what is needed for moral action or, stated another way, for doing the right thing.

Duty-Based Theories. Other normative value theories are not as heavily weighted toward producing good consequences. For example, duty-based theories, such as that of Immanuel Kant (1724-1804) and those of various religions (Judaism, Christianity, Islam), depend more on adherence to duties than on good consequences. Individuals are viewed as having certain duties that cannot be circumvented, even if deliberately avoiding the duty would result in good outcomes. For religions, these rules are imparted in some way by a divine being.

For Kant, our capacity to reason is what permits moral action. Moral reasoning has been proposed as a model for health promotion (Buchanan, 2006). Kant believed that lying is always wrong even if on some occasions it produces a good outcome. It is wrong because it is irrational to lie. If lying were widely practiced, we would lose our ability to trust what others tell us, and this would make effective communication impossible. Kant based his theory on the idea that what separates us from other life forms is our ability to make rules for ourselves using our ability to reason. His main rule, whereby each of us can determine for ourselves a moral course of action, is the categorical imperative. The categorical imperative was framed several different ways by Kant; however, the easiest to understand for current purposes is the following conceptualization, "I ought never to act except in such a way that I can also will that my maxim should become a universal law" (Kant, 1997/1785, p. 318). This could be stated alternatively as a question to ask oneself before acting, "Could any other person in the same or similar circumstances also take this action or refrain from this action?"

Limitations of Moral Theory

It is important to keep in mind that moral theories arise out of a particular perspective or philosophy about the world. They are conceptualized as a result of this perspective and within a historical and political context. The philosophical approach that evaluates value theories or ethical perspectives for their congruence and usefulness in human decision-making across

environments is metaethics. Philosophers interested in meta-ethical questions investigate where our ethical principles come from and what they mean. Are they merely social inventions? Do they involve more than expressions of our individual emotions? Metaethics allows us to critique the adequacy of ethical approaches for application across a variety of practice settings and cultural environments. Other sorts of metaethical questions posed by moral philosophers include the following: Are there such things as absolute ethical truths? If so, how do we go about discovering these? If not, what foundations should we use to guide our actions? What considerations are important? How do we know which actions are good? What is a valid moral theory? Should human values be congruent across settings and cultures?

Religiously based moral theories depend on the idea that good actions are those that obey the laws of a supreme being. However, because the foundational tenets of religions do not mirror each other, what constitutes a moral action from a Jewish perspective may well be morally prohibited from a Roman Catholic perspective. Moreover, even within a religion, the tenets of its different sects or branches may not always lead to the same conclusions about good actions. Nurses and other health care professionals need to recognize the influence of religion in persons' lives and not judge them on this account, because their duty to provide safe, competent, compassionate, and ethical care extends to an accommodation of religious and cultural values and practices (Reimer-Kirkham, 2009).

As a result of diverse religious and cultural values that affect health-promotion activities, there are divergent but strongly held views on what is the "good" for humans. Many contemporary philosophers have argued that there can be no single approach that permits the identification or resolution of all moral problems (Rachels & Rachels, 2011; Weston, 2010). Even the golden rule can be problematic from a cross-cultural perspective. For example, I might want to be treated as an autonomous being capable of making my own decisions, but a person from Thailand might be more used to family-centered decision-making. Treating my Thai friend as I would wish to be treated would be a mistake. An understanding of cultural beliefs is necessary for good action in such cases (Box 5-3: Diversity Awareness).

Additionally, utilitarian theories emerged out of a particular era and as a result of perceived injustices in societal arrangements in England during the turmoil of the industrial revolution. Utilitarians such as Jeremy Bentham (1748-1832) and John Stuart Mill (1806-1873) sought frameworks that would permit the rectification of unjust policy decisions and the vast economic inequities within their society. For this reason such theories have a tendency to privilege the good of the group over the needs of individuals.

Thus, we can see that it is not prudent to adopt one theory to guide actions in every situation related to health promotion. If moral theories are applied indiscriminately, it can lead to actions that are problematic for an individual and/or a group. Health-promotion activities mandate not only a general understanding of the nature of the problem or potential problem but also knowledge of the values, beliefs, needs, and desires of the person or population being served.

Self-Reflection

The increasingly multicultural society, multiple languages spoken, and diverse set of values presents health care providers with complex assessment and planning problems. Nurses and other health professionals are charged with facilitating optimal care for all, regardless of "personal attributes" and taking into account "the needs and values of all persons" (ANA, 2001, Provision 1 and interpretive statements). It is not possible to know details about every culture as well as the unique differences of each individual, family community, and group within each culture. There are strategies, however, that a health professional can employ to ensure that an individual's unique values and particular needs are the focus of health-promotion interventions. When a particular culture is part of your population base, opportunities should be pursued for learning individual differences in beliefs, values, and needs related to that culture. To facilitate your assessment, perhaps the most important undertaking is self-reflection. The following are self-reflection and other considerations for providing culturally sensitive care:

- Commitment to increasing knowledge and skill in sensitivity to cultural differences
- Self-awareness and awareness of one's own biases, beliefs, and values. Ask yourself:
  - What values and biases you bring to the relationship
  - How your background has influenced your beliefs
  - What knowledge and experience you have to draw on
  - What values you think you share with the client—validate with the client
  - How comfortable you are with who you are
  - What further information you need to facilitate culturally competent care
  - Who or what is the best resource for further information
- Awareness of the validity of different beliefs and values
- Attempts to understand the meaning behind client behavior
- Increased knowledge of the beliefs and values of other cultures
- Developing cultural skills through encounters with people from other cultures

BOX 5-4 INNOVATIVE PRACTICE

Nurses as Genetic Counselors

The genome project was completed by the International Human Genome Sequencing Consortium, led in the United States by the National Human Genome Research Institute and the Department of Energy, on April 14, 2003. This represents an important initial step in expanding our potential to understand the genetic contributors to disease and to formulate interventions. However, there are complex ethical issues associated with, and raised by, genetic advances.

Nurses are in an excellent position to position themselves for attaining advanced knowledge and skills related to serving as specialized genetic counselors. Although many health care professionals have the skills to counsel individuals about genetic testing issues, especially in their fields of expertise, genetic counselors are an increasingly important resource.

Genetic counselors are specially trained master's-prepared individuals. These professionals can obtain certification through the American Board of Genetic Counselors. Their professional society is the National Society of Genetic Counselors. Genetic counselors enter the field from a range of backgrounds including biology, genetics, nursing, psychology, public health, and social work.

The goals of the discipline are outlined in the society's *Code of Ethics*. Genetic counselors provide counseling services that are nondirective to avoid coercion or persuasion. Although there is controversy about how directive or nondirective advice should be based on the ethical ideals of autonomy, counselors strive to be nondirective while at the same time tailoring information to fit the specific

needs of persons. Andrews and colleagues (2002) note that nondirective methodology is a way for the genetic counseling community to avoid association with the eugenics movement. Because advances in embryo preimplantation genetic testing, as well as in utero fetal testing, permit screening for certain superior characteristics or the screening out of certain genetic diseases, the perceived need to distance the profession from this issue is understandable.

Ethical issues related to genetic counseling for screening purposes that apply both for genetic counselors and for other health care providers include the following:

- Understanding the wider context of genetic testing implications (privacy, discrimination, economics, health insurance denials, implications for family members, anxiety and apprehension, and eugenics [striving for perfection] and its associated implications for individuals and society)
- Assisting people to determine the risks and benefits of screening
- Assisting people to prepare for their future needs
- Assisting people with their procreative planning
- Understanding how cultural differences impact counseling needs
- Addressing societal issues related to genetic advances include determining research priorities, justice issues, and discrimination of the genetically disadvantaged

Sources: Andrens, L.B., Mehlman, M.J., & Rothstein, M.A. (2002). Genetics: Ethics, law and policy, St. Paul MN: West Group/Thompson; National Society of Genetic Counselors. (2004). *National Society of Genetic Counselors Code of Ethics*. Retrieved June 3, 2004, from www.nsgc.org/newsroom/code_of_ethics.asp.

Specific principles derived from ethical theories have proved useful because they highlight salient aspects of complex problems and help to examine implications of different proposed courses of action. Selection of pertinent principles, however, depends both on the context of the problem and on the beliefs and values of the individual or group for which action is needed. For example, a woman seeks assistance in deciding whether to undergo genetic testing for the breast cancer gene *BRCA2* because several members of her immediate and antecedent families have been diagnosed with breast or associated cancers. She tells her nurse practitioner that she is not sure whether it

would be beneficial to be tested. The nurse practitioner, in facilitating the woman's health-promotion efforts, understands that she must use clinical judgment to facilitate the woman's autonomous choice. Understanding the requirements of the principle of autonomy is important in helping the woman make her decision. It is not sufficient, however, to understand the meaning of autonomy and its limits; we also have to know something about the woman's life, values, beliefs, and relationships in order to provide her with the information and resources necessary for her decision. If the woman is screened and the results found positive for the gene, the woman not only must decide her next actions but also must consider the implications of the results (e.g., how the results affect her children or her decision to have children). Box 5-4: Innovative Practice presents information on genetic counseling. Individual principles of importance to decision-making in health care settings are explored in this chapter. They, along with associated ethical considerations such as professional, feminist, and virtue ethics, underpin a framework of moral decision-making for health promotion that is presented at the end of this chapter.

Feminist Ethics and Caring
Feminist Ethics

Feminist perspectives on ethics derive from the feminist movement's efforts to expose and rectify injustices to women. Feminist thought is not limited in its influence to the United States; it has also influenced societal changes in other countries. The feminist movement perspectives have broadened to include problems common to all oppressed groups. Feminist ethics, emerging as it has out of feminist thought and feminist philosophy, is not another ethical theory as such; rather it presents a viewpoint on moral problems in health care and other areas of life that have been historically neglected.

Feminist scholars have noted that traditional moral theories, and the principles derived from them, have been unable to adequately capture the nature and origins of health care problems. Feminist critics assert that moral decision-making must include an investigation of both hidden and overt power relationships implicit in ethical problems. Additionally, it is important to understand the contexts of situations and the interrelationships of those involved because human beings are not isolated individuals who may be viewed as totally independent of others. Thus, hidden power imbalances in various relationships and situations are an important element in moral decision-making. Feminist ethics, then, contributes a perspective that is often missing from traditional ethical approaches. This changes both the way problems are perceived and the way they are explored.

Characteristics of feminist ethics include the following:

- An understanding that human beings are inseparable from their relationships with others
- A focus on care and responsibility aspects of relationships, rather than application of abstract principles (Davis et al., 2010)
- A concern with the development of character and attitudes that result in caring actions reflective of a person who is related to rather than detached from context
- A concern for the rights and the equality of all individuals that is not limited to the oppression of women

Thus, feminist ethics allows for a critique of the treatment of individuals in the contexts in which they live. This approach to ethics often focuses on imbalances of power and oppression attributable to gender, sexual orientation, ethnicity, socioeconomics, politics, and other characteristics. For example, a punitive approach to perinatal substance abuse is not associated with improved outcomes for the fetus; in fact, the fetus may be at greater risk because it makes women fearful of accessing health services.

The feminist ethic of care is an important concept for health promotion because it focuses on the nature of health care professional–person relationships and on the context of people's lives. This approach to care has found increasing acceptance in nursing as both a virtue of the nurse and a responsibility of practice in which treatment is offered on a common ground basis that will support people within their relationships. Carol Gilligan's (1982, 2011) research, among that of others, has been instrumental in the acceptance of the concept of care as informing ethics in nursing practice.

The Ethic of Care

The ethic of care calls for a knowledgeable and skillful health professional to assume responsibility for unique needs of an individual in all of his or her complexities. Benner and colleagues (1998) define care as "the alleviation of vulnerability; the promotion of growth and health; the facilitation of comfort, dignity or a good and peaceful death," noting that care is "the dominant ethic found in [nurses'] stories of everyday practice" (p. 233). Many of the current conceptualizations of care, viewed as a responsibility of practice, have their origins in the work of Carol Gilligan. Gilligan (1982) was a graduate student and then colleague of Lawrence Kohlberg, a developmental psychologist. The main focus of Kohlberg's (1981, 1984) body of work was the nature of moral character development, which was informed by Piaget's work on the stages of cognitive development in children. Kohlberg's stages of moral development were derived from longitudinal studies of young men. These moral reasoning studies were designed around the idea that an ability to apply conceptions of justice, rules, and principles to difficult situations denoted the highest achievable level of moral development. Gilligan challenged the reliance on only males in the study of moral reasoning and implemented studies of women's experiences, discovering that women had a moral orientation based on the caring and nurturing of others. In this framework, interrelationships and contexts are critically important in understanding the complexities of a given situation (Paulsen, 2011).

One way to look at an ethic of care versus an ethic of justice is that justice demands that we treat people fairly and not focus on incidental differences in decision-making. Thus, justice is impartial and nondiscriminatory. An ethic of care, however, requires an understanding of situational particularities, ensuring that we try to understand a given individual's needs in the context of his or her life. Generally justice and care have been viewed as opposing concepts. Liaschenko (1999), however, presented a compelling argument for them to be viewed as interrelated concepts, in which justice policies concern individuals within a society, which in turn help to protect people's individual interests.

Limits of the Ethic of Care

One problem with using care as an ethic of health-promotion practice has to do with the issue of moral predictability or certainty (Nelson, 1992). If the emphasis is on relationships and there are no criteria for right and wrong actions, how can one be assured of the morally correct action in a given situation? An answer to this could be that a morally correct action emerges as a result of nursing judgment based on prior knowledge, experience, and an engaged relationship with the person. Thus the process of the interaction, coupled with the character, knowledge, experience, and intent of the moral agent, is the crucial factor that achieves the moral good for an individual. The action is right if the nurse possesses the right characteristics and the person's complex needs are met. When the solution to one person's problems affects others, however, the rightness of the action depends on more than the one-on-one caring relationship. The problem remains one of choosing between this person's needs and the needs of others who might be affected by the chosen actions. This problem is resistant to resolution via an ethic of care alone. The problem analysis framework described later combines the ethic of care with other considerations. Both an ethic of care and the principles derived from traditional moral theory may be needed for health promotion.

The purpose of ethical inquiry in health promotion is to gain clarity on actual or potential moral issues arising in the context of health-promotion endeavors and to understand what is expected of the health-promotion agent viewed as a moral agent. Ethical inquiry will not permit the resolution of all problems, because the environments in which health-promotion efforts are conceptualized are incredibly complex. It is impossible to foresee all possible consequences of action, but ethical reasoning can facilitate appropriate and in-depth data gathering, permit the uncovering of hidden agendas and interests, and focus on the most salient aspects of a particular problem, thus enhancing professional judgment.

Professional judgment and ensuing actions are integral to the goal of providing a good for the population of concern. Thus, health promotion is a moral endeavor requiring morally sensitive and knowledgeable agents. But what are the scopes and limits of a health care professional's obligations to anticipate, identify, and address morally problematic issues related to the promotion and protection of health for individuals, groups, and society? How do health care professionals balance their duties to individuals with a duty to the society? How are individuals' freedoms (autonomy) balanced with the collective responsibilities owed to society and future generations? The following section addresses these questions.

PROFESSIONAL RESPONSIBILITY

Accountability to Individuals and Society

Professions

Although this section focuses on the nursing discipline's mandate to promote health, the discussion can also be applied to the responsibilities of other health professionals who assume health-promotion responsibilities. Using the term *profession* to denote the status of nursing and other disciplines is controversial. Nursing is a profession insofar as it provides a service to society and is self-governing, and its members are accountable for their actions (Grace, 2001). One important characteristic of professions, especially those that provide crucial services to society, is that they have codes of ethics that provide essential elements of their promises of service to society. A significant consequence of professional status is that members can be held accountable for their practice formally by professional licensure boards. More importantly, they are morally accountable for practicing

according to their discipline's implicit or explicit code of ethics. Codes of ethics provide a normative framework for professional actions. A professional implicitly accepts these codes on acquiring membership in the discipline. Thus, each professional should establish a personal perspective on ethical practice within the broad framework of professional codes (Corey et al., 2011).

Trust

Service professions such as nursing, medicine, and teaching are in part defined by their relationships to those in need of services. This relationship is one of trust. The professional has the knowledge and skills to meet an individual's needs or the needs of a group. The potential recipients of services lack the knowledge or ability to anticipate or meet their own needs but trust that the professional will keep their best interests as the primary goal and will strive to meet their needs. For example, in the current health care environment in the United States, people may have trouble accessing a specialist provider because of their particular insurance coverage or the inability to afford health care insurance or to pay on their own.

Health care professionals are responsible not only for promoting health and healing but also for recognizing and addressing barriers to health-promotion activities. *Nursing's Social Policy Statement* (ANA, 2010) provides a detailed account of the nursing discipline's responsibilities, which describes the social contract between society and the nursing profession and emphasizes the nurse's responsibility to advocate for changes when health care services are threatened.

Codes of Ethics

Codes of ethics are examples of normative ethics in that they prescribe how members of a profession ought to act, given the goals and purposes of the profession related to individuals and society. In this sense the goals and purposes of the profession serve as foundational ethical principles. The provisions of the code provide direction and express "expectations of ethical behavior" (ANA, 2001, p. 5). They represent the profession's promises to society. "A code of ethics makes explicit the primary goals, values and obligations of the profession" (ANA, 2001, p. 5). Although the public is not directly involved in the formulation of such codes and, indeed, is for the most part not even aware of their existence, the profession is responsive to the evolving needs of a given society. It can be said that codes of ethics are the tentative end results of a discipline's political process in that they are not static but result from debate and discussion among the profession's scholars, leaders, and members over time.

When the nurse's strongly held values and beliefs are challenged by a nursing care situation, the nurse has the right to decide whether to participate. Decisions not to participate in a situation cannot be made trivially because of the trust relationship and a nurse's moral accountability for actions. The threat to the nurse's integrity must be serious and the person's well-being must not be jeopardized by the nurse's absence. Other arrangements must be made for care of the person in such circumstances. The nurse who encounters repeated threats to integrity has a responsibility to consider changing the situation in some way. Change efforts may be directed toward institutional policy or may require that an alternative work environment be considered.

Codes of ethics tend to offer guidelines not only about responsibilities for ensuring good care but also about responsibilities for recognizing and addressing barriers to service. The nursing profession in the United States, according to the ANA's *Code of Ethics,* proposes that "the nurse promotes, advocates for, and strives to protect the health, safety, and rights of the person" (ANA, 2001, Provision 3). This requires anticipation of future health needs and political activity when necessary to ensure health promotion. Codes of ethics represent the ideals of the profession and thus serve as general guides to action. The ANA *Code of Ethics* is nonnegotiable: that is, the goals and intent of the code may not be ignored, diluted, or downplayed by individuals or institutions employing nurses in the United States (ANA, 1994).

Advocacy

Advocacy, as an expectation of nurses, is strongly reinforced both in the *Code of Ethics* (ANA, 2001, 2008) and in innumerable scholarly articles. However, advocacy is also a controversial concept. The meaning of the term *advocacy* is derived from its use in law. In legal jurisprudence, advocacy is aggressive action taken on behalf of an individual, or perhaps a group viewed as an individual entity, to protect or secure that individual's rights. The individual lawyer does not have an opposing obligation to attend to social justice issues. This attention to broader questions of justice is the responsibility of other areas of the justice system.

Nurses and other health care professionals have a responsibility to speak up on behalf of people whose rights have been compromised or endangered. This is part of the nurse's role because people may not recognize either what is needed to meet their needs or when the care they are receiving is substandard. However, that is not the end of their responsibilities. They must also consider that specific actions they undertake in the name of advocacy may pose problems for other people who are relying on them for health care services.

For example, Juanita Rimmer, a nurse case manager, is assisting Jim Bailey to apply for services in a rehabilitation facility because he has residual hemiparesis secondary to a cerebro-vascular accident. There is a waiting list at the facility, but Juanita believes it is a priority for Jim to be treated there because he lives with his frail, elderly mother who will not be able to assist him with his activities of daily living. Because Juanita represents other people who will also benefit from rehabilitation, her decision to advocate for Jim must be weighed against the needs of these other people. A moral responsibility associated with advocacy in health care settings is that the effect of actions on others is considered. When advocating extra attention or specialized care for a given person, an injustice may be rendered simultaneously to other people in the nurse's care. Thus, professional advocacy requires a balancing of the health needs of the individual with the health needs of the population (Grace, 2001).

Advocacy is an ideal of health care professions that requires attention to individuals and to broader societal concerns. **Moral**

agency on the part of the nurse requires action and motivation directed to some moral end that is enacted through relationships. Being aware of one's self in relation to individual persons helps to establish the moral choice required to advocate for them (O'Keefe-McCarthy, 2009). Understanding the interdependent nature of individual and social needs facilitates preventive and health-promotion actions on the part of health care professionals both locally and globally. In the last decade, there has been a shift in global consciousness in both ethics and nursing, in which nursing views ethics in a much broader sense than just direct care to individuals (Tschudin, 2010). Advocacy may include political activity to address populations of concern. Preemptive and sociopolitical advocacy permits the source of the ongoing problems to be accurately identified and challenged. Nurses have moral obligations related to sociopolitical advocacy on behalf of their populations of concern. Juanita Rimmer's obligations include recognizing the problems caused by a chronic shortage of rehabilitation services. Her concerns include discovering the source of this problem and joining with others in an attempt to address it at this level. Strategies for solving seemingly intractable problems of health care include collaboration with specialty nursing, medical, or client advocacy groups, and communication of the issues in both professional and popular media.

Advocacy for health promotion is a concept with broad implications. It includes activities that are directed toward remedying socially-based inequities or inadequacies in the health care delivery system. Advocacy can be viewed as an ethic of practice that includes all activities directed toward the person's good. Advocacy carries risks, in that addressing or facilitating the good for individuals or groups may pit nurses against their peers or against potential adversaries who do not share the same professional goals.

The health care professional role of advocacy requires that professional knowledge and judgment be applied to a variety of situations, from the relatively simple to the complex. The 2010 Institute of Medicine (IOM) report *The Future of Nursing: Leading Change, Advancing Health* emphasized the need for advocacy in nurses through practicing to the fullest extent of their education and training and as full partners with physicians and other health care professionals in redesigning health in the United States (Institute of Medicine, 2010, p. 4). This process requires several steps. First, potential or real problems need to be identified and analyzed, often in collaboration with others. Second, appropriate actions need to be formulated and their likely consequences considered. Third, obstacles to action should be recognized and addressed. Finally, actions are carried out and evaluated. These basic steps are evident whether the object of health care or health promotion is an individual, a group, or society.

Problem-Solving: Issues, Dilemmas, Risks, and Moral Distress

The nature of health care environments makes it inevitable that difficult decisions will have to be made. However, many of the ethical problems encountered in health-promotion settings are issues rather than dilemmas. Daniel Chambliss (1996), a sociologist who studied nurses in acute care institutional settings, asserts that organizations such as hospitals often give rise to "practical problems, not individual dilemmas" (p. 91). These are nonetheless moral problems because they interfere with the goals of promoting health, well-being, or the relief of suffering. In both institutional and noninstitutional health care settings, obstacles to good care may be caused by health care system arrangements, interprofessional conflicts, and/or lack of resources. Dilemmas are ethical issues of a special sort. Ethical dilemmas are those situations in which a choice must be made between two or more equally undesirable options. Weston (2010) claims that true dilemmas are actually quite rare and that often options can be found by changing the way the situation is examined.

The goals of health promotion require that both issues and dilemmas be recognized and addressed. Neglected issues can become dilemmas. The situation that Graham Pink faced is an example of an ethical issue that became a dilemma. Mr. Pink was a charge nurse working on a geriatric ward in a British hospital. He had grave concerns about the treatment of individuals, especially during the night shift, which was chronically understaffed. First Mr. Pink went through the usual channels trying to get changes made. He notified his supervisors through verbal and written documentation but was unsuccessful in achieving change and the situation deteriorated further. He informed higher administration personnel that people were being neglected and endangered by the situation but was unsuccessful at all levels. Finally, his moral concerns were such that he decided to report the situation to the local newspaper, even though he knew that he might lose his position as a result. Mr. Pink was fired in September 1991 but was eventually exonerated (Wilmot, 2000).

As noted in the preceding example, advocacy carries risks. When a nurse is in danger of losing his or her position as a result of advocating for better conditions, it requires a balancing of foreseeable risks and benefits to the individual or group. The process of decision-making in this situation can lead to moral distress. Moral distress occurs when a nurse knows the ethically correct action to take but feels powerless to take that action (Epstein & Delgado, 2010). Nurses who are faced with ethical issues that seem to be irresolvable may experience guilt, frustration, and a sense of powerlessness, sometimes because they do not believe that they can adhere to their personal values (Rees et al., 2009). Moral distress can occur when the nurse's values and perceived obligations conflict with the needs and prevailing views of the work environment. The framework for making ethical decisions that is discussed later in the chapter includes considerations related to personal security along with preserving integrity.

Preventive Ethics

Preventive ethics, like preventive health care activities, aims to forestall ethical problems before they develop. Preventive ethics is an important requirement of health-promotion endeavors that includes individual action by the nurse, as well as social and political activism with other nurses or professional nursing organizations. Preventive ethics requires

the health promoter to envision potential problems and institute actions that halt their development. For example, it is possible to extend a dying person's life almost indefinitely using available technology and medications. Although a competent person has the right to refuse treatment and this right is legally recognized as a result of the Patient Self-Determination Act (PSDA) of 1991, many people become incapacitated before they are able to make their wishes known. Although all states recognize and honor advance directives, the legally recognized form varies from state to state (Box 5-5). Also, most people have not formulated advance directives. Much more work needs to be done on engaging people in discussion and planning for such eventualities while they are still well. Preventive ethics in this situation entails initiating communication with persons and families before a problem arises. This is often missing both in institutional and in primary care settings.

Preventive ethics using a feminist ethics perspective would encourage addressing institutional practices to provide more humanistic care and underlying social issues that lead people to overeat, smoke, or be inclined toward violence. For example, preventive ethics would require investigating why as a society we have trouble discussing death and dying, and why we find it so hard to have a peaceful or good death. Weston (2010) notes that much of the energy used on the polarized abortion debate could be more profitably put to use in determining why people who do not want to be pregnant nevertheless become pregnant. Weston suggests that it would be useful to reframe the question to ask "why pregnancy, or pregnancy at the wrong time, is so unacceptably burdensome for many women" (p. 43). We need to ask questions about lack of support, lack of education, poor or difficult-to-use birth control methods, resistance from spouses and lovers, lack of child care, and so on. Strategies for identifying potential ethical problems before they occur include examining problematic cases for their antecedents. We should ask fundamental questions about societal arrangements and influences on health trends.

On a local level, nurses and other health promoters need to employ clinical judgment in anticipating and forecasting problems before they arise. For example, unrecognized health literacy may affect an individual's understanding of his or her rights and entitlements (Marks, 2009). When a nurse observes that a person and family do not understand either the information that has been given to them or the implications of following a given course of action, the nurse engages in preventive ethics by supplying that information and ensuring that the information is understood. The nurse acts to prevent negative consequences that can arise as a result of poorly understood information. Many problems in health care occur as a result of poor communication or because information has been provided too late for reasoned decision-making (Box 5-6: Quality and Safety Scenario).

ETHICAL PRINCIPLES IN HEALTH PROMOTION

Although the tenets of nursing's codes of ethics and standards of practice provide some guidance about the nature

BOX 5-5   PREVENTIVE ETHICS: PATIENT SELF-DETERMINATION ACT AND ADVANCE DIRECTIVES

One fact that all people face is the uncertainty and fragility of life. Health-promotion endeavors can increase individual capacities to withstand the difficulties of life and even assist individuals to flourish while living with chronic illness. However, what often cannot be predicted is whether and when one will lose the ability to make our wishes for treatment and care known. Over the last 2 to 3 decades, great technological and therapeutic advances have been made, with the resulting ability to save the lives of people experiencing catastrophic illnesses and trauma. One effect of these advances, unfortunately, is that sometimes we are successful only in prolonging the dying process. Although it is now recognized that people have a right to refuse treatment to prolong life, it is not uncommon that critically ill people lose the ability to articulate their wishes for treatment. Advance directives are a way for people to ensure that when they become incapacitated the care and treatment they receive matches their predetermined wishes. At their best, advance directives also have the potential to relieve the strain felt by loved ones as they strive to make the "right" treatment choices for a friend or relative. They also guide health professionals in their decision-making regarding the person in question.

Types of Advance Directives

All states have advance directive laws. However, they differ regarding what is the legal form of advance directive and what is required to validate it. For example, in Massachusetts the legal advance directive is a health care proxy. It requires the designation of a person to make one's health care decisions in the event of incapacity. Two people have to witness the signature, neither of whom can be the designee.

- *Instructional.* A written document, this is also known as a living will or terminal care document. It can be very specific and tailored to order or may be a form document that can be downloaded from the Internet.
- *Health care proxy.* This is also known as a durable power of attorney for health care. It allows a competent person to designate a decision maker in the event of incapacity.

Fagerlin and Schneider (2004) found that living wills are the least effective advance directive in the absence of a health care proxy. The best advance directive is a combination of proxy and written directions.

The Patient Self-Determination Act (PSDA) of 1991, which was formulated in response to 2 decades of ambiguity and litigation involving right-to-die cases, represented an attempt to ensure that people's rights were honored. The PSDA required changes in public policy, public and professional education, institutional policy, and social awareness. The PSDA was expected to improve communication related to end-of-life care issues and preferences among individuals, health care providers, and proxy decision makers. It requires institutions that receive Medicare and Medicaid funds to:

- Give written information on admission to all (not just the Medicare and Medicaid) persons about their rights under the law to make their own treatment decisions.
- Inform people of their rights to complete state-allowed advance directives and provide written policies about those rights.
- Document when a person has an advance directive.
- Not discriminate or make care conditional on the presence or absence of an advance directive.
- Provide staff education about advance directives and personal rights.

Although the PSDA has great potential, it serves its purpose only to the extent that it is taken seriously as a responsibility of a given institution. All too frequently institutions fail to ensure that a suitably qualified person is available to impart the information or to request personal preferences. It is important for those involved in health promotion to understand, and therefore address, why people may be reluctant to make an advance directive, why institutions are not diligent in providing information and education, and why even in the presence of the PSDA most people do not have advance directives.

Impediments to the Use of Advance Directives

- Discussions with health care providers about the implications of desired choices have been inadequate.
- People do not want to talk about future incapacity or death. They may have cultural prohibitions about discussing the possibility of serious illness or death.
- Past encounters with the health care system have led to distrust.
- People cannot predict accurately their future preferences and they know too little about what constitutes life support.
- People may change their minds about what they will accept.
- The health care proxy may turn out to be a poor choice or may cause conflicts among other family members or loved ones. The person or family may ask for something that is morally unacceptable.
- Treatments may be specified to which the provider has conscientious objections.
- Documentation may be lost, misplaced, or not accessible in an emergency.
- Written instructions are too vague and open to divergent interpretation to be useful guides.
- Even the most diligent proxy cannot always know what the person would have wanted in the absence of a detailed treatment directive.
- The proxy may make a treatment choice contrary to the person's directive.
- The proxy may make a decision with which the institution or physician disagrees.

Adapted from Fagerlin, A., & Schneider, C. E. (2004). Enough. The failure of the living will. *Hastings Center Report, 34*(2), 30-42; Wolf, S. M. (2001). Sources of concern about the Patient Self-Determination Act. In W. Teays & L. M. Purdy (Eds.), *Bioethics, justice and health care* (pp. 411-419). Belmont, CA: Wadsworth/Thompson Learning.

of practice and the manner in which services will be provided, they often leave some ambiguity about the best course of action in morally troubling situations. The use of principles derived from a variety of ethical theories, along with feminist insights or an ethic of care, helps to provide further guidance in decision-making in morally problematic health situations. Beauchamp and colleagues (2007) noted that ethical principles provide an important starting point for moral judgment and policy evaluation, but that principles alone are not enough. In other words, principles such as autonomy,

beneficence, and justice often serve as helpful starting points in teasing out the tangled elements of complex issues, but taken alone they are usually insufficient for moral problem-solving in health care environments. One must decide which principles are important to consider in a given case or situation, and this requires an exploration of the case as discussed in the decision-making framework provided later in the chapter.

Additionally, tenets of the *Code of Ethics for Nurses* and other ANA position statements provide guidance regarding what a

BOX 5-6   QUALITY AND SAFETY SCENARIO
Patient-Centered Care

Recognize the patient or designee as the source of control and full partner in providing compassionate and coordinated care based on respect for the patient's preferences, values, and needs (http://qsen.org).

How Is Health Literacy Related to Ensuring Autonomy in Decision-Making for Persons?

Autonomy is an important ethical principle for health-promotion activities. In order to ensure autonomy in individual decision-making, it is important to assess the individual's health literacy skills. These skills relate to a person's ability to obtain, process, and act on basic health information. Think how difficult it would be for a person with low literacy skills to navigate today's complex health care system. Adequate health literacy is essential for accessing necessary health care services and for fostering effective decision-making.

In the process of implementing health-promotion activities, the nurse should first determine whether the person has adequate health literacy skills. This can be assessed with tools such as the Rapid Estimate of Adult Literacy in Medicine (REALM) or the Test of Functional Health Literacy in Adults (TOFHLA). It is important, however, not to base an approach to health promotion solely on the results of one of these tools, which may not reveal the extent to which health recommendations may be misunderstood. The nurse should take the time to establish a rapport with the individual that includes fostering a sense of trust and openness for the person to ask important questions.

Unrecognized health literacy may interfere with individuals' rights to autonomy in decision-making because they may make a decision based on inaccurate information or may automatically accept the decision of the health care provider without deciding for themselves whether the decision is appropriate for their individual situation. Thus, it is an ethical obligation of the nurse to make sure that effective communication is implemented. This can help to ensure that the person is in control and a full partner in health-promotion decisions that respect his or her preferences, values, and needs.

Data from Marks, R. (2009). Ethics and patient education: Health literacy and cultural dilemmas. *Health Promotion Practice, 10*(3), 328-332.

---

nurse's moral responsibilities are in a particular type of situation. Certain tenets address the responsibilities of the nurse in improving the larger health care environment. These obligations include facilitating "community, national, and international efforts to meet health needs" (ANA, 2001, p. 23).

Autonomy as Civil Liberty

In health-promotion settings and endeavors the concept of **autonomy** can be understood from two different perspectives. From the vantage point of public health, the extent of individual autonomy, or freedom of action, may be limited by the duty of protecting the health and safety of the society. From this perspective there is an age-old struggle between civil rights and public safety. Moral questions ask to what degree society is justified in regulating the health and safety of society at large. There is an inevitable tension associated with curtailing **civil liberties** in the name of safety or health. This tension arises from perceptions that, in most Western contexts, freedom of action is a prerequisite of human flourishing.

Currently there are many indirect threats to the health and safety of our society. Actions to resolve any of these have the potential to impinge on civil liberties including, but by no means limited to, bioterrorism and the spread of human immunodeficiency virus/acquired immunodeficiency syndrome (HIV/AIDS) and drug-resistant tuberculosis. Advances in genetic knowledge present the possibility of discrimination from a variety of sources. It will be difficult to maintain individual privacy, and discrimination based on class or gene profile will be made easier. Also, genetic enhancement may be used by select individuals who can afford it.

The current managed care environment, while having a stronger focus on inculcating healthy behaviors, can impinge on civil liberties. Prioritizing behavior change in health-promotion endeavors over the need to address underlying social concerns, such as poverty and other forms of disadvantage, has been criticized by those who feel that a focus on the social determinants

of health would permit more effective, less restrictive health promotion and protection (Marmot & Wilkinson, 2006).

Autonomy as Self-Determination

A second, related, sense of autonomy has to do with individual choice. Autonomy is the moral principle that underlies the concept of informed consent to treatment, interventions, and health-promotion efforts. In Western societies it is probably the most powerful moral principle underlying the treatment of individuals. This principle asserts that people have the ability to reason, and a consequence of the ability to reason is the capacity to make choices. These choices concern both one's own behavior and how one should act toward others (Atkins, 2006). Although the idea that the essence of being human is our ability to reason originated with Aristotle, Kant (1997/1785) developed this idea in meticulous detail in his work *Foundations of the Metaphysics of Morals*. According to Kant, only people are capable of conscious desires and goals and are free agents capable of making decisions and setting goals as guided by their own reason. This principle is still a salient consideration in health care settings: it underpins the health provider and promoter-person relationship and the issue of informed consent. However, there is limited agreement about the scope, limits, and strength of this principle (Beauchamp & Childress, 2008). When describing autonomy in the context of health or treatment choices, it is important to delineate what we mean by autonomy in the context of the problem under discussion. Feminist criticisms of an emphasis on autonomy highlight the problem that our choices necessarily affect others because we are contextual beings inseparable from our relationships with one another.

Generally, respecting autonomy requires that we permit individuals to make their own decisions, even when these decisions seem to others to be ill-informed. There are exceptions to this rule. Exceptions include those situations in which there is a high risk of serious injury or death and when it cannot be

Research on Ethics in the Care of Older Adults

The population of older adults is increasing globally, especially in Western countries. We know that older people are a vulnerable group in society and often have special health problems. What do we know about specific ethical issues that nurses confront in the care of older adults? A review of literature was carried out to analyze research studies that focused on ethics in the nursing care for older adults. After a search of MEDLINE and CINAHL databases, and a 4-stage process to ensure that the retrieved articles met established criteria, 71 research studies were included in the review.

Reviews of literature suggest that research on ethics in nursing care for older adults has not received sufficient attention. Research articles focused on important issues, such as autonomy, self-determination, and informed consent. Although the studies included a wide range of health care settings, most of them focused on care of older adults in institutions. There was little research that focused on care in sheltered housing facilities or at home. This is an important gap in the research at a time when the older population is increasing rapidly and there are strategic plans for reducing institutional care in favor of home care. A mismatch between resources and facilities and the needs of older persons is in itself an ethical problem. There is a lack of empirical research on ensuring sound ethical decision-making in this area.

Data from Suhonen, R., Stolt, M., Launis, V., & Leiono-Kilpi, H. (2010). Research on ethics in nursing care for older people: A literature review. *Nursing Ethics, 17*(3), 337-352.

determined whether the person's judgment is impaired. Thus, we make exceptions to the rule of autonomy when we suspect that an individual is not able to reason adequately. A person's reasoning ability may be impaired by psychological or physical conditions, or it may be impaired as a result of incorrect or incomplete information. Respect for human autonomy permits individuals to make and learn from their own mistakes.

In health-promotion activities, respect for autonomy requires that individuals be given the information they need to make choices. Choices can be considered autonomous only if certain criteria are met. The criteria that determine whether or not a person is actually capable of autonomous (voluntary) choice include cognitive maturity, possession of appropriate information to permit decision-making, intact mental capacities (the ability to reason logically), the absence of internal or external coercive influences, and the ability to appreciate the risks and benefits of alternative choices. This is quite a tall order. It is probably true that nobody acts totally autonomously at any given time because of the influences of entrenched beliefs and values that are derived, for the most part, from our cultural and environmental backgrounds. Some of these are under conscious control in the sense that we can recognize what values we hold and even revise them if they are dissonant with other values. However, some of these influences are not readily recognizable: they lie beneath the surface of consciousness and are hard to access even if we are willing to try. We all have blind spots; autonomy viewed as informed, uncoerced, and reasoned action is therefore an ideal. Many of us fall short of the ideal.

Informed Consent

Informed consent to research, treatments, or health-promotion endeavors is a process of ensuring that a person has all of the appropriate information necessary to reach a decision about participation that facilitates autonomous action. Beauchamp and Childress (2008) note that informed consent occurs when a person with substantial understanding, and without substantial control by others, intentionally authorizes a professional to intervene on his or her behalf. The key phrase is "with substantial understanding." It is important to understand that even after a consent form is signed, a person has the right to rescind

consent in light of additional information and/or changed consequences.

Components of the consent process include determining the person's competency to consent. There must be no physical or mental impairments that hinder the person in question from understanding and processing information. For example, a person with pneumonia who is febrile and confused probably is not capable of making an informed decision until the fever is reduced and the confusion has cleared. To be substantially informed, a person must be made aware of important details of the proposed intervention, including its nature, purpose, probability of success, and important risks, and must also understand what alternatives (if any) are available. Since this information must be tailored to meet the specific needs of an individual and this requires knowledge of the person, an ethic of care is important to understanding a person's unique needs. We can check understanding to a certain extent by asking the individual to articulate how the proposed intervention will facilitate his or her own values and goals. There must be no subtle or overt coercion by professionals or others. Finally, appropriate supports must be available to complete the proposed intervention.

Obtaining consent for any interventions, or for involvement in research, is best viewed as a process that entails ongoing assessment of the person's status and evaluation of needs for further information or support. People may not understand information well when they are in stressful situations or when the information is complex. Thus, we should assess for and validate understanding on an ongoing basis.

It is important to ensure that all individuals, regardless of age, make informed choices. While the life span increases in society, nurses must be aware of strategies for ensuring that older adults, who may be less apt to advocate for their own health needs, participate in informed decision-making. More research is needed on the ethical problems older adults face in the community (Box 5-7: Research for Evidence-Based Practice). Based on theoretical conceptions and findings from research (Dickey & Deatrick, 2000; Lind et al., 2003; Ross, 1997), adolescents 14 to 17 years of age are generally considered able of making decisions as well as adults. Involving adolescents fully in their own health care facilitates self-care agency (Box 5-8: Research

BOX 5-8   RESEARCH FOR EVIDENCE-BASED PRACTICE

Use of Advance Directives with Adolescents

Discussions related to advance directives for care should begin while people are healthy and should take place in an ongoing fashion as part of health maintenance activities. McAliley and colleagues (2000) took this idea one step further, noting that although "The American Academy of Pediatrics (AAP) supports giving children a voice in their health care decision-making, …how teens want to be involved in this is not known" (p. 471). To answer this question they conducted an interview study of 107 adolescents between the ages of 15 and 18 years related to having or making a living will.

Results of the study yielded a wide range of information about adolescents and advance directives. Participants were able to pass a test used for demonstrating decision-making competency. They were willing to answer questions related to their own health care treatments as they envisioned themselves in a coma, and those responses were similar to those reported for adults. The vast majority of participants felt it was "somewhat important" or "very important" for someone their age to have a living will. Most of the adolescent participants did not report feeling uncomfortable discussing these issues (McAliley et al., 2000, p. 471).

From McAliley, L. G., Hudson-Barr, D. C., Gunning, R. S., & Rowbottom, L. A. (2000). The use of advance directives with adolescents. *Pediatric Nursing, 26*(5), 471-482.

for Evidence-Based Practice). For nurse theorist Orem, whose focus on self-care agency includes developmental considerations, there is a relationship between the deliberate self-care activities of mature and maturing people and the ongoing optimal development and future functioning. Self-care is learned as a result of membership within family or other social groups. Although for the most part this includes some supervision by responsible adults, respect for an adolescent's developing autonomy facilitates health (Orem, 2001).

Most health-promotion activities do not require formal informed consent. However, it is important to integrate the underlying principles and supporting research related to informed consent to be sure that we use health-promotion strategies that best fit individuals' beliefs and values.

Exceptions to Autonomous Decision-Making

In some cases, proxy decision-making on behalf of the individual is required (Box 5-9). Proxy decision-making must take into account what is known about the person and must follow a path of action that is most likely to respect that individual's goals and values. Braun and colleagues (2008) studied the burdens of end-of-life decision-making in a sample of African American, Caucasian, and Hispanic surrogates. Another study by Vig and colleagues (2007) described what helps and hampers surrogate decision-making (Box 5-10: Research for Evidence-Based Practice). Certain populations are considered less than fully autonomous for a variety of reasons. People with Alzheimer's disease or other physical or psychological disruptions or deficits that prevent adequate comprehension may require proxy decision makers. It is important not to assume, however, that all persons with a diagnosis of Alzheimer's disease are incapable of providing informed consent, because many persons in early stages of the disease are capable of making decisions related to their care (Sorrell & Cangelosi, 2009). Incarcerated people are restricted in their choices and may be subject to subtle or not-so-subtle coercion. Children are considered less than fully autonomous because they are not developmentally mature. Additionally, in people with certain mental illnesses, such as psychoses or bipolar disorders, capacity for decision-making may fluctuate. The President's Commission (1982) was formed to study health care decision-making and noted that the minimal capacities needed for competent decision-making are: "(1) Possession of a set of values and goals; (2) the ability to communicate and to

BOX 5-9   PROXY DECISION-MAKING

1. Autonomy based: person's previously articulated desires
   A. Written
   Living will, advance directive
   Document details to varying degrees what the person will or will not accept
   B. Substituted judgment
   Individual appoints a proxy who is expected to honor previously expressed preferences
   Informal (nonappointed significant other)
2. Best interests
   A. Surrogate chooses the actions that will give the highest overall benefit—may or may not be based on a person's previously expressed desires; a quality of life determination based when possible on knowledge about the person (Beauchamp & Childress, 2008)
   B. Best interests may trump the proxy's choice; doubt about the proxy's motives possible
3. Reasonable person standard
   A. Based on the answer to, "What would a reasonable person want?"

understand information, and (3) the ability to reason and deliberate about one's choice" (p. 57). These criteria are generally accepted as a basic minimum (Beauchamp & Childress, 2008). It can be seen from these criteria that some children would be able to understand the implications of a given course of treatment, and adults with cognitive impairments may be deemed competent to make certain decisions. Competency to make autonomous choices is not an all-or-nothing capacity. Competency determinations are, as a rule, made for a given decision or task. Thus, a person may vacillate between competency and noncompetency, depending on either the task at hand (degree of difficulty or risk) or the physical or psychological status during the period when a decision must be made.

When advocating decision-making for a cognitively impaired person, it is important to consider the risks and benefits of allowing the individual to make his or her own decision. The benefits in terms of self-esteem may well outweigh the risks of many choices. However, if the risk of injury is high and it is obvious that the person is not able to reason effectively, autonomous decision-making may not be feasible. In this case, nurses can collaborate with the individual, family members, and other health professionals to arrive at a decision that is best for the individual.

BOX 5-10   RESEARCH FOR EVIDENCE-BASED PRACTICE

Surrogate Decision-Making

A majority of end-of-life health care decisions are made by surrogate decision makers who are under a great deal of stress over their seriously ill family member. Both surrogates and clinicians have varying degrees of preparation, knowledge, abilities, or comfort in working effectively with another in making very difficult decisions for someone else.

Vig and colleagues (2007) surveyed 50 designated surrogates with previous decision-making experience. Through semistructured telephone interviews, surrogates were asked to describe and reflect on their experiences of making health care decisions for others.

Four types of factors that made decision-making more or less difficult were identified:

- Surrogate characteristics and life circumstances (e.g., competing responsibilities and coping strategies)
- Surrogate social networks (e.g., interfamily thoughts and feelings about the "right decision")
- Surrogate-client relationships (e.g., including communications [or the lack of communications] about difficulties in honoring known preferences)
- Surrogate-clinician relationships (e.g., surrogate primarily communicating with one clinician "spokesperson")

The results suggest areas where clinicians can intervene to facilitate the processes of surrogate decision-making.

From Vig, E. K., Starks, H., Taylor, J. S., Hopely, E. K., & Fryer-Edwards, K. (2007). Surviving surrogate decision-making: What helps and hampers the experience of making medical decisions for others. *Journal of General Internal Medicine, 22*(9), 1274-1279.

When children are involved, it is often the parent or guardian to whom we turn for permission to treat. Nevertheless, in pediatric settings it is incumbent on people involved in health-promotion endeavors or in research with minors to gain assent from the child in addition to consent from the parent or guardian (Lambert & Glacken, 2011). For the child's assent to be meaningful, an assessment of level of maturity and comprehension is required, and information must be provided in language and terms that are appropriate for the developmental level. Conversely, when there is conflict between the decision of the parent and that of the child, the health care provider has a duty to ensure that the parental choice is in the child's best interest. Where there is serious doubt, it may be necessary to involve the courts.

Confidentiality

Autonomy is also the principle underlying **confidentiality**: "The ability to maintain privacy in one's life is an expression of autonomy" (Burkhardt & Nathaniel, 2007). People have the right to decide who can have access to information about them, thus limiting the negative use of personal information by others. In certain situations the status of confidentiality between a person and others, such as clergy, is considered a privilege and as such is shielded from exposure by the legal system. In health care, confidentiality does not carry as strong a status as clergy-supplicant or lawyer-client privilege (Grace, 2004). There may be occasions when health care providers have a duty to warn others who are unknowingly endangered. This duty was highlighted by the landmark Tarasoff case. On October 27, 1969, Prosenjit Poddar killed Tatiana Tarasoff. Poddar was receiving psychiatric care during this period. He had informed his therapist 2 weeks earlier that he was going to kill a certain girl, easily identifiable as Tarasoff, on her return from Brazil. At the time his therapist tried to have him committed. The police detained Poddar briefly but decided he was rational, so they released him. No one warned Tatiana of the danger. The courts concluded that "once a therapist does in fact determine, or under applicable professional standards reasonably should have determined, that a person poses a serious danger of violence to others, he bears a duty to exercise reasonable care to protect the foreseeable victim of that danger" (*Tarasoff v. Regents of University of California*, 1976). The court recognized the difficulty of predicting the degree of danger and the importance of maintaining confidentiality but determined that when the risk is high, confidentiality should be breached.

Health care professionals must strive to keep the person's personal information confidential so as to enhance trust within the health care professional–person relationship. Therefore, in health care settings there are strong sanctions against breaching confidentiality. In theory, the principle of confidentiality may be overridden only in situations in which extreme harm to self or others is imminent. In practice, this is difficult to enforce, because in medical settings many people have access to the person's information. Insurance companies demand access to information before payment for services is made. In outpatient settings, barriers to privacy may occur when personnel are personally acquainted with the individual. When health professionals are members of the community in which they practice, there may be confidentiality issues associated with the intimate nature of small communities. Nurses and other health-promotion professionals may find themselves being asked by friends and relatives of the person for details about that person's health status. It can be very difficult to respond diplomatically while maintaining the person's privacy. The ethical implications of these threats to confidentiality are many. Thus, it is important for nurses to be aware of potential breeches of confidentiality and to advocate for confidential treatment of information for those they serve.

The Privacy Rule

The **Privacy Rule** (45 Code of Federal Regulations Part 160, 164 subparts A & E) was developed as a result of the Health Insurance Portability and Accountability Act (HIPAA). Its intent was to ensure that individuals' health information is properly protected, while allowing the flow of information needed to provide and promote high-quality care (including using information about the person receiving care for research) and to protect the public's health and well-being. HIPAA was meant to protect the privacy of individually identifiable health information in the face of advances in electronic technology and to limit the ways in which "health plans, pharmacies, hospitals, clinics, nursing homes and other covered entities (any provider that conducts or conveys information in electronic form, e.g., physicians, nurse practitioners)" can use medical information (U.S. Department of Health and Human Services [USDHHS], Office for Civil Rights, 2004). "Covered entities" means those covered by the Privacy Rule. The limitations on use of medical information extend to any identifiable information, written, oral, or computerized. Although there are some legal guidelines about disclosure, nurses and others are responsible for using clinical judgment in deciding what level of detail to share (USDHHS, 2004). It is important to understand that the purpose of the rule is to protect individual rights while still facilitating important public health and epidemiological research. Health-promotion activities include empowering people to exercise these rights. The Privacy Rule ensures that individuals are given a copy of the privacy practices at a given institution. Additionally, under the rule individuals have the following rights:

- To access their own information
- To limit who may receive their information
- To request corrections for errors
- To receive an accounting of how their information has been used
- To request special confidential reporting of their information to them at a location of their choosing (this may be especially important for individuals at risk for intimate partner violence)
- To pursue complaints with the Department of Health and Human Services Office for Civil Rights

A rule of thumb for health professionals related to sharing information with others is to disclose only as much information as is pertinent to the situation and is necessary to provide optimal care. A decision about disclosure of a person's information requires balancing the risks of information sharing with the benefits of treatment.

Although the Privacy Rule was meant to help safeguard people's rights, some commentators and researchers are finding the rule overly restrictive and worry that it might discourage important research, especially genetic research, with its far-reaching implications for individual privacy. As Kulynych and Korn (2002, p. 310) write:

> Although the rule's drafters wisely opted not to create special standards for genetic information, the limits they have placed upon the use and disclosure of all "identifiable" health information will profoundly affect the conduct of genetic studies and many other forms of research. Research compliance efforts will become more costly and time consuming as institutions and individual providers who use or disclose health information for research confront new procedural requirements and new liability for failures to meet the privacy rule's intricate compliance obligations. Investigators who use health information, as well as the institutional committees that must review human subjects research proposals, will need to familiarize themselves with a confusing array of new terminology, ambiguous standards and burdensome required paperwork.

Adolescents: Special Considerations of Confidentiality

Adolescents often provide health professionals with very tricky confidentiality issues. As Bandman and Bandman (2001) note,

"the adolescent is torn between wanting to challenge authority and to assert independence while still needing the "help and support of effective parents" (p. 195). The results of risk-taking behavior, such as drug and alcohol experimentation and risky sexual activity, and their normal developmental needs make teenagers a health-promotion challenge. The task of health promotion is to maintain and facilitate the adolescent's emerging autonomy and confidentiality needs, while mediating between the peer and parental figures who feel that they have a right to information about the adolescent. It is easy to become caught in the tension "between the anger and perceived duties of the parent and the defensiveness and vulnerability of the adolescent" (Bandman & Bandman, 2001, p. 200).

Although federal and state laws, as well as ethical considerations, generally serve to protect the privacy and autonomy of adolescents, health promotion involves more than mere protection. It involves facilitating the adolescent's health. Thus, responsibilities include helping an adolescent to grasp his or her authentic options and rights, facilitating interaction between the adolescent and parents or guardians, maintaining trust, and preserving confidentiality.

On the other hand, clinical judgment (which includes ethical judgment) is important in determining risk. If the risk of preserving the adolescent's privacy is high, based on all pertinent and available evidence such as the presence of sexual or physical abuse, then it may be necessary to report this information to appropriate authorities. Mandatory reporting laws exist. Such laws are important for the general protection of a society's citizens. However, there may be rare occasions when a judgment must be made about whether upholding the legal obligation would cause more harm than good. In such circumstances there are two separate considerations. First, one must decide whether the risk to professional standing and licensure of not following the legally required path is something that the professional is willing to assume. The second consideration involves assessing the potential benefits and risks to the person resulting from failure to report. There is no easy resolution for these types of problems. If the situation is not an emergency, it is prudent to solicit appropriate advice from a peer, a counselor, or an ethics expert or resource. In any case, it remains the professional's ethical responsibility to handle the given situation in a manner that preserves trust and provides ongoing support.

Veracity

Veracity, or devotion to the truth, is another principle that supports health-promotion activities. People whose health is in question are to varying degrees reliant upon the person who possesses the knowledge and skills to bring these to bear on their behalf. The contemporary bioethics literature favors characteristics of "veracity, ...candor, honesty and truthfulness" (Beauchamp & Childress, 2008) as virtues to be nurtured in the development of health professionals. This represents a change from the paternalistic (the physician knows what is best) attitudes that prevailed earlier in this century and up to the late 1960s.

Veracity in giving people information about their health care needs facilitates autonomous choice and enhances personal decision-making. Health care professionals may be tempted to withhold certain details when this is seen as serving the person's best interests or when family members demand it. It is sometimes difficult to determine how much and what types of information will best serve a person's needs. Knowledge of the person's beliefs, values, and lifestyle preferences is essential to the process of supplying adequate information to support autonomous decision-making. Withholding information, or providing information that is misleading or incomprehensible, in an attempt to influence someone to agree to a treatment or intervention, conflicts with veracity. It may be tempting to avoid the longer route to resolving such problems (e.g., education, understanding people's motives).

Veracity has some cross-cultural implications, in that some cultures have not traditionally valued truth-telling in the case of terminal illness. Decision-making about whether to honor veracity in such cases must take into consideration what is known about the culture, the particular person, the strength of his or her personal and cultural beliefs, and whether there is evidence about what sorts of things the person would like to know. The absence of veracity may interfere with autonomous action. In the case of terminal illness it may deprive the person of the ability to plan the remainder of his or her life.

At first glance, veracity appears an easy concept to incorporate into health-promotion interventions. It may sometimes be difficult, however, in health education endeavors aimed at changing patterns of behavior in society. Should health professionals just present the facts or should they attempt to persuade? What are the limits of veracity? Is it permissible to exaggerate the dangers of certain behavior in the interests of the health of society? These questions cannot be answered within the confines of this chapter but are important to keep in mind when assessing the merits of proposed population-based interventions.

Nonmaleficence

Related to autonomy is the principle of nonmaleficence, which enjoins people not to harm other people. In general society, this principle constrains people from autonomous actions that are likely to harm others. In health care settings, it prohibits clinicians from harming those for whom they provide services. For health promotion, it means that in planning activities on an individual or societal level, possible harms must be minimized. It is often impossible to foresee all the risks of a given course of action but professionals who engage in health-promotion endeavors are responsible for foreseeing predictable adverse consequences and taking these into consideration. These responsibilities include addressing social or health care policies that are discovered to have unintended effects.

Carter and colleagues (2011) illustrate how a policy designed to address obesity through use of a mass-media program can have unintended negative health effects. They describe how the program titled *How Do You Measure Up?* can carry the message to people to trim waistlines and "turn their lives around." Although mass-media campaigns such as this are targeted at the population level, they may also have a deeply personal and emotional effect on individuals, stigmatizing individuals who feel incapable of making changes in their lives to lose weight.

Employer incentive programs that differentiate among individuals based on their success in changing behaviors such as smoking or weight loss also carry the possibility of discrimination when they provide financial benefits to the most successful individuals, in that some individuals face significantly greater difficulty than others in achieving desired outcomes (Madison et al., 2011; Rothstein & Harrell, 2009). Well-designed employer incentive programs, however, can help individuals overcome barriers they face in trying to avoid disease and disability. Systematic evaluation of incentive programs will enhance understanding of how to design programs to prevent discrimination and maximize equity.

Unintentional harm is a possibility for actions designed to promote health. Risks can be minimized by anticipating potential negative effects and implementing measures to control for them. Professionals are responsible for understanding the limits of their knowledge or the data to which they have access. A synthesis of reflection, critical thinking, and knowledge, along with an understanding of the details and context of a situation, is required before embarking on a course of action aimed at facilitating a person's health or well-being. The overall discomfort encountered by the individual must be the minimum possible to achieve the primary good intended. In other words, the health care provider is accountable for his or her judgment and for providing interventions most likely to bring about the desired result. Thus, more than just the intention not to do harm is required.

Nurses and other health professionals can do harm inadvertently through such behaviors as ignorance or incompetence, referral to a provider who is incompetent or inappropriate, or inadequate supervision or training of those under one's supervision. However, the duty of nonmaleficence does not mean that health care professionals are always accountable for foreseeing the consequences of their actions. For example, a course of exercise may be designed for a person who has had a thorough physical, but during an exercise session, the person faints and fractures his arm. Further testing reveals a previously undetected cardiac anomaly that is subsequently surgically corrected. This is not maleficence; the main objective of the agent was therapeutic and the event was, if not totally unforeseeable, not identified upon routine pre-exercise testing. Thus, both deliberate harm and harm caused by indifferent or incompetent decision-making should be considered maleficent, but when a competent practitioner evaluates a problem thoroughly in its appropriate context and intervenes with therapeutic intent, this does not violate the concept of nonmaleficence.

Beneficence

Beneficence is the quality or state of doing or producing "good." As a moral principle, beneficence presents us with the duty to maximize the benefits of actions while minimizing harms. There are two related aspects of the moral principle of beneficence in health-promotion settings: actions taken to further the overall health or well-being of the society in general and actions taken to promote the good of a particular individual.

When society formulates rules designed to protect people against the negative effects of their own actions, these rules

BOX 5-11   HOT TOPICS

Direct-to-Consumer Marketing: Drugs and Tests

Commercial industries have discovered a novel way to increase profits. Direct-to-consumer marketing (DTCM) can occur via print, the Internet, or television. It impacts health-promotion efforts in a variety of ways and has serious ethical implications. For example, DTCM of genetic testing is more likely to benefit the commercial enterprise and its stakeholders than the individuals to whom the advertising campaigns are directed, as illustrated by the exemplar below:

DTCM: Genetic Testing

In a workshop held in March 2003 sponsored by the National Human Genome Research Institute of the National Institutes of Health, various interested parties, including scientists, ethicists, company spokespersons, and consumers, discussed the pros and cons of DTCM to promote genetic testing. The workshop's summary report noted that although DTCM may increase public awareness about the availability of genetic tests, there are also risks in adopting this strategy. It was noted that, according to recent research, advertisements could increase consumers' awareness about diseases, but they often fail to accurately convey risk information including the implications of test results on the mental status of test takers and on related others. Additionally, the information may fail to reach those most at risk.

Problems Associated with DTCM of Genetic Testing*
- Resource allocation (in terms of the implications of misdirected testing on consumer and provider time and counseling requirements)
- Lack of utility of available interventions
- Consumer inability to deal with the complexity of the information: confusion, false hope, false anxiety
- Economic harm to consumer
- Missed opportunities to pursue other health interventions
- Professionals with working knowledge of genetic testing not available to advise about testing
- Provider education (or lack thereof) with regard to genetics, non-health implications within families, and how to communicate genetic information
- Lack of regulatory oversight for tests, existing oversight is technology driven rather than public health oriented, lack of validated tests, lack of consensus on methods for validating genetic tests
- Scant data about harms or benefits of tests
- Questionable scientific accuracy and validity of the advertisements
- Misinformation in public sector about genetics

Modified from the *Summary Report of the National Human Genome Research Institute*, March 23, 2004.
*Note: Some of these problems are also associated with genetic testing in general.

are considered beneficent. It is important to emphasize, however, that beneficence should be carried out in accordance with the person's own will or values, and respecting the person's autonomy (Braunack-Mayer & Louise, 2008; Kangasniemi, 2010; Keane, 2010). Sometimes rules designed to protect people are described as paternalistic because they override a person's autonomy to disobey them. For example, seat belt laws are paternalistic, as are rules governing the use of therapeutic or so-called recreational drugs. Paternalism is often justified by the assertion that the persons affected will be better off or protected from harm.

The principle of beneficence, when it overrides an individual's autonomous choice in order to serve that individual's interests, is appropriate when a person lacks the capacity to make personal decisions. Thus, any of the factors discussed earlier that interfere with rational decision-making may require the health care provider to beneficently override the individual's decisions. Generally, though, beneficence permits interference only when the risks of the individual's proposed actions are high. This is because autonomy is such a powerful principle in Western societies that a decision to override is not taken lightly. One may be justified in preventing a person from taking an overdose of sleeping pills or jumping off a cliff because the risks of not doing so are high and if the person succeeds there is no possibility of future autonomous actions.

Beneficence, unlike nonmaleficence, is not necessarily a moral requirement of action on the part of societal members toward each other (Grace, 2004). Whether beneficence is viewed as a moral requirement of societal members in everyday life very much depends on philosophical beliefs and the ethical theory or perspective (if any) recognized by the person. An individual is not necessarily morally required to go out of his

or her way to help someone unless the person is endangered and assistance would mitigate the danger. In that case, failing to offer assistance could be seen as violating the principle of nonmaleficence. Also, when an individual has responsibility for vulnerable others, such as when parents must use beneficence on behalf of their children, beneficence is required.

In contrast to ordinary members of society, health care professionals have duties of beneficence because their professional goals involve meeting health care needs and thus are aimed at providing good. For such reasons, beneficence is a moral expectation of health care professionals. Beneficence is often a difficult principle to use in health-promotion settings; however, because of the dual nature of health-promotion goals—health for individuals and health for communities. As noted earlier, there is often a tension between the two.

A paradox exists when we try to change unhealthy behaviors but do not address the underlying causes of those behaviors. For example, although smoking cessation programs assist some people to stop smoking, and restricting areas where people may smoke tends to persuade some people that it is becoming too inconvenient to continue, we also should address problems such as advertising campaigns that aim to gather new smoking recruits from among adolescents. Some advertising campaigns encourage adolescents to try flavored cigarettes through offering a variety of flavors and attractive packaging. But these tobacco cigarettes are addictive and dangerous. Education-based health-promotion programs without underlying societal changes are often doomed to fail. Thus, health professionals have obligations to address deep-rooted social problems that jeopardize health or are associated with health disparities. See Box 5-11: Hot Topics for discussions of direct-to-consumer marketing (DTCM) of genetic testing for examples of this.

Beneficence: Conflict with Autonomy

From the previous discussion it can be seen that the principles of beneficence and autonomy sometimes conflict. For example, seat belt rules are ostensibly created to protect people from injury, but they take away autonomous choice. Beneficence may justify overriding the decision of a febrile, confused person who refuses to take her antibiotics for pneumonia. What is the clinician's responsibility? Duties of beneficence seem to mandate medicating her against her will, ensuring that the good of health is facilitated although violating the principle of autonomy. The justification for this must include an assessment of her status related to capacity for autonomous decision-making. Preserving the person's life so he or she can make autonomous decisions in the future may be required by beneficence. However, it can be argued that beneficence takes precedence over autonomy only in those cases in which the choice cannot be considered autonomous. First, there has to be evidence that a choice has been made. In this case the choice was between accepting antibiotic treatment versus not accepting antibiotic treatment. Second, the reasonableness (or rationality) of the decision has to be discerned. It must be ascertained whether the person really has grasped the implications of refusing treatment. The reasons given for the treatment refusal, then, should illuminate gaps in information delivery or processing. Finally, it must be determined whether there are any external or internal coercion factors impinging on the decision. Perhaps the person feels she cannot afford the medicine (external) or perhaps she has a mistrust of antibiotics because of a previous experience (internal). When a decision cannot be said to be informed, the principle of beneficence directs us to decide treatment based on the person's best interests.

Justice

Justice is an ethical principle of major importance in health-promotion settings. There are various conceptions of justice, and the term is used in a variety of ways. For the purposes of this chapter the discussion is about social justice rather than criminal justice. Social justice includes formal or informal systems within a society that are concerned with disparities in socioeconomic conditions leading to poor health and fairness in the distribution of goods such as health, education, food, and shelter (Powers & Faden, 2008; Slomka et al., 2008). Buchanan (2000) notes that the concept of justice has been central to human understandings of socially significant values for a long time. Justice in health care is a major commitment of nursing and thus the discipline of nursing is becoming more focused on active engagement in social justice issues (Crigger, 2008).

There are two broad socially oriented ideas regarding justice. One perspective of justice views those who are more worthy of merit, or who contribute more, as deserving of better social benefits. The other perspective views justice as equalizing benefits across society, regardless of merit. This latter view is justice as fairness. The tendency when discussing the provision of health care for a society is to focus on justice viewed as fairness and as favoring equality. However, when the discussion turns to allocation of scarce resources, such as organs for transplant, one can detect in the discussion a justice standard that favors merit rather than equality.

The social justice arrangements in a society are indicative of what the society values (Coursen, 2009). In democratic societies, the requirements of social justice generally include equitable distribution of the benefits and burdens of societal life. "Justice as fairness" reflects the ideas behind Rawls' (1971, 1999) *A Theory of Justice.* Rawls identifies two "rules of justice that he argues will enable humankind to resolve disputes fairly and justly" (Buchanan, 2000, p. 156). "First: each person is to have an equal right to the most extensive liberty compatible with a similar liberty for others. Second: social and economic inequalities are to be arranged such that they are both (a) reasonably expected to be to everyone's advantage, and (b) attached to positions and offices open to all" (Rawls, 1971, p. 60). Rawls formulates these rules as a result of his hypothetical method for deciding how a society's institutions should be arranged in order to provide for fairness. Rawls proposes that these rules of justice would emerge as a result of an average person's reasoning from behind a "veil of ignorance" (ignorant about their place in society, personal assets, or handicaps) about what social arrangements they would prefer if they did not know what their personal impediments or assets were going to be.

Rawls' theory, although respected by ethicists, is subject to criticism on a variety of fronts. One significant criticism is that justice as fairness does not provide much guidance for some common social problems, such as abortion, welfare, and the righting of previous wrongs (e.g., affirmative action, the rights of native people), and ignores the problems of those without legal rights such as undocumented workers (Buchanan, 2000; MacIntyre, 2007). Dinkins (2011), however, suggests that the "veil of ignorance" thought experiment described by Rawls may help us realize that when we step out from the veil into the workplace being envisioned, we could be anybody—a single mother without insurance unable to access health care for her children, an elderly woman with a hoarding disorder who lives surrounded by piles and piles of decaying garbage, or any other vulnerable population in our society. Rawls suggests that we remain behind the veil of ignorance while we examine how we would like our society to work. In this way, we can learn to ask what problems need to be addressed. How is each individual being treated? Who seems to be the best off? Who seems to be the worst off, and how bad is their situation? Rawls argues that while we are behind the veil of ignorance, not knowing which role and situation we may step into, we are motivated to seek fairness for everyone as far as possible, that is, to *maximize the minimum* by ensuring that whoever is the worst off is as well off as possible, without sacrificing the overall success of the society as a whole.

An emphasis on justice in health care settings is sometimes called the impartialist perspective in that it considers the needs of all who fall under its umbrella. For example, within the prison system, this view of justice would mandate access to care for prisoners in need. Thus it would not permit arbitrary obstacles to access (such as requiring good behavior or favors) that might be presented by prison officers or by other prisoners who wish to exert physical or psychological control. Justice would also require improved access to care for the poor and underprivileged, in terms of both receiving care and having access to transportation or local availability of services.

Although justice might require consideration of the special needs of a disadvantaged group, it does so impartially: that is, it does not distinguish among the particulars of individuals. Each member within the group has an equal right to whatever is proposed. In an economically and profit-driven health care system, injustices occur both at the local and at societal levels. Because justice viewed as fairness is impartial about individual differences, that moral perspective considered alone is not a perfect tool with which to look at health care disparities and their causes.

Nurses and other health professionals need to move beyond thinking about 'doing no harm' to identifying and addressing adverse social influences on the health of underprivileged groups and the implications of their consequent poor health (Rogers & Kelly, 2011). The combination of justice, feminist concerns about power and oppression, and the acknowledged responsibilities of health care professionals to promote health permit a comprehensive view of problems associated with health protection and promotion. This view incorporates an ethical approach to problems both for society and for individuals within the society. Buchanan (2000) captures this necessary synthesis of perspectives well, noting "the mutually reinforcing relationships among justice, caring and responsibility" which will help health care professionals to "enable people to live well" (p. 167).

STRATEGIES FOR ETHICAL DECISION-MAKING

Locating the Source and Levels of Ethical Problems

Most health-promotion problems are moral or ethical issues in the sense that obstacles exist that prevent an individual from living life well or achieving personal goals related to health. Throughout this chapter discussions of both the larger (societal) and narrower (individual) perspectives have been emphasized and their relationships highlighted. Sometimes tensions between the two require mediation and may force the health promoter to decide which problem must be addressed first. For example, a nurse at a family practice clinic cares for a teenager who is morbidly obese. At the level of the individual, the nurse is charged with discovering underlying causes of the obesity (e.g., physical, psychological, contextual) and designing strategies with the individual to help resolve the problem. However, the nurse has responsibilities also to address the issue at the more political level with interested others.

To address health-promotion issues effectively, professionals need to possess not only their particular disciplinary expertise and an understanding of ethical language, principles, and perspectives, but also a willingness to understand their own values and preconceptions about health and people. Understanding personal philosophy, biases, and values permits one to control for these in the sense of being aware of the influences they have in our interactions with others.

Values Clarification and Reflection

Gaining confidence in moral decision-making is a slow process. The following are suggestions that will guide development related to recognizing and addressing ethical issues.

Examine Beliefs and Values

Cultivate the habit of examining how your personal values and beliefs relate to the human condition, justice, and responsibility. Be willing to revise your beliefs in line with your professional knowledge base, experiences, or current research findings. For example, how do beliefs that "people get what they deserve" correlate with what we know—for example, that those of lower socioeconomic status have lower levels of health and that poor health interferes with functioning and is associated with depression? How do our attitudes change when we try to place ourselves in the context of the other person's life?

This is not to say that maintaining personal integrity is not important—it is. Maintaining both personal and professional integrity is essential to good practice. Integrity has to do with a sense of wholeness of the self and consistency of actions with truly examined beliefs and values. "Nurses have both personal and professional identities that are neither entirely separate nor entirely merged, but are integrated" (ANA, 2001, p. 19). Tenet 5 of the ANA (2001) *Code of Ethics for Nurses with Interpretive Statements* validates the nurse's preservation of integrity in those situations in which he or she feels that personal integrity is compromised. It notes that "where a particular treatment, intervention, activity or practice is morally objectionable to the nurse…the nurse is justified in refusing to participate on moral grounds" (ANA, 2001, p. 20). When this involves risk to the individual, though, other arrangements must be made to safeguard individual care.

A true examination of beliefs and values requires a willingness to admit that these may not always be justifiable—they may be remnants from childhood indoctrination of various sorts. For example, one might believe that certain ethnic groups are inferior in some way, or that one should not question authority. An honest and ongoing examination of one's values and biases permits one to control for these beliefs when providing care to diverse persons.

The Influence of Personal Beliefs and Values

In addition to examining beliefs and values, it is important to think about the influence that these characteristics have on our practice. An understanding of how personal beliefs and values either are congruent or are liable to interfere with the task at hand is crucial to ethical problem-solving. In any given situation, the health professional must ask himself or herself, "What are my beliefs and biases in this situation? How are these likely to influence my actions?" For example, if the home health nurse believes his below-poverty level, depressed, obese, diabetic person who smokes is responsible for the poor healing of her leg ulcer, he may be less inclined to work with the person to discover and address the person's goals.

Reflection on Practice

A third helpful strategy is to reflect on situations afterward to discover what worked, what did not work, and what could be done differently in the future. It is often helpful to interact with peers or other experts after particularly difficult situations to discover alternative perspectives or resources for the purposes of future problem-solving.

Decision-Making Considerations

Decision-making in health-promotion settings has inescapable moral components. As noted earlier, the nurse has a professional responsibility to further the good for individuals and society. Thus, the careful exercise of experience, skill, and knowledge is warranted when trying to formulate the best course of action for a given individual or group, or in resolving societal health-promotion problems. This framework is offered as a way of ensuring clarity about a particular case or situation. Because of the diverse nature of health-promotion activities, no straightforward models of decision-making can realistically be applied in all situations. Additionally, decision-making is often an ongoing process and revisions to plans may be required in light of new information. The following are important facets of decision-making but do not necessarily occur in the order given.

Identify the Main Problem or Issue

What level of problem is this: social, group, or individual? If the location of the problem is societal, it will also impact individuals and groups and a decision has to be made about the order of interventions. Try to determine the main ethical principle involved or whether it is a problem of conflicting principles. For example, after identification of the problem you may determine that in order to provide benefit to the person the person's autonomy must be overridden. Is this a social justice issue? An autonomy issue? What factors led to the problem? Is there coercion or other power imbalances? Who has an interest in maintaining the power imbalances and who gains the most from the imbalance? These are the questions feminist ethics would ask.

Determine Who or What Created the Problem

Who has a stake in the issue and in how it will be resolved? Answering this question will permit a determination of whose input is crucial to the decision-making process. Who and what are important considerations (e.g., institutions, individuals, businesses, social policy)? Does this issue result from a failure to predict the consequences of certain social policies?

Determine the Prevalent Values

What are the values held by all the different players? Are there value conflicts? The value conflicts might be individual versus social, as in the case of a person with tuberculosis who refuses to take his medicines, thus putting at risk members of his family or of the community. Values conflicts might also be interpersonal among the health-promotion team or personal versus professional. As a general rule, more weight is assigned to the values of the individual who is most likely to be affected by a decision. It is important to consider the influence of culture on values when the issue involves health promotion for culturally diverse groups. It is also important to involve people who can help explain the cultural beliefs, especially when language difficulties are present. A knowledgeable but neutral interpreter may be helpful when liaison between groups is needed.

Identify Information Gaps

This is a good place to reflect upon whether the decision maker(s) are confident about what they do and do not know. This is not always an easy task. Information may exist that has not yet reached our awareness, or we might fail to ask a question that would reveal important information. How can we be confident about the scope and limits of our knowledge? Clinical judgment is a good tool but is not foolproof. When doubts exist or the decision is likely to have serious or risky consequences, we need to involve knowledgeable others or try to determine the best places to gain missing information.

Formulate Possible Courses of Action and Probable Consequences

Courses of action may involve further information gathering, brainstorming, and possibly collaboration with other experts or specialists. Although further data may be needed to resolve problems at the level of individuals or small groups, it is especially necessary to enlist additional help when the issue is one that requires political action to effect policy changes. It may be necessary to recruit community members and leaders or to enlist the political power of specialty groups. Finally, a determination must be made about which proposed courses of action will be the least harmful and the most beneficial.

Initiate the Selected Course of Action and Evaluate the Outcome

Does the actual outcome match the anticipated outcome? If not, what happened that was unexpected? Would this have been foreseeable given more data? Would you do things differently in another similar situation given what you have learned? Does the problem need to be addressed at a different level (institutional or public policy)?

Engage in Self-Reflection and Peer or Expert Group Reflection

What could you have done differently? Would consulting with others have altered your conception of the problem or your course of action? What insights can you or your peers glean from this that could be appropriate for similar situations in the future? How might continuing education opportunities help you or your peers more appropriately address similar problems in the future? Would an ethics resource (committee or consultant) be helpful in such situations? Could you use this case as a focused learning experience for your peers and collaborators?

ETHICS OF HEALTH PROMOTION: CASES

Some cases of special relevance to health promotion are presented next. They are followed by questions that can be answered by individual readers, but they also provide a good starting point for group discussion. Try using the decision-making strategies suggested throughout the chapter as you explore these problems. It is anticipated that you will want more information than is provided. Deciding what extra information would be helpful is an important part of the exercise.

Case 1: Addressing Health Care System Problems—Elissa Needs Help

Elissa is 38 years old. She recently moved 200 miles from her home to a small town (population 6000) and separated from her abusive husband to escape his continuing threats and to be near her childhood friend. She suffers from chronic, sometimes incapacitating, depression for which she has in the past received antidepressant medications and counseling, with temporary relief. She has been unable to work and has no private health insurance. She is eligible for the state's Medicaid program, however, and has recently discovered that Medicaid will cover her health care needs. Her friend refers her to the only primary care center in the area, where she is seen by Jill, one of the two nurse practitioners. As part of her evaluation, Jill discovers that Elissa was also abused as a child and has very poor self-esteem. Elissa affirms that her childhood friend is very supportive. Jill believes that longer term psychological counseling would benefit Elissa and facilitate her well-being, but she also knows that none of the counseling services within a 50-mile radius accepts Medicaid payment. Elissa has no transportation.

- What are Jill's options? Responsibilities?
- What actions might Jill pursue both on a local level and on a political level? What are her resources?
- What is the responsibility of the health-promotion disciplines in cases like this?

Case 2: She's My Client!—Lilly and "Jake" (a.k.a. Paul)

Shirley, a nurse practitioner, is at a conference when a physician colleague discusses a difficult case. One of his clients, "Jake," is HIV positive but refuses any treatment. The physician explains that Jake fears that his wife will discover and recognize the names of the medications, because he knows "these drug names are discussed on television all the time." Jake has not told, nor does he ever intend to disclose, his wife that he is HIV positive. Jake firmly believes his condition is his private information and, for now, the couple uses condoms for birth control. The physician is concerned that Jake will not tell his wife. The physician is

presenting this case to colleagues to highlight the public awareness campaigns that, to some extent, have affected client privacy. He argues, "Listen to how they call out your name and the drugs at the pharmacy counter."

Shirley recognizes bits and pieces of information and comes to the painful realization that Jake is really Paul, and Paul is the husband of one of her clients, Lilly. Lilly has begun to discuss with Shirley that she wants to get pregnant soon. The town is too small for Shirley to be mistaken. Or is it?

- Is it ethical for the nurse practitioner to ask the physician if Jake is Paul?
- Is it ethical for Shirley to tell Lilly she suspects Paul is HIV positive?
- Should this information change how Shirley counsels Lilly about a pregnancy?
- What is in Lilly's best interests?
- What resources are available?

Case 3: Don't Touch My Things! Mrs. Smyth and Autonomy

Mrs. Smyth, 78, had lived in the same home for 30 years. Never married, she cared for her disabled mother for 15 years. After her mother died, she lived alone on a small pension. She appeared to be well groomed and appropriately dressed when she left her house.

Mrs. Smyth was hospitalized for a bowel obstruction and Joe, a community health nurse, made a follow-up visit after discharge to her home. When Joe arrived at the house, he was overcome with the smell of rotting garbage, urine, and feces. Five small dogs ran back and forth among piles of garbage and magazines, overturned furniture, and discarded appliances. There was no running water and the bathroom was not functional. Joe told Mrs. Smyth that her living conditions were

CASE STUDY

Genetic Screening Programs

Knome, Inc., in Cambridge, Massachusetts, has been sequencing the DNA of 20 individuals. With the individuals' consent, the results will be made available to researchers. Each donor will be offered information about genetic variations that might indicate a higher-than-average likelihood of developing a life-threatening condition.

There are hopes that genetic screenings of large populations will change the practice of health care from a focus on treating diseases to preventing them. Some researchers predict the complete sequencing of each human genome will provide routine data to health care providers, as are the common measurements of blood pressure, pulse, temperature, and blood counts today.

Other research data show, however, that better predictors of determining the risk of diabetes are asking people about their family history of diabetes, their weight, and their age rather than sequencing their DNA.

At present, the genetic analyses for Knome, Inc., are performed by a laboratory in Beijing, China; they take 4 to 6 months to complete and cost $350,000 for each sequence of DNA.

Reflective Questions

Apply different concepts and theories of ethics in thinking about the following questions.

1. What are some of the ethical issues of these analyses?
2. What are the responsibilities of health care professionals in the genetic screenings of a population?
3. What additional components could a community health nurse add to the following plan of care for participants having their DNA sequenced?

Sources: Beery, T. A., & Shooner, K. A. (2004). Family history: The first genetic screen. *Nurse Practitioner: American Journal of Primary Health Care, 29*(11), 14–25; Kayton, A. (2007). Newborn screening—A literature review. *Neonatal Network—The Journal of Neonatal Nursing, 26*(2), 85–95; Kirsner, S. (2008). Innovation economy: Mapping out a nascent market. *Boston Globe,* G1–G5. August 10, 2008; Lashley, F. R. (2007). *Essentials of clinical genetics in nursing practice.* New York: Springer; Prue, C. E., & Daniel, K. L. (2006). Social marketing: Planning before conceiving preconception care. *Maternal and Child Health Journal, 10*(5), S79–S84; Sheridan, S. L., Harris, R. P., & Woolf, S. H. (2004). Shared decision making about screening and chemoprevention. A suggested approach from the U.S. Preventive Services Task Force. *American Journal of Preventive Medicine, 26,* 55–66.

unhealthy and that he would contact a community agency to help her clean her house. Mrs. Smyth became very angry and said no one had the right to take her things away.

- Is it ethical for Joe to overrule Mrs. Smyth's autonomy in decision-making?

- What action is in Mrs. Smyth's best interests?
- What action is in the community's best interests?
- What ethical issues are involved in caring for a client with a hoarding disorder, such as that seen in Mrs. Smyth's disorder?

◎ CARE PLAN

Genetic Screening Programs

The use of developments in genetics research, including genetic counseling, testing, and screening, as well as advanced therapeutic and reproduction choices, influences the health of both present and future generations throughout the world.

As previously addressed, health care professionals have many complex ethical responsibilities in the applications of genetic developments with local, national, and international communities, as well as with individuals and families.

In the following care plan, the community health nurse from the preceding case study addresses aspects of the ineffective management of genetic screenings in a community.

*NURSING DIAGNOSIS: Ineffective community therapeutic regimen management

Definition
Pattern in which a community experiences (or is at risk to experience) difficulty integrating a genetic screening program for the prevention/treatment of illness and reduction of risk

Defining Characteristics
Major: Community verbalizes desire to manage the genetic screenings and treatment of illness and prevention of sequelae; community verbalizes difficulty with regulation and integration of prescribed regimens for genetic screening and treatment of illness and its effects or prevention of complications.
Minor: Knowledge of risk factors for illness (expected or unexpected) is accelerated.

Related Factors
Treatment Related
- Complexity of genetic screening and therapeutic regimen
- Complexity of health care
- Financial costs
  - Actual cost of procedure
  - Potential cost (e.g., loss of health insurance)
- Side effects
  - Expected (e.g., anxiety)
  - Unexpected (e.g., despair)

Situation/Environment Related
- Health and health care needs, multiple and complex, especially for vulnerable population (e.g., unborn children)
- Presence of known and unknown environmental (including occupational) health hazards
- Availability of community resources for screening for risk factors of diseases
  - Less expensive (e.g., family health histories and physical exams); more expensive (e.g., genetic screenings)
  - Overall needs and financial resources

Expected Outcomes
- With the community health nurses' guidance community members will:
  - Evaluate the actual and potential (e.g., significant increases in birth rates) health problems and resources of the community.

- Identify community resources that are needed to promote health and prevent illness, including genetic screenings.
- Participate in program development as needed to improve the effectiveness of the therapeutic regimen management of genetic screening programs.

Interventions
- Complete a community assessment including:
  - Actual and potential health problems and needs
  - Actual and potential resources for health
  - Develop an overall program plan for genetic screenings.
  - Develop a specific program for the genetic screening of an individual, perhaps including the following components:
  - Complete initial interview, individual and family histories, and physical exam with appropriate laboratory studies.
  - Generally discuss the genetic screenings and informed consent, focusing on the concerns of the individual and/or family.
- Assess barriers to learning:
  - Physical condition
  - Sensory status (e.g., vision, hearing)
  - Intelligence, learning abilities/disabilities
  - Emotional state(s) (e.g., fears, guilt)
  - Stressors, concerns
- Provide information:
  - Explain needed knowledge and perhaps changes (e.g., lifestyle behaviors).
  - Discuss and add to individual's knowledge of the pros and cons of genetic screening.
  - Identify influencing factors to decision-making about individual's genetic screening.
- Perform screenings (e.g., depression, financial resources).
- Give time to integrate new information, perhaps having a second appointment to:
  - Readdress questions.
  - Develop informed consent, including policies on privacy.
- Perform actual genetic screening procedure.
- Explain results with genetic and reproductive counseling.
- Repeat and follow-up as necessary.
- Compare the diagnostic criteria for Ineffective Therapeutic Regimen Management with other differential diagnoses potentially present in the case study.

References
Beery, T., & Workman, L. L. (2011). *Genetics and genomics in nursing and health care.* Philadelphia: F.A. Davis.
Carpenito, L. J. (2009). *Handbook of nursing diagnosis* (13th ed.). Philadelphia: Lippincott Williams & Wilkins.
Gordan, M. (2008). *Assess notes. Nursing assessment and diagnostic reasoning.* Philadelphia: F.A. Davis.
Gulanick, M., & Myers, J. L. (2011). *Nursing care plans: Diagnoses, interventions, and outcomes* (7th ed.). St. Louis: Mosby.
Lashley, F. R. (2007). *Essentials of clinical genetics in nursing practice.* New York: Springer.

SUMMARY

Health promotion is a vast and complex practice area; consequently, the associated ethical challenges are diverse and multileveled. This chapter has outlined the nature and purpose of health care ethics and related this to the responsibilities of health care providers in health-promotion interventions. Health promotion should be viewed as a moral undertaking of health care providers. After reading this chapter, students will have knowledge of some of the tools and language needed to explore ethical issues, discuss these issues with others, and address problematic issues at both the individual and the societal levels. Perhaps the most important factor to consider is that ethical problems manifesting at the level of the individual almost always have their origins in the broader societal environment.

REFERENCES

American Nurses Association. (1994). *Position statement: The non-negotiable nature of the ANA code for nurses with interpretive statements.* Washington, DC: Author.

American Nurses Association. (2001). *Code of ethics for nurses with interpretive statements.* Washington, DC: Author.

American Nurses Association. (2008). *Guide to the code of ethics for nurses: Interpretation and application.* Washington, DC: Author.

American Nurses Association. (2010). *Nursing's social policy statement. The essence of the profession* (3rd ed.). Silver Spring, MD: Author.

Andrews, L. B., Mehlman, M. J., Rothstein, M. A. (2012). *Genetics: Ethics, law, and policy.* St. Paul, MN: West Group/Thompson.

Atkins, K. (2006). Autonomy and autonomy competencies: A practical and relational approach. *Nursing and Philosophy, 7*(4), 205–215.

Bandman, E. L., & Bandman, B. (2001). *Nursing ethics through the life span* (4th ed.). Upper Saddle River, NJ: Prentice Hall.

Beauchamp, T. L., & Childress, J. F. (2008). *Principles of biomedical ethics* (6th ed.). New York: Oxford University.

Beauchamp, T. L., Walters, L., Kahn, J. P., & Mastroianni, A. C. (2007). *Contemporary issues in bioethics* (7th ed.). Belmont, CA: Wadsworth.

Benner, P., Tanner, C. A., & Chesla, C. A. (1998). *Expertise in nursing practice: Caring, clinical judgment, and ethics.* New York: Springer.

Bennett, P., & Smith, S. J. (2007). Genetics, insurance and participation: How a citizen's jury reached its verdict. *Social Science & Medicine, 64*(12), 2487–2498.

Braun, U. K., Beyth, R. J., Ford, M. E., & McCullough, L. B. (2008). Voices of African American, Caucasian, and Hispanic surrogates on the burdens of end-of-life decision making. *Journal of General Internal Medicine, 23*(3), 267–274.

Braunack-Mayer, A., & Louise, J. (2008). The ethics of community empowerment: Tensions in health promotion theory and practice. *Promotion & Education, 15*(3), 5–8.

Buchanan, D. R. (2000). *An ethic for health promotion: Rethinking the sources of human well-being.* New York: Oxford University.

Buchanan, D. R. (2006). Moral reasoning as a model for health promotion. *Social Science & Medicine, 63*(10), 2715–2726.

Burkhardt, M. A., & Nathaniel, A. K. (2007). *Ethics and issues in contemporary nursing* (3rd ed.). Albany, NY: Delmar.

Carter, S. M., Rychetnik, L., Lloyd, B., Kerridge, I. H., Baur, L., Bauman, A., et al. (2011). Evidence, ethics, and values: A framework for health promotion. *American Journal of Public Health, 101*(3), 465–472.

Chambliss, D. F. (1996). *Beyond caring: Hospitals, nurses, and the social organization of ethics.* Chicago: University of Chicago Press.

Corey, G., Corey, M. S., & Callanan, P. (2011). *Issues and ethics in the helping professions* (8th ed.). Belmont, CA: Brooks/Cole.

Coursen, C. C. (2009). Inequalities affecting access to healthcare: A philosophical reflection. *International Journal for Human Caring, 13*(1), 7–15.

Crigger, N. J. (2008). Towards a viable and just global nursing ethics. *Nursing Ethics, 15*(1), 17–27.

Davis, A. J., Fowler, M. D., & Arosker, M. (2010). *Ethical dilemmas and nursing practice* (5th ed.). New York: Prentice Hall.

Dickey, S. B., & Deatrick, J. (2000). Autonomy and decision making for health promotion in adolescence. *Pediatric Nursing, 26*(5), 461–467.

Dinkins, C. S. (2011). Beyond patient care: Practicing empathy in the workplace. *Online Journal of Issues in Nursing, 16*(2). Retrieved January 22, 2012, from http://ana.nursingworld.org/MainMenu Categories/ANAMarketplace/ANAPeriodicals/OJIN/Columns/ Ethics/Empathy-in-the-Workplace.aspx.

Epstein, E. G., & Delgado, S. (2010). Understanding and addressing moral distress. *Online Journal of Issues in Nursing, 15*(3). Retrieved January 22, 2012, from http://ana.nursingworld.org/MainMenuCat egories/ANAMarketplace/ANAPeriodicals/OJIN/TableofContents/ Vol152010/No3-Sept-2010/Understanding-Moral-Distress.aspx.

Fagerlin, A., & Schneider, C. E. (2004). Enough. The failure of the living will. *Hastings Center Report, 34*(2), 30–42.

Gilligan, C. (1982). *In a different voice: Psychological theory and women's development.* Cambridge, MA: Harvard University Press.

Gilligan, C. (2011). *Joining the resistance.* Malden, MA: Polity Press.

Grace, P. J. (2001). Professional advocacy: Widening the scope of accountability. *Nursing Philosophy, 2*(2), 151–162.

Grace, P. J. (2004). Ethics in the clinical encounter. In S. Chase (Ed.), *Clinical judgment and communication in the nurse practitioner practice.* William F. Connell School of Nursing: Boston College.

Institute of Medicine. (2010). *The future of nursing: Leading change, advancing health.* Retrieved from http://books.nap.edu/openbook. php?record_id=12956.

International Council of Nurses. (2006). *The ICN Code of Ethics for Nurses.* Geneva, Switzerland: Author. Retrieved January 22, 2012, from www.icn.ch/about-icn/code-of-ethics-for-nurses/code-of-ethics-for-nurses.html.

Kangasniemi, M. (2010). Equality as a central concept of nursing ethics: A systematic literature review. *Scandinavian Journal of Caring Sciences, 24,* 824–832.

Kant, I. (1997). Foundations of the metaphysics of morals (Trans. L. W. Beck). In A. I. Melden (Ed.), *Ethical theories: A book of readings* (2nd ed., pp. 317–366). Englewood Cliffs, NJ: Prentice Hall (Original work published 1785).

Keane, M. (2010). Ethics as individual health interventions. *The American Journal of Bioethics, 10*(3), 36–38.

Kohlberg, L. (1981). *The philosophy of moral development: Moral stages and the idea of justice. Essays on moral development* (Vol. 1). San Francisco: Harper & Row.

Kohlberg, L. (1984). *The psychology of moral development: The nature and validity of moral stages. Essays on moral development* (Vol. 2). San Francisco: Harper & Row.

Kulynych, J., & Korn, D. (2002). Use and disclosure of health information in genetic research: Weighing the impact of the new federal medical privacy rule. *American Journal of Law & Medicine, 28*(2-3), 309–324.

Lambert, V., & Glacken, M. (2011). Engaging with children in research: Theoretical and practical implications of negotiating informed consent/assent. *Nursing Ethics, 18*(6), 781–801.

Liaschenko, J. (1999). Can justice coexist with the supremacy of personal values in nursing practice? *Western Journal of Nursing Research, 21*(1), 35–50.

Lind, C., Anderson, B., & Oberle, K. (2003). Ethical issues in adolescent consent for research. *Nursing Ethics, 10*(5), 504–511.

MacIntyre, A. (2007). *After virtue: A study in moral theory* (3rd ed.). Southbend, IN: Notre Dame University.

Madison, K. M., Volpp, K. G., & Halpern, S. D. (2011). The law, policy, and ethics of employers' use of financial incentives to improve health. *Journal of Law, Medicine & Ethics, 39*(3), 450–468.

Marks, R. (2009). Ethics and patient education: Health literacy and cultural dilemmas. *Health Promotion Practice, 10*(3), 328–332.

Marks, R., & Shive, S. E. (2007). "Health for all": An ethical imperative or unattainable ideal? *Health Promotion Practice, 8*(1), 28–30.

Marmot, M., & Wilkinson, R. G. (2006). *Social determinants of health* (2nd ed.). New York: Oxford University.

Mill, J. S. (2002). *Utilitarianism* (2nd ed.). Indianapolis, IN: Hackett (Originally published 1861).

Murphy, N. (2008). An agenda for health promotion. *Nursing Ethics, 15*(5), 697–699.

National Society of Genetic Counselors. (2011). Code of ethics. Retrieved January 9, 2013, from www.nsgc.org/Advocacy/NSGCCodeofEthics/tabid/ISS/Default.aspx.

Nelson, H. L. (1992). Against caring. *Journal of Clinical Ethics, 3*(1), 8–20.

O'Keefe-McCarthy, S. (2009). Technologically-mediated nursing care: The impact on moral agency. *Nursing Ethics, 16*(6), 786–796.

Orem, D. (2001). *Nursing concepts of practice* (6th ed.). St. Louis: Mosby.

Paulsen, J. E. (2011). Ethics of caring and professional roles. *Nursing Ethics, 18*(2), 201–208.

Powers, M., & Faden, R. (2008). *Social justice: The moral foundations of public health and health policy* (2nd ed.). New York: Oxford University Press.

President's Commission for the Study of Ethical Problems in Medicine and Biomedical and Behavioral Research. (1982). *Compensating for research injuries: The ethical and legal implications of programs to redress injured subjects.* Washington, DC: U.S. Government Printing Office.

Rachels, J., & Rachels, S. (2011). *The elements of moral philosophy* (7th ed.). New York: McGraw-Hill.

Rawls, J. (1971 and 1999). *A theory of justice.* Cambridge, MA: Harvard University.

Rees, J., King, L., & Schmitz, K. (2009). Nurses' perceptions of ethical issues in the care of older people. *Nursing Ethics, 16*(4), 436–452.

Reimer-Kirkham, S. (2009). Lived religion: Implications for nursing ethics. *Nursing Ethics, 16*(4), 407–417.

Rogers, J., & Kelly, U. A. (2011). Feminist intersectionality: Bringing social justice to health disparities research. *Nursing Ethics, 18*(3), 397–407.

Ross, L. F. (1997). Health care decision making by children. Is it in their best interest? *Hastings Center Report, 27*(6), 41–45.

Rothstein, M. A., & Harrell, H. L. (2009). Employer-sponsored health plans: Part II—Law and ethics. *Journal of Occupational and Environmental Medicine, 51*(8), 951–957.

Ruger, J. P. (2008). Ethics in American health 2: An ethical framework for health system reform. *American Journal of Public Health, 98*(10), 1756–1763.

Singer, P. (1993). *A companion to ethics.* Cambridge, MA: Wiley-Blackwell.

Slomka, J., Quill, B., DesVignes-Kendrick, M., & Lloyd, L. E. (2008). Professionalism and ethics in the public health curriculum. *Public Health Reports, 123*(Suppl 2), 27–35.

Sorrell, J. M., & Cangelosi, P. R. (2009). Respecting vulnerability: Informed consent in persons with Alzheimer's disease. *Southern Online Journal of Nursing Research, 9*(4). Retrieved January 22, 2012, from www.resourcceenter.net/images/SNRS/Files/SOJNR_articles2/Vol09Num04Art02.html.

Tarasoff v. *Regents of University of California.* (1976, July 1). California Supreme Court 131. *California Reporter, 14.*

Tschudin, V. (2010). Nursing ethics: The last decade. *Nursing Ethics, 17*(1), 127–131.

U.S. Department of Health and Human Services, Office for Civil Rights. (2004). *HIPAA privacy rule.* Retrieved January 22, 2012, from www.hhs.gov/ocr/hipaa/.

Vig, E. K., Starks, H., Taylor, J. S., Hopely, E. K., & Fryer-Edwards, K. (2007). Surviving surrogate decision-making: What helps and hampers the experience of making medical decisions for others. *Journal of General Internal Medicine, 22*(9), 1274–1279.

Weston, A. (2010). *A practical companion to ethics* (4th ed.). New York: Oxford University.

Wilmot, S. (2000). Nurses and whistleblowing: The ethical issues. *Journal of Advanced Nursing, 32*(5), 1051–1057.

UNIT 2
Assessment for Health Promotion

CHAPTER
6

Health Promotion and the Individual

Anne Rath Rentfro

 WEBSITE

http://evolve.elsevier.com/Edelman/
- Study Questions
- Glossary
- Website Resources
  6A: Functional Health Patterns Assessment for an Adult

OBJECTIVES

After completing this chapter, the reader will be able to:
- Define the framework of functional health patterns as described by Gordon.
- Describe the use of the functional health pattern framework to assess individuals throughout the life span.
- Illustrate health patterns of the functional, potentially dysfunctional, and actually dysfunctional categories of behavior.

- Identify risk factors or etiological aspects of actual or potential dysfunctional health patterns to consider with nursing diagnoses.
- Discuss planning, implementing, and evaluating nursing interventions to promote the health of individuals.
- Develop specific health-promotion plans based on an assessment of individuals.

KEY TERMS

Age-developmental focus	Functional health patterns	Nursing interventions
Culturally competent care	Health status	Pattern focus
Expected outcomes	Individual-environmental focus	Risk factors
Functional focus	Nursing diagnosis	

From U.S. Department of Health and Human Services. (2011). *Healthy People 2020 topics and objectives*. Retrieved January 7, 2012, from www.healthypeople.gov/2020/topicsobjectives2020/default.aspx.

THINK ABOUT IT

Assessment of Alcohol Consumption

*Women have different patterns of alcohol consumption and different thresholds for problem drinking than men. Instruments such as the CAGE detect alcohol dependence and would not be a sensitive enough measure for some women, in particular pregnant women, who are less likely than men to be alcohol dependent. The T-ACE instrument provides a measure of alcohol intake patterns more appropriate for women than that derived from the CAGE test (considered **Cutting** down on drinking, been **Annoyed** by criticism of drinking, feeling **Guilty** about drinking, and using alcohol as an **Eye** opener). The T-ACE test, developed for use with women, was the first validated screening tool for assessing drinking risk in pregnant women and continues to provide a highly sensitive tool for identifying risk drinking (Burns et al., 2010). Screening is a useful strategy in health-promotion assessment and intervention (see Chapter 9). A pattern of drinking is established using the following questions:*

T—*How many drinks does it **Take** to make you feel high?*
A—*Have you ever been **Annoyed** by people criticizing your drinking?*
C—*Have you ever felt you ought to **Cut** down your drinking?*
E—*Have you ever had a drink first thing in the morning (**Eye** opener) to steady your nerves or get rid of a hangover?*

Scores are calculated as follows:
- A reply of more than two drinks to question T is considered a positive response and scores 2 points, and an affirmative answer to question A, C, or E scores 1 point, respectively.
- A total score of 2 or more points on the T-ACE indicates evidence of risk drinking.
  - Why would a nurse tailor the assessments to individual characteristics of a population?
  - How effectively would this screening tool identify alcohol problems in women other than the pregnant women within the population? Why?

BOX 6-1   HEALTHY PEOPLE 2020

- Increase educational achievement of adolescents and young adults.
- (Developmental) Reduce the proportion of persons who did not receive a transfusion because of a blood product shortage.
- Increase the proportion of parents who use positive parenting and communicate with their doctors or other health care professionals about positive parenting.
- Increase the proportion of women with a family history of breast and/or ovarian cancer who receive genetic counseling.
- Decrease the tuberculosis (TB) case rate for foreign-born persons living in the United States.
- Increase the proportion of older adults who are up to date on a core set of clinical preventive services.
- Reduce the time necessary to activate designated personnel in response to a public health emergency.
- Increase the proportion of students in grades 9 through 12 who get sufficient sleep.
- Increase the proportion of adults who get sufficient sleep.

- Early and Middle Childhood
- Genomics
- Global Health
- Health Care–Associated Infections
- Health-Related Quality of Life and Well-Being
- Lesbian, Gay, Bisexual, and Transgender Health
- Older Adults
- Preparedness
- Sleep Health
- Social Determinants of Health

Nurses promote health by encouraging the use of processes in patterns that lead toward wellness. Health and illness within this context reflect changing patterns of the life process. Holistic nursing acts as a central unifying theme to connect pattern recognition to the examination of person-environment relationships throughout the life span. Disorganization or ineffective coping produces fluctuations in patterns that eventually result in illness. Patterns of strength, according to Newman's Theory of Health as Expanding Consciousness, redirect the individual toward more harmonious patterns of health promotion (Pharris, 2011).

In the United States the health-promotion initiative called *Healthy People 2020* establishes national goals and provides a framework for prevention (U.S. Department of Health and Human Services, 2011). *Healthy People 2020* publishes national health objectives that identify the most significant preventable threats to health. Communities use these objectives and associated indicators to evaluate progress toward the overall goals of attaining high-quality longer lives, decreasing health disparity, and creating environments that promote health and improve the quality of life for all (U.S. Department of Health and Human Services, 2011). *Healthy People 2020* added the following topics that were not part of the *Healthy People 2010* initiative:

- Adolescent Health
- Blood Disorders and Blood Safety
- Dementias, including Alzheimer's Disease

Most of these new topics concern primary prevention for individuals in some way. Selected examples of how *Healthy People 2020* (2011) objectives address these primary prevention areas for individuals are presented in Box 6-1: *Healthy People 2020*.

Long before this current focus on health promotion with the *Healthy People* initiatives in the United States, Florence Nightingale expressed the belief that laws of both health and nursing are similar and pertinent to both sick and well individuals (Selanders, 2010). The International Council of Nurses defines nursing as encompassing the "autonomous and collaborative care of individuals of all ages, families, groups and communities, sick or well and in all settings. Nursing includes the promotion of health, prevention of illness, and the care of ill, disabled and dying people. Advocacy, promotion of a safe environment, research, participation in shaping health policy and in patient and health systems management, and education are also key nursing roles" (International Council of Nurses, 2010). This broad definition provides a model for nursing globally using the nursing process: assessment, diagnosis, outcome criteria, process criteria (including planned interventions), implementation, and evaluation. The nursing process, in turn, establishes a useful framework for the health-promotion assessment of the individual.

Nurses typically use assessment strategies including health promotion that addresses interactions among individual's biophysical, psychosocial, and spiritual states and patterns with the environment. When assessing for primary prevention, techniques also include generalized health promotion and specific protection from disease, both of which fall within the scope of nursing practice. The active process of promoting health involves protection (immunizations, occupational safety, and environmental control) along with lifestyle, value, and belief system behaviors that enhance health.

With health promotion serving as the underlying theme, this chapter addresses nursing assessment of individuals. In most areas of nursing, tertiary care and prevention of further disease provide the assessment focus (Black & Lobo, 2008). This tertiary focus limits reflection to problem-solving, excluding assessment of overall general health and wellness. Most nursing diagnoses approved by the North American Nursing Diagnosis Association International (NANDA-I) are problem oriented. The NANDA-I definition of nursing diagnosis includes life processes as well as actual or potential health problems. One way to address nursing diagnoses in well individuals is to focus on human developmental or maturational tasks. Although most approved nursing diagnoses reflect a focus on deficit assessment and problem-solving, this inclusion of life processes provides a broad base for nursing diagnoses to use strength-based healthy responses or potential for healthy responses (Black & Lobo, 2008; Curwood et al., 2011; Haley, 2011; Herdman, 2008). Furthermore, concentrating on strengths in the health-promotion setting provides a foundation to help individuals move toward improved health. Nurses support and enhance the ability of healthy individuals to maintain or strengthen their health.

Current U.S. health care systems continue to use deficit assessment rather than the strength-based approach that is more appropriate for health-promotion settings. Mental health, social work, and nursing, however, embrace a strength-based approach to assessment within the health-promotion context. From using infant competencies to plan care and person-centered approaches for care of people with dementia, nurses incorporate strength-based assessment into their diagnostic process (Black & Lobo, 2008; Brazeau, 2011; Curwood et al., 2011; Marshall et al., 2010; Rawana, 2009; Skerrett, 2010). Although NANDA-I has stated that there is a need for work in this area of strength-based assessment and wellness, published material for using wellness diagnoses appears infrequently. The NANDA-I taxonomy, however, uses multiple dimensions of human response in the consideration of each diagnosis. These seven dimensions include the status of the diagnosis that considers whether the diagnosis is addressing wellness, risk, or an actual problem (Boldt et al., 2010). More work is necessary to develop and promote useful language for health-promotion and wellness diagnoses.

Gordon's framework, which uses a functional health patterns assessment, provides the foundation for the construction of the NANDA-I nursing diagnosis nomenclature (Boldt et al., 2010; Gordon, 2011). As NANDA-I continues to develop diagnoses for health promotion, Gordon's framework will most likely continue to provide the foundation for these diagnoses. This same framework is used throughout this chapter to demonstrate assessment approaches with the family and community

TABLE 6-1	ASPECTS OF A NURSING ASSESSMENT
DEFINITION	DELIBERATE AND SYSTEMATIC DATA COLLECTION
Components	Subjective data: Health history, including subjective reports and individual perceptions Objective data: Observations of nurse Physical examination findings Information from health record Results of clinical testing
Function	Description of person's health status
Structure	Organization of interdependent parts describing health, function, or patterns of behavior that reflect whole individual and environment
Process	Interview, observation, and examination
Format	Systematic but flexible; individualized to each person, nurse, and situation
Goal	Nursing diagnosis or problem identification Identification of areas of strengths, limitations, alterations, responses to alterations and therapies, and risks

(see Chapters 7 and 8). This chapter also discusses components of the nursing process as they relate to health promotion of the individual.

GORDON'S FUNCTIONAL HEALTH PATTERNS: ASSESSMENT OF THE INDIVIDUAL

Nursing assessment determines the health status of individuals. Table 6-1 demonstrates aspects of a complete nursing assessment. Assessment, in this case, refers to collection of data that culminates in problem identification or a diagnostic statement. Effective health assessment considers not only physiological parameters, but also how the human being interacts with the whole environment. Behavior patterns, beliefs, perceptions, and values form the essential components of health assessment when maximal health potential of the individual is considered by nurses. Pattern recognition supports our understanding of health of individuals and is reflected in nursing theories such as those initially developed by nursing theorists such as Newman (Pharris, 2011).

Historically, conceptual models in nursing have employed Gordon's health-related behaviors particularly in regard to formulating a framework to guide assessment (Boldt et al., 2010; Epstein et al., 2010; Flanagan & Jones, 2009). Gordon's (2011) 11 functional health patterns interact to depict an individual's lifestyle. Using this framework, nurses combine assessment skills with subjective and objective data to construct patterns reflective of lifestyles.

Functional Health Pattern Framework

Holism and the totality of the person's interactions with the environment form the philosophical foundations of Gordon's functional health patterns. This foundation provides a context

TABLE 6-2   TYPOLOGY OF 11 FUNCTIONAL HEALTH PATTERNS

PATTERN	DESCRIPTION
Health perception-health management pattern	Individual's perceived health and well-being and how health is managed
Nutritional-metabolic pattern	Food and fluid consumption relative to metabolic needs and indicators of local nutrient supply
Elimination pattern	Excretory function (bowel, bladder, and skin)
Activity-exercise pattern	Exercise, activity, leisure, and recreation
Sleep-rest pattern	Sleep, rest, and relaxation
Cognitive-perceptual pattern	Sensory, perceptual, and cognitive patterns
Self-perception–self-concept pattern	Self-concept pattern and perceptions of self (body comfort, body image, and feeling state); self-conception and self-esteem
Roles-relationships pattern	Role engagements and relationships
Sexuality-reproductive pattern	Person's satisfaction and dissatisfaction with sexuality and reproduction
Coping-stress tolerance pattern	General coping pattern and effectiveness in stress tolerance
Values-beliefs pattern	Values, beliefs (including spiritual), or goals that guide choices or decisions

Modified from Gordon, M. (2011). *Manual of nursing diagnosis* (12th ed.). Sudbury, MA: Jones & Bartlett.

for collecting data that provide information about the entire person and most life processes. By examining functional patterns and interactions among patterns, nurses accurately determine and diagnose actual or potential problems, intervene more effectively, and facilitate movement toward outcomes to promote health and well-being (Gordon, 2011). In addition to providing a framework to assess individuals, families, and communities holistically, functional health patterns provide a strong focus for more effective nursing interventions and outcomes. This stronger focus provides a solid position from which nurses participate as decision makers in health care systems at organizational, community, national, and international levels.

Definition

Functional health patterns view the individual as a whole being using interrelated behavioral areas. The typology of 11 patterns serves as a useful tool to collect and organize assessment data and to create a structure for validation and communication among health care providers. Each pattern described in Table 6-2 forms part of the biopsychosocial-spiritual expression of the whole person. Individual reports and nursing observations provide data to differentiate patterns. As a framework for assessment, functional health patterns provide an effective means for nurses to perceive and record complex interactions of individuals' biophysical state, psychological makeup, and environmental relationships.

Characteristics

Functional health patterns are characterized by their focus. Gordon (2011) uses five areas of focus: pattern; individual-environmental; age-developmental; functional; and cultural.

Pattern focus implies that the nurse explores patterns or sequences of behavior over time. Gordon's term *behavior* encompasses all forms of human behavior, including biophysical, psychological, and sociological elements. Pattern recognition, a cognitive process, occurs during information collection. Cues are identified and clustered while gathering information. Patterns emerge that represent historical and current behavior. Quantitative patterns such as blood pressure are readily identified, and pattern recognition is facilitated when baseline data are available. As the nurse incorporates a broader range of data, patterns imbedded within other patterns begin to emerge. Blood pressure, for example, is a pattern within both the activity and the exercise patterns. Individual baseline and subsequent readings may present a pattern within expected norms. Erratic blood pressure measurements indicate an absence of pattern. This lack of pattern forms its own type of pattern. Functional health pattern categories provide structures to analyze factors within a category (blood pressure: activity pattern) and to search for causal explanations, usually outside the category (excessive sodium intake: nutritional pattern) (Gordon, 2011).

Food intake examples illustrate the individual-environmental focus of Gordon's framework (Gordon, 2011). Reference to environmental influence occurs within many patterns in the form of physical environments within and external to the individual. Environmental influences in functional health patterns include role relationships, family values, and societal mores. Personal preference, knowledge of food preparation, and ability to consume and retain food govern the individual's intake. Cultural and family habits, financial ability to secure food, and crop availability also influence food intake. Additionally, the person who secures, prepares, and serves the food controls nutritional intake for the family.

Each pattern also reflects a human growth and age-developmental focus (Hockenberry & Wilson, 2010). As individuals fulfill developmental tasks complexity increases. These tasks, however, provide learning opportunities for the individual to maintain and improve health. Erikson's framework, which organizes specific health tasks for the individual to accomplish at each developmental phase of the life cycle, continues to serve as the framework to assess and plan care (Vogel-Scibilia et al., 2009). Erikson's eight stages provide the traditional developmental assessment nurses generally use to plan care (see Table 6-3 on p. 139). Each stage presents a central task or crisis that must be resolved before healthy growth can continue (Hockenberry & Wilson, 2010). Individuals develop their sense of autonomy in early childhood and struggle with the sense of shame and doubt. When this developmental level is achieved or resolved, the child moves on to develop initiative during the next stage.

Both age and developmental stage continue to provide the foundation for contemporary assessment of individuals' health status. Developmental tasks begin at birth and continue until death. By considering current epidemiological data and recommended health behaviors, Gordon's (2011) framework continues to be useful today for health promotion throughout the life span Therefore, Unit 4 uses Gordon's framework to explore developmental tasks and their related health behaviors for health promotion.

Functional focus refers to an individual's performance level. Other disciplines plan care using functional patterns, but assessment data vary among disciplines (Boldt et al., 2010). Physical therapists and occupational therapists, for example, focus on physical ability to perform activities of daily living and rely on assessments of independent ability to carry out personal activities of daily living to develop their plans. For physicians, genitourinary function refers to frequency or voiding patterns and characteristics of urine, such as color, odor, and laboratory analysis results. In addition to these factors of genitourinary function, nurses assess how the particular voiding pattern affects lifestyle, particularly how urinary frequency affects sleep patterns and the ability to perform activities such as shopping or socializing. Additional concerns might include the individual's ability to walk or climb stairs to the bathroom or to manage these activities safely at night. It has been suggested that all disciplines employ the *International Classification of Functioning, Disability and Health* to promote transdisciplinary communication about functional patterns that can be used along with the NANDA-I taxonomy (Boldt et al., 2010).

Culture, age, and developmental and gender norms, considered during assessment, influence development of health patterns. Leininger defines transcultural nursing concepts of cultural care, health, well-being, and illness patterns in different environmental contexts and under different living conditions (Andrews & Boyle, 2011). Culturally competent care is delivered with knowledge of and sensitivity to cultural factors influencing health behavior. Complex cultural patterns transmitted from former generations contribute to individuals' health behavior. Culturally competent care respects the underlying personal and cultural reality of individuals. Nurses provide more culturally competent care when they identify and use cultural norms, values, and communication and time patterns in their self-reflection and interpretation of assessment information (Bourke Bearskin, 2011).

Functional health patterns form a framework that centers on health and can account for cultural factors. Most nursing assessments use functional pattern assessment as a foundation to their practice. Although nursing theoretical and conceptual frameworks vary, the functional health pattern framework is relevant to most conceptual models. In fact, functional health patterns provide the structure used by NANDA-I to support nursing diagnosis nomenclature. Nursing classification of interventions and outcome nomenclature also use Gordon's functional patterns as a foundation (Boldt et al., 2010). Advantages of a functional health pattern framework specific to the practice of nursing include the following:

- Provides consistent nursing language through collecting, organizing, presenting, and analyzing data to determine nursing diagnoses.
- Allows flexibility to tailor content for individuals and situations.

- Suits diverse practice areas (e.g., home, clinic, institution) for assessment of individuals (adult/children), families, or communities.
- Supports theoretical components of nursing service, education, and research by organizing clinical knowledge using nursing diagnoses, interventions, and outcomes.
- Incorporates medical science data while retaining the focus on nursing knowledge and practice.

The Patterns

Each pattern reflects a biopsychosocial spiritual expression of the individual's lifestyle or life processes from the perspective of both the individual and the nurse. The following are revealed by this expression: a pattern or sequencing of behaviors; the role of the environment (physical surroundings, family, societal, and cultural influences); and developmental influences. The assessment of each pattern includes its status as functional (strengths/wellness), dysfunctional (actual), or potentially dysfunctional (risk) as well as an indication of the individual's level of satisfaction with the pattern (Boldt et al., 2010). Nurses assess reported problems in more depth to generate an explanation for the problem, to determine remedial actions to take, and to understand the perceived effect of these actions from the individual's perspective. An important goal when assessing each pattern is to determine the individual's knowledge of health promotion, the ability of the individual to manage health-promoting activities, and the value that the individual ascribes to health promotion using a strength-based approach to identify wellness diagnoses. Each pattern is presented in this chapter, with details for nurses to use to assess individuals and determine health-promotion diagnoses using a functional health pattern framework along with a discussion of nursing implications for use of the patterns in health-promotion practice.

Health Perception–Health Management Pattern

The health perception–health management pattern involves individuals' health status and health practices used to reach the current level of health or wellness with a focus on perceived health status and meaning of health (Gordon, 2011). When eliciting this information, nurses discover areas for further exploration under other functional health patterns. For example, if the individual reports shortness of breath when mowing the lawn, the nurse stores this information to retrieve later when assessing activity and exercise patterns or cognitive-perceptual patterns.

Health perception–health management patterns affect lifestyle and ability to function even when individuals do not perceive actual health problems, are unaware of necessary health promotion in the absence of problems, do not feel capable of managing their health, or believe activity on their part is useless to promote health. Health-promoting activities (e.g., adequate nutrition, activity and exercise, sleep and rest), routine professional examinations, self-examinations, immunizations, and safety precautions (e.g., auto safety restraints and locked medicine cabinets) provide this pattern's clues to improve or maintain optimal quality of life.

Assessment objectives for health perception–health management consist of obtaining data about perceptions, management, and preventive health practices (Gordon, 2011).

Exploring values identifies potential health hazards, such as lack of adherance to a prescribed medical or nursing regimen or ability to manage health effectively. In addition to these kinds of assessment cues, nurses identify unrealistic health and illness perceptions and expectations. The Transtheoretical Model (TTM) consists of five stages that can be useful in assessing an individual's readiness to change (see Chapter 10). These stages—precontemplation, contemplation, planning/ preparation, action, and maintenance—have been used widely in health-promotion programs for diverse populations and multiple age groups with topics ranging from prevention of injury to nutrition education programs (Kannan et al., 2010; Muir & Bennett, 2010).

Assessment includes the following parameters:
- Health and safety practices of the individual
- Previous patterns of adherence or compliance
- Use of the health care system
- Knowledge of health service availability
- Health-seeking behavior patterns
- Means to access health care (e.g., financial resources, health insurance, and transportation)

In addition to methods of health management, nurses explore health perceptions as individuals describe their current health status, past problems, and anticipation of future problems associated with health or health care. These findings reveal beliefs about health, perceived susceptibility, self-efficacy, and level of knowledge about health status, taking into account the influence of culture (Andrews & Boyle, 2011) (Box 6-2: Diversity Awareness). Health and illness perceptions significantly influence overall direction for care planning. Health beliefs, also discussed under the values-beliefs pattern, directly impact participation in care. Partnership with providers is also more likely to yield better attention to self-care, particularly in cultures that value collective responsibility (Gallant et al., 2010). In an integration of the literature regarding older Americans of African, Latin, Asian, and Native American Indian descent, Gallant, Spitze, and Grove (2010) indicate that these individuals from cultures valuing collectivism are more likely to engage in self-care measures when their cultural patterns and social support within families are considered.

Past health management serves as a predictor of future health management (Berentson-Shaw et al., 2009; Klinedinst et al., 2009). If adherence to a prescribed regimen has not occurred in the past, adherence now is unlikely unless the nurse is able to identify and remedy the causes of the discrepancies between provider recommendations and the individual's implementation of those recommendations. For example, an individual with high blood pressure who has failed to keep follow-up appointments, often forgotten to take medication, and eaten foods with high sodium content should be assessed to determine whether this evident nonadherence results from a conflict within the value system of the individual (health beliefs); inaccurate information; misunderstanding; inadequate ability to learn, retain, or retrieve information (knowledge deficit); denial of illness (health perception); or inability to access care and/ or resources. Variables such as financial resources, transportation difficulties, nutritional preferences, daily activities (individual and family patterns), ability to read written instructions

(literacy or visual acuity), and ability to manipulate numbers (numeracy) may affect the individual's behaviors.

Nutritional-Metabolic Pattern

Nutritional-metabolic patterns center on nutrient intake relative to metabolic need (Gordon, 2011). This pattern includes individuals' descriptions of food and fluid consumption (history) as well as evidence of adequate nutrition (physical examination). Nurses explore their satisfaction with current eating and drinking patterns, including restrictions, and their perceptions of problems associated with eating and drinking, growth and development, skin condition, and healing processes.

Intake and supply of nutrients to tissues and organs influence bodily functions and interact with lifestyle. Sufficient food and fluid intake provides energy for performance, which includes both internal physiological functioning and external body movements. Interruption in acquisition or retention of food or fluids offsets balance and significantly alters lifestyle. Nutrition and metabolism also govern the growth rates (Ball & Lewis, 2011; Hasnain, Connell, Menon, & Tranmer, 2011; Moodley & Bertrand, 2011; Villar-Loubet, Jones, Waldrop-Valverde, Bruscantini, & Weiss, 2011).

Assessment within this pattern includes data about typical patterns of food and fluid consumption and adequacy of consumption patterns, along with perceived problems associated with nutritional intake. Nurses attend to cues to conditions of overweight, underweight, overhydration, dehydration, or difficulties in skin integrity, such as breakdown or delayed healing. Individuals may also be at risk for developing these problems. Conversely, this pattern may exhibit strengths that can be used to support the health-promotion plan.

Parameters for assessment for this pattern fall into two broad categories of evaluation: nutrient intake and metabolic demand. Intake may be assessed with a 24-hour recall of food and fluid consumption; a listing of dietary restrictions, food allergies, vitamin supplements, and caffeine and alcohol ingestion (when not included in the medication history); and a schedule of eating and drinking patterns. Assessment includes screening for problems associated with swallowing or chewing.

With identified problems, focused assessments include food preferences, feelings about present weight, and eating habits. Intake may be affected when individuals eat alone. Frequent dining out may indicate the need for further exploration within the nutrition area or other functional patterns. Diets may consist of fast food. Consumption patterns may be deficient in essential vitamins or minerals. Food security may also be explored. Who purchases food? Is shopping preplanned with a grocery list? Are financial resources and food budgets adequate? Is food stored properly? Who prepares food? How is food prepared (fried, broiled, steamed, boiled, or baked)?

Metabolic demands vary from individual to individual and within the same individual during times of illness, stress, growth, high or low activity levels, healing, or recovery. Developmental and environmental conditions alter metabolic demands. Appetite and reported changes in weight, skin integrity, and general healing ability are explored during the interview or health history. Individuals may also report decreased tolerances for hot or cold weather.

Health Perspectives for Emerging Majority Groups in the United States

	TRADITIONAL DEFINITIONS		TRADITIONAL METHODS	
GROUP	HEALTH	ILLNESS	MAINTAIN/ PROTECT HEALTH	RESTORE HEALTH
American Indian and Alaska Native population	Total harmony with nature; Survive extremely challenging situations	Price paid for past/future; Details specific to nations; Results from presence of evil spirits; Contagious/generalized symptoms; Human body considered as whole, with harmony between origins and superficial structures; Integration within context of environment	Maintain positive relationship with nature; Treat body with respect; Purification acts using water/herbal remedies and rituals	Removal of external causative factor by traditional healer after special ceremony to determine cause; Drumming
Asian population	Total physical and spiritual harmony with universe; For majority religious traditions pose variations on cultural values; Examples: respect for life moderation; basic relationships: balance between evil and good	Human body considered as whole with harmony between organs and superficial structures; Integration of human body within context of environment; Imbalance of yin and yang	Body is gift from parents/ancestors; must be protected; Dietary practices; Formal daily exercise (tai chi); Amulets (Chinese)	Acupuncture applying poultices; Cupping; Bleeding; Massage; Herbal remedies; Other products; Use physicians; Women treat women; Use of immunizations; Important to keep body intact (Chinese); Amulets
African population	Process/energy force rather than a state; Consists of body/mind/spirit harmony with nature; Older adults held in high esteem	Harmony; illness attributed to demons and evil spirits; Pain as sign of illness; If no pain then illness is gone	Dietary practices; Rest; clean environment; Laxatives/cod liver oil taken internally; sulfur and molasses on back; Protective material of various substances (copper/silver/dried flesh); prayer	Voodoo and magic; Care for the entire community; Prayer; Use of healers; Pictures-Catholic saints/relics; Sugar and turpentine herbs, minerals, oral preparations including hot water and lemon garlic, flannel with camphorated oil
Hispanic population	Gift from God	Imbalance in body; punishment for wrongdoing; Imbalance between hot and cold/wet and dry (definitions vary); Dislocation of body parts; Magic or supernatural causes such as evil	Maintain equilibrium in universe through behavior, diet, and work	Prayer, dietary practices of hot/cold magic/religious rituals, artifacts; Frequently in Catholic and Pentecostal traditions such as offerings, confession, candles, laying of hands; Folk holistic healers using herbs, prayer, massage, social rapport, spiritual
Middle Eastern population	Holistic nature; Full-bodied person is considered healthier than one who is thin; Fatalistic acceptance: whatever happens is in accordance with God's plan	Goal to meet physical and spiritual needs; Myths and supernatural beliefs about illness as punishment; Traditional thoughts about causes of illness: exposure to cold/dampness, sudden fear, emotional upset/carelessness; associated with bad luck, poverty; Health is traditionally associated with good luck/wealth	Causes: supernatural (God or the devil), social (mal de ojo, the "evil eye"); Natural (cold or dirty environment); hereditary; Practices preventing ill health for newborns (father's role; placenta/umbilical cord disposal); medicine, food taboos	Authority of health provider is not generally questioned; Modesty, prayers, fasting, family involvement; Islam: religion followed by all Muslims, regardless of their country of origin; May wear religious charms to encourage God's protection; God is considered healer and afflictor

From Wilson, S. H., & Dorne, R. (2005). Impact of culture on the education of the geriatric patient. *Topics in Geriatric Rehabilitation, 21*(4), 282-294; Andrews, M. M., & Boyle, J. S. (2011). *Transcultural concepts in nursing care* (6th ed.). New York: Lippincott; Gallant, M., Spitze, G., & Grove, J. (2010). Chronic illness self-care and the family lives of older adults: A synthetic review across four ethnic groups. *Journal of Cross-Cultural Gerontology, 25*(1), 21-43.

Nurses' observations and perceptions play a vital role when assessing nutritional and metabolic patterns. Physical examination allows assessment of both nutrient supply to the tissues and metabolic needs of the individual. Objective findings serve as indicators to validate subjective reports concerning nutrient intake. Gross metabolic indicators include temperature, height, and weight. Physical examination focuses on skin, bony prominences, dentition, hair, and mucous membranes. Skin and mucous membranes, in particular, use nutrients rapidly and provide excellent indices of nutritional adequacy. Skin assessment includes color, temperature, turgor, and evaluation of any skin lesions, areas of dryness, scaliness, rashes, pruritus, or edema. Mucous membranes are examined for color, integrity, moisture, and lesions. Dentition is evaluated for structure. Are teeth erupted at normal stages of development? Are teeth firmly implanted? Do dentures fit properly? Additionally, decay and evidence of oral hygiene are evaluated. Healing is assessed when there is evidence of injury. The assessment also may include laboratory information such as levels of fasting glucose, lipids, blood urea nitrogen, creatinine, calcium, and vitamin D.

Although problem identification occurs after assessment of all 11 functional health patterns, a problem in any 1 area serves as a clue to dysfunction in others. Assessment of one pattern facilitates synthesis and analysis of data collected in other functional health patterns. Nutrition and metabolism influence patterns of health management, elimination, activity, sleep, cognition, roles, and stress tolerance. The values-beliefs pattern may significantly alter all other functional patterns. Sociocultural values and ethnic backgrounds play a major role in the determination of eating patterns. Other areas to consider include eating habits, food preferences, and patterns of nutrient supply and demand across the life span. Raw fruits and vegetables may be fun "finger food" for the toddler, but the older adult, especially one with loose dentures or arthritis of the temporomandibular joint, may find these foods intolerable. Older adults may also find gastrointestinal intolerances that develop over time and were not present in their youth.

A nutritional pattern focus emphasizes educational needs. Assessment aims to demonstrate strengths in functional patterns along with disclosing dysfunctional or potentially dysfunctional patterns. Nutritional health-promotion activities present a strength that provides impetus for similar activities in the other patterns. For example, if balanced nutritional intake improves functional level, individuals may extend their health-promoting behaviors to stress reduction or other behaviors. Understanding food/fluid intake and balance of body requirements helps individuals adjust caloric intake as growth slows in order to prevent overweight problems during the adult years.

Elimination Pattern

Elimination patterns include bowel, bladder, and skin function. Nurses determine regularity, quality, and quantity of stool and urine through subjective reports about methods used to achieve regularity or control and any pattern changes or perceived problems. Perspiration quantity and quality determine excretory skin function (Gordon, 2011).

Elimination pattern significance varies from individual to individual. Many people view elimination patterns as a measure of health and as a sensitive indicator of proper nutrition and stress level. Individuals' perceptions determine whether patterns become problematic or dysfunctional. Assessment concerns usual patterns. Misconceptions about regularity exist, particularly of bowel function, and self-treatment commonly occurs to correct perceived problems.

Elimination pattern dysfunction affects interpersonal interactions (Heath, 2009; Saunjoo et al., 2011). Lack of control affects body image (self-perception), activity level, socialization, and sleep patterns. Age, developmental levels, and cultural considerations direct the interview. Pediatric assessment includes toilet training methods, whereas adult assessment may focus on regularity and patterns of dysfunction (Heath, 2009; Hockenberry & Wilson, 2010; Kyle, 2011; Rogers, 2011). In addition to constipation, older adults may begin to develop urinary control problems (Heath, 2009; Kyle, 2011). Women past childbearing years often develop urinary stress incontinence (Busuttil-Leaver, 2011).

Assessment includes data about regularity and control of excreta (Gordon, 2011). Nurses investigate cues suggesting constipation patterns, diarrhea, or incontinence through focused assessment. Elimination pattern changes, pain, discomfort, and perceived problems receive attention. Data collection includes exploration into the individual's explanation of the problem, methods of self-treatment, and perceived results (Gordon, 2011).

Quantity, quality (color, odor, and consistency), frequency, and regularity of stool, urine, and perspiration determine the direction of further exploration. Nurses assess excretory mode, time patterns, and control. Nurses encourage discussion about pattern changes, perceived problems, and elimination habits. Examination includes gross screening of specimens, noting amount, consistency, color, and odor. Skin assessment includes careful observation and description of wound/fistula drainage.

Transition from nutrition to elimination pattern assessment can occur seamlessly. Fluid intake affects elimination. Dietary fiber affects bowel elimination patterns. Skin integrity heralds concerns about urinary incontinence, leading to additional discussion of elimination patterns. Direct questions about laxatives may be necessary because of the availability of over-the-counter treatments for constipation. Discrepancies between dietary intake and reported bowel regularity indicate the need for further questioning. Laxative dependency in the form of oral supplements, suppositories, or enemas may indicate knowledge deficits in the area of bowel elimination (Heath, 2009; Kyle, 2011). Health education about normal bowel function, nutritional guidelines to assist the individual in elimination, or implementation of an exercise program may significantly improve elimination pattern dysfunction. Urinary frequency requires health education as well. Research indicates that prolonged time between urinations is linked to urinary tract infections (Busuttil-Leaver, 2011; Heath, 2009). Evidence-based practice guides the nurse in establishing a more suitable elimination routine for the individual.

Activity-Exercise Pattern

The activity-exercise pattern centers on activity level, exercise program, and leisure activities. Parameters include movement capability, activity tolerance, self-care abilities, use of assistive devices, changes in pattern, satisfaction with activity and exercise patterns, and any perceived problems (Gordon, 2011). Limitations in movement capabilities or ability to perform activities of daily living significantly alter lifestyle and may affect every other functional health pattern. Movement and independent functioning in self-care are almost universally valued. Child-rearing practices demonstrate this value: parents boast about their infant who walks early, their toilet- trained toddler, and their preschooler who dresses without assistance.

Activity-exercise patterns provide effective indicators for commitment to health promotion and prevention (Figure 6-1). Exercise's impact on health status has been extensively documented with increased public awareness. Overweight and obesity, linked to sedentary lifestyle, has reached an epidemic state worldwide. More than 1 billion adults are overweight with one third of these designated as obese (World Health Organization, 2012). This problem extends from developing countries with undernourished populations to industrialized societies. Obesity prevalence has tripled since 1980 in many parts of the world including the United States, Europe, the Middle Eastern countries, Pacific Islands, Australia, Asia, and China (World Health Organization, 2012). Obesity is currently second only to cigarette smoking in mortality from preventable disease in both the United States and Australia (Dhaliwal & Welborn, 2009). Assessment and planning to prevent obesity has a major impact on global health and health promotion in the United States.

Activity-exercise patterns also indicate energy expenditure and activity tolerance levels. Movement directly affects activities of daily living along with control of the immediate environment. Environment contributes to mobility as well. For example, individuals living alone in high-crime areas may limit activity for fear of harm. Factors such as inclement weather, distance from public transportation, and negotiating stairways with a cane can also influence decisions about activity (Hutch et al., 2011). Environmental barriers significantly impair exercise activity patterns for individuals with neuromuscular or perceptual disturbances. Moreover, leisure activities provide clues to individuals' value systems (Boldt et al., 2010). For example, American work ethic, competitiveness, stage in career, and age influence how individuals perceive leisure and recreational activities.

The objective of assessment within the activity-exercise pattern is to determine the pattern of activities that require energy expenditure. Components reviewed are exercise, activity, leisure, and recreation (Gordon, 2011). The nurse seeks clues to discover strengths and weaknesses within the pattern. Decreased energy levels, perceived problems, coping strategies, changes within the patterns, and associated explanations for these changes are all important clues that require further exploration. Generally, individuals with respiratory or cardiac disease warrant in-depth assessment, and focused assessment is indicated for individuals with neuromuscular, perceptual, or circulatory impairments.

Dimensions to be described and assessed within the activity-exercise pattern include daily activities, leisure activities, and exercise. Daily activities include occupation (position, hours of work or school, and amount of physical exercise versus cognitive or sedentary activities); self-care abilities (feeding, bathing, grooming, dressing, and toileting); and home-management routines (cooking, cleaning, shopping, laundry, and outdoor activities) (Gordon, 2011). Problems within any of these areas require explanation. Is it a problem of energy expenditure, mobility limitations, or decreased motivation caused by depression, grieving, or incongruent values?

Exercise parameters include type, frequency, duration, and intensity of the individual's regular exercise. Nurses also assess the value the individual places on exercise as a part of determining their feelings about it. A 24-hour recall of the previous day's activities provides an initial picture of the pattern whereas each major component addresses specific elements. Weekly logs provide follow-up assessment for suspected problems (Gordon, 2011). In addition to weekly logs, focused assessments include details about modes of transportation. Is a car used for transportation? If public transportation is used, how far away is the route? Are elevators or stairs used more often? Factors interfering with exercise or mobility include dyspnea, fatigue, muscle cramping, neuromuscular or perceptual deficits, chest pain, and angina. As with other patterns, feelings of satisfaction and

FIGURE 6-1 (A, B) Activity-exercise patterns provide effective indicators for commitment to health promotion and prevention. **(B,** From iStockphoto/Thinkstock.)

perception of problems provide valuable indications of dysfunctional or potentially dysfunctional patterns.

Nurses evaluate subjective complaints, such as dyspnea, noting difficulty with breathing during the interview and physical examination. Examination includes circulatory, respiratory, and neuromuscular indicators. Assessment also includes skin color, skin temperature, apical heart rate, radial heart rate, and blood pressure, as well as respiratory rate, rhythm, depth of inspiration, and effort involved. Gait, posture, and balance are evaluated during ambulation. Muscle tone, strength, coordination, and range of motion provide useful clues to validate reports of activity and exercise. Assistive devices or prostheses are evaluated for proper use, proper fit, and degree of assistance or support provided (Osborn et al., 2010).

Information obtained during the interview is linked closely to the examination. Examination alone may not disclose the invaluable subjective reports of early morning pain and joint stiffness. When appropriate, the nurse may ask the individual to climb stairs or perform self-care activities under observation to assess impairment. Direct observation validates assessment findings. Various instruments have been designed to quantify level of ability or disability. For some individuals, a metabolic activity index, in which each activity is measured according to kilocalories of energy expended per minute, helps to quantify assessment results and plan care.

Developmental norms have been established for infants and toddlers. Milestones such as sitting, crawling, walking, running, and hopping determine a child's development (Hockenberry & Wilson, 2010). Careful assessment of ability, limitations, and interests helps to guide the nurse in a more holistic assessment. Problem identification is reserved for the conclusion of the assessment after all 11 patterns have been constructed. Useful clues within a pattern lead into other pattern areas; however, premature closure of a topic during the exam is avoided. At this point, only tentative diagnoses are possible. Often explanations of problems lie in other functional health patterns. For example, when the individual expresses an inability to perform exercise on a routine basis, barriers may be discovered in another pattern. Barriers may be associated with knowledge deficit, personal or family value system, overriding priorities, or low value placed on exercise. Is the inability to perform activities a result of general fatigue caused by inadequate or decreased sleep time associated with anxiety, nocturia, pain, or an infant waking every 3 hours for feeding? Are responsibilities associated with caring for several preschoolers and inadequate financial resources to secure a babysitter the cause? The assessment's purpose is to narrow the number of possible explanations.

Sleep-Rest Pattern

Perhaps the single most important factor assessed in the sleep-rest pattern is the perception of adequacy of sleep and relaxation. Subjective reports of fatigue or energy levels provide some indication of the individual's satisfaction. People make assumptions about the roles that sleep and rest play in preparing the individual for required or desired daily activities. This pattern becomes extremely important when sleep and rest are perceived as insufficient. Sleep serves a restorative function in most individuals. Sleep deprivation studies provide vivid demonstrations of the need for different types of sleep: light, deep, dream, and rapid eye movement sleep. Again, problems within this pattern may cause problems in other patterns. A person who has difficulty with sleep may be tense and irritable, unable to tolerate stress, more prone to infectious processes, and incapable of making health-promoting relationships. Appetite alterations, elimination difficulties, and activity intolerance will likely be experienced (Osborn et al., 2010). Some degree of cognitive dysfunction generally occurs.

The objective when assessing the sleep-rest pattern is to describe the effectiveness of the pattern from the individual's perspective (Coren, 2009; Gordon, 2011). Wide variation in sleep time (from 4 hours to more than 10 hours) does not necessarily affect functional performance; different individuals require different amounts of sleep. Pertinent information includes data suggestive of difficulties with sleep onset, sleep interruptions, and awakening. The nurse also evaluates disturbances such as dreaming and nightmares, sleepwalking, nocturnal enuresis, and penile tumescence. Counseling, institution of safety measures, or medical referral may be necessary. In addition to sleep, the nurse assesses rest and relaxation according to the individual's perceptions. Activities of the sedentary isolate type, such as reading or crocheting, may be relaxing for some individuals. Passive involvement, as with television viewing, may provide the only source of relaxation for the individual. Daily naps or relaxation exercises (meditation, yoga, or breathing exercises) may also be a part of this pattern.

Assessment parameters of the sleep dimension are divided into two parts: sleep quality and sleep quantity. Sleep quality includes the individual's perception of sleep adequacy, performance level, and physical and psychological state on awakening. Sleep quantity, in addition to focusing on the hours slept each day, is used to build a schedule of sleep times. The nurse assesses for regularity of the time of retiring, time of awakening, and additional periods of sleep throughout the day. Sleep onset, the number of awakenings, and reasons for awakening provide clues to problems. The dimensions of rest and relaxation include the parameters of type, frequency or regularity, and duration. The perceived effectiveness of methods used to promote rest is also assessed.

When problems exist, focused assessment that evaluates efficiency of sleep compared with actual sleeping time is warranted. Individuals are conditioned to sleep under certain circumstances, and maintaining bedtime rituals is a distinct advantage in sleep promotion. A person who expects to sleep usually will sleep if such routines are maintained. Nurses assess schedule and routine changes associated with bedtime. When assessing bedtime routines, rituals along with other aids to sleep, such as natural aids (warm milk) or medications (prescription and nonprescription), should be explored. Physical examination includes general appearance, behavior, and performance changes. As with pain, sleep is a subjective experience. Comprehensive examination may be performed (for example, with polysomnography), but discussion of this is beyond the scope of this text. Research indicates that subjective reporting of sleep quality and measures of sleep time closely approximate electroencephalographic findings.

Nursing care focuses on the need to identify evidence of sleep disturbances to design appropriate interventions before sleep deprivation occurs. Frequent awakenings do not necessarily imply sleep interruption. Many individuals awaken numerous times during the night but return to sleep within seconds. These awakenings occur in older adults who generally spend most of the night in stages of light sleep. The normal developmental pattern of aging does not include deep sleep; therefore, awakenings may not affect the sleep cycles. Older individuals, however, more often experience difficulty returning to sleep because they experience discomfort or anxiety. Biological rhythm and peak performance time may be helpful to the nurse when planning health education and return visits. Individuals commonly refer to themselves as morning people or night owls; therefore, patterns of retiring and arising provide clues. Patterns of sleep and rest in conjunction with subjective reports of physical and mental well-being help determine appropriate interventions.

Cognitive-Perceptual Pattern

Cognitive patterns include the ability of the individual to understand and follow directions, retain information, make decisions, solve problems, and use language appropriately. Auditory, visual, olfactory, gustatory, tactile, and kinesthetic sensations and perceptions determine perceptual and sensory patterns. Pain perception and tolerance are analyzed within this pattern area (Gordon, 2011). Capacity for independent functioning is considered a major role of thinking and perceiving. Compensation for cognitive-perceptual difficulties ensures safety. Health requires a balance between individual and environment. Decreased levels of cognition or perception require increased levels of environmental control. For example, mentally or sensory-impaired individuals may require sheltered work environments and supervised group living arrangements.

Interrelationships among the individual, the developmental stage, and the environment contribute to several patterns. For example, the behavior patterns of a 20-year-old high school "dropout" who works in a factory may differ from those of a 20-year-old second-year premedical student. Developmental stage plays a role in cognitive and perceptual abilities as well. Vision and hearing achieve full potential when children reach school age, with 20/30 vision considered normal in preschoolers. Developmental stage determines the ability to problem solve and conceptualize as described by the theorist Piaget (Hockenberry & Wilson, 2010). As adults mature, visual acuity, hearing, touch, and even taste decline. Cognitive function must be evaluated within the context of the environment (Gordon, 2011). Environmental complexity results in different levels of functioning.

Assessing cognitive-perceptual patterns includes evaluating language capabilities, cognitive skills, and perception related to desired or required activities (Gordon, 2011). Nurses address clues indicating potential problems, particularly sensory deficits, sensory deprivation or overload, and ineffective pain management. Cognitive dysfunction may cause impaired reasoning, judgment, or knowledge deficits related to health practices, as well as memory deficits.

Assessment parameters include hearing and vision test results. Changes in sensation or perception should be noted. In addition to decreased ability or acuity in hearing, vision, smell, and taste, evaluation includes other perceptual disturbances, such as vertigo; increased or decreased sensitivity to heat, cold, or light touch; and visual or auditory hallucinations or illusions. Use and perceived effectiveness of assistive devices, such as hearing aids, eyeglasses, and contact lenses, is also noted.

Discomfort and pain are evaluated further. Useful tools that use pain scales have been designed to record and quantify changes in pain perception (Liu et al., 2010). Location, type, degree, and duration of pain provide indicators of possible causes or sources. Relief measures used to control pain and their effectiveness provide data and a focus for health education. Medication, heat or cold applications, and relaxation are examples of relief measures that should be explored for their usefulness in a plan of care (Hsu et al., 2010; Smith & Grimmer-Somers, 2010). For all individuals, exploring tolerance to pain is appropriate, using questions such as "Do you feel you are particularly sensitive to pain?" and "What level of pain is associated with your (cut, sprain, broken bone, or labor contractions)?"

Other areas of cognitive patterning to be explored include educational level, recent memory changes, ease or difficulty in learning, and preferred method of learning. Even when no problems are apparent or suspected, the nurse may assess these areas in more detail to determine areas of strength for use with health teaching plans.

Objective data are accumulated throughout the interview or assessment process. This data collection begins with the nurse's perception of the individual's general appearance: hygiene and grooming, proper use of clothing, neatness and appropriateness of dress, and indication that these are appropriate to the individual's developmental stage. Language and vocabulary use, the ability to convey an idea with words or with actions when speech is impaired or not yet developed, and grammatical correctness provide clues to cognitive functioning. Amplitude and quality of speech, affect and mood, as well as attention and concentration are all indicative of the individual's mental status. For many individuals, this information is sufficient to relay a sense of the level of understanding, memory, and mentation. Problem-solving abilities usually can be determined when the individual is asked to relate any perceived problems, provide an explanation of the problems and/or actions taken to solve the problems, and describe results of the actions taken. Because this is a basic assessment in each functional health pattern, the nurse already has an idea of whether thought processes are logical, coherent, and relevant for this individual.

When problems within the cognitive realm do not surface, the information is recorded as part of the objective data or findings of the physical examination. Data to be noted include language; vocabulary; attention span; grasp of ideas; level of consciousness; orientation to person, place, and time; language spoken (whether primary or secondary); and behavior during the data collection process, including posture, facial expression, and general body movements.

When a problem is apparent or suspected based on age, hereditary factors, or inconsistencies in the assessment data, a focused assessment is essential. Coma scales or functional dementia scales may be appropriate. More commonly, a Folstein Mini-Mental Status Examination (MMSE) is performed to assess orientation, attention, calculation, language (ability to name objects, repeat abstract ideas, and follow commands), and recall (immediate, short-term, and long-term memory). Abilities to read, write, and copy designs can also be assessed (see Chapter 24: Older Adult). The examination of a sensory-perceptual pattern evaluates hearing, vision, and areas of pain at a screening level; comprehensive examinations are available and may be indicated. A full neurological assessment is warranted when specific sensory deficits are identified during the examination.

Although completing these assessment areas may seem overwhelming, the time required is generally less than that in most other pattern areas, perhaps because more information relevant to the cognitive-perceptual patterns becomes available as each pattern is assessed. Transition into the cognitive-perceptual pattern from other patterns may be facilitated by referring to a problem already described, with a question such as "Do you generally find it easy to solve problems effectively?" The self-perception pattern follows the cognitive pattern particularly well, because mental status measures include feelings and perceptions of the individual regarding self. Mood, affect, and responses to the interviewer, such as eye contact, are indications of self-esteem. Cognitive-perceptual ability greatly influences the ability to function (self-care) or manipulate within the environment (activity and exercise).

The placement of each of the patterns in a sequence suitable to each nurse, individual, or situation has been discussed. When the cognitive-perceptual pattern is dysfunctional, however, the individual is most likely unreliable as the historian; therefore, it is wise to consider this pattern early in the assessment process. Approaching this pattern early saves valuable time and permits the identification of patterns that can be assessed more reliably.

Every person has experienced temporary memory lapses at one time or another. These events alone are not a sufficient basis for judgments. Sequencing of behaviors and clustering of appropriate signals (defining characteristics) are necessary to determine any nursing diagnosis. Equally important is the need to assess all pattern areas before data analysis and problem identification.

Cognitive and sensory ability data guide the nurse in planning care, which is especially apparent in health teaching. Formulation of health teaching plans ideally reflects each individual's preferred method of learning. The effective plan considers the individual's demonstrated developmental level; the ability to store information, retrieve information, and compensate for deficits; and also the neuromuscular and sensory levels necessary for skills development. An individually tailored plan contains mutually developed goals and short-term objectives. Although self-care might be an outcome for any person newly diagnosed with diabetes mellitus, behaviors expected of an adult with diabetes will differ from those expected of a child.

Self-Perception–Self-Concept Pattern

The self-perception–self-concept pattern encompasses the sense of each individual's personal identity, goals, emotional patterns, and feelings about the self. Self-image and sense of worth stem from the individual's perception of personal appearance, competencies, and limitations, including the individual's self-perception and others' perceptions. The nurse assesses physical, verbal, and nonverbal cues (Gordon, 2011).

The significance of the sense of self to the whole person is best exemplified by personal experiences. Individuals who feel good about themselves look and act differently from those who feel unable to accomplish anything worthwhile. Patterns of eating, sleeping, and activity usually change if self-concept changes.

The individual's developmental level affects and is affected by this pattern. One of the tasks identified during the later phases of Erikson's developmental framework, described previously, is building wholesome attitudes toward oneself (self-esteem). Delays in self-esteem and self-concept development affect progress toward subsequent tasks (Hockenberry & Wilson, 2010) (Table 6-3).

Family climate and relationship patterns provide the environmental impact that influences the self-concept pattern (see Chapter 7). People who are closely associated with the individual affect that person's self-esteem. Most people care about what others think of them; therefore, the support of significant others affects the self-perception–self-concept pattern (Kutob et al., 2010; McMahon et al., 2011) (Figure 6-2).

Achieving a sense of "I" versus "we" is vital for the individual. A sense of "I" as a person, apart from the roles that the person may assume, is important. For example, the sense of "me" rather than roles such as mother, father, daughter, son, student, or nurse helps to establish self-perception (Hockenberry & Wilson, 2010).

The assessment objective in this pattern area is to describe each individual's patterns and beliefs about general self-worth and feeling states (Gordon, 2011). The nurse looks for clues that indicate identity confusion, altered body image, disturbances in self-esteem, and feelings of powerlessness. Anxiety, fear, and depression states can be identified and are responsive to nursing interventions (Harvey et al., 2012; Iloabachie et al., 2011; Porter et al., 2011; Samad et al., 2011; Surkan et al., 2012).

Erikson's framework describes sequential and healthy developmental patterns for each individual. Accomplishment of the wellness tasks may be apparent in other functional health patterns as well, providing additional indications of developmental level (see Unit 4) (Hockenberry & Wilson, 2010). Feelings about self contribute additional information for this pattern. Knowledge of individual strengths and limitations along with attitudes toward these strengths and limitations becomes important data when planning care (Rawana, 2009). To elicit this kind of information, questions are asked regarding personal appearance and capabilities in the cognitive, affective, and psychomotor domains. This portrayal provides evidence of a sense of identity and worth, self-image, and body image. A description of emotional patterns or a general feeling state concludes the history when no problems are indicated. A focused assessment may use specific tools, when necessary, to measure body image (Petti & Cowell, 2011).

The nurse notes general appearance and affect of each individual, which may have been assessed as part of a formal mental status examination. Low self-esteem may be indicated by

TABLE 6-3 RELATIONSHIP BETWEEN SELECTED DEVELOPMENTAL TASKS AND WELLNESS TASKS FOR EACH STAGE OF THE LIFE CYCLE

ERIKSON'S EIGHT LIFE STAGES	HAVIGHURST'S DEVELOPMENTAL TASKS	EXAMPLES OF MINIMAL WELLNESS TASKS FOR EACH DEVELOPMENTAL STAGE
1. Infancy (trust vs. basic mistrust)	Learning to walk Learning to take solid foods Learning to talk Learning to control elimination of body waste	Acquiring ability to perform psychomotor skills Learning functional definition of health Learning social and emotional responsiveness to others and to physical environment
2. Early childhood (autonomy vs. shame and doubt)	Learning gender difference and sexual modesty Achieving physiological stability Forming simple concepts of social-physical reality Learning to relate emotionally to parents, siblings, and others Learning to distinguish right from wrong and developing a conscience Learning physical skills necessary for ordinary games	Learning about proper foods, exercise, and sleep Learning dental hygiene Learning injury prevention (safety belts and helmets, sunscreen, smoke detectors, poisons, firearms, and swimming) Refining psychomotor and cognitive skills
3. Late childhood (initiative vs. guilt)	Building wholesome attitudes toward self as a growing organism Learning to get along with peers	Developing self-concept Learning attitudes of competition and cooperation with others Learning social, ethical, and moral differences and responsibilities
4. Early adolescence (industry vs. inferiority)	Learning appropriate gender identity: masculine or feminine role Developing fundamental skills in reading, writing, and calculating Developing concepts necessary for everyday living Developing conscience, morality, and scale of values Achieving personal independence Developing attitudes toward social groups and institutions	Learning that health is an important value Learning self-regulation of physiological needs—sleep, rest, food, drink, and exercise Learning risk taking and its consequences (injury prevention)
5. Adolescence (identity vs. role confusion)	Achieving new and more mature relations with peers and both genders Achieving gender identity Accepting physique and using body effectively Achieving emotional independence of parents and other adults Achieving assurance of economic independence Selecting and preparing for occupation Preparing for marriage and family life Developing intellectual skills and concepts necessary for civic competence Desiring and achieving socially responsible behavior	Learning economic responsibility Learning social responsibility for self and others (preventing pregnancy and sexually transmitted diseases) Experiencing social, emotional, and ethical commitments to others Accepting self and physical development Reconciling discrepancies between personal health concepts and observed health behaviors of others (use of alcohol, drugs, tobacco, firearms, and violence) Learning to cope with life events and problems (suicide prevention) Considering life goals and career plans and acquiring necessary skills to reach goals Learning importance of time to self and world
6. Early adulthood (intimacy vs. isolation)	Selecting and learning to live with a mate Starting a family; managing a home Taking on civic responsibility	Committing to mate and family responsibilities Selecting a career Incorporating health habits into lifestyle
7. Middle adulthood (generativity vs. stagnation)	Accepting and adjusting to physiological changes Achieving adult social responsibility Maintaining economic standard of living Assisting adolescent children	Accepting aging of self and others Coping with societal pressures Recognizing importance of good health habits Reassessing life goals periodically
8. Maturity (ego integrity vs. despair)	Adjusting to decreasing physical strength and health Adjusting to retirement and reduced income Adjusting to death of spouse Establishing an explicit affiliation with own age group Establishing satisfactory physical living arrangements	Becoming aware of risks to health and adjusting lifestyle and habits to cope with risks Adjusting to loss of job, income, and family and friends through death Redefining self-concept Adjusting to changes in personal time and new physical environment Adjusting previous health habits to current physical and mental capabilities

Modified from Hockenberry, M. J., & Wilson, D. (2010). *Wong's nursing care of infants and children* (9th ed.). St. Louis: Mosby; Osborn, K. S., Wraa, C. E., & Watson, A. B. (2010). *Medical surgical nursing: Preparation for practice.* New York: Pearson; U.S. Department of Health and Human Services, and Centers for Disease Control and Prevention. (2012). *The guide to community preventive services: What works to promote health.* Retrieved February 5, 2012, from www.thecommunityguide.org/index.html.

FIGURE 6-2 Most people care about what others think of them; therefore, the support of significant others, like a teacher to a student, affects their self-perception–self-concept pattern.

head and shoulder flexion, lack of eye contact, and mumbled or slurred speech. Anxiety or nervousness might be revealed through extraneous body movements such as foot shuffling or tapping, facial tension or grimace, rapid speech, voice quivering, twitches or tremors, and general restlessness or shifts in body position. Any of these indicators demands further exploration to determine underlying problems for each individual.

Self-concept influences each individual's interaction with others, including the nurse. Because the information in this pattern is personal, sharing the information may actually facilitate the process of goal setting and intervention planning when the nurse possesses strong communication skills and a caring attitude.

Roles-Relationships Pattern

The roles-relationships pattern describes the position assumed and the associations engaged in by the individual that are connected to that position. The individual's perception is a major component of the assessment, and exploration of the pattern includes each individual's level of satisfaction with roles and relationships.

The need for relationships with other people is universal. Dossey and colleagues (2012) have identified basic needs for communication, fellowship, and love in high-level wellness. The ability to communicate with other people in a meaningful way greatly affects the whole person. The concept of health as the harmonious balance between the individual and the environment indicates the major role that relationships with others play in health status (Dossey et al., 2012). The function development plays in health is also apparent (Hockenberry & Wilson, 2010). This series of hypotheses about readiness proposes that attainment of each stage is required to progress to the next stage. For example, a person can become immersed in a relationship of genuine intimacy only after self-identity has stabilized. Certain tasks for family development have been identified similarly by Duvall and Miller (Ward & Hisley, 2009) (see Chapter 7). The emphasis within these models is on the individual's relationships within the nuclear family.

The objective of the roles-relationships pattern assessment is to describe an individual's pattern of family and shared circumstances, with the associated responsibilities. The individual's perception of satisfaction with the established relationship contributes to this assessment. Loss, change, and threat produce the major problems within this pattern. Clues indicative of impaired verbal communication, social isolation, alterations in parenting, independence-dependence conflicts, dysfunctional grieving, and potential for violence are pertinent.

Assessment focuses on family, work, and community roles and relationships. Within the family, assessment parameters include the family structure, tasks performed, social support systems, and other dynamics, such as decision-making, power, authority, division of labor, and communication patterns. Parenting or marital difficulties and family violence issues are explored. The roles of student and employee are explored to determine specific occupation or position, along with work responsibilities and work environment. Parameters such as stress, safety, and health factors should be included (see the Case Study and Care Plan at the end of this chapter). Financial concerns, job security, and retirement plans are elicited. Activity-rest patterns elicit information about time commitments, leisure activities, and physical exercise; therefore, the assessment at this point addresses the impact of these factors on the roles-relationships pattern. Community roles and relationships indicate involvement within the neighborhood and other social groups, such as the level of socialization and the amount of social support available. Within all three components (family, work or school, and community) the individual is asked to describe the level of satisfaction with the roles and relationships.

Threat of change, actual change, and loss are areas to be explored further. In addition, family or work roles alone may not cause stress, but combining them may cause difficulties, as with the working mother or traveling husband and father.

Objective data for assessment within this pattern are usually unavailable unless the nurse makes a home visit or sees the individual in the company of significant others in some other capacity. Family interaction and communication patterns are noted whenever possible. Cognizant of meaningful relationships within the family, the nurse identifies potential problems, such as those that occur with the college student away from home, the individual who travels or moves frequently, and sole family survivors when older adults outlive their family members and friends (Hockenberry & Wilson, 2010; Ward & Hisley, 2009). The relationships among the functional health patterns are clearly apparent in light of the developmental stages. Difficulties within the self-concept pattern and difficulties with relationships often appear together (Curwood et al., 2011). Relationships affect the whole person; therefore, problems in the roles-relationships pattern may be exhibited in other areas such as sleep, appetite, and sexuality.

Sexuality-Reproductive Pattern

The sexuality-reproductive pattern describes the individual's sexual self-concept, sexual functioning, methods of intimacy, and reproductive areas. Data collection combines subjective information, nursing observations, and physical examination.

Normal development and perceived satisfaction combine to provide the elements of this pattern (Gordon, 2011).

Sexuality is the behavioral expression of sexual identity. The importance of this pattern area to the individual's life and health is closely related to the self-perception and the relationships patterns. Body image, self-concept, and role and gender identity are linked to sexual identity. This concept of sexual self and the individual's relationships pattern indicate the level and the perceived satisfaction of sexual functioning. Sexual functioning involves, but is not limited to, sexual relations with a partner. Reproductive patterns are equally significant to this pattern assessment, the whole individual, and the family and community (see Chapters 7 and 8).

As discussed, individual development influences reproductive capacities; these include secondary sex characteristics, genital development, ego integrity, and the family life-cycle stage (Hockenberry & Wilson, 2010; Ward & Hisley, 2009). Environment also plays a part in expression of the sexuality-reproductive pattern. Cultural and family norms may contribute to the expression of sexuality and combine with other factors, such as the family's financial stability, to influence reproductive patterns (Lev, 2010). Norms within society may create issues in expressions of sexuality.

One objective of assessment in this pattern is to describe behavioral problems or difficulties (Gordon, 2011). Equally important is assessing the individual's knowledge of sexual functioning and preventive health practices, such as breast and testicular self-examination, Papanicolaou smears, effective contraceptive use, and avoidance of infection. Clues are evaluated for potential or actual sexual dysfunction.

The following parameters are assessed: sexual self-concept, which may be derived from information collected in the self-perception–self-concept and the roles-relationships patterns; sexual functioning, with the nurse noting evidence of some form of intimacy, the level of sexual activity or libido, and the effect of health or illness on sexual expression; and reproductive patterns, in which the nurse collects data pertinent to health-promotion factors, such as feelings related to aging, preventive practices, and knowledge of sexual functioning. For women, reproductive pattern assessment would also include information about menstruation, such as onset, duration, frequency, date of last menstrual period, discomfort, and menopause, as well as information about reproductive stage, such as pregnancy history and birth control methods.

Level of satisfaction with sexual self-concept, sexual functioning, and reproduction is also explored. Difficulties such as ineffective or inappropriate sexual performance, discharges, infections, venereal disease, discomfort, and history of abuse are evaluated. Focused assessment to collect additional information is warranted with sexual dysfunction or trauma. Physical examination evaluates genital development and secondary sex characteristics. Signs of intimacy between partners, such as holding hands and hugging, are noted.

People may feel threatened by discussion of topics in this pattern; depth of exploration is governed in part by the individual's wishes. Dialogue is encouraged but may be postponed until a firm and trusting relationship is established.

A clear representation of the individual's knowledge and use of preventive practices facilitates planning for health promotion. Although sex education usually is associated with school programs, information and discussion about sexuality is just as important for adults of all ages. Sex education is a key element of parenthood classes. Improved understanding of sexuality and sexual function leads to discovery and increased satisfaction.

Coping-Stress Tolerance Pattern

Gordon (2011) describes the coping-stress tolerance pattern as a depiction of general coping and the individual's ability to effectively manage stress. This pattern includes the individual's ability to process life crises and to resist disruptive factors that will influence self-integrity of ego, mode of conflict resolution, stress management, and accessibility to necessary resources (Box 6-3: Quality and Safety Scenario).

The ability to manage stress effectively in life is a learned behavior. Stress is a necessary part of life; without it there is no motivation to grow. Stress becomes a problem when tolerance is weak and daily activities are affected (Dossey et al., 2012). Most stress comes not from great tragedies, but from an accumulation of minor irritations. Stress is not inherent in the event but in the individual's perception of that event. Whereas one individual may experience stress from missing a bus and can think only of being 10 minutes late, another will consider the same event an opportunity to spend 10 minutes reading the newspaper. This difference in perception may represent the different values used to identify sources of stress or it may represent coping strategies.

For purposes of assessing this pattern, coping, which is considered the individual behavioral response to stress, includes both problem-solving ability and use of defense mechanisms. Coping is viewed not as a single act but as a process incorporating many behaviors. The function of coping is to deal with the threat or emotional distress of an event. Coping effectiveness is assessed from the individual's perspective and from the nurse's observation of the individual's ability to function in the presence of actual or potential stressors in the environment.

The perception of stress and the ability to manage it depend on personal development, amount of stress previously experienced, current level of stress within the environment, and sources of social support. For example, an older adult may experience many stresses during life and manage them effectively, but now coping may no longer be possible because too many stressors are present, such as physical incapacitation, fixed income, fear of illness or injury, and lack of transportation. In addition, this person may no longer have a social support system, which has been associated with promotion of health (Haley, 2011; Muliira & Musil, 2010; Nordin et al., 2010; van Woerden et al., 2011). Determining individuals' stress tolerance and past coping patterns becomes the objective of assessment for this functional pattern. Clues to difficulties in managing past and current stressors and changes in the effectiveness of a coping pattern help to determine personal coping capacity.

The following assessment parameters are included: the coping task, including the physical, psychological, and socioeconomic stimuli with which the individual must cope; coping

BOX 6-3   QUALITY AND SAFETY SCENARIO
Sexuality and Aging Women: Common Myths

- Sexual desire and prowess wane during the climacteric for most women; therefore, menopause is the death of a woman's sexuality.
- Sexual activity is uncommon in older adults, particularly women.
- Older women are not likely to need treatment for sexually transmitted diseases.
- If the older woman is sexually active, sexual activity generally occurs less than once per month.
- Hysterectomy creates a physical disability that causes the inability to function sexually.
- Sex has no role in the lives of older adults except as perversion or remembrance of times past.
- Masturbation is an immature activity of youngsters and adolescents, not of older women.
- Sexual expression is unacceptable among older women.
- Older women are too frail to engage in sex.
- Sex is unimportant to the older woman.

- Older women do not wish to discuss their sexuality with professionals.
- Older adults' sexual expression has recently been greatly enhanced because of the availability of new drugs.
- Medical conditions do not affect sexual expression.
- Assessment Guide. Ask the woman to describe:
  - How she expresses her sexuality
  - Concerns she has about fulfilling her sexual needs
  - How her sexual relationship with her partner has changed with her age
- Use the PLISSIT Model:

P—Obtaining **Permission** from the individual to initiate sexual discussion

LI—Providing the **Limited Information** needed to function sexually

SS—Giving **Specific Suggestions** for the individual to proceed with sexual relations

IT—Providing **Intensive Therapy** surrounding the issues of sexuality for that individual

Updated with information from Hinchliff, S., & Gott, M. (2008). Challenging social myths and stereotypes of women and aging: Heterosexual women talk about sex. *Journal of Women & Aging, 20*(1-2), 65-81; Jeffers, L. A., & DiBartolo, M. C. (2011). Raising health care provider awareness of sexually transmitted disease in patients over age 50. *MEDSURG Nursing, 20*(6), 285-290; Miracle, A. W., & Miracle, T. S. (2009). Chapter 16: Sexuality in late adulthood. In B. R. Bonder, V. Dal Bello-Haas, & M. B. Wagner (Eds.), *Functional performance in older adults* (3rd ed., pp. 409-426). Philadelphia: F.A. Davis; Trudel, G., Villeneuve, L., Preville, M., Boyer, R., & Frechette, V. (2010). Dyadic adjustment, sexuality and psychological distress in older couples. *Sexual & Relationship Therapy, 25*(3), 306-315; Wallace, M. A. (2008). Assessment of sexual health in older adults. *AJN, American Journal of Nursing, 108*(7), 52-60. Try this: Best practices in nursing care to older adults from the Hartford Institute for Geriatric Nursing. (2010). Accessed on February 4, 2012, from http://hartfordign.org/practice/try_this/; Evidence based geriatric topics. (2008). Sexuality issues in aging: Nursing Standard of Practice Protocol. *Sexuality in older adults.* Accessed on February 4, 2012, from http://consultgerirn.org/topics/sexuality_issues_in_aging/want_to_know_more; and Office on Aging. (2012). *Aging and human sexuality resource guide.* Accessed on February 4, 2012, from www.apa.org/pi/aging/resources/guides/sexuality.aspx.

style, or the tendency to use a specific style, such as approach oriented, avoidance oriented, or nonspecific; coping strategies, including specifics; and coping effectiveness. Coping strategy may be divided into information seeking, direct action (fight or flight), inhibition of action, or use of social support. Coping effectiveness is best assessed by eliciting the individual resources and the individual's functional level (Dossey et al., 2012). Individual resources include the variety of coping mechanisms used by the individual, the flexibility of these mechanisms, and the health-promotion value associated with each.

Stress tolerance patterns elicit the amount of stress effectively processed in the past. Use of anticipatory coping is assessed along with whether the individual knows how to cope, but does not (production deficit), or simply does not know how to cope (skill deficit). Other indicators of value within this pattern are discussed under the self-perception–self-concept pattern. Objective data of concern include physical signs of restlessness, irritability, and nervousness, such as increased heart rate and blood pressure and perspiration. Evidence of coping ability and tolerance to stress are found in every other functional health pattern. Stress also affects the other patterns, thereby resulting in health problems such as insomnia, weight loss, and poor concentration (Dossey et al., 2012; Gordon, 2011).

Health can be promoted through early intervention to reduce stress. Coping patterns and stress tolerance in the past may uncover unhealthy behavior, such as smoking and drinking, that needs to be replaced by alternative coping strategies. Stress-reduction workshops would be helpful for most of the

population because the future undoubtedly holds stressful events, some of which may be overwhelming without coping strategies. Box 6-4: Innovative Practice includes information about a unique company that offers stress-management interventions. Dossey and colleagues (2012) offer categories for stress management: social engineering strategies, such as time management or planned change; personality engineering strategies, such as assertiveness training or cognitive rehearsal; and altered states of consciousness, such as meditation or relaxation. Planning based on the assessment of all functional health patterns to help determine a coping pattern should include these kinds of strategies.

Values-Beliefs Pattern

The values-beliefs pattern describes values, including the individual's spiritual values, beliefs, and goals. This pattern also includes perceptions of what is right, what is good, and conflicts that beliefs or values impart. Each of the 11 patterns addresses value systems of individuals, family, and society. Individual beliefs or values develop over time and govern life through personal experiences and family and societal influences (Elder et al., 2010; Epstein et al., 2010; Ho et al., 2010; Hockenberry & Wilson, 2010; Marshall et al., 2010; Schutz et al., 2011). The objective in assessing this pattern is to determine the basis for health-related decisions and actions (Gordon, 2011). Individuals engage in preventive health behavior when a threat to wellness or health status exists. Several other health belief models expand on this concept by including other motivations, such as

BOX 6-4   INNOVATIVE PRACTICE

The Humor Potential, Inc.

The Humor Potential, Inc., is a company that provides resources, products, and seminars for stress management with the use of humor. Company president Loretta LaRoche is an internationally recognized expert on stress management, emphasizing the importance of balancing daily living experiences with humor. The Humor Potential, Inc. offers seminars and lectures to health care professionals, schools, corporations, other organizations, and the general public. The corporation also produces television programs that have been televised nationally in the United States. One television program, *The Joy of Stress,* was nominated for a regional Emmy Award.

Books, prints, audiotapes and videotapes, and other products dealing with humor can be purchased from her website. The collection consists of audiotapes and videotapes that have been developed for corporate meetings and training. An example is *Lighten up!* This is a videotape and action guide that increases productivity by reducing stress. A catalog is available for e-mail, fax, phone, and mail orders.

Contact Information:

The Humor Potential, Inc.
Corporate Offices
50 Court Street
Plymouth, MA 02360
E-mail: www.lorettalaroche.com
Telephone: 800-99-TADAH (800-998-2324)

Based on data from the Humor Potential, Inc. Retrieved February 4, 2012, from www.lorettalaroche.com.

personal values and environmental influences. Clues to conflict within the individual's value system or between the person's value system and that of the family or society are explored.

Dimensions of assessment include the individual's values, beliefs, or goals that guide choices or decisions that are related to health. The nurse collects information while exploring each pattern, while summarizing, clarifying, and securing additional information. Specifically, values and beliefs about self, relationships, and society are appraised. Individuals' beliefs, goals, and purposes of life are reviewed, along with any conflicts, perceived philosophies, and philosophies of the family, culture, and society. Sources of strength, such as a higher being or significant individual practices, are explored, including religious beliefs and preferences. Past goals and expectations are assessed through the individual's satisfaction. The nurse must identify the individual's goals and expectations concerning health, clarifying to help the individual achieve them. To be effective, health-promotion interventions are based on the individual's value system and health beliefs (Dossey et al., 2012). The brevity of this discussion is no indication of the importance that the values-beliefs pattern plays in the assessment of the individual. Individual values play a role in all of the patterns.

INDIVIDUAL HEALTH PROMOTION THROUGH THE NURSING PROCESS

The nursing process—the systematic approach to reduce or eliminate the individual's health problem—is accomplished in several steps, the first being the collection of necessary data. With the individual, the nurse analyzes the data, identifies a nursing diagnosis, projects outcomes, prescribes interventions, and evaluates effectiveness. Reassessment, reordering of priorities, new goal setting, and revising the plan continue as part of the process toward outcome attainment (Carpenito-Moyet, 2010).

Collection and Analysis of Data

Assessment is a systematic technique for learning as much as possible about the individual. The main purpose in collecting data from a new individual is to see whether health problems exist and to identify the individual's health goals. An assessment of an adult based on the functional health patterns is presented in **Website Resource 6A.** Data collection includes biographical data, such as age, gender, and the purpose of the visit. This process is followed by assessment of the previously outlined 11 functional health patterns. Subjective reporting, nursing observations and perceptions, and the physical examination are assessed and recorded. The remaining discussion focuses on nursing diagnosis.

Problem Identification

Although the concept of problem identification has been debated in the past, most nurses now have distinguished *nursing diagnosis* as the problematic label. Diagnosis is a careful examination and analysis of the facts in an attempt to explain something. Nursing diagnosis is the naming of an individual's response to actual or potential health problems or life processes (Carpenito-Moyet, 2010; Gordon, 2011; North American Nursing Diagnosis Association International, 2011). Nursing diagnoses provide the basis for selection of nursing interventions to achieve outcomes for which the nurse is accountable (Gordon, 2011). Leadership from NANDA-I has provided standardization of the descriptions of human responses that nurses manage. The most recent revision of this taxonomy has been approved for clinical testing and has been endorsed by the American Nurses Association (ANA) (North American Nursing Diagnosis Association International, 2011).

Gordon (2011) proposed the accepted format of nursing diagnosis that lists the problem, etiology, and signs and symptoms, or defining characteristics, for each diagnosis accepted for clinical testing. The NANDA-I taxonomy uses a multiaxial framework for nursing diagnoses including diagnostic concept (e.g., parenting); acuity (e.g., altered); unit of care (e.g., individual); developmental stage (e.g., adolescent); potentiality (e.g., at risk for); and descriptor, or creation of the diagnostic statement (North American Nursing Diagnosis Association International, 2011). Box 6-5: Research for Evidence-Based Practice discusses how this nursing classification system compares to a non-nursing system.

In discussions of problems, the meaning of the problem must be clearly defined and identified. The concept as used in this text refers to Gordon's (2011) proposition that a health problem is defined as a dysfunctional pattern and that nursing's major contribution to health care is in preventing and treating these patterns. A pattern is dysfunctional when it represents a deviation from established norms or from the individual's previous condition or goals. (Normative behavior is further discussed in

Unit 4.) A dysfunctional pattern is a problem when it generates therapeutic concern on the part of the individual, others, or the nurse and when it is amenable to nursing therapies.

As patterns are assessed, the nurse proposes several hypotheses regarding functional or dysfunctional labeling. At the completion of the assessment, conclusions must be drawn. The possibility exists that all patterns are functional, that some are functional, and that others are dysfunctional or potentially dysfunctional. Functional refers to wellness and optimal health. Dysfunctional patterns, indicating some health problems, may be present in the absence of disease; that is, nursing care may be needed for health promotion and health maintenance, not health restoration. The case history of Frank Thompson in Chapter 1 effectively illustrates the multiple nursing care needs of an individual who is not ill. In potentially dysfunctional patterns, sufficient evidence exists or enough risk factors are present to indicate that a pattern dysfunction will likely occur if interventions are not made. Early identification of potential problems is possible through systematic data collection and analysis.

Contributing Etiological Factors

To plan care, the nurse must first determine what has caused the actual or potential health problem: its contributing etiological factors. The etiological factors of most dysfunctional patterns lie within another pattern or patterns. Although etiology is never an absolute within human sciences, the projection of outcomes or goals must be based on probable causes. Interventions then focus on mediating or resolving the probable causes. Most often, many factors are involved and problems are said to relate to rather than be a result of these factors. Potential problems are not actual problems but risk states; therefore, they have no specific cause and are identified when risk factors are present. Nursing intervention is directed toward risk reduction through education (classes or brochures) to improve nutrition, prevent accidents, and so forth. Risk estimate theory and potential health problems are developed further in Chapters 7 and 8 and Unit 4 (Box 6-6: Hot Topics).

Diagnostic Variables

The ability to arrive at an accurate diagnosis, even when comprehensive data are unavailable, is governed primarily by the nurse's clinical knowledge. Experience improves the effectiveness when nursing is performed as a scientific process. Nursing requires gathering information, interpreting it based on normative values, organizing and grouping information on the basis of healthy findings, identifying the problem, and then planning appropriate goals and interventions. Difficulties are encountered when there are no available norms, which occurs frequently in the psychosocial assessment components. Using the 11 interdependent functional health patterns helps to solve these difficulties. By focusing on each of these areas, recognizing whether a problem does or does not exist is easier. Any change within the pattern may be a sign of dysfunction or an unhealthy but stabilized behavior. For example, a sign of dysfunction might be a 2-year-old child who is still not walking; developmental growth is a major factor in activity patterns of infants, toddlers, and children.

The use of physiological parameters clearly demonstrates the idea of a stabilized dysfunctional pattern, but equal attention must be given to psychological development. For instance, a 26-year-old man who lives with his mother and gives no indication of independent decision-making should be evaluated. It should be apparent that assessment information primarily comes from the initial contact with the individual and the database, which is generally the case in health-promotion activities. However, in any acute situation or emergency, quick assessment of the major problems is given high priority on a hierarchy-of-needs basis and the full nursing assessment is postponed temporarily. For further understanding of the

---

BOX 6-5 RESEARCH FOR EVIDENCE-BASED PRACTICE

Classification Systems

The conceptual and practical relationships between two nursing diagnosis classification systems were compared for their use in nursing practice—the International Classification of Functioning, Disability and Health (ICF) and the North American Nursing Diagnosis Association International (NANDA-I).

The ICF and NANDA-I are two conceptually driven classification systems. Although ICF describes diagnostic terms, the NANDA-I system includes diagnostic criteria, and related etiologies in addition to the description. The authors conclude that although NANDA-I fulfills needs that are exclusively nursing, the ICF is useful to communicate nursing issues without health professionals using consistent nomenclature. These two systems should be used to enhance transdisciplinary quality of care.

From Boldt, C., Grill, E., Bartholomeyczik, S., Brach, M., Rauch, A., Eriks-Hoogland, I., & Stuckey G. (2010). Combined application of the International Classification of Functioning, Disability and Health and the NANDA-International taxonomy II. *Journal of Advanced Nursing, 66*(8), 1885-1898.

BOX 6-6 HOT TOPICS

Heart Disease in Women

Contrary to what many people think, coronary artery disease (CAD) is the leading cause of death in women in most developed countries. Women may not experience a typical pain pattern of angina and may delay care. In fact, if they do seek care, women may not be treated the same as men. Females may believe that CAD is uncommon in women, which is an idea embedded in both public and professional perceptions. One in three women in the United States has CAD, and postmenopausal rates of CAD are closely aligned to those of men. The vasodilation, antioxidant, and antiproliferation properties of estrogen are thought to protect a woman from cardiovascular disease before menopause. Stress test results may be equivocal in women, resulting in misdiagnoses. There is support for the perspective that women receive different treatment compared to men, and there are gender differences in responses and outcomes to treatment. Based on evidence from the literature, nurses can focus on five areas when educating women: (a) perception, (b) presenting symptoms, (c) prevention, (d) treatment, and (e) quality of life.

From Shirato, S., & Swan, B. A. (2010). Women and cardiovascular disease: An evidentiary review. *MEDSURG Nursing, 19*(5), 282-306; Wenger, N. K., Mischke, J. M., Schroeder, R., Schroeder, K., Collins, P., Grady, D., et al. (2010). Electrocardiograms of menopausal women with coronary heart disease are at increased risk for its occurrence. *American Journal of Cardiology, 106*(11), 1580-1587.

nursing diagnosis, the nurse is referred to books discussing the development of diagnoses, the diagnostic process, and specific details of each accepted diagnosis (Carpenito-Moyet, 2010; Gordon, 2011; North American Nursing Diagnosis Association International, 2011).

Planning the Care

In the nursing process, planning is the proposal of diagnosis-specific treatment to assist the individual toward the goal, or expected outcome, of optimal health. The individual's goals and the determined nursing diagnosis provide the basis for planning. Clear goals and diagnoses are critical to development of an effective plan of care. The nursing process identifies the following purposes of the planning phase: to assign priority to the problems diagnosed; to specify the behavioral outcomes or goals with the individual, including the expected time of achievement; to differentiate individual problems that can be resolved by nursing intervention, those that can be handled by the individual or family member, and those that should be handled with or referred to other members of the health team; to designate specific actions, the frequency of these actions, and the short-term, intermediate-term, and long-term results; and to list the individual's problems (nursing diagnosis) and nursing actions (frequency and expected outcomes, or goals) on the nursing care plan or blueprint for action (Carpenito-Moyet, 2010). This plan provides the direction for individual and nursing activities and is the guide for the evaluation. There are many research studies involving outcomes from which nurses can draw to improve effectiveness of the care they provide.

Implementing the Plan

Implementation is the completion of the actions necessary to fulfill the goals for optimal health; it is the enactment of the nursing care plan to elicit the behaviors described in the proposed individual outcome. The selection of a nursing intervention depends on several factors: the desired individual outcome; the characteristics of the nursing diagnosis; the research base associated with the intervention; the feasibility of implementing the intervention; the acceptability of the intervention to the individual; and the capability of the nurse (Carpenito-Moyet, 2010). A nursing interventions classification is being developed. As discussed in Unit 1, a critical component of effective communication is the accurate interpretation of the individual's information. This feedback process continues throughout all phases of the nursing process; the nurse continues to collect data to modify the plan as needed and does not blindly implement the care plan. As discussed in Unit 3, the most frequently used nursing interventions in health promotion are screening, education, counseling, and crisis intervention. All of these interventions require strong communication abilities from the nurse. Checklists and screening instruments may be used to document nursing assessment and help to ensure transmission of reliable and quality information for patients. Implementation requires transdisciplinary collaboration of the analysis and plan. Computerized data entry, information systems, and electronic medical records may facilitate communication; however, ongoing interaction with other health care providers is essential for collaboration.

Evaluating the Plan

The process of analyzing changes experienced by the individual occurs in the evaluation phase of the nursing process, with the nurse examining the relationships between nursing actions and the individual's goal achievement. Nursing process emphasizes that evaluation is always considered in terms of how the individual responds to the plan of action (Osborn et al., 2010). As discussed, the nursing diagnosis (or health problems) and the goal (or expected outcome) guide the evaluation of the nursing care plan. Many variables influence outcomes: the interventions prescribed by the health care providers, the health care providers themselves, the environment in which the care is received, the individual's motivation and genetic structure, and the individual's significant others. The task for nursing is to define which outcomes are sensitive to nursing care so as to identify the expected and attainable results of nursing care for each individual (North American Nursing Diagnosis Association International, 2011). All of these components of the nursing process are documented by the nurse on the individual's health care record (Osborn et al., 2010).

CASE STUDY

Spiritual Distress: Cindy

Cindy is a single 28-year-old woman. Cindy studies nursing and shares an apartment with two friends. She was having increasing difficulties with her course work and was placed on academic probation. Cindy became concerned about the effect of stress on her ability to finish her studies and on her future career. She grew increasingly nervous and began to ask, "Will I ever be okay?" and "Will I ever be able to finish school and function as a nurse?" Cindy expressed her fear of weakness and feelings of isolation, loneliness, helplessness, and loss of control. These feelings began to find expression in anger related to this major life disruption. She verbalized her anger at God for allowing this to happen to her. Her incapacity deprived her of her normal outlets for expressing and finding support for such concerns. Cindy was unable to participate in the practices of her faith, in which she previously had found strength in facing life's challenges. Her inability to concentrate and her growing feeling of lethargy added to her frustration. Expressing these fears and concerns was difficult for Cindy. The nurse, however, developed a trusting relationship with Cindy, permitting her to express her fears, anxieties, and concerns. Based on the nurse's assessment, the nursing diagnosis of spiritual distress was formulated.

Reflective Questions
1. What differential diagnoses should the nurse consider?
2. Describe other individuals you know who have experienced spiritual distress.

Sources: Carpenito-Moyet, L. J. (2010). *Nursing diagnosis: Application to clinical practice* (13th ed.). Philadelphia: Lippincott Williams & Wilkins; Ackley, B. J., & Ladwig, G. B. (2011). *Nursing diagnosis handbook: An evidence-based guide to planning care* (9th ed.). St. Louis: Elsevier.

CARE PLAN

Spiritual Distress: Cindy

*NURSING DIAGNOSIS: Spiritual Distress related to a threat to well-being, loss of meaningful role, and separation from religious and family ties

Defining Characteristics
- Experiences a disturbance in belief system.
- Demonstrates discouragement or despair.
- Chooses not to practice religious rituals.
- Shows emotional detachment from self and others.
- Expresses concern, anger, resentment, and fear, related to a major life disruption.

Related Factors
- Threat to well-being from change in role as a student and fear of failure
- Loss of meaningful role as a student
- Separation from religious and family ties

Expected Outcomes
- Person will verbalize a greater sense of purpose, meaning, and hope.
- Person will express feelings of anger verbally and will discuss anger with another person.

Interventions
- Take time to be present and available to listen to the individual.
- Convey a nonjudgmental attitude.
- Encourage the individual to verbalize feelings.
- Pray with the individual as indicated.
- Engage the individual in values clarification.
- Encourage the individual to acknowledge feelings of anger and to acknowledge and name any other feelings experienced.
- Reassure the individual that it is acceptable to feel anger toward a supreme being.
- Encourage honest dialogue with a peer whom the individual trusts.
- Offer consultation with an appropriate spiritual advisor.
- Inform the individual of religious resources.

*NANDA Nursing Diagnoses—Definitions and Classification 2012-2014, Herdman T.H. (ED). Copyright © 2012, 1994-2012 NANDA International. Used by arrangement with John Wiley & Sons Limited. In order to make safe and effective judgments using the NANDA-I nursing diagnoses it is essential that nurses refer to the definitions and defining characteristics of the diagnoses listed in this work.
Modified from Carpenito-Moyet, L. J. (2010). *Nursing diagnosis: Application to clinical practice* (13th ed.). Philadelphia: Lippincott Williams & Wilkins.

SUMMARY

Data relevant to the health-promotion activities of the individual focus primarily on the assessment of the current health status so that the nurse can identify problem areas, or areas of dysfunction, within the individual's health and lifestyle pattern. This process is a fundamental first step and precedes all other components of the nursing process. Without a clear picture of the problem, nursing activities are fruitless. Gordon's functional health pattern framework provides guidance for the individual assessment. The focus of each pattern includes the age-developmental influences exerted, cultural and environmental roles played, functional ability displayed, and behavioral patterns specific to each individual. The interaction between internal mechanisms and the environment is assessed through these 11 functional health patterns. When assessing each pattern, the nurse must understand the pattern definition, the significance of the pattern to the whole individual, the developmental influences, the environmental role, the assessment objectives, the assessment parameters and indicators, and the nursing implications. Assessment is essential to all components of the nursing process in health promotion for the individual.

REFERENCES

Andrews, M. M., & Boyle, J. S. (2011). *Transcultural concepts in nursing care* (6th ed.). New York: Lippincott.

Ball, J., & Lewis, M. (2011). "An altogether different approach": Roles of speech-language pathologists in supporting indigenous children's language development. *Canadian Journal of Speech-Language Pathology & Audiology*, 35(2), 144–158.

Berentson-Shaw, J., Scott, K. M., & Jose, P. E. (2009). Do self-efficacy beliefs predict the primiparous labour and birth experience? A longitudinal study. *Journal of Reproductive & Infant Psychology*, 27(4), 357–373.

Black, K., & Lobo, A. (2008). A conceptual review of family resilience factors. *Journal of Family Nursing*, 14(1), 33–55.

Boldt, C., Grill, E., Bartholomeyczik, S., Brach, M., Rauch, A., Eriks-Hoogland, I., & Stuckey, G. (2010). Combined application of the International Classification of Functioning, Disability and Health and the NANDA-International taxonomy II. *Journal of Advanced Nursing*, 66(8), 1885–1898.

Bourke Bearskin, L. (2011). A critical lens on culture in nursing practice. *Nursing Ethics*, 18(4), 548–559.

Brazeau, J. N. (2011). The strengths assessment inventory: Reliability of a new measure of psychosocial strengths for youth. *Journal of Child and Family Studies*, 18(6), 746–753.

Burns, E., Gray, R., & Smith, L. A. (2010). Brief screening questionnaires to identify problem drinking during pregnancy: A systematic review. *Addiction*, 105(4), 601–614.

Busuttil-Leaver, R. (2011). Urinary stress incontinence. *Practice Nurse*, 41(12), 32–38.

Carpenito-Moyet, L. J. (2010). *Nursing diagnosis: Application to clinical practice* (13th ed.). Philadelphia: Lippincott Williams & Wilkins.

Coren, S. (2009). Sleep health and its assessment and management in physical therapy practice: The evidence. *Physiotherapy Theory & Practice*, 25(5-6), 442–452.

Curwood, S. E., DeGeer, I., Hymmen, P., & Lehmann, P. (2011). Using strength-based approaches to explore pretreatment change in men who abuse their partners. *Journal of Interpersonal Violence*, 26(13), 2698–2715.

Dhaliwal, S. S., & Welborn, T. A. (2009). Central obesity and cigarette smoking are key determinants of cardiovascular disease deaths in Australia: A public health perspective. *Preventive Medicine*, 49(2-3), 153–157.

Dossey, B. M., Keegan, L., & Guzzetta, C. E. (2012). *Holistic nursing: A handbook for practice* (6th ed.). Boston, MA: Jones & Bartlett.

Elder, J. P., Arredondo, E. M., Campbell, N., Baquero, B., Duerksen, S., Ayala, G., Crespo, N., et al. (2010). Individual, family, and community environmental correlates of obesity in Latino elementary school children [corrected] [published erratum appears in *Journal of School Health 2010, 80*(3), 159]. *Journal of School Health, 80*(1), 20–30.

Epstein, S., Geniteau, E., Christin, P., Hermouet, P., Mok, E., Fournier, J., & Hankard, R. (2010). Role of a clinical nurse specialist within a paediatric multidisciplinary weight-management programme team. *Journal of Clinical Nursing, 19*(17), 2649–2651.

Flanagan, J., & Jones, D. (2009). High-frequency nursing diagnoses following same-day knee arthroscopy. *International Journal of Nursing Terminologies & Classifications, 20*(2), 89–95.

Gallant, M., Spitze, G., & Grove, J. (2010). Chronic illness self-care and the family lives of older adults: A synthetic review across four ethnic groups. *Journal of Cross-Cultural Gerontology, 25*(1), 21–43.

Gordon, M. (2011). *Manual of nursing diagnosis* (12th ed.). Sudbury, MA: Jones & Bartlett.

Haley, J. M. (2011). Revealing the strengths of Latino parent caregivers using a transcultural strength assessment tool. *Journal of Theory Construction & Testing, 15*(1), 10–16.

Harvey, S. T., Fisher, L. J., & Green, V. M. (2012). Evaluating the clinical efficacy of a primary care-focused, nurse-led, consultation liaison model for perinatal mental health. *International Journal of Mental Health Nursing, 21*(1), 75–81.

Hasnain, M., Connell, K. J., Menon, U., & Tranmer, P. A. (2011). Patient-centered care for Muslim women: Provider and patient perspectives. *Journal of Women's Health, 20*(1), 73–83.

Heath, H. (2009). The nurse's role in helping older people to use the toilet. *Nursing Standard, 24*(2), 43–47.

Herdman, T. H. (2008). Nursing diagnosis: Is it time for a new definition? *International Journal of Nursing Terminologies & Classifications, 19*(1), 2–13.

Ho, A., Berggren, I., & Dahlborg-Lyckhage, E. (2010). Diabetes empowerment related to Pender's Health Promotion Model: A meta-synthesis. *Nursing & Health Sciences, 12*(2), 259–267.

Hockenberry, M. J., & Wilson, D. (2010). *Wong's nursing care of infants and children* (9th ed.). St Louis: Mosby.

Hsu, C., BlueSpruce, J., Sherman, K., & Cherkin, D. (2010). Unanticipated benefits of CAM therapies for back pain: An exploration of patient experiences. *Journal of Alternative & Complementary Medicine, 16*(2), 157–163.

Hutch, D. J., Bouye, K. E., Skillen, E., Lee, C., Whitehead, L., & Rashid, J. R. (2011). Potential strategies to eliminate built environment disparities for disadvantaged and vulnerable communities. *American Journal of Public Health, 101*(4), 587–595.

Iloabachie, C., Wells, C., Goodwin, B., Baldwin, M., Vanderplough-Booth, K., Gladstone, T., Murray, M., et al. (2011). Adolescent and parent experiences with a primary care/Internet-based depression prevention intervention (CATCH-IT). *General Hospital Psychiatry, 33*(6), 543–555.

International Council of Nurses. (2010). *Definition of nursing.* Retrieved January 13, 2012, from www.icn.ch/about-icn/icn-definition-of-nursing/.

Kannan, S., Sparks, A. V., Webster, J. D., Krishnakumar, A., & Lumeng, J. (2010). Healthy eating and harambee: Curriculum development for a culturally-centered bio-medically oriented nutrition education program to reach African American women of childbearing age. *Maternal & Child Health Journal, 14*(4), 535–547.

Klinedinst, N. J., Gebhardt, M. C., Aycock, D. M., Nichols-Larsen, D., Uswatte, G., Wolf, S. L., & Clark, P. C. (2009). Caregiver characteristics predict stroke survivor quality of life at 4 months and 1 year. *Research in Nursing & Health, 32*(6), 592–605.

Kutob, R. M., Senf, J. H., Crago, M., & Shisslak, C. M. (2010). Concurrent and longitudinal predictors of self-esteem in elementary and middle school girls. *Journal of School Health, 80*(5), 240–248.

Kyle, G. (2011). Risk assessment and management tools for constipation. *British Journal of Community Nursing, 16*(5), 224–230.

Lev, A. I. (2010). How queer!—The development of gender identity and sexual orientation in LGBTQ-headed families. *Family Process, 49*(3), 268–290.

Liu, J. Y.W., Briggs, M., & Closs, S. J. (2010). The psychometric qualities of four observational pain tools (OPTs) for the assessment of pain in elderly people with osteoarthritic pain. *Journal of Pain and Symptom Management, 40*(4), 582–598.

Marshall, A., Bell, J. M., & Moules, N. J. (2010). Beliefs, suffering, and healing: A clinical practice model for families experiencing mental illness. *Perspectives in Psychiatric Care, 46*(3), 197–208.

McMahon, S., Felix, E., & Nagarajan, T. (2011). Social support and neighborhood stressors among African American youth: Networks and relations to self-worth. *Journal of Child & Family Studies, 20*(3), 255–262.

Moodley, R. (2011). The Toronto Traditional Healers Project: An introduction. *International Journal of Health Promotion & Education, 49*(3), 74–78.

Moodley, R., & Bertrand, M. (2011). Spirits of a drum beat: African Caribbean traditional healers and their healing practices in Toronto. *International Journal of Health Promotion & Education, 49*(3), 79–89.

Muir, N., & Bennett, C. (2010). Prevention of unintentional injury in the community setting. *Nursing Standard, 24*(42), 50–56.

Muliira, J. K., & Musil, C. M. (2010). Relationship between methods of coping, social support and receipt of preventive care procedures by primary grandmother caregivers. *Journal of Community Health, 35*(5), 479–486.

Nordin, M., Andersson, L., & Nordin, S. (2010). Coping strategies, social support and responsibility in chemical intolerance. *Journal of Clinical Nursing, 19*(15-16), 2162–2173.

North American Nursing Diagnosis Association International. (2011). *Nursing diagnoses: Definitions and classifications 2012-14 (NANDA International)* (9th ed.). Indianapolis, IN: Wiley.

Osborn, K. S., Wraa, C. E., & Watson, A. B. (2010). *Medical surgical nursing: Preparation for practice.* New York: Pearson.

Petti, Y. M., & Cowell, J. M. (2011). An assessment of measures of body image, body attitude, acculturation, and weight status among Mexican American women. *Journal of the American Academy of Nurse Practitioners, 23*(2), 84–91.

Pharris, M. D. (2011). Margaret A. Newman's theory of health as expanding consciousness. *Nursing Science Quarterly, 24*(3), 193–194.

Porter, K. N., Fischer, J. G., & Johnson, M. A. (2011). Improved physical function and physical activity in older adults following a community-based intervention: Relationships with a history of depression. *Maturitas, 70*(3), 290–294.

Rawana, E. (2009). Making the possible probable: A strength-based assessment and intervention framework for clinical work with parents, children and adolescents. *Families in Society, 90*(3), 255.

Rogers, J. (2011). Functional constipation in childhood. *Nurse Prescribing, 9*(7), 328–331.

Samad, Z., Brealey, S., & Gilbody, S. (2011). The effectiveness of behavioural therapy for the treatment of depression in older adults: A meta-analysis. *International Journal of Geriatric Psychiatry, 26*(12), 1211–1220.

Saunjoo, L. Y., Grundmann, O., Koepp, L., & Farrell, L. (2011). Management of irritable bowel syndrome (IBS) in adults: Conventional and complementary/alternative approaches. *Alternative Medicine Review, 16*(2), 134–151.

Schutz, B., Wurm, S., Ziegelmann, J. P., Warner, L. M., Tesch-Romer, C., & Schwarzer, R. (2011). Changes in functional health, changes in medication beliefs, and medication adherence. *Health Psychology, 30*(1), 31–39.

Selanders, L. C. (2010). The power of environmental adaptation. *Journal of Holistic Nursing, 28*(1), 81–88.

Shirato, S., & Swan, B. A. (2010). Women and cardiovascular disease: An evidentiary review. *MEDSURG Nursing, 19*(5), 282–306.

Skerrett, K. (2010). Extending family nursing: Concepts from positive psychology. *Journal of Family Nursing, 16*(4), 487–502.

Smith, C., & Grimmer-Somers, K. (2010). The treatment effect of exercise programmes for chronic low back pain. *Journal of Evaluation in Clinical Practice, 16*(3), 484–491.

Surkan, P., Gottlieb, B., McCormick, M., Hunt, A., & Peterson, K. (2012). Impact of a health promotion intervention on maternal depressive symptoms at 15 months postpartum. *Maternal & Child Health Journal, 16*(1), 139–148.

U.S. Department of Health and Human Services. (2011). *2020 topics and objectives.* Retrieved January 7, 2012, from www.healthypeople. gov/2020/topicsobjectives2020/default.aspx.

van Woerden, H. C., Poortinga, W., Bronstering, K., Garrib, A., & Hegazi, A. (2011). The relationship of different sources of social support and civic participation with self-rated health. *Journal of Public Mental Health, 10*(3), 126–139.

Villar-Loubet, O., Jones, D., Waldrop-Valverde, D., Bruscantini, L., & Weiss, S. (2011). Sexual barrier acceptability among multiethnic HIV-positive and at-risk women. *Journal of Women's Health, 20*(3), 365–373.

Vogel-Scibilia, S., McNulty, K. C., Baxter, B., Miller, S., Dine, M., & Frese, F. J., III (2009). The recovery process utilizing Erikson's stages of human development. *Community Mental Health Journal, 45*(6), 405–414.

Ward, S. L., & Hisley, S. M. (2009). Chapter 3: The evolving family. In *Maternal-child nursing care: Optimizing outcomes for mothers, children & families* (pp. 46–70). Philadelphia, PA: F.A. Davis.

Weeks, M. R., Liao, S., Li, F., Li, J., Dunn, J., He, B., He, Q., et al. (2010). Challenges, strategies, and lessons learned from a participatory community intervention study to promote female condoms among rural sex workers in southern China. *AIDS Education & Prevention, 22*(3), 252–271.

Wenger, N. K., Mischke, J. M., Schroeder, R., Schroeder, K., Collins, P., Grady, D., et al. (2010). Electrocardiograms of menopausal women with coronary heart disease or at increased risk for its occurrence. *American Journal of Cardiology, 106*(11), 1580–1587.

World Health Organization. (2012). *Global strategy on diet, physical activity, and health.* Retrieved January 26, 2012, from www.who. int/dietphysicalactivity/publications/facts/obesity/en/.

Health Promotion and the Family

Anne Rath Rentfro

 WEBSITE

http://evolve.elsevier.com/Edelman/
- Study Questions
- Glossary
- Website Resources
  7A: Developmental Tasks of the Family at Critical Stages
  7B: Eleven Functional Health Pattern Guidelines for Family Assessment
  7C: Newman's Definitions of Family Health
  7D: Examples of Family Nursing Diagnoses

OBJECTIVES

After completing this chapter, the reader will be able to:

- Describe various theoretical approaches to the study of families.
- Assess families throughout the life span using the functional health pattern framework.
- Describe examples of the clinical data to collect in each health pattern during each family developmental phase.
- Provide examples of behavioral changes (functional, potentially dysfunctional, and actually dysfunctional) within the health patterns of families.

- Describe developmental and cultural characteristics of the family to consider when identifying risk factors or etiological factors of potential or actual dysfunctional health patterns.
- Develop planning, implementing, and evaluating nursing interventions in health promotion with families.
- Evaluate a specific health-promotion plan based on family assessment, nursing diagnosis, and contributing risks or etiological factors.

KEY TERMS

Cultural competence	Family health status	Family strengths
Developmental theory	Family nursing diagnosis	Family structure
Ecomap	Family nursing interventions	Family theory
Family	Family pattern	Genogram
Family developmental tasks	Family resilience	Risk-factor theory
Family function	Family risk factors	Systems theory

A **family** consists of a group of interacting individuals related by blood, marriage, cohabitation, or adoption who interdependently perform relevant functions by fulfilling expected roles. Relevant family functions include practices and values placed on health. Family health practices, whether effective or ineffective, encompass activities performed by individuals or families as a whole to promote health and prevent disease. How families complete developmental tasks and how well families, including individuals within a family, generate health-promoting behaviors determine a family's potential for family health practices enhancement.

How family members relate to one another influences their understanding of behavior, which is demonstrated in the family's structural, functional, communicational, and developmental patterns (Committee on Hospital Care and Institute for Patient-and-Family-Centered Care, 2012; Flor-czak et al., 2010). Families provide the structure for many health-promotion practices; therefore, family assessment informs health-promotion and disease-prevention appraisal. Within families, children and adults are nurtured, provided for, and taught about health values by word and by example. Within families, members first learn to make choices to promote health. The American Academy of Pediatrics urges health providers to include families in decision-making and to encourage their presence and participation in all aspects of care from acute care to health promotion (Committee on Hospital Care and Institute for Patient-and-Family-Centered Care, 2012). Families influence children's lifestyle choices. *Healthy People 2020* views families as a means of providing important opportunities for health promotion and disease prevention (U.S. Department of Health and Human Services, 2011). Through family planning, parents assume responsibility of caring for their children. Prenatal care and breastfeeding give infants a healthy start. Nutritious diets support physical growth and development. Children first observe and learn behaviors within their family. Patterns of nutrition, activity, oral hygiene, and coping develop at early ages, supported by family members' example. Patterns of alcohol consumption and tobacco use are similarly established within families. Learning about human development fosters a healthy self-concept, including positive awareness of the family member's sexuality. Promoting self-esteem and reinforcing positive behaviors also strengthen the health of children. Primary care providers support positive behaviors by providing family members with scientifically sound health-promotion and clinical preventive services, such as anticipatory guidance

for developmental tasks, immunizations, screening for early detection, and appropriate counseling.

This chapter uses **family theory, systems theory, developmental theory,** and **risk-factor theory** to guide the nursing process with families. The 11 functional health patterns described in the previous chapter establish the structure for interview questions during data collection. The analysis phase of the nursing process categorizes these data within stages of family development and, from the analysis, nursing diagnoses are formulated. **Family health status** is considered functional, potentially dysfunctional (potential problem), or dysfunctional (actual problem) (Gordon, 2011). The planning phase begins when family goals and objectives are stated. The family, the nurse, or another health professional facilitates implementation. Later in this chapter, four types of interventions for health promotion and disease prevention are discussed: increasing knowledge and skills; increasing strengths; decreasing exposure to risks; and decreasing susceptibility. Nurses assume various roles throughout the stages of family development, and these roles are also presented. Evaluation of a family plan considers outcomes that are specific, objective, and measurable and that rely on the family's subjective interpretation of concerns and probability of success as well as that at the population level (Kaakinen et al., 2010; Lundy & Janes, 2010; Maurer & Smith, 2009).

THE NURSING PROCESS AND THE FAMILY

The nursing process with families is a two-level process that includes the family as a group and the interactions among family members (Ward & Hisley, 2009). The entire family is viewed as the care recipient that guides assessment from a holistic framework (Ward & Hisley, 2009). Home is a natural environment for health-promotion encounters, although the process may occur in other settings as well. Different age groups (infants, children, and older adults) are likely to be available in the home. Nurses observe physical surroundings firsthand during home visits. For example, household safety hazards are observed directly. Nurses also monitor family unit rituals, roles, and interpersonal interactions. Generally the nurse contacts the family and establishes an appointment time for visiting. Including each family member in the visit provides a broad perspective. During visits, the nursing process occurs mutually with families, not for families. Families collaborate with nursing in all phases of the process. Guidelines for home visits are presented in Box 7-1.

Comprehensive family assessment provides the foundation to promote family health (Kaakinen et al., 2010; Lundy & Janes, 2010; Ward & Hisley, 2009). Several factors influence family assessment, such as nurses' perceptions about family constitution; theoretical knowledge; norms; standards; and communication abilities during visits. In addition to factors that pertain to the nurse, familial factors also influence assessments, such as family cooperation, mutual agreement to work toward goals, and family ability to recognize the relevance of health-promotion plans. Useful health-promotion family assessments involve listening to families, engaging in participatory dialogue,

Planning the Visit
- Make arrangements with the family.
- Study information regarding the family from agency records, referral forms, and other sources.
- State the purpose of the visit.
- Obtain appropriate supplies and teaching aids for visits.

Making the Visit
- Offer an introduction and explain the purpose of the visit.
- Place the nurse's bag in an appropriate location.
- Include all family members in the discussion.
- Identify the family's request for assistance.
- Understand the situation from the family's perspective.
- Identify appropriate activities for health promotion and disease prevention.
- Identify how the home visit is to be financed.
- Make a contract with the family that states specific goals and objectives that the family wants to reach.
- Terminate the visit with specific instructions and information about the next visit: when it will occur, what will happen, who will be present, and what the family must accomplish before then.

- Assist the family in decision-making about lifestyle choices.
- Provide reinforcement for positive health-behavior practices.
- Provide health information to the family.
- Assist the family in learning behaviors to promote health and prevent disease.
- Assist the family in problem-solving and decision-making about health promotion.
- Serve as a liaison for referral or collaboration between community resources and the family.

Nurses use family theoretical frameworks to guide, observe, and classify situations. Nursing roles for families in various stages of development are presented in Table 7-3 on p.173.

FAMILY THEORIES AND FRAMEWORKS

Family theory stems from a variety of interrelated disciplines (Ward & Hisley, 2009). Family systems theory explains patterns of living among the individuals who comprise family systems. In systems theory, behaviors and family members' responses influence patterns. Meanings and values provide the vital elements of motivation and energy for family systems. Every family has its unique culture, value structure, and history. Values provide a means for interpreting events and information, passing from one generation to the next. Values usually change slowly over time. Families process information and energy exchange with the environment through values. For example, holiday food traditions may be changed slightly by a daughter-in-law whose own daughter may then adjust the traditional recipe within her own nuclear family.

System boundaries separate family systems from their environment and control information flow. This characteristic forms a family internal manager that influences and defines interactions and relationships with one another and with those outside the family system. Family forms a unified whole rather than the sum of its parts—an integrated system of interdependent functions, structures, and relationships. For example, one drug-dependent individual's health behavior influences the entire family unit.

Living systems are open systems. As living systems, families experience constant exchanges of energy and information with the environment. Change in one part or member of the family results in changes in the family as a whole. For example, loss of a family member through death changes roles and relationships among all family members. Change requires adaptation of every family member as roles and functions assume new meanings. Changes families make are incorporated into the system.

When the system is the family, issues can be clarified using family processes, communication interaction among family members, and family group values. In Bowen's Family Systems Theory, birth order is considered an important determinant of behavior (Ward & Hisley, 2009). In addition, family patterns of behavior differentiate one family from another (Ward & Hisley, 2009). When an individual family member expresses behaviors that differ from the learned family pattern, differentiation of self occurs. Interaction among family members and

recognizing patterns, and assessing family potential for active, positive change (Kaakinen et al., 2010; Lundy & Janes, 2010; Ward & Hisley, 2009).

The assessment phase of the nursing process seeks and identifies information from the family about health-promotion and disease-prevention activities. To obtain this information, nurses follow family progress through developmental tasks and identify strengths in the family's ability to generate low risk-taking behaviors associated with disease prevention. The approaches considered in this chapter include the developmental framework, strength-based assessment, and the risk-factor estimate. Developmental phases for families as proposed by Duvall and Miller (Kaakinen et al., 2010; Ward & Hisley, 2009), strength-based assessment as proposed by Wright and Leahy (Marshall et al., 2010), and risk-factor estimates as proposed in *Healthy People 2020* can be used to guide nurses through the steps of the nursing process when working with families (U.S. Department of Health and Human Services, 2011).

The Nurse's Role

Nurses collaborate with families using a systems perspective to understand family interaction, family norms, family expectations, effectiveness of family communication, family decision-making, and family coping mechanisms. The nurse's role in health promotion and disease prevention includes the following tasks:

- Become aware of family attitudes and behaviors toward health promotion and disease prevention.
- Act as a role model for the family.
- Collaborate with the family to assess, improve, enhance, and evaluate family health practices.
- Assist the family in growth and development behaviors.
- Assist the family in identifying risk-taking behaviors.

the transmission of these interaction patterns from one generation to the next provide the framework for the family systems approach (Ward & Hisley, 2009).

The framework for health promotion introduced by Pender and colleagues (2011) recognizes the family as the unit of assessment and intervention, because families develop self-care and dependent-care competencies; foster resilience among family members; provide resources; and promote healthy individuation within cohesive family structures. Furthermore, because family often provides the structure for implementing health promotion, family assessment becomes an integral tool to foster health and healthy behaviors (Pender et al., 2011).

THE FAMILY FROM A DEVELOPMENTAL PERSPECTIVE

Building on Erikson's (1998) theory of psychosocial development, Duvall and Miller (1985) identified stages of the family life cycle and critical family developmental tasks. Although Duvall's classification has been criticized for its middle class homogeneity and lack of diversity in family forms, this conceptual model helps to anticipate family events, and has formed the basis for more contemporary developmental models (Kaakinen et al., 2010; Lundy & Janes, 2010; Ward & Hisley, 2009). Knowing a family's composition, interrelationships, and particular life cycle helps nurses predict overall family pattern. Box 7-2 lists characteristics of healthy families. From Duvall's perspective, most families complete these basic family tasks. Each family performs these tasks in a unique expression of its personality. Progression through the stages occurs in a linear fashion; however, regression may occur and families may experience tasks in more than one stage at a time (Kaakinen et al., 2010; Ward & Hisley, 2009). Specific tasks arise as growth responsibilities during family development. Failure to accomplish a developmental task leads to negative consequences. For example, intimate partner violence or child abuse or neglect may result in intervention by police, welfare, health department, or other agencies. Life cycle tasks build upon one another. Success at one stage is dependent upon success at an earlier stage. Early failure may lead to developmental difficulties at later stages.

As families enter each new developmental stage, transition occurs. Families move through new stages as a result of events ranging from marriage (heterosexual, homosexual), gay and lesbian relationships, childbirth, single-led families, joint custody, or remarried families; to adolescents maturing into young adults and leaving the home; to the aging years.

Each new developmental stage requires adaptation with new responsibilities. Concurrently, developmental stages provide opportunities for families to realize their potential. Nurses anticipate change through analysis of progress through each stage. Each new stage presents opportunities for health promotion and intervention.

Family developmental stages, although reflective of traditional nuclear families and extended family networks, also apply to nontraditional family configurations (Kaakinen et al., 2010; Lundy & Janes, 2010; Ward & Hisley, 2009). For example, couples may marry and bring children from a previous marriage to

---

BOX 7-2 CHARACTERISTICS AND INDICATORS OF HEALTHY FAMILIES

- Maintains trust traditions and shares quality time.
- Evolves during crises and respects each member of the group.
- Communications are open and members listen to each other.
- Family table time and conversation occur regularly.
- Establishes patterns to promote mental health: interacting, communicating, and expressing affection, aggression, sexuality, and similar interactions.
- Maintains routines that promote health patterns of nutrition, hygiene, rest, physical activity, and sexuality.
- Maintains routines to promote safety and injury prevention; health protection; disease prevention; smoking, alcohol, or substance abuse; and/or violence.
- Maintains morale and motivation, rewarding achievement, meeting personal and family crises, setting attainable goals, and developing family traditions, loyalties, and values.
- Promotes strategies to make decisions about health and illness.
- Members act as interactive caregivers across the life span to socialize children and adolescents, to participate in the community, and to support members as they age.

Modified from Kaakinen, J., Gedaly-Duff, V., Coehlo, D. P., & Hanson, S. M. H. (2010). *Family nursing: Theory, practice and research* (4th ed.). Philadelphia: F.A. Davis.

---

a blended family that works toward achieving developmental tasks of couples along with family stages for the children. Both the couple and their children possess values and beliefs from the past that must integrate within the present union. Childless couples present developmental tasks that are different from those proposed for couples with children.

Nurses collect data to determine progress toward task attainment (Kaakinen et al., 2010; Lundy & Janes, 2010; Ward & Hisley, 2009). Assessment of family developmental stages entails using guidelines to analyze progress toward developmental tasks, family growth, and health-promotion needs. Family developmental task guidelines are summarized in **Website Resource 7A.**

THE FAMILY FROM A STRUCTURAL-FUNCTIONAL PERSPECTIVE

Families consist of both structural and functional components. Family structure refers to family composition, including roles and relationships, whereas family function consists of processes within systems as information and energy exchange occurs between families and their environment.

THE FAMILY FROM A RISK-FACTOR PERSPECTIVE

Family risk factors can be inferred from lifestyle; biological factors; environmental factors; social, psychological, cultural, and spiritual dimensions; and the health care system. As outlined in the Frank Thompson case study in Chapter 1, lifestyle habits such as overeating, drug dependency, high sugar and cholesterol intake, and smoking influence health outcomes. Biological risk factors may include the elements of genetic inheritance, congenital malformation, and mental retardation. To fully explore environmental risk factors that influence family function, nurses explore work pressures, peer pressure, stress, anxieties, tensions, and air, noise, or water pollution. Social and psychological dimensions such as crowding, isolation, or rapid and accelerated rates of change are areas to consider when assessing family risk factors. Cultural and spiritual aspects may include traditions of preventing illness such as daily prayer and meditation practices. Finally, health care system factors such as overuse, underuse, inappropriate use, or accessibility are considered in the family risk assessment.

To reduce risk factors, nurses help families focus on influencing health behaviors of their members. Society glamorizes many hazardous behaviors through advertising and mass-media promotions that minimize negative health consequences. Families influence their members to weigh consequences of risk-taking behavior. Awareness of risk factors may prompt families to reduce modifiable risk factors. Healthy behavior, including use of preventive health care services, is a significant area of family responsibility.

Traditionally, epidemiology has used levels and trends of mortality and morbidity rates as indirect evidence of health. Data such as infant mortality rates, stillbirth rates, and leading causes of death have long been used as indicators of collective community health. Healthy family functioning links the family life cycle stages with specific risk factors. Epidemiology often describes a disease association in terms of risk. Health risks can be physiological or psychological. Physiological risks arise from genetic background, whereas psychological risks include those related to low self-image. Risks also arise from environmental considerations, including physical environment and socioeconomic condition (Freudenberg et al., 2011). Risk-factor theory considers families a pivotal part of the environment and also an important support system used to decrease health risks for individuals. As young family members mature developmentally and seek more independence from the family, peers may influence risk to compete with family values.

Risk estimates calculate differences between two groups: one with the risk factor and one without. Frequency of deaths, illnesses, or injuries with some specific risk factor compared to another group without the risk factor, or the population as a whole, determines the risk estimate. Some diseases occur more frequently in certain families, such as sickle cell anemia in Black families and Tay-Sachs disease in Ashkenazi (East European) Jewish families (Hockenberry & Wilson, 2010). Other diseases such as iron deficiency anemia may not be attributed to specific genetic background. The natural history of a chronic disease predisposes family members to greater risk, but specific causes may be difficult to identify. Well siblings, particularly adolescents, may be affected (O'Haver et al., 2010). Lubkin and Larsen (2011) describe nine phases that individuals and families may experience as they progress through chronic illness adaptation from the time before the disorder is recognized through a stable adjustment phase to the final relinquishment of life interest and activities.

Probabilities of risk change may also change depending on the family's activities in health promotion and disease prevention. Stages of family development are used to classify risk factors. Age-specific developmental stages, along with their associated age-specific health risks, appear in Table 7-1, which displays periods during which families become most sensitive to certain problems with corresponding key times for health promotion and disease prevention. Risk behaviors highlighted include tobacco and alcohol use, faulty nutrition, overuse of medications, fast driving, stress, and relentless pressure to achieve. Habits learned in family settings help to develop individual lifestyle behaviors. In fact, 5 habits—nutrition, smoking, exercise, alcohol use, and stress—affect at least 7 of the 10 leading causes of death listed in the *Healthy People 2020* report (U.S. Department of Health and Human Services, 2011). See Box 7-3: *Healthy People 2020* for selected objectives related to families.

GORDON'S FUNCTIONAL HEALTH PATTERNS: ASSESSMENT OF THE FAMILY

Gordon's (2011) 11 functional health patterns help organize basic family assessment information (Kaakinen et al., 2010). Patterns form the standardized format for family assessment using a systems approach with emphasis on developmental stages and risk factors. Assessment includes evaluation of dysfunctional patterns within families with corresponding details in one or more of the other interdependent patterns (see Chapter 6).

The presence of risk factors predicts potential dysfunction. Developmental risk and risk arising from dysfunctional health patterns increase whole family risk (see Table 7-1). Gordon (2011) interprets risk states as potential problems. To formulate nursing diagnoses, nurses identify problems along with their associated and etiological factors. Influencing factors may precede or occur concurrently with the problem and are used to plan care. Interventions aim to modify influencing factors to promote positive change.

Family history begins with the health perception–health management pattern. Exploring issues within this pattern first provides an overview to help locate where problems exist in other patterns and to determine which ones may require more thorough assessment. Interviewing from the family's perspective helps families define situations. The roles-relationships pattern defines family structure and function. The remaining nine patterns address lifestyle indicators.

Health Perception–Health Management Pattern

Characteristics of family health perceptions, health management, and preventive practices are revealed with assessment of the health perception–health management pattern. The National Survey of Children's Health (www.childhealthdata.org) has been designed to contribute data to identify health-promoting behaviors of families. Data collected in this survey include information about frequency of family meals; attendance at religious services; characteristics of parental relationship with children; parental coping abilities while

TABLE 7-1   FAMILY STAGE: SPECIFIC RISK FACTORS AND RELATED HEALTH PROBLEMS

STAGE	RISK FACTORS	HEALTH PROBLEMS
Beginning childbearing	Lack of knowledge about family planning	Premature baby in family
	Adolescent marriage	Birth defects
	Lack of knowledge concerning sexual and marital roles and adjustments	Birth injuries
	Low-birth-weight infant	Accidents
	Lack of prenatal care	SIDS
	Inadequate nutrition	Respiratory distress syndrome
	Poor eating habits	Sterility
	Smoking, alcohol, and drug abuse	Pelvic inflammatory disease
	Unmarried status	Fetal alcohol syndrome
	First pregnancy before age 16 or after age 35	Mental retardation
	History of hypertension and infections during pregnancy	Child abuse
	Rubella, syphilis, gonorrhea, and AIDS	Injuries
	Genetic factors	Birth defects
	Low socioeconomic and educational levels	Underweight or overweight
	Lack of safety in home	
Family with school-aged children	Working parents with inappropriate use of resources for child care	Behavior disturbances
	Poverty	Speech and vision problems
	Abuse or neglect of children	Communicable diseases
	Generational pattern of using social agencies as way of life	Dental caries
	Multiple, closely spaced children	School problems
	Low family self-esteem	Learning disabilities
	Children used as scapegoats for parental frustration	Cancer
	Repeated infections, accidents, or hospitalizations	Injuries
	Parents immature, dependent, and unable to handle responsibility	Chronic diseases
	Unrecognized or unattended health problems	Homicide
	Strong beliefs about physical punishment	Violence
	Toxic substances unguarded in the home	
	Poor nutrition	
Family with adolescents	Racial and ethnic family origin	Violent deaths and injuries
	Lifestyle and behavior patterns leading to chronic disease	Alcohol and drug abuse
	Lack of problem-solving skills	Unwanted pregnancies
	Family values of aggressiveness and competition	Sexually transmitted diseases
	Family values rigid and inflexible	Suicide
	Daredevil risk-taking attitudes	Depression
	Denial behavior	
	Conflicts between parents and children	
	Pressure to live up to family expectations	
Family with middle-aged adults	Hypertension	Cardiovascular disease, principally
	Smoking	coronary artery disease and
	High cholesterol levels	cerebrovascular accident (stroke)
	Physical inactivity	Diabetes
	Genetic predisposition	Overweight
	Use of oral contraceptives	Cancer
	Sex, race, and other hereditary factors	Accidents
	Geographical area, age, and occupational deficiencies	Homicide
	Habits (i.e., diet with low fiber, pickling, charcoal use, and broiling)	Suicide
		Abnormal fetus
	Alcohol abuse	Mental illness
	Social class	Periodontal disease and loss of teeth
	Residence	Depression
Family with older adults	Age	Mental confusion
	Drug interactions	Reduced vision
	Metabolic disorders	Hearing impairment
	Pituitary malfunctions	Hypertension
	Cushing's syndrome	Acute illness
	Hypercalcemia	Infectious disease
	Chronic illness	Influenza
	Retirement	Pneumonia

TABLE 7-1   FAMILY STAGE: SPECIFIC RISK FACTORS AND RELATED HEALTH PROBLEMS— cont'd

STAGE	RISK FACTORS	HEALTH PROBLEMS
	Loss of spouse	Injuries such as burns and falls
	Reduced income	Depression
	Poor nutrition	Chronic disease
	Lack of exercise	Elder abuse
	Past environments and lifestyle	Death without dignity
	Lack of prevention for death	

Modified from U.S. Department of Health and Human Services. (2011). *Healthy People 2020 topics and objectives*. Retrieved July 7, 2011, from www.healthypeople.gov/2020/topicsobjectives2020/default.aspx.
SIDS, Sudden infant death syndrome.

BOX 7-3   HEALTHY PEOPLE 2020

Selected Examples of National Health-Promotion and Disease-Prevention Objectives for Families

- Provide patient and family referrals for hemoglobinopathies.
- (Developmental) Increase the proportion of persons with hemoglobinopathies who receive care in a patient/family-centered medical home.
- Increase the proportion of parents who read to their young child.
- Advocate for personal, family, and community health (skills).
- Decrease unhealthy dietary patterns.
- Increase the percentage of new single-family homes (SFH) constructed with radon-reducing features, especially in high-radon–potential areas.

Family Planning Objectives
- Increase the proportion of pregnancies that are intended.
- Reduce the proportion of females experiencing pregnancy despite use of a reversible contraceptive method.
- Increase the proportion of publicly funded family planning clinics that offer the full-range of FDA-approved methods of contraception, including emergency contraception, on-site.
- (Developmental) Increase the proportion of health insurance plans that cover contraceptive supplies and services.
- Reduce the proportion of pregnancies conceived within 18 months of a previous birth.
- Increase the proportion of females or their partners at risk of unintended pregnancy who used contraception at most recent sexual intercourse.
- Increase the proportion of sexually active persons who received reproductive health services.
- Reduce pregnancy rates among adolescent females.

- Increase the proportion of adolescents aged 17 years and under who have never had sexual intercourse.
- Increase the proportion of sexually active persons aged 15 to 19 years who use condoms to both effectively prevent pregnancy and provide barrier protection against disease.
- Increase the proportion of sexually active persons aged 15 to 19 years who use condoms and hormonal or intrauterine contraception to both effectively prevent pregnancy and provide barrier protection against disease.
- Increase the proportion of adolescents who received formal instruction on reproductive health topics before they were 18 years old.
- Increase the proportion of adolescents who talked to a parent or guardian about reproductive health topics before they were 18 years old.
- Increase the number of states that set the income eligibility level for Medicaid-covered family planning services to at least the same level used to determine eligibility for Medicaid-covered, pregnancy-related care.
- Increase the proportion of females in need of publicly supported contraceptive services and supplies who receive those services and supplies.
- Increase the proportion of women with a family history of breast and/or ovarian cancer who receive genetic counseling.
- Increase the proportion of adults who report having friends or family members whom they talk with about their health.
- Increase the proportion of children with special health care needs who receive their care in family-centered, comprehensive, coordinated systems.
- Increase the proportion of children with special health care needs who receive their care in family-centered, comprehensive, coordinated systems.

From U.S. Department of Health and Human Services. (2011). *Healthy People 2020 topics and objectives*. Retrieved July 7, 2011, from www.healthypeople.gov/2020/topicsobjectives2020/default.aspx.

---

raising children; and methods for handling family disagreements. The intent of the survey is to provide a data source to explore research questions related to *Healthy People 2020* and the variables correlate with drug use. However, such data have also been associated with eating disorders and risk behaviors other than drug use. These assessment indicators also provide data to guide the remaining functional health pattern assessment. Patterns overlap and findings in one pattern may encourage further assessment in another pattern. The following are some research questions that concern family health promotion:

- What are parents' chief concerns regarding their children's development, learning, and behavior?

- How do parents' health practices (physical activity and smoking behavior) relate to children's health status?
- What health-related behaviors, such as eating three meals a day at regular times, eating breakfast every day, exercising a minimum of 2 or 3 days a week, sleeping 7 to 8 hours each night, and abstaining from smoking, are practiced by the family?
- How safe are homes, schools, and neighborhoods from the perspective of parents?

Health practices vary from family to family. Families identify and perform health-maintenance activities based on their beliefs about health. Exploration during the assessment also includes the following areas:

- What is the family's philosophy of health? Does each family member hold similar beliefs? Do family members practice what they believe?
- In what negative behaviors or lifestyle practices, such as smoking, alcohol, and drug abuse, does the family engage?
- What chronic disease risk behaviors are exhibited within the family?
- Are risk factors present for infections, such as lack of immunization, lack of knowledge of transmittable diseases, and poor personal hygiene?
- Are risk factors for bodily injury, accidents, or substance abuse present in the home?
- Do older adult members know what medications they are taking and the reasons for using them?
- Does the family discard outdated medications or those not used?
- What unattended health problems exist?
- Is there a history of repeated infections and hospitalization?
- Is the home understimulating or overstimulating?
- Where does the family obtain health and illness care?
- Is the family engaged in a dental program?
- How does the family describe previous experiences with nurses and other health care professionals?

Nutritional-Metabolic Pattern

The nutritional-metabolic pattern depicts characteristics of the family's typical food and fluid consumption and metabolism (Gordon, 2011). Included are growth and development patterns, pregnancy-related nutritional patterns, and the family's eating patterns. Risk factors for obesity, diabetes, anorexia, and bulimia are identified.

Dietary habits, learned within the family context, involve behavioral patterns central to daily life. Keeping a diary of intake for a week provides a useful strategy for assessing family food and fluid intake patterns. Assessment notes both meals shared with the whole family as well as additional consumption by individuals. Recent research provides evidence that family meal sharing is associated with healthier eating habits (Kime, 2009). Frequency of family meals has also been inversely associated with other health behaviors and risk factors. For example, Kime (2009) determined that obese children were less likely to be eating meals with their family at regular times.

Exploration during nutrition pattern assessment includes the following areas:

- What kinds of foods are typically consumed?
- Who eats together at mealtimes?
- How is food viewed (reward/punishment)?
- Is there adequate storage and refrigeration?
- How is food purchased?
- How is food prepared?

Elimination Pattern

The elimination pattern describes characteristics of regularity and control of the family's excretory functions (Gordon, 2011). Bowel and bladder function and environmental factors such as waste disposal in the home, neighborhood, and community that influence family life are considered in this pattern.

Questions are phrased according to the age-specific developmental stage of the family. For example, in determining whether there is a problem in the preschool stage, it would be appropriate to ask whether the child is being toilet trained. In families with adolescents, the nurse may ask how often individuals have bowel movements and whether there have been any changes from usual patterns. The nurse may ask older adult members whether they have any problems with constipation. Issues that particularly concern older adults include constipation, diarrhea, polyuria, and incontinence, as well as use of antacids and anticonstipation agents. The nurse evaluates whether use of these agents is appropriate or possibly contributing to poor health.

Activity-Exercise Pattern

The activity-exercise pattern represents family characteristics that require energy expenditure (Gordon, 2011). The nurse reviews daily activities, exercise, and leisure activities. Families create settings for individual members to be physically active, sedentary, or apathetic toward physical activity. The quantity of sedentary activities such as television and video game screen time is explored.

Exploration during assessment of this pattern includes the following areas:

- How does the family exhibit its beliefs about regular exercise and physical fitness being necessary for good health?
- What types of daily activities include physical exercise and who does what with whom?
- What are the television viewing habits of children?
- How are other screen-viewing activities (computers, video games) incorporated into the daily routines?
- How often do children exercise?
- How are these activity and exercise factors related to children's health?
- What does the family do to have fun (Figure 7-1)?

Sleep-Rest Pattern

Rest habits characterize the sleep-rest pattern (Gordon, 2011). Without the restorative function of sleep, individuals exhibit decreased performance, bad temper, and decreased stress tolerance and may rely on substances such as alcohol or other chemicals to induce sleep. Regular, sufficient sleep patterns are linked to better mental status including learning and decision-making. Most families have sleeping patterns, although in some families these patterns may not be readily apparent. It is important to elicit the data about sleep and rest from the family's perspective.

Assessment of the sleep-rest pattern includes the following:

- What are the usual sleeping habits of the family?
- How suitable are they to the age and health status of the family members?
- What are the usual hours established for sleeping?
- Who decides when and how children go to sleep?
- Do family members take naps or have other regular means of resting or relaxing?
- How early does the family rise? What are the patterns related to bedtime and rising?

FIGURE 7-1 Family outings can be **(A)** leisurely and restful or **(B)** adventurous and exciting.

- Do all family members have the same general sleep-rest pattern?
- Is there a family member with sleep disruption?

Cognitive-Perceptual Pattern

The cognitive-perceptual pattern identifies characteristics of language, cognitive skills, and perception that influence desired or required family activities (Gordon, 2011). Specifically, this pattern concerns how families access information to make decisions, how concrete or abstract the thought processes are, and whether decisions focus on present or future issues. Decision-making in families is associated with power in family functioning. Highly educated families usually have greater repertoires for problem-solving. Power and ability to solve problems are linked to leadership; family leaders must be acknowledged if nursing interventions are to be implemented.

Cognitive-perceptual pattern assessment includes the following:

- How does the family access and interpret information, especially about health (e.g., newspaper, books, computer, television, or radio)?
- What are the usual family reading patterns and strategies used for ongoing learning (e.g., continuing education programs)?
- What kinds of materials does the family read to their children?
- How does the family usually make decisions about health promotion and disease prevention?
- How do members contribute to the decision-making process?
- How knowledgeable is the family about risk factors and developmental milestones?
- How are choices made regarding lifestyle?
- How knowledgeable are family members about correct information?
- How do family members acquire information?
- How accurate are the information sources used to make health-promotion choices?

- How do family members describe whether their health behavior is constructive or destructive?
- How do family members recognize signs and symptoms of deteriorating health?
- How do family members decide when medical attention is necessary?
- Who makes the decisions about when to seek health care?
- What factors contribute to delays from time of onset to time of treatment?
- How long do families wait before seeking care?
- What are some of the cues that signal to families that care is needed?
- How is professional care accessed?
- What type of health care is generally used (health maintenance for immunizations, well-child care or emergency/urgent care facilities)?
- How are decisions made about the use of over-the-counter medications or the use of alternative or traditional health practices?

Self-Perception–Self-Concept Pattern

The self-perception–self-concept pattern identifies characteristics that describe the family's self-worth and feeling states (Gordon, 2011). Rapport between the family members and the nurse facilitates disclosure. Families have perceptions and concepts about their image, their status in the community, and their competencies as a family unit. Families manifest these perceptions through shared aspirations, values, expectations, fears, successes, and failures. Relationships in families determine the amount of sharing that occurs. Situations affecting one member influence perceptions of the entire family group. How each member describes the family often gives clues to the family self-concept.

Exploration during assessment includes the following:

- How is this family similar to or different from other families?
- How does this family perceive itself to be similar to and different from other families?
- What special assets does each member contribute to the family?

- What changes would each member like to see occur in the family?
- What kinds of feelings do family members have for each other?
- Describe the general tone of feelings in the family. Is the tone indifferent, secretive, angry, or open?
- How does the family think it assimilates into the neighborhood and community?
- How does the family handle stress and crisis situations?
- How does the family experience changes in the way it feels about itself?
- How does the family describe the events that led to a change?

Roles-Relationships Pattern

The roles-relationships pattern identifies characteristics of family roles and relationships (Gordon, 2011). Both structural and functional aspects of the family are assessed. Structural aspects of families include each member's name, age, sex, education, occupation, and role in the family. Traditionally, families have been described as nuclear and extended. The traditional nuclear family consists of husband, wife, and children, with an extended family that would include aunts, uncles, cousins, and grandparents. Today there are many varieties of nuclear and extended families (Lev, 2010; Marken et al., 2010; Muliira & Musil, 2010). Ward and Hisley (2009) describe the various contemporary family structures: traditional nuclear family, extended families, single-parent families, stepfamilies, cohabiting families, gay and lesbian families, grandparent-headed families, foster families, and fragmentary families. Traditional nuclear family structure has been influenced by societal changes, such as the women's movement, employment of mothers, divorce, and remarriage. Exploration of family origin and genetic heritage completes family identification data collection. Cultural practices in the home may or may not reflect the family's genetic heritage; therefore, it is important to explore the diversity of cultural and ethnic practices (Andrews & Boyle, 2011).

The Academy of Pediatrics regards family as the most enduring link to health for children. The U.S. Census Bureau (2012) released information in 2011 from the *Annual Report of Families and Living Arrangements*. The number of young adults ages 5 to 34 who are living in their parents' homes has increased from 14% in 2005 to 19% in 2011 and has extended beyond the economic recession. Most children (69%) live with both parents. Children living with only one parent are likely to live with their mother. Grandparents live within 10% of the homes that have children less than 18 years of age. The number of children with stay-at-home mothers decreased from 24% in 2007 to 23% in 2011. There is also an overall trend of increasing numbers of individuals living alone in their home, from 13% in 1960 to 28% in 2011.

Schoon and colleagues (2012) suggest that children in the United Kingdom experiencing poverty for the duration of their first 5 years of life are at higher risk for impaired cognitive development than those who do not experience poverty. These data indicate the need to identify family structure for poverty-related factors to determine those families at risk (Table 7-2). Family

TABLE 7-2	VARIETY OF FAMILY STRUCTURES	
CONFIGURATION	**POSITIONS IN FAMILY**
Single parent (separated, divorced, or widowed)	Mother or father, sons(s), daughter(s)
Unmarried single parent (never married)	Mother or father
	Sons(s), daughter(s)
Unmarried couple	Two adults
Unmarried parents	Mother and father, sons(s), daughter(s)
Commune family	Mothers and fathers, shared son(s), daughters(s)
Stepparents	Son(s), daughter(s) from previous marriage
	Mother and father
Adoptive	Adopted son(s), daughter(s)
Family of choice	Adults with selected partners and family members
Married couple	Mother and father
Married parents	Mother and father, son(s), daughter(s)
Grandparent(s)	Grandmother and/or grandfather
	Grandchildren, son(s) and/or daughter(s)

structure and function influence family stability and pose a challenge to the nurse in health promotion and disease prevention.

Divorce and remarriage involve a complex transition that requires the disintegration of one family structure and reorganization to another (Lundy & Janes, 2010; Muliira & Musil, 2010; Ward & Hisley, 2009). Developmental levels of children, individual temperaments of children, and quality of environmental support for children all contribute to the family response (Hockenberry & Wilson, 2010; Lundy & Janes, 2010; Ward & Hisley, 2009). How parents cope during the situational crisis, as well as after the divorce, is a significant variable in long-term individual and family adjustment. See the Case Study at the end of this chapter for presentation of a stepfamily situation.

A family resilience framework may be useful to promote strategies for prevention efforts aimed at strengthening families as they face life challenges. Shin and colleagues (2010) explored family resilience in 171 divorced families in Korea with adolescent children. These researchers found positive beliefs about the parents' divorce to significantly predict the adolescents' adjustment. Children experiencing divorce, however, are on average 6 years old. Strachan and colleagues (2010) examined the psychometric properties of an instrument to measure children's perceptions of emotional security, positive parenting, negative parenting, and coparenting after divorce. This instrument was designed to provide more objective information for custody courts to facilitate placement by using a more objective and accurate depiction of a child's feelings and perceptions. The Structured Child Assessment of Relationships in Families (SCARF) instrument was used to assess 40 children experiencing court custody hearings in an attempt to provide voice to the children about their needs.

Family disruption has been associated with substance abuse and psychosocial maladjustment in adolescents and young adults. For example, Lehavot and colleagues (2011) used data from 224 participants with human immunodeficiency virus (HIV) to examine the moderating effects of social support. Their work provides evidence that family supports are associated with adherence and that substance abuse may decrease healthy social support systems. Moreover, both family dissolution and family disruption may be associated with substance abuse, alcohol consumption, and externalizing behaviors such as theft, property destruction, fighting, and assault (Kaakinen et al., 2010). Current literature provides support for the importance of the role-relationship patterns in the development of health-promoting behaviors (Kaakinen et al., 2010).

Family organization influences performance of health-promotion and disease-prevention functions. For example, a single parent without an extended family network may be in need of more community resources to help raise the children. A two-parent family living near its extended family may need less support to raise children, but members may need to know about growth and developmental stages and immunization schedules. Individuals may experience a variety of family structures in one lifetime. A person may be part of a nuclear family as an infant, a single-parent family after the parents are divorced, a stepparent family when the mother or father remarries, and an unmarried couple family when the person is one of two adults who share a household. The person brings the values and beliefs about health promotion and disease prevention that were practiced in previous unions to each new family configuration. Divergent values may result in conflicting expectations unless the new union forms a set of integrated values and beliefs. The current trend away from the nuclear family with extended family may influence the general direction of the health care system and the strategies used to promote health with other family configurations.

Certain health-promotion issues are of particular concern to the nurse while assessing family health promotion and disease prevention. Violence is a health problem that threatens the integrity of all families (Benzies & Mychasiuk, 2009). Family violence includes child abuse, spousal abuse, and elder abuse, with women being victimized more often during pregnancy. In fact, mortality in pregnancy is often associated with domestic violence (Kavanaugh et al., 2009). Health promotion and violence prevention require a complex set of skills. Nurses use approaches to reduce violence-related injuries and deaths by acquiring the role of advocate and helping to eliminate victim blaming (Box 7-4: Research for Evidence-Based Practice). Explorations to assess families for health promotion and violence prevention may include the following:

- What formal positions and roles does each of the family members fulfill?
- What roles are considered acceptable and consistent within the family's expectations?
- What kind of flexibility in roles takes place when needed?
- What informal roles exist? Who plays informal roles and with what consistency?
- What purpose do the informal roles serve?
- How are the family social support networks associated with health and development?
- Who were the role models for the couples or single people as parents?

BOX 7-4   RESEARCH FOR EVIDENCE-BASED PRACTICE

A Randomized Controlled Trial: Attempt to Decrease Victimization by Domestic Violence Through Skill Building and Empowerment

A total of 24 disadvantaged Pakistani women participated in an 8-week community-derived intervention consisting of 3 randomly assigned intervention groups (economic skill building [ESB] group, counseling group, and control group). The purpose of the study was to determine the differences in level of depression, domestic violence, self-efficacy, and employment between the three groups: women in adult literacy programs who receive a community health worker (CHW)–delivered 8-week counseling program; women who receive a CHW-delivered 8-week economic skill building program; and women who do not receive an intervention. The study was conducted in an inner-city slum area of Karachi, Pakistan (18 million residents), using a community-based participatory research approach. Three sets of two adjacent similar clusters were randomly assigned to the interventions of economic skill building, counseling, and control groups. Each cluster had several hundred adult women. The randomization took place maintaining the community-based participatory approach and the internal validity of the research remained strong. Depression, self-efficacy, and self-reported employment were measured. The skill building (ESB) group ($n = 9$) demonstrated significantly higher ($p < 0.05$) self-efficacy scores, as compared to the counseling ($n = 7$) and control groups of women ($n = 8$). There was also a trend, although not statistically significant, toward lower depression scores for the ESB group. The results provide support for using ESB interventions to promote family health and decrease violence in disadvantaged Pakistani women.

Data from Hirani, S. S., Karmaliani, R., McFarlane, J., Asad, N., Madhani, F., & Shehzad, S. (2010). Testing a community derived intervention to promote women's health: Preliminary results of a 3-arm randomized controlled trial in Karachi, Pakistan. *Southern Online Journal of Nursing Research, 10*(3), 5p.

- Who were the role models for marital partners and what were their characteristics?
- How does the family manage daily living? How are the household tasks divided?
- How are problems handled? How are problems with children handled?
- Who is employed outside the home?
- Who takes care of the children when both parents are employed outside the home?
- How does the family care for its ill members? How does it care for its older adult members?
- Are behaviors appropriate for family stages of development?
- Is decision-making allocated to the appropriate members?
- Does the family respond appropriately to its members' developmental needs?
- Is there fair distribution of tasks among family members?

Is the family's emotional climate conducive to growth and development? When this initial assessment reveals possible neglect, abuse, or violence, further assessment is warranted with a branched assessment that may include the following assessment parameters and questions:

- What cues are present to indicate chemical abuse?

BOX 7-5   **QUALITY AND SAFETY SCENARIO**

Domestic Violence: Intimate Partner Violence

If the person is still in the relationship:
- Think of a safe place to go if an argument occurs—avoid rooms with no exits (bathroom) or rooms with weapons (kitchen).
- Think about and make a list of safe people to contact.
- Keep a cell phone with you at all times.
- Memorize all important numbers.
- Establish a "code word" or "sign" so that family, friends, teachers, or coworkers know when to call for help.
- Think about what to say to partner if he/she becomes violent.
- Remind the individual that he/she has the right to live without fear and violence.

If the person has left the relationship:
- Change the phone number.
- Screen calls.
- Save and document all contacts, messages, injuries, or other incidents involving the batterer.
- Change locks, if the batterer has a key.
- Avoid staying alone.
- Plan how to get away if confronted by an abusive partner.
- If a meeting is necessary, do it in a public place.
- Vary the routine.
- Notify school and work contacts.
- Call a shelter.

If leaving the relationship or thinking of leaving, the individual should take important papers and documents to facilitate application for benefits or take legal action. Important papers include Social Security cards and birth certificates for self and children, marriage license, leases or deeds, checkbook, charge cards, bank statements and charge account statements, insurance policies, proof of income (pay stubs or W-2s), and any documentation of past incidents of abuse (e.g., photos, police reports, medical records).

The National Coalition Against Domestic Violence provides information to health care providers, a network of shelters, and counseling programs and operates a national hotline: 800-799-SAFE (7233); website: www.ncadv.org; address: One Broadway, Suite B210, Denver, CO 80203; phone: 303-839-1852; fax: 303-831-9251; telecommunication device (TTY): 303-839-1681; e-mail: mainoffice@ncadv.org.

Adapted from information on the National Coalition Against Domestic Violence. Retrieved from www.ncadv.org/.

- Who are the significant adult members of the household? (Determine presence of boyfriend/girlfriend.)

Nursing diagnoses and planning stem from a thorough assessment. High-quality evidence-based intervention is based on this systematic approach to assessment. For example, quality intervention for victims of intimate partner violence can be planned in advance to promote the safety and well-being of the victims (Box 7-5: Quality and Safety Scenario).

Genogram

A genogram, or family diagram, represents the family based on identification data that depict each member of the family with connections between the generations. This useful technique gathers data on at least three generations, including the current one; their parents, grandparents, aunts, uncles; and their children. The family genogram explores clues within family histories contributing to health problems. Figure 7-2 depicts accepted genogram symbols with a sample genogram of the fictional Graham family portrayed in Figure 7-3 (Stanhope & Lancaster, 2012). The Graham family genogram shows a variety of family structures, including changes resulting from marriage, divorce, death, and childbearing. This information highlights family health patterns to use for anticipatory health guidance; for example, in the case of the Graham family, hypertension, type 2 diabetes, cancer, and hypercholesterolemia. Family histories provide the unique perspective of family risk for inherited diseases as well as the family environmental contribution (Pender et al., 2011). Although *My Family Health Portrait* at www.familyhistory.hhs.gov takes a more traditional approach to family history, encouraging families to visit the website helps them explore their own family history. Nursing resources for this continuously evolving topic can be found at the National Human Genome Research Institute (www.genome.gov/17515679) and at an on-line educational program sponsored by The University of Cincinnati and the National Coalition for Health Professional Education in Genetics (http://bmihgjsd.cchmc.org:8081/gepnweb/c118/index.html). Health-promotion nursing relevance cannot be underestimated. Risk profiles and family risk can be ascertained by a nurse who has maintained competency in genetics.

Ecomap

The ecomap, which is similar to the genogram, uses pictorial techniques to document family organizational patterns with visual clarity. A genogram is constructed for a family or household. It begins with a circle in the center of the page. Outside the circle, smaller circles are drawn and labeled with the names of significant people, agencies, and institutions in the family's social environment. Lines are drawn from the family-household to each circle. Solid lines indicate strong relationships. Dotted lines reflect fragile or tenuous connections. Slashed lines signify stressful relationships. Arrows can be drawn parallel to the lines to indicate the direction for the energy flow or for resources (Kaakinen et al., 2010; Stanhope & Lancaster, 2012). Figure 7-4 shows an ecomap for the fictional Graham family. Both the genogram and the ecomap provide useful information and can be incorporated into family assessment (Correa et al., 2011; Ward & Hisley, 2009). The ecomap helps to overcome the issues of the genogram encountered when assessing nontraditional families. The ecomap uses a functional rather than a structural approach to the assessment of family roles and function.

Sexuality-Reproductive Pattern

Sexuality is the expression of sexual identity. The sexuality-reproductive pattern describes sexuality fulfillment (Gordon, 2011), including behavioral patterns of reproduction. This pattern also includes perceptions of satisfaction or disturbances in sexuality, sexual relationships, reproduction (including contraception), and developmental changes throughout the life span, such as menarche and menopause (Box 7-6: Hot Topics). The sexuality-reproductive pattern addresses transmission of information within the family about sexuality as well as sexuality for the couple, including their sexual relationship, perception of

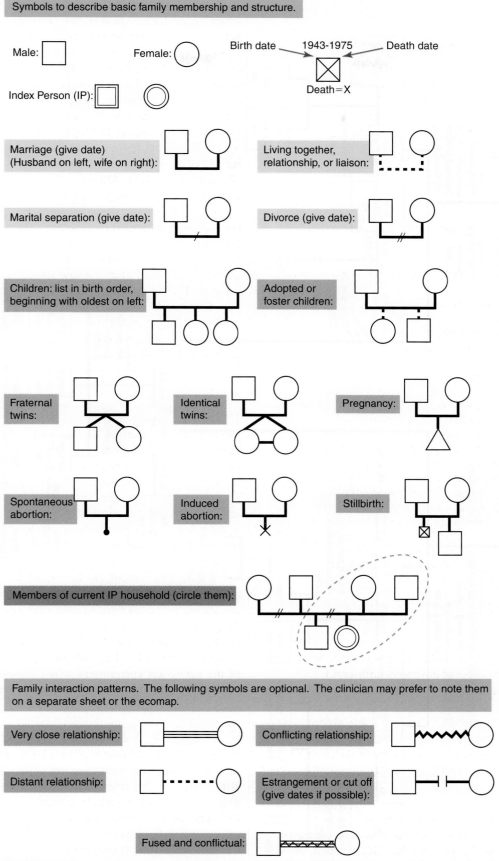

FIGURE 7-2 Genogram symbols. (Modified from McGoldrick, M., Gerson, R., & Petry, S. [2008]. *Genograms: Assessment and intervention* [3rd ed.]. New York: Norton.)

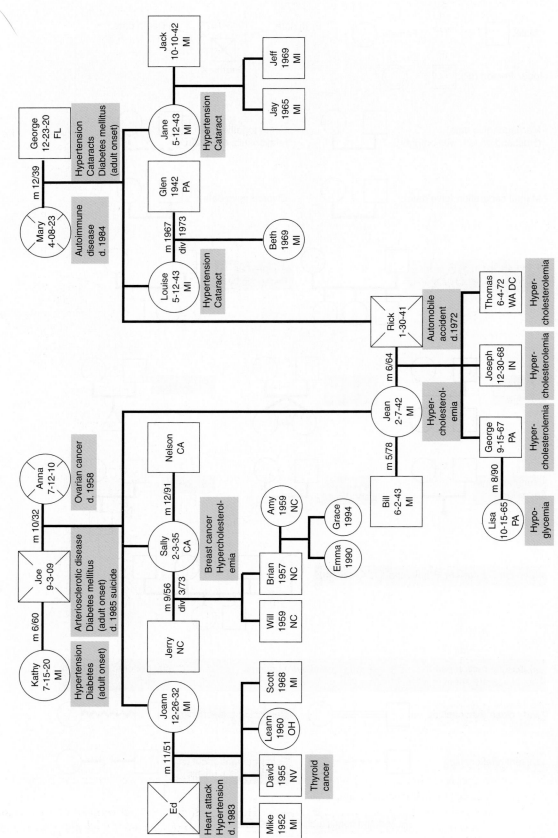

FIGURE 7-3 Genogram of the Graham family. (From Stanhope, M., & Lancaster, J. [2012]. *Public health nursing: Population-centered health care in the community* [8th ed., p. 634]. St. Louis: Mosby.)

FIGURE 7-4 Ecomap of the Graham family. (From Stanhope, M., & Lancaster, J. [2012]. *Public health nursing: Population-centered health care in the community* [8th ed., p. 636]. St. Louis: Mosby.)

problems, manner in which problems are handled, and actions taken to solve problems (Gordon, 2011). Information transmission during childhood is an important area to explore to better understand how issues related to sexuality and gender identity are addressed within the family (Gordon, 2011).

Topics to explore during the assessment may include the following areas:

- How do the adults in the family communicate needs to each other?
- How do family members commit to, love, and care for each other, as well as fulfill their obligations and responsibilities toward one another?
- How do the adults in the family view marriage, parenthood, and their relationship as lovers?

> **BOX 7-6   HOT TOPICS**
>
> ***Television, Aggressive Behavior, Sexuality, and Obesity***
>
> Television is one of the most pervasive influences in American society. During formative stages of development, children and adolescents view thousands of hours of television. This sedentary activity involves viewing scenes that depict violence and sexual relationships that are rapid, casual, and frequent. These scenes often convey status without depicting responsibility or consequences of actions. Although more research is needed, evidence shows that mass media influence aggressive behavior as well as beliefs about sexual behavior. In addition, as time viewing television programs increases, physical activity levels decrease.
>
> The American Academy of Pediatrics (AAP) has described the negative health effects of television viewing on children and adolescents. Among these effects are aggressive behavior, substance use, sexual activity, obesity, poor body image, and worse school performance. The AAP Committee on Public Education recommends that health professionals remain informed about these issues and use the resources available from AAP, such as the AAP Media Matters campaign and Media History Form. Strategies to ensure appropriate entertainment options should be available in agency waiting rooms and play rooms.
>
> In addition, body fat mass plays a role in accelerating puberty; therefore it is clear that prepubertal activity and nutrition contribute to sexual maturation at some level. These issues are essential to consider while evaluating the activity-exercise pattern.

From American Academy of Pediatrics (AAP). (2012). Media and children. Retrieved from http://www.aap.org/en-us/advocacy-and-policy/aap-health-initiatives/Pages/Media-and-Children.aspx; Huang, B., Biro, F. M., & Dorn, L. D. (2009). Determination of relative timing of pubertal maturation through ordinal logistic modeling: Evaluation of growth and timing parameters. *Journal of Adolescent Health, 45*(4), 383-388; Strasburger, V. C. (2009). Children, adolescents, and the media: What we know, what we don't know and what we need to find out (quickly!). *Arch Dis Child*, 94, 655-657.

- How does the family address family planning and birth control?
- How do family members participate in choice of family planning and contraceptives used?

When needed, complete pregnancy histories include sexual practices and partners, number and ages of children, number and outcome of pregnancies (including live births, miscarriages, spontaneous/therapeutic abortions), and birth control methods used. Nurses also observe comfort levels the adults demonstrate when discussing their own sexuality, or if an adult seems uninformed when discussing sexual subjects with children. Because of the impact that sexual relationships within the family have on children, exploring the variety of sexual practices within heterosexual, homosexual, and bisexual relationships in the family is an important part of health-promotion assessment (Hockenberry & Wilson, 2010; Lev, 2010; Lundy & Janes, 2010).

Coping-Stress Tolerance Pattern

The coping-stress tolerance pattern helps to depict the family's adaptation to both internal and external pressures (Gordon, 2011). On a daily basis family members generate energy to face evolving needs. Society continually compels families to adapt to new situations. Survival and growth depend on coping mechanisms as families face external demands required to move from one developmental stage to the next. The family's ability to cope with everyday living demands determines family success. Family relationships support coping or generate more stress. Life events, such as divorce, moving, or developmental stages of the life cycle, and economic hardships, such as loss of a job, provoke stress and mobilize family coping strategies. Exploration of coping and stress tolerance includes the following assessment areas:

- How does the family cope with stressful life events?
- What experiences have family members had with chemical abuse?
- What strengths does the family have and use to counterbalance the stresses?
- What stressful family situations are experienced?
- How does the family view the association between stress and children's health and development?
- How does the family make appraisals of the situations, and are they realistic?
- Describe the family's resources. How do family members use knowledge or links to family networks or community resources?
- What kinds of dysfunctional adaptive strategies are used, such as chemical abuse or violence?

Values-Beliefs Pattern

The values-beliefs pattern characterizes the family's perspective and attitudes about life meanings, values, beliefs, and spirituality and the way these issues affect behavior (Gordon, 2011). Assessment, diagnosis, and intervention are based on these attitudes. Assessment of this pattern enhances the interpretation of family behavior. Exploration of values and beliefs includes the following assessment areas:

- What are the values and beliefs held by the family?
- How flexible are rules?
- How do family members interact (calm, aggressive, competitive, or rigid)?
- How do family members view spirituality?
- Describe the cultural or ethnic group with which the family identifies. What family practices are consistent with the norms of that ethnic group? How are the practices inconsistent with these norms?
- What are the family's traditions and practices?
- How do the significant cultural beliefs affect health or illness?
- Describe the role that religion plays in the family on a regular basis and during times of stress. How does the family rely on religious practices?
- How does the family perceive its competency during crisis?
- What are the family goals and do members perceive that they are attaining these goals?
- How are value conflicts demonstrated within the family?
- How do identified family values affect the health status of the family?

Spirituality, defined as life purpose and connection with others, affects health. The metaphysical and transcendental phenomenon of spirituality as well as the religious and non-religious systems of belief within families should be assessed (Kaakinen et al., 2010). How well families communicate their unconditional love and forgiveness for injury or betrayal may contribute to physical symptoms within families. According to Kaakinen and colleagues (2010), spirituality and social skills promote health and prevent disease.

Data collected in the 11 functional patterns reveal ideas about family health-promotion and disease-prevention practices. Risks to healthy family functioning may be identified in each pattern. Risk factors may be found in more than one area. For example, passive smoke from one family member's cigarettes may be identified as an environmental risk factor in the home. However, the family's reaction to passive smoking determines their perceived susceptibility, their perceived severity of the problem, and whether they will make a change in the environment to promote family health. The pattern indicates high risk if chronic asthma is described during the family history. In this situation, several other pattern areas support the finding. The nurse determines each risk behavior along with its effects on the others.

ENVIRONMENTAL FACTORS

Environment also influences family health and well-being. Home, neighborhood, and community comprise the family environment. Assessment includes exploration of the following home environment areas (Figure 7-5):
- What type of dwelling is it (condominium, single dwelling, low-income apartment, or temporary shelter)?
- How has the family acquired their home (purchase, rental)?
- What is the condition of the home (interior/exterior: glass, trash, broken stairs, peeling paint, inadequate insulation, inadequate lighting on stairs, or broken fixtures)?
- Are the number and type of rooms adequate for the size of the family?
- How satisfactory are the furnishings to meet the needs of the family (enough chairs, beds, and a kitchen table)?
- How comfortable is the temperature (warm in winter and cool in summer, insulated)?
- How adequate is lighting for reading, sewing, and other activities?
- How adequate is the water supply (sufficient/clean/fluoridated/polluted)?
- Does the family have access to a telephone and are emergency numbers available?
- How safe are the kitchen sanitation and refrigeration capabilities?
- How adequate are the bathroom sanitation facilities, water supply, toilet, and towels and soap?
- Are sleeping arrangements adequate for family members, considering age, gender, relationships, and spatial needs?
- How adequate is the plan for escape in an emergency (smoke detectors/escape route/plan inside the home)?
- What are the arrangements and knowledge about first aid (directions posted for poisons, burns, lacerations, and other first-aid needs)?

FIGURE 7-5 Assessment of home includes environmental assessment of yard.

- What signs of rats, mice, or cockroaches are present inside or outside the home?
- What are the family's impressions about their home? How do they describe the adequacy of their living space for privacy, their own interests, and status?
- How are chemicals stored in the home (out of reach of children)?
- How is safety ensured in the home? What safety issues are evident?

Areas to explore for neighborhood assessment are as follows:
- What is the condition of the dwellings and streets (maintenance/deterioration)?
- How and when is the garbage collected?
- What is the incidence of violent crime, burglaries, and auto accidents?
- What kinds of industry are nearby and do they produce air pollution or toxic waste?
- What are the social class and ethnic characteristics of the neighborhood?
- What are the occupations and interests of the families in the neighborhood?
- What is the population density?
- How available and accessible is public transportation? Why is public transportation not used if it is available?

Exploration during assessment of the community includes the following areas:
- What resources, such as schools, church, transportation, shopping, and recreational facilities, are available for family use?
- How accessible are the health facilities, such as physician's office, clinic, hospital, gym, swimming pool, natural food store, and weight-reduction clinic?

By driving or walking around the area, the nurse can obtain neighborhood and community data. Other sources of information include the family, health professionals, teachers, business people, and others who work in the area. Official resources, such as the reports from the U.S. Census Department (www.census.gov/) or statistics from the city or state health departments and libraries, are also helpful in describing a neighborhood and community.

ANALYSIS AND NURSING DIAGNOSIS

Analyzing Data

After completing the data collection, the nurse and the family analyze the data. Several approaches are used to analyze health data, including systems theory, developmental theory, and risk-estimate theory. A systems approach categorizes families as open or closed, with permeable or rigid boundaries determining both structural and functional components of family systems. The 11 functional patterns organize baseline assessment data (**Website Resource 7B**).

Developmental theory approaches families from the perspective of tasks and progression through cycles. Nurses analyze data to identify accomplishment of family life cycle stages and family tasks needed to function successfully. Family developmental needs are determined considering the wide variety of family structures and functions in society. Although most family models are based on nuclear family structures, additional family structures should be explored as indicated by current population trends (Kaakinen et al., 2010; Maurer & Smith, 2009). Stages of family development guide the baseline data analysis. Identification of gaps, missing data, or conflicting information is obtained and clarified.

Couple Family

The first stage of family development begins when adults define themselves as a family regardless of the legal status. When individuals move from their family of origin to a new couple relationship, adaptation to role expectations of a partner becomes a developmental task for each individual. Establishing a mutually satisfying adult relationship that converges with the kinship network is one family developmental task. Adjustment for couples includes learning how to weave together two personalities, two life histories, and two aspirations of growth. Decisions in this stage include whether adults are gainfully employed, how money is managed, where they live, how they socialize with friends and other family members, patterns of sexual activities, and whether the couple has decided to have children. Determining how to divide household tasks of cooking, washing, cleaning, and shopping occurs either consciously or subconsciously.

Developmental tasks that integrate health practices and habits into the couple's lifestyle require consideration during analysis. Health behavior constitutes particular actions to promote health and prevent disease. Examples of health-promotion and disease-prevention activities may include maintaining well-balanced rest, exercise, diet, contraception; attending smoking-cessation classes; wearing seat belts; and directing activities toward self-actualization. Each individual brings values and beliefs to the relationship. Practices from the family of origin and values from personal experiences combine to form the adult beliefs of the individual. Achieving mutually satisfying relationships depends also on couples' conflict management. Strategies that stem from congruent value systems facilitate couple's adjustment. When couples use divergent strategies, problem-solving tends to be less effective.

Childbearing Family

Decisions about adding children to the family commit couples to more complex long-term responsibility. Family development and primary health needs change to focus on additional members. To analyze learning needs of pregnant couples, nurses consider aspects of decisions and motivations involved with the pregnancy. With single-parent families (usually mothers) becoming increasingly common through divorce, death, adoption, or the choice to have a child out of wedlock, analysis addresses these family structures (Kaakinen et al., 2010; Maurer & Smith, 2009).

Attitudes and practices in society regarding sexuality have influenced the incidence of sexually transmitted diseases such as genital herpes, gonorrhea, and syphilis. Acquired immunodeficiency syndrome (AIDS), first described in 1981, poses a threat to the family and society, in addition to affected individuals. Human immunodeficiency virus (HIV) is transmitted through heterosexual, homosexual, or oral sexual intercourse, as well as through direct contact with infected blood, shared needles during intravenous drug use, and perinatal transfer from infected mothers to their infants. Prevention of HIV transmission requires abstinence and modification of relevant behaviors.

Risk factors associated with sexuality include lack of knowledge about safe sexual practices, the reproductive system, and personal hygiene; lack of prenatal care; pregnancy before age 16; pregnancy after age 35; a history of hypertension or infection during pregnancy; and unplanned or unwanted pregnancy.

Risk factors for premature pregnancies and unsatisfying marriage consist of ignorance about, or values regarding, family planning; adolescent age; and sexuality and role adjustment problems. In unplanned pregnancies, adolescent parents put themselves and their developing child at risk. Lack of knowledge about prenatal care, childbirth, and childrearing practices compounds risks for both the mother and the child. Parents who are unable to perform parenting roles risk an unsatisfying relationship and inappropriate developmental growth for this beginning stage of the family life cycle. If couples decide to remain childless, learning needs include information about contraception.

Birth or adoption of a child begins a new family unit. Family members adjust to new roles as the unit expands in function and responsibility. As described more fully in the cultural competence section of this chapter (see Formulating Family Nursing Diagnosis), parents' history as a dyad and their experiences in other groups, particularly their families of origin, influence the development of the triad (Box 7-7: Diversity Awareness). Accommodating new members disrupts family equilibrium. As a group, families explore ways to meet each other's needs, to minimize differences, and work together. First-time parents

BOX 7-7 DIVERSITY AWARENESS

Preconception Care

Preconception care is a significant health-promotion opportunity for the whole family. The importance of this care has been recognized by *Healthy People 2020*, the Institute of Medicine, and the Public Health Services Expert Panel on the Content of Prenatal Care.

One important area of preconception care is evaluating a couple's genetic history as documented on the standard family genogram. Further evaluation should be considered for couples who are related outside marriage or who have ethnic backgrounds such as Mediterranean, Black, or Ashkenazi Jew, and for women older than 35 years of age or younger than 16 years of age who have preexisting medical conditions. Couples who have family histories of any of the following health problems should be referred for further genetic testing and counseling: cystic fibrosis, hemophilia, phenylketonuria, Tay-Sachs disease, thalassemia, sickle cell disease or trait, birth defects, or mental retardation.

often feel a lack of emotional support during the first several months of parenthood. Some, but not all, new parents have available family leave policies that may facilitate this transition. Without a family network or friends, the first days after the birth or adoption may be difficult. Parents may care for the child proficiently, but may need assistance to grow in the parenting role. If parents are both employed outside the home, they may encounter difficulty with the routines of baby care and being confined to the house more for child care. Anxiety about the adequacy of income may cause parents to increase work hours to increase income. Exhaustion for both parents is common from working full-time while providing child care as the infant develops. Single parents, usually mothers, carry these same burdens alone. Emotional support may be limited, particularly if one has not found satisfaction in parenthood. Families of origin or other support systems, such as self-help groups, neighbors, or friends, assist family members as they struggle to adapt to a new member (Kaakinen et al., 2010; Lundy & Janes, 2010). Nurses facilitate this process to promote health in the newly formed family unit.

Some parents thrive during the period when an infant needs almost constant care and nurturing. These parents find support in a network of family and friends. Couples who find satisfaction in parenthood seem to realize that parental influence begins at birth and is the single most important factor in the child's physical, emotional, and cognitive development. The parents' ability to assume responsibility depends on a complex array of factors: their own maturity; how they were nurtured as children; their conceptions about self, culture, social class, and religion; their relationship with each other; their values and philosophy of life; their perceptions of and experiences with children and other adults; and the life stresses they have experienced.

In analyzing needs of childrearing families, nurses consider many factors, including providing for physical health, economic support, and nurturing actions that are vital to learning and social development of children. In analyzing couples' needs during this stage, nurses recognize the importance of interactions among the triad. Observing decision-making helps nurses determine family functioning, member roles, and effectiveness

of family members. Risks associated with role relationships include working parents with insufficient resources for child care, abuse or neglect of children, multiple closely spaced children, low family self-esteem, children used as scapegoats for parental frustration, immature parents who are dependent and unable to handle responsibility, and strong beliefs about physical punishment or obedience.

Family with Toddlers/Preschool Children

Families may have more than one child, each growing and developing at an individual pace. Preschool children place great demands on families. Families adjust to each new member with space and equipment for expansion. Needs and interests of preschool children influence home environments. Nurses assess the quality of the home environment for whether children have healthy amounts of stimulation-promoting opportunities. Safety balanced with exploration by the child results in health-promoting home environments. Rather than removing children from the kitchen or garden, finding ways to include them in a cooking or planting activity provides learning experiences. Other environmental influences affecting the child's rate and style of development include religious practices, ethnic background, education, and discipline techniques.

Evidence increasingly demonstrates the link between environment and health. Home environments that contain contaminated air, water, or food increase health risks. For example, lead poisoning, a preventable disease that continues to affect thousands of children, often results from lead paint and other factors in the home. Although restrictions exist in the United States to limit lead-based paint to exteriors, many homes have lead within the interior. Both homes and automobiles are considered possible sources of exposure to the poisonous agent carbon monoxide. Nurses also review data for home safety, including storage of dangerous materials, such as detergents, insecticides, and medications.

Health-promotion needs for young children include proper foods, adequate exercise and sleep, and dental hygiene. Parents teach children through modeling and use of positive reinforcement. Family developmental tasks include adjusting to fatigue resulting from parenting demands. Nurses explore alternatives to relieve parents. Parents need time for themselves, individually and as a couple (e.g., to exercise, socialize), while knowing their children are safe with a responsible person. Economic restraints may limit relaxation time away from the children. Sharing child care with friends and family provides one source of support for new parents.

Family with School-Aged Children

A family with children in school may have reached its maximal size in numbers and interrelationships. The parents' major problem during this stage is the dichotomy between pursuing self-interests and finding fulfillment in producing the next generation. Family developmental tasks revolve around goals of reorganization to prepare for the expanding world of school-aged children. School achievement becomes a critical task for socialization. Viewing social and educational goals from the perspective of family culture and parents' defined goals becomes

FIGURE 7-6 School-age girl learns about her family heritage and presents this information through a school project.

particularly important during this developmental stage. For example, many opportunities for health education exist in schools, including influencing healthy beliefs and behaviors. However, school health programs focus on problems such as tobacco and substance abuse with messages aimed at problems and crises rather than healthy behaviors. Families influence health at home and in school both by teaching children ways to assess and manage risky situations and by describing the benefits to expect when healthy behaviors are practiced.

As children's activities broaden away from the home, another important developmental task for both parent and child becomes "letting go." Parents become involved in community groups such as the parent-teacher association, scout groups, sports teams, and other volunteer organizations. Encouraging children to join in family discussions to learn about their heritage can foster understanding of self within the family network (Figure 7-6). Children exposed to unsafe home environments are at risk for behavior disturbances, school problems, and learning disabilities. Parents who cannot manage their children in growth-promoting ways soon experience energy depletion and may turn to dysfunctional relief from parenting (e.g., drug and alcohol abuse).

Family with Adolescents

Parents with adolescent children may experience a late pregnancy, resulting in care for an infant while other children in the family are in school. A new family member at this stage may be a source of joy or frustration for the family. The overall goal with adolescent members is to loosen family ties to allow greater responsibility and freedom in preparation for releasing young adults. Although each member of the family strives to achieve individual developmental tasks in the midst of social pressures, the family as a whole has tasks to accomplish. Strengthening

the marital relationship to build a foundation for future family stages is a critical task during this time.

Open communication is often difficult during this stage, partly because of the differing developmental tasks of adolescents and adults. Adolescents seek their own identity, and adults attempt to facilitate adolescent decision-making processes. Choices about values and lifestyles may differ. Adolescents may challenge family values and standards. Although parents maintain some authority, adolescents tackle their own desires and needs. Adolescents want to do what their friends do, have their own cars, and make their own money to spend in ways that they see fit. Parents who give adolescent members opportunities to experience social, emotional, and ethical situations with others are providing learning opportunities to enhance their sense of autonomy and responsibility. As adolescents become mature and emancipated, families face balancing freedom with responsibility. Health problems in this age group include violent deaths including suicide, injuries, and alcohol and drug abuse. Contributing risk factors involve lack of problem-solving skills, family values of aggressiveness and competition, socioeconomic factors, peer relationships, rigid and inflexible family values, daredevil risk-taking attitudes, and conflicts between parents and children. Environmental risk-related violent deaths and injuries are influenced by the highway system, automobile manufacturers, and the legislation of standards of safety. Families rely on public health officials and nurses' efforts as advocates to reduce environmental risks.

Families support adolescents in this stage of development by including them in decision-making and ensuring that they experience the positive and negative consequences of their choices. Family values of winning at all costs, aggressiveness, and competition may need to be explored during this period. Adolescents may discard these values if they are no longer applicable. Considerable change in adolescent values produces conflict and poses a threat to family cohesiveness. Families may place pressure on adolescents to conform to family values. In matters of life and death—for example, in regard to driving rules—parents must stay firm.

Families with adolescents experience identity crises for the adolescent, the adults, and the family as a whole. Adolescents move from childhood to adulthood while adults progress beyond parenthood. Adolescents struggle to find independent identities that remain connected to their family. Adults, in midlife, must resolve their own adolescent fantasies to move toward an identity for their remaining life.

Family with Young Adults

Families with young adults act as a launching center when children begin to leave home. As children leave home, parents relinquish their parenting roles of many years to return to the marital dyad. The couple builds a new life together while maintaining relationships with aging parents, children, grandchildren, and in-laws. Couples focus on redefining relationships during this stage. For a woman, the role as mother changes, because children no longer need their mother in the same way as during childhood. When mothers devote years to raising children, they must realize a changed role and purpose within the family. Transition from a life with children as the priority to new or renewed interests (e.g., career, community service) may require assistance and support for both parents. Careers for both parents at this stage may become more stable. Developmental tasks at this stage for both adults require focus on future prospects. In addition to individual changes occurring within couples, families with young adults may experience other pressures. Aging parents and adult children may require financial or emotional support. Financial and emotional responsibilities to other family members hinder the couple's ability to focus on the marital relationship during this developmental phase. Health-promoting activities to focus on during this stage include coping with pressures of social roles and occupational responsibilities, maintaining health tasks to promote healthy aging, and reassessing life goals.

Family with Middle-Aged Adults

Families consisting of only two members are able to enhance self-concept and support the marital relationship during middle age. Usually children have left home and parents experience a sense of freedom and well-being. Some marriages, by this stage, have reached a level of security and stability; husband and wife meet each other's needs. Parenting pressures diminish, allowing them to enjoy the accomplishments of their children and grandchildren. Couples have acquired a network of friends. Long-time acquaintances seek participation from the couple in neighborhood rituals and events. Economic security and personal self-esteem may be at a peak.

In contrast, some marriages falter at this time. Departed children create a quiet house with less activity, known as the "empty nest." When unprepared for this stage, individuals might seek opportunities to enhance self-concept from outside of the marriage. The couple, thinking that their parenting role is now complete, may develop feelings of inadequacy or begin a new relationship, start a new family, or resort to substance abuse. In addition, this life phase may include becoming grandparents; parenting grandchildren; coping with the needs of middle-aged children; and caring for older adults (children, siblings, or parents).

Health tasks in this developmental stage require new awareness of susceptibility or vulnerability to health problems. Couples adjust their lifestyle and habits to cope with health risks. Losses promote health problems, and at this stage couples begin to cope with deaths among family and friends, along with declining income. If either member has developed physical or mental illness, the other adjusts to resultant physical and mental impairments, redefining self-concept.

Middle-aged families face a host of risk factors leading to three prevalent causes of death: (1) heart disease, (2) cancer, and (3) cerebrovascular accident (stroke). Family lifestyle may decrease risks by placing a high value on being physically active, refraining from smoking, maintaining adequate and sound nutritional habits, and consuming moderate amounts of alcohol. Lifestyle habits that are transmitted through role modeling have a greater influence on the younger members of the family than any verbal edict. Middle-aged members positively influence their health if they are able to choose environments low in water and air pollution and free from crippling stress factors such as excessive noise, traffic, and overcrowding. Family members can also apply pressure on key members of the community to decrease risks in the environment.

Family with Older Adults

Retirement affects many aspects of life for couples and each individual in the family and their relationships with others. Besides decreased work hours, retirement also means reduction in income and fixed incomes for most people. Adjusting living standards to retirement income and being able to supplement this income with wage-earning activity is one task of the family with older adults. Other tasks during this stage include ensuring a safe and comfortable home environment, preparing for end of life, and adjusting to the loss of a spouse (Kaakinen et al., 2010). Surviving spouses often look to their family for support and satisfaction (Kaakinen et al., 2010). Illness may create further dependence on family members (Kaakinen et al., 2010).

Health promotion aims to maintain functional ability, limit effects of disabling conditions, and maintain quality of life. Older adults may fear becoming helpless, feeling useless, and being incapable of caring for themselves. When analyzing risk factors in the aging family, nurses look for the couple's ability to function well enough to carry out normal roles and responsibilities. As with all people, older adults hope for a state of well-being that will allow them to function at their highest capacity physically, psychologically, socially, and spiritually (Figure 7-7). Many older adults remain in their own homes, and most of these individuals are vigorous and completely independent (Kaakinen et al., 2010).

Ego integrity (the union of all previous phases of the life cycle) is the challenge in this stage and demands successful aging through continued activity. Having gone through the various stages of family development, the couple accepts what they have done as their own. At this time, they may need family or professional support to pursue other interests or maintain former activities to feel needed and useful.

The nurse and family jointly analyze the information comparing the family's data to documented norms of health promotion and disease prevention in older adults. Norms or expected values can be derived from the family's baseline information of 11 functional pattern areas, knowledge of growth and development for all age groups and the family as a whole, risk-factor estimates, and population norms. Population norms specify normal ranges for these groups. For example, age is associated with various risk factors; some disorders are so common that they are referred to as diseases of the older person. In certain diseases, such as lung cancer, there is a long period of exposure. Risk increases with cumulative exposure; therefore, the incidence and prevalence of diseases increase with age.

Sexuality. Because of the popular perception that older adults are asexual, their sexual concerns may be disregarded (Miracle & Miracle, 2009). Strength of sexual desire of the older women may be more influenced by age, education, and attitude than by biomedical factors (Jeffers & DiBartolo, 2011; Miracle & Miracle, 2009; Trudel et al., 2010; Wallace, 2008).

FIGURE 7-7 As with all people older adults hope for a state of well-being that allows them to function at their highest capacity physically.

General population norms for values, beliefs, self-perception, or role relationships may be less available than physical population norms. Cultural, ethnic, and religious factors contribute to values and beliefs about health. Family baseline information provides important comparative criteria for analysis. Family records provide useful information when available. The first contact assessment provides baseline information for subsequent comparison and evaluation of progress. Whether the family perceives situations to be problematic should also be considered in the analysis phase. Nurse and family perceptions about problems may differ (Trudel et al., 2010). Newman's definitions of family health, presented in **Website Resource 7C,** provide a framework to view increased awareness or consciousness of a family's health (Pharris, 2011; Smith, 2011).

Formulating Family Nursing Diagnoses

Writing a family nursing diagnosis helps families promote health throughout the life cycle and prevents disease through decreasing risk-taking behaviors. Nurses derive diagnoses from assessed validated data. As a concise summary statement of a problem or potential problem, diagnoses provide direction for outcomes and interventions by identifying negative health states and factors to change to alleviate or prevent the problem (see Chapter 6). Examples of family nursing diagnoses using developmental and risk-factor approaches are presented in **Website Resource 7D.** Describing health and validating potential or actual health problems with families facilitates cooperation. Assessment and negotiation continue until agreement occurs and a plan for resolution develops.

Cultural competence and respect for familial beliefs forms a foundation for the nursing process of assessing, determining nursing diagnoses, planning, intervening, and evaluating (refer to Chapter 2 for more detail). With changing trends in families and shifts in heritage within society, cultural competence becomes a priority within nursing practice and should take an organizational approach to addressing the issue of organizational responsiveness to diversity as well as professional competence (Leever, 2011). Cultural values, such as those connected to nutrition, influence most health-promotion practices (Kime, 2009). As globalization occurs, diversity will also expand and competent care for indiginous populations and migrating populations will be needed (Andrews & Boyle, 2011; Moodley, 2011; Sidumo et al., 2010). Cultural competence increases efficacy of health promotion for all families, particularly families from within vulnerable populations (Andrews & Boyle, 2011; Kaakinen et al., 2010).

PLANNING WITH THE FAMILY

Intervention planning stems from complete assessment, analysis, and nursing diagnosis. The plan's purpose aims for behavioral change in families to promote health or prevent dysfunction. As in the assessment phase, family members play an active role in the planning process. Family responsibility for personal health status enhances success of behavioral change outcomes. The planning process involves several steps, with the nurse and family identifying the following:

- Order of priority for problems or potential problems
- Items that can be handled by the nurse and the family and items that must be referred to others
- Actions and expected outcomes

The nursing plan provides direction for implementation and the framework for evaluation (see the Care Plan at the end of this chapter).

As mentioned, a family's health status can be diagnosed as functional, potentially dysfunctional, or dysfunctional. Functional family health status warrants verification by the nurse with a plan for periodic reevaluation that is formulated jointly. Plans to continue healthy living behaviors are reinforced. The nurse provides specific information requested by the family, such as immunization schedules, growth and development milestones, and recommended dietary allowances. In working with healthy families, the nurse controls the assessment and analysis phases of the nursing process. If the health status is judged functional, then planning health education materials, scheduling periodic examinations, and providing accessibility of the nurse remain professional responsibilities. Implementation and evaluation of health-promotion activities become family responsibilities.

In health-promotion and disease-prevention settings, life-threatening situations rarely occur; however, when such situations do occur they become the highest priority for intervention. For other identified potential or actual problems, the nurse relies on the family to decide which problem or potential problem to approach. After the ordering of priorities is established, the family and nurse determine who will work on the problem. Problems or potential problems to be resolved by the nurse are identified separately from those requiring referral or family intervention. Problems for the family to handle or those the family is already addressing are considered strengths and are acknowledged and supported by the nurse. For example, when there is consistency among values and actions, physical fitness, weight management, and ability to cope with stress, the family is already taking informed and responsible action in these areas. The extent to which family members can provide their own health promotion and disease prevention will depend on their knowledge, skills, motivation, and orientation toward health.

Problems that need medical, legal, or social attention are referred to appropriate agencies. The nurse should have a directory of resources in the community when referrals are needed. Nursing intervention requires clearly stated actions that are purposeful, moral, capable of being accomplished, and adapted to the particular life situation, beliefs, and expectations of the family.

Goals

Goals are statements describing desired outcomes. Family outcome statements include expected family behaviors, circumstances for exhibited behaviors, and criteria for determining performance. Health-promotion goals reflect a desire to function at a higher level of health and to grow beyond maintaining health or preventing disease.

IMPLEMENTATION WITH THE FAMILY

The implementation phase is dynamic. As the nurse and family work together, new information is used to adapt and change the plan as necessary. Family nursing interventions aim to assist families in carrying out functions that members cannot perform for themselves. In health promotion and disease prevention, nurses assist families to improve their capacity to act on their own behalf (Kaakinen et al., 2010).

Families may know that they take risks by smoking, drinking, and engaging in a stressful lifestyle. As the nurse explains the rationale behind proposed changes, families may choose to deny how they jeopardize their future health and continue their risk-taking behaviors. Factors that the nurse has not considered may cause the family's resistance. For example, families may have more pressing basic needs such as food, clothing, and housing. The Affordable Healthcare Act (2010) addressed some of these health care issues of the family by permitting parents to retain children on their health insurance plans until the age of 26 years, regardless of their marital status, living situations, or employment (unless in some cases where health insurance is an employee benefit). New insurance plans must cover preventive benefits such as well-child visits and immunizations without additional cost to the insured. Although the Patient Protection and Affordable Care Act (PL 111-148) became law on March 23, 2010, and was amended by the Health Care and Education Reconciliation Act of 2010 (HCERA, PL 111-152), the statute was brought before the U.S. Supreme Court beginning March 26, 2012, as unconstitutional, citing four major arguments (requiring the Individual Mandate, applying the Anti–Injunction Act, lacking a Severability Clause, and expanding Medicaid). The Supreme Court ruled in favor of the statute in June 2012.

Health promotion and disease prevention may not have been part of the family's life experiences, giving the nurse the educational task to try to change attitudes and values by expanding the options for families to consider health promotion. Four types of nursing interventions appear in health-promotion and disease-prevention planning: increasing knowledge and skills; increasing strengths; decreasing exposure; and decreasing susceptibility. Increasing knowledge and skills to improve family capacity for health-promotion and disease-prevention behavior may be the primary strategy. Use of this strategy helps families make informed choices about healthful lifestyle behaviors and to eliminate harmful environmental influences that affect health. Improved knowledge aims to create awareness as the nurse and family work together to uncover actual or potential problems. Nurses recognize particular families at risk and move toward motivating and supporting behavioral change in these families. Box 7-8: Innovative Practice presents an example of one program that provides education and support to people with cancer and their families.

Family strengths or forces that contribute to family unity and solidarity foster the development of inherent family potential (Kaakinen et al., 2010). These factors include the following:

- Physical, emotional, and spiritual factors
- Healthy childrearing practices and discipline
- Meaningful and clear communication
- Support, security, and encouragement
- Growth-producing relationships and experiences
- Responsible community relationships
- Growth with and through children
- Self-help and acceptance of help
- Flexibility in family functions and roles
- Mutual respect for individuality
- Crisis as a means for growth
- Family unity and loyalty and intrafamily cooperation
- Adaptability of family strengths

In recent years, a shift of family health care from an illness or problem and deficiency focus to a strength-based focus has occurred (Rawana, 2009). Multiple models in nursing view families as systems and base their assessment and nursing process on strengths rather than deficits (Kaakinen et al., 2010; Marshall et al., 2010). These models of nursing provide the framework to assess and plan care using family strengths and resources (Kaakinen et al., 2010). Kaakinen and colleagues (2010) describe how family members develop and maintain health-promoting behaviors by using commitment, appreciation, affection, positive communication, time together, a sense of spiritual well-being, and ability to cope with stress and crisis. Multiple assessment tools are available for nurses to use to generate discussion among family members about their strengths. Marshall and colleagues (2010) identify corresponding nursing interventions to support and further develop the family dynamics of socialization, support, and nurturance. Additionally, Kaakinen and colleagues (2010) describe the importance of understanding the significance of family legacy to a family's health and related health practices.

Families with significant strengths may need to learn new, unfamiliar skills for mastering a specific technique such as meditation and to apply new tools for decision-making. These

✳ BOX 7-8   INNOVATIVE PRACTICE

The Wellness Community and Gilda's Club

The Wellness Community, which was founded in the 1982 by Dr. Harold Benjamin in California, has many local chapters throughout the United States. Comedian Gilda Radner attended the Wellness Community during her battle with ovarian cancer and shared her experiences in her book, *It's Always Something*. After her death, Joel Siegel and Mandy Patinkin began Gilda's Club and opened the first club house in New York in 1991 with the support of her spouse Gene Wilder. These two organizations shared 45 years of offering free educational and support programs for people with cancer and their families on both coasts. Emphasis is placed on family to acknowledge that no person with cancer makes their journey alone. Weekly support groups help family members support one another, explore new ways of coping with the stresses of cancer, and learn ways to become the most effective partners possible with their health care teams. These two organizations now have partnered to continue their vision with the Cancer Support Community to "ensure that all people impacted by cancer are empowered by knowledge and strengthened by action, and sustained by community."

These communities now offer a wide variety of workshops and programs (Gentle Strength and Stretch, Meditation and Guided Imagery, Nutrition Matters, Nutrition and the Immune System, Nutrition at Midlife: Preventing Heart Disease and Osteoporosis, Tai Chi, Yoga, Mindfulness, and Feng Shui). Social events are organized (Comfort Food Potluck Dinner, Couples Networking Groups, Singles Networking Group, Family and Friends Networking Group). Although chapters generally do not charge for their services, donations are appreciated and necessary to help serve the thousands of people living with cancer and their families.

Contact Information:
Cancer Support Community
1050 17th Street, NW
Suite 500
Washington, DC 20036
Phone: 202-659-9709
Toll Free: 888-793-9355
Fax: 202-659-9301
E-mail: http://cancersupportcommunity.org/Functional-Menu/Contact-Us.html
Website: http://cancersupportcommunity.org/default.aspx

families rarely require ongoing supervision or support of sustained interventions aimed at changing their coping patterns, communication, or role behavior. They may be highly capable of seeking and using information. Assisting functional families may simply involve providing information in terms that can be understood and offering opportunities to ask questions and clarify information. Unit 3 contains individual chapters devoted to many of the strategies commonly employed in health-promotion intervention, such as health teaching and counseling.

Decreasing exposure to risk factors may include enhancing parents' ability to assess and adjust their behavior to their child's temperament. Parents with limited literacy may need assistance to learn to respond constructively to their child's communication attempts. Health promotion includes teaching parents to avoid exposure to risks—for example, to use adequate restraints in automobiles, to protect their toddler from wandering into dangerous streets, and to supervise children to avoid falls and hazardous materials.

Although no substitute can be found for continuous supervision of a child, homes can be made safer by moving common hazards out of children's reach. This effort includes storing all cleaning solutions and medications beyond children's reach; erecting barriers in front of exposed heaters, high windows, and stairways; keeping pots and pans turned inward on the stove; fencing in a yard or a swimming pool; and teaching children to avoid dangerous areas. Becoming aware of peeling paint and toxic chemicals that parents might carry home from the job on their clothing can also protect the child.

Decreasing susceptibility means educating families about prevention principles. Families who realize how diseases are spread are better able to avoid transmission from person to person; through air, water, and food; and by insects and the rodents on which insects live. Health promotion includes emphasizing the role of personal hygiene and cleanliness to avoid infection. Families who know signs and symptoms that require medical attention and how to treat minor illnesses are better able to maintain healthy environments.

Pender and colleagues (2011) cite research that demonstrates how perceived susceptibility predicts preventive behavior. Perceived susceptibility is the family's estimated subjective probability that a specific health problem will be encountered. Family perceptions of health risks and their susceptibility to them will determine how they change their behavior. If the overweight family believes obesity is a threat to the health of their family, they are more likely to react positively to the changes suggested by the nurse than a family who perceives no health threat. Nurses who introduce threat as a motivator to action are morally obligated to reduce the threat by meaningful and purposeful interventions. Table 7-3 lists various nursing roles used in the implementation stage.

EVALUATION WITH THE FAMILY

The purpose of evaluation is to determine how the family has responded to the planned interventions and whether these interventions were successful. Goals and objectives that are stated in specific behavioral terms will make evaluation much easier than when they are given in general terms. Criteria used to evaluate interventions, such as weight change, increased lung capacity from an exercise program, and lower pulse rate as a result of relaxation exercises, are simple to measure. Other results of health promotion and disease prevention are not as easy to measure but must be considered in the evaluation step of the nursing process. When considering such factors as values, beliefs, self-perceptions, or role relationships, the nurse may base the evaluation on whether the family indicates that the interventions were successful. Additionally, the family's baseline data are used as comparative criteria in evaluation. The nurse reassesses the situation and compares the new information with that on the original assessment to determine whether change has occurred.

The following five measures of family functioning can be used to determine the effectiveness of interventions: changes in interaction patterns; effective communication; ability to express emotions; responsiveness to needs of members as individuals;

TABLE 7-3	POSSIBLE NURSE'S ROLES IN HEALTH PROMOTION AND DISEASE PREVENTION THROUGH STAGES OF FAMILY DEVELOPMENT
STAGE	**POSSIBLE NURSING ROLE**
Couple	Counselor on sexual and role adjustment
	Teacher of and counselor on family planning
	Teacher of parenting skills
	Coordinator for genetic counseling
	Facilitator in interpersonal relationships
Childbearing family	Monitor of prenatal care and referrer for problems of pregnancy
	Counselor on prenatal nutrition
	Counselor on prenatal maternal habits
	Supporter of amniocentesis
	Counselor on breastfeeding
	Coordinator with pediatric services
	Supervisor of immunizations
	Referrer to social services
	Assistant in adjustment to prenatal role
Family with preschool or school-age children	Monitor of early childhood development; referrer when indicated
	Teacher of first-aid and emergency measures
	Coordinator with pediatric services
	Counselor on nutrition and exercise
	Teacher of dental hygiene
	Counselor on environmental safety in home
	Facilitator in interpersonal relationships
Family with adolescents	Teacher of risk factors to health
	Teacher of problem-solving issues regarding alcohol, smoking, diet, and exercise
	Facilitator of interpersonal skills with adolescents and parents
	Direct supporter of, counselor on, or referrer to mental health resources
	Counselor on family planning
	Referrer for sexually transmittable disease
Family with young or middle-age adults	Participant in community organizations involved in disease control
	Teacher of problem-solving issues regarding lifestyle and habits
	Participant in community organization involved in environmental control
	Case finder in home and community
	Screener for hypertension, Pap smear, breast examination, cancer signs, mental health, and dental care
	Counselor on menopausal transition
Family with older adults	Facilitator of interpersonal relationships among family members
	Referrer for work and social activity, nutritional programs, homemakers' services, and nursing home
	Monitor of exercise, nutrition, preventive services, and medications
	Supervisor of immunization
	Counselor on safety in home
	Counselor on bereavement

and problem-solving ability. Using these measures, the nurse returns to the original assessment of the family's functioning and compares current observations with previous data. These characteristics of family functioning continue to provide a useful framework even today, when family structures are becoming more diverse and the nuclear family less prevalent (Kaakinen et al., 2010).

When, during the planning phase of the nursing process, the nurse has identified the criteria (norms and standards) for the desired outcomes, these outcomes are the basis of evaluation. Data from the family that describe their behavior relative to the desired outcomes determine whether the nursing care was successful. With the criteria stated, the goals and objectives outline how the family can demonstrate a successful outcome and the behavior change expected to result from nursing intervention. The more objective and measurable the desired outcome is, the more reliable the results of evaluation will be.

After the goals and objectives are reached, the problem no longer exists. If evaluation shows the nursing actions did not achieve the goals or objectives, the nurse must review the nursing process to determine whether there were gaps in the assessment data, errors in analysis or nursing diagnosis, or alternative interventions that might have been considered. The nurse also needs to review the process with the family to determine whether they have contributed to outcome failure. Finally, the agency employing the nurse may be another factor; if intervention is costly or a shortage of staff exists, then health promotion and disease prevention may have low priority.

CASE STUDY

Family Member with Alzheimer's Disease: Mark and Jacqueline

Mark and Jacqueline have been married for 30 years. They have grown children who live in another state. Jacqueline's mother has moved in with the couple because she has Alzheimer's disease. Jacqueline is an only child and always promised her mother that she would care for her in her old age. Her mother is unaware of her surroundings and often calls out for her daughter Jackie when Jacqueline is in the room. Jacqueline reassures her mother that she is there to help, but to no avail. Jacqueline is unable to visit her children on holidays because she must attend to her mother's daily needs. She is reluctant to visit friends or even go out to a movie because of her mother's care needs or because she is too tired. Even though she has eliminated most leisure activities with Mark, Jacqueline goes to bed at night with many of her caregiving tasks unfinished. She tries to visit with her mother during the day, but her mother rejects any contact with her daughter. Planning for the upcoming holidays seems impossible to Mark, because of his wife's inability to focus on anything except her mother's care. Jacqueline has difficulty sleeping at night and is unable to discuss plans even a few days in advance. She is unable to visit friends and is reluctant to have friends visit because of the unpredictable behavior of her mother and her need to attend to the daily care.

Reflective Questions
1. How do you think this situation reflects Jacqueline's sense of role performance?
2. How do you think that Jacqueline may be contributing to her own health?

◎ CARE PLAN

Family Member with Alzheimer's Disease: Mark and Jacqueline

*NURSING DIAGNOSIS: Risk for Ineffective Role Performance related to caring for a family member with Alzheimer's disease

Defining Characteristics
- Feeling exhausted
- Inability to complete tasks
- Feeling loss of usual or expected relationship with care receiver
- Increased stress or nervousness about the future
- Preoccupation with care routine
- Withdrawal from social contacts or change in leisure activities

Related Factors
- Illness severity of care receiver
- Increasing needs of care receiver
- Addiction or codependency of caregiver or care receiver
- Conflicting role demands
- Caregiver health impairment
- Unpredictable illness course or instability in the care receiver's health
- Psychological or cognitive problems in the care receiver
- Caregiver not developmentally ready for caregiving role
- Developmental delay or retardation of the care receiver or caregiver
- Marginal family adaptation or dysfunction before caregiving situation began
- Marginal coping patterns of caregiver
- Providing direct, ongoing in-home care
- History of poor relationship between caregiver and care receiver
- Care receiver who exhibits deviant, bizarre behavior
- Incontinence in the care receiver

Expected Outcomes
- Caregiver distinguishes obligations that must be fulfilled from those that can be controlled or limited.

- In conjunction with the nurse, the caregiver develops a plan of care for the individual.
- Caregiver receives and accepts appropriate levels of support from family members, friends, and others.
- Caregiver describes help available from informal and formal support systems in the community and takes steps to obtain help.

Interventions
- Assess the level of the caregiver's stress.
- Assist the caregiver in developing a realistic plan of care, considering the care receiver's abilities and limitations; the plan will require modification as the person decompensates.
- Instruct the caregiver to encourage the person to participate, to the greatest extent possible, in social and self-care activities such as bathing, dressing, dining out with friends, and playing cards.
- Facilitate a family meeting to help the primary caregiver seek assistance from other family members.
- Support the caregiver and family members as they adjust to the degenerative nature of the disease; be aware that over time the stress associated with caring for the person increases.
- Identify community resources that may offer the caregiver relief from constant supervision of the individual (home health aides, respite care, and adult day care).
- Help the caregiver contact informal sources of support, such as church groups, extended family, and community volunteers.
- Encourage the caregiver to attend an Alzheimer's support group.
- Refer the caregiver to the Alzheimer's Association.

* *NANDA Nursing Diagnoses—Definitions and Classification 2012-2014*, Herdman T.H. (ED). Copyright © 2012, 1994-2012 NANDA International. Used by arrangement with John Wiley & Sons Limited. In order to make safe and effective judgments using the NANDA-I nursing diagnoses it is essential that nurses refer to the definitions and defining characteristics of the diagnoses listed in this work.
Modified from Carpenito-Moyet, L. J. (2010). *Nursing diagnosis: Application to clinical practice* (13th ed.). Philadelphia: Lippincott Williams & Wilkins.

SUMMARY

Learning about health promotion and disease prevention begins at birth, with the family providing the stimulus for incorporating health in the value system of its members. From a systems perspective, the family has both structure and function; relevant functions include values and practices related to health. The effective execution of health-related functions involves the family's progression through its developmental tasks and its ability to generate low risk-producing behaviors associated with disease prevention.

Developmental and risk-estimate theories can be applied effectively to the nursing process with the family. The nurse uses functional patterns (an inherent part of both theories) to collect data for assessment. After organizing information on family life cycle stages for analysis with the family, the nurse writes the nursing diagnosis and plans, implements, and evaluates the interventions used to promote health and prevent disease in the family.

REFERENCES

American Academy of Pediatrics (AAP). (2012). *Media and children*. Retrieved from http://www.aap.org/en-us/advocacy-and-policy/aap-health-initiatives/Pages/Media-and-Children.aspx.

Andrews, M. M., & Boyle, J. S. (2011). *Transcultural concepts in nursing care* (6th ed.). New York: Lippincott.

Benzies, K., & Mychasiuk, R. (2009). Fostering family resiliency: A review of the key protective factors. *Child & Family Social Work*, 14(1), 103–114.

Carpenito-Moyet, L. J. (2010). *Nursing diagnosis: Application to clinical practice* (13th ed.). Philadelphia: Lippincott Williams & Wilkins.

Committee on Hospital Care and Institute for Patient-and-Family-Centered Care. (2012). Patient- and family-centered care and the pediatrician's role. *Pediatrics*, 129(2), 394–404.

Correa, V. I., Bonilla, Z. E., & Reyes-MacPherson, M. (2011). Support networks of single Puerto Rican mothers of children with disabilities. *Journal of Child & Family Studies*, 20(1), 66–77.

Duvall, E., & Miller, B. (1985). *Marriage and family development* (7th ed.). New York: Harper Collins.

Erikson, E. H. (1998). *The life cycle completed*. New York: W.W. Norton.

Florczak, K. L., Falkenstern, S. K., & Baumann, S. L. (2010). A glimmer into the understanding of family. *Nursing Science Quarterly*, 23(2), 105–112.

Freudenberg, N., Pastor, M., & Israel, B. (2011). Strengthening community capacity to participate in making decisions to reduce disproportionate environmental exposures. *American Journal of Public Health*, S123–130.

Gordon, M. (2011). *Manual of nursing diagnosis* (12th ed.). Sudbury, MA: Jones & Bartlett.

Hirani, S. S., Karmaliani, R., McFarlane, J., Asad, N., Madhani, F., & Shehzad, S. (2010). Testing a community derived intervention to promote women's health: Preliminary results of a 3-arm randomized controlled trial in Karachi, Pakistan. *Southern Online Journal of Nursing Research*, 10(3), 5p.

Hockenberry, M. J., & Wilson, D. (2010). *Wong's nursing care of infants and children* (9th ed.). St. Louis: Mosby.

Huang, B., Biro, F. M., & Dorn, L. D. (2009). Determination of relative timing of pubertal maturation through ordinal logistic modeling: Evaluation of growth and timing parameters. *Journal of Adolescent Health*, 45(4), 383–388.

Jeffers, L. A., & DiBartolo, M. C. (2011). Raising health care provider awareness of sexually transmitted disease in patients over age 50. *Medsurg Nursing*, 20(6), 285–290.

Kaakinen, J., Gedaly-Duff, V., Coehlo, D. P., & Hanson, S. M.H. (2010). *Family nursing: Theory, practice and research* (4th ed.). Philadelphia: F.A. Davis.

Kavanaugh, V. M., Fierro, M. F., Suttle, D. E., Heyl, P. S., Bendheim, S. H., & Powell, V. (2009). Psychosocial risk factors as contributors to pregnancy-associated death in Virginia, 1999-2001. *Journal of Women's Health*, 18(7), 1041–1048.

Kime, N. (2009). How children eat may contribute to rising levels of obesity: Children's eating behaviours: An intergenerational study of family influences. *International Journal of Health Promotion & Education*, 47(1), 4–11.

Leever, M. G. (2011). Cultural competence: Reflections on patient autonomy and patient good. *Nursing Ethics*, 18(4), 560–570.

Lehavot, K., Huh, D., Walters, K. L., King, K. M., Andrasik, M. P., & Simoni, J. M. (2011). Buffering effects of general and medication-specific social support on the association between substance use and HIV medication adherence. *AIDS Patient Care & STDs*, 25(3), 181–189.

Lev, A. I. (2010). How queer!—The development of gender identity and sexual orientation in LGBTQ-headed families. *Family Process*, 49(3), 268–290.

Lubkin, I. M., & Larsen, P. D. (2011). *Chronic illness: Impact and interventions* (8th ed.). Sudbury, MA: Jones & Bartlett.

Lundy, K. S., & Janes, S. (2010). *Community health nursing: Caring for the public's health* (2nd ed.). Sudbury, MA: Jones & Bartlett.

Marken, D. M., Pierce, D., & Baltisberger, J. A. (2010). Grandmother's use of routines to manage custodial care of young children. *Physical & Occupational Therapy in Geriatrics*, 28(4), 360–375.

Marshall, A., Bell, J. M., & Moules, N. J. (2010). Beliefs, suffering, and healing: A clinical practice model for families experiencing mental illness. *Perspectives in Psychiatric Care*, 46(3), 197–208.

Maurer, F. A., & Smith, C. M. (2009). *Community/public health nursing practice: Health for families and populations* (4th ed.). St. Louis: Saunders Elsevier.

Miracle, A. W., & Miracle, T. S. (2009). Chapter 16: Sexuality in late adulthood. In B. R. Bonder, V. Dal Bello-Haas, & M. B. Wagner (Eds.), *Functional performance in older adults* (3rd ed., pp. 409–426). Philadelphia: F.A. Davis.

Moodley, R. (2011). The Toronto Traditional Healers Project: An introduction. *International Journal of Health Promotion & Education*, 49(3), 74–78.

Muliira, J. K., & Musil, C. M. (2010). Relationship between methods of coping, social support and receipt of preventive care procedures by primary grandmother caregivers. *Journal of Community Health*, 35(5), 479–486.

O'Haver, J., Moore, I. M., Insel, K. C., Reed, P. G., Melnyk, B. M., & Lavoie, M. (2010). Parental perceptions of risk and protective factors associated with the adaptation of siblings of children with cystic fibrosis. *Pediatric Nursing*, 36(6), 284–291.

Pender, N. J., Murdaugh, C. L., & Parsons, M. A. (2011). *Health promotion in nursing practice* (6th ed.). Upper Saddle River, NJ: Pearson.

Pharris, M. D. (2011). Margaret A. Newman's theory of health as expanding consciousness. *Nursing Science Quarterly*, 24(3), 193–194.

Rawana, E. (2009). Making the possible probable: A strength-based assessment and intervention framework for clinical work with parents, children and adolescents. *Families in Society*, 90(3), 255.

Schoon, I., Jones, E., Cheng, H., & Maughan, B. (2012). Family hardship, family instability, and cognitive development. *Journal of Epidemiology and Community Health*, 66, 716–722.

Shin, S. H., Choi, H., Kim, M. J., & Kim, Y. H. (2010). Comparing adolescents' adjustment and family resilience in divorced families depending on the types of primary caregiver. *Journal of Clinical Nursing*, 19(11-12), 1695–1706.

Sidumo, E. M., Ehlers, V. J., & Hattingh, S. P. (2010). Cultural knowledge of non-Muslim nurses working in Saudi Arabian obstetric units. *Curationis*, 33(3), 48–55.

Smith, M. C. (2011). Integrative review of research related to Margaret Newman's theory of health as expanding consciousness. *Nursing Science Quarterly*, 24(3), 256–272.

Stanhope, M., & Lancaster, J. (2012). *Public health nursing* (8th ed.). St. Louis: Mosby.

Strachan, A., Lund, M. E., & Garcia, J. A. (2010). Assessing children's perceptions of family relationships: An interactive instrument for use in custody disputes. *Journal of Child Custody*, 7(3), 192–216.

Strasburger, V. C. (2009). Children, adolescents, and the media: What we know, what we don't know and what we need to find out (quickly!). *Arch Dis Child*, 94, 655–657.

Trudel, G., Villeneuve, L., Preville, M., Boyer, R., & Frechette, V. (2010). Dyadic adjustment, sexuality and psychological distress in older couples. *Sexual & Relationship Therapy*, 25(3), 306–315.

U.S. Department of Health and Human Services. (2011). *2020 topics and objectives*. Retrieved July 7, 2011, from www.healthypeople.gov/2020/topicsobjectives2020/default.aspx.

United States Census Bureau. (2012). Retrieved February 26, 2012, from www.census.gov/newsroom/releases/archives/families_households/cb11-183.html.

Wallace, M. A. (2008). Assessment of sexual health in older adults. *AJN, American Journal of Nursing*, 108(7), 52–60.

Ward, S. L., & Hisley, S. M. (2009). Chapter 3: The evolving family. In *Maternal-child nursing care: Optimizing outcomes for mothers, children & families* (pp. 46–70). Philadelphia: F.A. Davis.

Health Promotion and the Community

Anne Rath Rentfro

OBJECTIVES

After completing this chapter, the reader will be able to:

- Describe the 11 functional health patterns and explain how they are used for data collection to assess communities.
- Evaluate community characteristics that indicate risk.
- Identify developmental aggregates of potential or actual dysfunctional health patterns.
- Explain methods of community data collection and sources of information.
- Describe a method of planned change for the community.
- Discuss planning, implementing, and evaluating nursing interventions in health promotion with communities.
- Develop a health-promotion plan based on community assessment (including resources), nursing diagnoses, and other contributing factors.

KEY TERMS

Advocate	Community risk factors	Measurement data
Ambient	Demography	Observation data
Community	Developmental theory	Policy decision-making
Community diagnosis	Focus groups	Risk-factor theory
Community evaluation	Function of a community	Structure of a community
Community health promotion	Interview data	Systems theory
Community nursing intervention	Key informants	Windshield survey
Community outcomes	Lobbying	
Community pattern	Lobbyist	

Teenagers: Drinking and Driving

In a small rural community, seven teenagers have died in alcohol-related car accidents within the past 3 months. Alcohol and drug education is taught during the first year at the local high school, but driver's education classes are not offered because the school cannot afford the program. Parents within this community are extremely concerned.

- *What other information must be acquired before making a diagnosis?*
- *What health-promotion ideas could be recommended based on the information provided?*

Over the last few decades, several social trends in the United States have increased public interest in health promotion and disease prevention. The *Healthy People 2020* initiative shifts the focus of health care from reactive to proactive with its emphasis on disease prevention and health promotion (U.S. Department of Health and Human Services, 2011). By stating national health objectives as population-specific risks to good health, this venture guides community strategies to promote health, thereby reducing disease risk factors. Box 8-1: *Healthy People 2020* highlights the emphasis this initiative takes with environmental context and community.

Another social trend creating interest for health promotion is the changing population of the United States (see Chapter 2). The U.S. Census Bureau estimates that between 2000 and 2010, for example, the older population increased faster than the total population (Werner, 2011). During this same time, the population of older men increased (Figure 8-1). Although women continue to outnumber men in the older age groups, that difference is decreasing (Werner, 2011). Older people tend to have more chronic diseases and consume larger portions of health care resources than people in other age groups. This aging population will require more home services than previous generations because of increased lifespan and the concurrences of health problems (including altered levels of functioning).

The term community is used in various contexts with various meanings, depending on the frame of reference. Nursing generally adopts a broad sense of community that includes the concepts of groups of people that share social relationships, generally live within the same geographical location, and share common interests (Kaakinen et al., 2010). A broad definition of community encompasses a wide variety of settings, such as school, workplace, and the international community.

Nurses in the nation's schools serve youth and provide access to community resources. Linking school nurses with communities can increase access to resources to improve health-promoting behaviors (de Heer et al., 2011). *Healthy People 2020* addresses this issue: "ECBP-5: Increase the proportion of the Nation's elementary, middle, and senior high schools that have a full-time registered school nurse-to-student ratio of at least 1:750" (U.S. Department of Health and Human Services, 2011). In 2006, the Health Indicators' Warehouse (www.healthindicators.gov/) reported that 40.6% (CI=35.3% to 45.9%) of U.S. schools had the specified full-time registered nurse-to-student ratio (1:750). The next evaluation of this indicator is scheduled for 2012.

Selected Examples of National Health-Promotion and Disease-Prevention Objectives for Communities

- Offer surveillance and health-promotion programs.
- Provide transition planning.
- Discourage use of inappropriate medications.
- Encourage participation in social, spiritual, recreational, community, and civic activities.
- Reduce number of nonfatal unintentional injuries requiring medical care.
- Provide preschool health education.
- Provide school health education courses on personal growth and wellness.
- Encourage participation in employer-sponsored health-promotion programs.
- Offer community-based primary prevention services.
- Offer culturally appropriate community health programs.
- Increase the proportion of persons served by community water systems who receive a supply of drinking water that meets the regulations of the Safe Drinking Water Act.
- Increase the proportion of Council on Education for Public Health (CEPH) accredited schools of public health, CEPH-accredited academic programs, and schools of nursing (with a public health or community health component) that integrate Core Competencies for Public Health Professionals into curricula.

From U.S. Department of Health and Human Services. (2011). *2020 topics and objectives.* Retrieved July 7, 2011, from www.healthypeople.gov/2020/topicsobjectives2020/default.aspx.

People are integral to any concept of community; human beings give each community shape, character, and form. The diversity within a community and the diversity among various communities contribute to the health of that community. Individual health is reflected in each community through each person's contribution to its statistical rates and cultural and psychological makeup. Conversely, the context of the community is reflected in the individual through similar modes of expression (Pender et al., 2011).

This chapter focuses on the application of the nursing process to the community with independent, interdependent, and dependent nursing activities. Globalization has affected communities. Swift methods of travel and Internet communication impact community health (Maurer & Smith, 2009). Communities in all corners of the Earth are exposed to diseases such as severe acute respiratory syndrome (SARS), human immunodeficiency virus (HIV)/acquired immunodeficiency syndrome (AIDS), and pandemics of tuberculosis and influenza (Maurer & Smith, 2009). Disparities in health across the world are associated with poverty, industrialization, violence, social disruption, education, food access, and maternal health. Even in developed countries with health resources, disparity occurs. Health may be different in urban versus rural geographical areas. Compared to urban Americans, rural people have increased levels of all of the following: infant and maternal morbidity, chronic illness, industrial health problems, stress-related disorders, and mental illness. Furthermore, rural individuals are less likely to have insurance with pharmaceutical coverage, therefore spending more on their medications (Maurer & Smith, 2009).

Methods of data collection and sources of information about communities differ from individual sources. Systems theory,

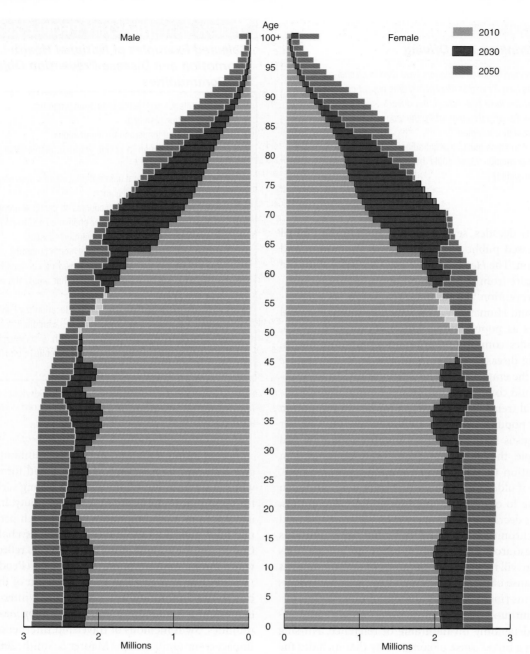

FIGURE 8-1 Age and gender structure of the population for the United States: 2010, 2020, 2030. (From U.S. Census Bureau, 2008.)

developmental theory, and risk-factor theory guide nursing process. Developmental theory refers to a variety of explanations of phases of human development—physical, psychosocial, cognitive, and spiritual dimensions—based on descriptive research studies. Similarly, risk-factor theory identifies human characteristics and behaviors that increase the likelihood of the manifestation of health problems. Diverse communities require comprehensive assessment techniques that gather information about the unique characteristics of the population (e.g., cultural health practices or herbal remedies).

Gordon's (2011) functional health patterns provide the assessment framework for this text. Although other community assessment strategies exist, Gordon's (2011) patterns are useful to align community assessment findings with those of families and individuals to plan health promotion. An example of a data collection guide patterns is presented to facilitate the comprehension, synthesis, and application of observation data, interview data, focus groups, and measurement data. An example of data analysis, nursing diagnosis, planning, implementation, and evaluation follows along with a description (Table 8-1).

THE NURSING PROCESS AND THE COMMUNITY

Community nursing stems from a theoretical base that recognizes the impact of systems on health. General systems theory (described in Chapter 7) provides a foundation for most methods community nurses use to assess, plan, and evaluate (Maurer &

TABLE 8-1   IMPLEMENTATION OF COMMUNITY HEALTH PLANS WITH OBJECTIVES AND RATIONALE

NURSING DIAGNOSIS: Potential for increasing the incidence of fatal motor vehicle accidents in high school population related to alcohol use and driving.

GOAL: North High School population will have reduced incidence (at least 20%) of fatal motor vehicle accidents related to alcohol use and abuse by December.

OBJECTIVE	PLANS	RATIONALE
1. Community will have access to information about incidence of fatal motor vehicle accidents and drunken driving arrests of its high school population for past 5 years by March.	Interview local police about incidence of fatal auto accidents and substance abuse in community. Interview parents of deceased high school students, students, teachers, physicians, clergy, and emergency room personnel about incidence of the problem and suggested measures for decreasing incidence; suggest that interviews be broadcast over high school station. Have several people write to community newspaper, commenting on the broadcast and the problem.	*Unfreezing:* For change to occur, community has to become dissatisfied with status quo and sense a need for change. *Empiric-rational strategy:* People are rational; discussion of facts can result in support for change. Important elements for preventing the problem include educating the public and having key community leaders discuss their views; concern lends credibility and is necessary for action. People tend to listen to those with informal power. Keeping the issue before the community can raise consciousness.
2. Community will take action to inform population at risk about responsible drinking and driving by June.	Suggest to school principal and school board the creation of a task force of community residents to plan a health program on individual responsibility and alcohol use in high school. Conduct focus groups with the task force and develop collaborative group goals and strategies. Task force should include teachers, students, parents, clergy, police, nurses, and physicians. Task force will examine ways to determine and teach content, integrate it into curriculum, and recommend that community members, such as a nurse, be involved in teaching content.	*Changing:* Moving to a new level; community involvement will influence acceptability of changes. Community residents like to be involved in decision-making. It is important to establish trust and collaboration among community groups; this opens communication channels between adolescents and the health community. Community involvement facilitates acceptance of change.
3. Community will implement an educational program for its high school population related to use of alcohol and individual responsibility.	Implement educational plans.	*Refreezing:* Moving to level of change brought about by community forces. Educational strategies built around concept of individual responsibility are essential elements in promoting health of young adults.

Smith, 2009). Because nursing theories often address self-care and individual-environment interaction, nurses are well-prepared to function in this setting. Public health theory uses a population focus with risk identification to assess communities. Assessing aggregates is therefore an important part of community nursing assessment (Maurer & Smith, 2009).

The approach to community nursing assessment addresses each community as unique and provides the rationale for the assessment. The community nurse may use a comprehensive needs-assessment approach that includes all aspects of the community and is the traditional rigorous approach (Maurer & Smith, 2009). Other approaches that may be used include the problem-oriented approach, the single-population approach, and the familiarization approach (Maurer & Smith, 2009). These approaches determine the data to collect. In strength-based approaches and Gordon's functional pattern approach, positive factors play a consistent role in the information gathering.

Gordon's (2011) health-related patterns provide a useful guide to collect observation, interview, and measurement data. Health-related patterns depend on community settings, assessment focus, and the preference of each community. Assessing all pattern areas provides a basic data set to analyze and use for comparison during evaluation (see Chapter 6).

Risk factors and development also influence health patterns. For example, health concerns may occur in one pattern area, such as the increased age-related factor of teenage pregnancy (sexuality-reproductive pattern). Data from other areas may reveal that parental opposition (values-beliefs pattern) tends to restrict sex education and limit sex education in schools (coping-stress tolerance pattern). Attempting to restrict sex education or "ignoring" it in school and primary care may place the community at risk for unwanted pregnancy in its young people of childbearing age. Factors from several pattern areas may form clusters of risk for certain groups (see Chapter 6).

THE NURSE'S ROLE

Community health nursing combines nursing practice and public health concepts to promote the health of populations without limitation to any particular individual or group of individuals (Maurer & Smith, 2009). Nursing concerns become community's responses to existing and potential health-related problems, including such health-supporting responses as monitoring and teaching population groups. Nurses supply educational information to at-risk communities to develop health-oriented skills, attitudes, and related behavioral changes.

Community nurses also develop essential relationships aimed at accomplishing community's health-related missions. Complex and dynamic communities, with their increasing public involvement in health and health policy, highlight the importance of human interactions inherent in nurses' responses to potential health problems, needs, and expectations. For example, active participation in environmental issues (such as decreasing the use of plastics) and contributions to passage of the Safe Cosmetics Act of 2011 (HR2359) and the Safe Cosmetics Amendment of 2011 (HR 4395 IH) may provide a role for some community health nurses. Concern about harmful effects of environmental contaminants includes decreased fertility in women, demasculization of men exposed to plastics, and premature maturation of the reproductive tract with a trend toward earlier sexual maturation. Community nursing practice, therefore, requires a broad knowledge base derived from the natural, behavioral, and humanistic sciences with application of intellectual, interpersonal, and technical skills using the nursing process.

Influencing Health Policy

The primary responsibility of the nurse is to the individual, family, group, or community served. A major portion of the nurse's role is to advocate not only for the individual but also for justice in health care delivery. Nurses need to be aware of issues that have an effect on the health of the American people and know how to influence necessary change.

Health and environment are integrally connected; therefore, nurses who engage in all planning aspects facilitate the health potential of those communities they serve. Involvement that includes attention to policy decisions and political action affects broader aspects of environmental, biophysical, and socioeconomic conditions of homes, schools, workplaces, communities, and health care delivery. For example, nurses could take active roles in how plastics impact population health (http://-envirn.org/pg/groups/3755/environmental-health-scope-and-standards-of-practice), and in safeguarding natural resources. One organization, the Alliance of Nurses for Healthy Environments (ANHE), has created a website called the Knowledge Network (http://envirn.org/) to facilitate nurses' participation and competence in environmental health issues. In 2010, ANHE and the American Nurses Association (ANA) joined forces to develop ANA's *Scope and Standards of Practice for Nurses* (2010). By virtue of their numbers, nurses, who comprise the largest group of health care providers in the United States, have tremendous potential to influence decision-making.

Participation in policy decision-making requires that nurses take a proactive stance to determine needs before a problem arises. Policy development and change take place on many levels, from within the nurse's agency or work group to the community, state, and national levels. At the institutional level, clinical decisions influence policy, as do management issues. The nurse examines rationales that underlie existing or planned policy and determines their current relevance. Nurses, by virtue of their education and experience, develop communication skills and apply change theory to influence policy.

Health-related decision-making often results from legislation at the local, state, or national level. Laws—rules enforced by a ruling authority by which society is governed—and regulations—agency or department rules developed to implement laws—define services offered. Politics influence change and

provide an arena for nursing to participle in shaping the future of health care. Political involvement may include voting, communicating with local representatives, supporting candidates, contributing time or financial support, and running for city, county, state, or national office. Voting, after becoming well-informed on current issues and candidates, and serving on local and state committees are important ways for nurses to be actively involved.

In addition, knowing local representatives, informing them about health care issues, and advising them as to their constituents' needs are other ways nurses become involved. Legislators are influenced by the information that they receive and by the sources of that information. Nurses have a wealth of knowledge about health care. The process of seeking to influence legislators' views and votes is called lobbying. When an individual is employed to lobby they are known as a lobbyist and are required to register as the representative of a special interest group. The American Nurses Association (ANA), located in Washington, DC, employs nurse lobbyists as do many states. Individual nurses, however, can support colleagues who represent nursing's interests and who run for political office. The ANA Nurses Strategic Action Team (N-STAT) network is an organized grassroots effort by nurses to help elect endorsed candidates and to inform legislators about policy issues of concern to nurses. When nurses join N-STAT they receive alerts and updates detailing specific legislative issues. Financial contributions to Nurses for Political Action Coalition (N-PAC), ANA's political arm, increase the power base of nurses. Membership in professional and community groups provides nurses with the collective voice to influence legislators.

Communicating with a legislator is essential and can be done by phone, writing a letter, personal visits, or e-mail correspondence. Legislators have staffs of experts in various areas, and each legislator is assigned to committees. To understand the legislative process, the nurse needs to follow the progress of a bill. Thousands of bills are introduced at both the state and federal levels and must be passed within 2 years or die by default. Once a bill is introduced, it is referred to committee, and the committee chairperson determines which bills will be considered. Hearings are then held on the considered bills. When finished in committee, a bill is "reported out" at the federal level to the floor of the Senate or House of Representatives for a vote. Both the Senate and the House must pass identical versions of the bill and, once passed by both chambers, it is forwarded to the President for signing. If signed, it is enacted into law (Willmann, 2011). It is important for nurses to lobby, to inform legislators of new issues, and to give expert testimony on introduced bills. Nurses who are politically aware extend the collective nursing voice to its full potential (Box 8-2: Hot Topics).

Unfortunately, nursing's collective voice is rarely heard. Only a small proportion of nurses are members of the American Nurses Association or the ANA constituent nursing organizations (Sportsman et al., 2010). Other health care professionals, like the American Medical Association, have more united professional organizations with large memberships, providing a united voice and political clout that influences health

BOX 8-2   HOT TOPICS

The Future of Nursing: Leading Change, Advancing Health

This landmark report was published in 2011 and calls for the transformation of nursing, the health profession with the most members. The report justifies that the four key actions should be completed:

- Nurses should practice to the full extent of their education and training (Chapter 3).
- Nurses should achieve higher levels of education and training through an improved education system that promotes seamless academic progression (Chapter 4).
- Nurses should be full partners, with physicians and other health professionals, in redesigning health care in the United States (Chapter 5).
- Effective workforce planning and policy making require better data collection and an improved information infrastructure (Chapter 6).

Each of these recommendations has implications for the future of community health nurses. Soon after publication, U.S. nurses organized to establish a campaign for action. In the first year, groups gathered in almost all of the 50 states and 2 U.S. territories, and 36 of these have proposed recommendations. Nursing garnered support from businesses and organizations to facilitate the integration of the recommendations into the business and professional sectors. For example, the American Red Cross designed a new health services community response model that uses nurses to the extent of their scope of practice. Marketing to promote action to meet the recommendations also began. The AARP formed a nursing coalition of non-nursing organizations to encourage action on the recommendation.

From Institute of Medicine. (2009). *The future of nursing: Leading change, advancing health*. Washington, DC: The National Academies Press; Robert Wood Johnson Foundation. (2011). *Future of nursing: Campaign for action*. Retrieved March 6, 2012, from http://thefutureof nursing.org/highlights.

care policy and law. Nurses have multiple professional organizations. With high membership dues, nurses likely join only a few groups and may gravitate toward their specialty organization. Without a single national organization with the majority of nurses as members, nursing's voice is diluted. When organizations promote an issue, the collective voice of the group rather than the individual sends a more powerful message to influence policymakers. Without a collective voice, nursing's influence on shaping health care policy is weakened.

To strengthen nursing's collective voice, ANA has undergone significant reorganization with emphasis on increasing membership, by collaborating with their state constituent organizations, specialty organizations, and non-nursing health organizations. Engaging students in these strategies early in legislative processes will help to provide more well-informed practicing nurses. Well-informed, empowered professional nurses play significant roles in supporting legislative initiatives that promote and protect the health of the public (see Box 8-2: Hot Topics). Other ways for nurses to be involved in policy change are to support candidates and run for office. Volunteering during campaigns to help a specific candidate or to encourage voter registration and voting are ways that nurses can influence policy. Many nurses now represent their local constituencies and have increasing visibility at the state and national levels. For

example, four nurses joined the U.S. 112th Congress in 2012 to raise the total number of nurses serving in Congress to seven.

Community nurses' roles include the interaction of independent, interdependent, and dependent functions. Independent functions include assessing, analyzing, diagnosing, planning, implementing, and evaluating communities for health promotion and health education. Interdependent functions include collaboration with community members and interdisciplinary teamwork functions that are crucial to effective community health. Dependent functions include implementing the therapeutic plans of team members.

Community health promotion includes all of the following (U.S. Department of Health and Human Services, 2011):

- Community participation, with representatives from multiple community sectors including government, education, business, faith organizations, health care, media, voluntary agencies, and the public
- Assessment guided by a community-planning model to determine health problems, resources, perceptions, and priorities for action
- Targeted and measurable objectives to address health outcomes, risk factors, public awareness, services, and protection
- Comprehensive, multifaceted, culturally relevant interventions that have multiple targets for change
- Monitoring and evaluation of objectives and strategies used

METHODS OF DATA COLLECTION

Nurses obtain community assessment data through observation, interviews (including focus groups), and measurement. These three methods are used most frequently in various combinations to ensure the validity of the information. Obtaining data through observation—often referred to as the windshield survey approach to assessment—includes the use of the senses (sight, touch, hearing, smell, and taste) to determine community appearances. These appearances include types and condition of residential dwellings and their people and also physical and biological characteristics, such as animal and plant life, temperature, transportation, sounds, and odors. Some communities have a characteristic "flavor." Community's physical characteristics influence health. What type of space is available? Children need space to run and play; young and middle-aged adults require space for recreation and exercise. What spatial barriers exist? Where is this space located in relation to traffic and schools? What does the air feel and smell like? What does the water taste like?

Community nurses obtain abundant subjective data by simply walking or riding around a community. Data obtained by observation provide important clues about the community, its actual or potential health problems, and its strengths. Technological advances such as the use of geographic information systems (GIS) enhance nurses' ability to assess communities. For example, Fisher-Hoch and colleagues (2010) used GIS to show the geographical distribution of 810 participants by household incomes for their cohort study of a community with a high prevalence of diabetes along the Texas-Mexico border of the United States. In their sample, the lower socioeconomic group had a higher prevalence of undiagnosed diabetes. Analysis of observation data generates hypotheses to explore further using interview, focus group, and measurement data.

Interview data, the most common source of information from people, include verbal statements from community residents, key community officials, health care personnel, and various community agency staff. **Key informants** provide useful ways to learn how members perceive their community. Key community leaders often provide important information about community health concerns, necessary health resources, and community strengths along with particular health beliefs and community health goals. Community residents provide useful information about their perceptions of health, health concerns, and needs as well as of the availability, accessibility, and acceptability of health services. Health agency personnel provide data about health resources, population served, availability, and perceptions of concerns and needs. Developing a basic set of questions in advance enhances the relevance of interview data.

Community partners can be approached in groups to participate in assessment, planning, intervention, and evaluation (Andrews et al., 2012b). Community nurses who have expertise in building partnerships engage the community in assessment, planning, choosing effective strategies, and evaluation. Andrews' research team has used this strategy for multiple community issues and health-promotion projects. They have developed a toolkit for assessing partnerships (Andrews et al., 2011). Access to the toolkit is available at http://academicde partments.musc.edu/nursing/cchp/toolbox.htm. Strategies initiated by engaged community members empower community partners and enhance the ability to transfer evidence-based strategies into their unique communities (Andrews et al., 2011).

Measurement data use instruments to quantify data during information collection. Measurement data include population statistics, pollution indices, morbidity and mortality rates, census statistics, and epidemiological data. These data can be accessed by Internet or locally in community libraries; health departments; environmental protection agencies; schools; police and fire departments; local health system agencies; and town, city, or state planning offices. Publicly supported agencies share their information, and community nurses readily use such data.

SOURCES OF COMMUNITY INFORMATION

Census information located at www.census.gov and also found in libraries and public agencies is the most complete source for population information. Because the U.S. Census is completed once every 10 years at the beginning of a decade, data for most communities become less accurate as the decade progresses. Community agencies and local planning commissions project statistics and developmental trends that nurses use to understand population patterns and dynamics. Many communities and states also have databases available for public use.

Environmental measurement data can be obtained fron the local branch of the U.S. Environmental Protection Agency.

Generally, local health departments monitor water, food, and sanitation systems. Nurses may be called upon to facilitate safeguarding of natural resources protecting communities from industrial toxins. For examples of community issues related to environmental issues, see *Gasland* (www.gaslandthe movie.com/). Health departments along with school nurses and administrators provide school health information. Town, city, or county administrators provide information about land use, boundaries, housing conditions, utilities, and community services. Community newspapers supply information about community dynamics, health-related concerns, cultural activities, and community decision-making. Documentation techniques for community observation, interview, and measurement data are similar to those used for individuals and families. A triple-column format that separates the data of each method facilitates recording.

COMMUNITY FROM A SYSTEMS PERSPECTIVE

Systems theory provides an overall framework to connect and integrate community data. Systems consist of interrelated, interacting parts or components within boundaries that filter both the type and the rate of input and output (Andrews et al., 2011; Maurer & Smith, 2009; Newman et al., 2011). Similar to how families form systems (see Chapter 7), communities viewed as systems have both structure and function. Assessment of communities includes exploration of aspects of the population within specific geographical areas.

Structure

The **structure of a community** system or subsystem consists of a formal or informal arrangement of parts, including both animate and inanimate properties. Nursing, which operates within the context of the health system, can be considered within the context of community systems. Figure 8-2 shows the hierarchical arrangement of a community system. The suprasystem, often a county or state, shapes the larger part of the system that encompasses numerous subsystems. Community's structural parts form the subsystems, each of which is in itself a system. Health agencies, schools, fire departments, and governmental bodies are examples of structural parts. Arrangement and organization of a community, such as age distribution and types of health-promotion/protection programs, change over time. Parts fluctuate depending upon environmental processes occurring locally and within the larger environment.

Community leadership provides direction for both health-promotion and health-protection activities; therefore, community assessment includes exploration of various community systems as they relate to health. The practice of viewing community structure as a population (collection of people) and considering the arrangement of community's health care parts (existing health services) plays an important role in the assessment process.

The study of populations is referred to as **demography.** A population is a group defined as an aggregate of people who share similar personal or environmental characteristics. Demography provides information about population characteristics—such

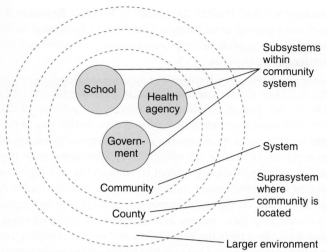

FIGURE 8-2 Hierarchical nature of a community system.

as size and racial composition, along with the distribution of age, gender, marital status, nationality, language, religious affiliations, education, and occupation. Demographic data provide the basis for analysis and a means to identify groups who may have high risk for health concerns. Such information also provides direction for health strategies. For example, examining age distribution over several years reveals important population shifts with associated needs for additional health-promotion activities. The increasing numbers of individuals older than age 65 require changes in community health priorities that reflect this group's needs. Comparing population characteristics statistically enables nurses to make inferences about the community. Comparisons are made among three systems: the town, which is a part of the county; the county, which is a part of the larger system; and the state. Comparisons between affluent and poor communities, rural and urban communities, and diverse and homogeneous communities may provide important information for planning.

Function

The function of a community refers to the process of dynamic change with adaptation in the system's parts and the ways that community systems and subsystems interact. Decision-making and allocation of health-promotion and health-protection resources are important considerations for community assessment. As health educators, nurses interact with communities to promote health. Community health promotion involves a complex array of responsibilities. Nurses act as advocates using proactive planning and collaboration with other disciplines and agencies. As a community liaison, the nurse establishes priorities for programming; matches resources with needs determined by a community needs assessment; empowers community members; and facilitates social, environmental, and political change. These multifaceted functions require expertise in communication and interpersonal relations that involve a deliberate approach. Using such an intentional process, while maintaining the community's vision, can produce effective change (Andrews et al., 2011; Newman et al., 2011).

Interaction

Through dynamic interaction with the environment, systems exchange matter, energy, and information (in such communication forms as verbal and behavioral) to make decisions. Interaction also contributes to community systems' survival ability, as well as to protect and promote the health of its members. Through environmental interactions, community systems use adaptation mechanisms. Nurses determine how communities apply these mechanisms toward health services. For example, policy that removes soft drink and candy sales from schools must consider lost revenue from these unhealthy but lucrative structures within the school system.

Various health-related patterns emerge from these interactions. For example, certain human-activity patterns negatively alter natural environmental patterns, which in turn influence human health patterns. Gordon's (2011) assessment framework focuses on 11 health-related functional patterns that assume community and environment interaction from a systems perspective.

COMMUNITY FROM A DEVELOPMENTAL PERSPECTIVE

A framework based on developmental theory can also be used to identify existing or potential health problems for particular age groups in communities. Community nurses, focusing on the total community population, use a developmental, age-correlated approach to identify health-promotion and health-protection activities.

Nurses identify age-related risks at each life stage, taking steps to maximize wellness and health promotion as a lifelong concern (U.S. Department of Health and Human Services, 2011). For example, adolescent single mothers of infants, at risk both emotionally and physically, require parenting skills. Accidents are the greatest threat to children's health; therefore, accident-prevention activities become a priority for communities with a young population and with adolescent mothers. Age-related risk factors (see Chapters 6 and 7) associated with individuals and families can be extended to include community groups based on the demographics of the community.

COMMUNITY FROM A RISK-FACTOR PERSPECTIVE

Risk factors associated with disease, illness, and death rates, although not causally associated, predict the likelihood of a particular adverse health condition in communities of interest (U.S. Department of Health and Human Services, 2011). Risk factors include a combination of demographic, psychological, physiological, and environmental characteristics (or they may include a single characteristic). For example, age, gender, race, geographical location, consumption pattern, or lack of health services may be considered risk factors, because one or more may contribute to disease or death and place the population sharing them at risk (Box 8-3: Research for Evidence-Based Practice). The influence of various risk factors differs from person to person and group to group because of genetic

BOX 8-3 RESEARCH FOR EVIDENCE-BASED PRACTICE

Associations Among Parent/Peer Relationships and Individual Characteristics of Children

This study uses socioecological theory as a foundation to explore associations among parent/peer relationships and individual characteristics. A total of 3 rounds of data were collected over 3 years in this sample of 667 children. Each round consisted of a 45- to 90-minute interview with the guardian of the child. Instruments were used to measure internalization of problems, externalization of problems, exposure to community violence, exposure to family violence, attachment to parents, attachment to friends, delinquency of friends, self-reported competence, moral disengagement (justification for the use of aggression), household dysfunction, and mental health of guardians. The consent process explained that counseling services would be available and child abuse would be reported. Stepwise hierarchical linear regression was used to analyze the data. High exposure to violence was associated with little protection from normally protective factors (e.g., attachment to parents) compared to low exposure to violence. In the low exposure to violence setting, peer protective factors (e.g., friends) were effective. Less internalizing of problems was independently associated with individual competence. Externalizing problems was independently associated with variables from all domains, and exposure. Parent attachment and other protective factors were associated with decreased problems, whereas increased problems were associated with risk factors, such as a friend's delinquency. Community violence reduction, health-promotion, and health-prevention programs that emphasize and promote protective factors with parents and peers may decrease adverse behavioral outcomes in urban adolescents.

From Salzinger, S., Rosario, M., Feldman, R. S., & Ng-Mak, D. S. (2011). Role of parent and peer relationships and individual characteristics in middle school children's behavioral outcomes in the face of community violence. *Journal of Research on Adolescence: The Official Journal of the Society for Research on Adolescence, 21*(2), 395-407. doi:10.1111/j.1532-7795.2010.00677.x.

composition, geographical location, lifestyle patterns, resources, socioeconomic status, education level, or environmental variation. Some groups may be at high risk from a single risk factor such as insufficient immunizations or exposure to asbestos. A combined potential for adverse health effects exists when many risk factors are present, because they interact in multiple ways and synergistically influence each other.

Communities, therefore, experience substantial variability in health conditions in regard to both incidence and susceptibility. Risk-factor theory views health and disease as multifactorial with etiology attributed to no single risk factor. For example, risk factors such as air pollution, smoking, and forms of radiation in various combinations may be related to high rates of lung cancer, emphysema, and bronchitis in a community. The potential to control risk factors and to provide relevant health-related resources forms the basis for health-promotion and health-protection activities.

GORDON'S FUNCTIONAL HEALTH PATTERNS: ASSESSMENT OF THE COMMUNITY

A variety of functional health pattern assessments are used with communities. Nurses use Gordon's (2011) functional health reference assessment as exemplified in this chapter or other assessments described in the literature **Website Resource 8A** contains a general description of Gordon's 11 functional health patterns with guidelines for posing questions in interviews and pertinent observations.

Health Perception–Health Management Pattern

The health perception–health management pattern identifies data about community health status, health-promotion and disease-prevention practices, and community members' perceptions of health (Gordon, 2011). Residents may perceive a substance abuse problem in adolescents or a high rate of unwanted pregnancies, breast cancer, or sexually transmitted disease as concerns. Valuable information can be elicited by conducting focus groups and interviewing key community members about their health concerns and issues. Mortality and morbidity statistics and other public health information sources provide measurement data (see Chapter 2).

Nutritional-Metabolic Pattern

The nutritional-metabolic pattern identifies data relevant to community consumption habits as reflected in accessibility and availability of food stores and subsidized food programs for infants, children, and older adults. Community well-being, which depends on adequate dietary habits, food intake, and supply of nutrients, is influenced by culture, the presence or absence of kitchen facilities, and adequate plumbing.

Community assessment includes collecting data by driving or walking through the community while employing all five senses; it provides information about grocery stores, fast-food establishments, ethnic shopping facilities, and street corner vendors. Even in affluent developed countries, pockets of areas without adequate access to food or "food deserts" can be found. Examining communities for the presence of community gardens or farmers' markets provided data about access to local produce. In rural areas, small stores may dictate eating choices (C. Gordon et al., 2011; Scarpello et al., 2009). Cummins and colleagues (2010) examined 15 fruit and vegetable item prices in 310 stores in 10 diverse areas of Scotland and found the smaller stores compared to large supermarkets sold fruits and vegetables at higher prices than larger supermarkets. Government programs, private soup kitchens, and food donations by houses of worship also provide information about nutritional patterns of communities.

Elimination Pattern

The elimination pattern identifies environmental factors, including exposure to pollutants in the community through contaminated soil, water, air, and the food chain. This pattern further classifies environmental factors into the two broad categories—physical and biological. Alterations in environmental processes threaten the health and integrity of communities, necessitating health-promotion and health-protection activities.

Physical agents include geological, geographical, climatic, and meteorological aspects of the community. Certain population groups are particularly susceptible to acute respiratory disease and aggravated asthmatic episodes when the air quality

FIGURE 8-3 The activity-exercise pattern identifies a community's physical activities and recreational options.

is poor (e.g., when schools are located in high-pollution or high-traffic areas). Geographical locations of communities and major waterways, highways, or mountains located within communities act as barriers to access of health facilities. Inaccessibility of health care services also hinders health in at-risk groups. Knowledge of climatic conditions provides clues to susceptibility to illness resulting from temperature or humidity in certain populations.

Biological agents include living things—such as plants, animals and their waste products, disease agents, microbial pathogens, and toxic substances—that can be hazardous to health. For example, Lyme disease, viral hepatitis, pneumonia, influenza, and the large number of diseases associated with childhood continue to be threats to community health. Observation, focus groups and interviews with key community members reveal information concerning elimination patterns. The Environmental Protection Agency (www.epa.gov/) and Centers for Disease Control and Prevention (www.cdc.gov/) provide excellent resources for community health nurses.

Activity-Exercise Pattern

The activity-exercise pattern identifies physical activities and recreational options within communities. Science and technology have increasingly influenced productivity while simultaneously reducing or eliminating physical work. Consequently, physical activity no longer occurs during the work day for most community members, leaving leisure time as the only time for physical activity. Physiological evidence demonstrates that physical activity improves many biological measures associated with health and psychological functioning. Regular physical activity and musculoskeletal fitness are important to healthy, independent living as people grow older. Physical activity reduces the risk of many diseases, including obesity, heart disease, hypertension, cancer, osteoporosis, and diabetes mellitus.

Observation, focus groups, and interviews provide clues to a community's ability to provide cultural and recreational activities (Figure 8-3). Furthermore, noting whether the community has evidence of recreational facilities or is a "built community" with physical activity options (such as bike/walking trails), assessing transportation options, and observing community

development that encourages walking should be included in the community assessment of the activity-exercise pattern.

Sleep-Rest Pattern

The sleep-rest pattern identifies a community's rhythm of sleeping, resting, and relaxing. Some towns never close, with stores, traffic flow, and recreational facilities operating during both day and night hours. This ongoing activity produces unpleasant disturbances, such as unwanted noise that may be harmful to community well-being. Excessive noise from highways or airplanes produces physiological or psychological problems eliciting responses ranging from mild irritation to pain or permanent hearing loss. Although noise cannot be eliminated, efforts to minimize and control it are possible. Observation, focus groups, and interviews provide clues to this pattern.

Cognitive-Perceptual Pattern

The cognitive-perceptual pattern identifies information about problem-solving and decision-making within communities. Systems depend on decision-making and resource allocation processes for survival. Communities require functional decision-making bodies to ensure adherence to rules and goals' attainment. Individual patterns and environmental patterns connect with important implications for community health. Community assessment includes appraisal of interaction with the environment along with effectiveness of strategies used to meet health concerns and needs (Maurer & Smith, 2009).

One strategy, bargaining, offers communities a plan to exchange resources for health service. For example, a community that owns a mammography machine but has no primary care facility might negotiate with another community to provide mammography for primary care services in return. Strategies using outside authority (legal bureaucratic methods) ensure compliance through rules and structures. In this case, states may mandate that communities maintain certain health standards. For example, a law may require all school children to be immunized against specific diseases before entering public school. Cooperative strategies promote health when members share common goals (Andrews et al., 2012a; Andrews et al., 2012b; Newman et al., 2011). For example, community residents may unite to oppose a chemical landfill that is a health hazard.

Convincing people to comply because they hold some loyalty in the situation or relationship is another method that mobilizes communities. For example, community residents might expend a great deal of effort and money to retain a particular health clinic because of loyalty to the agency. Identifying decision-making patterns used by communities provides clues about health priorities and values, as well as matches and mismatches between existing circumstances, health goals, and planning strategies. Data can best be obtained by observation, focus groups and interviews.

Self-Perception–Self-Concept Pattern

The self-perception–self-concept pattern identifies self-worth and personal identity of communities. Characteristics such as image, status, and perceived competency with problem-solving indicate community self-concept. Housing conditions, buildings, and cleanliness reflect community image. School systems, crime rates, accidents, and opinions about whether the community is considered a good place to live suggest community perception of self-worth. Competency with social and political issues as well as community spirit creates positive self-evaluation. Community pride facilitates development of innovative health programs. Emotional tone (fear, depression, or positive emotional outlook) relates to findings in other pattern areas. For example, tensions in the cognitive-perceptual pattern (conflict between groups concerning health issues) may explain a general feeling of fear among the residents. Data are obtained through observation, focus groups, and interviews.

Roles-Relationships Pattern

The roles-relationships pattern identifies communication styles along with formal and informal relationships. Of particular concern are roles and relationships affecting community ability to realize health potential. Patterns of crime, racial incidents, and social networks form indices of human relationships in communities. Publicizing health promotion becomes more effective when using patterns of official communication. Health program success depends upon support from prominent community members. Community members involved in health programs help identify other key community leaders. Use of media and other mass information programs improves communication, the flow of health information, and the number of community members reached. Interviews, television, the Internet, and newspapers are examples of ways to obtain and convey information.

Sexuality-Reproductive Pattern

The sexuality-reproductive pattern identifies reproductive data of communities, which is reflected in live birth statistics, mothers' ages, ethnicity, and marital status. This information provides clues to the health-promotion needs of a particular community group. Premature infant rates, low-birth-weight infants, abortion rates, as well as neonatal, infant, and maternal death rates reflect reproductive patterns of communities. Such information identifies at-risk groups based on particular characteristics associated with these rates. Mismatches between existing health services, health education, and community health statistics also indicate health concerns. Availability of sex education in schools; levels of spousal and child abuse; and number of sex-related crimes also indicate health-promotion issues. Minutes of meetings, health records, statistical data, and public documents provide sources for these data.

Coping-Stress Tolerance Pattern

The coping-stress tolerance pattern identifies the community's ability to cope or adapt. Communities respond to stress in different ways, some of which might threaten their integrity. Community responses reveal the group coping patterns. Communities develop abilities to exchange goods, services, goals, values, and ideals to survive and to promote community health. Community efforts to obtain goods from the environment, contain goods within the environment, retain goods within the community, and dispose of goods play significant roles to influence health. Examples of goods that communities obtain from the environment to promote health include local, state, or federal funding; health services; health-related workforce personnel; new knowledge; and technological advances. Some communities obtain abundant health care services; however, primary services often remain inadequate or nonexistent. Lack of available health services, or lack of ability to obtain them, characterizes community health need. Examples of goods communities may attempt to control include sex-related crimes, diseases, substance abuse, industry, hazardous waste in the water supply, and noxious chemicals in the air.

Community coping patterns aim to retain certain health-protection services, such as immunization services for children and adequate health facilities. Coping efforts may also include strict zoning laws and housing codes or certain values such as sex education within the home. Expendable goods of communities include industrial and human wastes. Data can be obtained through minutes of meetings, public documents, health surveys, statistical data, and health records.

Values-Beliefs Pattern

The values-beliefs pattern identifies the community values and beliefs. Such information provides clues for health-promotion and health-protection efforts valued by the community. Values underlie decisions about community health education and tax support for schools, hypertension screening for the public, disease prevention programs, or well-child clinics. Traditions, norms, and cultural and ethnic groups share values and beliefs in communities. Data can be obtained through focus groups and throughinterviews with key community members and health-related personnel.

ANALYSIS AND DIAGNOSIS WITH THE COMMUNITY

Analysis refers to data categorization and pattern determination. Data synthesis and organization occur to ascertain patterns of health activities and trends. An example of a clinical scenario about a particular community is presented in the Case Study and Care Plan at the end of this chapter. Decision-making and judgment inherent in the nursing process become most important during the analysis and diagnostic phases. Table 8-2 presents an example of one way to organize community data using Prochaska's stages of change (Pender et al., 2011).

Organization of Data

Charts, figures, and tables graphically display population distributions, morbidity and mortality data, or vital statistics to pinpoint significant community concerns with actual or potential health problems along with health-related responses to these concerns. Another valuable organizational technique—mapping—facilitates data analysis. For example, a series of maps gathered using technology such as GIS can be used to display data that change over time. Analysis of several variables simultaneously occurs. Overlap of locations of environmental hazards, densely populated areas, health-promotion services, and major highways

TABLE 8-2   STAGES OF CHANGE

STAGES	INTERVENTIONS
Precontemplation	Provide information (identify risk factors)
	Raise doubts about current behaviors and future outcomes
Contemplation	Discuss risks of not changing
	Discuss benefits of changing
Planning or preparation	Help plan phases of change
	Help implement phases of change
Action	Help develop strategies to prevent relapse, emphasizing self-efficacy
	Offer encouragement
Maintenance	Highlight past successes and future benefits

Modified from Pender, N. J., Murdaugh, C. L., & Parsons, M. A. (2011). *Health promotion in nursing practice* (6th ed.). Upper Saddle River, NJ: Pearson.

becomes apparent. Poor environmental conditions; distribution of illness, disease, and death rates; and accessibility of health-protection and health-promotion activities for the population appear at a glance with dotted scatter maps. Use of maps requires knowledge about the community's population base. Less-populated rural areas with fewer health facilities or fewer neonatal deaths in a community with fewer women of childbearing age are examples of how population statistics influence interpretation of mapping techniques. Using theoretical frameworks for community health and Gordon's (2011) 11 pattern areas facilitates analysis of community data. Several guidelines, presented next, help community nurses analyze population data. Analysis often supports the need for further data collection.

Guidelines for Data Analysis
Check for Missing Data
Complexity, size, and number of community characteristics prohibit gathering all possible facts about the health-related pattern areas; however, missing or insufficient data that indicate areas for further assessment should be identified. Additional assessment may determine specific approaches or a particular community diagnosis. Examples of missing data in community assessment include pollution indices, links between health resources and population groups, accessibility to resources, and morbidity statistics. Dates for census data used should be noted.

The nurse examines community data for incongruities and conflicting information. For example, a key community official might deny the existence of pollutants in the water supply, whereas newspaper reports of health department water analysis findings indicate otherwise. The nurse evaluates such inconsistencies before identifying existing or potential health concerns.

Identify Patterns
Clues about a community pattern emerge from subjective and objective data gathered. During this stage, community nurses make decisions, begin to formulate diagnostic hypotheses (ideas and tentative judgments about possible health concerns), identify community groups that might be at risk, and establish probable causes or relationships. Ideas generated from this

activity direct the search for additional clues in the data to confirm, reject, or revise hypotheses. Judgments about hypotheses continue to support patterns in the data.

To narrow the huge list of possible community health-promotion and health-protection concerns, community nurses formulate broad problem statements based on the health-related pattern areas (Gordon, 2011). For example, the community nurse differentiates among elimination problems (e.g., noxious chemicals), coping and stress-tolerance problems, and health perception–health management problems (e.g., high teenage mortality rate from motor vehicle accidents). Developing these general categories facilitates analysis.

Apply Theories, Models, Norms, and Standards
Analyzing community data requires extensive knowledge about developmental, age-related risks as well as theories and concepts of nursing, public health, and epidemiology. Such a broad foundation enables nurses to identify additional clues in health-related patterns that contribute to community nursing diagnoses and intervention. Developmental approaches form a basis to identify groups with potential health concerns. Age groups vary in susceptibility; therefore, nurses examine community resources directed toward highly susceptible groups. For example, community data that show increases in the number of live births among older women indicate a need for health-promotion services for this group. If community data show increasing numbers of aging citizens, nurses explore the availability and accessibility of existing health services for this older group.

Analysis of data for common personal or environmental characteristics also occurs. For example, select groups may be at risk based on a shared health concern, such as substance abuse, lack of immunizations, unsafe housing conditions, high exposure to asbestos or noxious chemicals, or inadequate health services. Shared characteristics, such as race or ethnicity, provide clues to susceptibility and need for screening activities. For example, Black populations warrant screening for hypertension. Also, if a fluoridated water supply is unavailable, additional intervention to prevent dental caries in children is justified. In addition, community literacy contributes to health-promotion activity development methods used by nurses to establish educational programs. Literacy level limits the ability to use all available resources.

Environmental information is readily available on the Internet. Databases and search engines provide useful information about environmental hazards and other environmental problems in communities. Prevention of disease worldwide depends on the dissemination of global environmental health information (U.S. Department of Health and Human Services, 2011). Analysis of data relies on standards developed nationally or globally. For example, community data regarding air quality can be compared with state or national ambient air quality standards to determine health. In this context the term ambient refers to outside air in a town, city, or other defined region. In the United States, air-monitoring stations are generally located in urban and rural areas within each state. One source for air quality information is the CHARTing Health Information website (https://sph.uth.tmc.edu/charting/) maintained by The University of Texas Health Science Center at Houston School of Public Health. The goal of this center is to serve as a resource in Texas for publicly available data to use for analysis and research. Data and links to other sites are continually monitored and updated (The University of Texas Health Science Center at Houston, 2012). Current information about community resources enables more effective strategies to prevent risk factors and avoid health problems. Internet access facilitates identification of gaps in health-promotion and health-protection services.

Identify Strengths and Health Concerns

Interpretation of community data occurs with regard to community concerns, community strengths, and feasibility studies. Community nurses make judgments and inferences about community health, community responses to health situations, and population needs. One approach assumes health concerns exist unless assessment data indicate otherwise (Gordon, 2011). Other systems of assessment base decisions on community strengths. With the problem-focused assessment of health concerns, nurses make diagnoses based on summarized data using the nursing process, which results in one or more of the following determinations:

- No problem exists, but providing health-promotion or health-protection services may address a potential health concern. For example, providing health education in a high school could offset a potential for increased sexually transmitted disease in the high school population.
- A problem exists but is recognized by community members or health-related professionals with effective strategies for problem-solving; for example, flu immunizations.
- A problem exists that the community recognizes, but resources are inadequate or the community has not responded. Assistance is needed; for example, highway traffic noise.
- A problem exists that the community recognizes but cannot cope with at this time, such as a lack of fluoridated water systems. Dentists, nurses, and nutritionists could be assigned to assist the community in resolving actual problems of dental caries.
- A problem or potential health concern exists that needs further study; for example, lack of sidewalks.

Using strength-based approaches to assessment emphasizes strengths and integrates health-promotion and health-protection activities into their plans. For example, a community may have nutritional feeding programs for older adults, women, and children that are underutilized. Community members may not use them because communication is inadequate. Examples of community strengths and concerns are shown in Table 8-3.

Identify Causes and Risk Factors

Data are examined for factors or characteristics that contribute to identified potential and existing health-related concerns. Nurses make inferences about population groups and identify risk factors. Identifying risk factors guides community nursing actions. Some risk factors signify immediate health concerns, such as polluted water supply, whereas other risk factors indicate

TABLE 8-3   EXAMPLES OF COMMUNITY STRENGTHS AND CONCERNS

STRENGTHS	CONCERNS
Well-child clinic available	Unavailable
Feeding program accessible to older adults	Inaccessible
Sex education in schools acceptable	Unacceptable
Family planning services accessible	Inaccessible
Fluoridated water system	Nonfluoridated water system
Open communication	Dysfunctional communication
Interagency cooperation	Dysfunctional transactions
Adequate kitchen and plumbing facilities	Inadequate
High interest of key leaders in health promotion	Lack of interest

BOX 8-4   DIVERSITY AWARENESS

Comparing Poverty Rates by Racial and Ethnic Categories

The United States uses the Current Population Survey (CPS) to assess labor force, but this survey also provides a broad-based database that includes demographic data facilitating comparison among groups (U.S. Census Bureau, 2010). The poverty rate in 2010 (15.1%) increased from that in 2009 (14.1%). This trend has continued since 2007. The poverty rate for non-Hispanic Whites increased from 9.4% to 9.9% from 2009 to 2010. Poverty rates for the Black population increased from 25.8% to 27.4%. The Hispanic population followed this same trend with an increase in the poverty rate from 25.3% to 26.6% (U.S. Census Bureau, 2010). Only the Asian population exhibited little variation from 2009, with a 2010 poverty rate of 12%. Overall, poverty in 2010 was higher than that in any other year since 1993. More people (46.2 million) lived in poverty in 2010 than at any other time since these estimates have been published. Furthermore, disparity exists among different age groups. Rates of poverty in children and adults to age 64 increased by about 1% each; however, the poverty rate for adults older than age 65 did not change substantially.

From U.S. Census Bureau. (2010). *Current population survey.* Retrieved March 7, 2012, from www.census.gov/cps/.

potential problems, such as lack of knowledge about childhood disease prevention. Nurses consider whether community risk factors can be altered, eliminated, or regulated through nursing actions. Nurses modify factors when possible by using strategies such as health education (Box 8-4: Diversity Awareness).

Community Diagnosis

Community assessment, as previously described, culminates in nursing diagnoses. The following components are included in the community diagnosis process: community situations or states within a population or population group; data collection using some combination of observation, focus groups, interview, and measurement; a framework; existing or potential health concerns; risk factors related to health concerns; and potential solutions through nursing actions. Diagnoses form the basis for planning, implementing, and evaluating solutions to health concerns (Gordon, 2011; Maurer & Smith, 2009).

BOX 8-5 QUALITY AND SAFETY SCENARIO

Workplace Violence

Targets for violent acts may be places where people work to support their families. Workplace violence was once considered isolated, unplanned incidents that fell under the jurisdiction of the federal Occupational Safety and Health Administration (OSHA). Currently, workplace violence prevention and preparation often also include external threats of terrorism. The following are some recommendations to minimize workplace violence:

- Encourage public awareness campaigns.
- Develop workplace policies and plans.
- Employ preventive law enforcement policies.
- Study government agencies that make workplace violence a priority.
- Provide proper training for employees.
- Ensure protection of the abused person when domestic violence or stalking occurs in the workplace.
- Develop and distribute clear and comprehensive legal and legislative guidelines.
- Evaluate programs and strategies after they have been implemented.

Suggestions for approaches included the following strategies:

- Educational efforts should reflect cooperative efforts by government agencies, major corporations, unions, and advocacy groups, with OSHA acting as a facilitator and coordinator.

- Enact multidisciplinary no-threats/no-violence policies and prevention plans.
- Violence prevention training should occur regularly and include practicing the plan.
- Work space and policies should provide a physically secure work environment.
- Preventive measures should be established, including documenting incidents, planning antiviolence strategies, and conducting threat assessments.
- Systems should be developed for monitoring incidents of workplace violence.
- Resource lists should be maintained and include social service, mental health, legal, and other agencies that provide assistance.
- Training programs should extend community policing concepts to workplace violence. Government or private organizations should develop training materials for small employers. Employers should keep the abuser out of the workplace (e.g., screening telephone calls, making the victim's work space physically more secure, instructing security guards or receptionists).
- Employers should provide resources for emotional, financial, and legal counseling. Clear, comprehensive, and uniform legal guidelines should be distributed widely.
- Incentives for employers should be identified and instituted.

From Occupational Safety and Health Administration. (2012). *Workplace violence.* Retrieved March 7, 2012, from www.osha.gov/SLTC/workplace violence/.

Box 8-5: Quality and Safety Scenario and Box 8-6: Innovative Practice provide an overview of how workplace violence contributes to quality and safety and how leaders might intervene to prevent or diffuse violence.

Community diagnoses facilitate communication among community health professionals, team members, and community members through the use of clear and concise nomenclature with development of diagnostic categories specific to community nursing (Maurer & Smith, 2009). Diagnoses may be written or stated according to the structural and functional aspects of a community.

Structural aspects include those related to the population, such as the demographic characteristics of groups with similar characteristics (preschool children, adolescents, or a high school population). Functional aspects include those related to the psychosocial, physiological, or spiritual health patterns, such as decision-making (cognitive-perceptual pattern) or communication links among health care resources (roles-relationships pattern). Functional health patterns guide data collection about health concerns and risk factors. Structural and functional aspects of the community provide a framework for diagnostic statements (see Chapter 6).

PLANNING WITH THE COMMUNITY

Community health planning begins with nursing diagnoses. Nurses design goals to resolve existing or potential health concerns. For example, high rates of childhood diseases in the community require goals aimed to decrease rates. Identifying specific or potential health concerns with planned actions to achieve desired **community outcomes** provides the framework and data for **community evaluation.**

BOX 8-6 INNOVATIVE PRACTICE

Intervention Techniques to Prevent and Diffuse Workplace Violence

Recognize warning signs, which include changes in mood, personal hardships, mental health issues (e.g., depression, anxiety), negative behavior (e.g., untrustworthy, lying, bad attitude), verbal threats, and history of violence. Do not limit at-risk behavior to a standard profile. Environments should be designed to detect signs of impending violence and to prevent violence with security cameras, key card access, administrative controls, and behavioral strategies. Reporting systems should be confidential and seamless.

Utilize intervention techniques:

- Stay calm; create a relaxed environment and speak calmly.
- Separate the individual from the group, if possible.
- Use nonthreatening body language; build trust and strengthen the relationship.
- Keep your verbal communication simple, clear, and direct; be open and honest.
- Reflect on the person's message to allow time for clarification, allow the person to verbalize, listen attentively, and stop what you are doing and give full attention.
- Ask for examples to help illustrate the points that are being made. Carefully define the problem, exploring with open-ended questions.
- Silence allows the individual time to clarify thoughts.
- Monitor the tone, volume, rate, and rhythm of your speech.
- Seek opportunities for agreement.
- Be creative and open to new ideas.

From Occupational Safety and Health Administration. (2012). *Workplace violence.* Retrieved March 7, 2012, from www.osha.gov/SLTC/workplace violence/.

Purposes

The following are major purposes of the planning phase:

- Prioritization of problems and identification of diagnoses through assessment
- Differentiation of problems resolved through nursing actions from those best resolved by others
- Identification of immediate, intermediate, and long-term goals, as well as behavioral objectives oriented to the community derived from the goals and specific actions to achieve objectives
- Formalization of a community nursing care plan (see the Care Plan at the end of this chapter) that includes written problems, actions, and expected behavioral outcomes

The planning phase culminates in a nursing plan that provides the framework for evaluation. Once developed, the plan is implemented. Costs associated with delivery of health services and personnel, as well as financial resources available, influence priorities for implementation. Community values and the nurse's philosophy about people, health, the community, and nursing also influence implementation. High-priority issues often include infectious agents, sexually transmitted disease, alcohol and drug use, smoking, inadequate nutrition, inadequate infant and child care, high death rate from motor vehicle accidents, and unwanted teenage pregnancies.

Community participation in health planning facilitates effective assignment of priorities. As health service recipients, community members strive for reasonably priced, high-quality services. Residents aim to acquire appropriate benefits for the needs and concerns of the population. Communication and rationale for designating priorities help to resolve differences in opinion.

During the planning phase, nurses determine those problems most amenable to community nursing intervention, behavior implemented by the nurse to fulfill a health goal of the community. Community nurses differentiate problems nursing can resolve from those health concerns that could best be managed by community members, referred to health-related professionals, or handled with community support. Nurses refer problems related to presence of rodents, poor sanitation conditions, or absence of community recreational facilities to appropriate community leaders or agencies.

Community nurses focus on determining goals, developing measurable behavioral objectives, and designating actions to achieve expected outcomes. Nurses describe specific behaviors intended to reach projected outcomes. Evaluation includes appraisal of the effectiveness of nursing actions. Health planning emphasizes promoting and protecting population health; therefore, problems, solutions, and actions are defined at the group level. Community nurses plan and implement health plans for groups, such as school-aged children, and facilitate development of health-promotion services for all residents. Nurses frequently act as change agents by taking responsibility for influencing health patterns and behavior. Decisions about health interventions stem from community nurses' appreciation of human behavior and principles of planned change. **Website Resource 8B** offers guidelines for interventions with one population group: ethnic elders.

Planned Change

Planned change results from efforts by individuals or groups and involves fundamental shifts in behavior (Pender et al., 2011). Individuals act as agents of their own health conditions. Community health objectives often depend upon active decisions by individuals to change their lifestyles (reducing alcohol consumption or quitting smoking). Efforts to influence and reinforce changes in community health behavior become the central focus of effective risk reduction programs.

Studies attempt to explain why some groups of people effectively participate in certain health programs or make lifestyle changes, whereas others do not. Early work by Rosenstock, who developed the Health Belief Model, has evolved to models such as those by Pender and Prochaska used to explain and change health-promotion behaviors (Pender et al., 2011). These models identify critical concepts for understanding how individuals change their health behavior. Rosenstock's model includes the following four steps:

- Perceiving behavior as a health threat in terms of susceptibility and seriousness
- Believing the behavior is a threat to their personal health
- Taking action to adopt preventive health behaviors
- Reinforcing the new behavior

In Rosenstock's model, community members take a passive role at first, and then transition from passive to active between steps two and three (belief to action). Ultimately, to improve community health through risk reduction programs, community members assume more responsibility for their own health, become more active in adopting healthy lifestyles, and monitor resources in the community to gain healthy behaviors. In planning health-promotion activities, nurses consider effective strategies to motivate and support community transition from a passive to an active state.

Plans guide nursing actions. Nurses make additions and changes based on community problems, resources, and problem resolution to maintain a viable plan. Table 8-1 on p. XXX provides one example of a community-oriented, health-promotion plan based on the goals recommended by the Surgeon General's report about health promotion and disease prevention. The report's general goal generates several specific objectives. Nursing diagnoses guide the direction of the objectives including risk factors to address. Examples of various rationales in Table 8-1 show how nurses incorporate important concepts of planned change into community-based health-promotion plans.

Communicating plans to other health professionals, community members, and key officials remains an essential aspect of planning. Unification of care systems and linkages through shared data entry, computerized documentation, and electronic medical records contribute to more streamlined and transparent communication and collaboration. Local newspapers, local bulletins, and school correspondence to parents provide avenues to communicate with the community about health-promotion plans. Other community-based actions, such as those for nursing involvement in prevention of alcohol abuse in the community, can be employed (Box 8-7). The various plans have been categorized according to the health patterns to show that a community problem can be approached

BOX 8-7 PLAN OPTIONS FOR COMMUNITY-BASED ACTION: ALCOHOL ABUSE

Coping-Stress Tolerance Pattern
- Identify community alcohol treatment resources.
- Develop local alcohol control laws oriented toward prevention of abuse; develop consistent state regulation and control laws.

Roles-Relationships Pattern
- Increase communication among community control agencies, schools, residents, and health-related agencies.
- Restrict community advertisements for alcohol in local newsletters and newspapers.

TABLE 8-4 POTENTIAL SOURCES OF RESISTANCE TO HEALTH-PROMOTION PROGRAMS, WITH AGENT RESPONSES

SOURCE OF RESISTANCE	RESPONSE
Lack of communication about implementation of program	Communicate through community newsletter, newspapers, high school radio station, and posters
Misinformation regarding time and place of healthy activity	Disseminate valid information
Fear of unknown	Inform and encourage
Need for security	Clarify intentions and methods
No desired need to change behaviors	Demonstrate opportunity for change
Cultural or religious beliefs or vested interests threatened	Enlist key community leaders in planning change
Inaccessibility	Focus activities near largest target population and in an area accessible by public transportation

from multiple directions. Feasible plans that are well formulated facilitate implementation (U.S. Department of Health and Human Services, 2011).

IMPLEMENTATION WITH THE COMMUNITY

Implementation of the nursing process begins based on the health-promotion and health-protection plans. In collaboration with community members or other health team members, the nurse tests feasibility and implements the plan. Involving key community members in the assessment and planning process is crucial for success. To ensure involvement, activities must be accessible. For example, schedule meetings in accessible areas, offer child care services, and provide light refreshments.Identify clearly what the community perceives as health-promotion needs. Maintain open communication—clear and correct information at regular intervals.

Intellectual, interpersonal, and technical skills of the community members facilitate the collaborative contribution. Community nurses often prepare community members with development of technical skills of community engagement and empowerment. Success also depends on overcoming expected resistance to change. Resistance to new health-promotion and health-protection activities, however, provides useful feedback to improve planning. People generally resist change to defend values that appear to be threatened by the change. Collaborating with communities initially facilitates change during the implementation phase. Table 8-4 lists factors that deter community participation. Informed nurses collaborate with community members throughout the process.

Community nurses implement health-promotion and health-protection plans in multiple community settings (schools, industry, public and private health agencies, and ambulatory care settings) where population groups experience relatively good health. Nursing centers provide nursing faculty, staff, and students unique opportunities to assess health and plan, implement, and evaluate care (including holistic health promotion and primary health care) to individuals, families, and communities with unmet health care needs (Harvey et al., 2012; Maurer & Smith, 2009). Community assessment includes observation of reciprocal interaction between the individual and his or her environment, similar to those techniques used for individual and family health promotion assessment (see Chapters 6 and 7, respectively). Community assessment also commonly uses factors related to self-efficacy and Bandura's Social Learning Theory to explain relationships between human behavior and the environment. Complexity of health actions varies from one community to another. As plans evolve, nurses learn more about the community and their own responses, strengths, limitations, and abilities to cope or adapt (Newman et al., 2011). Although implementation takes an action focus, it also includes assessment, planning, and evaluation activities to monitor actions taken to resolve, reduce, eliminate, or control the health concern.

EVALUATION WITH THE COMMUNITY

During the evaluation phase of the process, community nurses learn whether planned actions achieved desired outcomes. Communities and nurses determine progression toward goal achievement (Maurer & Smith, 2009). Nurses take overall responsibility for the process; however, collaborating with community members and health team members in the process produces the most valid results. For example, if implemented plans intend to reduce the incidence of fatal motor vehicle accidents, nurses guide the process to obtain community indicators and outcomes data, requisite community actions, and expected outcomes achieved from joint collaboration with community stakeholders.

Nursing plans, which include nursing diagnoses, expected outcomes, and interventions, provide the evaluation framework. With a community focus, goals and objectives define the evaluation, considering how the community responded to planned actions. For example, if childhood disease rate reduction is expected to result from certain nursing actions, community responses before the actions are compared to those after the actions. Comparison determines the level of effectiveness (complete, partially effective, or ineffective) of the nursing actions to achieve the goal.

Community nurses approach the dynamic process of evaluation in a purposeful, goal-directed manner (Maurer & Smith, 2009; U.S. Department of Health and Human Services, 2011). Determining effectiveness of nursing actions evaluates the degree to which goals are achieved. Frequency of evaluation depends on situations, changes expected, and objectives. For example, an individual who is bleeding may need evaluation at frequent intervals, whereas behavioral changes in community groups occur slowly and require long-term evaluation methods. Evaluation intervals vary depending upon immediate, intermediate, and long-range goals. The evaluation process continues until community goals are realized.

Evaluation results indicate need for reassessment, revision, or modification of plans. Community nurses reassess situations, plan new approaches, and implement and evaluate revised plans, creating the continual cycle of the nursing process. Self-evaluation determines strengths and weaknesses as well as ways the nursing plan could have been more effective or efficient. The quality of community health-promotion and health-protection efforts depends on the professional qualities of those providing services along with effective use of the nursing process.

Workable, cost-effective programs of community health promotion are needed. Nurses play an important role in providing evidence to support effective community health plans. Historically, documentation of effective health-promotion activities has been limited (Maurer & Smith, 2009; Pender et al., 2011). Effectiveness is determined through research studies that include analyses and outcomes evaluation of home-based and community-centered nursing interventions designed to meet needs of high-risk families, geographical communities, and vulnerable populations. For example, in a study of 679 women eligible for the Special Supplemental Nutrition Program for Women, Infants and Children (WIC), health-promotion strategies of nutrition, physical activity, and social support were employed to reduce depressive symptoms (Surkan et al., 2012). These researchers were able to demonstrate that health-promotion interventions delivered through home visits and telephone calls reduced depressive symptoms at 15 months' postpartum among low-income, ethnically diverse women (Surkan et al., 2012). Such evidence-based practice and research helps to garner support for community health-promotion programs. *Healthy People 2020* objectives include examples of national and state partnerships establishing health objectives and sustaining the initiatives (U.S. Department of Health and Human Services, 2011).

CASE STUDY

Community Efforts to Decrease Adolescent Pregnancy Rates

The community health nurse is facilitating a grassroots community group that is determined to decrease the adolescent pregnancy rate in the city. The community population hovers around 100,000. It is a community that lies on the Mexican border of the United States. The population is predominantly Mexican American, and there is a high poverty rate.

The schools offer health courses twice between seventh and twelfth grades. The only formal sex education provided occurs within the context of these two health courses. There is community opposition to increasing the amount of sex education in the curriculum. A community group that has researched the problem has decided to use a social marketing approach because of this community resistance.

Most of the materials reviewed do not address the cultural needs of the region. Many of the Spanish language materials use Spanish from countries other than Mexico. The situations posed in the audiovisual materials show people who the adolescents will perceive as different from themselves.

Reflective Questions

1. How could the community group approach their goal to decrease the adolescent pregnancy rate in a manner that will be culturally competent?
2. How might the community group approach this issue without the support of the school district?

CARE PLAN

Community Efforts to Decrease Adolescent Pregnancy Rates

*NURSING DIAGNOSIS: Risk for Ineffective Community Coping related to increased levels of teen pregnancy

Defining Characteristics
- Absence of education or support for sexually active teenagers
- Absence of programs for pregnancy testing, counseling, or teaching young women to care for infants
- Absence of sex education in the home, school, and community
- Community conflicts over what to teach adolescent and preadolescent children about sex
- Failure of teenagers to perceive long-term effects of having babies
- High incidence of infants who are born prematurely or with health problems
- High rate of teen pregnancy
- Lack of access to birth control pills or devices for teenagers
- Lack of community support for preventive sex education

Related Factors
- Community members' lack of knowledge about causes and contributing factors in teen pregnancy
- Inadequate community resources for preventing teen pregnancy
- Lack of adequate communication patterns and community cohesiveness regarding strategies to prevent teen pregnancy

Interventions
- Assess teenagers' knowledge about sex and sexuality to determine their educational needs.
- Work with schools to develop pregnancy prevention programs that provide adolescents with information about the risks, problems, and complications of early pregnancy.
- Work closely with individual adolescents who are pregnant to assess their needs and provide care.
- Implement an outreach and health-promotion program to raise community members' awareness of the need to approach teen pregnancy as a community problem. Consider taking the following five steps:
  1. Work with teachers, school psychologists, counselors, school nurses, students, and the parent-teacher association to determine the extent of the teen pregnancy problem.

CARE PLAN

Community Efforts to Decrease Adolescent Pregnancy Rates—cont'd

2. Encourage local youth groups, churches, and social service organizations to feature presentations on pregnancy prevention at their meetings.
3. Contact representatives of local corporations to ask for funding for educational programs.
4. Help community members (school nurses, counselors, and teachers) recognize adolescent girls who need counseling regarding such issues as peer pressure to be sexually active and the long-term consequences of pregnancy. Remind community members of the importance of listening attentively and remaining nonjudgmental.
5. Provide education on birth control measures (including abstinence from sex) and make this information available at school.

- Establish clubs for adolescent girls in the community. The goal of these clubs is to foster self-esteem. During club meetings, members should have the opportunity to openly discuss difficult questions, such as why girls consider a baby a status symbol and how to respond to peer pressure to be sexually active. Improved self-esteem has been found to be the most effective way to reduce teen pregnancy rates.
- Encourage adolescents to participate in peer support networks where they can openly discuss social and dating pressure and other issues related to teen pregnancy, to allow them an opportunity to express their feelings openly and obtain support from peers.
- Encourage community members to establish school-based clinics in which teens can have access to reproductive system models, pregnancy tests, and nonprescription birth control measures to support the teenagers who make the decision to protect themselves from unwanted pregnancies.

- Develop a list of referrals for teenagers, such as hospitals with human sexuality courses, charities that provide prenatal care and childbirth services, women's clinics, and Planned Parenthood, to compensate for restricted access to information in the adolescent's home or school.
- Encourage community members to implement an information campaign to educate adolescents, parents, and community members about the problems associated with teen pregnancy.
- Work with community members to evaluate the effectiveness of the teen pregnancy prevention program and assist in modifying it as needed to ensure its effectiveness and promote the program as a model for preventive health.
- Collect statistical data from the schools to analyze the teen pregnancy rates, to help evaluate the effectiveness of the prevention program.

Expected Outcomes
- Community members express awareness of the seriousness of the high adolescent pregnancy rate in their community.
- Community members express the need for a plan to reduce the prevalence of teen pregnancies.
- Community members develop and implement plans to prevent teen pregnancy.
- Community members evaluate the success of the plan in meeting goals and objectives.
- Community members continue to revise the plan to prevent teen pregnancy as necessary.

*NANDA Nursing Diagnoses—Definitions and Classification 2012-2014, Herdman T.H. (ED). Copyright © 2012, 1994-2012 NANDA International; used by arrangement with John Wiley & Sons Limited. In order to make safe and effective judgments using the NANDA-I nursing diagnoses it is essential that nurses refer to the definitions and defining characteristics of the diagnoses listed in this work.
Modified from Sparks, S. M., & Taylor, C. M. (2010). *Sparks and Taylor's nursing diagnostic reference manual* (8th ed.). Philadelphia: Lippincott Williams & Wilkins.

FIGURE 8-4 Communities come together for the enjoyment of one of their traditional holidays. (From iStockphoto/Thinkstock.)

SUMMARY

Risk factors, injury, and disease are not inevitable events experienced equally among a community's members. Effective community nurses understand the dynamic and complex nature of communities (Figure 8-4). Nurses use various theoretical frameworks to assess health-related patterns, health concerns, and health action potential and to implement the nursing process within communities. Collection and analysis of community data identify susceptible subpopulations. Planning contributes to the development of effective and efficient health-promotion and health-protection services. The nursing process enhances the efficacy of planning activities.

Many communities experience obvious deficiencies in health services that warrant health planning action. Community nurses play a significant role in health planning directed toward reducing risks associated with disease, premature death, and injury as well as health promotion among community members. Nurses use principles of planned change to increase community awareness of health, promote healthy behaviors, and encourage participation in preventive health services. Complexity varies from one community or geographical area to another. Community nurses connect health-promotion actions to specific community phenomena, providing scientific evidence to support nursing actions in the community.

REFERENCES

American Nurses Asssociation (ANA). (2010). *ANA scope and standards of practice* (2nd ed.). Silver Spring, MD: ANA.

Andrews, J. O., Cox, M. J., Newman, S. D., & Meadows, O. (2011). Development and evaluation of a toolkit to assess partnership readiness for community-based participatory research. *Progress in Community Health Partnerships: Research, Education, and Action, 5*(2), 183–188.

Andrews, J. O., Newman, S. D., Meadows, O., Cox, M. J., & Bunting, S. (2012a). Partnership readiness for community-based participatory research. *Health Education Research, 27*(4), 555–571. Retrieved from www.ncbi.nlm.nih.gov/pubmed/20837654.

Andrews, J. O., Tingen, M. S., Jarriel, S. C., & Caleb, M. (2012b). Application of a CBPR framework to inform a multi-level tobacco cessation intervention in public housing neighborhoods [online first]. *American Journal of Community Psychology, 50*(1–2), 129–140.

Cummins, S., Smith, D. M., Aitken, Z., Dawson, J., Marshall, D., Sparks, L., et al. (2010). Neighbourhood deprivation and the price and availability of fruit and vegetables in Scotland. *Journal of Human Nutrition & Dietetics, 2*(5), 494–501.

de Heer, H. D., Koehly, L., Pederson, R., & Morera, O. (2011). Effectiveness and spillover of an after-school health promotion program for Hispanic elementary school children. *American Journal of Public Health, 101*(10), 1907–1913.

Fisher-Hoch, S. P., Rentfro, A. R., Salinas, J. J., Pérez, A., Brown, H. S., Reininger, B. M., et al. (2010). Socioeconomic status and prevalence of obesity and diabetes in a Mexican American community, Cameron county, Texas, 2004-2007. *Preventing Chronic Disease, 7*(3), A53. Retrieved from www.cdc.gov/pcd/issues/2010/may/09_0170.htm.

Gordon, M. (2011). *Manual of nursing diagnosis* (12th ed.). Sudbury, MA: Jones & Bartlett.

Gordon, C., Purciel-Hill, M., Ghai, N. R., Kaufman, L., Graham, R., & Van Wye, G. (2011). Measuring food deserts in New York City's low-income neighborhoods. *Health & Place, 17*(2), 696–700.

Harvey, S. T., Fisher, L. J., & Green, V. M. (2012). Evaluating the clinical efficacy of a primary care–focused, nurse-led, consultation liaison model for perinatal mental health. *International Journal of Mental Health Nursing, 21*(1), 75–81.

Institute of Medicine. (2009). *The future of nursing: Leading change, advancing health.* Washington, DC: The National Academies Press.

Kaakinen, J., Gedaly-Duff, V., Coehlo, D. P., & Hanson, S. M.H. (2010). *Family nursing: Theory, practice and research* (4th ed.). Philadelphia: F.A. Davis.

Maurer, F. A., & Smith, C. M. (2009). *Community/public health nursing practice: Health for families and populations* (4th ed.). St. Louis: Saunders Elsevier.

Newman, S. D., Andrews, J. O., Magwood, G. S., Jenkins, C., Cox, M. J., & Williamson, D. C. (2011). Community advisory boards in community-based participatory research: A synthesis of best processes. *Preventing Chronic Disease, 8*(3), A70.

Pender, N. J., Murdaugh, C. L., & Parsons, M. A. (2011). *Health promotion in nursing practice* (6th ed.). Upper Saddle River, NJ: Pearson.

Robert Wood Johnson Foundation. (2011). *Future of nursing: Campaign for action.* Retrieved March 6, 2012, from http://thefutureofnursing.org/highlights.

Salzinger, S., Rosario, M., Feldman, R. S., & Ng-Mak, D. S. (2011). Role of parent and peer relationships and individual characteristics in middle school children's behavioral outcomes in the face of community violence. *Journal of Research on Adolescence: The Official Journal of the Society for Research on Adolescence, 21*(2), 395–407. doi:10.1111/j.1532-7795.2010.00677.x.

Scarpello, T., Poland, F., Lambert, N., & Wakeman, T. (2009). A qualitative study of the food-related experiences of rural village shop customers. *Journal of Human Nutrition & Dietetics, 22*(2), 108–115.

Stanhope, M., & Lancaster, J. (2012). *Public health nursing: Population-centered health care in the community* (8th ed.). St. Louis: Elsevier.

Sparks, S. M., & Taylor, C. M. (2010). *Sparks and Taylor's nursing diagnostic reference manual* (8th ed.). Philadelphia: Lippincott Williams & Wilkins.

Sportsman, S., Wieck, K. L., Yoder-Wise, P., Light, K. M., & Jordan, C. (2010). Creating tomorrow's leaders today: The emerging nurse leaders program of the Texas Nurses Association. *Journal of Continuing Education in Nursing, 41*(6), 259–266.

Surkan, P., Gottlieb, B., McCormick, M., Hunt, A., & Peterson, K. (2012). Impact of a health promotion intervention on maternal depressive symptoms at 15 months postpartum. *Maternal & Child Health Journal, 16*(1), 139–148.

The University of Texas Health Science Center at Houston. (2012). *CHARTing health information for Texas.* Retrieved March 7, 2012, from https://sph.uth.tmc.edu/charting/.

U.S. Census Bureau. (2010). *Current population survey.* Retrieved March 7, 2012, from www.census.gov/cps/.

U.S. Department of Health and Human Services. (2011). *2020 topics and objectives.* Retrieved July 7, 2011, from www.healthypeople.gov/2020/topicsobjectives2020/default.aspx.

Werner, C. A. (2011). *2010 census briefs: The older population* (Government No. C2010BR-09). Washington, DC: United States Census Bureau (Older Population Census). Retrieved from www.census.gov/prod/cen2010/briefs/c2010br-09.pdf.

Willmann, J. (2011). Understanding the legislative process is key to success. *Texas Nursing Voice, 5*(1), 7–8.

CHAPTER

9

Screening

Elizabeth Kudzma and Suzy Harrington

evolve WEBSITE

http://evolve.elsevier.com/Edelman/
- Study Questions
- Glossary

OBJECTIVES

After completing this chapter, the reader will be able to:
- Discuss screening and its role in secondary prevention and health promotion.
- Analyze the criteria that determine a screenable disease.
- Identify health care and economic issues and resulting ethical implications related to the screening process.

- Discuss how a collaborative community and national partnerships and policies assist in the development and implementation of a screening program.
- Describe the nursing role in the screening process.

KEY TERMS

Affordable Care Act (ACA)
Agency for Healthcare Research and Quality (AHRQ)
Asymptomatic pathogenesis
Community assessment
Community guide
Community resources
Cost-benefit ratio analysis
Cost-effectiveness analysis
Cost-efficiency analysis
Disability Adjusted Life Year (DALY)
Efficacy
Efficiency
Epidemiology
False-negative test results
False-positive test results

Five A's (Ask, Advise, Assess, Assist, Arrange) of Tobacco Cessation
Five star rating
Group or mass screening
Iatrogenic
Incidence
Individual screening
Interobserver reliability
Intraobserver reliability
Key community individuals
Lead agency
Morbidity
Mortality
Multiple test screening
National Prevention Strategy (NPS)
One-test disease-specific screening
Prevalence

Quality Adjusted Life Year (QALY)
Quality of life
Quantity of life
REACH (Racial and Ethnic Approaches to Community Health) (Centers for Disease Control [CDC])
Reliability
Secondary prevention
Sensitivity
Significance
Specificity
Stakeholders
Target community
U.S. Preventive Services Task Force (USPSTF)
Validity

Botkin, J., Goldberg, A. J., Rothwell, E., Anderson, R. A., & Huckaby, M. (2013). Use of residual newborn screening bloodspots. *Pediatrics*, 131(1):120-7.

THINK ABOUT IT

Screening Then and Now

In the 1920s, educators were introduced to the concepts of intelligence quotient, lower intelligence, and mental handicaps. Intelligence categories were quantified and cretin was a medical term used to describe one of the lower levels of intelligence. Neonatal hypothyroidism (cretinism) was more common in mountainous inland areas away from sources of sea salt iodine. It is very rare in the modern world because of the required screening of all infants at birth (blood tests measure levels of thyroid-stimulating hormone and thyroxine, or T_4). Screening testing of mothers during pregnancy and of infants shortly after birth with dried blood spot (DBS) technology allows treatment and lifetime monitoring before the serious signs of thyroxine deficiency occur. This disorder and others (e.g., phenylketonuria) are health screenings' modern success stories. Neonatal hypothyroidism has virtually disappeared in the developed world as a result of the screening of babies (target population) followed by appropriate treatment for affected individuals. However, the storage and research use of DBS technology raises significant controversy over lack of parental knowledge and consent for research activities; in some states privacy laws may inhibit retention of DBS samples without explicit parental knowledge (Botkin et al., 2013).

Very recently biotechnology companies have developed tests that aim to screen an individual's DNA (deoxyribonucleic acid) for genes associated with diseases or population subgroups. DNA testing examines a person's genetic code to provide information about genealogy or ancestry that may be helpful in assessing a person's risk for disease. Personalized DNA testing kits are available to help consumers discover their risks for disorders (such as Alzheimer's disease, diabetes, and breast cancer). An over-the-counter home test for human immunodeficiency virus (HIV) was approved by the Food and Drug Administration and was marketed to consumers in 2012. The availability of screening options that may be novel, but unproven, raises new questions about information provided to the public and the reliability and validity of screening methods and associated counseling assistance.

- Why has the newborn period been identified as an important time to require screening tests?
- Each government regulates a list of mandated screening for newborns. Do you know what your government/state/ministry of health requires?
- The availability and feasibility of screening tests is constantly changing. How are new screening tests evaluated and added to the mandated requirements?
- What characteristics about screening tests have to be considered for neonates? Individuals of any age?
- How is the margin of error further defined for screening tests/ instruments?
- What aspects of screening program development should nurses participate in? Assessment, data analysis, implementation, evaluation of health outcomes?

"Evidence-based preventive services are effective in reducing death and disability, and are cost-effective or even cost-saving. Preventive services consist of screening tests, counseling, immunizations or medications used to prevent disease, detect health problems early, or provide people with the information they need to make good decisions about their health. While preventive services are traditionally delivered in clinical settings, some can be delivered within communities, work sites, schools, residential treatment centers, or homes" (National Prevention Council, 2011, p. 18, www.healthcare.gov/prevention/nphpphc/strategy/report.pdf).

Clinical and community preventive services are vital to health promotion and disease prevention. Identified as such, they have become one of the four *Strategic Directions of the National Prevention Strategy*, which will be discussed later in the chapter. Adults may not be up-to-date on a core set of clinical preventive services and the proportion of older adults who are current or unwilling diminishes as more screening strategies are added (Bolen et al., 2007; Bynum et al., 2012; Shenson et al., 2007). Screening is an important component of clinical preventive services, because it is a valuable tool for health care professionals to identify chronic conditions and risk factors before the condition becomes costly both in financial terms and in quality of life. This is particularly important as the health care paradigm shifts from a medical and volume-based model of care to a health-promotion and value-based model of care. Although health education about screening is categorized as part of the rubric of primary prevention, the actual process of screening is part of secondary prevention.

The primary goal of screening is to detect risk factors and a disease or condition early, to prevent or treat it, and to deter its progression. An important assumption underlying the concept of screening is that detection during the early asymptomatic period allows treatment at a time when the eventual course of the disease can be altered significantly. Similarly, identifying risk factors assists in identifying the populations needing screening and points to the needed behavior change before the disease develops. The screening concept and process is based on the principle that the selected disease is preceded by a period of asymptomatic pathogenesis or latency (disease origin or development before symptoms first appear) when risk factors predisposing a person to the disease are building toward full manifestation of the disease. Screening takes advantage of the prepathogenic state and the early pathogenic state—identifying risks relating to disease in the earliest and most treatable stages. Administration of screening tests, some of which might be fairly simple and relatively inexpensive when compared to the burden of disease, provides value in improved quality of care and decreased health care costs. Screening is not generally a diagnostic measure, nor is it curative. It is a preliminary step to identify individuals who need more diagnostic workup to prevent further development of the condition or disease and to ameliorate adverse disease outcomes. More importantly, it is a step towards empowering individuals to make more informed choices about their health and health behaviors. A second, but equally important, objective of screening is to reduce the costs of managing the disease by avoiding more intensive interventions required in later disease stages. A cost-conscious approach to health care mandates that health care professionals, at all levels, acquire a basic understanding of the screening process and its application. Screening activities can occur every day or be conducted by individuals, offices, or a large public community.

ADVANTAGES AND DISADVANTAGES OF SCREENING

Advantages

Some screenings can be very simple and performed at home (blood pressure, heart rate, weight). Nurses are involved in promoting and educating their use. This chapter, however, will focus more on the efficacy and efficiency of clinical, procedural, and lab-based tests. Screening tests offer several advantages. Although some screening procedures are simple and relatively inexpensive, others are expensive and may not be cost-effective. The simplicity of the screening procedure decreases the time and cost of involved health care personnel and enables less skilled technicians to administer the test, especially when compared to the cost of treating the disease after symptoms appear.

A second advantage is the ability to apply the screening process to both individuals and large groups. In an individual screening program, one person is tested by a health professional who has designated the individual as high risk (such as prior hypertension). The practitioner can make this selection independently; the health care agency can define a specific policy; or legislative bodies can require the screening by law as in the case of neonatal hypothyroidism, phenylketonuria (PKU), or lead-screening programs in children. As electronic health records become more sophisticated, a proactive flag notification during health care visits ideally alerts the provider when the care recipient should have a recommended screening. Group or mass screening occurs when a target population is selected on the basis of an increased incidence of a condition or a recognized element of high risk within an identified group. For example, the target population may be invited to a central location on a designated day to be tested for the selected disorders (elevated levels of lipids and cholesterol, hypertension, osteoporosis, blood glucose level).

A third advantage is the ability to provide one-test specific screening or multiple test screenings. A one-test disease-specific screening is the administration of a single test that searches for a characteristic that indicates a high risk of developing a disorder. An example of this would be blood pressure screening to evaluate hypertension. Multiple test screening is the administration of two or more tests to detect more than one disease. In some cases, one sample can be used to evaluate the possibility of several conditions, saving time and money and making the process efficient and economical. For example, a blood sample can be assessed for many components including elevated glucose and cholesterol levels. The combination of the relatively low-cost screening test and flexibility makes screenings adaptable to all levels within the health care delivery system. Other screenings of importance are for substance abuse, mental health disorders and depression, and sexually transmitted infections (STIs).

A final advantage of screening is that it creates an opportunity for providing health education to a group of individuals who may not otherwise receive it. In some situations, it is possible to establish a clinical relationship during the screening process that leads to preventive visits and includes educating people about healthy lifestyles, risk reduction, developmental needs, activities of daily living, and preventive self-care. Many

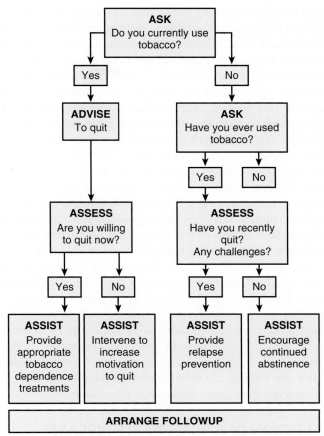

FIGURE 9-1 Five A's of tobacco cessation.

of today's chronic illnesses are a result of individual health behaviors. Awareness is the first step in prevention. Although it requires more than awareness to change behaviors, it is still necessary to embrace the concept of prevention. If awareness is combined with health-education and health-promotion tools, individuals would have a better opportunity to manage their own risks. Taking advantage of a potential teachable moment should never be overlooked.

An example is the standard 6-month dental screening or "check-up" covered by many insurance companies. Although the individual is at the dentist's office to be screened for cavities and cancer of the mouth and to have teeth cleaned to avoid gum disease, the hygienist provides reminders on the correct way and the necessity to brush and floss correctly, while frequently providing a sample toothbrush to be taken home. Another example is the Five A's (Ask, Advise, Assess, Assist, Arrange) of Tobacco Cessation (Agency for Healthcare Research and Quality [AHRQ], n.d.) recommended screening and counseling for successful tobacco intervention (AHRQ, 2009 (Figure 9-1). It is not enough to simply screen with the question, "Do you use tobacco?" Readiness to quit should also be determined, combined with cessation treatment assistance and counseling through "Assist and Advise" (Fiore et al., 2009).

Disadvantages

The primary disadvantages of screening stem largely from the imperfection of modern science, which results in a range of error for many screening tests. When effectiveness depends on the screening program's ability to distinguish those who probably do have the disease from those who do not, any margin of error can result in serious consequences. Some individuals who do not have the condition will be referred for further tests and some who do have the disease will not. Those incorrectly referred (false positive) suffer needless anxiety and more unnecessary medical interventions while awaiting more definitive diagnosis (e.g., high levels of prostate-specific antigen [PSA]). Mammography screening for breast microcalcifications identifies a significant number of women (who may be false positives) to more specific follow-up testing and medically invasive breast biopsies (Kudzma, 2008). False-positive osteoporosis screens can mean unnecessary bone building medication treatment that may also have adverse effects. Care recipients also bear the burden of the follow-up visits, costs, lost time, and inconvenience.

The effects on those whose diseases have been overlooked (false negative) are even more important. These individuals have a false assurance of health that will be shattered eventually, and they lose the opportunity to receive early treatment that could prevent irreversible damage. The difficulty of balancing the benefits to some against the losses to others may be an ethical issue underlying many screening programs. The significance of this disadvantage can vary; therefore, it should be assessed for each screening program, disease, and population.

SELECTION OF A SCREENABLE DISEASE

The selection of a screenable disease goes beyond examination of the disease alone. The selection process must also encompass less tangible factors, such as the emotional (human immunodeficiency virus [HIV]) and financial impact (osteoporosis) (Nayak et al., 2011) of the disease's detection on the screened population. Even after gathering data and reviewing the critical issues, the final decision of whether to screen must often be reached with incomplete evidence or with answers that raise ethical issues, on an epidemiological and a personal level.

The potential uncertainties confounding the decision emphasize the need to conduct an analysis of available material to obtain a decision that is as objective and scientific as possible. The answers to the following three questions provide a basis for designating a disease as screenable or nonscreenable:

- Does the significance of the disorder warrant its consideration as a community problem?
- Can the disease be detected by screening?
- Should screening for the disease be done?
  - What are the health benefits? For example, can it be treated?
  - What are the tangible and intangible costs?

As simplistic as these questions may appear, the answers or lack of answers may expose numerous complex issues that determine whether a well-informed decision can be made on screenability.

Significance

The significance of a disease refers to the level of priority assigned to the disease as a public health concern. Although the opinions of political and public interest groups may influence the evaluation, significance generally is determined by incidence and prevalence, and by the quantity and quality of life affected by the disorder (Max & Lynn, Interactive Textbook, n.d.).

According to the Centers for Disease Control and Prevention (CDC), epidemiology is the "study of the distribution and determinants of health-related states in specified populations, and the application of this study to control health problems (and is used to) plan and evaluate strategies to prevent illness and as a guide to the management of patients in whom disease has already developed" (CDC, 2004). Health information on both morbidity and mortality may be used to identify the most important diseases affecting populations. The term morbidity refers to a diseased state or disability from any cause; however, the concept of morbidity can be broader, including a range or degree of the illness that affects the person. Information on mortality (deaths) in a given population can be easier to use as end outcome indices as long as statistical collection measures are accurate.

Key factors in assessing the need for screening criteria are quantifying measures of disease frequency. Two measures most used in epidemiology are incidence and prevalence (Lundy & Janes, 2009). Incidence is the rate of a new population problem and estimates the risk of an individual developing the specific disease or condition during a specific period or over a lifetime. Prevalence is the proportion of a given population with the disease or condition at any one point in time. It provides the best estimate of whether a person is likely to become ill during a specific period of time. Usually chronic conditions are measured by their prevalence (generally existing), whereas acute conditions are assessed by their incidence (rate of occurrence). Both are used in assessing the need for community services and screenings, and help form the foundation of many evidence-based practice screening guidelines to include the age at which screening should be performed, the frequency and manner of screening, and the person who should perform the screening. The greater the physical and psychological harm experienced by the population, the greater is the need to designate the disease as a priority health problem. The first step in assessing screening feasibility is evaluation of this significance to decide if the disorder warrants the time, effort, and financial resources that must be allocated.

Estimating the quality of life affected by a disease presents problems but is a necessary step. The perception of quality of life is subjective and individual evaluations may differ. For example, not all people equally perceive the disability resulting from a disease; some make adjustments and cope, whereas others do not. Those who do not may be more likely to say that the quality of their lives is significantly lower than that of other people.

A Quality Adjusted Life Year (QALY) is a measurement of quality of life. It is defined as perfect health minus the Disability Adjusted Life Year (DALY). The QALY assumes that 1 year of excellent health is 1 QALY (1 year of life times 1 utility value equals 1 QALY). It also assumes that 1 year spent in a less perfect state of health or with disease (or comorbidities) is worth less. A determination of the QALY value involves multiplying the utility value associated with a state of health by the years lived in that state of health. Following this thinking, half a year lived in excellent health is 0.5 QALY (0.5 year of life times 1 utility value), which is the same as 1 full year of life lived in a disease state (immobile, fractured hip) (1 year times 0.5 utility value).

The Disability Adjusted Life Year (DALY) is a year spent in less than healthy life. It is a measure of the burden of disease and measures the gap between the current health status and excellent health status. It also accounts for life lost and life quality diminished through disability. Both the QALY and DALY concepts may be used depending on whether the outcome of the screening measure is intended to maximize health or minimize disability (Airoldi & Morton, 2009; Hirskyj, 2007).

Recently, there has been greater focus on quantifying measurements of health outcomes in order to weigh the costs of screening, treatment, and effects on populations. The QALY incorporates morbidity and mortality in a single arithmetic measure. It allows for computation, estimation, and comparisons of screening decisions; however, the estimation of formulas association with utility and disability is difficult. QALYs do bridge the gap between strict treatment decisions and their economic costs, informing public health decision-making (Hirskyj, 2007). By contrast, measures of the quantity of life affected by the disease are more readily obtainable. In addition to prevalence and incidence rates, disease-specific mortality rates present another picture. Disease-specific mortality may be linked to the severity of an incident occurring or the longtime health burden cost associated with management of the disease. There is some evidence that mandatory screening of athletes reduces the incidence of sudden cardiac death in athletes who are supposedly young and fit (Shephard, 2011); a death in a young fit person is a very severe event. With other diseases, the prevalence of the disorder may not be great, but the problem requires disproportionate amounts spent on maintenance or management after the condition is fully expressed. For phenylketonuria (PKU), a case undetected at birth means a lifetime of case management.

Detection

With the relative significance of the disease established, the next step is to determine if health professionals can screen for the disease. Do well-documented diagnostic criteria for the disorder exist? Is there a valid and reliable screening instrument? Are sufficient community resources and treatment modalities available to support a screening program?

Diagnostic Criteria

Detection of a disease requires knowledge of characteristics that indicate its presence or, as in screening, its early pathogenic, asymptomatic state, and is often based on risk factors such as heredity, age, gender, and family history. For example, screening tests may be recommended for men or women (USDHHS, 2011a,b; Womenshealth.gov, 2012). Selected disease diagnostic criteria should be well documented and defined and not be merely accepted as commonly used indicators. The impact of uncertainty in detecting disease is amplified when considering the application of the screening design. Some diseases, such as sickle cell anemia or phenylketonuria (PKU), are defined by the presence or absence of a single, isolated gene or chemical. Other conditions, such as high blood glucose levels (diabetes), are measured according to numerical values for which a normal range has been set. Although there may be some disagreements over normal parameters, diabetes is a serious disease and early treatment has been shown to decrease the incidence of morbidity and mortality particularly attributable to vascular diseases and stroke.

Screening Instruments

The next step is to determine if methods exist to detect the disease during early pathogenesis. If instruments are available, a careful analysis should determine if any of them fulfill the requirements for the screening process: available, easy to administer, safe with minimal discomfort, cost-effective, and accurate. Ultimately the decision to use a screening test will depend on how well the instrument can distinguish those individuals who probably do not have and will not develop the condition from those who are likely to develop the condition. The variables that aid in a screening instrument's evaluation include reliability, validity, and reproducibility, which are a measure of the accuracy of the instrument.

Reliability is an assessment of the reproducibility of the test's results when different individuals with the same level of skill perform the test during different periods and under different conditions. The instrument or measure should yield consistent or stable results over time. If the same result emerges when two individuals perform the test, interobserver reliability is shown. If the same individual is able to reproduce the results several times, intraobserver reliability is demonstrated.

From these data, health professionals can determine the amount of training that is required for health care technicians or personnel who administer the test. For example, if interobserver reliability is low, additional training might be required to work toward a more consistent method of test delivery. This is frequently necessary in cuff hypertension screening or in weight measurements where the scale may not function properly. If intraobserver reliability is low, the health professional might surmise that the instrument, and not the individual, is at fault. Other screening measures are even more qualitative; for example, intraobserver reliability may be necessary in substance abuse or mental health/depression screening. Finally, for a screening test to be valid, which is the next concept, it must first be reliable, but reliability is only a necessary condition, but not entirely sufficient for validity.

Validity reflects the accuracy or truthfulness of the test or instrument itself. In a controlled setting, validity is evaluated by testing the instrument on a group of individuals who have positive or negative results. A valid test correctly categorizes individuals who have preclinical disease from those without preclinical disease. The ideal result is to have the instrument identify 100% of the diseased individuals (positive reactions) and 100% of the nondiseased individuals (negative reactions). There are also ranges of measurement for disease reliability and validity. Perfectly accurate categorization of validity rarely occurs in practice; therefore, the measure of validity has been divided into two more components that quantify the margin of error in screening instruments.

Sensitivity measures the first component. This refers to the proportion of people with a condition who correctly test positive when screened. If a test has good sensitivity, the number of individuals with the disease who are missed through inaccurate categorization as false negatives will decrease. Conversely, a test with poor sensitivity will overlook individuals with the condition and there will be a large number of false-negative test results; individuals actually have the condition but were told they are disease-free or negative.

Specificity is the second component. Specificity measures the test's ability to recognize negative reactions or nondiseased individuals. A test with excellent specificity will rarely be positive if the disease is not present. A test with poor specificity could result in false-positive test results. Individuals with false-positive test results are told that they have a disease or condition when in actuality they do not.

In a perfect world, tests would be highly sensitive and highly specific; however, usually that is not the case and there is some balance reached between the two concepts. For some tests, there may also be an indeterminate zone in which the individual does not test strictly negative or positive. In these tests, the numerical cut-off may be subject to interpretation or a more arbitrary decision. A cut-off decision may be made so that the screening instrument is less likely to miss actual cases of disease at the cost of identifying some erroneously having the disease (false positives) that will need more diagnostic work, which may be expensive and invasive.

Consider the issues that a public health nurse must face when using a newly developed screening test with low specificity and moderate sensitivity. Low specificity means few true-negative and more false-positive test results. The nurse and other health professionals (also health advocacy groups, such as those involved in breast cancer awareness) must then consider the cost, inconvenience, and psychological stress experienced by the people with false-positive reactions during the period after their incorrect screening test, the unnecessary additional referrals, and the ability of the existing follow-up services to meet these needs. With only moderate sensitivity, a number of false-negative results could occur, which may ignore individuals who could benefit from treatment. Medical, economic, and ethical issues could be involved; that is, should a screening program be implemented when it is known that the tests deliver false-positive and false-negative results?

A broader issue concerns large health fair screening programs, for example, where a targeted population such as older adults is sought for a mass screening. The efficiency and efficacy of such programs must be analyzed. The following are examples of questions that address efficiency and efficacy: Is the targeted population prepared in an appropriate way before engaging in the screening tests? Are the health care practitioners who are administering the test educated (and certified) according to the standard protocols of test administration? And, are follow-up measures and appropriate referral access instituted in the program? There are times when an older adult lacks the cognitive ability or finances to follow-up on positive screening results.

Answers to these questions challenge health care providers in the development, implementation, and follow-up processes identified so that screening efficiency and efficacy is enhanced.

Very recently, a number of for-profit genomic and biotechnology companies have marketed genetic tests to identify genes and ancestry associated with risk factors and diseases. A number are available on the Internet. One of the most widely known, 23andme (www.23andme.com), reports that their DNA analysis can provide information about 100 health disorders and traits including carrier risk, drug response, and disease risk (e.g., Parkinson's disease, cholesterol levels, presence of diabetes). Another DNA prenatal test (Verinata Health, 2012, www.verinata.com) reports that their test can identify neonatal chromosomal abnormalities including Down syndrome at 10 weeks' gestation with a simple blood test in the physician's office; this test would be less invasive than amniocentesis. These tests are highly marketed, becoming common and dramatically less expensive. They can involve issues of standardization, cost, and privacy, and may fail to make reports fully explainable or understandable to the consumer.

Issues emerging from full investigation of screening instruments demonstrate the significant influence they have on the entire process. Data on the reliability and validity of individual tests and screening programs in general provide valuable information to evaluate, anticipate, and ideally control these influences, enabling the program to work effectively toward its goal and positive care outcomes.

Primary Care and Community Screening Resources

Screening is often done in an outpatient primary care setting. Screenings are also often based in the community with the assistance of a public health nurse, in the worksite by an occupational health nurse, and in schools by a school health nurse. Since funding for traditional public health nursing roles is declining, some of the responsibility for screening will fall to nurses in other basic and advanced practice roles. Implementing a screening program depends on availability of appropriate community resources, such as funds, health care workers, and follow-up services including access, treatment sources, and administrative personnel. Judicious organization of the overall program is key to its success. Knowledge of the disease's characteristics and the screening instrument is useless without financial and organized human support to apply it. The overall approach is complex, requiring intense efforts in the area of partnership development.

A lead agency or group may be identified to oversee the development process of the community health program. Origins of the lead agency vary from a community service organization to local public health departments responding to regulations or a mandate from the state. Regardless of its origin, the agency must perform a self-evaluation to compare its level of expertise with what is required to supervise the process of the screening effort. Early identification of the lead agency, along with potential partnerships, allows for the effective use of talents and the division of labor.

Some screening programs may involve intricate legal issues. HIV screening and testing is highly recommended in high-risk persons—those who have injected steroids or drugs, those who have unprotected sex (especially men who have sex with men), and those diagnosed with other STIs or comorbidities (e.g., hepatitis caused by hepatitis C infection). States have their own procedures about HIV testing and identification of cases. To protect individual identities, consumer-controlled home screening kits are available (CDC, 2011b, http://hivtest.cdc.gov/faq.aspx#tested). In 2012, the Food and Drug Administration (FDA, 2012) approved the first over-the-counter HIV test (www.fda.gov/forconsumers/byaudience/forpatientadvocates/hivandaidsactivities/ucm117922.htm). This test, OraQuick, requires a fluid specimen from the mouth at the gum line and gives preliminary results in 30 minutes.

For the lead agency to develop and oversee the development process of any community health program such as the delivery of a screening program, partnerships and coalitions are essential. The agency must contact and organize necessary stakeholders. Stakeholders are individuals or groups who have a legitimate interest in the topic. Examples of stakeholders include key community individuals, hospitals, health and social service agencies such as primary health care centers, and community organizations including houses of worship, community centers, schools, transportation agencies, and volunteer organizations. Key community individuals are those people who are considered leaders within the community. The primary rule is to never assume that what is appropriate and effective for one community will be appropriate and effective for another.

The members of the partnership carry out the community assessment together. A community assessment is a systematic method of data collection that provides a detailed account, first identifying need and subsequently determining the type, quantity, and quality of resources. Reviewing demographic, vital statistics, and morbidity and mortality data may identify the assessed need. Resources might come from an eclectic variety of support to include government entities such as public health departments, social services, and even safety and transportation in cases of car seat safety screenings. Schools, private businesses, churches, and places of social gatherings might provide resource support, either in screening support or in the actual administration of the screening.

After completing the assessment, the data analysis will reveal the target community or high-risk population, the available health care resources, and the health needs of the high-risk population. The identified partners collaborate, review, and analyze the data, leading to the development of health improvement strategies (in this case a screening program), with methods of implementation to move the target population smoothly through the screening process. Finally, monitoring and evaluating outcomes is essential to determine the effectiveness of the program and the achievement of stated goals. Evaluation includes monitoring the entire process, including the successful workings of the partnership. Figure 9-2 presents a model of collaborative partnership: community health program development.

Constraints affecting the operation of a screening program include financial concerns, political issues, cultural constraints, follow-up and referral services, and accessible treatment

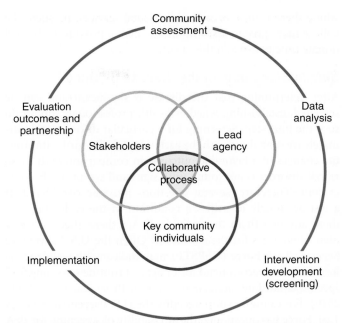

FIGURE 9-2 Collaborative partnership: community health program development.

facilities. All partners are aware that responses from the target community are affected partly by their experience with other screening programs, such as the means used to inform them, the accessibility of the location, the availability of transportation, the convenience of the program's hours, and the cultural sensitivity of the delivery and design of the program. A public health nursing approach identifies the necessary community resources and defines how these resources interact and may be mobilized to achieve maximal benefits and positive outcomes. Financial support of the screening program is a constraint that can influence all points in the system. Although some programs are delivered entirely on a voluntary basis, organizers of others must submit grant proposals to local, state, or federal departments when consideration of medical and economic ethics is involved. Planners must look beyond the screening day and investigate financial resources for follow-up care and treatment.

In addition to financial accessibility, follow-up services need to be accessible in terms of convenient locations and open hours. For example, an evening clinic may reach those who are reluctant or financially unable to miss work. An efficient referral system links the follow-up resources to the screening program, providing continuity of care. A method must be devised to encourage the participant to take positive action on the referral. Public health nurses will facilitate this process with a variety of communication techniques, such as telephone or in-person counseling, mailings, and home visits.

Another example is that the local college of health sciences provides a health fair screening day. Pharmacists screen for medical use of inappropriate or contraindicated medications. Nursing students and medical students manage physical assessments and laboratory screenings. Social workers may assess for mental health issues. However, there must be a plan for continuation of care if disease issues and risks are identified; for example, persons needing immediate dental care in an area where there is little or no public dental services. As such, the college may agree to assist in finding dental providers who will donate time to assist in this effort.

Should Screening for the Disease Be Done?

After determining that the disease is significant and can be screened, establishing whether health professionals should do so is the final step. Screening for a particular disorder and ultimately treating those with the early-identified disorder improve the chances of a favorable outcome in comparison with those whose disorder is not found until signs and symptoms become evident. Therefore, several questions must be considered. If a test accurately identifies a condition in the early stages, is there any benefit to the individual? Are there effective treatment modalities for the condition? Often the U.S. Preventive Services Task Force (USPSTF) may indicate "the evidence is insufficient to recommend for or against routine screening for" specific conditions because of some of these issues (USPSTF, 2010). For example, more recently the U.S. Preventive Services Task Force has questioned the advisability of screening for PSA (prostate-specific antigen). The USPSTF has determined that there is insufficient evidence to assess the balance of benefits and harms of prostate cancer screenings in men younger than age 75 (www.uspreventiveservicestaskforce.org/uspstf/uspsprca.htm). It is necessary for the health care provider to keep abreast of changes in critical health screening guidelines. The nurse needs to be aware of screening guidelines for the most common disabilities.

Screening is based on the disease's asymptomatic period; therefore, adequate information must exist concerning the optimal time for screening, specific intervention during this time, and knowledge regarding the effect of early detection and treatment on the prognosis. Without this knowledge, health care professionals are unable to explain how the consequences of the detected disease differ from those of persons with undetected disease. They can neither evaluate nor explain the health benefits derived from the screening program.

Follow-up is critical to determine if intervention strategies prescribed are in fact taking place. Should screening be done if there is no follow-up in terms of medical or social services? A prescribed follow-up regimen may be very broad and include a wide variety of intervention strategies such as diet, exercise, and drug therapy. Follow-up services may include an evaluation and review of the literature that discusses evidence-based practice pertaining to a particular drug, as well as the identification of intervention characteristics that impair follow-up, such as cost, inconvenience, or side effects. Consideration must also be given to those factors that enhance follow-up. For example, nurses can provide ongoing counseling and education about a medication and assist individuals in a lifestyle transformation that includes health-promoting behaviors.

The safety of the intervention is a concern when considering the widespread application of further medical interventions or invasive diagnostic tests after a screening program. Risks or harmful side effects can be costly in terms of human health and the increased medical care required to correct iatrogenic or interventional effects resulting from the intervention.

Health care professionals must decide if these risks significantly diminish the success of the treatment and outweigh the benefits derived from the treatment.

The bottom line is that to be effective, a high-quality, cost-effective, research/evidence-based screening tool or technique is needed that identifies a real or potential "problem" and provides a real and workable "solution," in which the tangible and intangible costs of the screening are less than the risk of the disease or condition and the health benefit.

ETHICAL CONSIDERATIONS

A step taken toward improving health usually is deemed a just and moral act within the health care system's values. However, health care recommendations must be approached with a more critical eye and it is necessary to realize that not all the results of a well-intended practice are beneficial, and there is a need to balance the benefit against potential detrimental effects. The resulting decision process then becomes a value judgment and an ethical issue.

Health Care Ethics

A screening program is in a category separate from interventions offered for established disease processes. Rather than receiving those who have performed a self-assessment and elected to enter the system, a screening program invites seemingly well individuals to be tested to determine disease risk and the need for follow-up. The request for participation implies that a health benefit will be derived, although at this stage nothing is said about what it will be or what the consumer must do to obtain it. Program planning that attempts to clarify this implication and inform participants of the issues develops the basis for an ethically sound project and enhances the screenability of the disease.

Most screening programs are named by the disease being screened, such as hypertension screening or diabetes screening; therefore, it is not surprising that participants enter screening programs assuming the results received are diagnostic and will classify them as disease-free or disease-laden. This is untrue, because the screening goal is only to identify and refer individuals at risk or who may need further follow-up or evaluation. The initial presentation of and contact with the program implies a benefit not being delivered. To alleviate this problem, the planning committee should develop a method of informing participants of the meaning and limitations of the results. Participants need to know whether the ultimate benefit is preventive, ameliorative, or curative and, most importantly, what responsibility they must assume to secure this outcome.

Misinterpretation caused by the screening instrument is of even greater ethical concern than human misperception. As the information on sensitivity and specificity indicates, false-positive and false-negative results occur with any screening instrument. One of the more difficult ethical issues in screening is to evaluate whether the benefits received by those who receive correct results are worth the problems experienced by those who receive incorrect results. What obligation does the project have to the latter? What is an acceptable number of people with false-negative test results, all of whom will both miss the benefit of early treatment and be misled about the need for tests in the near future? What will be the response of an individual who has a false-positive test? Answers to these questions are value judgments that may vary according to the disease.

Additional issues that confound the medical ethics of screening are cut-off points for the screening instrument and borderline cases. How precisely do the instrument's numerical values define the high-risk disease state? The goal of a screening program, identifying an individual as high risk or not high risk, depends on this numerical value. When the parameter for this distinction is not clear, a cut-off point is set. Above this point, the person is considered disease-positive; below this point, the individual is disease-negative. Consequently, readjusting the cut-off point becomes a highly controversial issue, because it controls the percentage of positive and negative results. If the disease were potentially life threatening, an increase in false-positive results (lower cut-off point) would be preferred to missing individuals who may have the disease. In addition, if a disease is relatively benign in terms of potential stigmatization, anxiety, and problems with treatment, lowering the cut-off point could again be safe and ethical.

A problem closely related to the cut-off point is defining a policy for borderline cases. Hypertension is a common disease in which a variance of 5 to 10 mm Hg can make the difference in identifying a person as high risk. Lipid and cholesterol level cut-offs and ratios are always subject to further examination. Osteoporosis standards for men are debated (USPSTF, www.uspreventiveservicestaskforce.org/uspstf10/osteoporosis/osteors.htm). Guidelines constantly change as new research emerges and new special interest groups change the definitions, but it is helpful to look at the whole picture and see it as a great opportunity for health education whether the individual is high risk or borderline. A more sophisticated approach may be taken to discriminate between a borderline case that should be referred and one that should not. The health professional can specify other risk factors associated with hypertension or lipid evaluation, such as family history, diet, and smoking, as criteria for deciding whether to refer an individual. With the increasing interest in and knowledge of risk factors, the effectiveness of this method has improved.

The medical ethics of screening will continue to demand review of the same questions and issues; however, the answers may change as more is discovered about the various conditions and their treatments. An updated literature review is imperative before reviewing these issues in relation to a particular screenable disease.

Economic Ethics

Associating a monetary value with health care outcomes generally disputes the ideal ethic of professionals involved in health care. In the past, the tendency was to place no limits on the cost of promoting a healthy, disease-free, or disease-controlled status, resulting in a philosophy that all care should be given to all people at all costs. This philosophy has evolved to one of conscious recognition of the costs of screening events. Allocating community funds to a large screening event could result

in a lack of funds for other projects. Those benefiting from a screening test will be countered by those suffering from a lack of service for other medical or social needs. These trade-offs result in ethical decisions demanding careful analysis by the screening administration (Box 9-1: Hot Topics).

Screening can be a costly project for both organizers and consumers. Initial operational costs must be considered, including buying or renting the screening instruments, renting floor space, and engaging professionals or technicians to administer the tests and interpret the results.

These costs are encountered again when people are referred for further evaluation. Consumer costs include follow-up visits, treatment, time, and income that are lost while complying with each. Given the combined operational and consumer costs, several questions are raised. Do the costs result in the desired health outcome to the individual, group, or community? Are the benefits reaped worth the expenditures required? The answer is determined partly by what values (other than monetary ones) are attributed to the benefit, such as saving a life. A strictly economic approach, however, generally eliminates the intangible variables, demanding the use of more objective data for decision-making.

When program designs are being considered with screening, three main approaches may be used to evaluate the economic resources affected: cost-benefit ratio, cost-effectiveness, and cost-efficiency analyses. Once far from the thoughts of health care workers, the current relevance and use of such concepts require a basic understanding of their role in the selection of a screenable condition. Although presented here in successive fashion, they are entirely separate methods and most frequently are used independently of one another.

Cost-Benefit Ratio

Cost-benefit ratio analysis is performed first, because it allows the comparison of various outcomes in monetary terms (Hankins, 2009). This comparison is necessary in health planning when the initial consideration is dependent upon whether the expected health outcome (such as reduction in cardiovascular disease, decrease in infant mortality, or reduction of a visual problem) will be most beneficial to the community at the most reasonable cost. The cost of the screening versus the cost of chronic care management must also be considered. For example, what is the cost-benefit ratio of blood pressure screenings, compared to the medical and financial cost of a stroke caused by undiagnosed hypertension, to the individual, the community, and the health care system? The cost of screening may also have to be weighed against other factors such as the cost and feasibility of vaccination programs, as in the case of screening for human papillomavirus for cervical cancer prevention (Maine et al., 2011). Resources are becoming much more available because of the advancement of electronic data gathering tools, such as the Centers for Disease Control and Prevention *Chronic Disease Cost Calculator* (CDC, 2011a, www.cdc.gov/chronicdisease/resources/calcula tor/index.htm), which estimates state Medicare expenditures for certain diseases.

Cost-Effectiveness

If the reduction of cardiovascular disease is chosen as the desired outcome, the next step is a cost-effectiveness analysis, which determines the optimal use of resources to reach a predetermined, constant end point or the desired health outcome. The outcome remains the same; the best method of deriving it is the issue. For example, considering the selected health outcome, such as the reduction of cardiovascular disease, various methods might be used. These methods include screening for hypertension, performing electrocardiograms on all individuals ages 25 or older who are admitted to the hospital, screening young athletes for cardiovascular disease, beginning an antismoking campaign, or obtaining nutrition counseling. Implementation of all these options would be ideal, but with limited resources a choice must be made.

Cost-Efficiency

The last approach to help bring the economic resources into perspective is cost-efficiency analysis. The purpose is to be efficient and budget a limited amount of money toward achieving as much of the desired outcome as possible. The funds are the central issue, not the health benefit.

SELECTION OF A SCREENABLE POPULATION

The selection of a screenable population is as important as the selection of a screenable disease and is often based on incidence and prevalence. The objective is to identify a high-risk group that, when tested, will yield a significant number of diseased individuals. With such results, the efforts and cost of screening the population are minimized and the health benefit received is maximized. The main criterion used to define an appropriate population is the definitive presence of risk factors related to the disorder. To ensure a thorough examination of possible risk

---

BOX 9-2   RESEARCH FOR EVIDENCE-BASED PRACTICE

Population-Based Research Optimizing Screening Through Personalized Regimens (PROSPR)

The National Cancer Institute has developed PROSPR (Population-based Research Optimizing Screening through Personalized Regimens) to support research on the community-based screening processes to include experiences and outcomes for breast, colon, and cervical cancer. The overall aim is to develop coordination between the research practices carried out in multiple sites. It reviews recruitment, screening, diagnosis, referral, and treatment rates. It focuses on research translation and implementation, addressing issues such as the controversy regarding breast cancer screening and mammography by studying the comparative effectiveness and outcomes of existing and emerging research. In September 2011, the National Cancer Institute funded seven research centers and one statistical site as part of this integrated research screening program. Be on the lookout for similar new programs because the Prevention Fund supported by the Affordable Care Act supports the development of other such opportunities to discover and support evidence-based health-promotion and disease-prevention activities.

From National Cancer Institute (NCI). (2011). *PROSPR*. Retrieved June 23, 2012, from http://applied research.cancer.gov/networks/prospr/.

---

factors, both person-dependent and environment-dependent factors should be reviewed (Box 9-2: Research for Evidence-Based Practice).

Person-Dependent Factors

The person's age is increasingly important because of age-dependent changes in levels of risk factors throughout the population. Practice has always placed a high priority on screening the vulnerable, at-risk infant population, partly because of the health outcomes that affect the child's growth and development. As the average life span increases, however, the effects of longer-range risk factors are becoming apparent, making certain prevalent and costly chronic conditions equally important to control. Middle-aged adults have been a targeted group for certain conditions, such as hypertension, diabetes, breast cancer, glaucoma, and heart disease, which have commonly appeared during this period, but are requiring earlier screening since they are becoming apparent in early adulthood and even teenage years. Older-aged adults may be screened for Alzheimer's disease, although screening for the asymptomatic elderly is controversial because of lack of effective Alzheimer's disease treatment. Routine genetic screening is also not recommended for a gene risk factor involved in Alzheimer's disease, *APOE-e4*, which apparently repairs connections between brain neurons, because there are various copies of the gene and multiple factors may cause the disease (Alzheimer's Association, 2008).

Gender has obvious implications for screening programs. For example, women are tested frequently for two conditions: breast cancer and cervical cancer (Figure 9-3) (WomensHealth. gov, 2012).

A population representing a particular ethnic or racial group is also appropriate to consider. Some disorders occur more frequently in certain racial or ethnic groups. For example, African American women are more than 35% more likely to die from breast cancer than White women, but are diagnosed 10% less frequently (CDC, 2010). Vietnamese American women have the highest rates of cervical cancer than any other racial or ethnic group in the United States, and are five times higher than the rates among non-Hispanic White women (CDC, 2010). Nurses can lobby and advocate for specific groups to have more targeted screenings, particularly in communities that have large numbers of ethnic or racial minority women (Box 9-3: Diversity Awareness).

Income level has been associated repeatedly with the presence or absence of a healthy state, and it underlies many health disparities. According to a 2010 Gallup poll, "Low-income Americans are more likely than their high-income counterparts to say they have been diagnosed with each of the chronic conditions…the differences are largest for depression, high blood pressure, and diabetes…the high level of obesity among low-income Americans is likely a contributing factor in these differences" (Mendez, 2010). In addition to driving higher uninsured rates, "Low-income Americans are less likely to report healthy eating and frequent exercise compared with those with higher incomes. Smoking is nearly three times as common among low-income as among high-income Americans" (Mendez, 2010). Low-income Americans can least afford access to the necessary preventive care, effective treatment, and health education to improve their health and well-being.

Personal behavioral characteristics related to lifestyle may suggest the need to screen a particular individual or group. When health care practitioners consider lifestyle, they are looking at

FIGURE 9-3 Mammography screening. (From John Foxx/Stockbyte/Thinkstock.)

BOX 9-3   DIVERSITY AWARENESS

Eliminating Health Disparities Among Ethnic Groups

The United States has been referred to frequently as a population melting pot. Diversity is acknowledged as a strength of the United States, but it is apparent that disparities exist among the various racial and ethnic groups in the attainment and maintenance of health. The minority populations of the United States include African Americans, Hispanics, Asian/Pacific Islanders, American Indians, and Alaskan Natives. These categories oversimplify the reality of the multicultural nature of assessing health status, screening, and making plans to improve health. These particular racial groupings are not absolute, because there are subgroups within each.

These disparities and factors such as access to care need to be taken into consideration when planning screening programs. In order to plan, implement, and evaluate a screening program that targets a specific population, the provider must have an awareness of the target population that includes components such as lifestyle, socioeconomic characteristics, education, heredity, environmental factors, values, religious and cultural beliefs, communication style, and language. Partnering with key individuals and organizations in the community through the entire process is important for any screening program to be successful, as the following scenario illustrates.

Hospital administrators in a town located outside a city in the Northeast are concerned about the health status of a new immigrant population. Recent census data indicate that the number of immigrants from Guatemala has grown. The census data also reveal that this population is primarily young adults, male and female. The officials of the town and the hospital are aware that most of the men are day laborers, many of whom gather each morning in the town square to be transported to their jobs. The young women are mothers who work in small, privately owned businesses or are hired by local house-cleaning services.

Based on these data, the hospital officials decide to plan a health and screening day for this population. The hospital distributes flyers in the community in the primary native language of the target population. The day of the screening arrives and the number of participants is very low. The hospital officials are very concerned. They had good intentions. They do not know what to do next.

- What critical actions did the hospital officials perform that might be considered positive in the planning of the health and screening day?
- What critical actions did the hospital officials not perform that might have contributed to the poor turnout at the health and screening function?
- What might the hospital officials consider in their planning for the next health and screening day?
- How might they engage the community and the target population in planning the health and screening day?
- What local community agencies and groups might be invited to participate as partners when planning and implementing the health and screening day?
- Can you identify any creative ways to bring the health and screening day to the targeted population, making the program more accessible?

daily habits that affect health and wellness, such as nutrition, fitness level, tobacco use, alcohol and drug use, sexual practices (HIV), stress management, adequate rest, immunizations, periodic exams, use of seat belts, and other safety factors. Engaging in some of these behaviors while avoiding others is essential for living a healthy life. Therefore screening for personal behavioral characteristics that are considered risky assesses the likelihood of a longer, disease-free life. Once screening suggests risky behaviors, the development of healthy behaviors via programming and a conscious transformation in lifestyle is key. Health care providers bear a responsibility to educate and empower individuals about the next step in the evaluation of their potential condition once a screening is completed. Those being screened bear a responsibility to seek treatment and follow-up services, and ultimately engage in behavioral change toward a healthy lifestyle if the screening is to serve a purpose.

Regional disparities exist and incorporate many of the previously mentioned disparities. These disparities are of great concern, but identifying the cause is complex. Research is being done on interrelationships between the determinants of health, to include biology and genetics, individual behaviors, the social environment, the physical environment, and health services (access and quality). The **Centers for Disease Control and Prevention REACH (Racial and Ethnic Approaches to Community Health,** www.cdc.gov/reach/) program addresses this and is demonstrating success by empowering residents to "seek better health; help change local health care practices; and mobilize communities to implement evidence-based public health programs that address their unique social, historical, economic, and cultural circumstances" (CDC, 2010). Proper screening is integrated into this program.

Environment-Dependent Factors

The area of environmental health and protection has expanded over the years and is becoming more complex. Environmental health and protection has been defined as the science that is concerned with elements of the environment that influence people's health and well-being. These factors include conditions of the workplace, home, and communities including chemical, physical, and psychological forces (Allender et al., 2009). Environment-related risk factors relevant to screening designs are derived from an individual's surroundings. Areas that may be considered include overpopulation; indoor and outdoor air pollution; water pollution; safe drinking water; noise pollution; radiation exposure; biological pollutants; hazardous waste management and disposal of garbage; vector and pesticide control; deforestation, wetlands destruction, and desertification; energy depletion; inadequate housing; contaminated food and foods with toxic additives; safety in the home, worksite, and community; and psychological hazards (Allender et al., 2009; Roelofs et al., 2010).

In occupational health, a legitimate population for screening includes those in high-risk work areas, where harmful chemicals, airborne particles, or high-decibel machinery put the workers at risk of cancer, respiratory conditions, or auditory problems. At the other extreme is the sedentary executive work life, where the lack of exercise is prevalent, placing the worker at risk for obesity and obesity-related conditions such as diabetes. The use of an occupational health nurse to provide individual and mass screening for such problems, in addition to routinely recommended screening, is recognized as an integral role by both the health professions and the business world.

National Guidance and Health Care Reform
Healthy People 2020

Many national organizations are guiding and promoting evidence-based care and screening. *Healthy People 2020* has been establishing benchmarks and monitoring progress on goals and objectives to "Encourage collaborations across sectors, guide individuals toward making informed health decisions, and measure the impact of prevention activities" (healthypeople.gov, 2011). This newest version also includes resources for implementing community programs that support its goals and objectives, including screening. For more specific objectives related to screening, see Box 9-4: *Healthy People 2020*.

Recommended Screenings of the USPSTF

More specifically, the U.S. Preventive Services Task Force (USPSTF), part of the Department of Health and Human Service's **Agency for Healthcare Research and Quality (AHRQ),** identifies the following categories in their *Guide to Clinical Preventive Services:* cancer; heart, vascular, and respiratory disease; infectious diseases, injury, and violence; mental health conditions and substance abuse; metabolic, nutritional, and endocrine conditions; musculoskeletal conditions; obstetrics and gynecological conditions; vision disorders; and a section on recommendations for children and adolescents (USPSTF, 2011a). The recommendations evolve as new scientific evidence becomes available, so this text will not provide specific details on the recommended screenings, because they can be quickly obtained on the AHRQ/USPSTF website (www.uspreventiveservicestaskforce.org/recommendations.htm). Boxes 9-5, 9-6, and 9-7 list the USPSTF recommended services for adults (USPSTF, 2011b), women (including pregnant women), and children and adolescents at the time of publication.

The Affordable Care Act and Prevention Incentives

The passing of the **Affordable Care Act (ACA)** in 2010 catalyzed a public health movement towards prevention and health promotion, with incentives and policies, including the development of the *National Prevention Strategy*. One result is that preventive services are required to be covered by new health insurance plans or policies, as an incentivized quality program for Medicare recipients. When covered by a network provider, insurance plans or policy services (signified with asterisks in Box 9-6) must provide certain preventive services without a requisite copayment or co-insurance (see www.healthcare.gov/news/factsheets/2010/07/preventive-services-list.html).

Medicare now covers new annual wellness visits to include a personalized prevention plan according to the recommendations of the USPSTF, which are based on an individual's age and health status; these visits can be conducted by a variety of practitioners, including nurse practitioners, clinical nurse specialists, and certified nurse midwives. According to the Center for

BOX 9-4 HEALTHY PEOPLE 2020

Objectives Related to Screening

- (Developmental) Increase the proportion of persons with a diagnosis of hemoglobinopathies who receive early and continuous screening for complications.
- Increase the proportion of women who receive a cervical cancer screening based on the most recent guidelines.
- Increase the proportion of adults who receive a colorectal cancer screening based on the most recent guidelines.
- Increase the proportion of women who receive a breast cancer screening based on the most recent guidelines.
- Increase the proportion of adults who were counseled about cancer screening consistent with current guidelines.
- Increase the proportion of elementary, middle, and senior high schools that provide school health education to promote personal health and wellness in the following areas: hand washing or hand hygiene; oral health; growth and development; sun safety and skin cancer prevention; benefits of rest and sleep; ways to prevent vision and hearing loss; and the importance of health screenings and check-ups.
- Stress the importance of health screenings and check-ups.
- Ensure children are screened for hearing loss no later than age 1 month.
- Reduce the proportion of children diagnosed with a disorder through newborn blood-spot screening.
- Reduce the proportion of children who experience developmental delay requiring special education services but have not received help.
- Increase appropriate newborn blood-spot screening and follow-up testing.
- Increase the number of states and the District of Columbia that verify through linkage with vital records that all newborns are screened shortly after birth for conditions mandated by their state-sponsored screening program.
- (Developmental) Increase the proportion of children with a diagnosed condition identified through newborn screening who have an annual assessment of services needed and received.
- Increase depression screening by primary care providers.
- (Developmental) Increase the proportion of adults who received an oral and pharyngeal cancer screening from a dentist or dental hygienist in the past year.
- Increase the number of level I and level II trauma centers and primary care settings that implement evidence-based alcohol screening and brief intervention (SBI).
- Hold screenings in health care settings.
- Increase tobacco screening in office-based ambulatory care settings.
- Increase tobacco screening in hospital ambulatory care settings.
- (Developmental) Increase tobacco screening in dental care settings.
- (Developmental) Increase tobacco screening in substance abuse care settings.
- Increase the proportion of preschool children aged 5 years and under who receive vision screening.

USDHHS. (2012). *Healthypeople.gov. Topics and objective index (Healthy People 2020* objectives in spreadsheet format download). Retrieved November 20, 2012, from www.healthypeople.gov/2020/topicsobjectives2020/default.aspx.

BOX 9-5 COVERED PREVENTIVE SERVICES FOR ADULTS

- **Abdominal Aortic Aneurysm** one-time screening for men of specified ages who have ever smoked
- **Alcohol Misuse** screening and counseling
- **Aspirin** use for men and women of certain ages
- **Blood Pressure** screening for all adults
- **Cholesterol** screening for adults of certain ages or at higher risk
- **Colorectal Cancer** screening for adults older than 50
- **Depression** screening for adults
- **Type 2 Diabetes** screening for adults with high blood pressure
- **Diet** counseling for adults at higher risk for chronic disease
- **HIV** screening for all adults at higher risk
- **Immunization** vaccines for adults—doses, recommended ages, and recommended populations vary:
  - Hepatitis A
  - Hepatitis B
  - Herpes Zoster
  - Human Papillomavirus
  - Influenza
  - Measles, Mumps, Rubella
  - Meningococcal Pneumonia
  - Pneumococcal Pneumonia
  - Tetanus, Diphtheria, Pertussis
  - Varicella
- **Obesity** screening and counseling for all adults
- **Sexually Transmitted Infection (STI)** prevention counseling for adults at higher risk
- **Syphilis** screening for all adults at higher risk
- **Tobacco Use** screening for all adults and cessation interventions for tobacco users

Medicare Advocacy, Inc. (2012), the wellness "visit may include health education or preventive counseling services designed to reduce risk factors that have been identified during the visit. Examples of such education and counseling services include those designed to promote self-management and wellness, including weight loss, physical activity, smoking cessation, fall prevention and nutrition" (see www.medicareadvocacy.org/InfoByTopic/PartB/10_09.09.WellnessVisit.htm).

Among other incentives, Medicare has developed a five star rating guide for Medicare Advantage programs, incentivizing four and five star "quality" health plans with up to a 10% bonus. Many of the criteria that determine the star rating are preventive services to include screenings. This will help drive quality and will also help seniors identify quality insurance plans that cover preventive services and provide the necessary follow-up access and care needed, much like the star ratings for many consumer products and services on-line.

National Prevention Strategy

In addition to increasing the funded coverage of preventive services and screenings, the ACA also created the National Prevention Council (NPC), comprised of "17 heads of departments, agencies, and offices across the Federal government who are committed to promoting prevention and wellness. The Council provides the leadership necessary to engage not only the federal government but a diverse array of stakeholders, from state and local policy makers, to business leaders, to individuals, their families and communities, to champion the policies and programs needed to ensure the health of Americans prospers" (NPC, 2011, p. 3) (Box 9-8: Innovative Practice).

BOX 9-6   COVERED PREVENTIVE SERVICES FOR WOMEN, INCLUDING PREGNANT WOMEN

- **Anemia** screening on a routine basis for pregnant women
- **Bacteriuria** urinary tract or other infection screening for pregnant women
- *BRCA* counseling about genetic testing for women at higher risk
- **Breast Cancer Chemoprevention** counseling for women at higher risk
- **Breast Cancer Mammography** screenings every 1 to 2 years for women older than 40
- **Breastfeeding** comprehensive support and counseling from trained providers, as well as access to breastfeeding supplies, for pregnant and nursing women*
- **Cervical Cancer** screening for sexually active women
- *Chlamydia* **Infection** screening for younger women and other women at higher risk
- **Contraception:** Food and Drug Administration–approved contraceptive methods, sterilization procedures, and patient education and counseling, not including abortifacient drugs*
- **Domestic and Interpersonal Violence** screening and counseling for all women*
- **Folic Acid** supplements for women who may become pregnant
- **Gestational Diabetes** screening for women 24 to 28 weeks' pregnant and those at high risk of developing gestational diabetes*
- **Gonorrhea** screening for all women at higher risk
- **Hepatitis B** screening for pregnant women at their first prenatal visit
- **Human Immunodeficiency Virus (HIV)** screening and counseling for sexually active women*
- **Human Papillomavirus (HPV) DNA Test:** High-risk HPV DNA testing every 3 years for women with normal cytology results who are age 30 or older*
- **Osteoporosis** screening for women older than age 60 depending on risk factors
- **Rh Incompatibility** screening for all pregnant women and follow-up testing for women at higher risk
- **Sexually Transmitted Infection (STI)** counseling for sexually active women*
- **Syphilis** screening for all pregnant women or other women at increased risk
- **Tobacco Use** screening and interventions for all women, and expanded counseling for pregnant tobacco users
- **Well-Woman Visits** to obtain recommended preventive services for women younger than 65*

*Note: Services marked with an asterisk must be covered with no cost-sharing in plan years starting on or after August 1, 2012.

BOX 9-7   COVERED PREVENTIVE SERVICES FOR CHILDREN AND ADOLESCENTS

- **Alcohol and Drug Use** assessments for adolescents
- **Autism** screening for children at 18 and 24 months
- **Behavioral** assessments for children of all ages
- **Blood Pressure** screening for children
- **Cervical Dysplasia** screening for sexually active females
- **Congenital Hypothyroidism** screening for newborns
- **Depression** screening for adolescents
- **Developmental** screening for children younger than age 3, and surveillance throughout childhood
- **Dyslipidemia** screening for children at higher risk of lipid disorders
- **Fluoride Chemoprevention** supplements for children without fluoride in their water source
- **Gonorrhea** preventive medication for the eyes of all newborns
- **Hearing** screening for all newborns
- **Height, Weight, and Body Mass Index** measurements for children
- **Hematocrit or Hemoglobin** screening for children
- **Hemoglobinopathies** or sickle cell screening for newborns
- **HIV** screening for adolescents at higher risk
- **Immunization** vaccines for children from birth to age 18—doses, recommended ages, and recommended populations vary:
  - Diphtheria, Tetanus, Pertussis
  - *Haemophilus influenzae* type b
  - Hepatitis A
  - Hepatitis B
  - Human Papillomavirus
  - Inactivated Poliovirus
  - Influenza
  - Measles, Mumps, Rubella
  - Meningococcal Pneumonia
  - Pneumococcal Pneumonia
  - Rotavirus
  - Varicella
- **Iron** supplements for children ages 6 to 12 months at risk for anemia
- **Lead** screening for children at risk of exposure
- **Medical History** for all children throughout development
- **Obesity** screening and counseling
- **Oral Health** risk assessment for young children
- **Phenylketonuria (PKU)** screening for this genetic disorder in newborns
- **Sexually Transmitted Infection (STI)** prevention counseling and screening for adolescents at higher risk
- **Tuberculin** testing for children at higher risk of tuberculosis
- **Vision** screening for all children

☀ BOX 9-8   INNOVATIVE PRACTICE

Health Information Technology (IT) and Newborn Screening

Health information technology will allow health care to better assess and manage quality health care with the streamlining of efficient and effective information. The Office of National Coordinator for Health Information Technology highlights the ability to share newborn screening (NBS) information and long-term follow-up information within the clinical research community on "all newborn screening orders, results, and information associated with an order or result. Result information may include normal, abnormal, out of range, and confirmatory results within the domains of hearing, hemoglobin, metabolic, and pulmonary/genetic screening tests" electronically sharing and exchanging information between "related to newborn screening among ordering clinicians, pediatric clinicians, consumers, Public Health, testing laboratories, and audiology service providers" (p. 6).

- What benefits do you see for the clinicians? For the person seeking care? For public health?
- Where else do you think health care could benefit from similar abilities?
- What do you think is necessary for this to happen (think about differences in data collection requirements)?

From USDHHS, Office of National Coordinator for Health Information Promotion. (2008). *Newborn screening AHIC detailed use case December 31, 2008*. Retrieved June 25, 2012, from http://healthit.hhs.gov/portal/server.pt/community/use_cases_and_requirements_documents/1202/newborn_screening/15660.

Pender's Health-Promotion Model

A health care provider's responsibility is to assess, plan, implement, and evaluate a screening program. Part of this responsibility includes teaching individuals, families, and populations about the importance of participating in these programs and ultimately engaging in safe behaviors promoting health. The health-promotion model is a useful guide for practice (Pender et al., 2011). The model presents the interrelationship among behavior-specific cognitions and affective factors and individual characteristics and experiences that motivate individuals to engage in behaviors that promote health and decrease unsafe habits and practices. The health care provider may find that the application of this model in practice influences the relationship between the provider and the individual in a positive way. The model is a framework that assists the provider in assessing factors believed to influence health behavioral changes. Once the provider has an accurate assessment, obtained via questions, decisions may be made concerning factors that inhibit health-promoting behaviors and, ultimately, potential interventions to assist individuals in achieving positive health outcomes. This information will assist the provider to develop appropriate teaching methods.

Health-Promotion Assessment Questions
- How do you define health?
- What does health mean to you?
- How would you describe your health now?
- Do the choices you make and actions you take affect your health?
- Can you give examples when choices and actions created a positive change in health for you?
- Can you give examples when choices and actions created a negative or unsafe change in health for you?
- What factors facilitated choices and actions that created a positive change in health?
- What factors created barriers to choices and actions that led to a negative or unsafe change in health?
- Are there any supportive personal influences in your life that would assist you in choices and actions that would create a positive change in your health (i.e., family, friends, and health care providers)?
- Are there any supportive situational influences, such as more than one plan of action, pertaining to the health change available to you?

Modified from Pender, N., Murdaugh, C., & Parsons, M. A. (2011). *Health promotion in nursing practice* (6th ed.). Upper Saddle River, NJ: Prentice Hall.

The resulting *National Prevention Strategy (NPS)* was released in June 2011 and "recognizes that good health comes not just from receiving quality medical care, but also from clean air and water, safe outdoor spaces for physical activity, safe worksites, healthy foods, violence-free environments and healthy homes. Prevention should be woven into all aspects of our lives, including where and how we live, learn, work and play. Everyone—businesses, educators, health care institutions, government, communities and every single American—has a role in creating a healthier nation" (www.cdc.gov/Features/PreventionStrategy/) (Box 9-9: Quality and Safety Scenario).

The following is a list of the four strategic directions:
- Healthy and Safe Community Environments: Create, sustain, and recognize communities that promote health and wellness through prevention.
- Clinical and Community Preventive Services: Ensure that prevention-focused health care and community prevention efforts are available, integrated, and mutually reinforcing.
- Empowered People: Support people in making healthy choices.
- Elimination of Health Disparities: Eliminate disparities, improving the quality of life for all Americans.

Under the second strategic direction, the strategy identifies six recommendations including a focus on improving cardiovascular health, incorporating screenings, using payments and reimbursement to encourage clinical preventive services, and reducing access barriers to community preventive services (NPC, 2011) (Figure 9-4).

THE NURSE'S ROLE

The need for nursing involvement exists at all levels of the collaborative partnership process. As one of the important stakeholders (IOM, 2010), nurses play a role in every aspect of the screening program development process, including assessment, data analysis, planning, implementation, evaluation of the health outcomes, and evaluation of the process (including the workings of the partnership). One aspect of this health process is the development and implementation of screening programs for targeted groups. As nurses become more involved in decision-making and are used optimal levels of their education and expertise (IOM, 2010), they will be faced with the question, "Should this condition be screened for or not?" In the role of decision maker and planner, the nurse is responsible for reviewing all the issues concerning a screenable disease, including the criteria specific to the disease, the medical and economic ethics, and the community resources that are affected. If the choice is to screen, the participation of nurses and other partnering groups is essential in the development of a care plan. The last step is the planning and development of an efficient referral system to enhance continuity of care and to ensure follow-up.

Because many preventive care services are provided through insurance coverage (www.healthcare.gov/law/features/rights/preventive-care/index.html), the nurse can collaborate with other health providers to ensure that preventive services, along with the required education and counseling, are available through primary care or community services such as a primary care clinic, person-centered medical home, or community health center or even at the worksite, such as:
- Blood pressure, diabetes, and cholesterol tests
- Many cancer screenings, including mammograms and colonoscopies
- Counseling on such topics as quitting smoking, losing weight, eating healthy, treating depression, and reducing alcohol use
- Routine vaccinations against diseases such as measles, polio, or meningitis
- Flu and pneumonia shots
- Counseling, screening, and vaccines to ensure healthy pregnancies
- Regular well-baby and well-child visits, from birth to age 21

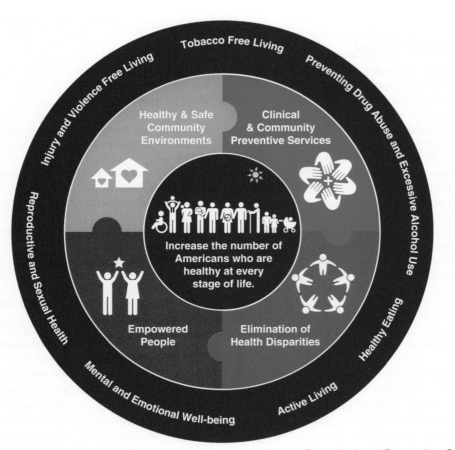

FIGURE 9-4 America's plan for better health and wellness. (From National Prevention Council. [2011]. *National prevention strategy*. Retrieved June 29, 2012, at www.healthcare.gov/prevention/ nphpphc/strategy/report.pdf.)

Nurses have long been responsible for screening individuals and educating persons about healthy lifestyles and decreased risks, in the ordinary office intake assessment process. Questions concerning nutrition, coping, and self-care are all assessment or screening questions, leading to moments of opportunity or "teachable moments" for health promotion. Although these are not evidence-based tools (proven valid and reliable), these moments are invaluable in assessment. As in any nursing intervention, adequate knowledge of the method of administration and the potential side effects is needed. Teaching individuals the meaning and limitation of the test results is an important element of this role, as is informing them of their part in obtaining the implied benefit.

Nursing staff, at all levels, are important in applying preventive services to include screening and education. The concept of the person-centered medical home encourages using each member of the primary health care team to the full level of their professional and licensing abilities. The combined health educator and screener component means that the nurse continues to educate individuals about risk factors and teach them ways to alter and reduce risks generally through lifestyle changes, such as proper diet, exercise, and stress management, and by limiting the use of alcohol, drugs, and tobacco. The role as educator is essential in the screening process, because nurses provide individuals with the information

necessary for choices they will make regarding healthy behavioral change. The nurse is actually practicing primary prevention interventions, but it is in coordination with a secondary preventive role.

COMMUNITY GUIDE

On the community level, many on-line resources currently exist and are being continually developed according to best practice guidelines, to support the nurse in providing optimal preventive services. One excellent resource is the *"Community Preventive Services"* community guide. It is a "free resource that uses systematic reviews to help you choose programs and policies to improve health and prevent disease in your community" (www. thecommunityguide.org/index.html). It helps the nurse identify effective program and policy interventions, determine their cost and return on investment, and decide how to choose an intervention based on individual communities. Topics include adolescent health, alcohol abuse, asthma, birth defects, cancer, diabetes, health communication, HIV/AIDS, STIs, pregnancy, mental health, motor vehicle safety, nutrition, obesity, oral health, physical activity, social environment, tobacco use, vaccines, violence, and worksite injuries. In addition to providing support in the planning of preventive programs or services, it also offers guidance in policies, funding, research, education, and general use.

CDC REACH U.S.

Another excellent resource is the CDC REACH U.S. community website (www.cdc.gov/chronicdisease/resources/publications/AAG/reach.htm). It supports effective community-level programs to reduce health disparities in minority communities across the United States. Data from the REACH Risk Factor Survey, focusing on breast and cervical cancer prevention, cardiovascular health, and diabetes management, have shown that changing health behaviors in these communities has improved health and reduced community disparities. Although the community guide provides guidance on the preventive programs themselves, REACH U.S. has identified "key principles and supporting activities for effective community-level work to reduce health disparities in racial and ethnic minority communities across the United States" to support success through true community engagement and collaboration, for the nurse to remember while building a preventive services community program (Box 9-10).

BOX 9-10   REACH (RACIAL AND ETHNIC APPROACHES TO COMMUNITY HEALTH) U.S KEYS TO SUCCESS

Trust: Build a Culture of Collaboration with Communities that Is Based on Trust

- **Empowerment.** Give individuals and communities the knowledge and tools needed to create change by seeking and demanding better health and building on local resources.
- **Culture and History.** Design health initiatives that are grounded in the unique historical and cultural context of racial and ethnic minority communities in the United States.
- **Focus on Causes.** Assess and focus on the underlying causes of poor community health and implement solutions that will stay embedded in the community infrastructure.
- **Community Investment and Expertise.** Recognize and invest in local community expertise and motivate communities to mobilize and organize existing resources.
- **Trusted Organizations.** Enlist organizations within the community that are valued by community members, including groups with a primary mission unrelated to health.
- **Community Leaders.** Help community leaders and key organizations forge unique partnerships and act as catalysts for change in the community.
- **Ownership.** Develop a collective outlook to promote shared interest in a healthy future through widespread community engagement and leadership.
- **Sustainability.** Make changes to organizations, community environments, and policies to help ensure that health improvements are long-lasting and community activities and programs are self-sustaining.
- **Hope.** Foster optimism, pride, and a promising vision for a healthier future.

From www.cdc.gov/chronicdisease/resources/publications/AAG/reach.htm.

CASE STUDY

Screening

Mrs. C. is a 77-year-old white widowed female. Six years ago she moved from her house into a one-bedroom apartment. She is "on Medicare." She maintains her apartment and does all of her errands without assistance, all of which she is very proud. She reports that occasionally she has fallen, probably because of some degree of decreasing vision especially when moving from direct sunlight into shadows and when walking at night. The only medications she takes are an analgesic for pain management of osteoarthritis, an antihypertensive agent, and a daily vitamin and cranberry supplement.

Today, she is going to her annual "check-up" with nurse practitioner (NP) Kelly, who is part of a new practice of "integrative medicine." The collaborative practice of RNs, NPs, and MDs emphasizes health promotion, including screenings. While Kelly is assessing Mrs. C.'s health status, she is also reflecting on how to better care for the practice's ever enlarging older adult population.

Reflective Questions

1. What data will nurse practitioner Kelly collect to assess Mrs. C.'s health? Why?
2. What risk factors will Kelly most likely evaluate? Why?
3. What screening tests will Kelly suggest? Why?
4. Propose several possible nursing diagnoses for Mrs. C. What possible etiological factors from Mrs. C., her family, and her community might be involved?
5. What questions will Kelly ask to evaluate Mrs. C.'s health status?
6. Compare and contrast these different (individual, family, and community) approaches to health promotion, emphasizing screening and cost-effectiveness.
7. Discuss your thoughts and feelings about screening older adults.

CARE PLAN

Health Promotion, Emphasizing Screenings of Older Adults: Mrs. C.

Caring for older adults is challenging and rewarding. New ways of caring need to be developed especially considering the increasing number of the older "baby boomer generation" in America.

*NURSING DIAGNOSIS: Effective Community Therapeutic Regimen Management

Definition

The pattern in which an individual, family, and/or community experiences (or is at risk to experience) difficulty integrating screening programs for the promotion of health and reduction of risk factors

Defining Characteristics

Major
- Individual, family, and/or community verbalizes desire to manage health promotion with assistance of family and community including nurse practitioner.
- Individual and family verbalize inadequate knowledge of health-promotion strategies, especially risk factors identified through screening methods.

Minor
- What are Mrs. C.'s health-promotion needs?
- What is Mrs. C's understanding of aging and of accelerated risk factors for illness?

Related Factors
- Complexity, including discomfort, of some screenings (e.g., mammograms, osteoporosis testing)
- New ways of thinking about and delivering health promotion, including periodic screening recommended for older adults

- Shifts of resources and costs from individual providers to the community and family (e.g., self-screenings, transportation)

Interventions
- Promote attitudes of openness to new health information.
- For elevated blood pressure readings, repeat blood pressure screening on three different visits.
- Develop a more detailed activity/experience log with special attention to physical safety (falls) and vision problems.
- Explore nutritional and activity strategies that are more appealing to each individual.
- Begin program slowly.
- Follow-up on additional risk factors.
- Offer resources to support goals and interventions.

Expected Outcomes
- The person may experience anxiety.
- The person may experience despair.

Mrs. C., her family, and her community will:
- Verbalize a full understanding of health promotion, especially screenings.

Mrs. C. will:
- Identify and discuss her own risk factors and other data yielded from screenings.
- Establish appropriate goals to decrease the unhealthy findings of her screenings.
- Design and implement a modification program to fulfill these goals.
- Evaluate the efficacy of this care plan with nurse practitioner Kelly.

*NANDA Nursing Diagnoses—Definitions and Classification 2012-2014, Herdman T.H. (ED). Copyright © 2012, 1994-2012 NANDA International. Used by arrangement with John Wiley & Sons Limited. In order to make safe and effective judgments using the NANDA-I nursing diagnoses it is essential that nurses refer to the definitions and defining characteristics of the diagnoses listed in this work. *Retired NANDA Nursing Diagnosis.*

SUMMARY

As a method of preclinical secondary prevention, screening is the administration of a test to distinguish individuals who may have a condition from those who probably do not have it. It can be an effective, efficient tool in preventive health care if used for conditions applicable to the screening model and directed toward an at-risk population. A unique characteristic and significant advantage of screening is that it can be applied to individuals or groups.

Implementing screening programs requires consideration and planning and provides numerous roles for nurses, especially in the currently evolving health care environment. Nurses can provide individuals, communities, and populations valuable preventive, health-promotion, and health-education support in the care of healthy individuals and populations.

REFERENCES

Agency for Healthcare Research and Quality (AHRQ). (n.d.). *The 5 A's: Treating tobacco dependence as a chronic disease.* Retrieved June 29, 2012, from www.ahrq.gov/clinic/tobacco/tobaqrgfig1.htm.

Agency for Healthcare Research and Quality (AHRQ). (2009). *Treating tobacco use and dependence, quick reference guide for clinicians.* Retrieved June 29, 2012, from www.ahrq.gov/clinic/tobacco/tobaqrg.htm.

Airoldi, M., & Morton, A. (2009). Adjusting life for quality or disability: Stylistic difference or substantial dispute? *Health Economics, 18*(11), 1237–1247.

Allender, J., Rector, C., & Warner, K. (2009). *Community health nursing: Promoting and protecting the public's health* (7th ed.). New York: Lippincott.

Alzheimer's Association. (2008). *Genetic testing.* Retrieved June 25, 2012, from www.alz.org.

Bolen, J., Adams, M., & Shenson, D. (2007). Routine preventive services for women: A composite measure highlights gaps in delivery. *Journal of Women's Health, 16*(5), 583–593.

Broder, M. (2012). *Communities' attitudes toward cancer screenings shed light on cultural differences.* Retrieved June 29, 2012, from http://sph.berkeley.edu/pubs/magazine/mag_sp06/pdf/cancer_screening.pdf.

Bynum, S. A., Davis, J. L., Green, B. L., & Katz, R. V. (2012). Unwillingness to participate in colorectal cancer screenings: Examining fears, attitudes, and medical mistrust in an ethnically diverse sample of adults 50 years and older. *American Journal of Health Promotion, 26*(5), 295–300.

Centers for Disease Control and Prevention (CDC). (2004). *Excite, epidemiology in the classroom.* Retrieved November 20, 2012, from www.cdc.gov/excite/classroom/intro_epi.htm.

Centers for Disease Control and Prevention (CDC). (2010). *Reach U.S. finding solutions to health disparities: At a glance 2010.* Retrieved November 20, 2012, from www.cdc.gov/chronicdisease/resources/publications/AAG/reach.htm.

Centers for Disease Control and Prevention (CDC). (2011a). *Chronic disease cost calculator.* Retrieved November 19, 2011, from www.cdc.gov/chronicdisease/resources/calculator/index.htm.

Centers for Disease Control and Prevention (CDC). (2011b). *National HIV and STD testing resources.* Retrieved November 20, 2012, from http://hivtest.cdc.gov/faq.aspx#tested.

Center for Medicare Advocacy, Inc. (2012). *Affordable Care Act expands Medicare coverage for prevention and wellness.* Retrieved November 20, 2012, from www.medicareadvocacy.org/InfoByTopic/PartB/10_09.09.WellnessVisit.htm.

Fiore, M. C., Jaén, C. R., Baker, T. B., et al. (2009). *Treating tobacco use and dependence: 2008 update. Quick reference guide for clinicians.* Rockville, MD: U.S. Department of Health and Human Services, U.S. Public Health Service.

Food and Drug Administration (FDA). (2012). *HIV testing: OraQuick rapid HIV-1 antibody test questions and answers.* Retrieved July 5, 2012, from www.fda.gov/forconsumers/byaudience/for patientadvocates/hivandaidsactivities/ucm117922.htm.

Hankins, S. (2009). The necessity of accurate costs. *American Journal of Preventive Medicine, 37*(3), 258–259.

Healthcare.gov. *Preventive care.* Retrieved June 29, 2012, from www.healthcare.gov/law/features/rights/preventive-care/index.html.

HealthCare.gov. *Preventive services covered under the Affordable Care Act.* Retrieved June 29, 2012, from www.healthcare.gov/news/factsheets/2010/07/preventive-services-list.html.

Healthy People.gov. (2011). *Cancer.* Retrieved June 29, 2012, from http://healthypeople.gov/2020/topicsobjectives2020/overview.aspx?topicId=5.

Hirskyj, P. (2007). QALY: An ethical issue that dare not speak its name. *Nursing Ethics, 14*(1), 72–82.

Institute of Medicine (IOM). (2010). *The future of nursing: Leading change, advancing health.* Retrieved June 29, 2012, from www.iom.edu/Reports/2010/The-Future-of-Nursing-Leading-Change-Advancing-Health.aspx/.

Kudzma, E. (2008). Breast microcalcifications: How to answer womens' questions. *Nursing for Women's Health, 12*(1), 38–45.

Lundy, K., & Janes, S. (2009). *Community health nursing: Caring for the public's health* (2nd ed.). Boston: Jones & Bartlett.

Maine, D., Hurlburt, S., & Greeson, D. (2011). Cervical cancer prevention in the 21st century: Cost is not the only issue. *American Journal of Public Health, 101*(9), 1549–1555. doi:10.2105/AJPH.2011.300204.

Max, M., & Lynn, J. (Eds.). (n.d.). *Symptoms research methods and opportunities: Interactive textbook.* Retrieved November 20, 2012, from http://painconsortium.nih.gov/symptomresearch/chapter_19/sec2/cihs2pg1.htm.

Mendez, E. (2010). *In U.S., health disparities across incomes are wide-ranging.* Retrieved June 29, 2012, from www.gallup.com/poll/143696/health-disparities-across-incomes-wide-ranging.aspx.

National Cancer Institute. (2011). *PROSPR: Population-based Research Optimizing Screening through Personalized Regimens.* Retrieved June 29, 2012, from http://appliedresearch.cancer.gov/networks/prospr/.

National Prevention Council. (2011). *National prevention strategy.* Retrieved July 5, 2012, from www.healthcare.gov/prevention/nphpphc/strategy/report.pdf. Washington, DC: U.S. Department of Health and Human Services, Office of the Surgeon General.

Nayak, S., Roberts, M., & Greenspan, S. (2011). Cost-effectiveness of different screening strategies for osteoporosis in postmenopausal women. *Annals of Internal Medicine, 155,* 751–761.

Roelofs, C., Shoemaker, P., Skogstrom, T., Acevedo, P., Dendrick, J., & Nguyen, N. (2010). The Boston safe shops model: An integrated approach to community environmental and occupational health. *American Journal of Public Health, 100*(Suppl. 1), S52–S55. doi:10.2105/AJPH.2009.176511.

Shenson, D., Bolen, J., & Adams, M. (2007). Receipt of preventive services by elders based on composite measures, 1997-2004. *American Journal of Preventive Medicine, 32,* 11–18.

Shephard, R. (2011). Mandatory ECG screening of athletes: Is this question now resolved? *Sports Medicine, 41*(12), 989–1002.

U.S. Department of Health and Human Services (USDHHS), Office of National Coordinator for Health Information Technology. (2008). *Newborn screening AHIC detailed use case December 31, 2008.* Retrieved June 25, 2012, from http://healthit.hhs.gov/portal/server.pt/community/use_cases_and_requirements_documents/1202/newborn_screening/15660.

USDHHS Office on Women's Health. (2011a). *Screening tests for men.* Retrieved June 25, 2012, from www.womenshealth.gov/publications/our-publications/screening-tests-for-men.pdf.

USDHHS Office on Women's Health. (2011b). *Screening tests for women.* Retrieved June 25, 2012, from www.womenshealth.gov/publications/our-publications/screening-tests-for-women.pdf.

USDHHS. (2012). *Healthypeople.gov. Topics and objective index (Healthy People 2020 objectives in spreadsheet format download).* Retrieved November 20, 2012, from www.healthypeople.gov/2020/topicsobjectives2020/default.aspx.

USPSTF. (2010). *USPSTF A and B recommendations.* Retrieved November 12, 2011, from www.uspreventiveservicestaskforce.org/uspstf/uspsabrecs.htm.

USPSTF. (2011a). *Child and adolescent recommendations.* Retrieved June 29, 2012, from www.uspreventiveservicestaskforce.org/tfchildcat.htm.

USPSTF. (2011b). *Recommendations for adults.* Retrieved June 29, 2012, from www.uspreventiveservicestaskforce.org/adultrec.htm.

Verinata Health (2012). *DNA prenatal testing.* Retrieved June 25, 2012, from www.verinata.com.

Womenshealth.gov. (2012). *Screening Tests and Vaccines.* Retrieved June 29, 2012, from www.womenshealth.gov/screening-tests-and-vaccines/screening-tests-for-women/.

23and me. *DNA testing.* Retrieved June 25, 2012, from www.23andme.com.

CHAPTER

10

Health Education

Susan A. Heady

volve WEBSITE

http://evolve.elsevier.com/Edelman/
- Study Questions
- Glossary

OBJECTIVES

After completing this chapter, the reader will be able to:
- Analyze the goals of health education.
- Discuss learning principles that affect health education.
- Apply teaching and learning concepts to teaching.
- Describe the Health Belief Model and behavior change process.
- Describe the use of the Transtheoretical Model in planning for health teaching.
- Explain the steps in preparing a health teaching plan.
- Propose learning strategies appropriate to each learning domain.
- Discuss the importance of evaluating the educational process.

KEY TERMS

Behavior change	Health education	Self-efficacy
Empowerment	Health literacy	Social cognitive theory
Health behaviors	Health promotion	Social marketing
Health Belief Model	Internet	Transtheoretical (Stages of Change)
Health counseling	Noncompliant	Model (TTM)
Health disparities	Quality and safety	

? THINK ABOUT IT

The Challenges of Health Education

An analysis of a nursing assessment often leads to a nursing diagnosis related to the individual's lack of knowledge in the areas of health promotion or health-promotion strategies. The nurse may recognize certain risk factors in a person, such as a lack of knowledge, possession of incorrect knowledge, misinterpretation of information, or reliance on harmful myths and folk medicine. Additionally, the individual may demonstrate little or no interest in learning, a lack of motivation to learn, or a cognitive or perceptual inability to learn.

The success of any health activity or goal will depend on the individual's perception of the situation and responsiveness to teaching. The success of health teaching depends on a person's ability to learn and process information and the motivation to change behaviors to improve the present condition or move toward better health. The nurse assists each person in a process of self-understanding and self-direction, so the individual will experience the desire and motivation to change. Frequently, major life decisions need to be made in the process of learning. If through education and counseling the nurse can elicit logical and clear thinking, then the individual's decision-making abilities and progress in meeting life's needs will be developed further. To encourage critical thinking by an individual, the nurse may pose some of the following questions:

- What do you know about the health problem or concern?
- What were you told?
- What do you think will help you deal with the problem or concern?
- How do you explain this problem or concern to yourself?
- How do you see yourself in 6 months?

- What types of efforts have worked for you in the past with this problem or concern?
- How does the problem or concern affect your daily life?
- What one aspect would indicate an improvement in your condition?
- How much control do you think you have over this situation?
- What is one goal that you would like to set for yourself?

Scenario

Ronald is a successful executive in a local business. In his annual physical examination, an irregular heartbeat was noted on the electrocardiogram. Ronald's father died of a heart attack at age 50; therefore, the physician scheduled Ronald

for a thallium stress test. The stress test indicated a need for further evaluation with a cardiac catheterization. A 60% blockage in one artery was detected during this process. Ronald's condition will be handled conservatively at this point. He recognizes that some lifestyle changes are necessary. He is overweight and eats in restaurants frequently. He has not been active in regular exercise. He and his wife live in a condominium. They have grown children and grandchildren. One of their sons has a serious drug problem, so they have not seen him for several years and hear from him only rarely.

- How might the nurse begin working with Ronald?
- How likely is he to be motivated to learn and change?
- What are some barriers to change in his behaviors?

Health education is a vital component in promoting individual and community health. Individual behaviors such as diet, physical activity level, and substance abuse play a significant role in health outcomes.

Lifestyle changes should not be viewed as only primary prevention. Cardiovascular disease, prostate and breast cancer, diabetes, and obesity account for 75% of health care costs. Intensive lifestyle changes can be effective not only in preventing chronic diseases but also in reversing their progression and significantly reducing health care costs (Ornish, 2009).

Health education to promote positive behavior change, along with policies and programs that address the social determinants of health, can reduce the rates of chronic illness and disability in this country. The *Healthy People 2020* national health objectives emphasize priorities to improve the health of individuals, groups, and communities in the United States. These priorities involve promoting positive health behaviors, increasing health literacy, and reducing health disparities (U.S. Department of Health and Human Services [USDHHS], 2010). Achievement of these objectives provides challenges and opportunities for health promotion.

Although many health goals are affected by individual lifestyle practices, health is influenced significantly by social, economic, physical, and political factors. The 2020 vision for health education includes a commitment to providing early health literacy and prevention education beginning with preschool, then continuing throughout the K-12 education continuum and beyond. This involves an approach to developing healthy citizens not only by delivering basic health-promotion and disease-prevention concepts and encouraging risk-reduction behaviors, but also by demonstrating the value of interrelatedness and the connection between individual and community health (Koh et al., 2011). Box 10-1: *Healthy People 2020* includes objectives related to educational programs.

Nursing, with its unique contributions to health care, represents a professional resource that can help facilitate these changes through health education strategies. Nurses, in partnership with other health care professionals, can be the link between the philosophy of *Healthy People 2020* and the people who need to hear its messages and act on those messages.

NURSING AND HEALTH EDUCATION

Nurses as educators play a key role in improving the health of the nation. Educating people is an integral part of the nurse's role in every practice setting—schools, communities, work sites, health care delivery sites, and homes. Health education involves not only providing relevant information but also facilitating health-related behavior change. The nurse, using health education principles, can assist people in achieving their health goals in a way that is consistent with their personal lifestyles, values, and beliefs.

Nursing: Scope and Standards of Practice describes health teaching and health promotion as primary nursing responsibilities. This includes educating people about healthy lifestyles, risk reduction, developmental needs, activities of daily living, and preventive self-care (American Nurses Association [ANA], 2010a). ANA's *Social Policy Statement* also addresses health teaching and health counseling (ANA, 2010b). This responsibility to teach individuals is balanced by their right to receive information about their health status, risks, and ways to reduce their risks. The nurse provides health teaching and health counseling based on individual interests and decisions to enable individuals to make informed decisions about their health.

Nurses usually function as health care coordinators for individuals in their care. Depending on the interests and needs of a person, nurses establish a partnership to guide the individual in the selection and use of relevant health services. Principles of health education provide the nurse with strategies and tools for assessing an individual's readiness for health teaching, with technical information, and with help in practicing health care techniques at home. These strategies also help the nurse facilitate behavior change, while satisfying the person's right to relevant health information and the freedom for people to make decisions about their own health. Health education encourages self-care, self-empowerment, and, ultimately, less dependence on the health care system.

Nurses have long been involved in public health education, taking on the full-time role of coordinating the educational services provided by a health agency or institution. As a health educator, the nurse may use marketing strategies to enhance the effectiveness of health education programs that are focused on certain target populations. The health education specialist

♥ **BOX 10-1 HEALTHY PEOPLE 2020**

Selected Health-Promotion and Disease-Prevention Objectives Related to Educational and Community-Based Programs (ECBP)

Goal: To increase the quality, availability, and effectiveness of educational and community-based programs designed to prevent disease and injury, improve health, and enhance quality of life

School Setting

- Increase the proportion of preschool programs that provide health education to prevent problems in these areas: unintentional injury; violence; tobacco use; alcohol and other drug use; unhealthy dietary patterns; and inadequate physical activity, dental health, and safety.
- Increase the proportion of elementary, middle, and senior high schools that provide comprehensive health education to prevent problems in these areas: unintentional injury; violence and suicide; tobacco use; alcohol and other drug use; unintended pregnancy and sexually transmitted infections; unhealthy dietary patterns; and inadequate physical activity.
- Increase the proportion of elementary, middle, and senior high schools that have health education goals or objectives that address the knowledge and skills articulated in the National Health Education Standards (high school, middle, elementary).
- Increase the proportion of elementary, middle, junior high, and senior high schools that have a nurse-to-student ratio of at least 1:750.

- Increase the rate of completion of high school.
- Increase the proportion of college and university students who receive information for the institution of each of the six priority health-risk behavior areas listed in the preceding fourth bulleted objective.

Work Setting

- Increase the proportion of work sites that offer an employee health-promotion program to their employees.
- Increase the proportion of employees who participate in employer-sponsored health-promotion activities.

Community Setting and Select Populations

- Increase the proportion of tribal and local health service organizations that provide population-based primary prevention services in these areas: injury and violence prevention; mental illness; tobacco use; substance abuse; unintended pregnancy; chronic disease programs; nutrition; physical activity.
- Increase the proportion of local health departments that establish culturally appropriate and linguistically competent community health-promotion and disease-prevention programs.

Modified from U.S. Department of Health and Human Services. (2010). *Healthy People 2020: Improving the health of Americans*. Washington, DC: Author. Available at www.healthypeople.gov.

helps other nurses and health professionals improve their skills in developing and delivering teaching plans.

Definition

Health education is "any combination of planned learning experiences based on sound theories that provide individuals, groups, and communities the opportunity to acquire the information and the skills needed to make quality health decisions" (Joint Committee on Health Education and Promotion Terminology, 2002, p. 6). This process involves several key components. First, health education involves the use of teaching-learning strategies. Second, learners maintain voluntary control over the decision to make changes in their actions. Third, health education focuses on behavior changes that have been found to improve health status.

Health education facilitates the development of health knowledge, skills, and attitudes through the application of theories or models. Two commonly used theories, behavioral theory and social cognitive theory, will be discussed later in this chapter. Generally, health education strategies help ensure that individuals, as consumers of health services, are satisfied and have received the health care that is most relevant to their problems. From a public health perspective, health education programs are intended not only to enhance individuals' abilities to make positive lifestyle changes but also to support social and political actions that promote health and quality of life in communities.

The following scenario is an example of a therapeutic situation in which a health education approach may be used to meet an individual's health needs.

Sada Thompson, a 21-year-old university senior, visits university health services because she wants to change her method of birth control. She has experienced side effects from the birth control pill that she has been taking for the past year and knows little about other options. She has recently started dating John after breaking up with Steven 3 months ago. Having decided to be sexually active with John, Sada is feeling uncertain about what she needs to do to take care of herself and how to discuss this uncertainty with John. She is aware of all the talk about acquired immunodeficiency syndrome (AIDS) on campus and she knows that John is popular and has dated several other women in school, which concerns her.

Sada needs to learn new information, she may need to acquire new skills, and she needs to clarify any feelings or attitudes that affect her decision to use a new birth control method and ensure her continued safety. After recording her health assessment history and arranging for a gynecological examination and laboratory tests, the nurse develops a teaching plan. Selecting one or more strategies for helping Sada review all the birth control options, the nurse establishes an environment in which Sada can choose to try a new method or request a change in her prescription for oral contraceptives. Together they identify actions that Sada can take to use the method properly. They also anticipate and identify ways that Sada can solve problems of adjusting to the new method.

The nurse answers Sada's immediate questions about safe sex, gives her several pamphlets written for college students about this topic, and suggests that she participate in the peer counseling night on sexually transmitted diseases that will be held on campus in 2 weeks. The peer counseling hotline number and drop-in hours are given to Sada. The nurse explains that these students are trained to help other students talk about and deal with this important issue. The nurse invites Sada to call or come back to the office for additional help, information, and problem-solving discussion.

This example illustrates that educational interventions, in addition to direct health services, are necessary to meet the individual's goal. Although health care providers and nurses prefer

BOX 10-2   QUALITY AND SAFETY SCENARIO

Strategies to Promote Health Literacy

Create a Shame-Free Environment
- Encourage questions.
- Show respect, helpfulness, and a caring attitude.
- Orient to surroundings, nursing care routines, and people on unit.
- Provide "frequently-asked questions" handout and review orally.
- Convey empathy and reassurance.
- Assist in completing forms.
- Speak slowly and distinctly.
- Ensure the person's privacy when talking.
- After physician's visit, ask care recipient to share information and clarify.
- Teach care recipients to ask:
  - What is my main problem?
  - What do I need to do about the problem?
  - Why is it important for me to do this?
- Invite a family member or friend.
- Offer note pad and pencil.
- Simplify self-care and treatment regimens as much as possible.
- Be positive and supportive

Use Clear, Purposeful Communication
- Intentionally speak clearly, distinctly.
- Use plain, everyday language.
- Avoid medical and technical jargon.
- Limit key points to three or fewer.
- Face person when speaking.
- Put information in a familiar context.

- Repeat and review key points.
- Avoid medical concepts and categorical words.
- Be specific and concrete; avoid words that require inferences.
- Use vocabulary that is familiar to the person.
- Define new health care and medical terms.
- Consistently use same terms.
- Conclude with a summary of key points.

Communicate in a Person-Centered Manner
- Identify person's personal motivators.
- Assess unique interests and activities.
- Address person's main concern.
- Link new information to past experiences.
- Assess what is already known.
- Be sensitive to age and cultural mores.
- Use active voice and personalize the message.
- Accommodate visual, hearing, and cognitive changes in the elderly.

Reinforce the Spoken Word
- Use a variety of methods: photographs, audio, and drawings.
- Select or create only highly readable written materials.
  - Summarize key points in the first paragraph.
  - Put a heading before each section.
  - Use 14 point, plain font with uppercase and lowercase letters.
  - Use short sentences of fewer than eight words.

From Speros, C. I. (2011). Promoting health literacy: A nursing imperative. *Nursing Clinics of North America, 46,* 321-333. http://dx.doi.org/10.1016/j.cnur.2011.05.007.

that people choose to take actions that will promote health and not detract from it, the individual controls the at-home application of health recommendations.

Goals

The goal of health education is to help individuals, families, and communities achieve, through their own actions and initiative, optimal states of health. Health education facilitates voluntary actions to promote health. Another important goal of health education is improving health literacy.

Health literacy is defined as "the degree to which individuals have the capacity to obtain, process, and understand health information and services needed to make appropriate health decisions" (Selden et al., 2000). Simply stated, "Health literacy is about communicating health information clearly and understanding it correctly" (Osborne, 2013, p. 1). Health literacy includes the ability to read, write, speak, listen, compute, and comprehend, and to apply those skills to health situations.

According to the 2003 National Assessment of Health Literacy study, only about 12% of U.S. adults had proficient health literacy. More than one third of U.S. adults have only basic or below basic health literacy. This means they would have difficulty with common health tasks, such as following directions on a prescription drug label or adhering to a childhood immunization schedule using a standard chart. Although half of adults without a high school education had below basic health literacy skills, even high school and college graduates can have limited

health literacy. The more vulnerable members of our communities—those with lower education levels, racial/ethnic minorities, the uninsured and publicly insured, and the elderly—have the lowest levels of health literacy (USDHHS, 2008).

The ability to communicate clearly with people from all literacy levels is an important component of person-centered **quality and safety** in health education. Using strategies to promote health literacy can have a significant impact on the outcomes of health care recipients (Box 10-2: Quality and Safety Scenario).

Nurses, through their unique responsibility for the majority of care recipient, caregiver, and community health education and communication, can also contribute to improving health literacy by assuming a lead role in reviewing and revising all types of forms and educational materials intended for care recipients, examining these materials for relevance, clarity, cultural appropriateness, and clinical accuracy (Baur, 2011).

Addressing health literacy and providing culturally sensitive health education are critical to reducing health disparities and achieving health equity. **Health disparities** are systematic, potentially avoidable health differences that adversely affect socially disadvantaged groups. Groups affected are those with characteristics such as race/ethnicity, skin color, religion, language, or nationality; socioeconomic resources or position; gender, sexual orientation, or gender identity; age; physical, mental, or emotional disability or illness; geography; political or other affiliation; or other characteristics that have been linked historically to discrimination or marginalization (Braverman et al., 2011).

BOX 10-3 HOW TO FACILITATE LEARNING

- Use methods that stimulate a variety of senses.
- Involve the person actively in the learning process.
- Establish a comfortable, appropriate learning environment.
- Assess the readiness of the learner, which may be affected by physical, social, emotional, and financial factors.
- Make the information relevant by connecting with the existing needs and interests of the learner.
- Use repetition. Review and reinforce concepts several times in a variety of ways.
- Make the learning encounter positive. Structure it to achieve progress recognizable by the individual and provide frequent, positive feedback.
- Start with what is known and proceed to what is unknown, moving from simple to complex.
- Apply the concepts to several settings to facilitate generalization.
- Pace the learning appropriately for the individual.

Health education encourages positive, informed changes in lifestyle behaviors that prevent acute and chronic disease, decrease disability, and enhance wellness. Another goal of health education that may foster successful changes in health behavior is empowerment. People who believe that they can make a difference in health and who are involved in decision-making are more likely to make changes (Anderson et al., 2008).

Changes in health behaviors that are related to health education help prevent disease and disability. Two main objectives of health education and counseling are to change health behaviors and to improve health status. Information alone does not change behavior.

Health education and health counseling are mutually supportive activities. Health educators often use one-to-one and group counseling techniques as strategies for active health learning. Counselors may refer people to health education resources or assist them in acquiring information pertinent to solving a health problem. The following example helps illustrate the goals of health education. The general principles of learning that are found in Box 10-3 are fundamental to the planning of successful health education programs.

Kate Hanson, age 22, visits the local family health center for fatigue and symptoms similar to influenza. During the assessment with the nurse, Kate discloses that she has missed her last two periods.

The physical examination, the laboratory tests, and the health assessment pattern confirm Kate's suspicions of pregnancy. Psychosocial evaluation reveals that Kate works part-time as a secretary for a temporary agency and lives in an apartment with her recently unemployed husband, Jim. Further interviewing reveals that Kate has minimal knowledge of prenatal care; she has a diet of take-out food that is high in fat, sodium, and sugar, with infrequent consumption of fresh fruits or vegetables; and she has three or four beers on the weekends. Kate has never taken vitamins, she leads a sedentary lifestyle, and she obviously is overwhelmed by the news that she is pregnant.

The nurse first takes steps to create a safe and trusting atmosphere in which Kate can feel free to share her concerns and apprehensions. When Kate expresses concerns about telling her husband about the pregnancy, the nurse discusses this with her. Kate is then taught the importance of taking a multiple vitamin with an iron supplement daily, discontinuing the use of alcohol, checking with her physician before taking medications, and making time for more rest during the day. Sensing that this is all that can be accomplished at this time, the nurse gives Kate two pamphlets on prenatal care and makes an appointment for her to return in a week with her husband. Kate acknowledges that she understands the instructions, and the nurse documents the teaching and recommendations in Kate's chart.

During the next visit, the nurse meets with Kate and Jim, explores the meaning of the pregnancy in their lives, and helps them identify actions they will need to take. The recommendations that were made during Kate's first visit are reviewed and reinforced. The nurse then details specifics of dietary changes, reinforces the need for proper rest and exercise, and helps the couple solve problems while they adjust to these new responsibilities. Most importantly, the nurse gives them information on the clinic's weekly prenatal classes and explains that because the classes are partially covered by local community funding, the charge is minimal. The classes include information about physical changes, psychosocial changes, and nutritional needs during the pregnancy, the labor and delivery period, and the newborn and postpartum periods. A nurse practitioner conducts the classes at the clinic, which are given in a group format to facilitate social support and problem-solving among expectant parents.

The nurse gives Kate and Jim several other pamphlets to read at home, makes an appointment for Kate to see the physician in a couple of weeks, and encourages her to call if she has questions or concerns in the interim. A schedule of the prenatal classes is reviewed and a date for the next session is made. The couple is encouraged to meet with the social worker to explore their financial needs and options because Jim was recently laid off. Kate and Jim acknowledge that they understand what they need to do, and the nurse documents what was taught and discussed in Kate's health care record.

This example illustrates the goal of health education: to help individuals achieve optimal health and well-being through their actions and initiative. Through health education, individuals can learn to make informed decisions about personal and family health practices and to use health services in the community. The individual in this example receives educational assistance from the nurse that will promote better health and well-being for herself and her baby.

Learning Assumptions

Individual chapters in this text address the factors to consider when teaching different age groups and the learners' respective characteristics to consider when developing a teaching plan.

The nurse considers the developmental stage, cognitive level, and interests of the individual. The level of information to be conveyed and the skills and abilities of the individual will guide the methods and resources used.

Family Health Teaching

The family plays an important role in health and illness. Because the family is the unit within which health values, health habits, and health risk perceptions are developed, organized, and performed, individual's health, understanding, and intervening with the family is essential to promoting health and reducing health risks in individuals and communities (Anderson et al., 2008). Skills in family interviewing and assessment are valuable tools for nurses. Family health

FIGURE 10-1 School-aged children engaged in checking their travel bags with school books.

assessment and health teaching are closely related. The assessment model in the chapter on family health promotion (see Chapter 7) provides a comprehensive approach to identifying problems, strengths, and health education needs. The goal is to help the members achieve optimal states of health while guiding them through problem-solving and decision-making. This process empowers them. Members believe they can make a difference in their own health.

In clarifying the health teaching needs of a family, the nurse might ask herself/himself the following questions: "Who is in this family? What health-related tasks are they performing? How are they functioning and how are they meeting each other's needs? How well are they communicating? What does this family need to know? What do they need to know now? What do they think they need to know? How can they learn what they need to know?"

The nurse sets a broad health-promotion goal for the family but directs the health teaching toward a more specific area. It is essential that the family agrees with the goal and teaching needs. As the family participates in the assessment interview, perhaps members can identify their own health teaching needs. Health teaching includes all family members, with learning activities appropriate for each individual. The general teaching goal will be the same for all members, but the approaches and specific goals for each member or subsystem will be different. Children, adolescents, and elderly members pose special challenges to the nurse, who may be geared toward teaching young or middle-aged adults (Figure 10-1).

Health Behavior Change

The process of health education directs people toward voluntary changes of their health behaviors. This section examines: the use of the Health Belief Model to analyze the probability that a person will make changes to improve health or prevent disease, the application of social cognitive theory to clarify environmental and social factors that affect learning of new health behaviors, and the use of the stages of change, or the Transtheoretical Model, in planning health teaching.

Beliefs, attitudes, values, and information contribute to motivation and behavior and are underlying factors in making any decision to change behavior (Richards & Digger, 2008).

Health behaviors are any activities that an individual undertakes to enhance health, prevent disease, and detect and control the symptoms of a disease. Identifying and teaching people about lifestyle behaviors that need to be changed is only the first step in the process of assisting individuals in moving from knowledge to action. The nurse uses the Health Belief Model and social learning theory as subsequent steps in formulating an action plan that meets the needs and capabilities of each person in making healthy behavior changes.

Health Belief Model

The Health Belief Model is a paradigm used to predict and explain health behavior. The Health Belief Model was developed to describe why people failed to participate in programs to detect or prevent disease. The model has been expanded to explain responses to symptoms, disease, prescribed treatments, and potential health problems (Champion & Skinner, 2008). The Health Belief Model and social learning theory assist the nurse in formulating an action plan that meets the needs and capabilities of the individual making health behavior changes.

The following components of the Health Belief Model provide guidelines for nurses to analyze factors that contribute to a person's perceived state of health or risk of disease and to the individual's probability of making an appropriate plan of action:

- Individual perceptions or readiness for change
- The value of health to the individual compared with other aspects of living
- Perceived susceptibility to a health problem, disease, or complications
- Perceived seriousness of the disease level threatening the achievement of certain goals or aims
- Risk factors to a disease attributed to heredity, race or culture, medical history, or other causes
- Perceived benefits of health action
- Perceived barriers to promotion action (Becker, 1974; Janz & Becker, 1984; Rosenstock et al., 1988)

The Health Belief Model does not specify the interventions that will influence an individual's likelihood of taking action; rather, it explains the role of values and beliefs in predicting treatment outcomes and adherence, while generating data that guide nurses in choosing effective educational strategies. The most appropriate interventions for a particular person need to be negotiated between the individual and the health care professional.

Social Cognitive Theory

Social cognitive theory is another model that adds to the understanding of the determinants of health behavior. Bandura (1997) emphasizes the influence of self-efficacy, or efficacy beliefs, on health behavior. Self-efficacy refers to an individual's belief in being personally capable of performing the behavior required to influence one's own health (see the Case Study and Care Plan at the end of this chapter.) Social cognitive theory also describes the roles of reinforcement and observational learning in explaining health behavior change. Modeling, or providing opportunities for imitating the behavior of others, can be used to demonstrate the desired behavior.

Transtheoretical Model of Change

The Transtheoretical Model (TTM), or the stages of change model, is useful for determining where a person is in relation to making a behavior change. The model, developed by Prochaska and DiClemente (1984), is based on extensive research with smoking cessation. Health-related behavior change is proposed to progress through the following five stages regardless of whether quitting or adopting a behavior:

- Precontemplation: The person is not thinking about or considering quitting or adopting a behavior change within the next 6 months (not intending to make changes).
- Contemplation: The person is seriously considering making a specific behavior change within the next 6 months (considering a change).
- Planning or preparation: The person who has made a behavior change is seriously thinking about making a change within the next month (making small or sporadic changes).
- Action: The person has made a behavior change and it has persisted for a period of 6 months (actively engaged in behavior change).
- Maintenance: The period beginning 6 months after action has started and continuing indefinitely (sustaining the change over time) (Prochaska & DiClemente, 1984).

The TTM is useful in determining the person's readiness for learning in relation to changing a behavior so that health education or behavior change interventions can be matched to the stage. Self-efficacy is a key construct in this model. The TTM has been used by health professionals in planning interventions with a wide variety of persons at risk.

Regardless of the quality of nurses' assessment methods and educational strategies, experience in the area of health education indicates that people do not always make the choices recommended to them by health professionals. Nurses often label these people noncompliant, a negative term that suggests that the individual has not followed their instructions. Naturally health professionals want people to choose the recommended course of action, but each individual has the right to choose not to follow advice. Enlisting the individual's partnership or cooperation rather than compliance achieves better results.

Attempts to influence a person's behavior through education are not always successful. Attempting to persuade people to change their behavior to something that might make them, their friends, and their family healthier can be discouraging and sometimes futile. An individual's values, beliefs, and life stresses may present obstacles to these changes. Effective health education requires an understanding of the influential factors affecting the individual's decision-making (values, beliefs, attitudes, life stresses, religion, previous experiences with the health care system, and life goals). Another key factor in the ability to comply with health education is financial constraints. The individual may not have the resources to pay for medications or a proper diet, or may not have transportation to appointments.

Many health professionals tend to view a person's cooperation with the health care regimen as a single choice, when this cooperation often involves many choices every day. For example, following a low-fat, low-cholesterol diet involves constant, and often inconvenient, choices throughout the day. The expectation is that people will do this every day for the rest of their lives, even when the nurse cannot guarantee freedom from angina, myocardial infarctions, or other complications.

Ultimately, the nurse needs to respect a person's right to choose. However, nurses can increase an individual's motivation and capabilities to change by involving the individual in planning and goal setting, providing information that is understandable and acceptable, and assisting the person in developing new skills.

After clarifying behaviors that a person is willing to change, the nurse can use the following framework based on a cognitive behavioral approach for developing interventions for behavior change:

- Assess the behavior.
- Educate about the need for and benefits of change.
- Motivate using personalized messages.
- Assess and increase self-efficacy.
- Assess and offer resources to decrease barriers to change.
- Modify behavior.
- Maintain behavior change (Saarmann et al., 2002).

Theories of health behavior change are at the heart of health education. The theories presented in this section help the nurses to assess an individual's stage in the behavior change process and to develop appropriate teaching plans. The goals of the teaching plans and the strategies selected will differ depending on the factors affecting the individual's readiness to learn and to change.

Ethics

Applying principles of respect, autonomy, justice, and beneficence, nurses have an active role as advocates in empowering care recipients to make their own informed decisions about their health and care. The nurse works as partner, facilitator, and resource for the person and family (Burkhardt & Nathaniel, 2008). However, when planning health education to promote health, nurses experience several ethical dilemmas.

Nurses have an active role as advocates in empowering individuals to make their own informed decisions about their health and care (Burkhardt & Nathaniel, 2008). Although the focus of health education may be on the behavior change process, the nurse needs to exercise caution in using tools of persuasion in communication with people because of the potential for manipulation and coercion, particularly when addressing different cultural or minority groups (Simons-Morton et al., 2012).

Choices about health care practices belong to individuals, not health care providers. All competent persons have the right to autonomous choice. Nurses should respect decisions made by persons and families, even when the choice is not what the nurse might do or suggest or is considered "unhealthy," and the nurse should avoid labeling these persons as noncompliant. The nurse and family should work together on a mutually agreed upon plan that incorporates these individual and family values and beliefs (Burkhardt & Nathaniel, 2008). When health promotion focuses on individual behavior, disregarding other social factors that may contribute significantly to the problem, this can inadvertently lead to victim blaming. Defining a problem as simply an individual problem suggests the individual is responsible for both the problem and the solution (Simons-Morton et al., 2012).

※ BOX 10-4 INNOVATIVE PRACTICE

Workplace Intervention

To address health disparities in a vulnerable U.S. population, an innovative workplace intervention was developed to reduce cardiovascular risk in a group of Hispanic women employed as housekeeping staff at a southern Texas university. A nursing research team conducted a descriptive study evaluating the effects of a culturally sensitive cardiac health education program provided to 21 low-income, Hispanic immigrant women at their workplace. The majority of the women were Catholic, first-generation immigrants born in Mexico who spoke only Spanish, and were "Mexican oriented." Almost half of the group had less than an eighth grade education. A significant percentage of the women were overweight and had blood pressure readings in the pre-hypertensive or hypertensive range.

The program was based on three educational goals: "(1) to provide information that matched the assessed objective needs of the participants; (2) to develop culturally sensitive interventions; and (3) to teach at least one skill as part of each educational session" (p. 219). Two graduate nursing students and one graduate kinesiology student worked with the housekeeping supervisor in developing the classes to ensure that they were culturally appropriate. All classes were presented in Spanish by a bilingual, bicultural nursing graduate student. The educators incorporated three concepts central to the Hispanic culture—personalismo (progression of a relationship from formal to personal), respeto (mutual respect), and dignidad (understanding and respect for cultural behaviors)—in their approach and development of rapport with the housekeepers.

A series of three 45-minute classes were presented during regularly scheduled staff meetings. Class one focused on reducing salt in the diet, class two on increasing physical activity, and class three on lowering fats in the diet. Examples of low-cost foods were used. Blood pressure measurements were taken before each class to provide participants' information about their cardiac risk.

A survey 4 months after the class indicated that more than 80% of the respondents (17 of the 21 participants) were reading food labels and determining the fat content of meat before buying when grocery shopping, using less salt, and incorporating healthier fat in their diets; however, fewer than half of the respondents were practicing the exercises. Comments indicated that they were interested in continuing health education classes at the workplace. Additional classes on cardiac risk reduction were added and the blood pressure clinics were extended. At 17 months from baseline, both systolic and diastolic blood pressure measurements were significantly improved.

This project demonstrates the value of providing assessment-based, culturally sensitive cardiac risk reduction education in the workplace. Basing the program on relationship concepts important to Hispanics showed potential in improving outcomes. Although the concepts of personalismo, respeto, and dignidad appear simple, the authors indicate they take some time to develop.

Data from Zarate-Abbott, P., Etnyre, A., Gilliland, I., Mahon, M., Allwein, D., Cook, J., et al. (2008). Workplace health promotion: Strategies for low-income Hispanic immigrant women. *AAOHN Journal, 56*(5), 217-222.

The role of the nurse is to facilitate a communicative environment in which people can exercise their right to make informed free choices. Individuals need to participate in the decision-making process when their lives may be influenced by a change.

Although each person's state of health affects family members and the community, individuals are responsible for their own health maintenance. Health professionals need to accept and welcome individual differences in meeting this responsibility. By selecting interventions that create an environment of open communication and risk-taking, individuals can better develop the problem-solving skills to direct their own growth and development.

Diversity and Health Teaching

The increasing racial and ethnic diversity of the U.S. population, as well as the challenge to eliminate disparities in the health status of people of diverse backgrounds, demands that we provide culturally appropriate health education and health promotion. Individuals' cultural groups influence their beliefs about health, perceptions of disease and illness, help-seeking behaviors, and attitudes toward health providers, and play a role in their use of traditional and complementary healing practices. Prevention strategies must address each group's unique culture, experiences, language, age, gender, and sexual orientation and be culturally and linguistically appropriate in order to be effective (Perez & Luquis, 2008).

Another challenge for health professionals is to apply health education strategies with people from diverse cultural backgrounds, people who do not speak English as their native language, and people who cannot read at elementary levels (Box 10-4: Innovative Practice). Nurses also need to provide a welcoming environment for the lesbian, gay, bisexual, and transgender (LGBT) community. This involves, but is not limited to, using inclusive language (such as partner rather than spouse and relationship status instead of marital status), not making assumptions, and respecting each person's sexual self-identity (Perez & Luquis, 2008).

The health professional needs to take the time to assess cultural beliefs that influence social and health practices and make an effort to analyze educational interventions that are acceptable and satisfying to the individual. Social marketing processes discussed in the next section help identify characteristics, interests, and concerns of target populations.

When teaching people of different cultural, racial, and ethnic groups, the nurse endeavors to provide culturally sensitive education. Nurses recognize that the person's or group's background, beliefs, and knowledge may differ significantly from their own and seek to understand and show respect for these differences (Degazon, 2008) (Box 10-5: Diversity Awareness).

SOCIAL MARKETING AND HEALTH EDUCATION

When nurses begin to teach groups of people, they automatically enter a program planning and administrative process. When an organization wants to offer an ongoing health education program for a target population, social marketing provides a strategy for reaching members of the group and implementing a service that will satisfy these members as consumers. Principles of social marketing and health education strategies are

BOX 10-5   DIVERSITY AWARENESS
Cultural Aspects of Health Teaching

When There Is a Language Barrier
- Use courtesy and a formal approach.
- Address the person by his or her last name.
- Introduce yourself, pointing to yourself as you give your name.
- Project a friendly attitude with a smile and a handshake.
- Speak with a moderate tone and volume.
- Attempt to use words in the person's language, which indicates respect for the individual's culture.
- Use simple, everyday words rather than complex words, medical jargon, or colloquialisms.
- Use hand gestures to help the person understand.
- Instruct the person in small increments.
- Have the person demonstrate understanding of the message.
- Provide written instructions for the person to take home.
- When available, use flash cards and phrase books in other languages.
- Use qualified health care interpreters.*

Areas to Consider in Cultural Assessment
- Individual's identification with a particular cultural group
- Habits, customs, values, and beliefs
- Language and communication patterns
- Cultural sanctions and restrictions
- Healing beliefs and practices
- Cultural health practices
- Kinship and social networks
- Nutritional beliefs, food preferences, and restrictions
- Religious beliefs and practices related to health
- Attitudes, values, and beliefs about health†

*For specific requirements of The Joint Commission (2012), see www.languageline.com/main/files/wp_joint_commission_012411.pdf.
†From Andrews, M. M., & Boyle, J. S. (2008). *Transcultural concepts in nursing care* (5th ed.). Philadelphia: Wolters Kluwer/Lippincott.

BOX 10-6   STEPS IN THE TEACHING-LEARNING PROCESS

1. Assessment
   A. Learner characteristics
   B. Learning needs
2. Development of expected learning outcomes
3. Development of a teaching plan
   A. Content
   B. Teaching strategies, learning activities
4. Implementation of the teaching plan
5. Evaluation of expected outcomes
   A. Achievement of learning outcomes
   B. Evaluation of the teaching process

by social marketing strategies will improve the nurse's ability to develop effective educational interventions.

TEACHING PLAN

Preparation for teaching a group program, such as a seminar or course, begins after the marketing and administrative plans are well underway. These activities ensure that there are enough participants for the program, and they provide the structure for developing the teaching plan—the program objectives, available time, human and material resources, and so on. When the marketing and administrative functions have been provided by others and when educational strategies are developed for one person at a time, the nurse can concentrate efforts on developing the teaching plan.

A health teaching plan may emphasize a phase of the behavior change process that is related to the individual's health-promotion needs or problems. The written teaching plan represents a package of educational services provided to a consumer or student. The plan is written from the learner's point of view (Box 10-6).

The process of generating a teaching plan helps the nurse recognize and use methods of learning that involve the individual as an active participant. The plan includes a list of specific actions or abilities that the person may perform at intervals during and at the end of the educational intervention. Teaching plans help nurses clarify these outcomes. Preparing a teaching plan involves the steps of the teaching-learning process outlined in Box 10-6.

Assessment

Assessment, the first step in the process, involves determining the characteristics of the learner and identifying learning needs. The following characteristics of the learner are important for the nurse to identify and consider in planning:
- Age, developmental stage in the life cycle, and level of education
- Health beliefs
- Motivation and readiness to learn
- Health risks and problems
- Current knowledge and skills
- Barriers and facilitators to learning

combined to promote population-based changes in behavior to improve health.

Social marketing is defined as "the application of commercial marketing technologies to the analysis, planning, execution, and evaluation of programs designed to influence the voluntary behavior of target audiences in order to improve their personal welfare and that of their society" (Andreasen, 1995, p. 7). The primary objective of social marketing is to change behavior.

Key attributes of a social marketing approach are the offering of benefits and the reduction of barriers to influence the target group's behavior. Social marketers attempt to modify the attractiveness of specific behavioral options to favor one choice over competing alternatives. The systematic approach to understanding and responding to specific audience characteristics makes the messages more appealing (Storey et al., 2008). For example, social marketing strategies could be used in designing smoking-cessation programs for ethnic minorities. Health-related social marketing offerings may include physical goods such as nutritious lunches, services such as stress-management workshops, or ideas and concepts such as encouraging safer sex or preventing heart disease (Bensley & Brookins-Fisher, 2009). Any information about the target population that is generated

The reader is encouraged to refer to the chapters about individual development (see Unit 4).

Assessment of the learner can be accomplished by answering the following five questions:

- What are the characteristics and learning capabilities of the individual?
- What are the learner's needs for health promotion, risk reduction, or health problems?
- What does the person already know and what skills can the person already perform that are relevant to the health needs?
- Is the learner motivated to change any unhealthy behaviors?
- What are the barriers to and facilitators of health behavior change?

When preparing a teaching plan for one person in a primary care setting, the nurse may learn background information about the individual from that person's record and agency reports that include descriptions of the person's population group. Nurses often agree to teach health classes that others have organized. In this case, the nurse asks for project reports that provide marketing and needs-assessment information about the students who are expected to attend the classes (see the Care Plan at the end of the chapter).

Determining Expected Learning Outcomes

To determine the expected learning outcomes of a health education intervention, the nurse answers the following questions:

- What broad public health and social goals guide the proposed educational program?
- What are the participant's learning goals?
- What does the learner need to know, do, and believe to progress through the behavior change process?

Program Goals

The program goals of a health education project reflect the desire to facilitate improvement in some health problem or social living condition. Program goals are broad statements on long-range expected accomplishments that provide direction; they do not have to be stated in measurable terms (Miller & Stoeckel, 2011).

Learning Goals

Learning goals are best established when the student and the nurse work together. These goals reflect the health behavior or health status change that the person will have achieved by the end of an educational intervention. Learning goals relate to the program goals.

Learning Objectives

Learning objectives indicate the steps to be taken by the individual toward meeting the learning goal and may involve the development of knowledge, skill, or change in attitude. Objectives are most useful when stated in behavioral terms and when they contain these components: the learner and a precise action verb that indicates what the learner will be able to do; the conditions under which the task is performed; and the level

of performance expected (Bastable & Doody, 2008). Learning objectives guide the selection of content and methods and help narrow the focus of a teaching plan to more achievable steps; they also aid in setting standards of performance and suggesting evaluation strategies.

Selecting Content

To select appropriate content for a health education program, the nurse considers what information, skills, and attitudes need to be taught and the level of learning to be achieved.

Three Domains of Learning

Content is commonly divided into three domains: cognitive; psychomotor; and affective. Cognitive learning refers to the development of new facts or concepts, and building on or applying knowledge to new situations. Psychomotor learning involves developing physical skills from simple to complex actions. Affective learning alludes to the recognition of values, religious and spiritual beliefs, family interaction patterns and relationships, and personal attitudes that affect decisions and problem-solving progress.

To learn or change a health behavior, a person may need to acquire new information, practice some physical techniques, and clarify the ways in which the new behavior may affect relationships with others. The nurse's role is to select a combination of content from the three domains that is appropriate to meet the behavioral objective. To find samples of content for a teaching plan, the nurse researches resource materials, such as books, teaching guides, journal articles, pamphlets, and flyers created by nonprofit agencies and professional organizations. The nurse is careful about giving students materials with technical vocabulary that is too complex for the audience.

Examples of Learning Objectives

In writing learning objectives, the nurse selects action verbs from the taxonomies previously mentioned that indicate observable learning. In Table 10-1 examples are given for objectives in each domain of learning. The first objective listed for each domain is incorrect because the verb does not indicate observable learning. The second example for each domain is measurable because the verb used (indicated in boldface type) allows the learning to be observed.

Levels of Learning

The level of learning to be achieved depends on how the nurse anticipates that the content will be used. Taxonomies developed by Bloom and others (Bloom et al., 1956; Krathwohl et al., 1964) are widely accepted as the standard tools for arranging levels of learning objectives according to type and complexity. For example, in the cognitive domain, levels of learning include the following:

- Knowledge: Person recalls facts and the concept.
- Comprehension: Person understands the meaning of the concept.
- Application: Person uses the concept.
- Analysis: Person can examine or explain the concept.

TABLE 10-1	EXAMPLES OF NONMEASURABLE AND MEASURABLE OBJECTIVES	

DOMAIN	OBJECTIVES
Cognitive	**Not Measurable:** Dan will understand the correct food choices for following a diabetic diet. **Measurable:** Dan will correctly **select** food choices based on his diabetic meal plan.
Affective	**Not Measurable:** Dan will demonstrate the importance of regular blood glucose monitoring by checking his blood glucose level before each meal and at bedtime. **Measurable:** Dan will **verbalize** the importance of checking his blood glucose level before each meal and at bedtime.
Psychomotor	**Not Measurable:** Dan will know how to correctly give himself an insulin injection. **Measurable:** Dan will **demonstrate** proper technique and dosage when giving an insulin injection to himself.

TABLE 10-2	DOMAINS OF LEARNING, TEACHING STRATEGIES, AND EXAMPLES OF DESIRED OUTCOMES RELATED TO A BEHAVIOR CHANGE	

DOMAIN OF LEARNING	TEACHING STRATEGIES	EXAMPLES OF DESIRED OUTCOMES RELATED TO A BEHAVIOR CHANGE
Cognitive (thinking)	Lecture One-to-one instruction Discussion Discovery Audiovisual or printed materials Computer-assisted instruction	Describes and/or explains information relevant to the behavior change
Affective (feeling)	Role modeling Discussion Role playing Simulation gaming	Expresses positive feeling, attitudes, values toward changing the behavior
Psychomotor (acting)	Demonstration Practice Mental imaging	Demonstrates performance of skills related to the behavior change

- Synthesis: Person integrates the concept with other learning.
- Evaluation: Person judges or compares the concept (Bastable & Dart, 2008).

When preparing a teaching plan, the nurse differentiates between information the individual needs to know and information considered helpful to know to develop appropriate learning objectives. This process provides cues to the nurse for planning effective strategies for the necessary level of learning. As the level of learning to be achieved becomes complex, the educational strategies and methods selected involve the individuals in more active application and analysis of the content.

Designing Learning Strategies

Designing the learning strategies for an educational intervention involves selecting the methods and tools and structuring the sequence of activities. The teaching plan to this point provides the foundation on which to base the activity selection and sequence. The following questions guide the design of learning strategies:

- What are some basic considerations for selecting teaching methods for health education programs?
- How does the nurse, as instructor, establish and maintain a learning climate?
- What actions can the nurse perform to increase the effectiveness of the learning methods?
- What are the appropriate methods for each learning domain?
- What methods tend to promote behavior change?

Teaching Strategies

Numerous strategies for teaching are available (Table 10-2). A few of those most commonly used are listed and described here.

Lecture is a well-known method in which the teacher verbally presents information and instructions to the person or audience. Lecture provides a way to present a large amount of information to a number of people in a nonthreatening way. This can be an effective method if active learning strategies such as questioning are integrated. Discussion involves interaction between the nurse educator and the individuals. The nurse prepares questions in advance to guide the discussion. This method allows an opportunity for the nurse to gain a better perception of the individuals' understanding of the topic and to clarify the information.

Demonstration and practice is used in learning psychomotor skills such as giving oneself an injection, changing a dressing, or performing exercises. The nurse demonstrates the expected behavior while the person observes. Then the nurse watches and provides feedback and encouragement while the person performs the behavior. Using the actual equipment that the individual will use in their home facilitates successful performance. For complex tasks, teaching a few steps at a time, in sequence, aids skill development.

Simulation gaming may involve computer learning, board games, or role play. Obviously, computer learning games are dependent on the availability of hardware and software appropriate for the individual and the topic. Simple board games can be developed for cognitive learning. An example might be developing a bingo game based on the food pyramid. Role play involves acting out a potential scenario. This allows individuals to practice appropriate responses to challenging situations. For example, a person restricted to a low-fat diet can act out a response to being offered dessert by an insistent family member or friend played by the nurse. Or a grandmother, unsure of what to do when her grandson's blood glucose level is high, might practice making calls to the physician and giving the necessary information.

Considerations for Selecting Methods

The nurse's first consideration is to promote an environment and use methods that foster self-directed learning. An active participant usually learns more.

There will be many learning styles in a group audience; therefore, the nurse varies the teaching methods used in a given session. Taking into consideration the characteristics of the population (developmental stage, age, and knowledge of the topic), the nurse selects teaching methods that best support the goals and theme of the educational program. The order of content proceeds from simple ideas and skills to the more complex concepts, from known material toward lesser-known data. The nurse is sensitive to the energy level and anxiety of the audience when presenting content that requires strong concentration or causes anxiety.

Learning Climate

For group presentations, the nurse addresses several activities when seeking to establish an environment that is conducive to health behavior change. The first activity is creating a sense of preparedness and organization by providing physical facilities with adequate furnishings and suitable audiovisual materials and handouts. Even the instructor's appearance will lend credibility or distraction to the presentation.

The second activity involves anticipating the needs of the group and communicating information about the schedule and the facilities. This action alleviates the group's apprehension and makes them more comfortable.

The third activity focuses on the nurse's assessment of the individual and group learning needs, possibly through questions and dialogue. Members of the group need to believe that the program will be beneficial and relevant to their situations. The instructor watches for and reinforces signs of motivation to participate in the experience.

Fourth, having established a positive learning climate, the nurse seeks to maintain a high level of motivation, a sense of individualized attention, and a progression. As a reality check, the nurse might ask for periodic feedback from the group about the effectiveness of the program and its relevance to group needs.

Finally, the nurse works with the group to maintain the learning climate. This process involves observing group interactions, helping individuals to participate, intervening to help the group deal with controlling its members, and remaining cognizant of dynamics in the group process that will facilitate or inhibit learning.

Teaching for Each Learning Domain

As mentioned, teaching is directed toward one or more of three learning domains: cognitive, psychomotor, and affective. Examples of appropriate teaching strategies for each domain and the expected outcomes in relation to behavior change are summarized in Table 10-2.

Evaluating the Teaching-Learning Process

The teacher can evaluate the learning, or measure achievement of learning objectives, in all domains through the use of written or oral testing, demonstrations, observation, self-reports, and self-monitoring. Teaching methods for one domain may overlap those for another domain.

The nurse can incorporate written, verbal, and nonverbal techniques into the teaching plan for obtaining feedback about teaching performance. End-of-program questionnaires are the usual method for obtaining written feedback. The nurse may ask for verbal feedback at various times from the group, from individual students, and from observers of the class. Nonverbal communication cues from participants may indicate their satisfaction, fatigue, or frustration with the educational intervention.

The overall process of the teaching-learning experience needs to be evaluated. The procedures used to organize and promote an educational program can affect its ultimate success. The nurse (or a program administration committee) records activities such as advertising, registration, fee collection, and availability and repair of equipment and materials. This evaluative information can then be used to improve subsequent programs. Surveys by telephone or by questionnaires help obtain the consumer's opinion about these implementation procedures. Word-of-mouth referrals to future programs and support from other community agencies and professionals may also indicate approval of the program format.

Occasionally the nurse is asked to justify a health education program in terms of its effect on the community's public health goals or social problems. Health promotion involves a combination of health-protection activities, preventive health services, and health education programs; therefore, drawing a direct correlation between an educational intervention and the statistical improvement of the health problem can be difficult.

Nurses often can describe the theoretical influence of an educational intervention on health behaviors, health problems, and social problems. Statistics such as the number of people served each year, the percentage of the target population reached, the number of service providers used, and the number and cost of programs are important and need to be preserved. As these statistics change over time, the data will provide cues to program successes and problems.

Referring Individuals to Other Resources

The end of a teaching plan includes resources for people to use for continuing education, counseling, peer support, and health services. Nurses encourage people to view health education as a lifelong learning process. Each person has different developmental needs and health concerns through the life cycle. Moreover, any one educational intervention may help a person move only from one phase of the behavior change process to the next. Additionally, the Internet as a health education tool may influence a person's health practices (Box 10-7: Hot Topics).

BOX 10-7 HOT TOPICS

The Internet as a Health Education Tool

The availability of health information on the **Internet** has far-reaching implications for health education. The Internet provides access to information from numerous sources on a broad range of topics to an increasing number of individuals and families. Examples of these topics include well-child care, women's health, nutrition, and information regarding disease treatment and provision of home care for the terminally ill.

Consumers have access to a wealth of valuable information, but they may be overwhelmed by the number and types of resources. Some resources may be useful and accurate; others may be biased, inaccurate, misunderstood, and potentially problematic. Nurses need to develop skill in using the Internet as an education tool for care recipients and in guiding individuals' selection of health information sources.

Guidelines are available for selecting sources. One that is useful is *Evaluating Health Information on the Internet*. This can be found on the National Cancer Institute's website at www.cancer.gov/cancertopics/factsheet/Information/Internet.

In addition, the Health On the Net Foundation (HON) code on a website indicates that it is a recognized nongovernmental source of "reliable, understandable, relevant, and trustworthy" medical and health information based on eight principles (Health On the Net Foundation, 2008).

Before recommending Internet sources, nurses determine if the source is reputable and reliable and if the information is current, accurate, understandable, and appropriate for the target audience. The nurse identifies sites that may be useful to the target group and checks them before recommending them. Encouraging people to discuss information obtained from Internet resources is essential to establish an opportunity to clarify their understanding and direct them to sources that are more appropriate, when necessary.

The following are some websites that provide access to general health information:

www.mayoclinic.com
www.healthfinder.gov
www.intelihealth.com
www.medlineplus.gov
www.health.gov
www.aoa.gov
www.nutrition.gov

The Internet may also serve as an avenue of accessibility to an abundance of information for persons from rural areas or for individuals who are homebound. Although Internet access is expanding rapidly, it is important to recognize that not everyone has access in their homes. This is particularly true for those with lower levels of income or education.

BOX 10-8 RESEARCH FOR EVIDENCE-BASED PRACTICE

Comparison of Narrative and Traditional Health Information

In a study of African American women ($n = 489$) age 40 and older recruited from low-income neighborhoods in St. Louis, Missouri, the effect of personal narratives about mammography and breast cancer was compared with a traditional informational approach.

The women were randomly assigned to watch a narrative video comprised of African American breast cancer survivors or an informational video with equivalent content. Outcomes were measured immediately following the video, and at 3- and 6-month follow-up intervals.

The women who watched the narrative video ($n = 244$) compared to the informational video ($n = 245$) experienced stronger negative and positive affect responses immediately. Narratives were found to increase persuasion by reducing counterarguing, and also by increasing risk perceptions and fear. These findings may indicate that narrative messages, by reducing counterarguing and increasing engagement and cognitive rehearsal (talking to others), may increase acceptance and motivation to act on health information. Results suggest that narratives have several advantages over traditional information and may be more effective in cancer control in a high-risk population.

Modified from Kreuter, M., Holmes, K., Alcaraz, K., Kalesan, B., Rath, S., Richert, M., et al. (2010). Comparing narrative and informational videos to increase mammography in low-income African American women. *Patient Education & Counseling*, 81(S6-14). http://dx.doi.org/10.1016/j.pec.2010.09.008.
Modified from McQueen, A., Kreuter, M., Kalesan, B., & Alcaraz, K. (2011). Understanding narrative effects: The impact of breast cancer survivor stories on message processing, attitudes, and beliefs among African American women. *Health Psychology: Official Journal of the Division of Health Psychology, American Psychological Association*, 30(6), 674-682.

TEACHING AND ORGANIZING SKILLS

To develop teaching and organizing skills in health education, the nurse often needs to learn new behaviors. A systematic guide can be used for learning these professional skills. To perform these steps, the nurse does the following:

- Seeks self-assessment opportunities.
- Identifies, lists, and prioritizes learning needs.
- Begins to identify the resources that are available for reading, instructor training, and practice teaching.
- Drafts an initial set of learning goals.
- Selects the target population and the general topic.
- Works through steps of the teaching-learning process, including the development of a teaching plan.
- Identifies other people or a project team to help.

After implementing the educational intervention, the nurse sets time aside to discuss what took place. Did the program go as planned? What changes were made in the teaching plan? What can be changed for the next program? The nurse reviews the self-developed learning goals and determines new ones.

In addition, health education research evaluates teaching interventions. This contributes to the evidence base from which nurses can implement new teaching strategies or question the effectiveness of traditional approaches. For an example of a study comparing the effects of using narrative information versus traditional information to teaching a high-risk group, please see Box 10-8: Research for Evidence-Based Practice.

As additional programs on either an individual or a group basis are provided, the nurse will be able to clarify specific instructor teaching and organizing skills that come naturally.

CASE STUDY
Albert

Albert Mitchell is a 36-year-old man who will be traveling to Dubai to give a business presentation in 3 months. Although he has traveled widely in the United States as a consultant, this is his first trip to the Middle East. He requests information regarding immunizations needed before his trip. Albert states that since he will only be in Dubai for a few days, he is unlikely to contract a disease in such a short time and therefore believes that it is illogical to obtain immunizations. Albert states that he has heard that the side effects of the immunizations might be worse than the diseases they prevent. He is also concerned about leaving his wife at home alone because she is 6 months' pregnant.

Reflective Questions
1. How would you address Albert's beliefs?
2. What learning would be needed in each domain?
3. What learning theories would you consider?
4. How might his family concerns be addressed?

◎ CARE PLAN
Preparing a Teaching Plan

*NURSING DIAGNOSIS: Deficient Knowledge (Specify Area)

Defining Characteristics
- Verbalization of inadequate information or an inadequate recall of information
- Verbalization of misunderstanding or misconception
- Request for information
- Instructions followed inaccurately
- Inadequate performance on a test
- Inadequate demonstration of a skill

Related Factors
- Pathophysiological states
- Sensory deficits
- Memory loss
- Intellectual limitations
- Interfering coping strategies (denial or anxiety)
- Lack of exposure to accurate information
- Lack of motivation to learn
- Inattention
- Cultural or language barriers

Expected Outcomes
- The individual will express an interest in learning.
- The individual will correctly state the information on the specific topic.
- The individual will correctly demonstrate skills needed to practice health-related behavior.
- The individual and family will explain how to incorporate new information into their lifestyle.
- The individual will modify health behavior based on the acquisition of new knowledge.
- The individual will list resources for more information or support.

Interventions
- Provide accurate and culturally relevant information related to the specific topic.
- Select teaching techniques appropriate to the individual's learning needs.
- Explore the individual's interpretation of the information and its meaning in the context of the person's life.
- Demonstrate and then have the individual practice new skills.
- Assist the person in identifying and implementing alternative strategies when initial choices are not successful.
- Include the family or significant others as appropriate.
- Provide names and telephone numbers of resource people or organizations.

*NANDA Nursing Diagnoses—Definitions and Classification 2012-2014, Herdman T.H. (ED). Copyright © 2012, 1994-2012 NANDA International. Used by arrangement with John Wiley & Sons Limited. In order to make safe and effective judgments using the NANDA-I nursing diagnoses it is essential that nurses refer to the definitions and defining characteristics of the diagnoses listed in this work.

These skills tend to improve a program's effectiveness and enable the logistics to run smoothly. The teacher is first a learner; this is true in health education and any other form of education.

SUMMARY

Of all health professionals, nurses spend the most time in direct contact with individuals; they have many opportunities to recognize a need for knowledge and a readiness to learn new information and behaviors. Nurses often coordinate group programs. The more accurate the analysis of the educational aspects of a health-promotion program and the assessment of characteristics and learning needs of the target audience, the more effective an educational intervention will be in influencing health behaviors.

The principles of health education form a generic basis for implementing a variety of health topics, such as accident prevention and use of first aid, expectant parent education, hypertension education, nutrition and fitness, stress management, substance abuse, sex education, and education in areas including diabetes and arthritis. The two scenarios described in this chapter provide insights into the nurse's role in conducting educational interventions about family planning and prenatal care.

Planning to teach one person is different from planning to teach a group. One-to-one interventions tend to follow a counseling or problem-solving approach. Group interventions can range from guided discussions on concerns that evolve from the group to a more structured learning experience involving presentations, skill practice, and attitude-awareness exercises. The range of health education strategies provides nurses and all health care professionals with techniques and methods applicable in health service settings, schools, work sites, and other community facilities.

REFERENCES

American Nurses Association. (2010a). *Nursing: Scope and standards of practice* (2nd ed.). Silver Spring, MD: The Association.

American Nurses Association. (2010b). *Nursing's social policy statement.* Washington, DC: The Association.

Anderson, D. G., Ward, H., & Hatton, D. C. (2008). Family health risks. In M. Stanhope, & J. Lancaster (Eds.), *Public health nursing: Population-centered health care in the community* (7th ed.). St. Louis: Mosby Elsevier.

Andreasen, A. R. (1995). *Marketing social change: Changing behavior to promote health, social development, and the environment.* San Francisco: Jossey-Bass.

Andrews, M. M., & Boyle, J. S. (2008). *Transcultural concepts in nursing care* (5th ed.). Philadelphia: Wolters Kluwer/Lippincott.

Bandura, A. (1997). *Self-efficacy: The exercise of control.* New York: W.H. Freeman.

Bastable, S. B., & Dart, M. A. (2008). Developmental stages of the learner. In S. B. Bastable (Ed.), *Nurse as educator: Principles of teaching and learning for nursing practice* (3rd ed.). Sudbury, MA: Jones & Bartlett.

Bastable, S. B., & Doody, J. A. (2008). Behavioral objectives. In S. B. Bastable (Ed.), *Nurse as educator: Principles of teaching and learning for nursing practice* (3rd ed.). Sudbury, MA: Jones & Bartlett.

Baur, C. (2011). Calling the nation to act: Implementing the national action plan to improve health literacy. *Nursing Outlook, 59*(2), 63–69. doi: 10.1016/jouylook.2010.12.003.

Becker, M. H. (1974). *The Health Belief Model and personal health behavior.* Thorofare, NJ: Charles B. Slack.

Bensley, R. J., & Brookins-Fisher, J. (2009). *Community health education methods: A practical guide* (3rd ed.). Sudbury, MA: Jones & Bartlett.

Bloom, B. S., Englehart, M. S., Furst, E. J., Hill, W. H., & Krathwohl, D. J. (1956). *Taxonomy of educational objectives: The classification of educational goals—Handbook 1: Cognitive domain.* White Plains, NY: Longman.

Braverman, P. A., Kumanyika, S., Fielding, J., LaVeist, T., Borrell, L. N., Manderscheid, R., et al. (2011). Health disparities and health equity: The issue is justice. *American Journal of Public Health, 101*(Suppl. 1), S149–S155.

Burkhardt, M. A., & Nathaniel, A. K. (2008). *Ethics and issues in contemporary nursing* (3rd ed.). Clifton Park, NY: Delmar Cengage Learning.

Champion, V. L., & Skinner, C. S. (2008). The Health Belief Model. In K. Glanz, B. K. Rimer, & K. Viswanath (Eds.), *Health behavior and health education: Theory, research, and practice* (4th ed.). San Francisco: Jossey-Bass.

Degazon, C. E. (2008). Cultural diversity in the community. In M. Stanhope, & J. Lancaster (Eds.), *Public health nursing: Population-centered health care in the community* (7th ed.). St. Louis: Mosby Elsevier.

Health On the Net Foundation. (2008). Retrieved from www.hon.ch/HONcode/Conduct.html.

Janz, N. K., & Becker, M. H. (1984). The Health Belief Model: A decade later. *Health Education Quarterly, 11*(1), 1–47.

Joint Committee on Health Education and Promotion Terminology. (2002). Report of the 2000 Joint Committee on Health Education and Promotion Terminology. *Journal of School Health, 72*(1), 3–7.

Koh, H. K., Nowinski, J. M., & Piotrowski, J. J. (2011). A 2020 vision for educating the next generation of public health leaders. *American Journal of Preventive Medicine, 40*(2), 199–202.

Krathwohl, D. R., Bloom, B. S., & Masia, B. B. (1964). *Taxonomy of educational objectives: The classification of educational goals—Handbook 2: Affective domain.* New York: David McKay.

McQueen, A., Kreuter, M., Kalesan, B., & Alcaraz, K. (2011). Understanding narrative effects: The impact of breast cancer survivor stories on message processing, attitudes, and beliefs among African American women. *Health Psychology: Official Journal of the Division of Health Psychology.* American Psychological Association, *30*(6), 674–682.

Miller, M. A., & Stoeckel, P. R. (2011). *Client education: Theory and practice.* Sudbury, MA: Jones & Bartlett.

Ornish, D. (2009). Intensive lifestyle changes and health reform. *The Lancet Oncology, 10*(7), 637–639.

Osborne, H. (2013). *Health literacy from A to Z: Practical ways to communicate your health message* (2nd ed.). Burlington, MA: Jones & Bartlett Learning.

Perez, M. A., & Luquis, R. R. (2008). *Cultural competence in health education and health promotion.* San Francisco: Jossey-Bass.

Prochaska, J. O., & DiClemente, C. C. (1984). *The transtheoretical approach: Crossing traditional boundaries of change.* Homewood, NJ: Dow Jones-Irwin.

Richards, E., & Digger, K. (2008). Compliance, motivation, and health behaviors of the learner. In S. B. Bastable (Ed.), *Nurse as educator: Principles of teaching and learning for nursing practice* (3rd ed.). Sudbury, MA: Jones & Bartlett.

Rosenstock, I. M., Strecher, K. J., & Becker, M. H. (1988). The social learning theory and Health Belief Model. *Health Education Quarterly, 15,* 175–183.

Saarmann, L., Dougherty, J., & Riegel, B. (2002). Teaching staff a brief cognitive-behavioral intervention. *MEDSURG Nursing, 11*(3), 114–151.

Selden, C. R., Zorn, M., Ratzen, S., & Parker, R. M. (2000). *Health literacy: January 1990 through 1999.* NLM publication #CBM 2000-1, Bethesda, MD: National Library of Medicine. Retrieved February 4, 2012, from www.nlm.nih.gov/archive//20061214/pubs/cbm/hliteracy.html.

Simons-Morton, B. G., McLeroy, K. R., & Wendel, M. L. (2012). *Behavior theory in health promotion practice and research.* Burlington, MA: Jones & Bartlett Learning.

Speros, C. I. (2011). Promoting health literacy: A nursing imperative. *Nursing Clinics of North America, 46,* 321–333. doi: 10.1016/j.cnur.2011.05.007.

Storey, J. D., Saffitz, G. B., & Rimon, J. G. (2008). Social marketing. In K. Glanz, B. K. Rimer, & K. Viswanath (Eds.), *Health behavior and health education: Theory, research, and practice* (4th ed.). San Francisco: Jossey-Bass.

U.S. Department of Health and Human Services (USDHHS). (2008). *America's health literacy: Why we need accessible health information. An issue brief from the U.S. Department of Health and Human Services.* Available from www.health.gov/communication/literacy/issuebrief/#intro.

U.S. Department of Health and Human Services (USDHHS). (2010). *Healthy People 2020.* Washington, DC: Author. Available at www.healthypeople.gov.

Zarate-Abbott, P., Etnyre, A., Gilliland, I., Mahon, M., Allwein, D., Cook, J., et al. (2008). Workplace health promotion: Strategies for low-income Hispanic immigrant women. *AAOHN Journal, 56*(5), 217–222.

Nutrition Counseling for Health Promotion

Toni Tucker

 WEBSITE

OBJECTIVES

After completing this chapter, the reader will be able to:
- Identify *Healthy People 2020* nutrition and food safety objectives.
- Analyze the leading nutrition-related causes of illness and death in the United States and identify both common dietary factors associated with them and those specific to each.
- Summarize the basic nutrition recommendations contained in the *Dietary Guidelines for Americans.*

- Compare the number of servings and serving sizes recommended in MyPlate with serving sizes featured currently in the marketplace.
- Compare the current MyPlate with other suggested versions of daily nutrition requirements.
- Analyze U.S. food aid programs for the poor and older adults.
- Plan a 1-day menu that is consistent with recent dietary guidance for a person at any stage of the life cycle (older than age 2 years).

KEY TERMS

Body mass index (BMI)
Botanicals
Cancer
Cardiovascular disease
Cholesterol
Cirrhosis
Coronary heart disease (CHD)
DASH
Diabetes mellitus
Dietary Guidelines Advisory Committee (DGAC)
Dietary Guidelines for Americans
Dietary reference intakes (DRIs)

Dyslipidemia
Fats
Fiber
Food insecurity
Heart disease
Hemolytic uremic syndrome
Hemorrhagic colitis
Herbals
High-density lipoprotein (HDL)
Human immunodeficiency virus (HIV)
Hyperglycemia
Hyperlipidemia
Hypertension

Incidence
Lacto-ovo vegetarian
Low-density lipoprotein (LDL)
Macronutrients
Metabolic syndrome
Micronutrients
MyPlate
MyPyramid
Nutrition screening
Obesity
Osteoporosis
Overweight
Pre-diabetes

KEY TERMS—cont'd

Pre-hypertension	Stroke	Triglyceride
Prevalence	Sugar	Type 2 diabetes
Salmonellosis	Teratogenic	Underweight
Serving sizes	Trans fatty acids (trans fat)	Vegan

? THINK ABOUT IT

How Healthy Is My Own Plate?

Begin thinking about your food and health and the food and health of people around you. Check each statement that describes the way you usually eat. Add up the number of statements that you have checked and compare that number with the scores listed after the questions.

The way I **usually** eat:

- I take the time to fully enjoy my food as I eat it, so that I am not distracted and tempted to eat too much or too fast. I pay attention to hunger and fullness cues so that I recognize when to eat and when I have had enough.
- I know how to balance calories between my portions and my activity level as a first step to manage my weight for someone of my age, size, and activity level. (Stop and check out www.ChooseMyPlate.gov or **Website Resource 11A** to find out, if not sure.)
- I avoid oversized portions by using any of the following: using a smaller bowl, plate, or glass at home; portioning out my plate before I eat; or choosing a smaller size option, sharing a dish, or taking home part of a meal when I eat out.
- Most days of the week, I make vegetables, fruits, whole grains, and fat-free or 1% milk or dairy products (or their nondairy equivalents) the foundation for my meals and snacks.
- Either I eat small servings of meat, poultry, and fish (no larger than the size of a deck of cards) or I do not eat meat and substitute other protein sources such as eggs, beans, legumes, or nuts/seeds.
- I make fruits and vegetables half of my plate at most meals with a variety of types and colors when available.
- I have switched to drinking 1% or skim milk or the equivalent substitute (almond, soy milk) or eating low-fat or fat-free dairy products or equivalent substitutes daily.
- I eat grains daily (such as bread, cereal, pasta, rice) and normally make half of them whole grains (such as substituting whole-wheat bread for white bread or brown rice for white rice).
- I use small amounts of unsaturated liquids such as olive, canola, safflower, or corn oils or tub margarine (without trans fat or partially hydrogenated oil) and low-fat salad dressing, when needed, rather than butter, stick margarine, lard, or regular salad dressing.
- I substitute water or unsweetened beverages for sugary drinks (soda, energy drinks, and sports drinks).
- I compare sodium levels in foods by reading ingredients or using the *Nutrition Facts* label to choose lower sodium versions of soup, bread, and frozen meals or canned products.
- I do not drink alcohol or I drink no more than 1 to 2 beers, 1 to 2 glasses of wine, or 1 to 2 mixed drinks daily.

Number of Statements Checked

Score: 9 to 12. Evaluation: Great job! Recommendation: While reading this chapter, you will be reminded of all the things you are doing that contribute to your healthy lifestyle. Check out if there is anything you want to tweak a little. You are an excellent role model for others. Keep it Up!

Score: 5 to 8. Evaluation: You are on the right track! Recommendation: You do make some good choices. On a scale of 1 to 10 (with 1 being lowest and 10 highest), what would it take to move up another step or two? As you read, think about your family risk factors and what might be motivating to you. Check out popular websites such as Spark.com or www.MyPlate.gov or popular cooking magazines that help you get healthy, tasty food on the table without a ton of money or time in the kitchen.

Score: 0 to 4. Evaluation: You are on the wrong track! Recommendation: The first steps toward better eating habits are the hardest to take, but making healthy choices is an investment in yourself. On a scale of 1 to 10 (with 1 being lowest and 10 highest), what would it take to move up another step or two? As you read, think about your family risk factors and what might be motivating to you. Make a list of the pros and cons of changing. Think about one small step you could take in the next 6 months and surround yourself with others who are also trying to improve their health. You deserve it!

NUTRITION IN THE UNITED STATES: LOOKING FORWARD FROM THE PAST

Classic Vitamin-Deficiency Diseases

Food and nutrition have always been vitally important to health. Until as recently as the 1940s, many nutrient-deficiency diseases, such as rickets, pellagra, scurvy, beriberi, xerophthalmia, and goiter, were still prevalent in the United States (Carpenter, 2000). Although these conditions still persist in developing countries, they have virtually disappeared from developed areas of the world. Why? The availability of an abundant food supply, the fortification of some foods with critical nutrients, and the implementation of better methods of determining and improving the nutrient contents of foods have contributed to the decline of nutrient-deficiency diseases.

The introduction of iodized salt in the 1920s, for example, contributed greatly to eliminating iodine-deficiency goiter as a public health problem. Similarly, pellagra disappeared after the discovery that inadequate niacin levels contribute to the condition. Today, nutrient deficiencies rarely are reported in the United States. The few cases of protein-energy malnutrition that are listed annually as causes of death generally occur as secondary results of severe illness or injury, premature birth, child neglect, problems of the homebound aged, alcoholism, or some combination of these factors. Although undernutrition still occurs in some groups of people in the United States, including those who are isolated or poor, these once-prevalent diseases of nutritional deficiency have been replaced by diseases of dietary excess and imbalance (Table 11-1).

TABLE 11-1 HEALTH PROBLEMS RELATED TO POOR NUTRITION

HEALTH PROBLEM*	CONTRIBUTING LIFESTYLE AND NUTRITION PRACTICES†
Anemia	Diet with inadequate iron, folate, or vitamin B_{12} intake (depending upon type of anemia)
Cancer (breast, cervical, and colon)	Excessive calorie intake, belly fat; low fiber intake
Cirrhosis	Excessive alcohol intake
Constipation	Inadequate fiber or fluid intake; high fat intake; sedentary lifestyle
Dental caries	Excessive, frequent consumption of concentrated sweets or sugar-sweetened beverages; lack of fluoride; poor dental hygiene
Type 2 diabetes	Excessive calorie intake; excessive fat intake (in particular saturated fat, trans fat); sedentary lifestyle
Cardiovascular/heart disease	Excessive calorie intake; excessive fat intake (in particular saturated fat, trans fat); excessive sodium, inadequate fiber intake; sedentary lifestyle
Hypertension	Excessive sodium and insufficient potassium intake; excessive calorie intake; possible excess alcohol intake; sedentary lifestyle
Obesity	Excessive calorie intake; excessive fat intake; sedentary lifestyle
Osteoporosis	Low calcium intake; low vitamin D intake; excessive intake of protein, sodium, and caffeine; sedentary lifestyle; excessive alcohol intake
Underweight and growth failure	Inadequate calorie intake; poor diet

*A number of health problems are caused or exacerbated by poor nutrition. Health care professionals strive to prevent or delay these health problems.
†Not all may apply in every case.

Dietary Excess and Imbalance

Problems resulting from overconsumption now rank among the leading causes of illness and death in the United States. As stated in 2010 by the U.S. Department of Agriculture and U.S. Department of Health and Human Services (USDA/USDHHS) in their *Dietary Guidelines for Americans:*

> "On average, American men, women, and children consume too much sodium, solid fats (the major source of saturated and trans fatty acids), added sugars, and refined grains. Men consume too much cholesterol, which also is found in some solid fats. In addition, some people consume too much alcohol."

Four leading causes of death directly associated with diet are coronary heart disease (CHD), some types of cancer, stroke, and diabetes mellitus. Four more major causes of death—accidents, cirrhosis of the liver, suicide, and homicide—are associated with excessive alcohol intake.

Indirectly, overweight and obesity also play a huge role. Current statistics show that two in three American adults and one in three children are either overweight or obese (Flegal et al., 2010). Although adult levels of overweight/obesity are alarming on their own, excess weight among the young has been linked with health problems that until now were only seen in adults: high blood pressure, type 2 diabetes, and high cholesterol levels (White House Task Force on Childhood Obesity, 2010). Former Surgeon General Richard Carmona testified before Congress about the critical issue, stating, "Because of the increasing rates of obesity, unhealthy eating habits and physical inactivity, we may see the first generation that will be less healthy and have a shorter life expectancy than their parents" (The Growing Obesity Epidemic, 2004).

The number of American children who are obese is currently 18.1% among 12 to 19 year olds, 19.6% among 6 to 11 year olds, and 10.4% among 2 to 5 year olds (average = 1%) compared with 10.5%, 11.3%, and 7.2%, respectively, from 1988 to 1994 (National Center for Health Statistics [NCHS], 2010).

Reducing the incidence of obesity (in both young and old) is an important public health goal (Flegal et al., 2010). Although excess weight or obesity is commonly viewed as an imbalance between energy intake and expenditure, other factors need to be considered. For example, genes are involved in the process of energy balance as well as differences in fat distribution by gender and age (Bray & Champagne, 2007). Besides these influences, other societal factors contribute to the current obesity epidemic (as well as other chronic diseases). During the release of the *Dietary Guidelines for Americans* in January 2011, both secretaries of the USDA and the USDHHS emphasized

> "…All sectors of society, including individuals and families, educators and health professionals, communities, organizations, businesses, and policymakers, contribute to the food and physical activity environments in which people live. We all have a role to play in reshaping our environment so that healthy choices are easy and accessible for all." (See Box 11-1: Innovative Practice for examples.)

Encouraging healthy choices in diet, exercise, and weight control is one of the major themes of *Healthy People 2020* (USDHHS, 2010a) (Figure 11-1). It also includes a new framework to include additional emphasis on health disparities and health inequities as well as focus on future preventive measures to help healthy choices be the easy choices wherever people live, work, learn, and play.

Because dietary factors contribute substantially to the burden of preventable illness and premature death, *Healthy People 2020* is aimed at directing American dietary patterns toward current dietary recommendations, especially the *Dietary Guidelines for Americans* (USDA/USDHHS, 2010).

HEALTHY PEOPLE 2020: NUTRITION OBJECTIVES

The Nutrition and Weight Status objectives for *Healthy People 2020* (Box 11-2: *Healthy People 2020*) reflect strong science supporting the health benefits of eating a healthful diet and maintaining a healthy body weight. The objectives also emphasize that efforts to change diet and weight should address both individual behaviours and policies and environments that support these behaviors in settings such as schools, worksites, health care organizations, and communities.

The report also contains 12 topics with leading health indicators, a small set of high-priority health issues that provide a way for the nation, states, and local communities to assess and monitor their current health status for key areas and follow them over time. "Nutrition, Physical Activity, and Obesity" is 1 of the 12 topics. Although the importance of physical activity will be discussed in Chapter 12, combining physical activity with nutrition and obesity as one topic illustrates how physical activity, healthy weights, and nutrition are interrelated. See the details of the leading nutrition health indicators listed in Box 11-2.

✳ BOX 11-1 INNOVATIVE PRACTICE

Summary of Recommended Community Strategies and Measurements to Prevent Obesity in the United States Related to Healthy Foods*

Strategy 1
Communities should increase availability of healthier food and beverage choices in public service venues.
Suggested Measurement
A policy exists to apply nutrition standards that are consistent with the *Dietary Guidelines for Americans* (USDA/USDHHS, 2010) to all food sold (e.g., meal menus and vending machines) within local government facilities in a local jurisdiction or on public school campuses during the school day within the largest school district in a local jurisdiction.

Strategy 2
Communities should improve availability of affordable healthier food and beverage choices in public service venues.
Suggested Measurement
A policy exists to affect the cost of healthier foods and beverages as defined by the Institute of Medicine (IOM, 2005) relative to the cost of less healthy foods and beverages sold within local government facilities in a local jurisdiction or on public school campuses during the school day within the largest school district in a local jurisdiction.

Strategy 3
Communities should improve geographic availability of supermarkets in underserved areas.
Suggested Measurement
The number of full-service grocery stores and supermarkets per 10,000 residents located within the three largest underserved census tracts within a local jurisdiction.

Strategy 4
Communities should provide incentives to food retailers to locate in and/or offer healthier food and beverage choices in underserved areas.
Suggested Measurement
Local government offers at least one incentive to new and/or existing food retailers to offer healthier food and beverage choices in underserved areas.

Strategy 5
Communities should improve availability of mechanisms for purchasing foods from farms.
Suggested Measurement
The total annual number of farmer-days at farmers' markets per 10,000 residents within a local jurisdiction.

Strategy 6
Communities should provide incentives for the production, distribution, and procurement of foods from local farms.

Suggested Measurement
Local government has a policy that encourages the production, distribution, or procurement of food from local farms in the local jurisdiction.

Strategies to Support Healthy Food and Beverage Choices

Strategy 7
Communities should restrict availability of less healthy foods and beverages in public service venues.
Suggested Measurement
A policy exists that prohibits the sale of less healthy foods and beverages (as defined by IOM [2005]) within local government facilities in a local jurisdiction or on public school campuses during the school day within the largest school district in a local jurisdiction.

Strategy 8
Communities should institute smaller portion size options in public service venues.
Suggested Measurement
Local government has a policy to limit the portion size of any entree (including sandwiches and entree salads) by either reducing the standard portion size of entrees or offering smaller portion sizes in addition to standard portion sizes within local government facilities within a local jurisdiction.

Strategy 9
Communities should limit advertisements of less healthy foods and beverages.
Suggested Measurement
A policy exists that limits advertising and promotion of less healthy foods and beverages within local government facilities in a local jurisdiction or on public school campuses during the school day within the largest school district in a local jurisdiction.

Strategy 10
Communities should discourage consumption of sugar-sweetened beverages.
Suggested Measurement
Licensed child care facilities within the local jurisdiction are required to ban sugar-sweetened beverages, including flavored/sweetened milk and limit the portion size of 100% juice.

Strategy to Encourage Breastfeeding

Strategy 11
Communities should increase support for breastfeeding.
Suggested Measurement
Local government has a policy requiring local government facilities to provide breastfeeding accommodations for employees that include both time and private space for breastfeeding (or pumping of milk) during working hours.

From U.S. Department of Agriculture and U.S. Department of Health and Human Services (USDA/USDHHS). (2010). *Dietary guidelines for Americans* (7th ed.). Washington, DC: U.S. Government Printing Office; Institute of Medicine (IOM). (2005). *Preventing childhood obesity: Health in the balance.* Washington, DC: The National Academies Press.
***Note:** The entire report includes 24 total strategies and measurements to include those related to physical activity. Because physical activity is discussed in Chapter 12, this excerpt includes nutrition advice only. For those who might be interested in specifics of how to get involved or to see the background evidence that informed these specific strategies/measurements, see Khan et al. (2009 in references). Recommended community strategies and measurements to prevent obesity in the United States.

FIGURE 11-1 Learning nutritional food choices starts at a young age. (From Jochen Sand/Thinkstock.)

Nutrition-Related Health Status

A variety of diet-related factors exact a heavy toll on the U.S. population as the following key facts illustrate (Food Research and Action Center [FRAC], 2011; National Prevention Council [Healthy Eating section], 2011). The following statements give a broad-based view of the health status of Americans:

- Fewer than 15% of adults and 10% of adolescents eat the recommended amounts of fruits and vegetables every day.
- A total of 63% of adults and 84% of adolescents consume at least one sugar-sweetened drink (e.g., soda, sport drinks, fruit drinks and punches, low-calorie drinks, sweetened tea) each day.
- Most American adults consume more than twice the recommended average daily sodium intake level (for healthy people). Nearly 80% of this sodium originates from packaged, processed, and restaurant foods.
- More than two thirds of the adult population is overweight or obese. Approximately one in five children is overweight or obese by the time he or she reaches age 6 and more than half of obese children become overweight at or before age 2.
- Low-income women are more likely than their higher-income counterparts to return to work earlier after

---

♥ BOX 11-2 HEALTHY PEOPLE 2020

Objectives Related to Nutrition and Food Safety, Healthier Food Access

- Increase the number of states with nutrition standards for foods and beverages provided to preschool-aged children in child care.
- Increase the proportion of schools that offer nutritious foods and beverages outside of school meals.
- Increase the number of states that have state-level policies that incentivize food retail outlets to provide foods that are encouraged by the *Dietary Guidelines.*
- (New Developmental Objective) Increase the proportion of Americans who have access to a food retail outlet that sells a variety of foods that are encouraged by the *Dietary Guidelines.*

Health Care and Worksite Settings

- Increase the proportion of primary care physicians who regularly measure the body mass index of their care recipients (both adults and children/adolescents).
- Increase the proportion of physician office visits that include counseling or education related to nutrition or weight (by diagnosis such as cardiovascular disease, diabetes, hyperlipidemia, or obesity).
- (New Developmental Objective) Increase the proportion of work sites that offer nutrition or weight-management classes or counseling.

Weight Status

- Increase the proportion of adults who are at a healthy weight.
- (New Developmental Objective) Prevent inappropriate weight gain in youth and adults.

Food Insecurity

- Eliminate very low food security among children.
- Reduce household food insecurity and in so doing reduce hunger.

Food and Nutrient Consumption

- Increase the contribution of fruits to the diets of the population aged 2 years and older.
- (Leading Health Indicator) Increase the variety and contribution of vegetables to the diets of the population aged 2 years and older (increase the contribution of total vegetables including dark green vegetables, orange vegetables, and legumes).
- Increase the contribution of whole grains to the diets of the population aged 2 years and older.
- Reduce the consumption of calories from solid fats and added sugars in the population aged 2 years and older.
- Reduce the consumption of saturated fat in the population aged 2 years and older.
- Reduce the consumption of sodium in the population aged 2 years and older.
- Increase the consumption of calcium in the population aged 2 years and older.
- Reduce iron deficiency among young children and females of childbearing age (children aged 1 to 2 and aged 3 to 4, females aged 12-49).
- Reduce iron deficiency among pregnant females.

Objectives for Selected Diseases with Nutrition Components
Heart Disease and Stroke

Goal: Increase overall cardiovascular health in U.S. population and reduce CHD and stroke deaths.

- Reduce the proportion of adults with high total blood cholesterol levels.
- Reduce the mean total blood cholesterol levels among adults (for adults aged 20 years and older).
- (New Developmental Objective) Increase the proportion of adults with prehypertension who meet the recommended guidelines (for nutrition: BMI, saturated fat consumption, sodium intake, and moderate alcohol consumption).

Continued

♥ **BOX 11-2   HEALTHY PEOPLE 2020**

Objectives Related to Nutrition and Food Safety, Healthier Food Access—cont'd

- (New Developmental Objective) Increase the proportion of adults with hypertension who meet the recommended guidelines (for nutrition: BMI, saturated fat consumption, sodium intake, and moderate alcohol consumption).
- (New Developmental Objective) Increase the proportion of adults with elevated low-density lipoprotein (LDL) cholesterol who have been advised by a health care provider regarding cholesterol lowering management including lifestyle changes (such as cholesterol lowering diet, weight control) and, if indicated, medication.
- (New Developmental Objective) Increase the proportion of adults with elevated LDL cholesterol who adhere to the prescribed LDL cholesterol lowering management lifestyle changes (such as cholesterol lowering diet, weight control) and, if indicated, medication.
- (New Developmental Objective) Increase the proportion of adults with coronary heart disease or stroke who have their LDL cholesterol level at or below recommended levels.

Obesity
- (Leading Health Indicator) Reduce the proportion of adults who are obese (to 30.6% from 34%).
- (Leading Health Indicator) Reduce the proportion of children and adolescents (age categories 2 to 5, 6 to 11, 12 to 19) who are considered obese (to 14.6% from almost 17%).

Diabetes
- Improve glycemic control among the population with diagnosed diabetes.
- Improve lipid control among persons with diagnosed diabetes.
- Increase the proportion of the population with diagnosed diabetes whose blood pressure is under control.
- Increase the proportion of people with diabetes who receive formal diabetes education.
- Increase prevention behaviors in persons at high risk for diabetes with pre-diabetes.

Objectives for Food Safety
- Reduce the number of outbreak-associated infections due to Shiga toxin–producing *E. coli* O157, or *Campylobacter, Listeria,* or *Salmonella* species associated with food commodity groups (beef, dairy, fruits and nuts, leafy vegetables, and poultry).

Key Food Safety Practices
- Increase the proportion of consumers who follow key food safety practices (Clean: wash hands and surfaces often; Separate: do not cross-contaminate; Cook: cook to proper temperatures; Chill: refrigerate promptly).
- (Developmental) Improve food safety practices associated with food-borne illness in foodservice and retail establishments.

Source: *Healthy People 2020.* Retrieved from www.healthypeople.gov/2020/default.aspx.

childbirth and to be engaged in jobs that make it challenging for them to breastfeed. Babies who are breastfed may be less likely to become obese (USDHHS, 2011).

- Almost 50 million households (15%) experience **food insecurity** at least occasionally during the year, meaning that their access to adequate food is limited by a lack of money and other resources. Individuals and families who experience food insecurity may be more likely to be overweight or obese, potentially because the relatively lower cost of junk foods (i.e., foods low in nutrients but high in calories) can promote overconsumption of calories.
- Among all households during the years from 2008 to 2010, 8.2% of Gallup poll respondents (of 1 million) reported that it was "not easy to get affordable fresh fruits and vegetables" (FRAC, 2011).
- Those in the aforementioned Gallup poll with annual household incomes less than $24,000 reported problems accessing affordable fresh fruits and vegetables 2.5 times more frequently than those with annual incomes between $60,000 and $89,999 (13.8% versus 5.7%).
- Each year, approximately 1 in 6 Americans (48 million people) becomes ill. Of those who are sick, 128,000 are hospitalized and 3000 die of food-borne diseases. Reducing the number of people affected by food-borne illness by 10% would prevent illness in approximately 5 million Americans each year.

Nutrition Objectives for the United States

As can be seen already, a considerable gap exists between public health recommendations and consumers' practices. The overarching goal for nutrition in the second decade of the millennium is that food intake change in the direction of the targeted goals recommended in *Healthy People 2020,* the 2010 *Dietary Guidelines for Americans,* and the USDA/CNPP (Center for Nutrition Policy and Promotion)'s MyPlate (formerly MyPyramid) food guidance system.

FOOD AND NUTRITION RECOMMENDATIONS

Food and nutrition guidelines are introduced in this chapter, with the intent of motivating the reader to achieve three principal goals. The first goal is both to peak individual interest in the health-promoting power of good nutrition and to promote self-evaluation and comparison of one's own food habits and choices against the dietary recommendations presented here. The second goal is to understand the many systemic factors that have contributed to the current nutrition-related health issues, problems so pervasive that many health authorities believe a multisectored approach, beyond traditional education about healthy food choices, is required to redirect the country in a positive direction. A final goal is to define the kinds and amounts of food that are generally acknowledged as essential for obtaining the necessary energy and nutrients required by a healthy person. The following reports provide the foundation for national nutrition recommendations that have been translated into law, policy, programs, and many consumer messages.

- Dietary reference intakes (National Research Council, 2006, 2010)
- *Dietary Guidelines for Americans,* seventh edition (USDA/USDHHS, 2010)
- **MyPlate,** a revised food guidance system introduced by the USDA in 2010 (USDA/CNPP [Center for Nutrition Policy and Promotion], 2010)

BOX 11-3 DIETARY REFERENCE INTAKE (DRI) COMPONENTS AND DEFINITIONS

Estimated Average Requirement (EAR)

EAR is the (median) intake that meets the estimated nutrient needs of one half of the individuals in a particular life stage and gender group. It is used as a basis for developing the RDA and is especially useful for evaluating adequacy of nutrient intake of a group (or groups) and for planning how much the group(s) should consume.

Recommended Dietary Allowance (RDA)

RDA is the average dietary intake level that is sufficient to meet the nutrient requirement of nearly all (97% to 98%) healthy individuals in a particular life stage and gender group. It is computed using the EAR. In the past, the RDA of most nutrients represented the levels needed to prevent deficiency diseases. Now an RDA also includes the goal of preventing chronic diseases (e.g., heart disease or osteoporosis, where applicable). As a variety of IOM DRI publications note, the RDA should not be used to assess or plan nutrient intake for groups but may be useful in some individual applications (Taylor, 2008).

Adequate Intake (AI)

An AI is set to fill the gap (e.g., infants) when there is not enough scientific evidence to determine the RDA. The AI is based on estimates of observed or experimentally determined mean nutrient intake eaten by a group (or groups) of healthy people and assumes that the amount consumed is adequate to promote health. The level is set to meet or exceed the needs of almost all people in a particular life stage and gender group. This is the most controversial component in the DRIs.

Tolerable Upper Intake Level (UL)

This is the highest average daily intake that can be safely eaten continuously and still be considered safe for almost all healthy individuals in a specified group. UL is not intended to be a recommended level of intake. No established benefit exists for individuals to consume nutrients at levels above the RDA or AI. As intake increases above the UL, the potential risk of adverse health effects increases. For most nutrients, the UL would include total intakes from any of the following (alone or in combination): food, fortified food, and nutrient supplements. It is important to note that ULs are only set when there is a strong pool of scientific data. In cases where the evidence is limited or inconclusive, a UL will not be established. In that case, eating levels close to the RDA or AI (as applicable) is not advised.

Acceptable Macronutrient Distribution Range (AMDR)

This is the range of intake for a particular energy source (e.g., carbohydrate, fat, and protein) that is associated with reduced risk of chronic disease while providing intakes of essential nutrients for a healthy person within an identified life stage and gender group. An intake outside of the AMDR carries the potential of increased risk of chronic diseases and/or insufficient intakes of essential nutrients. For example, the AMDR for carbohydrates for a 19-year-old woman (in the life stage and gender group of female, 19-30 years old) is 45% to 65% of calories.

Estimated Energy Requirement (EER)

This is the average dietary energy intake predicted to maintain energy balance in a healthy adult of a specific life stage and gender group using a reference weight, height, and level of physical activity that is consistent with good health.

Adapted from U.S. Department of Agriculture. (2010). *Dietary guidelines for Americans* (7th ed.). Appendix 16: Glossary of terms. Washington, DC: U.S. Government Printing Office. Retrieved from www.cnpp.usda.gov/Publications/DietaryGuidelines/2010/PolicyDoc/PolicyDoc.pdf; Institute of Medicine (IOM). (2008). *Framework for DRI development: Components "known" and components "to be explored."* Background paper. Washington, DC: Institute of Medicine National Academies. Retrieved from http://www.iom.edu/Activities/Nutrition/SummaryDRIs/~/media/Files/Activity%20Files/Nutrition/DRIs/New%20Material/11Bckgrd%20PaperFramework%20for%20DRI%20Devel.pd.

Dietary Reference Intakes (DRIs)

The original dietary reference intakes (DRIs) were developed by the Institute of Medicine of The National Academies in 1997 to reflect the latest understanding about nutrient requirements based on optimizing health in individuals and groups. They replaced previously issued recommended dietary allowances (RDAs), which were focused on the minimal amounts of nutrients needed to protect against nutrient deficiency.

In contrast to the old RDAs, which were one value, the DRIs were developed to reflect a range of values with lower and upper limits to mitigate "risk" of adverse effects. The concept of probability was also introduced to address limited knowledge in evidence (particularly in research relating to infants). In the case of micronutrients such as vitamins and minerals, the DRIs include four categories of reference intakes. For macronutrients, which typically provide calories (energy) such as carbohydrates, protein, and fat, two additional DRI components were added (Taylor, 2008). See Box 11-3 for details on these components and suggested uses.

DRIs are intended to serve as a guide for good nutrition and for establishment of nutrition and health policy. As such, they are widely used for planning and assessing diets of individuals and groups and provide applicable scientific basis for food guidelines, such as the U.S. *Dietary Guidelines for Americans* and the guidelines developed in Canada. However, it is important to note, that in contrast to the routine 5-year review of the *Dietary Guidelines for Americans*, the DRIs are only updated when deemed necessary. In 2008, the U.S. and Canadian governments decided there were enough new studies as well as concern about vitamin D, in particular, to warrant development of new DRIs for vitamin D and calcium. The latest updates were published in late 2010. The revision of the vitamin D and calcium DRIs since 1997 demonstrates that DRIs continue to be researched and revised as more information and high-quality studies are available.

There are some controversies over DRIs that are worth mentioning. As one might already infer from the preceding discussion, there may be limited data relating to genetic diversity in the population or specific groups such as children, pregnant women, and the elderly. The DRIs are created when even limited data are deemed better than no guidance at all. As such, they are a good starting point based on best available evidence and probability of harm or benefit.

As a health care provider, keep in mind that DRIs are intended to be applied to healthy people. Thus, it is possible that a provider might override the dietary reference intake for a specific value based on clinical judgment and recommend more or less for a particular care recipient. Also, it is helpful to remember that while DRIs may be used for individuals, ideally they are guidelines for population groups and apply over time.

So, if an individual does not meet the recommendation for a specific nutrient, such as vitamin C, on a certain day, that is not a cause for alarm. It is the trend that matters (except in the event of an acute mega dose).

Although the DRIs are established by different committees of experts, the values have been compiled into a single listing for easy viewing. A summary guide has also been developed to help users of the DRIs understand the values and their applications. In addition, focused in-depth publications have been made available to help users understand the important considerations in applying the values for assessing and planning diets.

Dietary Guidelines for Americans

After discussing DRIs, the twentieth century anthropologist Margaret Mead's statement that "People eat food, not nutrition" seems particularly apt. Nutrition recommendations stated in terms of ranges or milligrams of vitamin C are useless unless people are advised as to what types and quantities of foods should be consumed to obtain the recommended nutrients. Enter the *Dietary Guidelines for Americans.* In 1980 the *Dietary Guidelines* were the federal government's response to the public's desire for authoritative, consistent guidance on diet and health. Critics of the *Dietary Guidelines* might argue that this objective has not been accomplished because of food politics. However, the intent has been to translate science-based nutrition recommendations into healthy eating guidelines that can be adopted by the public to maximize healthy habits and minimize chronic disease.

Since their inception, the influence of the *Dietary Guidelines* has been wide-ranging, affecting millions of Americans each day. They form the foundation for U.S. nutrition policy, helping policymakers in the design and implementation of nutrition-related programs, including federal nutrition programs for families, children, and the elderly. These guidelines also provide nutrition education initiatives for the general public of adults and children 2 years of age and older.

As mandated by Congress, every 5 years the U.S. Department of Agriculture (USDA) and the U.S. Department of Health and Human Services (USDHHS) must jointly review, update (as needed), and publish a new *Dietary Guidelines for Americans.* Readers appreciate the evolution from the science to the final report more clearly when they understand that the departments juggle balancing scientific rigor with politics. The guidelines have far-reaching impacts on many sectors of business and agriculture. Thus, the review and updating process includes three steps: An appointed external scientific committee, the **Dietary Guidelines Advisory Committee (DGAC)**, conducts an analysis of relevant new scientific information (Box 11-4: Research for Evidence-Based Practice) and writes a report summarizing its findings. Upon completion, the general public and federal agencies have an opportunity to provide feedback before the process moves to stage 2. The departments write the policy document, using the DGAC's report with consideration of comments received. The departments develop materials and messages to communicate the dietary guidelines to the public (also known publicly first as the Food Guide Pyramid, then MyPyramid, and now MyPlate) (Figure 11-2).

Several important changes occurred during step 1 of the process for the 2010 update to the *Dietary Guidelines.* The advances included greater use of systematic reviews with support from USDA's new nutrition evidence library (www.nel.gov) and increased transparency in early developmental stages.

Key recommendations from the 2010 DGAC include to:
- Reduce the **incidence** and **prevalence** of overweight and obesity of the U.S. population by reducing caloric intake and increasing physical activity.
- Shift food intake patterns to a diet that emphasizes more vegetables, cooked dried beans, fruits, whole grains, nuts, and seeds. In addition, increase seafood and fat-free and low-fat milk and milk products and consume only moderate amounts of lean meats, poultry, and eggs.
- Reduce the intake of added sugars and solid fats significantly. In addition, reduce sodium intake and lower intake of refined carbohydrates that are coupled with added sugar, solid fat, and sodium.
- Meet the 2008 National Physical Activity Recommendations (discussed in Chapter 12).

To support these focus areas, the resulting recommendations of the 2010 *Dietary Guidelines for Americans* are grouped into key messages and presented next. For the first time, the 2010 *Dietary Guidelines for Americans* have an entire chapter devoted to addressing the impact of the broader food and physical environment on the public's food, drink, and activity choices using the social-ecological model (Figure 11-3). The guidelines acknowledge the importance of a coordinated, system-wide approach that engages all sectors of influence. As a part of that focus, there is an appendix table listing key consumer behaviors and potential strategies that nursing professionals can use to help implement the *Dietary Guidelines for Americans* (see **Website Resource 11C**). In summary, the following is a list of the principal messages for consumers.

Balancing Calories
- Enjoy your food, but eat less.
- Avoid oversized portions.

Foods to Increase
- Make half your plate fruits and vegetables.
- Make at least half your grains whole grains.
- Switch to fat-free or low-fat (1%) milk.

Foods to Reduce
- Compare sodium in foods such as soup, bread, and frozen meals and choose the foods with lower numbers.
- Drink water instead of sugary drinks.

Other topics addressed in detail include guidance for specific population groups: children and adolescents, women capable of becoming pregnant, pregnant women, breastfeeding women, older adults, and adults at high risk of chronic disease. A discussion of how to build healthy eating patterns embraces USDA eating patterns with **lacto-ovo vegetarian, vegan,** and **DASH** variations provided at various caloric levels also. (For details, access www.dietaryguidelines.gov and see Appendices 8, 9, and 10, respectively.) For nursing professionals interested in helping

BOX 11-4   RESEARCH FOR EVIDENCE-BASED PRACTICE

Dietary Guidelines Advisory Committee (DGAC) Conclusion Grading Chart Used to Evaluate the Strength of the Body of Evidence Supporting Conclusion Statements

ELEMENTS	STRONG	MODERATE	LIMITED	EXPERT OPINION ONLY	GRADE NOT ASSIGNABLE
Quality					
Scientific rigor and validity. Study design and execution	Studies of strong design. Free from design flaws, bias, and execution problems	Studies of strong design with minor methodological concerns OR only studies of weaker study design for question	Studies of weak design for answering question OR inconclusive findings because of design flaws, bias, or execution problems	No studies available. Conclusion based on usual practice, expert consensus, clinical experience, opinion, or extrapolation from basic research	No evidence that pertains to question being addressed
Consistency					
Consistency of findings across studies	Findings generally consistent in direction and size of effect or degree of association, and statistical significance with very minor exceptions	Inconsistency among results of studies with strong design OR consistency with minor exceptions across studies of weaker design	Unexplained inconsistency among results from different studies OR single study unconfirmed by other studies	Conclusion supported solely by statements of informed nutrition or medical commentators	NA
Quantity					
Number of studies. Number of study participants	One large study with a diverse population or several good quality studies. Large number of subjects studied. Studies with negative results have sufficiently large sample size for adequate statistical power	Several studies by independent investigators. Doubts about adequacy of sample size to avoid type I and type II errors	Limited number of studies. Low number of subjects studied and/or inadequate sample size within studies	Unsubstantiated by published research studies	Relevant studies have not been done
Impact					
Importance of studied outcomes. Magnitude of effect	Studied outcome relates directly to question. Size of effect is clinically meaningful. Significant (statistical) difference is large	Some doubt about statistical or clinical significance of effect	Studied outcome is an intermediate outcome or surrogate for true outcome of interest OR size of effect is small or lacks statistical and/or clinical significance	Objective data unavailable	Indicates area for future research
Generalizability					
Generalizability to population of interest	Studied population, interventions, and outcomes are free from serious doubts about generalizability	Minor doubts about generalizability	Serious doubts about generalizability because of narrow or different study population, intervention, or outcomes studied	Generalizability limited to scope of experience	NA

Criteria adapted from the American Dietetic Association Evidence Analysis Library and based upon Greer, N., Mosser, G., Logan, G., & Wagstrom Halaas, G. (2000). A practical approach to evidence grading. *The Joint Commission Journal on Quality Improvement, 26,* 700-712. (Explanation of Grades and Grading Chart).

themselves or others balance calories, Chapter 2 is particularly helpful. Just like *Healthy People 2020,* the report includes an emphasis on consumer aspects of food safety.

Representing the best and most current scientific evidence and advice from nutrition experts, these guidelines are intended

FIGURE 11-2 Learn about healthy eating at ChooseMyPlate.gov. (From U.S. Department of Agriculture/Center for Nutrition Policy and Promotion [USDA/CNPP]. [2010]. *MyPlate.* Retrieved November 3, 2011, from www.choosemyplate.gov/.)

to reduce the nation's major diet-related health problems such as CHD, certain cancers, diabetes, high blood pressure, obesity, osteoporosis, and stroke (U.S. Department of Agriculture & Food and Nutrition Service, 2011).

Nursing professionals play a key role in promoting the *Dietary Guidelines of Americans* as one component of healthful lifestyles. For further study, information can be found at http://health.gov/. The report is an excellent source of background information for nursing professionals. For more information about the articles and reports used to inform the development of the *Dietary Guidelines for Americans,* refer to the *Report of the Dietary Guidelines Advisory Committee on the Dietary Guidelines for Americans, 2010,* and the related Nutrition Evidence Library website (see www.nutritionevidencelibrary.gov).

FOOD GUIDANCE SYSTEM

Historically, in the process of developing *Dietary Guidelines,* step 3 includes translating nutrition recommendations into terms that consumers understand, which can form the basis for nutrition education messages for adults and children. For those who have followed either the 1992 Food Guide Pyramid or the 2005 MyPyramid icons, these were created to visually show graphic representations of dietary balance and variety for the general population 2 years old and older.

The MyPyramid updated the Food Guide Pyramid by adding recommendations for physical exercise as well as a more personalized, stepwise, and flexible approach. Several tools, one for adults and one for children, allowed users to evaluate

FIGURE 11-3 Social-ecological framework for nutrition decisions. (From U.S. Department of Agriculture, & U.S. Department of Health and Human Services. [2010]. *Dietary guidelines for Americans* [7th ed.]. Washington, DC: U.S. Government Printing Office. Retrieved November 1, 2011, from www.health.gov/dietaryguidelines/dga2010/documents/.)

their personal diet and physical activity and "track" against suggested *Dietary Guidelines*. The USDA also introduced a Spanish language version of MyPyramid with traditional ethnic foods to emphasize eating patterns of this diverse cultural group. The latest MyPlate food icon revision has retained the on-line tracker tools (now called SuperTracker for adults and BlastOff for kids) as well as Spanish language versions of educational materials.

USDA unveiled MyPlate in June 2011 in keeping with the 2010 White House Child Obesity Task Force's call for action to provide the U.S. public easy to understand and useful advice. MyPlate visually "reminds" consumers what a healthy "plate" looks like using a familiar place setting (see Figure 11-2). It is not meant to stand alone as a teaching tool. Consumers and health professionals are directed to the website (www.ChooseMyPlate.gov) for details. As with the previous MyPyramid, consumers are

encouraged to start with small steps and can pick topics of interest for more information. The new food guidance system puts four of the food groups on the plate (grains, vegetables, fruits, and protein group [which replaced meat and bean group]) with dairy (including milk and dairy substitutes) on the side.

Although the USDA's MyPlate food guidance system reflects general eating patterns of Americans, it has enough flexibility for different cultural traditions and eating patterns including vegetarian (see Box 11-5: Diversity Awareness). Recognizing that in recent years almost 15 million adults and children have found it difficult to obtain enough food to meet their needs, the ChooseMyPlate website includes an emphasis on resources for eating on a budget and how to access nutrition assistance programs. The USDA also has resources available in Spanish. Updates to the website continue to be made so it is worth checking periodically.

BOX 11-5 DIVERSITY AWARENESS
Food and Culture

The reasons why people eat the ways they do are numerous. Although it is true that without food people cannot survive, food is much more than a tool of survival. Food is also a source of pleasure ("Let's eat out tonight"), a source of comfort ("Right now, I could use some of my mother's chicken soup"), a symbol of hospitality ("Please come to my house for brunch on Sunday"), and an indicator of social status (consider an expensive T-bone steak versus a hamburger). Food has ritual significance, also. Drinking champagne to celebrate an important event, the bride and groom saving the top layer of their wedding cake, or people of the Jewish faith sharing challah (braided bread) at their Sabbath (Friday evening) meal are examples.

To a large extent, the environment determines what people typically eat. For example, wheat that is plentiful in the heartland of the United States is the principal grain in North America, whereas rice enjoys a similar status in Asian countries. Typical wheat-based staples in the United States and Canada include a slice of wheat bread, a bowl of wheat cereal, wheat crackers, pastries made from wheat flour, and pasta made from wheat. Rice-based foods form the backbone of the Chinese diet.

Every culture has its particular food ways, or activities related to food. Food ways include the activities that surround procuring, distributing, storing, consuming, and disposing of food, all of which define what is fit to eat, or what is edible. Factors that affect everyone's food choices and factors that affect food selections of new arrivals to a community should be examined. It is important to remember, however, that just because a person is from a specific culture it does not mean the person follows his or her cultural food patterns. These general guidelines are helpful as a starting point, but do not assume—ask questions to clarify specific eating habits with individuals and families.

Among traditional Chinese people, health and disease are believed to relate to the balance between the forces of yin and yang in the body. Diseases that are caused by yang forces may be treated with yin forces to restore balance. Yin foods include low–caloric density, low-protein foods, such as fresh fruits and vegetables. Yang foods are high in calories, cooked in oil, and irritating to the mouth, or are red, orange, or yellow in color. Examples include most meats, chili peppers, tomatoes, garlic, ginger, and alcoholic beverages. The hot-cold theory in Puerto Rico follows the same basic principles as do yin and yang, but the food groupings differ somewhat.

Religious beliefs affect the food choices of millions of people worldwide. Many religions, including Buddhism, Hinduism, Islam, Judaism, and Seventh

Day Adventism, specify the foods that may be eaten and how they should be prepared. The following is a very basic summary of the principal dietary practices of these five major world religions (adapted from Barer-Stein [1979] and Kittler and Sucher [2000]).

Many Buddhists practice vegetarianism. Foods of plant origin are viewed as the most appropriate for consumption, except pungent foods (garlic, leeks, scallions, chives, and onions), which are believed to generate lust when eaten cooked and to cause rage when eaten raw. For most Buddhists, however, dietary rules such as these are observed on a voluntary basis. What characterizes all Buddhists is the belief that all forms of life share a common link and are thus sacred. Therefore, rather than the specific type of food eaten, more important is the attitude of the person receiving the food and the person's sincere gratitude for the lives of the plants and animals contained in the meal that have served to sustain and further enhance the life of the individual.

Many Hindus practice vegetarianism, but those who originate from the cold northern areas of India usually eat meat (except for beef, which is considered sacred and prohibited).

Many Muslims follow Islamic food laws, which include foods that are Halal (permitted), Haram (prohibited), and questionable (Mashbooh). Foods believed to be unclean, or Haram, are animals that are improperly slaughtered or already-dead animals such as carrion, swine/pork and its by-products (bacon, lard, shortening), carnivorous animals with fangs (dogs, cats, and lions), birds of prey, and land animals without ears (frogs and snakes). Alcohol and intoxicants are also prohibited. Halal certified products are used.

Conservative Jews follow Judaic food laws, which prohibit the consumption of swine/pork, carrion, carrion eaters (scavengers), shellfish, animals with a cloven (split) hoof and do not chew their cud (horses), and animals not slaughtered by the appropriate ritual method or Kosher (fit). According to Jewish Kosher dietary laws, meat (beef, lamb, veal, and poultry), fish, and meat products (eggs) cannot be served at the same meal or be cooked or eaten in the same vessels as dairy products. Kosher certified products are used.

The dietary practices of Seventh Day Adventists focus on health, so many Seventh Day Adventists practice vegetarianism as the foundation of their dietary standard. They also abstain from alcohol and many do not drink caffeine-containing beverages.

DIETARY SUPPLEMENTS AND HERBAL MEDICINES

In recent decades, the popularity of supplemental vitamins, minerals, proteins, fiber, and herbs has earned a high profile in the health field. It was the explosion of use of single-component dietary supplements in the 1980s that helped to spur the change from the old RDAs to the DRIs. New evidence showed that perhaps ranges of nutrients could be used that were higher than the old "one size fits all" RDAs. At the same time, there appeared to be a point at which a nutrient could pose more risk than advantage. The tolerable upper limit (UL) guidelines were developed for specific life stages, ages, and gender as a result (Taylor, 2008).

According to the National Institutes of Health Office of Dietary Supplements (NIH ODS, 2012), most U.S. adults take one or more dietary supplements either daily or occasionally. Almost 18% take other natural products such as fish oil, echinacea, flaxseed oil, and ginseng (National Center for Complementary and Alternative Medicine [NCCAM], 2010). The 1994 Dietary Supplement Health and Education Act expanded the definition of dietary supplement to include any product intended for ingestion as a supplement to the diet. Today's dietary supplements include vitamins, minerals, herbals and botanicals, amino acids, enzymes, and many other products. Dietary supplements are available in a variety of forms: traditional tablets, capsules, and powders, as well as drinks and energy bars. Popular supplements include vitamins D and E; minerals such as calcium and iron; herbs such as echinacea and garlic; and specialty products such as glucosamine, probiotics, and fish oils.

People use supplements as if they were drugs; they are marketed in the same manner as over-the-counter medications. Often they are sold in the pharmaceutical section of retail stores in a variety of forms (tablets, capsules, powders, soft gels, gel caps, and liquids) that make them resemble drugs. To distinguish a dietary supplement from an over-the-counter drug, the words *dietary supplement* must appear on the product label. The labels may carry certain types of structure-function claims about certain common conditions associated with aging, pregnancy, menopause, and adolescence that do not relate to disease. These include health maintenance claims ("maintains a healthy circulatory system"), other nondisease claims ("for muscle enhancement" or "helps you relax"), and claims for common, minor symptoms associated with life stages ("for common symptoms of premenstrual syndrome" or "for hot flashes"). Such a claim must be followed by the words (FDA, 2008): "This statement has not been evaluated by the Food and Drug Administration. This product is not intended to diagnose, treat, cure, or prevent any disease."

Because the FDA is the federal agency that oversees both dietary supplements and drugs, it might be easy to assume the federal regulations for supplements and drugs are similar. However, they are not. Dietary supplements are unregulated by the FDA in the sense that they do not require pre–market review or approval by the FDA. Although a supplement company is responsible for showing evidence that their products are safe

and their label claims are truthful and not misleading, they do not have to provide that evidence to the FDA before marketing.

Once a dietary supplement is on the market, the FDA monitors information on the product's label and package insert to make sure that information about the supplement's content is accurate and that any claims made for the product are truthful and not misleading. If the FDA finds a product to be unsafe or otherwise unfit for human consumption, it may take enforcement action to remove the product from the marketplace or work with the manufacturer to voluntarily recall the product. Some supplements have had to be recalled because of proven or potential harmful effects. Reasons for these recalls include microbiological, pesticide, and heavy metal contamination; absence of a dietary ingredient claimed to be in the product; or the presence of more or less than the amount of the dietary ingredient claimed on the label.

The federal government can take legal action against companies and websites that sell dietary supplements when the companies make false or deceptive statements about their products, if they promote them as treatments or cures for diseases, or if their products are unsafe. Although laws exist to help protect the consumer, the reality is that it is a "buyer beware" environment because of historically low funding and resources for the FDA, along with political pressure and lack of scientific study on the overwhelming majority of supplements available in the United States (Nestle, 2002).

The NCCAM and the NIH ODS are two federal offices promoting and conducting the scientific study of the benefits and risks of dietary supplements, including medicinal herbs, in health maintenance and disease prevention.

Low-dose supplements that contain the recommended intakes for micronutrients (vitamins and minerals) appear to be generally safe. Although the desirable way for the general public to obtain recommended levels of nutrients is by eating a variety of foods, when people take dietary supplements they should avoid taking them in excess of the UL of the DRI for those nutrients for their age and gender group to preclude possible adverse effects (**Website Resource 11B**). For other types of supplements, such as herbals or botanicals, caution is also advised. Natural is not always better. For example, the National Center for Complementary and Alternative Medicine cautions against use of products such as comfrey or kava, which can be toxic to the liver.

When health care professionals are asked, "Should I take a nutrient supplement?" here are some further considerations for times when supplements may be toxic and when they may, in fact, be helpful. The discussion focuses on vitamins and minerals because they are widely used.

Vitamin and Mineral Toxicity

Toxic levels of certain micronutrients can cause a host of health problems. For example, it is important to advise individuals not to overuse vitamins of the fat-soluble class (vitamins A, D, E, and K). Of particular concern is vitamin A, an excess of which may be teratogenic during pregnancy or may increase the risk of lung cancer for current or former smokers (American Dietetic Association, 2009). On the other hand, water-soluble vitamins such as vitamin C and the B-complex vitamins pose less danger, because the body is able to excrete them through the urine.

Nutrient imbalances and toxicities are less likely to occur when nutrients are derived from foods. Most nutrient toxicities occur through supplementation, and in some cases with a combination of supplementation and fortification of foods (e.g., older women, who may be at risk at the 95th percentile of UL for calcium). Estimated toxic doses for daily oral consumption of vitamins and minerals by adults are as low as 5 times the recommended intake for selenium, and as high as 25 to 50 times or more the recommended intakes for folic acid and vitamins C and E. The toxicities of high doses of nutrients such as vitamin A, vitamin B_6, vitamin D, niacin, iron, and selenium are well established. Iron supplements intended for other household members are the most common cause of pediatric poisoning deaths in the United States (National Library of Medicine [NLM], 2011).

Large doses of vitamin A may be teratogenic. Because of this risk, supplementation with preformed vitamin A should be avoided during the first trimester of pregnancy unless there is evidence of deficiency (see Box 11-6: Quality and Safety Scenario). Excess preformed vitamin A (more than 10,000 international units [IU]) during the first trimester of pregnancy has been linked to birth defects of the eyes, lungs, skull, and heart (Office of Dietary Supplements, 2012). Such a risk in early pregnancy raises a need for caution about general vitamin and mineral supplement use by women of childbearing age.

Besides problems with direct toxicity of some individual nutrients, nutrient supplementation can cause problems related to nutrient imbalances or adverse interactions with prescribed medication. Many problems associated with high doses of a single nutrient may reflect interactions that result in a relative deficiency for another nutrient (American Dietetic Association, 2009). Some examples follow:

- High doses of vitamin E can interfere with vitamin K action and enhance the effect of Coumadin as one of the anticoagulant drugs. Examples such as this are one of the reasons that health care providers may ask about supplement use before surgery and recommend discontinuing certain supplements for 1 week before and 1 week after surgery.
- Large amounts of calcium inhibit absorption of iron and possibly other trace elements.
- Folic acid can mask hematological signs of vitamin B_{12} deficiency, which, if untreated, can result in irreversible neurological damage. Folic acid can also interact adversely with anticonvulsant medications.
- Zinc supplementation can reduce copper status, impair immune responses, and decrease levels of high-density lipoprotein cholesterol ("good" cholesterol).

Nursing professionals can help persons who suspect an adverse supplement effect by reporting the event to the FDA, or by encouraging the individual to file a report. It should be done as soon as possible when there is a suspected problem. Information on how to do this is available at www.cfsan.fda.gov/~dms/ds-rept.html. Another avenue is to alert the product's manufacturer or distributor of any serious side effects through the address or phone number listed on the supplement's label.

BOX 11-6 QUALITY AND SAFETY SCENARIO

Supplements/Vitamin A

Adele is a 32-year-old married African American female with no children and a history of one miscarriage. She and her husband have been trying to conceive for the past 4 years and have recently started talking about going to a fertility clinic. Always one to try the "natural way" first, she read that vitamin A is important for normal fetal development and decides to take a multivitamin supplement with 25,000 IU of preformed vitamin A. Adele knows that she can get vitamin A from food but she also makes an effort to read nutrition labels and choose fortified foods that have 20% or more vitamin A content. She comes into the physician's office for a regular routine visit. It is common knowledge that she and her husband are trying to have a baby.

Reflective Questions
- Why is it important to discuss use and type of supplements (and potentially fortified food use) during preconception/pregnancy?
- What is the vitamin A DRI recommendation for a woman of her age?
- How can learning about simple changes in her eating habits/supplement use affect her risk for a spontaneous abortion or a birth defect in the event of pregnancy?
- What would your next step be in this situation?

*Note: 1 retinol activity equivalent (mcg RAE) = 1 mcg of all-trans-retinol = 3.33 IU from retinol = 2 mcg of supplemental all-trans-β-carotene = 12 mcg of dietary all-trans-β-carotene = 24 mcg of other dietary provitamin A carotenoids.

By law, dietary supplement firms are required to forward reports they receive about serious adverse effects to the FDA within 15 days.

Circumstances When Nutrient Supplementation Is Indicated

Nutrient supplements or fortified foods, or sometimes a combination of both, are sometimes necessary for specific populations to obtain desirable amounts of particular nutrients (National Research Council, 2010; USDA/USDHHS, *Dietary Guidelines for Americans*, 2010). Some examples follow:

- Folic acid (400 micrograms [mcg]) from fortified enriched grains or supplements in addition to folate-rich foods for females who could become pregnant, to help prevent neural tube defects
- Iron supplements during pregnancy
- Calcium and vitamin D supplements in older postmenopausal women to reduce their risk for osteoporosis (levels should not exceed UL of 2000 mcg for calcium or 4000 mcg for vitamin D through either supplements or a combination of foods and supplements)
- Vitamin D for those who do not meet recommended DRI intake (without exceeding DRI UL of 4000 IU or 100 mcg by a combination of food, supplement, and fortified food)
- Vitamin B_{12} through food fortified with the crystalline form or B_{12} supplements for individuals older than 50 years (who often may have a reduced ability to absorb naturally occurring vitamin B_{12}). In addition, vegans should ensure adequate intake of vitamin B_{12} through fortified foods or supplements.

FOOD SAFETY

Americans spend more than 1 trillion dollars on food each year, with nearly 50% of food consumption occurring outside the home (Congressional Research Service, 2011). The combined efforts of the food industry and the regulatory agencies often are credited with making the U.S. food supply among the safest in the world. Nonetheless, the Centers for Disease Control and Prevention (CDC) reports that each year an estimated 1 in 6 Americans—a total of 48 million people—becomes sick from food-borne illnesses caused by contamination from any of a number of microbial pathogens. Of these, an estimated 128,000 people require hospitalization and 3000 people die (CDC, 2011a). Food-borne illnesses are estimated to cost the United States 77.7 billion dollars annually, not including costs to the food industry or public health agencies.

Attention to food-borne illnesses is becoming increasingly important with the globalization of the world's food supply. New disease-causing organisms have emerged and food imports from countries without the same safety standards as the United States are on the rise. Furthermore, more consumers are demanding fresh produce and more seafood be available throughout the year as well as accessibility to less-processed foods, such as raw milk and fresh juices that are not cooked or pasteurized to kill bacteria. Consumers may also ignore warnings about unsafe food habits because of preferences for foods such as raw oysters, rare hamburgers, fresh juices, unpasteurized cheese, and runny egg yolks, which all carry higher risks of contamination.

To protect the public from numerous sources of food contamination (physical, chemical, biological), private industry and numerous federal, state, and local agencies share responsibilities for regulating the safety of the U.S. food supply. On the food industry side, one example of initiatives are food processors who are working on programs to better trace products through the supply chain and monitor temperatures in trucks from remote locations. In late 2010, Congress passed sweeping food safety legislation called the Food Safety Modernization Act (FSMA). The FSMA gives the FDA new powers to police food safety and focus its efforts on preventing food contamination. Subject to adequate funding, it allows the FDA to heighten its inspection of imported food, set safety standards for fresh produce, force companies to recall tainted products, and require companies to keep better production records.

When the safeguards built into this system fail, however, consumers themselves must serve as the final and sometimes most important guardian against unsafe food. Therefore it is essential to be informed and educated about the potential dangers of food-borne illness and ways to avoid contaminated food products.

Causes of Food-Borne Illness

A food-borne illness is classified according to the source of its contamination (the unintended presence of harmful substances or microorganisms). Food contaminants may be categorized as biological, chemical, or physical. Biological contaminants include bacteria, viruses, parasites, and fungi (yeasts and mold). Chemical contamination refers to the presence of pesticides, kitchen cleaning supplies, and toxic chemicals in food that have been leeched out of worn metal cookware and equipment. Physical contamination includes dirt, glass chips, crockery, wood, splinters, stones, hair, jewelry, and metal shavings from dull can openers. Another unintended physical contaminant may be an unintended allergen added to a food product that typically does not include that ingredient (such as peanuts) during food processing in the same location.

Examples of Common Food-Borne Pathogens

The safety of the U.S. food supply is so important that there are specific objectives tied to monitoring of common pathogens in *Healthy People 2020*. These include outbreak-associated infections attributable to Shiga toxin–producing *Escherichia coli* O157, or *Campylobacter, Listeria,* or *Salmonella* species associated with food commodity groups (e.g., beef, dairy, fruits and nuts, leafy vegetables, and poultry). Two common types are discussed next.

Salmonellosis

According to the USDA, the most frequently reported cause of food-borne illness is *Salmonella* bacteria. Each year in the United States, approximately 40,000 cases of salmonellosis are reported and 400 persons die from acute salmonellosis (CDC, 2010). The actual number of infections may be closer to 1.4 million since milder cases are often not diagnosed or reported. Salmonellosis is an infection caused by *Salmonella,* a bacterium discovered more than 100 years ago by Dr. Daniel E. Salmon, an American veterinarian-pathologist. *Salmonella* is a gram-negative microscopic germ that passes from the feces of people or animals to other people or other animals. Although the *Salmonella* family includes more than 2300 serotypes of the bacterium, the most common in the United States are *Salmonella enteritidis* and *Salmonella typhimurium*.

The typical way humans are exposed to salmonellosis is by eating foods contaminated with animal feces. Foods of animal origin such as beef, poultry, milk, and eggs are often the source of infection. However, *all* foods, including seafood from polluted water and vegetables, may become contaminated. Contamination may also occur from unsanitary handling of foods and utensils by infected food handlers and contact with the feces of some pets, especially those with diarrhea. Symptoms of Salmonellosis (CDC, 2004) include abdominal cramping, mild to severe diarrhea, nausea, vomiting, and fever within 8 to 72 hours after infection. Symptoms may resolve within 4 to 7 days without treatment; however, infections can become life threatening for people with weakened immune systems as well as infants, young children, pregnant women, and older adults. Antibiotics usually are not necessary unless the infection spreads from the intestines. To prevent salmonellosis, avoid uncooked egg dishes, undercooked meat, shellfish, and unpasteurized milk and juice. Adherence to sanitary regulations as well as proper food handling is necessary to control salmonellosis outbreaks.

Escherichia coli O157:H7 Infection

The *Escherichia coli* bacterium was first discovered in the human colon in 1885 by Theodor Escherich, a German pediatrician. A particularly virulent strain of the bacterium *Escherichia coli* know as *E. coli* O157:H7 was first identified in 1982 as a food-borne pathogen during an investigation of an outbreak of persons suffering from severe bloody diarrhea attributable to ingestion of contaminated hamburgers. As a leading cause of food-borne illness, *E. coli* O157:H7 can produce a powerful toxin causing severe illness and damage to the intestinal lining (CDC, 2011a). The illness is characterized by severe abdominal cramping, watery to bloody diarrhea, dehydration, nausea, and vomiting with or without low-grade fever. Hemorrhagic colitis is usually self-limited and lasts for an average of 8 days. The majority of *E. coli* O157:H7 infections (CDC, 2004) are food-borne and associated with undercooked or raw ground beef. Outbreaks have also involved unpasteurized fruit juices and milk, alfalfa sprouts, lettuce, spinach, and water. Moreover, outbreaks can be caused by secondary person-to-person contamination in homes, day care centers, nursing homes, and hospitals. Another mode of transmission of *E. coli* O157:H7 is by hand-to-mouth contact with animals or contaminated surfaces at petting zoos and agricultural fairs. Although all people are included in *E. coli* O157:H7 target populations, children and older adults are more susceptible. In cases confirmed in children, infection may develop into hemolytic uremic syndrome (HUS), leading to permanent loss of kidney function.

Food Safety Practices

Just the few examples already cited demonstrate how devastating food-borne illness can be. Individuals in their own homes can reduce contaminants and keep food safe to eat by following safe food handling practices. Four basic food safety principles work together to reduce the risk of food-borne illness—**Clean, Separate, Cook,** and **Chill.** These four principles are the cornerstones of Fight BAC!®, a national food safety education campaign (www.fightbac.org). There are so many that *Healthy People 2020* included a key food safety objective designed to increase the proportion of consumers following them. As you can see by the results of a 2006 National Food Safety survey below, there is significant room for improvement (USDHHS, *Healthy People 2020*, FS-5.1-5.4 details).

- **Clean:** Wash hands, utensils, and cutting boards before and after contact with raw meat, poultry, seafood, and eggs. (33% of surveyed population does not) (USDA National Evidence Library [NEL] statistics, 2012)
  - Wash all parts of hands thoroughly with running warm water with soap and friction for about 20 to 30 seconds. Teach children to sing the happy birthday song twice. If no water is available use alcohol-based (≥60%) hand sanitizers.
  - Clean all surfaces with warm, soapy water often (including all appliances, knobs, and handles) and clean spills immediately. A solution of 1 tablespoon of unscented, liquid chlorine bleach per gallon of water can be used to sanitize surfaces.

- At least once a week, discard refrigerated foods that should no longer be eaten. Cooked leftovers should be discarded after 4 days; raw poultry and ground meats, 1 to 2 days.
- **Separate:** Do not cross-contaminate. Keep raw meat and poultry separated from foods that will not be cooked while shopping, preparing, or storing foods. (11% does not)
  - Rinse fresh fruits and vegetables thoroughly with running water before eating, cutting, or cooking (unless prepackaged). Scrub firm surfaces (e.g., cantaloupes and cucumbers) with produce brush. Commercial cleaners are unnecessary.
- **Cook:** Cook to proper temperatures and use a food thermometer. You cannot tell if food is cooked safely by its appearance. (63% does not)
  - Seafood, meat, poultry, and egg dishes should be cooked to the recommended safe minimum internal temperature to destroy harmful microbes.
  - When cooking using a microwave, foods should be stirred, rotated, and/or flipped periodically to help them cook evenly.
- **Chill:** Refrigerate food promptly within 2 hours, or in 1 hour for environments that are 90° F or hotter. This includes groceries, food being prepared, and leftovers and takeout foods. Keep the refrigerator at 40° F or less and the freezer at 0° F or less and monitor temperatures with a thermometer. (12% does not)
  - Keep hot food hot (140° F or higher) and cold foods cold (32° to 40° F). Between these temperatures is the danger zone in which harmful bacteria can grow rapidly, even exponentially.
  - Thaw properly to avoid any bad bacteria: in the refrigerator; in cold water such as in a leak-proof bag, changing with cold water every 30 minutes; or in the microwave.

These guidelines also apply to carryout meals, restaurant leftovers, and home-packed meals to go. If in doubt, throw it out.

Making a food safe after it has been handled improperly may not always be possible. Therefore the best practice is to discard food when there is a doubt as to the safety of food preparation, service, or storage. For example, certain bacteria found in food that has been left at room temperature too long may produce a heat-resistant toxin that cannot be destroyed by cooking. Therefore the principal point is to be careful in preparing food, including cooking foods to the right temperatures, keeping track of the time food is exposed to certain temperatures, and being vigilant when eating out. If there is any doubt about the safety of the food, caution is urged; it is better not to eat it.

Without exception, everyone should exercise their best judgment and care when eating out, when handling their own food, or when handling the food of others. Prevention through education is the key to promoting healthy lives that are unscathed by the potentially severe and life-threatening effects of food-borne illness. People who do not have healthy immune systems (individuals with various health problems and many older adults) and infants with immune systems that are not fully developed are at the greatest risk of developing food-borne illnesses.

On a more positive note, normal healthy adults with healthy immune systems are able to ward off most of the contaminants from the environment and from food without much effort most of the time. Nevertheless, everyone should follow standard safety procedures when handling food and when eating out.

FOOD, NUTRITION, AND POVERTY

As already noted in the discussion of *Healthy People 2020* previously (Figure 11-1), a current focus is on attempting to reduce health disparities and health inequities, as well as focus on future preventive measures to help health choices be the easy choices wherever people live, work, learn, and play.

Healthy People 2020 Goal: Promote health and reduce chronic disease risk through the consumption of healthful diets and achievement and maintenance of healthy body weights.

- Eliminate very low food security among children (from 1.3% of households with children in 2008 to 0.2% in 2020).
- Reduce household food insecurity (from 14.6% in 2008 to 6% in 2020) and in doing so reduce hunger.

Poverty and Income Distribution

For most people in the United States, income has risen over time, providing more options for personal consumption expenditures, including those on food. However, growth in income has not increased equally for all households. Moreover, in recent tough economic times, people who normally have never needed help have flooded food banks and other federal and community resources (USA Today Supplement, *A Hunger Free America*, 2010).

According to the U.S. Census, in 2010 alone, 15.1% of the U.S. population (or 46.2 million people) lived below the poverty level set by the government to determine eligibility for various types of government programs. This was the largest number in 52 years, since the beginning of poverty surveys. Of those people, about one out of three (35.5%) was a child. Close behind this statistic were those with disabilities (28%) and older Americans (25%) at about one in four persons. Regionally, poverty is concentrated in the South, followed by the West, Midwest, and Northeast. It also appears higher in cities than in rural areas (Nord et al., 2010; U.S. Census, 2011).

In 2010, groups with particularly high poverty rates included Hispanics and African Americans, with statistically equivalent poverty rates of 20.6% and 24.3%, respectively. Food assistance programs, as discussed next, are one mechanism to provide a limited safety net to keep people from falling further into poverty (Nord et al., 2010).

Food Assistance for the Poor

Most Americans are **food secure,** having enough money and resources to eat enough food for active, healthy lives. However, for the minority who are poor, obtaining a nutritious diet without assistance can be a challenge. Low-income families spend one third more on food than other families, often with less access to healthier options such as fresh fruits and vegetables (FRAC, 2011). A variety of federal, state, and local governments and private charitable organizations work to reduce hunger in

the United States. The primary responsibility at the federal level falls to the USDA, which administers 15 nutrition assistance programs through the Food and Nutrition Service (FNS) using a combination of federal funding and farm commodities. Programs target the diverse needs of different subgroups of low-income persons by providing supplemental assistance through a variety of forms and settings. In 2011 federally funded outlays for nutrition assistance programs resulted in amounts as detailed in the following list (USDA, FNS, 2011a):

- Supplemental Nutrition Assistance Program (SNAP)—formerly known as Food Stamps: $71 billion (Rosenbaum, 2012)
- Child Nutrition Program (includes National School Breakfast Program [NSBP], National School Lunch Program [NSLP], Special Milk Program, Child/Adult Care Food Program, and Summer Food Service Program): almost $19.4 billion
- Supplemental Nutrition for Women Infants and Children (WIC): more than $7 billion
- Commodity Supplemental Food Programs (e.g., to Native American communities, Nutrition Service Incentive Program [NSIP], The Emergency Food Distribution Program [TEFP], Farmer's Market Programs): almost $153 million

One in six people in the United States receives federally funded food assistance at some point every year. SNAP, NSLP, NSBP, WIC, and Older American Act programs, administered by the Agency on Aging through the USDHHS, are the main programs that provide domestic food and nutrition assistance. With tightening federal and state budgets, these programs are already targeted for significant cuts. Even so, Table 11-2 contains information on identifying low-income people who need help getting enough food and referring them to the appropriate program(s) that can evaluate their eligibility.

SNAP (Supplemental Nutrition Assistance Program, formally known as Food Stamps)

SNAP supplements the food-buying power of eligible low-income households and is the foundation of the nations' nutrition safety net. Benefits are provided through an electronic benefit transfer (EBT) card that participants use to purchase food at authorized stores. It is designed to help low-income families and individuals purchase nutritionally adequate foods. Households can use their EBT card to purchase any food or food product for home consumption as well as seeds and plants for use in home gardens. Restaurants can be authorized to accept EBT cards from qualified homeless, older, or disabled people in exchange for low-cost meals. Items that recipients cannot buy with EBT cards include alcoholic beverages, tobacco, hot ready-to-eat foods, lunch-counter items, foods to be eaten in the store, vitamins, medicines, and pet foods.

Although there is no requirement that the EBT card be used to purchase high-quality food, the goal of the SNAP nutrition education program is to increase the likelihood that recipients will make healthy food choices within their limited food budget. SNAP uses multiple strategies to facilitate healthy food choices and active lifestyles. These include providing nutrition

TABLE 11-2 REFERRAL GUIDE FOR FEDERAL NUTRITION ASSISTANCE PROGRAMS

PROGRAM	TARGET POPULATION	INDICATORS OF NEED	WHERE TO CALL
Child and Adult Care Food Program (CACFP)	Children from low-income family; adults ages 60 years or older or functionally impaired persons	Low-income, poor nutritional status	Local social service office
SNAP	Eligible low-income people and family	Economic stress	Local SNAP offices
		Low-income, poor nutritional status	Find at www.fns.usda.gov/snap/outreach/default/htm
			Local school district
School Nutrition Program (both breakfast and school lunch)	Eligible low-income children and those already in SNAP	Eligible low-income children	Contact local school or school district
Summer Food Service Program	Children of school age who live in low-income neighborhoods	Eligible low-income children	Local school district
Women, Infants and Children (WIC)	Low-income pregnant, breastfeeding, and non-breastfeeding postpartum women; infants and children up to age 5	Risk of existing health or nutritional problems	Local social services office / Local health department or community action agency

Adapted from USDA Food and Nutrition Service. (January 2012). *Eat right when money's tight.* Retrieved from www.nal.usda.gov/snap/EatRightWhenMoneysTight.pdf.

education programs; encouraging more farmers' markets, small urban markets, and bodegas to participate in the program; and offering a demonstration project to examine the impact of incentives on participant purchases of fruits and vegetables.

The program is administered nationally by the Food and Nutrition Service (FNS) and locally by state and welfare agencies in all 50 states, the District of Columbia, Guam, and the U.S. Virgin Islands. Eligibility is based on financial factors such as income and expenses available to the household, as well as 5 years in legal immigrant status, if applicable. SNAP requires most able-bodied adults between 16 and 60 (with few exceptions) to register for work, to take part in employment/training programs referred by the SNAP office, and to accept or continue suitable employment. Households may own certain limited resources. In addition to income, the EBT allotment is also based on family size. In contrast to public perception, fewer than 10% of households received cash welfare in 2009 and the latest statistics from 2010 showed 40% of households had at least one wage earner. In addition, according to FNS data, most households advance from SNAP in less than 1 year (Rosenbaum, 2012). In 2011, 92% of SNAP funding went directly to 40.3 million people: 48% children, 44% adults, and 8% age 60 or older. The average monthly benefit per person was approximately $134 and almost $290 per household (USDA, FNS, 2011b).

With passage of the 2012 Farm Bill, approximately 4.5 billion dollars will be cut from SNAP with an estimated loss of 500,000 possible recipients and almost 90 dollars less in benefits per household.

Child Nutrition Program

Collectively called the "Child Nutrition Program," these programs provide cash reimbursement and commodity support for meals served to children in schools, child care facilities, and summer settings. They include the National School Lunch (NSLP) and Breakfast Programs (NSBP), the Child and Adult Care Food Program (CACFP), the Summer Food Service Program, and the Special Milk Program. The general purpose of

these programs is to help ensure the health and well-being of all the nation's children. The two biggest and most well-known programs are described next.

National School Lunch Program (NSLP). The federally funded NSLP is administered by the FNS. On the state level, the NSLP usually is administered by the U.S. Department of Education, which contracts with local public, nonprofit private, and residential child care centers and schools to provide balanced, low-cost or free lunches. In 2010 the NSLP reached about 31.6 million children each school day (FRAC, 2011), including the following:

- Children from families with incomes at or below 130% of the federal poverty level guidelines are eligible for free school meals.
- Children from families with incomes above 130% to 185% of the poverty level are eligible for reduced-price school meals.
- Children from families with incomes more than 185% of the poverty level are eligible for full-price school meals.

Schools that choose to take part in the lunch program must implement wellness policies that promote healthy eating, address obesity, and encourage physical activity. Schools are provided with cash subsidies and approved agricultural commodities from the USDA as a supplement. Up to January 2012, free, reduced-price, or full-price lunches had to meet these federal minimum pattern requirements:

- Must provide one third of the recommended nutrient intake of 1989 RDAs
- To the extent possible, be consistent with the *Dietary Guidelines for Americans* recommendations for reducing sugar, salt, and fat intake

Under the Healthy Hunger-Free Kids Act of 2010, the USDA gained authority to set policy and nutrition criteria for all child nutrition standards, including the NSLP. New meal standards were published in 2012 based on the 2009 Institute of Medicine (IOM) recommendations to move subsidized meals into line with the 2010 *Dietary Guidelines for Americans* and the DRIs

(Stallings et al., 2010; USDA, FNS, 2011). The new rules stipulate a doubling of previous amounts of fruits and vegetables served in schools, set limits on trans fats and salt levels, increase the amount of whole grains served, make 1% and fat-free milk the norm, and establish suitable ranges for daily caloric intake. They also require free drinkable water in food service areas and increase subsidies to schools following the new guidelines. Even with changes, the NSLP budget projections are less than the current budget by eliminating the meat/meat substitute requirement at breakfast, allowing a phase-in period for fruits and vegetables, honoring requests to take smaller portions, and discontinuing price supports for meals including separately priced items.

National School Breakfast Program (NSBP). The School Breakfast Program was designed to make it possible for all schoolchildren to receive a nutritious breakfast every day. Skipping breakfast can adversely affect children's performance in math and reading. A study of low-income elementary school students indicated that children who participated in the National School Breakfast Program (NSBP) had greater improvements in standardized test scores and reduced rates of absence and tardiness than did children who qualified for the program but did not participate (CDC, 2011). The School Breakfast Program provides assistance to states to initiate, maintain, or expand nonprofit breakfast programs in eligible schools and residential child care institutions. Any child attending a participating school may receive a free, reduced-price, or full-price breakfast based on the same income criteria used by the NSLP. In the 2010 to 2011 school year, 11.7 million children in almost 88 thousand schools were fed every day (FRAC, 2011).

WIC (Supplemental Nutrition for Women, Infants and Children)

WIC supplies free nutritious supplemental food, nutrition counseling, breastfeeding support, and health and social service referrals to eligible low-income pregnant or postpartum women and to children younger than 5 years old who are at nutritional risk. Congress funds WIC every year for a specific amount as a federal grant program to be administered by FNS and 90 "state" agencies (including 50 states, 34 tribes, the District of Columbia, and 5 U.S. territories). Services are offered in a wide variety of settings: county health departments, hospitals, mobile clinics, community centers, schools, public housing sites, Indian reservations, migrant health centers and camps, and Indian Health Service facilities.

Eligibility is based on the following factors. Income must be ≤185% of the U.S. poverty income guidelines (about $41,000 for a family of four in 2009) and participants must meet one of two major types of nutritional risk:
- Medically based risks, such as anemia, underweight, maternal age, history of pregnancy complications, or poor pregnancy outcome
- Diet-based risks, such as inadequate dietary pattern as determined by 24-hour recall, food frequency questionnaire, or diet history

Those who qualify usually receive monthly checks or vouchers to buy specific foods designed to augment their diet with specific nutrients. In addition, a growing number of state agencies issue an electric benefit card (like a debit card), and some distribute WIC foods through warehouses or deliver WIC foods to recipients' homes. The foods vary depending upon an individual's specific food package designation but can include iron-fortified infant cereal, iron-fortified adult cereal, fruit or vegetable juice rich in vitamin C, eggs, milk, cheese, and peanut butter or dried beans. WIC recognizes and promotes breastfeeding as the optimal source of nutrition for infants. For women who do not fully breastfeed, WIC provides iron-fortified infant formula. Special infant formulas and medical foods may be provided when prescribed by a physician for a specified medical condition. In 2009 new foods were added and specific food packages were reformulated to improve variety, to increase flexibility for diverse cultures, and to align with the *Dietary Guidelines* and American Academy of Pediatrics infant feeding practice guidelines. These foods include soy-based beverages, tofu, fruits and vegetables, baby foods, whole-wheat bread, and other whole-grain options.

Each WIC participant receives vouchers with maximum monthly allowable amounts of specific components specially designed for the following categories: fully breastfeeding mother; pregnant or partially breastfeeding mother; postpartum, fully formula feeding mother; fully breastfed baby; partially breastfed baby; full formula-fed baby; children 1 to 5 years old (California WIC Association, 2009).

Of the 9.17 million people who received WIC benefits each month in 2011, approximately 4.86 million were children, 2.17 million were infants, and 2.14 million were women (USDA, FNS, 2011a).

Financial constraints preclude WIC from serving all eligible people; therefore, a system of priorities has been established for filling program openings. After a local WIC agency has reached its maximum caseload, traditionally vacancies have generally been filled in the order of the following priority levels:
- Pregnant women, breastfeeding women, and infants determined to be at nutritional risk from serious medical problems
- Infants up to 6 months of age whose mothers participate in WIC or are eligible to participate and have serious medical problems
- Children up to age 5 years at nutritional risk from serious medical problems
- Pregnant or breastfeeding women and infants who are at nutritional risk from dietary problems
- Children up to age 5 years at nutritional risk from dietary problems
- Non-breastfeeding postpartum women with any nutritional risk
- Individuals at nutritional risk only because they are homeless or migrants and current participants who would likely continue to have medical or dietary problems without WIC assistance

Projected federal cuts in 2013 will undoubtedly impact the WIC caseload. Only time will tell what priorities will survive.

For state agencies that apply for a grant, the WIC Farmers' Market Nutrition Program (or WIC FMNP) gives additional coupons to persons to use for purchasing fresh fruits and vegetables at participating farmers' markets. The WIC FMNP has two goals: to provide fresh, nutritious, unprepared, locally grown fruits and vegetables from farmers' markets to WIC participants, and to expand consumers' awareness and use of farmers' markets.

The overall statistics on WIC demonstrate it is effective in improving the health of its participants. Medicaid costs for women who participate in the program during pregnancy and their infants are lower than those for women who do not participate. WIC participation is also linked to longer gestation periods, higher birth weights, and lower infant mortality rates (USDA, FNS, 2012).

Food and Nutrition Programs for Older Adults

At the other end of the life cycle, a significant number of older people face special obstacles to obtaining an optimal diet. Of particular concern are adults older than 75 who are frail, alone, or restricted to a limited budget. Life changes such as the loss of a spouse/significant other; sensory changes in taste or smell; physical inability to obtain food; and decreasing caloric needs can make acquisition of an adequate diet challenging.

A variety of nutrition assistance programs are available to this population. They include the USDA programs Supplemental Nutrition Assistance Program (SNAP), Senior Farmer's Market Nutrition Program (SFMNP), Child and Adult Care Food Program (CACFP), The Emergency Food Assistance Program (TEFAP), and the Commodity Supplemental Food Program (CSFP). However, the programs that most people may be familiar with are some of those provided under the Older Americans Act (OAA), collectively called the Elderly Nutrition Services Program, which are managed by the Administration on Aging (AoA) through the USDHHS. They are designed to help older adults access nutritionally sound meals, obtain nutritional services and other health-promotion services (including nutrition screening and counseling), and reduce the social isolation that may occur in old age. Priority is given to older persons with the greatest social and economic need: low income, minorities, those with limited English proficiency, rural location, and frail seniors at risk for institutionalization (USDHHS, AoA, 2009).

The Older Adults Nutrition Services Program. These programs include the Congregate Nutrition Services Program (CNSP); the Home-Delivered Nutrition Services Program (i.e., "Meals on Wheels"); and the Nutrition Services Incentive Program (NSIP), which gives states, territories, and Indian Tribal Organizations (ITOs) the ability to purchase food or to cover the cost of commodities from the USDA for the CNSP and the Home-Delivered Nutrition Services Program. AoA provides funds to states, territories, and ITOs, and they award money to Area Agencies on Aging for coordination with area food sites such as senior centers, faith-based sites, community centers, adult day care, and schools. For NSIP, money or commodity allocation is determined by the share of population who received meals under CNSP or Meals on Wheels in the preceding year.

By law, age is the only factor used in determining eligibility. People 60 years or older and their spouses, regardless of age, are eligible for benefits. ITOs may select an age younger than 60 for defining an older person for their tribes because of a shorter life expectancy and higher chronic illnesses. Additionally, disabled people who live in elder care housing facilities, people who accompany older participants to congregate feeding sites, and volunteers who assist in the meal service may also receive meals. For those in the home-delivered services, spouses of any age and disabled persons may also participate as long as they live with the homebound elder.

Also by law, there is no income requirement for meals. Each recipient may contribute as much as desired toward the cost of the meal, but meals are free to people who cannot make any contribution. As of 2011, federal money only contributed about 42% of money for these programs; 15% came from state funding with the balance coming from local, private, or participant contribution (Congressional Research Service, 2011). In recent years, many states have shifted allowable money from congregate feeding sites into Meals on Wheels or other nutrition/health-promotion programs to help keep older adults in their communities. Even so, long waiting lists for Meals on Wheels are not uncommon and volunteers to help deliver meals to stretch limited dollars are always needed. This situation is not likely to improve with continuing federal and state budget constraints.

In 2010, 92.5 million meals, or about 40% of total meals, were served in congregate settings to just less than 1.69 million meal participants. A 2009 report by the Administration on Aging showed 57% of those people were ≥75 years old, 48% lived alone, 13% had annual incomes of $10,000 or less, and 57% stated the meal provided half or more of their daily food intake. Participants also said they saw friends more often because of meals (87%). Of 10 meals, 6 were delivered to homebound elderly for a total of 149.2 million home-delivered meals to about 880,000 meal participants. Of those older persons, 70% were ≥75 years old, 56% lived alone, 25% had an annual income of $10,000 or less, and 59% said the meals provided half or more of their daily food intake. Four out of ten persons needed help with at least one activity of daily living and 85% needed help with shopping, housework, and ambulating.

NUTRITION SCREENING

Nutrition screening is the process of discovering characteristics or risk factors that are known to be associated with dietary or nutrition problems. Its primary purpose is to identify individuals (such as older adults and the poor) who are potentially at high risk from complex and involved problems that relate to nutrition. To serve this purpose, screening criteria must be simple, relatively straightforward, and easy to administer. Screening is also helpful in establishing priorities for the most efficient use of valuable time and money.

The single largest demographic group at disproportionate risk of malnutrition is older Americans. Nutrition screening holds a tremendous preventive health potential for older adults. The nurse should assess need for nutrition counseling or a referral to a registered dietitian for an older person who has food-related problems that are impacting eating pleasure and quality of life (American Dietetic Association, 2010a). The pendulum has shifted to reduce unnecessary therapeutic diets for those at risk of unintentional weight loss and undernutrition. There is also controversy about the benefit of weight loss for obese older Americans among experts. A dietitian or community nutrition program might be appropriate if any of the following are identified in the individual:

- Inappropriate or inadequate food intake
- Desire by obese elderly person to lose weight—tailoring to provide adequate calories, protein, and physical activity to preserve lean body mass
- Need for nutrient/disease-specific counseling with specific food preferences, cultural taboos, or environmental constraints
- Serum cholesterol level of more than 240 mg/dL with desire to change eating pattern
- Functional dependency for eating or for food-related activities of daily living

The health care professional should refer the individual to a physician when there has been an involuntary decrease in weight of more than 10 pounds during the previous 6 months. Additional anthropometric measurements suggesting malnutrition include the following:

- Triceps skin-fold thickness less than 10th percentile
- Midarm muscle circumference less than 10th percentile
- Serum albumin level less than 3.5 g/dL
- Evidence of osteoporosis or mineral deficiency (indicated by a history of bone pain or fractures, particularly in housebound older women)
- Evidence of vitamin deficiency (indicated by chronic inadequate fruit and vegetable intake; angular stomatitis, glossitis, or bleeding gums; or pressure sores in bedridden individuals)

NUTRITION RISK FACTORS

This section examines the role of nutrition in the etiology and prevention of the leading nutrition-related chronic diseases—heart disease, stroke, some forms of cancer, osteoporosis, obesity, and type 2 diabetes—and in the early treatment of people who were recently diagnosed with human immunodeficiency virus (HIV).

Cardiovascular Diseases

Cardiovascular diseases (CVDs), principally CHD and stroke, are among the nation's leading killers of both men and women among all racial and ethnic groups. Approximately one fourth of the nation's population has some form of CVD, including high blood pressure, CHD, and stroke.

Cardiovascular disease prevention is so important that *Healthy People 2020* has specific objectives specifically targeted to meet the goal to improve cardiovascular health and quality of life through prevention, detection, and treatment of risk factors for heart attack and stroke. Specific objectives are listed in Box 11-2 under Heart Disease and Stroke.

Heart Disease
Diet Intervention

In an attempt to reduce CVD, the American Heart Association (AHA) recommends that people over the age of 2 years adopt a well-balanced diet, achieve and maintain a healthy body weight, and reach optimal levels for cholesterol, HDL, LDL, blood pressure, and blood glucose (Lichtenstein et al., 2006). (The AHA did not set guidelines for those under 2 years of age.)

Generally, the 2006 *AHA Diet and Lifestyle Recommendations* mimic the 2010 *Dietary Guidelines for Americans* key recommendations (**Website Resource 11C**). All key suggestions apply with a few changes. Specifically:

- Eat two or more servings of fish (about 8 ounces) every week, preferably oily varieties rich in eicosapentaenoic acid (EPA) or docosahexaenoic acid (DHA) such as canned light tuna, salmon, pollock, and catfish.
- Limit intake of saturated fat to <7% of energy by choosing lean meats and vegetable alternatives, and fat-free (skim) or low-fat (1% fat) dairy products.
- When eating food prepared outside of the home, follow these *Diet and Lifestyle Recommendations:*
  - (More Specific) Reduce salt intake by comparing the sodium content of similar products (e.g., different brands of tomato sauce) and choosing products with less salt or sodium; choosing versions of processed foods, including cereals and baked goods, that are reduced in salt or sodium; and limiting condiments (e.g., soy sauce, ketchup).
  - Neither antioxidant vitamin supplements nor other supplements such as selenium are recommended.

Many children, adolescents, and adults who already have undesirable levels of lipids in their blood should receive nutrition counseling when their total cholesterol level is elevated (Grundy et al., 2004). In children ages 2 to 20, an acceptable level of cholesterol is less than 170 mg/dL.

Individuals with low-density lipoprotein (LDL) cholesterol levels that are higher than 200 mg/dL—the National Cholesterol Education Program (NCEP) targets for primary or secondary prevention—should be advised to reduce their intake of dietary saturated fat and cholesterol to levels below those recommended for the general population (Expert Panel on Detection, Evaluation, and Treatment of High Blood Cholesterol in Adults, 2001). The upper limit for these individuals is less than 7% of the total energy for saturated fat and less than 200 mg of cholesterol per day. In both cases, however, even lower intake levels can be of further benefit in reducing LDL cholesterol levels. After the program is outlined, follow-up sessions are scheduled to monitor lipid levels and dietary compliance. If acceptable lipid levels have not been achieved, then the individual should be referred to a registered dietitian or for drug therapy (Fazio, 2008).

The NCEP develops new guidelines periodically, as warranted by research advances. The most recent set of guidelines, the *Third Report of the NCEP Expert Panel on Detection, Evaluation, and Treatment of High Blood Cholesterol in Adults,* also known as the Adult Treatment Panel III (ATP III) (Table 11-3), was updated in 2004. The changes in options for more intensive cholesterol reduction treatment for high-risk and moderate-risk individuals were based on the review of five clinical trials

TABLE 11-3	ATP III CLASSIFICATION OF SERUM LIPID LEVELS* IN ADULTS AGE 20 AND OLDER†			
CLASSIFICATION	LDL CHOLESTEROL (mg/dL)	TOTAL CHOLESTEROL (mg/dL)	TRIGLYCERIDES (mg/dL)	HDL CHOLESTEROL (mg/dL)
Optimal/desirable	<100 Optional <70 for very high-risk persons	<200	<150	≥60
Near-optimal/above normal	100-129	—	—	—
Borderline high	103-159	200-239	150-159	—
High	160-189	—	200-499	—
Very high	≥190	≥240	≥500	—
Low	—	—	—	≤40

From Expert Panel on Detection, Evaluation, and Treatment of High Blood Cholesterol in Adults. (2001). Executive summary of the third report of the National Cholesterol Education Program (NCEP) Expert Panel on Detection, Evaluation, and Treatment of High Blood Cholesterol in Adults (Adult Treatment Panel III). *Journal of the American Medical Association, 285,* 2486-2497. Information about the update of the ATP III guidelines retrieved July 17, 2012, from www.nhlbi.nih.gov/guidelines/cholesterol/upd-info_prof.htm.
*Measured in milligrams (mg) of lipid per deciliter (dL) of blood.
†Includes 2004 update for LDL for very-high-risk individuals. Very high risk is defined as those with (a) recent heart attack, (b) cardiovascular disease with diabetes, or (c) cardiovascular disease plus severe or poorly controlled risk factors such as current smoking or metabolic syndrome.
ATP, Adult Treatment Panel; *HDL,* high-density lipoprotein; *LDL,* low-density lipoprotein.

of cholesterol-lowering statin treatment. The update did not change the ATP III recommendations for people at moderate or lower risk. As of late 2012, the ATP IV guidelines in development have not been released.

The current ATP guidelines recommend that healthy adults have a lipoprotein analysis once every 5 years. A lipoprotein profile measures levels of LDL, total cholesterol, high-density lipoproteins (HDL), and triglycerides (another fatty substance in the blood). The level at which low HDL becomes a major risk factor for heart disease is less than 40 mg/dL for men and less than 50 mg/dL for women.

In addition to a low high-density lipoprotein (HDL) level, there are other major risk factors for CHD:

- Clinical forms of atherosclerotic disease (peripheral arterial disease, abdominal aortic aneurysm, and symptomatic carotid artery disease)
- Age (55 for men and >65 for women)
- Cigarette smoking
- Hypertension (blood pressure [BP] higher than 140/90 mm Hg or taking antihypertensive medication)
- Diabetes (fasting blood glucose level higher than 110 mg/dL)
- Family history of premature heart disease (heart disease in a first-degree relative at age less than 55 for men or at age less than 65 for women)

HDL cholesterol level greater than 60 mg/dL is considered a negative risk factor.

Therapeutic Lifestyle Changes (TLC) Treatment Plan

The TLC treatment plan of nutrition, physical activity, and weight control is recommended for treating people who present with type 2 diabetes, elevated levels of LDL, or metabolic syndrome.

Metabolic syndrome describes the presence of a cluster of risk factors that often occur together, which dramatically increases the risk for coronary events. The syndrome is diagnosed when an individual has three or more of these factors:

- Excessive abdominal fat, as indicated by too large a waist measurement (>35 inches or 88 centimeters in women and >40 inches or 102 centimeters in men)
- Elevated blood pressure (higher than 130 mm Hg systolic or 85 mm Hg diastolic)
- Low HDL level (lower than 40 mg/dL)
- Elevated triglyceride level (higher than 150 mg/dL), which is significantly linked to the degree of heart disease risk (The guidelines recommend treating even borderline high triglyceride levels with therapy that includes weight control and physical activity.)

The dietary component of the TLC includes the following daily intake:

- Less than 7% of calories from saturated fat
- Less than 200 mg of dietary cholesterol
- Up to 35% of calories from total fat, provided most of the fat is from unsaturated fat, which does not raise cholesterol levels (A higher fat intake may be needed by some individuals with high triglyceride levels or a low HDL level, or both, to keep their triglyceride levels or HDL status from worsening.)
- Intake of certain foods to boost the diet's LDL-lowering power: 2 g/day of plant stanols and sterols found in cholesterol-lowering margarines and salad dressings, and 10 to 25 g/day of foods high in soluble fiber, such as cereal grains, beans, peas, legumes, and many fruits and vegetables

A primary treatment goal of the TLC is reducing an elevated LDL level to:

- Less than 100 mg/dL with a therapeutic option of <70 mg/dL in the presence of CHD or other forms of atherosclerotic disease
- Less than 130 mg/dL with a therapeutic option of <100 mg/dL in the presence of two or more risk factors for CHD
- Less than 160 mg/dL in the presence of fewer than two risk factors for CHD

The final goal of the TLC includes weight control (to enhance LDL level lowering and raise HDL level) and physical activity that lasts at least 30 minutes, expending at least 200 calories per day on most days (to improve HDL and, for some, LDL levels).

Removing Barriers to Treatment Goals

To improve an individual's compliance to ATP III goals, treatment barriers can be eliminated by developing protocols to encourage long-term individual adherence and follow-up, such as establishing clinic policy and developing computerized databases for those seeking care, establishing management algorithms, reinforcing and rewarding adherence, and enhancing third-party reimbursement. The nurse uses behavioral theories to identify a person's level of readiness to change and focus on counseling strategies to match that level of readiness (Snetselaar, 2004).

Hypertension

Blood pressure, the force of blood against the walls of arteries, is recorded as the systolic pressure (as the heart beats) over the diastolic pressure (as the heart relaxes between beats). The measurement is written with one number above (or before) the other, with the systolic blood pressure (SBP) listed first and the diastolic blood pressure (DBP) listed second. For example, a blood pressure measurement of 120/80 mm Hg (millimeters of mercury) is expressed verbally as "120 over 80." Normal blood pressure is less than 120 mm Hg systolic and less than 80 mm Hg diastolic. *The Seventh Report of the Joint National Committee on Prevention, Detection, Evaluation and Treatment of High Blood Pressure (JNC 7)* (National High Blood Pressure Education Program, 2003) added a pre-hypertension classification defined as a SBP range of 120 to 139 mm Hg or a DBP range of 80 to 89 mm Hg to highlight increased risk for progression to frank hypertension and cardiovascular disease (NCEP, 2003). *Healthy People 2020* added a new developmental objective related to pre-hypertension (see Box 11-2).

Epidemiology

In 2008 hypertension contributed to the deaths of approximately 348,000 Americans out of 2.4 million people. Approximately 44% were men and 56% were women (Roger et al., 2012). Using a definition of hypertension as a BP higher than 140/90 mm Hg, as many as 76.5 million adult Americans, or nearly one in three of all adults in the United States, has high blood pressure. Data from NHANES 2005-2008 show that one in three people with hypertension is unaware of his/her condition and over 50% in that survey do not have controlled high blood pressure (Egan et al., 2001). Untreated hypertension can damage arteries and increase the risk of stroke and congestive heart failure. High blood pressure is also responsible for many cases of kidney failure requiring dialysis and increases the risk of kidney failure in people with diabetes.

Non-Hispanic Black and non-Hispanic White Americans are more likely to suffer from high blood pressure than are Hispanic Americans although the rates for all ethnicities are significant. More women than men (3 out of 4) have high blood pressure at age 75 and older. It appears to affect more people with lower educational and income levels, although this fact may be related to other factors.

Diet Intervention

The modifiable nutrition-related risk factors for stroke include high blood pressure, obesity, habitual high alcohol intake, and high intake of sodium (CDC, 2011f; Lloyd-Jones et al., 2010; Appel et al., 2006). No certain method exists for identifying susceptible people or ascertaining how many of them become hypertensive as a result of excessive salt intake; therefore, the conservative preventive health approach recommends a salt intake limited to 6 grams (g) or less per day for adults. Sodium chloride is approximately 40% sodium by weight; therefore, a diet with 6 g of salt contains about 2300 mg of sodium. This amount is regarded as mild sodium restriction. Ideally, the recommendations are to reduce sodium intake to about 1500 mg but it is very difficult with the current prevalence of sodium in packaged and restaurant foods. More than 45 national health organizations and 20 restaurant and food packaging companies have joined in the National Salt Reduction Initiative so far, started by New York City mayor Michael Bloomberg in 2008; the initiative will aim to reduce the sodium level in food by 25% over a specified period of time. The following are the three major sources of sodium in the U.S. diet, in order of predominance:

- Salt added by food processing companies as an ingredient in almost all processed foods (including many foods that do not taste salty, such as baked goods); most processed foods are high in sodium content (80%)
- Salt added by consumers to food during cooking or at the table (5% to 6% each)
- Salt from all animal products, which are a natural source of sodium

The following recommended food tips are designed to reduce salt and sodium intake:

- Sodium occurs naturally in many foods and is also added to most processed foods; therefore, add salt only sparingly in home cooking and at the table.
- Consume fewer foods that have high sodium levels, such as many cheeses; processed meats; most frozen dinners and entrees; packaged mixes; most canned soups and vegetables; salad dressings; and condiments such as soy sauce, pickles, olives, catsup, and mustard.
- Rinse canned vegetables first before warming.
- Eat salty, highly processed salty, salt-preserved, and salt-pickled foods infrequently.
- Check labels for the amount of sodium in foods and choose products lower in sodium (free: <5 mg per serving; low: <140 mg per serving; reduced or less: 25% less than standard-reference food; healthy: <480 mg per serving).

DASH Eating Plan

Clinical studies show that blood pressure can be lowered by following the *Dietary Approaches to Stop Hypertension* (DASH) eating plan. The National Heart, Lung and Blood Institute (NHLBI), with additional support by the NIH, funded the DASH research with final results appearing in the *New England*

Journal of Medicine in 1997. The DASH eating plan makes consuming less salt and sodium easier because the plan includes abundant fruits and vegetables, which are lower in sodium than other foods. The plan also includes more fat-free or low-fat milk and milk products, whole grains, fish, poultry, beans, seeds, and nuts, but contains less sweets, added sugars and sugar-containing beverages, fats, and red meats than the average typical American diet.

The plan is rich in magnesium, potassium, calcium, protein, and fiber. At approximately 2100 calories a day, the nutrients include 4700 mg of potassium, 500 mg of magnesium, and 1250 mg of calcium. These totals are approximately two to three times the amounts most Americans receive.

Based on DASH clinical studies, a combination of the eating plan and reduced sodium intake can reduce elevated levels of blood pressure. When blood pressure is normal, the DASH eating plan may help prevent blood pressure problems. If blood pressure is only slightly elevated, then the plan may actually eliminate the need for medication. For more severe high blood pressure, the plan may allow a reduction in medication. Other steps to control or prevent hypertension should continue to be encouraged, including exercising, losing excess weight, not smoking, and limiting alcohol. DASH may improve health in other ways, also. Fruits and vegetables may reduce the risk for some cancers; the calcium in dairy products can lower the risk for osteoporosis; and a diet low in saturated fat and cholesterol can reduce CVD risk. The complete DASH eating plan entitled *Your Guide to Lowering Your Blood Pressure with DASH* (USD-HHS, 2005) can be accessed at the website www.nhlbi.nih.gov/health/public/heart/hbp/dash/index.htm. Specific calorie level plans ranging from 1200 to 3100 kilocalories are also available in Appendix 10 (p. 83) of the 2010 *Dietary Guidelines*, available at www.dietaryguidelines.gov.

Cancer
Epidemiology

The National Cancer Institute estimates that almost one in two (41%) women and men will be diagnosed with some type of cancer in their lifetime. As of 2009, cancer remained the second leading cause of death in the United States (Miniño, 2011). For cancer mortality, lung cancer ranks number one for both men and women with an incidence of 25%. Next, for men, leading causes of death include prostate cancer at 10% followed by cancer of the colon and rectum. After lung cancer, breast cancer ranks number two for women. More men than women die from cancer, irrespective of race or ethnicity. However, African American men have the highest death rate followed by Caucasians, Hispanics, American Indians/Alaska Natives, and then Asian Americans/Pacific Islanders. Overall, Blacks were more likely to develop cancer than were people of any other racial or ethnic group (American Cancer Society, 2008). The incidence of breast cancer in women is highest among White women. Black women have the highest incidence rates of colon and rectal cancer (23.7 per 100,000) and lung and bronchial cancer (46.2 per 100,000) followed by Whites, Asian Americans, Hispanic Americans, and Native Americans. Blacks are approximately 33% more likely to die of cancer than Whites and are

two times more likely to die of cancer than Asian Americans, Native Americans, and Hispanic Americans.

Approximately one third of cancer deaths among men and women are related to diet and sedentary lifestyle factors. The introduction of a healthy diet (Figure 11-4) and exercise practices at any time from childhood to old age can promote health and likely reduce cancer risk.

Diet Intervention for Risk Reduction

Many dietary factors can affect cancer risk: types of foods, food preparation methods, portion sizes, food variety, and overall caloric balance. An overall dietary pattern that balances caloric intake and physical activity for weight management along with inclusion of a high proportion of plant foods (fruits, vegetables, whole grains, and beans) and limited amounts of processed or red meats, dairy products (for men), and high-calorie/low nutritional value foods and beverages can reduce the risk of cancer. Food appears to have a protective effect by itself that dietary supplements, in particular supplements that exceed DRIs, do not provide.

Based on its review of the scientific evidence, the American Cancer Society (ACS) updated its nutrition and physical activity guidelines in 2011 (Kushi et al., 2012). The ACS recommendations are very consistent with the messages of the 2010 *Dietary Guidelines for Americans,* the MyPlate guidelines, and the dietary recommendations of other national agencies for general health promotion and prevention of other diet-related chronic conditions. Although no diet can guarantee full protection against any disease, the ACS believes that the following recommendations offer the best nutrition information currently available to help Americans.

For national, state, and local community action:

Apply policy and environmental changes that increase access to affordable, healthy foods in all places where adults and children live, work, go to school, or play and decrease access and marketing of foods and drinks of low nutritional value, particularly to youth.

For individuals:

Choose most of the foods you eat from plant sources. Choose fewer and smaller portions of high-fat or calorie-dense

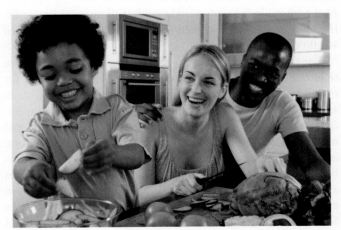

FIGURE 11-4 Choosing healthy options starts at home. (From Jupiter Images.)

foods and beverages. Eat at least 2½ cups of a variety of fruits and vegetables every day. Choose whole-grain breads, cereals, pastas, brown rice, and beans. Limit processed meat (bacon, sausage, luncheon meats) and red meats such as beef, pork, or lamb. For those who do eat meat, choose leaner cuts and small portions, not more than ¼ of plate (similar to MyPlate) or, at most, ⅓ of plate (New MyPlate). Many scientific studies show that eating fruits and vegetables (especially green and dark yellow or orange vegetables, foods in the cabbage family, soy products, and legumes) can protect against cancers at many sites, particularly for cancers of the gastrointestinal and respiratory tracts. Consumption of at least five servings of fruits and vegetables among both smokers and non-smokers seems to reduce risk of lung cancer. Grains are also an important source of many vitamins and minerals, such as folate, calcium, and selenium, which have been associated with a lower risk of colon cancer in some studies. Beans (legumes) are especially rich in nutrients that may protect against cancer. Consumption of meat, particularly red and processed meats, has been associated with an increased risk of cancer at several sites, most notably the colon and prostate.

Since 1991 the "5 A Day for Better Health Program" (now "Fruits and Veggies—More Matters®") has raised public awareness about the importance of fruits and vegetables in disease prevention. The program is jointly sponsored by the Centers for Disease Control and Prevention (CDC) and the Produce for Better Health Foundation (a nonprofit consumer education foundation representing the fruit and vegetable industry). Through its unique national public-private partnership, Fruits and Veggies—More Matters seeks to increase consumption of fruits and vegetables to five or more servings each day. The program focuses on moms as the gatekeepers for families and provides information, recipes, and materials for both consumers and partner organizations. It gives Americans a simple, positive message: eat more, start small, and all types of fruits and vegetables can fit.

Be physically active: Achieve and maintain a healthy weight. Being overweight or obese, by itself or in combination with excess belly fat, increases risk for cancers at several sites, such as the colon and rectum, prostate, endometrium, breast (among postmenopausal women), and kidney. Both increasing physical activity and balancing food intake to maximize nutrient density within calorie needs are essential. Keeping a normal BMI without being underweight is ideal. If overweight, avoiding more weight gain or even losing as little as 5% to 10% of weight can be beneficial.

For those who drink alcohol, limit consumption. No more than one drink per day for women or two drinks per day for men is recommended. Alcoholic beverages, along with cigarette smoking and the use of snuff and chewing tobacco, contribute to cancers of the oral cavity, esophagus, and larynx. The combined use of tobacco and alcohol leads to a greatly increased risk of oral and esophageal cancers; the effect of tobacco and alcohol combined is greater than the sum of their individual effects. Studies also have shown an association between alcohol consumption and an increased risk of breast cancer (American Cancer Society, 2009). The mechanism of this effect is not known, but the association may be related to carcinogenic actions of alcohol or its metabolites, to alcohol-induced changes in levels of

hormones such as estrogens, or to some other process. Regardless of the mechanism, studies show that the risk of breast cancer increases with an intake beginning at only a few drinks per week. Reducing alcohol consumption is a good way for women who drink regularly to reduce their risk of breast cancer. Women at highest risk for breast cancer may want to consider refraining from any alcohol consumption.

Nurses may find that it is helpful to refer to the sections in the nutrition and physical activity guidelines (Kushi et al., 2012) that refer to other aspects of food intake relating to prevention of cancer. They include more specific suggestions for particular cancers, evidence specific to nutrient supplementation, and answers to other frequently asked questions. It is available free for download (subject to copyright if used) at http://onlinelibrary.wiley.com/doi/10.3322/caac.20140/full.

Osteoporosis
Epidemiology
Osteoporosis, a bone disease characterized by low bone mass leading to fragile bones and an increased risk of hip, spine, and wrist fractures, is a major public health risk for an estimated 44 million individuals in the United States, or 55% of people age 50 or older (National Osteoporosis Foundation, 2011). Ten million people already have been diagnosed with osteoporosis and 34 million more people have low bone mineral density (BMD), placing them at increased risk for osteoporosis. Of the 10 million Americans estimated to have osteoporosis, 80% are women and 20% are men. Of those with hip fractures, 24% die within a year, men twice as often as women and African American women more often than Caucasian women. Direct financial expenditures for management of osteoporotic fracture alone were estimated at $19 billion in 2005 and will likely rise to about $25.3 billion by 2025. These figures underestimate significantly the true costs of osteoporosis, because they fail to include the costs of treatment for individuals without a history of fractures or the indirect costs of lost wages or productivity of either the individual or the caregiver.

The National Osteoporosis Foundation recognizes the following risk factors for osteoporosis:
- Older age: as age increases, risk increases
- Female gender
- Personal history of osteoporosis or fracture as an adult
- Family history of osteoporosis or broken bones
- Low levels of sex hormones: in women, early estrogen deficiency (younger than 45 years) or low estrogen levels during menopause, missing periods (amenorrhea); in men, low levels of testosterone and estrogen
- Diet: low in calcium or vitamin D intake; high intake of protein, sodium, and caffeine
- Sedentary lifestyle
- Use of oral corticosteroid therapy for 3 or more months
- Smoking (active or passive)
- High alcohol intake (three or more drinks per day)
- Specific medicines (steroids, some anticonvulsants, and others)
- Some diseases and conditions (anorexia nervosa, rheumatoid arthritis, gastrointestinal diseases including celiac disease, sickle cell anemia, and lupus)

Although the prevalence of osteoporosis and the incidence of fracture do vary by gender and race/ethnicity, there is a significant risk for all groups even with differences in bone mass density. The latest available facts (NIAMS, 2012a,b) indicate that an estimated 20% of non-Hispanic Caucasian/Asian women, 10% of Hispanic women, and 5% of non-Hispanic Black women 50 years or older have osteoporosis already. Low bone density is even higher in the same groups: 52%, 49%, and 35%, respectively. Currently, risk is rising most rapidly in Hispanic women although the reasons are unknown. Among men 50 years and older, an estimated 7% of non-Hispanic Caucasian/Asian men, 4% of non-Hispanic Black men, and 3% of Hispanic men have osteoporosis. Low bone density is higher in the same groups: 35%, 19%, and 23%, respectively (NIAMS, 2012a,b). There is limited information on other ethnic/racial groups so those data are not included.

Pathophysiology

Osteoporosis is a slowly developing condition that causes loss of bone mass and fractures, especially in the wrist, hip, and spinal areas. Osteoporosis is defined as a skeletal disorder characterized by compromised bone strength predisposing to an increased risk of fracture. Bone strength reflects the integration of two main features: bone density and bone quality. Bone mineral density (BMD) is expressed as grams of mineral per area or volume and, in any given individual, is determined by peak bone mass and amount of bone loss. Bone quality refers to architecture, turnover, damage accumulation (micro fractures), and mineralization. Osteoporotic bone fractures more easily than normal bone; therefore, osteoporosis is a significant risk factor for fracture.

Factors Involved in Building and Maintaining Skeletal Health Throughout Life. The bone mass attained early in life, 85% to 90% of which is reached by age 18 for girls and age 20 for boys, is perhaps the most important determinant of lifelong skeletal health. Individuals with the highest peak bone mass after adolescence have the greatest protective advantage when the inevitable declines in bone density associated with increasing age, illness, and diminished sex steroid production take their toll.

Genetic factors exert a strong and perhaps predominant influence on peak bone mass, but physiological, environmental, and modifiable lifestyle factors can also play a significant role. Among these factors are adequate nutrition and body weight, exposure to sex hormones at puberty, and physical activity (particularly weight-bearing activity). Therefore maximizing BMD early in life presents a vital opportunity to reduce the effect of bone loss related to aging. Childhood is a critical time for development of lifestyle habits conducive to maintaining good bone health throughout life. Additionally, cigarette smoking, which usually starts in adolescence, may have a deleterious effect on bone mass.

Prevention

Once thought to be a natural part of aging among women, osteoporosis is no longer considered age dependent or gender dependent and is largely preventable, thanks to the recent progress in the understanding of its causes, diagnosis, and treatment. Optimization of bone health is a process that must occur throughout the life span in both men and women. Factors that enhance bone health at all ages are essential to prevent osteoporosis and its devastating consequences. Calcium is the nutrient most important for attaining peak bone mass and for preventing and treating osteoporosis.

Good nutrition is essential for normal growth. A balanced diet, adequate calories, and appropriate nutrients are the foundation for developing all tissues, including bone. Adequate and appropriate nutrition is important for all individuals, but not everyone follows a diet that is optimal for bone health.

Table 11-4 suggests dietary calcium (and vitamin D) intake recommendations for various stages of life. Factors contributing to low calcium intake are restriction of dairy products because of food preferences or lactose intolerance, a generally low level of fruit and vegetable consumption, and a high intake of low-calcium beverages such as soft drinks. Lactose and vitamin D enhance calcium absorption and exercise enhances calcium balance. Calcium is absorbed best from dairy foods. It is the only source of the disaccharide lactose.

Vitamin D is a fat-soluble vitamin technically encompassing two molecules—vitamin D_2 (ergocalciferol) and vitamin D_3 (cholecalciferol). Vitamin D_3 is the form of vitamin D that best supports bone health. Vitamin D is synthesized in the body when the skin is exposed to the ultraviolet rays of the sun. Commonly added to milk, other food sources of vitamin D include fatty fish (salmon and mackerel); margarine; eggs; and some fortified, ready-to-eat cereals. Most infants and young children in the United States have adequate vitamin D intake from the supplementation and fortification of milk. During adolescence, when consumption of dairy products decreases, vitamin D intake is likely to be inadequate, which may affect calcium absorption adversely. Other nutrients have been evaluated relative to bone health. High dietary protein, caffeine, phosphorous, and sodium intake can adversely affect calcium balance; however, their effects appear to be offset in individuals with adequate calcium intakes.

Food should be selected to provide adequate calcium, paying special attention to that eaten by adolescents, who normally have high mineral requirements, and by women, who are susceptible to inadequate dietary calcium because of low caloric intake. Women of all ages should be concerned about adequate calcium intake. A means for increasing individual consumption of calcium includes educating consumers to eat more calcium-rich foods, including calcium-fortified foods such as orange juice, and recommending dietary supplements in some cases. Individuals who wish to increase their calcium intake can consume more low-fat or non-fat dairy products or fortified food products. Supplementation with calcium tablets may be appropriate for people at high risk of health problems from inadequate calcium intake. However, it is particularly important for older women to be vigilant about the levels of calcium they obtain from dietary sources, supplements, and

TABLE 11-4   DIETARY REFERENCE INTAKES (DRIS) FOR CALCIUM AND VITAMIN D

	CALCIUM			VITAMIN D		
LIFE STAGE GROUP	EAR (mg/Day)	RDA (mg/Day)	UL (mg/Day)	EAR (IU/Day)	RDA (IU/Day)	UL (IU/Day)
Infants birth to 6 months	—	—	1000	—	—	1000
Infants 6-12 months	—	—	1500	—	—	1500
1-3 years	500	700	2500	400	600	2500
4-8 years	800	1000	2500	400	600	3000
9-13 years	1100	1300	3000	400	600	4000
14-18 years	1100	1300	3000	400	600	
19-30 years	800	1000	2500	400	600	4000
31-50 years	800	1000	2500	400	600	4000
51-70 year-old males	800	1000	2000	400	600	4000
51-70 year-old females	1000	1200	2000	400	600	4000
>70 years	1000	1200	2000	400	800	4000
14-18 years, pregnant or lactating	1100	1300	3000	400	600	4000
19-50 years, pregnant or lactating	800	1000	2500	400	600	4000

Adapted from *Report brief on intakes for calcium and vitamin D.* Retrieved from http://iom.edu/~/media/Files/Report%20Files/2010/Dietary-Reference-Intakes-for-Calcium-and-Vitamin-D/Vitamin%20D%20and%20Calcium%202010%20Report%20Brief.pdf.
EAR, Estimated average requirement; *RDA,* recommended dietary allowance; *UL,* tolerable upper intake level.

medications such as antacids because they are at the greatest risk of exceeding the UL of any age/gender group (National Research Council [NRC], 2010). Men may also be wise to limit calcium supplementation and not exceed normal dietary levels because of an association with increased risk of prostate cancer (Kushi et al., 2012).

For those who do choose calcium supplements, calcium carbonate (40% elemental calcium), calcium citrate (24%), calcium lactate (14%), and calcium gluconate (9%) are preferred. (Dolomite and bone meal are not recommended, because they may be contaminated with lead.) Calcium supplement absorption is most efficient for individuals with adequate gastric acid production at individual doses no greater than 500 mg when taken between meals.

Individuals need to be encouraged to increase their consumption of calcium-rich foods. Milk and dairy products deliver the most calcium of any food group, but they are also among the richest sources of fat in the American diet. Low-fat (1%) and fat-free milk, low-fat yogurt, and low-fat cheeses are the dairy products of choice. Other good sources of calcium include sardines, canned salmon (if the bones are eaten), and some dark green leafy vegetables, especially collard greens. Orange juice and milk fortified with calcium are also good sources. The calcium and vitamin D contents of some common foods are summarized in **Website Resource 11D.**

Anyone younger than age 25 who ingests less than the recommended DRI for calcium should be urged to develop strategies for increasing it. Children, particularly girls between the ages of 9 and 18 years old, are at highest risk for deficiency (NRC, 2010). By modeling appropriate behaviors, health care professionals can help prevent or delay the onset of osteoporosis in themselves, their families, and the people who are in their care.

Obesity

As almost everyone working in the U.S. health care industry knows, a paradox exists in modern America. On the one hand, many people who do not need to lose weight are trying to do so, and on the other hand, many who actually need to lose weight are not trying; those who are trying are unsuccessful in losing the weight and maintaining their weight loss.

Overweight (defined under the Body Mass Index section) can seriously affect health and longevity and is associated with the leading nutrition-related causes of death in the United States: type 2 diabetes mellitus, CVD, and some cancers. Obesity (also defined under the Body Mass Index section) is also associated with gout and gallbladder disease and may contribute to the development of osteoarthritis in the weight-bearing joints.

Epidemiology

Overweight and obesity are found worldwide and the prevalence of these conditions in the United States ranks high in comparison with that of other developed nations. As already mentioned, two thirds of American adults are overweight or obese (Flegal et al., 2010), with one third of children in those categories. Numerous factors contribute, such as lifestyle, genetics, hormonal factors, and social-ecological factors.

The prevalence of being overweight has increased steadily over the years among nearly all racial and ethnic groups. From 1960 to 2000 the prevalence of overweight increased from 31.5% to 33.6% in adults in the United States. The prevalence of obesity during this same period increased from 13.3% to 30.9%—a relative increase of more than 50%, with most of this increase occurring during the 1990s. The prevalence of overweight and obesity increases with advancing age until people reach their sixties, when it starts to decline.

Obesity is more common in women than in men. Among men there is a modest ethnic variation in the prevalence of being overweight, the greatest difference occurring between Black men (67%) and Hispanic American men (74.6%). Among women, the ethnic variation is substantial. Almost 57.6% of White women are overweight; Hispanic American and Puerto Rican women have a greater prevalence of being overweight (73%) than their White counterparts; and more than 79.6% of Black women are overweight (National Center for Health Statistics, 2011). Potential contributing factors often associated with the greater propensity for adult Black women to become obese include lower level of physical activity, higher caloric intake, and lower level of education and social economic status as well as broader acceptance of a larger body size within the African American community (Hawkins, 2007; Sanchez-Johnson et al., 2004).

Body Mass Index for Adults

Based on an adult's height and weight, **body mass index (BMI)** (weight/height^2) is a helpful indicator of underweight, normal weight, overweight, and obesity (USDHHS, 2010b). A person's BMI can be determined by referring to the CDC's on-line BMI calculator (www.cdc.gov/nccdphp/dnpa/bmi/calc-bmi.htm), or by using a hand-held calculator and the following formulas:

Body Mass Index Formulas

English Formula

BMI = weight in pounds ÷ height in inches
÷ height in inches × 703

Example: For a 6-foot-tall person weighing 210 pounds: BMI = 210 pounds divided by 72 inches divided by 72 inches multiplied by 703 = 28.5.

Metric Formulas

BMI = weight in kilograms ÷ (height in meters)^2

and

BMI = (weight in kilograms ÷ height in centimeters ÷ height in centimeters) × 10,000

Example: For a person who is 182.9 centimeters tall and weighs 95.3 kilograms: BMI = 95.3 kilograms divided by 182.9 centimeters divided by 182.9 centimeters and multiplied by 10,000 = 28.5.

BMI is a good indicator of body fat, but it cannot be interpreted as a specific percentage of body fat. Age and gender influence the relationship between fat and BMI. For example, women are more likely to have a higher percentage of body fat than men have for the same BMI. At the same BMI, older people have more body fat than do younger adults (Gallagher et al., 2000). BMI is used to screen and monitor a population to detect the risk of health or nutritional disorders. In an individual, other data must be used to determine whether a high BMI is associated with increased risk of disease and death for that person; use of BMI value alone is not diagnostic. Waist circumference is also an indicator of risk. For more detail, see USDHHS, 2010b.

BMI ranges are based on the effect body weight has on disease and death. A BMI value from 19 to 25 is a healthy target range for adults. BMI values higher than 25 are associated with increasing risks for developing CVD, gallbladder disease, high blood pressure, and non–insulin-dependent diabetes mellitus (type 2 diabetes).

BMI values for adults are expressed with one number, regardless of age or gender, using the following guidelines established by the World Health Organization *Classification of Body Weight* (2006):
- Underweight: BMI less than 18.5
- Healthy weight: BMI of 18.5 to 24.9
- Overweight: BMI of 25 to 29.9
- Class 1 obese: BMI of 30 to 34.9
- Class 2 obese: BMI of 35 to 39.9
- Class 3 obese (morbid obesity): BMI of 40 or higher

Body Mass Index Growth Charts for Children

Growth charts have been used by pediatric health care providers since 1977, with the newest ones released in 2000 by the CDC to more accurately reflect the nation's cultural and racial diversity. Charts are used widely by pediatricians, nurses, and nutritionists to track growth and development in children and adolescents through age 20 to assist in signaling potential developmental and weight problems earlier in childhood/adolescence. They consist of a series of percentile curves that illustrate the distribution in growth of children across the United States.

The charts include an assessment of BMI. The BMI is an early warning signal that is helpful as early as age 2 years to help identify children who have the potential to become overweight. Early identification of obesity risk gives parents the opportunity to modify their family eating and activity patterns before their children develop a weight problem.

The CDC's charts are based on data gathered through the National Health and Nutrition Examination Survey, the only survey that collects data from actual physical examinations on a cross-section of Americans from all over the country. This survey shows that since the 1980s the number of overweight children and adolescents has doubled. The growth charts indicate that, in general, children are heavier today than in 1977, but height has remained virtually unchanged. The charts are available on the CDC website at www.cdc.gov/growthcharts.

Diet Intervention

"Please help me lose weight" is one of the most common requests heard in the health field. As discussed, a balanced diet is important and must include the appropriate **serving sizes** for the recommended daily intake of each food group. Additionally, exercise is particularly necessary from the outset, because with exercise there is less need to restrict food intake. Exercise also favors long-term maintenance of body weight (as described in Chapter 12).

Nurses make referrals to supervised or unsupervised programs as appropriate. People expect this type of advice on maintaining their health. Therefore nurses can play an important role, although not supervising individuals' weight loss efforts directly. For more information on obesity among adults, see references including the *White House Task Force Report on Childhood Obesity* (2010), *The Surgeon General's Vision for a Healthy and Fit Nation* (USDHHS, 2010b) and *Community Strategies and Measurements to Reduce Obesity* (Khan et al., 2009).

There are many positive effects of only relatively small amounts of weight loss (5% to 10% of body weight) for people who are obese, including the following:

- Decreased blood pressure (decreased risk of a heart attack and stroke)
- Reduced abnormally high levels of blood glucose associated with diabetes
- Reduced elevated levels of cholesterol and triglycerides associated with CVD
- Reduced sleep apnea (irregular breathing during sleep)
- Decreased risk of osteoarthritis in the weight-bearing joints
- Decreased depression
- Increased self-esteem

The acronym LEARN has been suggested as a mnemonic device for health professionals. LEARN refers to the steps nurses can take to help the person who needs to improve health-related behavior (Brownell, 2000). LEARN is particularly useful as a guideline for communicating with the clinically obese individual who has indicated dissatisfaction with current weight:

L—Listen with sympathy and understanding to the person's perception of the problem.
E—Explain personal perceptions of the problem.
A—Acknowledge and discuss differences and similarities.
R—Recommend treatment.
N—Negotiate an agreement.

In 1998 an NIH-sponsored technical support conference identified the following characteristics of voluntary weight loss and weight control in the United States (USDHHS, 2010b):

- Obesity is a chronic disease.
- Obesity has many causes.
- Cure is rare; palliation is realistic.
- Weight loss is slow.
- Recidivism is common.
- Weight regain may be slow, but it is often rapid.
- Management is often more frustrating than the underlying disease.

The conference noted significant adverse effects for obese dieters who regain lost weight:

- Repeated weight gain and loss may have adverse psychological and physical effects; for example, evidence suggests that mildly to moderately overweight women who are dieting may be at risk for binge eating.
- Although data on the health effects of repeated weight gain and loss (weight cycling) are also inconclusive, weight cycling appears to affect energy metabolism and may cause faster regaining of weight.
- Depression and decreased self-esteem occur.

Fad diets do not provide the best way to lose weight and should be avoided. However, recognizing that people will do almost anything to lose weight when desperate, it is helpful to be able to discuss current fads intelligently and to guide individuals as needed. A good source for credible, current information that is often updated is the Academy of Nutrition and Dietetics website (www.eatright.org) under the public section in the subsection titled healthy weight loss.

As already mentioned previously, a new prevention-focused model of health care that includes many facets is needed to avoid and treat obesity among adults and children in the United States. On an individual basis, for people who cannot or do not choose to maintain a BMI less than 30 as priority, the paradigm *Health at Any Size* (Spark, 2001) is described in Box 11-7: Hot Topics.

FDA-approved weight loss medication can play a helpful role in assisting individuals to lose weight and keep it off. As of early 2012, currently orlistat (also known as Xenical by prescription or Alli over-the-counter) is the only approved general weight loss drug. It is important to help those using it to recognize the warning signs and see a health provider if they have certain symptoms. Other non–FDA-approved weight loss supplements available are generally not recommended because of safety concerns.

Diabetes
Prevalence and Incidence

Diabetes is becoming more prevalent. The numbers of existing cases (**prevalence**) and new cases (**incidence**) are increasing, and most of this increase is not a result of aging of the U.S. population. The CDC's diabetes maps appear to be mirroring the trends seen in state obesity maps. An estimated 25.8 million Americans (8.3% of the U.S. population) had the disease in 2010 (CDC, 2011b). Among those, older adults and minorities were disproportionately affected. Almost 27% (or 10.9 million) of adults 65 years and older have diagnosed diabetes. After adjusting for population age differences, 2007 to 2009 national survey data of adults (ages 20 and older) showed the risk of diagnosed diabetes was 18% higher among Asian Americans, 66% higher among Hispanics, and 77% higher among non-Hispanic Blacks compared to non-Hispanic White adults. Among Hispanics compared to non-Hispanic White adults, the risk of diagnosed diabetes was about the same for Cubans and for Central and South Americans, 87% higher for Mexican Americans, and 94% higher for Puerto Ricans. In the Native American population, just among those served by the Indian Health Service (IHS), the prevalence is 16.1%, almost twice the national average. Rates vary by region from 5.5% among Alaska Native adults to 33.5% among Native American adults in southern Arizona.

Previously called non–insulin-dependent diabetes mellitus or adult-onset diabetes, type 2 diabetes accounts for 90% to 95% of all diagnosed cases of diabetes. Risk factors include the following: having pre-diabetes (impaired glucose tolerance [IGT] and/or impaired fasting glucose [IFG]), being older than 45, being overweight or obese, not exercising regularly, having a family history of diabetes or a personal history of gestational diabetes, or giving birth to a baby of at least 9 pounds; other risk factors include high blood pressure, low HDL cholesterol level, high triglyceride level, and race/ethnicity (Nesto, 2005).

Type 2 diabetes is the seventh leading cause of death among Americans and the leading cause of new cases of blindness, kidney failure, and lower extremity amputations; it also greatly increases a person's risk for a heart attack or stroke. In 2007,

---

🔥 BOX 11-7 HOT TOPICS

Health at Any Size: The Size Acceptance Nondiet Movement

This paradigm (Spark, 2001) has replaced the question, "How can fat people lose weight?" with the question, "How can fat people be healthy?" The following tenets are the foundation of the movement:

- Good health is a state of physical, mental, and social well-being. People of all sizes and shapes can reduce their risk of poor health by adopting a healthy lifestyle, which includes (1) eating a variety of healthy foods, (2) being physically active because it is fun and feels good, and (3) appreciating the body as it is.
- Human beings come in a variety of sizes and shapes; size diversity is a positive characteristic of the human race. Respect the bodies of others, although they might be quite different.
- There is no ideal body size, shape, BMI, or body composition that every individual should strive to achieve.
- Self-esteem and body image are strongly linked. Helping people feel good about their bodies and about who they are can help motivate and maintain healthy behaviors.
- People are responsible for care of their own bodies.
- Appearance stereotyping is wrong. Their weight notwithstanding, all people deserve to be treated equally in the job market and on the job, to be treated equally in the media, and to receive competent and respectful treatment by health care professionals.

How to Become a Size-Sensitive Health Professional

- On the intake form, include a question asking whether the person is satisfied with his or her body size. If the answer is "yes," then try to avoid the issue in the future.

- When the person asks not to be weighed, the request is acknowledged without complaint and automatically taken into account on follow-up office visits. (There are a few cases in which weighing is necessary, such as when administering certain medications, chemotherapy, or anesthetics.)
- A size-sensitive health care professional does not necessarily avoid mentioning weight but should avoid making an issue of weight, avoid lectures and humiliation, and respect the individual's wishes with regard to weight discussions.
- When weight contributes to a problem, the professional mentions this situation but also considers other diagnoses and recommends tests to determine the actual diagnosis when appropriate. If weight loss is a recommended treatment for a problem, the compassionate professional may mention this, but at minimum, and recommend and prescribe other treatments. Accept the individual's wish not to use weight loss as a treatment.
- Some health care professionals believe that overweight and obesity are not necessarily unhealthy. However, other professionals who believe that fat is unhealthy may acknowledge that weight loss is usually ineffective or that individuals have the right to direct their own treatment.
- Ideally, the waiting area, examining suite, and consultation room are equipped with armless chairs, large blood pressure cuffs, large examination gowns, and other equipment suitable for large people. If this is not the case, then the office staff acknowledges the importance of these items when told.

BMI, Body mass index.

---

diabetes accounted for more than $174 billion in direct and indirect medical costs and lost productivity (CDC, 2011b). Much of the burden of diabetes can be prevented or delayed with early detection, improved delivery of care, and better education on disease self-management (American Diabetes Association, 2012).

Type 2 Diabetes in Children

Although diabetes mellitus in children and adolescents was believed to be exclusively type 1, type 2 diabetes in children and adolescents is now considered a sizeable and growing problem among Native Americans and an emerging public health problem among other North American ethnic groups. The epidemic of obesity among children and adolescents, the decreasing level of physical activity during adolescence, and the increased exposure to diabetes in utero are likely contributors to the increase in prevalence of type 2 diabetes during childhood and adolescence.

Although some children and adolescents are symptomatic, others do not enter the clinical arena until they are in severe ketoacidosis and may have a transient insulin requirement. Diabetic complications (**dyslipidemia** and hypertension) have been observed among Pima Indians as early as the teenage years. No evidence-based guidelines for treatment of type 2 diabetes in children and adolescents are available, and oral agents have not been tested or approved for this age group. Generally, children and adolescents with type 2 diabetes have poor glycemic control. Population mobility, lack of symptoms, denial, absence of family support, and inadequate health care insurance coverage

have all been identified as major barriers to adherence to treatment and follow-up and to successful clinical management. Because of a longer duration of disease (from earlier onset) and because glucose control and compliance are challenging during the teenage years, the lifetime complications (microvascular and macrovascular diseases and decreased quality of life) in this population will probably be considerable (Fagot-Campagna et al., 2000).

Diet Intervention

Medical nutrition therapy (MNT) is the most critical and pivotal component of diabetes care. At the minimum, MNT involves the team efforts of a physician, a registered nurse or registered dietitian, and, in some practice settings, a mental health professional. The purpose of MNT for people with type 2 diabetes is to delay or prevent the development of diabetic complications (blindness, CHD, nephropathy, and neuropathy). No single diabetic diet or American Diabetes Association diet exists. The recommended diet can be defined only as a nutrition prescription based on assessment and treatment goals and outcomes. Nutrition advice for people with type 2 diabetes is essentially the same as that for the general population: follow the *Dietary Guidelines for Americans*. MNT for people with diabetes should be individualized, with consideration given to usual eating habits, culture, and other lifestyle factors. Nutrition recommendations are then developed and implemented to meet treatment goals and desired outcomes. Monitoring metabolic parameters, including blood glucose levels, glycosylated hemoglobin levels, lipid values, blood pressure, body weight, renal function (when appropriate), and quality of life, is crucial to ensure successful outcomes. The American Diabetes Association further recommends ongoing nutrition self-management education for these individuals.

For people with hyperglycemia, hyperlipidemia, obesity, or suboptimal nutrition, start with this nonpharmacological management:

- Together with the person seeking care, determine an appropriate, tailored meal plan. Decide daily energy needs based on body weight goals (moderate weight loss, weight maintenance, weight gain) and then use the individual's daily energy needs to determine the appropriate number of choices from the food groups in MyPlate, the new food guidance system.
- Encourage regular aerobic exercise.
- Evaluate the individual using the outcome measures listed in Table 11-5. People who have been counseled regarding diet and exercise but who have not responded satisfactorily after 4 to 6 weeks should be referred to a registered dietitian or a nurse who is a registered diabetes educator. Refer an individual with acute complications of diabetes, such as hypoglycemia, exercise-related problems, renal disease, autonomic neuropathy, hypertension, or CVD, to a physician.

Nurses learn as much as possible about the individual and the condition of the individual before writing a nutrition prescription. (This requirement is comparable to the physician's need to complete a physical and medical assessment before writing a medication prescription.) The nutrition prescription may be general, but it should reflect the person's therapy goals. The following are some sample orders the nurse might write for the dietitian:

- Individualized diabetic meal plan to achieve clinical goals of diabetes MNT
- MNT to achieve as near-normal blood glucose levels as possible
- Individualized meal plan to improve diabetes control and blood lipid levels
- Diet for improved glycemia and blood pressure measurements

The prescription may be defined further by the registered dietitian with a summary of the planned nutrition intervention. For example, the dietitian might write:

- Weight-reduction meal plan based on general eating guidelines, 1200 to 1500 calories, 3 meals, and 1 snack
- 2300 mg sodium meal plan with weight maintenance
- Carbohydrate-counting meal plan, adjusting carbohydrate and meal timing to achieve target glucose goals

TABLE 11-5 GOALS AND RECOMMENDATIONS OF MEDICAL NUTRITION THERAPY (MNT) FOR INDIVIDUALS WITH TYPE 2 DIABETES

INDEX	GOAL	RECOMMENDATION
A_{1C} (also known as glycated hemoglobin or HbA_{1C})	*For diagnosis must have:* ≥6.5% using method that is NGSP-certified and standardized to DCCT assay	A_{1C} is preferred test to diagnose diabetes in nonpregnant adults; other tests listed below may also be used
FPG (fasting plasma glucose)	≥126 mg/dL (7.0 mmol/L) Fasting is defined as no caloric intake for at least 8 hr	The FPG test detects diabetes and prediabetes. It is most reliable when given in the morning.
2-hr plasma glucose	≥200 mg/dL (11.1 mmol/L) during OGTT	May also be used with WHO-approved method and glucose load of 75 g of anhydrous glucose dissolved in water
Random plasma glucose	≥200 mg/dL (11.1 mmol/L)	In people with classic hyperglycemia or hyperglycemic crisis
A_{1C}	Reasonable A_{1C} goal for many nonpregnant adults is A_{1C} <7%; individualize to ≤6.5% or up to 8% depending on factors such as level of hypoglycemia, life expectancy, duration of disease, and level of CVD	Perform A_{1C} test at least 2 times a year in individuals who are meeting treatment goals and who have stable glycemic control. Lowering A_{1C} is associated with reduction of microvascular complications of diabetes and possibly macrovascular disease
Weight change	For most overweight/obese persons (<35 BMI) recommend modest weight loss (5-7% body weight)	Modest weight loss has been shown to reduce insulin resistance Structure program to emphasize lifestyle changes including education and regular physical activity
MNT	Individuals who have pre-diabetes or diabetes should receive individualized MNT as needed to achieve treatment goals, preferably provided by registered dietitian familiar with components of diabetes MNT; meet body's daily nutritional needs and minimized risk for chronic disease	Modify macronutrient composition to individual and medical condition while meeting DRIs for micronutrients; a variety of meal patterns work (Mediterranean, a lower fat, lower carbohydrate pattern; or vegetarian); saturated fat intake should be <7% of total calories; intake of trans fat should be minimized
Physical activity	If no medication limitations, physical activity distributed over at least 3 days/week with no more than 2 consecutive days without physical activity; encourage person to perform resistance training at least 2 times/week	Physical activity level gradually increased and sustained at target goal To improve glycemic control, assist with weight maintenance, and reduce risk of CVD, at least 150 min/week of moderate-intensity aerobic physical activity (50-70% of maximum heart rate)

Data from American Diabetes Association. (2012). Standards of medical care in diabetes. *Diabetes Care, 35*(1), S11-S63. doi: 10.2337/dc12-s011. Retrieved from http://care.diabetesjournals.org/content/35/Supplement_1/S11. Reprinted with permission from the American Diabetes Association. *BMI,* Body mass index; *CVD,* Cardiovascular disease; *DCCT,* Diabetes Control and Complications Trial; *DRI,* dietary reference intake; *MNT,* medical nutrition therapy; *NGSP,* National Glycohemoglobin Standardization Program; *OGTT,* oral glucose tolerance test.

Human Immunodeficiency Virus (HIV) and Acquired Immunodeficiency Syndrome (AIDS)

Epidemiology

According to the CDC in 2011, 1.2 million adults and adolescents in the United States are living with HIV infection, more than ever before (CDC, 2011e). Approximately 50,000 people are diagnosed with HIV each year. However, reports of new cases have stayed fairly stable because more people are aware they have the virus (80%) and at least 95% appear to modify behaviors that increase risk of transmission. In 2009 approximately 32,000 infected persons progressed to a diagnosis of AIDS, as a result of HIV weakening their immune systems. While many more people are diagnosed earlier, still as many as one third wait until it is too late for effective prevention or treatment and advance to AIDS within 12 months. Just more than 1 million people have been diagnosed with AIDS and nearly 600,000 have died since the beginning of the epidemic. The latest statistics show that 16,000 people died in 2008 alone.

The most severely affected groups include men who have sex with men (MSM), Blacks/African Americans, and Hispanics/Latinos. MSM accounted for 61% of the new cases of HIV infections in 2009 and represented 49% of people living with HIV in 2008 (the most recent prevalence data year). Heterosexuals accounted for 27% of the new diagnoses in 2009, followed by injection drug users at 9%. By gender and race/ethnicity, Black men are the most severely affected (1 in 16), followed by Latino men, and then White men. Among women, Black women have the highest risk (1 in 30), then Latino, and then White. Although all regions of the United States are affected, HIV/AIDS appears to be more prevalent in urban settings with populations greater than 500,000 and in cities such as Miami; Jacksonville, Florida; Baton Rouge, Louisiana; New York; and Washington, DC.

Diet Intervention

Attention to nutrition in early HIV intervention is essential for several reasons. People can now live for decades with HIV/AIDS as long as they are diagnosed and treated early. Even for those people who are HIV positive but diagnosed late, it may still take up to 1 year before most will progress to AIDS. Eating well can improve the sense of well-being, minimize disease symptoms and medicine side effects, and reduce risk of other diseases. For people who are asymptomatic, following the *Dietary Guidelines* recommendations for meal planning and food safety is suggested. Implementation of good dietary habits early in the disease may have benefits for end-stage developments such as severe weight loss. The person diagnosed as HIV positive usually becomes depressed. Depression can lead to loss of appetite; therefore, attention to nutrition is critical as soon as a diagnosis is made.

An initial nutritional assessment is necessary, suggesting the extent to which nutrition counseling is needed and providing valuable baseline information for evaluating the progression of the disease (American Dietetic Association, 2010b). Involving the person's significant others in early discussions of optimal nutrition and food safety is important. A nutrient-dense, protein-rich, well-balanced diet in line with the 2010 *Dietary Guidelines for Americans* should be stressed but also include a vitamin and mineral supplement. Evidence suggests that micronutrient deficiencies are common (zinc, iron, selenium, and vitamin B_{12}) and that those affected persons not taking vitamin supplementation have increased morbidity and mortality (American Dietetic Association, 2010b). Fair evidence also shows that people with HIV infection and their caregivers do not understand how to best avoid food-borne illness. Giving them practical tips as well as reasons to avoid certain foods is helpful (Hoffman et al., 2005). Because of a compromised immune system, persons with HIV/AIDS will become more ill when exposed to food-borne organisms.

The aims of nutrition therapy and counseling specifically for asymptomatic persons who have HIV/AIDS are individualized and based on the following questions:

- Determine how the person appeared physically before becoming HIV positive. Was the person obese or heavily muscled? Was the person a "couch potato" or an athlete? Was the person eating a balanced diet high in vitamins and minerals?
- How many calories does the person need to achieve or maintain a healthy weight? Is the person consuming enough high-quality protein to help maintain or gain healthy muscle mass?
- What does the person know about nutrition and its effect on the disease? What does the person know about food and water safety?
- Does the person know how to use food to ease some of the gastrointestinal side effects of medications (if any)?
- Does the person know or understand the importance of maintaining eating and medication schedules to ensure maximal absorption of medication?

Assess current knowledge when the individual has diabetes or dyslipidemia, and refer as appropriate for teaching about how to manage these conditions within the context of HIV/AIDS.

Breastfeeding should be avoided to prevent vertical transmission of HIV from mother to child. This objective is fairly easy to implement in the United States, which has a long history of safe breast milk substitutes in the form of milk-based and soy-based infant formulas. In many developing countries, however, the risks attached to feeding an infant with something other than breast milk are greater than the 20% risk of vertical transmission of the virus that causes AIDS.

Obesity/Overweight: Estella

Estella is a 34-year-old Hispanic single mother of three sharing a small apartment with her 68-year-old mother in inner-city Los Angeles. She is a full-time laborer in a local manufacturing facility and attends night classes to obtain her medical assistant's license. She is receiving some government assistance but is raising her children, ages 4, 7, and 10, on a meager income. Most days she arrives home too tired to prepare a well-balanced meal for her family and admits to eating a lot of fast foods. Her mother, despite declining vision, works part-time evenings at a local fast food restaurant to help with financial difficulties. Her mother is responsible for most of the preparation of meals. Their diet consists mainly of inexpensive carbohydrates: flour tortillas, breads, pasta, cheese, and potatoes. The family budget does not allow for much fresh fruit or vegetables or expensive meats; therefore, bologna and hot dogs are frequently served.

Estella has recently been hired at a county hospital as a nursing assistant. A required pre-employment physical revealed several health risks. At 5 feet, 4 inches, she weighs 185 pounds. Her resting heart rate and blood pressure are also elevated above normal levels. She has a family history of diabetes and heart disease, her father is deceased from a heart attack at age 55, and her mother has diabetes that requires daily insulin injections. She was referred to her primary care physician, who recommended immediate lifestyle changes including walking 30 minutes per day, 4 to 5 days per week, as well as dietary counseling.

Reflective Questions
1. What is Estella's understanding of healthy eating?
2. How can learning about simple changes in her eating habits affect Estella's weight and risk for type 2 diabetes?
3. What local resources promote inexpensive programs to help Estella lose weight?

Obesity/Overweight: Estella

NURSING DIAGNOSIS: Alteration in current weight related to diet modification and weekly monitoring

Defining Characteristics
* Single mother works full-time and attends night school. Is raising three children and supporting mother on limited income. Income falls into poverty level for family of five.
* Is a divorced woman with limited support system and resources.
* Current weight is 185 pounds at 5 feet, 4 inches tall (84.1 kg, 162.6 cm). Her body mass index calculates to 31.8, including her in the obesity category.
* Resting blood pressure is 164/87 mm Hg and pulse rate is 88 beats/min.
* Father died at age 55 from a massive heart attack.
* Mother is overweight and has type 1 diabetes and high blood pressure.
* Diet consists of processed foods and a high-fat diet with little fresh fruit or vegetables.
* Recent job change requires her to be on her feet, walking, lifting, and transporting care recipients.
* Inner-city neighborhood is unsafe to walk alone or allow children freedom to play outdoors.
* Single mother of three small boys; she realizes the need to improve own health to be able to care for and enjoy her children.

Expected Outcomes
* Estella's overall health will improve by reducing all of the following: weight, BMI, resting pulse rate, and blood pressure measurement.
* Establish realistic goals with Estella to improve quality of meals on a limited income.
* Develop realistic exercise plan that is inexpensive and not time-consuming.

Interventions
* Teach meal planning strategy to include *Dietary Guidelines* basic recommendations for a healthy diet and (as deemed appropriate) refer to a certified diabetes educator or registered dietitian if resources permit.
* Teach Estella easy menus to prepare that substitute more whole grains, fruits, and vegetables and less processed or fast foods. (Resources might include USDA's *CNPP Recipes and Tips for Healthy, Thrifty Meals*.)
* Encourage regular exercise program, beginning with a walking program of 30 minutes per day four to five times per week. Gradually increase pace and distance to intensify aerobic benefits.
* Investigate safe options, such as neighborhood YMCA or park program, for family activities; refer to SNAP or WIC as appropriate; or offer other community resources such as *Share Our Strength's Cooking Matters* courses for low-income adults and children.

SUMMARY

This chapter introduces a wide range of subjects, including the *Healthy People 2020* and *Dietary Guidelines for Americans 2010* nutrition objectives, the most current diet recommendations to reduce the risks of developing nutrition-related diseases, FDA regulations for food labeling, government nutrition assistance programs for the poor and older Americans, and primary and secondary prevention strategies related to the most common nutrition-related chronic diseases. Many more primary prevention strategies are being discussed as an adjunct to secondary prevention in an effort to make all strategies more successful. Together these topics form the basis of what is known as preventive nutrition, a requisite for the promotion of the nation's public health. All of the topics examined in this chapter can be studied further using the Internet. High-quality, up-to-date materials and continuing nutrition education literature for professionals are free and on-line. **Website Resource 11E** discusses the varied sources of nutrition information.

REFERENCES

American Cancer Society. (2009). *Breast cancer facts and figures 2007-2008.* Retrieved from www.cancer.org/downloads/STT/BCFF.final.pdf.

American Diabetes Association. (2012). Standards of medical care in diabetes—2012 (Position Statement). *Diabetes Care, 35*(Suppl. 1), doi: 10.2337/dc12-s011. Retrieved on February 7, 2012, from http://care.diabetesjournals.org/content/35/Supplement_1/S11.

American Dietetic Association. (2009). Position of the American Dietetic Association: Nutrient supplementation. *Journal of the American Dietetic Association, 109,* 2073–2085.

American Dietetic Association. (2010a). Position of the American Dietetic Association: Individualized nutrition approaches for older adults in health care communities. *Journal of the American Dietetic Association, 110,* 1549–1553. Retrieved from doi: 10.1016/j.jada.2010.08.022.

American Dietetic Association. (2010b). Position of the American Dietetic Association: Nutrition intervention and human immunodeficiency virus infection. *Journal of the American Dietetic Association, 110,* 1105–1119.

Appel, L. J., Brands, M. W., Daniels, S. R., Karanja, N., Elmer, P. J., & Sacks, F. M. (2006). Dietary approaches to prevent and treat hypertension: A scientific statement from the American Heart Association. *Hypertension, 47,* 296–308.

Barer-Stein, T. (1979). Multiculturalism and nutrition counselling. *Journal of the Canadian Dietetic Association, 40*(2), 112–116.

Bray, G. A., & Champagne, C. M. (2007). The complexity of obesity: Beyond energy balance. In E. D. Schlenker & S. Long (Eds.), *William's essentials of nutrition & diet therapy* (9th ed.). St. Louis: Mosby.

Brownell, K. (2000). *The LEARN program for weight management 2000.* Dallas: American Health Publishing.

California WIC Association. (2009). *Changes in the WIC food packages: A toolkit for partnering with neighborhood stores.* Co-produced with Public Health Law & Policy (now Change Lab Solutions). Retrieved January 5, 2012, from http://changelabsolutions.org/publications/tool kit-changes-wic-food-packages.

Carpenter, K. J. (2000). *Beriberi, white rice, and vitamin B: A disease, a cause, and a cure.* Berkeley, CA: University of California Press.

Centers for Disease Control and Prevention (CDC). (2004). Diagnosis and management of foodborne illnesses: A primer for physicians and other health care professionals. *Morbidity and Mortality Weekly Report, 53*(RR04), 1–33.

Centers for Disease Control and Prevention (CDC). (2010). *Salmonella.* Retrieved January 31, 2012, from www.cdc.gov/salmonella/general/index.html.

Centers for Disease Control and Prevention (CDC). (2011a). *CDC estimates of foodborne illness in the United States. CDC 2011 findings.* Retrieved January 31, 2012, from www.cdc.gov/foodborneburden/2011-foodborne-estimates.html.

Centers for Disease Control and Prevention (CDC). (2011b). *National diabetes fact sheet: National estimates and general information on diabetes and prediabetes in the United States, 2011.* Atlanta, GA: U.S. Department of Health and Human Services, Centers for Disease Control and Prevention.

Centers for Disease Control and Prevention (CDC). (2011c). *Adult obesity fact sheet, 2011.* Atlanta, GA: U.S. Department of Health and Human Services, Centers for Disease Control and Prevention. Retrieved January 4, 2012, from www.cdc.gov/obesity/data/adult.html.

Centers for Disease Control and Prevention (CDC). (2011d). *Basics about child obesity fact sheet, 2011.* Atlanta, GA: U.S. Department of Health and Human Services, Centers for Disease Control and Prevention. Retrieved January 4, 2012, from www.cdc.gov/obesity/childhood/basics.html.

Centers for Disease Control and Prevention (CDC). (2011e). *HIV in the United States: An overview. Divisions of HIV/AIDS prevention.* Retrieved May 22, 2012, from www.cdc.gov/hiv/topics/surveillance/resources/factsheets/pdf/HIV-US-overview.pdf.

Centers for Disease Control and Prevention (CDC). (2011f). Usual sodium intakes compared with current dietary guidelines—United States, 2005-2008. *Morbidity and Mortality Weekly Report, 60*(41), 1413–1417.

Congressional Research Service. (2011). *Johnson, Renee. The federal food safety system: A primer.* Retrieved January 31, 2012, from www.fas.org/sgp/crs/misc/RS22600.pdf.

Egan, B. M., Zhao, Y., Axon, R. N., Brzezinski, W. A., & Ferdinand, K. C. (2001). *Circulation, 124*(9), 1046–1058.

Expert Panel on Detection, Evaluation, and Treatment of High Blood Cholesterol in Adults. (2001). Executive summary of the third report of the National Cholesterol Education Program (NCEP) Expert Panel on Detection, Evaluation, and Treatment of High Blood Cholesterol in Adults (Adult Treatment Panel III). *Journal of the American Medical Association, 285*(19), 2486–2497.

Fagot-Campagna, A., Pettitt, D. J., Engelgau, M. M., Burrows, N. R., Geiss, L. S., Valdez, R., et al. (2000). Type 2 diabetes among North American children and adolescents: An epidemiologic review and a public health perspective. *Journal of Pediatrics, 136*(5), 664–672.

Fazio, S. (2008). Management of mixed dyslipidemia in patients with or at risk of cardiovascular disease. *Clinical Therapeutics, 30*(2), 294–306.

Flegal, K. M., Carroll, M. D., Ogden, C. L., et al. (2010). Prevalence and trends in obesity among U.S. adults, 1999-2008. *Journal of the American Medical Association, 307*(5), 491–497. doi: 10.1001/jama.2012.39.

Food and Drug Administration (FDA). (2008). *FDA 101-Dietary supplements.* Retrieved February 2, 2012, from www.fda.gov/consumer/updates/supplements080408.html.

Food and Nutrition Service (FNS), & U.S. Department of Agriculture (USDA). (2011). Nutrition standards in the national school lunch and school breakfast programs. Thursday, January 13, 2011/Proposed Rules, *Federal Register, 76*(9). Retrieved January 9, 2012, from http://federal.eregulations.us/fr/notice home/01/13/2011/2011-485.html.

Food Research and Action Center (FRAC). (2011). *A half-empty plate: fruit and vegetable affordability and access challenges in America.* Retrieved January 3, 2011, from http://frac.org/pdf/half_empty_plate_dec2011.pdf.

Gallagher, D., Ruts, E., Visser, M., Heshka, S., Baumgartner, R. N., Wang, J., et al. (2000). Weight stability masks sarcopenia in elderly men and women. *American Journal of Physiology, Endocrinology and Metabolism, 279*(2), E366–E375.

Greer, N., Mosser, G., Logan, G., & Wagstrom Halaas, G. (2000). A practical approach to evidence grading. *The Joint Commission Journal on Quality Improvement, 2000*(26), 700–712.

Grundy, S. M., Cleeman, J. I., Merz, C. N., et al. (2004). Implications of recent clinical trials for the National Cholesterol Education Program Adult Treatment Panel III Guidelines. *Circulation, 110*(2), 227–239.

Hawkins, B. (2007). African American women and obesity: From explanations to prevention. *Journal of African American Studies, 11,* 79–93. doi: 10.1007/s12111-007-9014-5.

Hoffman, E. W., Bergmann, V., Shultz, J. A., Kendall, P., Medeiros, L. C., & Hillers, V. N. (2005). Application of a five-step message development model for food safety education materials targeting people with HIV/AIDS. *Journal of the American Dietetic Association, 105,* 1597–1604.

Institute of Medicine, Koplan, J. P., Liverman, C. T., & Kraak, V. I. (2005). *Preventing childhood obesity: Health in the balance.* Washington, DC: The National Academies Press.

Keener, D., Goodman, K., Lowry, A., Zaro, S., & Kettel Khan, L. (2009). *Recommended community strategies and measurements to prevent obesity in the United States: Implementation and measurement guide.* Atlanta, GA: U.S. Department of Health and Human Services, Centers for Disease Control and Prevention.

Khan, L. K., Sobush, K., Keener, D., Goodman, K., Lowry, A., Kakietek, J., et al. (2009). Recommended community strategies and measurements to prevent obesity in the United States. *Morbidity and Mortality Weekly Report, 58*(RR07), 1–26. Retrieved November 11, 2011, from www.cdc.gov/mmwr/preview/mmwrhtml/rr5807a1.htm?s_cid=rr5807a1_e.

Kittler, P. G., & Sucher, K. P. (2000). *Cultural foods: Traditions and trends.* Belmont, CA: Wadsworth.

Kushi, L. H., Doyle, C., McCullough, M., Rock, C. L., Demark-Wahnefried, W., Bandera, E. V., et al. (2012). American Cancer Society guidelines on nutrition and physical activity for cancer prevention. *CA: A Cancer Journal for Clinicians, 62,* 30–67. Retrieved January 11, 2012, from http://onlinelibrary.wiley.com. doi/10.3322/caac.20140/full.

Lichtenstein, A. H., Appel, L. J., Brands, M., Carnethon, M., Daniels, S., Franch, H. A., et al. (2006). *Diet and lifestyle recommendations revision 2006: A scientific statement from the American Heart Association Nutrition Committee.* Retrieved January 3, 2012, from http://circ.ahajournals.org/cgi/content/full/4304635102.

Lloyd-Jones, D., Adams, R. J., Brown, T. M., et al. (2010). Heart disease and stroke statistics—2010 update. A report from the American Heart Association Statistics Committee and Stroke Statistics Subcommittee. *Circulation, 121,* e1–e170.

Miniño, A. M. (2011). *Death in the United States, 2009.* NCHS data brief, No 64. Hyattsville, MD: National Center for Health Statistics.

National Center for Complementary and Alternative Medicine (NCCAM). (2010). *Using dietary supplements wisely.* Retrieved February 1, 2012, from www.nccam.nih.gov/health/supplements/wiseuse.htm.

National Center for Health Statistics, & Health E-Stat. (2010). *Prevalence of obesity among children and adolescents: United States, trends 1963-1965 through 2007-2008.* Retrieved November 2, 2011, from www.cdc.gov/nchs/data/hestat/obesity_child_07_08/obesity_child_07_08.htm/.

National Center for Health Statistics. (2011). *Health, United States, 2011.* Hyattsville, MD: Author.

National High Blood Pressure Education Program. (2003). *The seventh report of the Joint National Committee on Prevention, Detection, Evaluation, and Treatment of High Blood Pressure.* Retrieved February 12–17, 2012, from www.nhlbi.nih.gov/guidelines/hypertension/jnc7full.pdf.

National Institute of Arthritis and Musculoskeletal and Skin Diseases (NIAMS). (2012a). *Osteoporosis and African American women.* Retrieved January 20, 2012, from www.niams.nih.gov/Health_Info/Bone/Osteoporosis/Background/default.asp.

National Institute of Arthritis and Musculoskeletal and Skin Diseases (NIAMS). (2012b). *Osteoporosis and Hispanic women.* Retrieved January 20, 2012, from www.niams.nih.gov/Health_Info/Bone/Osteoporosis/Background/hispanic_women.asp.

National Institutes of Health, & Office of Dietary Supplements (NIH ODS). (2012). Reliable resources for information about dietary supplements. Retrieved December 14, 2012, from http://ods.nih.gov/News/ ODS-update.aspx.

National Library of Medicine. (2011). *Iron.* Retrieved February 1, 2012, from http://www.nlm.nih.gov/medlineplus/druginfo/natural/912.html.

National Osteoporosis Foundation. (2011). *About osteoporosis: Fast facts.* Retrieved January 20, 2012, from www.nof.org/node/40/.

National Prevention Council. (2011). *National prevention strategy (Healthy Eating section).* Washington, DC: U.S. Department of Health and Human Services, Office of the Surgeon General. Retrieved November 3, 2011, from http://www.healthcare.gov/prevention/nphpphc/strategy/healthy-eating.pdf.

National Research Council. (2006). *Dietary reference intakes: The essential guide to nutrient requirements.* Washington, DC: The National Academies Press. Retrieved February 1, 2012, from www.nap.edu/catalog.php?record_id=11537#toc.

National Research Council. (2010). *Dietary reference intakes for calcium and vitamin D.* Washington, DC: The National Academies Press. Retrieved February 1, 2012, from www.nap.edu/catalog.php?record_id=13050.

Nestle, M. (2002). In *Food politics. Chapter 11: Making health claims legal: The supplement industry's war with the FDA.* Berkeley, CA: University of California Press.

Nesto, R. W. (2005). Beyond low-density lipoprotein, addressing atherogenesis lipid trial in type 2 diabetes mellitus and the metabolic syndrome. *American Journal of Cardiovascular Drugs, 5*(6), 379–387.

Nord, M., Coleman-Jensen, A., Andrews, M., & Carlson, S. (2010). *Household food security in the United States, 2009.* ERR-108, U.S. Department of Agriculture, Economic Research Service. Retrieved January 19, 2012, from www.ers.usda.gov/media/122538/err108_reportsummary_1_.pdf.

Office of Dietary Supplements, & National Institutes of Health. (2012). *Health professional vitamin A fact sheet.* Retrieved July 5, 2012, from http://ods.od.nih.gov/factsheets/VitaminA-Health Professional/.

Ogden, C. L., Carroll, M. D., Curtin, C. L., et al. (2010). Prevalence of obesity and trends in body mass index among U.S. children and adolescents, 1999-2010. *Journal of the American Medical Association, 307*(5), 483–490. doi: 10.1001/jama.2012.40.

Roger, V. L., Go, A. S., Lloyd-Jones, D. M., Benjamin, E. J., Berry, J. D., et al. (2012). On behalf of the American Heart Association Statistics Committee and Stroke Statistics Subcommittee. Heart disease and stroke statistics—2012 update: A report from the American Heart Association. *Circulation.* Published online before print December 15, 2011, at 10.1161/CIR.0b013e31823ac046.

Rosenbaum, D. (2012). SNAP is effective and efficient. *Center on Budget and Policy Priorities.* Retrieved January 15, 2012, from www.cbpp.org/files/7-23-10fa.pdf.

Sanchez-Johnson, L. A.P., Fitzgibbon, M. L., Martinovich, Z., et al. (2004). Ethnic differences in correlates of obesity between Latina-American and Black Women. *Obesity Research, 12,* 652–660.

Snetselaar, L. (2004). Counseling for change. In L. K. Mahan, & S. Escott-Stump (Eds.), *Krause's food, nutrition, and diet therapy* (11th ed., pp. 519–532). St. Louis: Elsevier.

Spark, A. (2001). Health at any size: The size acceptance nondiet movement. *Journal of the American Medical Women's Association, 56*(2), 69–72.

Stallings, V. A., Suitor, C. W., & Taylor, C. L. (2010). *School meals: Building blocks for healthy children*. Washington, DC: Institute of Medicine, National Academies Press.

Taylor, C. L. (2008). *Framework for DRI development: Components "Known" and components "To Be Explored." Background paper*. Washington, DC: Institute of Medicine National Academies. Retrieved February 1, 2012, from http://www.iom.edu/Activities/Nutrition/SummaryDRIs/~/media/Files/Activity%20Files/Nutrition/DRIs/New%20Material/11Bckgrd%20PaperFramework%20for%20DRI%20Devel.

U.S. Census. (2011). Areas with concentrated poverty: 2006-2010. *ACSBR/10-17*. Retrieved December 4, 2012 from http://www.census.gov/prod/www/abs/pop-acs.html.

USA Today Supplement. (2010). *A hunger free America*. Media Planet, September 2010. Retrieved December 4, 2011, from http://doc.mediaplanet.com/all_projects/5537.pdf.

U.S. Department of Agriculture and U.S. Department of Health and Human Services (USDA/USDHHS). (2010). *Dietary guidelines for Americans* (7th ed.). Washington, DC: U.S. Government Printing Office. Retrieved November 1, 2011, from www.health.gov/dietaryguidelines/dga2010/documents/.

U.S. Department of Agriculture, & Center for Nutrition Policy and Promotion (USDA/CNPP). (2010). *MyPlate*. Retrieved November 3, 2011, from www.choosemyplate.gov/.

U.S. Department of Agriculture, & Food and Nutrition Service. (2011a). *WIC nutrition program facts*. Retrieved May 1, 2012, from www.fns.usda.gov/wic/wic-fact-sheet.pdf.

U.S. Department of Agriculture, & Food and Nutrition Service. (2011b). *SNAP basics fact sheet*. Retrieved May 1, 2012, from www.fns.usda.gov/snap/outreach/toolkits/2011/resources/SNAP_Basics_FactSheet.pdf.

U.S. Department of Agriculture, & Food and Nutrition Service. (2011). *July 21, 2011 Audit hearing on farm bill's nutrition programs to House Subcommittee on Nutrition & Horticulture*. Retrieved January 6, 2012, from http://agriculture.house.gov/farmbill/Questionnaire_Nutrition.pdf.

U.S. Department of Agriculture, Food and Nutrition Service, Office of Research and Analysis. (2012). National survey of WIC participants II: Participant characteristics report, by D. M. Geller et al. Project officers: S. G. Kamara, K. Castellanos-Brown, Alexandria, VA. Retrieved May 1, 2012, from www.fns.usda.gov/ora/menu/published/wic/FILES/NSWP-II.pdf.

U.S. Department of Agriculture, & Center for Nutrition Policy and Promotion. (2012). *Evidence Library*. Retrieved December 14, 2012 from http://www.cnpp.usda.gov/NELhtm.

U.S. Department of Health and Human Services. (2010a). *Healthy People 2020*. Retrieved November 2, 2011, from www.healthypeople.gov/2020/topicsobjectives2020/default.aspx.

U.S. Department of Health and Human Services. (2010b). *The Surgeon General's vision for a healthy and fit nation*. Rockville, MD: Author. Retrieved January 4, 2012, from www.surgeongeneral.gov/library/obesityvision/obesityvision2010.pdf.

U.S. Department of Health and Human Services. (2011). *The Surgeon General's call to action to support breastfeeding*. Washington, DC: Author. Retrieved January 5, 2012, from www.surgeongeneral.gov/topics/breastfeeding/calltoactiontosupportbreastfeeding.pdf.

U.S. Department of Health and Human Services, & Administration on Aging. (2009). *Elderly nutrition program fact sheet*. Retrieved May 5, 2012, from www.aoa.gov/AoARoot/Press_Room/Products./pdf/fs_nutrition.doc.

U.S. Department of Health and Human Services, National Institutes of Health, National Heart, & Lung and Blood Institute. (2005). *Your guide to lowering your blood pressure with DASH*. Retrieved from www.nhlbi.nih.gov/health/public/heart/hbp/dash/index.htm.

U.S. Food and Drug Administration. (2008). *FDA 101. Dietary supplements*. Retrieved February 2, 2012, from www.fda.gov/consumer/updates/supplements080408.html.

White House Task Force on Childhood Obesity. (2010). *Solving the problem of childhood obesity within a generation: The White House Task Force on Childhood Obesity Report to the President. May 2010*. Retrieved October 28, 2011, from www.letsmove.gov/sites/letsmove.gov/files/TaskForce_on_Childhood_Obesity_May2010_FullReport.pdf.

World Health Organization. (2006). *Global database on body mass index*. Retrieved from www.who.int/bmi/index.jsp?introPage=intro_3.html.

12

Exercise

Kevin Chui, Gary Austin, Roseanne Prunty, Michael Fortin, and Brian Pecchia

evolve WEBSITE

http://evolve.elsevier.com/Edelman/
- Study Questions
- Glossary
- Website Resource
  12A: Major Coronary Risk Factors

OBJECTIVES

After completing this chapter, the reader will be able to:
- Explain the physical activity and fitness goals of *Healthy People 2010* and *Healthy People 2020*, and the progress made toward these goals.
- Describe how physical activity positively influences physical and psychological health.
- Identify the benefits of physical activity throughout the aging process.
- Evaluate the prescriptions for and benefits of daily physical activity, aerobic exercise, and resistance training.
- Explain the interventions to promote exercise adherence and compliance.

KEY TERMS

Aerobic exercise
Anaerobic exercise
Borg Scale
Cardiorespiratory fitness
Cool-down period
Cross-training
Exercise

Fat mass
Fibromyalgia syndrome
Flexibility
Muscular fitness
Obesity
Osteoporosis
Physical activity

Physical fitness
Relaxation response (RR)
Resistance training
Rheumatoid arthritis (RA)
Tai chi
Warm-up period
Yoga

? THINK ABOUT IT

Knowing Versus Doing

Having the knowledge about the benefits of exercise does not correlate well with long-term exercise compliance. Confidence in the ability to exercise and a sense of the meaning and purpose (core desire) of exercise in life ensure better success.

- What motivates putting the effort into developing and maintaining an active lifestyle?
- Why is being active and physically fit important?

Regular physical activity and exercise enhance both physical and psychological health. Generally people who exercise regularly, or those who naturally include physical activity in their daily routine, feel better mentally and physically, improve their health profiles, and safeguard their functional independence as they go through the aging process. A holistic approach to physical activity involves exercise for cardiorespiratory health (endurance), exercise for musculoskeletal health (strength, flexibility, and bone density), and body awareness. Body awareness and mindfulness during exercise facilitate self-inquiry and self-acceptance, helping to relieve psychological stress and preventing physical injury (Box 12-1). Not only is an active lifestyle an important component of primary prevention, but regular physical activity is also an essential modality in the treatment of chronic disease, which establishes the potential for benefit in all aspects of the biopsychosocial and spiritual model of health.

DEFINING PHYSICAL ACTIVITY IN HEALTH

To fully understand the *Healthy People 2020* objectives regarding exercise, the following definitions will be used:

Physical activity: body movement that is produced by the contraction of skeletal muscles and that substantially increases energy expenditure; includes transportation and vocational and leisure-time activity. Leisure-time activity can be further categorized into sports, recreational activities, and exercise training (Figure 12-1).

Exercise (exercise training): planned, structured, and repetitive body movement performed to improve or maintain one or more components of physical fitness.

Aerobic exercise: activity that uses large muscle groups in a repetitive, rhythmic fashion over an extended period to improve the efficiency of the oxidative energy-producing system and improve cardiorespiratory endurance; uses stored adipose tissue as a major fuel source.

Anaerobic exercise: high-intensity, short-duration activity that improves the efficiency of the phosphocreatine and glycolytic energy-producing systems and increases muscle strength, power, and speed of reactivity; uses phosphagens and glucose-glycogen as major fuel sources.

Physical fitness: a set of attributes (cardiorespiratory fitness, muscular fitness, and flexibility) that people have or achieve that relates to the ability to perform physical activity without undue fatigue or risk of injury.

Muscular fitness: the strength and endurance of muscles that allows for participation in daily activities with low risk of musculoskeletal injury.

Flexibility: adequate muscle length and joint mobility to allow free and painless movement through a wide range of motion (ROM).

HEALTHY PEOPLE 2020 OBJECTIVES

Unfortunately, only 23% of the adult population performs enough regular, sustained exercise to gain any significant health benefit, and slightly more than 10% of the population exercises at an intensity necessary to promote cardiorespiratory fitness. According to the Physical Activity and Fitness section (focus area) of *Healthy People 2020*, overall 36.2% of adults 18 years and older report no leisure-time physical activity (U.S. Department of Health and Human Services [USDHHS], 2010). Furthermore, the percentage of adults who report no leisure-time physical activity varies by race and ethnicity, gender, educational level, geographical location, disability status, age group, and presence or absence of arthritis symptoms. The tendency to be sedentary, unfortunately, continues to increase with age and affects all of the body's systems such as the cutaneous, cardiovascular, respiratory, gastrointestinal, and urinary systems. As a result of being sedentary,

---

BOX 12-1 HEALTH IMPACT OF PHYSICAL ACTIVITY

- Improves quality of life
- Improves mood and promotes a sense of well-being
- Improves flexibility
- Builds muscle strength
- Increases endurance
- Increases the efficiency of the heart
- Increases bone density
- Helps with weight reduction
- Decreases risk of stroke
- Decreases risk of heart disease
- Decreases risk for diabetes

FIGURE 12-1 Some people choose more vigorous types of exercise.

♥ BOX 12-2   HEALTHY PEOPLE 2020

Objectives for Physical Activity

- Reduce the proportion of adults who engage in no leisure-time physical activity.
- Increase the proportion of adults who meet current federal physical activity guidelines for aerobic physical activity and for muscle-strengthening activity.
- Increase the proportion of adolescents who meet current federal physical activity guidelines for aerobic physical activity and for muscle-strengthening activity.
- Increase the proportion of the nation's public and private schools that require daily physical education for all students.
- Increase the proportion of adolescents who participate in daily school physical education.
- Increase regularly scheduled elementary school recess in the United States.
- Increase the proportion of school districts that require or recommend elementary school recess for an appropriate period of time.
- Increase the proportion of children and adolescents who do not exceed recommended limits for screen time.
- Increase the number of states with licensing regulations for physical activity provided in child care.
- Increase the proportion of the nation's public and private schools that provide access to their physical activity spaces and facilities for all persons outside of normal school hours (that is, before and after the school day, on weekends, and during summer and other vacations).
- Increase the proportion of physician office visits that include counseling or education related to physical activity.
- (Developmental) Increase the proportion of employed adults who have access to and participate in employer-based exercise facilities and exercise programs.
- (Developmental) Increase the proportion of trips made by walking.
- (Developmental) Increase the proportion of trips made by bicycling.
- (Developmental) Increase legislative policies for the built environment that enhance access to and availability of physical activity opportunities.

From U.S. Department of Health and Human Services. (2010). Washington, DC.

the risk of premature morbidity, mortality, impairment, functional limitation, and disability increases.

The goal of the Physical Activity and Fitness focus area is to "improve health, fitness, and quality of life through physical activity" (USDHHS, 2010). In 2008, the USDHHS released the first-ever publication of national guidelines for physical activity, *Physical Activity Guidelines for Americans* (PAG) (USDHHS, 2008). The *Guidelines* provide an evidence-based approach to assist Americans to improve their health status. They recommend that children be active at least 60 minutes daily and advise adults to perform at least 150 minutes of moderate-intensity or 75 minutes of vigorous activity per week. More than 80% of adults do not meet the guidelines for both aerobic and muscle-strengthening activities. The importance of physical activity in the nation's health is reflected in the 15 physical activity and fitness objectives (USDHHS, 2010), a number of objectives which now emphasize traditional and nontraditional partnerships. These objectives take into account the demonstrated relationship between physical activity and an improvement in the biological markers associated with health, and they identify the reasons for the trend toward a more sedentary lifestyle. The National Physical Activity Plan has a vision that all Americans will be physically active in all aspects of their life, which include work and play (National Physical Activity Plan, 2010). Box 12-2: *Healthy People 2020* provides a summary of the updated physical activity objectives set for 2020.

Physical Activity Objectives: Making Progress

The review of *Healthy People 2010* (USDHHS, 2010) provides evidence of the progress that has been made toward achieving the original objectives. According to the *State Indicator Report on Physical Activity, 2010* (Behavioral Indicators), the U.S. national weighted percentage of adults who reported no leisure-time activity is 25.4%, for those physically active it is 64.5%, and for those highly active it is 43.5% (CDC, 2010a). Data from students in grades 9 to 12 indicate that 17.1% are physically active

and 30.3% have daily physical education. However, despite solid gains (indicating that the message regarding the benefits of physical activity is reaching some segments of the population), the improvements fall short of the objectives set for the year 2010. The new goals set for *Healthy People 2020* reflect the work that remains (USDHHS, 2010).

The prevalence of overweight children and adolescents and overweight and obese adults has increased in the United States and is considered an epidemic. Children and adolescents are categorized as being overweight if their body mass index (BMI), expressed as weight/height^2, is equal to or greater than the 95th percentile of age- and gender-specific BMI growth charts. According to results from the 2009-2010 National Health and Nutrition Examination Survey (NHANES), which is conducted by CDC's National Center for Health Statistics, 12.1%, 18.0%, and 18.4% of children and adolescents 2 to 5, 6 to 11, and 12 to 19 years of age, respectively, were overweight, which represents 5.5 million girls and 7 million boys (Ogden et al., 2012). These recent data are similar to data from 2003 to 2004 in which 13.9%, 18.8%, and 17.4% of children and adolescents 2 to 5, 6 to 11, and 12 to 19 years of age, respectively, were overweight (Flegal et al., 2006). While there was no change in the prevalence of obesity among children and adolescents from 2007-2008 to 2009-2010 for either gender, there is a significant increasing linear trend from 1999-2000 to 2009-2010 for boys but not girls.

Adults, those 20 years of age or older, are considered overweight if their BMI is 25.0 to 29.9, obese if their BMI is 30.0 or higher, and extremely obese if their BMI is 40 or higher. According to results from the 2009-2010 NHANES, 35.7% of adults age 20 or older were obese, which represents 40.6 million women and 37.5 million men (Ogden et al., 2012). This represents an increase from the 2003-2004 NHANES data in which 32.9% of adults 20 years or older were obese (Ogden et al., 2006). In the 2009-2010 NHANES data there was a significant increasing linear trend by age (for both genders) with 32.6%, 36.6%, and 39.7% of adults 20 to 39, 40 to 59, and 60 years and older, respectively, being obese (Ogden et al., 2012). There was also a significant increasing linear trend in obesity for women with increasing age. While there was no change in the prevalence of obesity among adults from 2007-2008 to 2009-2010 for either gender, there is a significant increasing linear trend from 1999-2000 to 2009-2010 for men but not women.

The number of adults who combine good dietary practice with regular physical activity in an attempt to attain an appropriate body weight has decreased. This decidedly negative trend may be related to the decline in physical activity in the schools. According to the CDC (2010a) 33.3% of adolescents participated in daily school physical education in 2009 (see objectives PA-5) and the target for *Healthy People 2020* is 36.6% (USDHHS, 2010).

In a study that tracked physical activity over time using data from the Trois-Rivières Growth and Development Study, there was a significant but weak correlation between adult and childhood physical activity (Trudeau et al., 2004). In a similar type of study based on data from the National Longitudinal Study of Adolescent Health, increased physical activity during adolescence decreased the likelihood of young adults being overweight (Menschik et al., 2008). Using data from the Canadian Physical Activity Longitudinal Study, researchers reported that previous cardiorespiratory fitness (Vo$_2$max) and previous BMI measurements are significant predictors of future weight gain and obesity in adults (Brien et al., 2007). Finally, a recent meta-analysis explored the different mechanisms through which physical activity during adolescence benefits adult health, such as reducing morbidity (Hallal et al., 2006).

If a standard is to be set for the importance of physical activity throughout the life span, it needs to start with children, who have the potential to develop lifelong healthy habits.

As the health care system moves toward a preventive model, primary care providers must facilitate a wellness attitude in their care recipients, which involves not only encouraging individuals to be physically active but also leading by example. Recommending regular exercise and espousing the benefits from personal experience can have a significant influence on individual involvement. Health care practitioners are in a position to inquire about and provide counseling for exercise habits of their care recipients. For example, for each of the *Preferred Physical Therapist Practice Patterns* (musculoskeletal, neuromuscular, cardiovascular/pulmonary, and integumentary), the first corresponding pattern is primary prevention/risk reduction. Although some progress has been made in providing preventive care to reduce risk, data indicate a shortfall in reaching the goal set for 2010 of 50% of the population (USDHHS, 2006). Although there has been some improvement in some areas, overall the proportion of the population reporting physical activity has remained essentially unchanged and progress is limited. Obviously the progress that has been made toward physical activity objectives for the year 2010 does not reflect a significant shift in the attitude of the general population or the health care profession. There are still populations at greater risk for obesity based on race/ethnicity (Whitson et al., 2011); school type, public versus private (Li & Hooker, 2010); and socioeconomic status (Balistreri & Hook, 2011; Scharoun-Lee et al., 2009) (Box 12-3).

Aging

The biological changes attributed to aging closely resemble the effects of physical inactivity. The list for both aging and inactivity includes an increase in body fat and a decrease in all of the following: aerobic capacity, muscle mass (sarcopenia), metabolic rate, strength and flexibility, bone mass, sexual function, mental performance, immune function, and sleep quality.

Among older adults, exercise can improve health, prevent disability and hospitalizations, improve blood lipid profiles, and reduce body fat. According to the 2010 United States census, the 65 and older population has grown to 40.3 million people, an increase of 15% since 2000 (U.S. Census Bureau, 2011). By 2030, the number of people 65 years or older in the United States will reach 71 million (CDC, 2008). Exercise is especially important for older women, who comprise the majority of the older population, because it may help prevent osteoporosis (Hamilton et al., 2010) and reduce fracture risk as part of a multidimensional approach (Perry & Downey, 2012).

By exercising, older people can improve levels of cardiovascular, cardiopulmonary, and metabolic functions, including muscle performance and aerobic capacity. Several researchers have reported significant improvements in strength (Candow et al., 2011), physical performance such as gait speed (Chou et al., 2012), flexibility (Marquard et al., 2012), self-efficacy (Park et al., 2011), quality of life (McGrath et al., 2010), balance (Rose & Hernandez, 2010), continence (Shamliyan et al., 2008), and the ability to live independently (Cowan et al., 2009). Additional resources are available that discuss exercise prescription considerations and guidelines for the older adult (American College of Sports Medicine, 2009; Chodzko-Zajko et al., 2009; Elsawy & Higgins, 2010; Liu et al., 2011; McDermott & Mernitz, 2006; O'Donovan et al., 2010).

Older adults in particular need to be concerned with their nutritional status since the potential for malnutrition, a common problem for older adults, is associated with a decline in muscle strength and thus poorer outcomes, such as decreased function (Bauer et al., 2008; Henwood et al., 2012; Jones et al., 2009; Morgan, 2012; Tarnopolsky, 2008; Walrand et al., 2011).

The health of the musculoskeletal system depends on movement and activity. Bone is a dynamic tissue, constantly changing and adapting to the stresses to which it is subjected. Bone strength depends on stresses applied by muscular and weight-bearing activity (mechanical stress during active movement). Exercise may improve or maintain bone mineral density (BMD), but recent meta-analytic data suggest that the effects of exercises on BMD may depend on the mode of exercise, body part, combination of exercises (mixed loading), and other (e.g., pharmacological, tai chi) concurrent treatments (Alperson & Berger, 2011; Guadalupe-Grau et al., 2009; Howe et al., 2011; Martyn-St James & Carroll, 2009). To stay healthy, joints must do what they are designed to do—move and bear weight. The health of the cartilage covering the joint surfaces is vital for maintaining proper joint function. The only way the cartilage can receive nourishment is through the manufacture and distribution of synovial fluid, which delivers nutrients, removes waste products, and lubricates joint surfaces. Movement is vital for creating this environment of blood and lymph in and out of joint structures and the adjacent soft tissues. Without the stress of weight-bearing activity, normal bone and cartilage metabolism and repair become dysfunctional, resulting in injury and disease.

Effects of Exercise on the Aging Process

Everyone needs physical activity to be healthy. Human physiology has evolved in preparation for physical exertion. Until recently, survival through the vigor of daily living depended on a moderate degree of physical fitness. However, with mechanization and the style of living in today's society, daily life has become too sedentary. A lifestyle of inactivity places the population at risk for mortality and morbidity, and the literature supports exercise as an essential element of health.

Regular physical activity can help maintain functional independence and improve the quality of life throughout the aging process (Figure 12-2). Physical and psychological benefits of increased physical activity have been documented widely in healthy and in chronically ill older adults (Arne et al., 2009; CDC, 2011; Dogra, 2011; Lin et al., 2010; Liu-Ambrose et al., 2010). Unfortunately, less than 20% of older adults engage in physical activity (USDHHS, 2008). According to the CDC (2011), older adults require at least 2 hours and 30 minutes of moderate-intensity aerobic activity weekly, as well as muscle strengthening on 2 or more days a week. Considerable research has tested interventions to increase activity by younger adults and by populations of all ages. Interventions' research with older adults is being reported more frequently. The most common interventions are self-monitoring, general health education, goal setting, supervised center-based exercise, problem solving, feedback reinforcement, and relapse prevention education. A few studies have examined multicomponent cognitive-behavioral group intervention (Rixt Zijlstra et al., 2009; Zijlstra et al., 2009). Lifestyle activity in an older adult recommends the accumulation of minutes of physical activity spread over the entire day. Some evidence suggests the potential beneficial effects of lifestyles activity and the probability that

FIGURE 12-2 In some countries bicycles are the main source of transportation and exercise.

some aging adults may be more receptive to lifestyle activity changes that include episodic exercise (Rixt Zijlstra et al., 2009).

CARDIAC RISK FACTORS

The literature strongly demonstrates that the risk of coronary heart disease (CHD) decreases as physical activity increases and that a plausible relationship between the decreased risk and a number of potential physiological and metabolic mechanisms exists (Berger et al., 2008; Keller et al., 2007):

- Increasing levels of high-density lipoprotein (HDL) cholesterol
- Decreasing levels of low-density lipoprotein (LDL) cholesterol
- Decreasing serum triglyceride (TRG) levels
- Decreasing high blood pressure
- Improving glucose tolerance and insulin sensitivity
- Decreasing obesity; altering distribution of body fat
- Reducing the sensitivity of the myocardium to the effects of catecholamines, thereby decreasing the risk of ventricular arrhythmias
- Enhancing fibrinolysis and altering platelet function

See **Website Resource 12A** for descriptions of major coronary risk factors.

High-Density Lipoprotein and Serum Triglyceride Levels

Exercise has a major influence on lipoprotein metabolism, primarily affecting plasma levels of HDL and TRG. There is a strong negative correlation between CHD and plasma HDL levels. Increases in HDL level lower the total cholesterol-to-HDL ratio, thereby reducing CHD risk. Exercise, a common part of treatment for hypertriglyceridemia, may have a lowering effect on TRG levels (Oh & Lanier, 2007; Pejic & Lee, 2006; Yuan et al., 2007). A recent meta-analysis of randomized controlled trials examined the effects of progressive resistance training on adults and found significant reductions in total cholesterol levels; the ratio of total cholesterol to HDL level; and the levels of non-HDL, LDL, and TRG (Kelley & Kelley, 2009). A similar systemic review examined exercise in obese children and found that aerobic exercise improved LDL and TRG concentrations and combined exercise (aerobic fitness, strength, and flexibility training) improved the HDL concentration (Escalante et al., 2012). In another study of obese children, exercise significantly lowered total cholesterol, TRG, LDL, very-LDL, and insulin levels and significantly increased HDL levels when compared to the (nonexercising) control group (Zorba et al., 2011).

The effect of exercise on lipid metabolism may be related more to the volume (duration and frequency) than to the intensity of the exercise. In a recent systematic review by Tambalis and colleagues (2009), the authors reviewed the literature for responses in the levels of blood lipids to a variety of modes and volumes of exercise. Moderate-intensity aerobic exercise training (less than 60% Vo$_2$max or six metabolic equivalents [METs]) appears to have the greatest effect on HDL levels. However, stronger evidence supported that high-intensity aerobic training promotes significant increases in HDL levels. This was observed among a wide range of 90 to 200 minutes per week. Resistance training supported a marked reduction in LDL levels, followed by a significant reduction in total cholesterol levels. The review found combining resistance and aerobic exercise can lead to remarkable improvements in LDL levels, significant increases in HDL levels, and significant decreases in total cholesterol levels (Tambalis et al., 2009).

Hypertension

The American College of Sports Medicine (ACSM, 2009b) and the American Heart Association (Braith & Stewart, 2006) recommend resistance training in the prevention and treatment of hypertension (HTN) (Box 12-4). Furthermore, the American College of Sports Medicine (Pescatello et al., 2004) summarizes evidence, of varying degrees, that supports the use of physical activity, dynamic aerobic training, dynamic exercise, and resistance training to decrease blood pressure in adults. Their summary of the evidence supports regular endurance exercise to decrease blood pressure in older adults. There was no evidence to support a different blood pressure response to exercise between genders and different ethnicities.

ACSM recommends endurance training to include aerobic activities with use of large muscle groups on most days of the week for 30 minutes or more (ACSM, 2009b). Low- to moderate-intensity aerobic exercise also appears to be effective in lowering blood pressure (Cornelissen et al., 2009; Hua et al., 2009; Roussel et al., 2009). Mechanisms underlying the exercise-training effect on lowering blood pressure are not completely clear but may involve attenuation of sympathetic nervous system activity. This attenuation results in the dilation of peripheral blood vessels, which decreases systemic vascular resistance. Decreasing sympathetic nervous system activity may have a beneficial effect on the insulin resistance that is often observed in hypertensive people. The literature has also uncovered significant effects of both interval and continuous training between 45 and 60 minutes on systolic and diastolic blood pressure measurements (Lamina, 2010). A recent study by Fagard (2011) performed a review of the current literature and found

inconclusive evidence about exercise intensity and its effect on blood pressure. This study observed two exercise groups, low intensity (33% of heart rate reserve) and high intensity (66% of heart rate reserve), performed three times a week for 1-hour sessions each. The results revealed that systolic blood pressure decreases with both intensities but diastolic blood pressure decreases significantly after higher intensity exercise (Fagard, 2011).

Hyperinsulinemia and Glucose Intolerance

Hyperinsulinemia and glucose intolerance account for the various types of diabetes. Diabetes mellitus (DM) encompasses a group of metabolic disorders that have in common an increase in blood glucose levels and associated metabolic dysfunction. Type 1 involves elevated blood glucose levels that are a result of a deficiency of circulating insulin caused by destruction of the pancreatic β cells, and type 2 diabetes involves elevated blood glucose levels from insulin resistance (decreased insulin sensitivity)—largely in skeletal muscles—or impaired insulin secretion. Approximately 90% to 95% of those with diabetes have type 2 diabetes. In addition, adiposity and poor fitness are linked with insulin resistance (Larson-Meyer et al., 2010). Complications of diabetes include heart disease and stroke, peripheral arterial disease, retinopathy, nephropathy, peripheral neuropathy, and lower-extremity amputation (Deshpande et al., 2008).

Exercise, in addition to diet, represents a first-line intervention for diabetes (Gulve, 2008). A recent randomized control trial by Belli and colleagues (2011) examined the effects of 12-week overground walking training in persons with type 2 diabetes. The exercise group performed walking at the ventilatory threshold velocity. When compared to the control group, the exercise group had significant improvements in hemoglobin A$_{1C}$ (HbA$_{1C}$) levels (glycemic control), body composition (body mass and BMI), and exercise capacity (peak oxygen uptake and exercise duration). Marcus and colleagues (2008) compared the effects of aerobic exercise with a combination of aerobic and high-force eccentric resistance exercise over the course of 16 weeks in persons with type 2 diabetes. Both groups had a significant decrease in HbA$_{1C}$ levels, decrease in amount of intramuscular fat, and increase in 6-minute walk distance, with no between-group differences. The aerobic and high-force eccentric resistance exercise group also had a significant gain in lean tissue and greater decrease in BMI when compared to the aerobic exercise group (Box 12-5: Diversity Awareness).

In addition, several recent meta-analyses examined the effects of different modes of exercise on glycemic control. Strasser and colleagues (2010) examined the effect of resistance training with abnormal glucose metabolism and found significant improvements in glycemic control with a mean HbA$_{1C}$ reduction of 0.48%. Irvine and Taylor (2009) found the following results in persons with type 2 diabetes: progressive resistance exercise resulted in a significant reduction in HbA$_{1C}$ level of 0.3% when compared to a (nonexercising) control group; there was no difference in HbA$_{1C}$ levels between resistance and aerobic exercise groups; and progressive resistance exercise resulted in significant improvements in strength when compared to aerobic and control groups. Chudyk and Patrella (2011) reported

BOX 12-4   RESISTIVE TRAINING EXERCISES

Chest Press (Figures 1 and 2)

a. Lie on bench with feet flat on bench, or lie on the floor with knees bent and feet flat, whichever is more comfortable.

b. Hold weights near shoulders with elbows out and palms facing away from body.

c. Exhale while extending arms straight up, following an "A" pattern with weights touching at peak.

d. Slowly lower weights back to original position while inhaling.

e. Repeat 8 to 12 times.

Chest Fly (Figures 3 and 4)

a. Lie on bench with feet flat on bench, or lie on the floor with knees bent and feet flat, whichever is more comfortable.

b. With palms facing each other, extend arms above chest, keeping elbows slightly bent at all times.

c. Inhale and lower arms perpendicularly away from body until arms are out of peripheral vision.

d. Exhale while returning to starting position by visualizing arms hugging a barrel that is lying on the chest.

e. Repeat 8 to 12 times.

Bent Over Row (Figures 5 and 6)

a. Bend at waist while supporting body with one hand (on table, bench, etc.) and holding weight with other in an overhand grip.

b. Keep knees bent while weight is hanging perpendicular to torso.

c. Slowly pull weight up to chest as if starting a lawn mower, exhaling and keeping elbow away from body.

d. Slowly lower weight back to starting position while inhaling.

e. Repeat 8 to 12 times on each side.

Dumbbell Curl (Figures 7 and 8)

a. Stand or sit with weights held at sides in an underhand grip, keeping elbows close to body and upper arms stationary.

b. Curl weight to chin or upper chest while exhaling.

c. Inhale while slowly lowering weights.

d. Keep back straight through duration of motion.

e. Repeat 8 to 12 times.

BOX 12-4   RESISTIVE TRAINING EXERCISES—cont'd

Triceps Extension (Figures 9 and 10)

a. While seated or standing in neutral back position, lift hand holding weight straight above head and in alignment with ear.

b. Keeping upper arm tight, slowly bend elbow to lower weight between shoulder blades.

c. Use free hand to support elbow and to prevent movement in upper arm.

d. Raise weight back to its original position by straightening arm and exhaling.

e. Repeat 8 to 12 times on each side.

⊕ BOX 12-5   DIVERSITY AWARENESS

Walk Away from Ethnic Glucose Intolerance

The Pima Indians of the Gila River Indian Community in Arizona have the highest documented incidence rates of type 2 diabetes in the world. On the island of Mauritius in the southwest Indian Ocean, all four ethnic groups (Hindu and Muslim Asian Indians, African Creoles, and Chinese) have unusually high rates of type 2 diabetes. In the United States, type 2 diabetes is 30% more prevalent in Blacks than in Whites. The presence of type 2 diabetes in each of these ethnic groups provides strong support for the existence of one or more modifiable risk factors in the cause of the disease.

Excessive weight gain is a strong independent predictor of type 2 diabetes. The development of type 2 diabetes (characterized by insulin resistance, hyperinsulinemia, and glucose intolerance) is related to weight gain in adults, particularly to fat accumulation around the waist, abdomen, and upper body (android or apple shape). This type of fat distribution is also associated with a higher risk of developing CHD. Adipose tissue is a major site for insulin insensitivity, and most obese individuals have increased insulin resistance or some degree of glucose intolerance, or both.

Physical activity has an important role in the prevention and treatment of type 2 diabetes. By helping to maintain a proper lean-to-fat body mass, either by losing weight or by preventing weight gain, physical activity may indirectly protect against the development of type 2 diabetes. The modulating effect of physical activity on fat stores helps to improve insulin sensitivity and glucose tolerance. Additionally, physical activity may directly affect glucose metabolism. The acute effect of exercise can lower plasma glucose levels by enhancing the effect of insulin; long-term exercise improves insulin action and glucose tolerance.

Epidemiological studies of ethnic groups indicate that physical inactivity is also a risk factor for type 2 diabetes. In the United States, Blacks and Native Americans have a disproportionate number of poor, unemployed, and disadvantaged individuals who lack access to the health care system. The least active individuals within these populations should be given the most attention, because they have the most to gain. The methods and programs that are used to relay information to the public on the importance of physical activity need to be varied, depending on the socioeconomic and cultural factors specific to ethnic populations. Promotion of physical activity by schools, communities, and government and health agencies, with these factors in mind, will significantly help achieve the goal of improving lifestyles and decreasing the incidence of type 2 diabetes.

that aerobic exercise alone or combined with resistance training significantly reduced HbA$_{1C}$ levels, systolic blood pressure readings, and triglyceride levels in persons with type 2 diabetes. Furthermore, waist circumference was significantly reduced only when aerobic exercise and resistance training were combined.

During physical activity, contracting skeletal muscles work with insulin to enhance glucose uptake into the cells (Turcotte & Fisher, 2008). Insulin resistance impedes glucose mobilization into cells, increasing plasma glucose levels and setting the potential for developing type 2 diabetes. Although insulin resistance in skeletal muscles may be the primary defect, the development of disease appears to be related to elevated insulin levels, a result of the body's response to the need to mobilize glucose into the cells. Additionally, this syndrome often also involves elevated TRG levels and HTN, which contribute to the potential for disease. Exercise increases insulin sensitivity, improves the inherent effect of endogenous insulin, decreases obesity, and plays a role in lowering TRG levels and blood pressure; therefore, it is recommended

in the management of type 2 diabetes (Gulve, 2008; Polikandrioti & Dokoutsidou, 2009; Waryasz & McDermott, 2010; Weltman et al., 2009). With diet, weight control, and exercise, preventing or decreasing the need for oral antiglycolytic agents and insulin is possible while maintaining normal blood glucose levels. Physical activity may be most beneficial in preventing the progression of type 2 diabetes during the earlier stages of the disease process, before insulin therapy is required. Overall, physical activity has a significant positive effect on a chronic disease that is associated with a high risk of developing CHD.

OBESITY

Overweight and **obesity** are conditions of excess body fat (adipose tissue). Adults are considered overweight if their BMI is 25.0 to 29.9 and obese if their BMI is 30.0 or higher. Furthermore, the ACSM (Wallace & Ray, 2009) considers those with a BMI of 40 or higher as being extremely obese.

Obesity may also be defined as body weight that is equal to or greater than 120% to 125% of the ideal body weight. Fat mass (body fat percentage) is also important in determining the ideal body weight. The recommended body fat levels for men and women are approximately 15% to 16% for men and 23% to 24% for women (ACSM, 2009b). The average American man and woman tend to exceed the recommended body fat level. An increase in fat mass and the development of obesity occur when energy intake exceeds total daily energy expenditure for a prolonged period. Decreased physical activity may be both a cause and a consequence of weight gain over a lifetime.

The prevalence of obesity, as well as overweight and extreme obesity, is typically reported based on BMI values, as is the case with the National Health and Nutrition Examination Survey (NHANES). Unfortunately, the prevalence of obesity in the United States remains high and has been increasing. According to the most recent NHANES (Ogden et al., 2012), in the 2009 to 2010 timeframe, the age-adjusted prevalence of obesity was 35.5% in men and 35.8% in women. And in the United States, no state has met the nation's *Healthy People 2010* goal to lower obesity prevalence to 15%. The number of states with an obesity prevalence of 30% or more has actually increased from none in 2000 to nine states in 2009, including Alabama, Arkansas, Kentucky, Louisiana, Mississippi, Missouri, Oklahoma, Tennessee, and West Virginia (CDC, 2010b).

According to the 2009-2010 National Health and Nutrition Examination Survey, the prevalence of obesity in women exceeds that of men in ethnic groups of Non-Hispanic Black, Hispanic, and Mexican American. Furthermore, the prevalence of obesity differs by racial/ethnic group for female adults only. That is, adult females of Mexican American (44.9%), Hispanic (41.4%), and non-Hispanic Black (58.5%) racial/ethnic backgrounds have a greater prevalence of obesity than do those of non-Hispanic White (32.2%) background. In contrast, the prevalence of obesity is comparable for males of Mexican American (36.6%), Hispanic (37.0%), non-Hispanic Black (38.8%), and non-Hispanic White (36.2%) racial/ethnic backgrounds.

Several studies have related increased fat mass and reduced physical activity to risk of cardiovascular disease and overall mortality (Larson-Meyer, 2010). Both obesity and decreased activity are related to insulin resistance, elevated blood pressure, and elevated total and LDL cholesterol concentrations; all of which improve with weight loss and fitness (Larson-Meyer, 2010). Nevertheless, obesity should be considered an independent target for intervention in health promotion. Being overweight and obese are major contributors to many preventable causes of death. On average, higher body weights are associated with higher death rates (USDHHS, 2000).

Maintaining fitness and health is closely related to controlling weight. Literature supports the positive influence that physical activity has on body weight and obesity. A recent meta-analysis concluded that exercise produced weight loss in people who were overweight or obese (Shaw et al., 2006). In fact, when compared to a control group (no treatment), the meta-analytic data show that exercise alone produced favorable changes in body weight, BMI, diastolic blood pressure, serum triglycerides, serum HDL, and fasting serum glucose. A more recent meta-analysis examined the effect of exercise on body composition in menopausal women (Yeh et al., 2011). Results showed a significant improvement (decrease) in weight, BMI, and body fat measures in menopausal women who exercised.

Physical activity does the following:
- Promotes a negative energy balance (burns calories)
- Increases metabolic rate for an extended period after the activity
- Increases metabolic efficiency for burning calories by increasing lean body mass
- Helps counteract the decrease in metabolic rate associated with low-calorie diets by preserving lean body mass
- Is a good alternative to eating when eating is a response to stress rather than to hunger

Unfortunately, most overweight people ignore exercise as a means of weight loss or they exercise at rates below federal health guidelines (CDC, 2010a).

Management of obesity involves a comprehensive program of nutrition management, behavior modification, and physical activity or exercise. The key to normalizing body fatness is long-term adherence and permanent lifestyle changes, not dieting or short-term exercise trials.

Increasingly sophisticated obesity treatments that demonstrate the best outcomes emphasize five components: behavioral techniques, cognitive strategies, social support, nutrition, and exercise. The effectiveness of physical activity is related to the frequency and duration of each activity session and the longevity of the activity program. Recommended ACSM guidelines for exercise include the following (Wallace & Ray, 2009):
- A program of low-impact aerobic exercise, increase in daily activities, and resistance training
- A frequency of 5 to 7 times a week
- A length of 40 to 60 minutes a day or 20 to 30 minutes twice daily

As long as calorie expenditure is similar, moderate lifestyle activity may be as effective as structured exercise. Moderate intensity appears to be most effective for total and fat calorie consumption during the activity.

Women tend to have a 5% to 10% lower resting metabolic rate than men and a higher percentage of body fat than men of similar weight. Consequently, women have a lower percentage of lean body mass and may not be as metabolically active as are men during exercise. Women may expend up to 40% fewer calories than do men during the same exercise protocol at the same relative intensity (Tremblay et al., 1985).

Fat in men is stored primarily in the upper body or upper abdominal region. Fat in women is primarily stored in the lower half of the abdomen, the hips, and the thighs. Adipose tissue metabolism tends to be different in various regions. The fat-metabolism response to exercise appears to be less in the femoral-gluteal region than in the upper body–abdominal region. Femoral-gluteal adipose tissue serves as an important source of energy during lactation. Women may not lose fat as easily as do men in response to exercise, because genetic differences are related to where and how fat is stored and metabolized.

Consequently, women who need to lose weight may need to be more diligent about increasing the duration of their exercise training sessions and making resistance training a priority to facilitate maximal energy expenditure.

Several studies have examined parental awareness of weight status in children. A survey by the American Academy of Child and Adolescent Psychiatry of parents, 23% of whom had overweight children, reported that only 10.5% of parents with overweight children perceived their children's weight accurately compared with 59.4% of other parents (American Academy of Child and Adolescent Psychiatry, 2004). In a study by He and Evans (2007), 29.9% of the children examined were overweight or obese. However, based on the parent's perception of their children's weight, only 18.3% were overweight or obese. Factors such as the child's gender, ethnicity, and mother's weight contributed to the parent's inability to recognize weight status. In a study by Huang and colleagues (2007), 61% of parents correctly identified their child's weight status and these parents were also able to correctly identify the weight status of unrelated children in 58% of reviewed photographs. Results indicate that the parent's ability to correctly identify their child's weight status depends on their child's age and weight status. And in a study by Moore and colleagues (2012), researchers examined factors that influenced parental concern about their child's weight. Their results indicate that parents were significantly more likely to be concerned about their child's weight if the child was female, they believed the child to be overweight or obese, or the child was overweight or obese based on BMI.

OSTEOPOROSIS

Osteoporosis, or porous bone, is the most common bone disease. It is characterized by low bone mass and structural weakness of bone tissue, leading to bone fragility and increased risk of fractures (National Institutes of Health, Osteoporosis and Related Bone Disease—National Resource Center, 2011; Smith et al., 2009). Osteoporosis is a major health threat for 44 million Americans, or 55% of those older than 50 years of age (National Osteoporosis Foundation, *Fast Facts,* 2011). In the United States, an estimated 10 million people have osteoporosis and 34 million more, given their low bone density, have an increased risk for developing osteoporosis. Eighty percent of those affected are women (National Osteoporosis Foundation, 2011).

Some loss of bone occurs naturally after age 30. Twenty to thirty percent of bone mass development is regulated by environmental factors, such as nutrition and physical activity. In addition to the importance of optimizing physiological intake of calcium and vitamin D (Kalyani et al., 2010), and maintaining normal menstrual cycles for maximizing peak bone mass, physical activity plays a significant role in developing bone mass during childhood and adolescence and in maintaining skeletal mass into adulthood and old age. Using environmental changes and lifestyle modification during the third and fourth decades of life, women can increase their bone mass and effectively retard osteoporosis.

Physical activities, those that involve weight-bearing in particular, increase bone mineral density (BMD) (Borer, 2005) and provide support for a stronger skeletal foundation throughout aging. Additionally, systematic reviews examining the effects of different exercises in menopausal and postmenopausal women suggested that an active lifestyle and strength training may help to reduce fracture risk and preserve BMD, specifically spine and hip BMD, in osteopenic and osteoporotic women (Howe et al., 2011; Hurley & Armstrong, 2012; Martyn-St James et al., 2009; Zehnacker et al., 2007). Inadequate calcium intake during growth has implications for peak bone mass, which may occur as early as the late teenage years or as late as the mid-thirties, and may have implications for bone health later in life (Theobald, 2005). Unfortunately, Caucasian females in North America ages 4 to 8, 9 to 18, 19 to 50, and older than 51 years intake 105%, 64%, 74%, and 55% of the recommended amount of calcium, respectively (Borer, 2005). Although dietary sources are the preferred means of achieving adequate calcium intake, foods fortified with calcium are becoming more prevalent and are manufactured to provide approximately 300 mg of calcium in each serving (see Chapter 11).

Bone mass increases during childhood and adolescence and peaks during the third decade of life. When a person reaches approximately age 30, age-related bone loss occurs throughout the skeletal system, in all races and in both genders. However, there are significant differences in bone loss patterns between the genders, with the female gender being a risk factor for osteoporosis. Women have less bone mass than men at all ages and by their mid-thirties can expect age-related bone loss at approximately 1% annually. The rate of bone loss accelerates rapidly during the first 5 postmenopausal years, with annual losses of 3% to 5% common. By the fifth decade, or during their forties, women can anticipate a 10% loss of vertebral bone mass. Cumulative bone loss can approach 40% of peak bone mass over a woman's lifetime. Unfortunately, a loss of at least 30% in bone mass is required for detection on plain film radiographs (McKinnis, 2010). Therefore it is important to detect women at risk early in the natural course of the disease and to target interventions toward lifestyle-oriented health promotion. Additional risk factors for osteoporosis include Caucasian/Asian race, family history, low body weight for height, premature menopause, lack of physical activity, chronic smoking, and excessive alcohol consumption among others (Smith et al., 2009). In addition, risk factors for osteoporotic fractures attributable to falls include sensory and coordination deficits, living situation, older age, musculoskeletal weakness, diminished reflexes, medication use, and associated diseases (Kessenich, 2007).

The American College of Sports Medicine recommends that osteoporotic people should engage in weight-bearing and impact exercises to promote strengthening and cardiovascular conditioning, as well as flexibility, coordination, and balance training to improve quality of life, maintain an active lifestyle, and decrease risk of falls (Kohrt et al., 2004) (Box 12-6: Hot Topics). Maintenance of bone mass may be related to the intensity of the physical activity and the degree to which the activity stresses the bone. Weight-bearing actions that stress the skeleton (walking, stair climbing, floor calisthenics, and aerobic

BOX 12-6   HOT TOPICS

Prevalence of No Leisure-Time Physical Activity

Fact: Physical inactivity is associated with obesity and increased risk for chronic diseases (e.g., cardiovascular disease, certain cancers, and diabetes mellitus) and premature mortality. A national health objective for 2020 is to reduce the prevalence of no leisure-time physical activity.

Fact: Women, older adults, and most racial/ethnic minority populations have the greatest prevalence of leisure-time physical inactivity.

Fact: The findings in this report indicate that, in 2002, the overall prevalence of no leisure-time physical activity in 35 states and Washington, DC, was at the lowest level in 15 years.

Fact: Despite the recent decline in no leisure-time physical activity, the prevalence of overweight and obese people has increased (Ogden et al., 2012). This disparity might be explained, in part, by nationally representative data indicating an increase in the caloric intake of the overall U.S. population (Centers for Disease Control and Prevention, 2004). In addition, the declines in leisure-time physical inactivity might not have been accompanied by increases in physical activity sufficient to maintain or lose weight.

State and local public health departments and other organizations are encouraged to promote physical activity by teaching evidence-based strategies recommended by the Task Force on Community Preventive Services: community-wide campaigns; signs near elevators and escalators encouraging stair use; individually adapted health-behavior changes; and creation of, or enhanced access to, physical activity sites combined with informational outreach activities.

Data from Centers for Disease Control and Prevention. (2004). *Trends in intake of energy and macronutrients—United States, 1971-2000; Morbidity and Mortality Weekly Report, 53*, 80-82; Ogden, C. L., Caroll, M. D., Kit, B. K., & Flegal, K. M. (2012). *Prevalence of obesity in the United States, 2009-2010. NCHS data brief, No 82.* Hyattsville, MD: National Center for Health Statistics.

BOX 12-7   RESEARCH FOR EVIDENCE-BASED PRACTICE

Resistance and Agility Training Reduce Fall Risk in Women Ages 75 to 85

Objectives: To compare the effectiveness of group resistance and agility training programs in reducing fall risk in community-dwelling older women with low bone mass.

Design: A randomized, controlled, single-blind 25-week prospective study with assessments at baseline, midpoint, and trial completion.

Setting: Community center.

Participants: Community-dwelling women ages 75 to 85 with low bone mass.

Intervention: Participants were randomly assigned to one of three groups: resistance training ($n = 32$), agility training ($n = 34$), and stretching (sham) exercises ($n = 32$). The exercise classes for each study were held twice weekly.

Measurements: The primary outcome measure was fall risk (derived from weighted scores from tests of postural sway, reaction time, strength, proprioception, and vision), as measured using a Physiological Profile Assessment. Secondary outcome measures were ankle dorsiflexion strength, foot reaction time, and Community Balance and Mobility Scale Score.

Results: Attendance at the exercise sessions for all three groups was excellent: resistance training (85.4%), agility training (87.3%), and stretching program (78.8%). At the end of the trial, Physiological Profile Assessment fall-risk scores were reduced by 57.3% and 47.5% in the resistance and agility training groups, respectively, but by only 20.2% in the stretching group. In the resistance and agility groups, the reduction in fall risk was mediated primarily by improved postural stability, where sway was reduced by 30.6% and 29.2%, respectively. There were no significant differences between the groups for the secondary outcomes measures. Within the resistance training group, reductions in sway were significantly associated with improved strength, as assessed using increased squat load in the exercise sessions.

Conclusion: These findings support the implementation of community-based resistance and agility training programs to reduce fall risk in older women with low bone mass. Such programs may have particular public health benefits because it has been shown that this group is at increased risk of falling and sustaining fall-related fractures.

From Liu-Ambrose, T., Khan, K. M., Eng, J. J., Janssen, P. A., Lord, S. R., & McKay, H. A. (2004). Resistance and agility training reduce fall risk in women aged 75 to 85 with low bone mass: A 6-month randomized, controlled trial. *Journal of the American Geriatrics Society, 52*(1): 657-665.

dance) have a positive effect on bone density. Weight-bearing exercise, which increases mechanical stresses on the skeleton, is an important component of reducing osteoporosis risk. These exercises should be performed for 20 to 30 minutes or more, at least three to five times per week (Smith et al., 2009). Recent intervention trials and meta-analyses suggest that low-to-moderate impact weight-bearing exercises combined with resistance and/or agility training facilitate the most effective gains in BMD, prevention of bone loss, and functional capacity in older men and women (Nikander et al., 2010). Aerobic exercise and resistance training have also been advocated for people with osteoporosis (Iwanto et al., 2010) and may give affected individuals more desire to participate in daily activities, promoting a more active lifestyle (Lirani-Galvao & Lazaretti-Castro, 2010). In younger women the goal of exercise is to increase bone density; in older women who are already 30 to 40 years postmenopause a more realistic goal would be to decrease the risk of fractures

through fall prevention (Box 12-7). With respect to reducing fall risk in older postmenopausal women, Lirani-Galvao and Lazaretti-Castro (2010) found that tai chi may play a role in preventing osteoporotic fractures because of improvements in muscle strength and balance and decreased risk for falling; however, research has shown that tai chi does not support increases in BMD. Furthermore, it was found that the incidence of fragility fractures was noticeably lower in middle-aged to older men and women who participated in 3 to 4 days per week of moderate to vigorous physical activity (Nikander et al., 2010) (Box 12-7: Research for Evidence-Based Practice).

ARTHRITIS

Arthritis upsets the balance of joint health. Although rheumatoid arthritis and osteoarthritis have different causes and attack different parts of the joint, impaired joint function is the result.

Cartilage is destroyed and irregularities occur in the bone ends. As proper joint alignment changes, normal ROM is decreased, normal muscle balance and activity are altered, and disfigurement and dysfunction occur; and ultimately normal movement patterns are altered. Although there is an ongoing progression in arthritis that cannot be reversed by exercise, physical activity nevertheless helps to restore health to synovium and cartilage, improve strength and flexibility, decrease joint vulnerability, and delay the onset of dysfunction. Most importantly, exercise has been shown to reduce pain and joint stiffness, reduce fatigue, and improve function and psychological well-being in persons with arthritis (Cooney et al., 2010; Kujala, 2009). Further evidence is needed to determine if postponing exercise is appropriate during exacerbations of rheumatoid arthritis (Cooney et al., 2010); however, vigorous exercise is typically contraindicated in persons with acute joint inflammation (ASCM, 2009b).

Using exercise to counteract the effects of inactivity associated with arthritis is certainly a component to effective management (ACSM, 2009b). Although researchers have concluded that regular exercise cannot improve or cure arthritis, exercise has the following quality-of-life benefits for people with arthritis (ACSM, 2009b; Cooney et al., 2010; Kujala, 2009; Nieman, 2000):

- Improvement in joint function and ROM
- Increase in muscle strength and aerobic fitness that enhance daily activities of living
- Improvement in psychological state
- Decrease in loss of bone mass, and may promote increased bone mineral density
- Decrease in the risk of chronic disease

Consequently, exercise programs based on individual needs and interests should emphasize exercises to develop joint ROM and flexibility (performed before aerobic or strength activities) and should also include muscle-strengthening (two to three times per week) and aerobic exercises (5 to 10 minutes with progression to 30-minute session 3 to 5 days per week) and be functionally based (ACSM, 2009a).

The collective evidence strongly and consistently suggests that exercise is beneficial for persons with osteoarthritis. The specific aspects of exercise prescription for persons with osteoarthritis have been studied to differing extents. In terms of the different modes of exercise, various forms of exercise have been shown to be effective for osteoarthritis. A systematic review of studies of the effect of aquatic exercise on osteoarthritis concluded that aquatic exercise produces short-term beneficial effects on function and quality of life and, to a lesser extent, pain management (Bartels et al., 2007). With respect to fall risk, available evidence produces mixed results with use of aquatic exercise to reduce fall risk in individuals with hip and/or knee osteoarthritis, supporting the use of aquatic exercise in conjunction with fall risk education to effectively reduce fall risk, but not with use of aquatic exercise alone (Arnold et al., 2010; Hale et al., 2012). Lastly, an 18-week trial comparing aquatic exercise with land-based exercise found that although both modes of exercise improved function and pain management, the aquatic exercise group demonstrated a significantly greater reduction in pain level (Silva et al., 2008). Long-term effects have not been shown to date; thus we suggest aquatic exercise either be incorporated into a broader exercise program or be modified and progressed regularly to promote adaptation to and avoid accommodation to the training stimulus.

With respect to non–aquatic-based exercise, an umbrella review found high-quality evidence supporting the beneficial effects of exercise on pain and function in persons with osteoarthritis of the knee (Jamtvedt et al., 2008). Similarly, a systematic review of the effects of strength training alone, exercise therapy alone, and a combination of exercise with manual therapy in persons with osteoarthritis of the knee concluded that these modes of treatment improved function and reduced pain to a small degree, with the addition of manual therapy into treatment producing a moderate effect on pain (Jansen et al., 2011). Lastly, a systematic review incorporating adults and older adults with knee osteoarthritis supported progressive resistance exercise and aerobic exercise as having modest benefit on strength, pain, and function (Keysor & Brembs, 2011).

Available evidence may also support a small but positive benefit to education and self-management programs as complements to exercise to improve self-efficacy (May, 2010). Furthermore, additional evidence suggests that increased belief that physical activity can be beneficial to manage arthritis leads to higher levels of participation in physical activity (Ehrlich-Jones et al., 2011) and is significantly associated with decreased pain and fatigue, increased function, and self-perceived positive effect (Bezalel et al., 2010; Hewlett et al., 2011; Pisters et al., 2010). Exercise intensity is another important consideration for exercise prescription in persons with osteoarthritis (OA); however, unlike mode of exercise, intensity has received little attention. There is limited research available that compares the outcomes in persons with OA to intensity of training; however, some evidence supports both high- and low-intensity training to be of equal benefit in persons with knee OA with respect to pain, strength, and function without difference in rate of unfavorable effects. More research is needed to determine optimal parameters for exercise in persons with osteoarthritis, and an impairment-based, patient-centered approach with consideration of comorbidities and accessibility is required (Bennell & Hinman, 2011).

Two related arthritic conditions that have begun to be studied more are **rheumatoid arthritis (RA)** and **fibromyalgia syndrome.** Evidence suggests that aerobic exercise in persons with fibromyalgia can increase function and reduce some symptoms (Busch et al., 2008). However, evidence pertaining to the effectiveness of strength training to produce similar effects in individuals with fibromyalgia is of low quality (Kujala, 2009). In addition to evidence supporting the use of a combination of aerobic and strength exercises to improve outcomes in those with rheumatoid arthritis (Cooney et al., 2010), the use of tai chi as a form of activity in persons with RA has also been considered. A case series study of the use of tai chi in persons with RA supported significant improvement in swelling of joints and improvement in strength and endurance as measured by the "timed sit to stand test," and suggests practicing tai chi may help persons with RA increase their level of physical activity (Uhlig et al., 2010). Importantly, although the evidence has not shown that tai chi reduces pain or other symptoms of RA, it does not appear to exacerbate these symptoms (Han et al., 2004). In addition, a recent meta-analysis of the effects of cardiorespiratory aerobic exercise in individuals with rheumatoid arthritis demonstrated small but meaningful effects on quality of life, function, and pain (Baillet et al., 2010).

Again, further evidence is needed to determine if postponing exercise is appropriate during exacerbations of rheumatoid arthritis (Cooney et al., 2010). A review of the studies of the effects of aerobic exercise and strength training on individuals with fibromyalgia syndrome concluded there is evidence supporting benefits of exercise in this population to improve function and well-being, and decreased pain (Busch et al., 2007; Kujala, 2009). Aerobic activities such as stepping and walking and strengthening exercises such as lifting weights or using resistance exercise machines can be utilized in addition to stretching for flexibility. Although exercise is part of the overall management of fibromyalgia syndrome, the review by Busch and colleagues (2007) examined the effects of exercise when used separately or combined with other strategies such as education programs, biofeedback, and medications. In this review, aerobic exercises were done for at least 20 minutes once a day (or twice for 10 minutes), 2 days a week. Strength training was done 2 to 3 times a week and with at least 8 to 12 repetitions per exercise. The exercise programs lasted between 2½ and 24 weeks. In a study by Sanudo and colleagues (2010), aerobic exercise was compared to combined exercise (aerobic, muscle strength, and flexibility exercises) and control (nonexercising) groups. Both exercise groups demonstrated significant improvements on the Fibromyalgia Impact Questionnaire and the Beck Depression Inventory. When compared to the aerobic exercise and control groups, the combined exercise group had significantly better outcomes on the SF-36 physical function, body pain, vitality, and mental health subscales and on range-of-motion (shoulder and hip) measurements and grip strength. In a more recent study, Sanudo and colleagues (2012) examined the effect of whole-body vibration exercise on balance in women with fibromyalgia. The control group received an exercise training program and the experimental group received the same exercise training program plus whole-body vibration exercises. The results indicated that the group with whole-body vibration demonstrated significantly better balance, as measured by the Medio-Lateral Stability Index, when compared to the control group.

LOW BACK PAIN

Low back pain is a common medical and social problem frequently associated with disability and absence from work. Low back pain is a multifactorial disorder that is unlikely to be caused by a single factor. Obesity is associated with an increased risk of low back pain as well as an increased likelihood of seeking care for subacute and chronic low back pain (Shiri et al., 2010). Contrary to commonly held opinion, there is a lack of evidence that a sedentary lifestyle is a risk factor for the onset of low back pain (Chen et al., 2009). However, higher levels of muscular and aerobic fitness are associated with a decreased risk for low back

pain (Heneweer et al., 2012). Roffey and colleagues (2010a) in a systematic review found strong evidence that there is no relationship between awkward occupational postures and low back pain. Specifically, it is unlikely that occupational bending and twisting (Wai et al., 2010a), occupational sitting (Roffey et al., 2010b), occupational standing or walking (Roffey et al., 2010c), occupational lifting (Wai et al., 2010b), occupational pushing or pulling (Roffey, et al., 2010d), occupational carrying (Wai et al., 2010c), and occupational manual handling and individual assistance (Roffey et al., 2010e) are independent risk factors for low back pain.

Exercise can, however, have a positive influence on low back pain. There is some evidence to support overground walking more than treadmill walking in the management of low back pain (Hendrick et al., 2010). A recently conducted systematic review concluded that exercise can effectively reduce pain and improve function in persons with chronic low back pain; however, there was no clear advantage to any one form of exercise (van Middelkoop et al., 2010). Staal and colleagues (2004) concluded that graded activity was more effective than usual care in reducing the number of days of absence from work because of low back pain. Hilde and colleagues (2007) concluded in their systematic review that although the best current evidence suggests that activity alone has minimal benefits for individuals with low back pain, the risk of harm is small. Given the acknowledged detriments of bed rest, staying active is good advice for individuals with low back pain. A recently updated Cochrane Review found that exercise therapy for acute low back pain may be effective at reducing pain and improving function in persons with chronic low back pain and improving absenteeism in persons with subacute low back pain (Hayden et al., 2005). A recent Cochrane Review found moderate evidence that exercise following treatment for low back pain may reduce recurrent episodes of low back pain (Choi et al., 2010).

The spinal column is composed of 24 vertebrae stacked vertically, forming natural curves that allow the bony column to function with the resiliency of a spring. The intervertebral disks help with mobility and shock absorption. The health of the bony vertebrae and the cartilaginous disks depends on movement. The cartilage receives its nutrients from cyclical compression and decompression as a function of weight-bearing and non–weight-bearing movement. Similarly, repeated weight-bearing and non–weight-bearing activity stimulates vertebral bone integrity.

Muscles are intimately involved in the support and function of the spinal column. Maintaining the proper curves (anterior and posterior convexities) of lordosis in the cervical and lumbar vertebrae and kyphosis in the thoracic vertebrae is vital for sustaining the spring and shock-absorption qualities of the spine. The lumbar curve is especially influenced by three sets of muscles that are attached to the pelvis and the lumbar vertebrae. By altering the tilt of the pelvis, these muscles can increase (iliopsoas muscle) or decrease (abdominal and hamstring muscles) the lumbar curve. In addition, the deep muscles of the back (paraspinal muscles) work in controlled synergistic and antagonistic fashions to control spinal planes of motion; they are also influential in supporting the spinal curves in posture. Weakness or shortening of any of these muscles can adversely impact posture and increase stress on the back. The result can be back pain from muscle strain, altered joint function (facet joints), and abnormal force on the intervertebral disks.

In a systematic review, Hayden and colleagues (2005) concluded that in persons with various levels of low back pain exercise was beneficial in terms of reducing pain, improving function, and decreasing absenteeism. The American Pain Society and American College of Physicians have also jointly stated that there is good evidence for the effectiveness of exercise in reducing chronic low back pain (Chou & Huffman, 2007). Specific types of exercise that have been shown to be effective in persons with low back pain include training of the deep and superficial paraspinal muscles as well as unweighted or suspended exercise. The only systematic review of the effects of unweighted movement on persons with chronic low back pain concluded that there was consistent and strong evidence to support unweighted exercise to decrease pain and improve function (Slade & Keating, 2007). Exercise targeting specific lumbar paraspinal muscles has been shown to substantially reduce pain and restore function (Hides et al., 2001; Koumantakis et al., 2005; Shaughnessy & Caulfield, 2004). Although walking appears to be effective in the management of low back pain, Rasmussen-Barr and colleagues (2009) found that graded exercises target both deep and superficial muscles that support and control the lumbar spine and pelvis and were more effective in the long term at reducing disability and the need for recurrent treatment and improving pain self-efficacy.

The goal of exercise programs for individuals with low back pain is to prevent debilitation as a result of inactivity and to improve endurance, strength, and flexibility, allowing for a return to usual functional activities. Exercise recommendations and progression of activity are highly individualized based on origin, duration, and severity of pain. Strengthening exercises for trunk and extremity musculature have been demonstrated to benefit people with low back pain. Aerobic conditioning, such as walking, swimming, and stationary bicycling, is recommended to maintain endurance and prevent debilitation from inactivity (ACSM, 2006).

Advanced age, osteoporosis, arthritis, and low back pain are not reasons to exclude exercise from anyone's lifestyle. In fact, the opposite is true. These conditions are reasons to remain as physically active as possible to facilitate the ability to function throughout the aging process.

A referral to a physical therapist is warranted in most, if not all, cases of low back pain to allow for proper comprehensive management, which may include exercise as well as other safe and effective interventions.

IMMUNE FUNCTION

The relationship between exercise and immune function has a fairly long history of study, and the interest that grew out of the human immunodeficiency virus (HIV) epidemic continues to stimulate investigations in this area. Several studies demonstrate that people with impaired immune function can exercise safely without risk to their health status and can enhance their physiological and psychological well-being with regular exercise (Fillipas et al., 2006; Galantino et al., 2005; Sax, 2006; Terry et al., 2006). A recent systematic review concluded that progressive resistive exercise may increase body weight and limb girth and aerobic exercise may improve adipose levels and lipid profiles in individuals living with HIV (Filipas et al., 2010). Furthermore, two recently updated meta-analyses suggest that aerobic exercise, either alone or in conjunction with progressive resistance exercise, can be safely performed by adults living with HIV/acquired immunodeficiency syndrome (AIDS) and may improve fitness, body composition, and well-being (O'Brien et al., 2009, 2010). Recommended parameters include exercising at least three times per week for 20 minutes over a period of 5 weeks or more (O'Brien et al., 2010).

The effect of exercise on immune system markers (e.g., CD4 levels, CD4/CD8 ratio, or viral load) in people with HIV/AIDS is unclear. Reviews discuss the effects of exercise on immune function in individuals with HIV/AIDS and report conflicting findings (Anderson, 2006; Dudgeon et al., 2004). A meta-analysis compared aerobic exercise groups with nonexercising groups and found no significant differences in CD4 count, CD4 percentage, or viral load (Nixon et al., 2005). Similarly, meta-analytic data compared the combination of aerobic and progressive resistance exercise groups with nonexercising groups and found no significant differences in CD4 count (O'Brien et al., 2004). Despite the fact that the CD4 count did not differ between exercising and nonexercising groups, there were significant beneficial changes in depressive symptoms, mean body weight, mean arm and thigh girth, and maximum heart rate for those in the exercising groups (Nixon et al., 2005; O'Brien et al., 2004).

Evidence suggests that regular exercisers and athletes are less likely to become ill than sedentary women (Nieman, 1994) and middle-aged men and women (Matthews et al., 2002). In direct contrast, evidence also suggests that athletes are also at increased risk for infection during increased periods of training or after competition (Nieman, 1994; Nieman et al., 1990; Pedersen & Bruunsgaard, 1995; Peters-Futre, 1997).

Epidemiological studies indicate that a J-curve relationship may exist between the intensity of exercise and the risk of upper respiratory tract infection (URTI) (modified from Nieman [1994] and Pedersen and colleagues [1998]) (Figure 12-3). That is, in theory, moderate exercise may decrease the risk of URTI below that of a sedentary individual, but high-intensity exercise may raise the risk above average. In direct contrast, Lee and colleagues (1992) concluded that immune function was not linked to the risk for URTI in a group of cadets during basic training and Pyne and colleagues (1995) reported similar rates of URTI between elite swimmers under intense training and age- and gender-matched sedentary controls. Factors that confound studies on the relationship between exercise and URTI include failure to distinguish between new infection and the clinical manifestations of a dormant infection (Gleeson et al., 2002) and failure to distinguish between airway hyperresponsiveness and URTI (Langdeau & Boulet, 2001).

Immune system changes that are apparently related to the intensity of exercise have been identified. Moderate-endurance

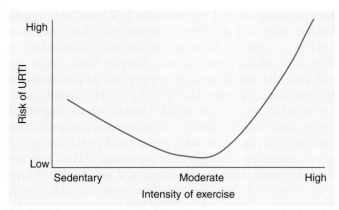

FIGURE 12-3 Relationship between exercise and the risk of upper respiratory tract infection (URTI). This relationship is often referred to as a J curve. (Modified from Nieman, D. [1994]. Exercise, upper respiratory tract infection, and the immune system. *Medicine & Science in Sports & Exercise, 26*, 128-139.)

exercise stimulates the neuroendocrine system, which causes changes in the function and numbers of various immune system cells, such as the NK, CD4, and CD8 cells as mentioned. Evidence also indicates that moderate exercise is associated with a prolonged improvement in the killing capacity of neutrophils (one of the most efficient phagocytes). Several immune marker changes suggest increased risk for illness in those who engage in high-intensity exercise, including a low level of salivary immunoglobulin (antibodies), low serum complement levels, low lymphocyte count, depressed NK cell activity, low helper and suppressor T-cell ratio, and decreased neutrophil phagocytic capacity (Mackinnon, 1992; Nieman, 1994; Pedersen & Ullum, 1994).

Changes in immune cell counts and activity may be related to hormonal immunoregulation. Moderate exercise increases the release of immunostimulatory hormones, such as growth hormone and endogenous opiates (β-endorphin and methionine-enkephalin). The increase in β-endorphins with exercise seems to have a positive effect on NK cell activity. Conversely, intense exercise is associated with increases in catecholamine and corticosteroid (cortisol) levels, which have immunosuppressive characteristics (Mackinnon, 1992). High-intensity exercise is also associated with muscle cell damage and inflammation. The immune system is involved in tissue repair. It is theorized that while immune cells are busy with the repair process, host protection may suffer. A window of opportunity for infection during recovery from high-intensity exercise appears to exist. Accordingly, rest is recommended after vigorous exercise to allow the body to recover, and moderate exercise may be the better choice for enhancing health and well-being.

There is convincing evidence that low-level exercise and physical activity have a significant protective effect on the gastrointestinal system, and, in particular, colon cancer (Martin, 2011). Additionally, growing evidence suggests that low-level physical activity may also have a protective effect on gastric and pancreatic cancer (Martin, 2011). Evidence also suggests that physical activity is a modifiable risk factor for breast cancer (Bardi, 2007). Physical activity appears to lower the risk for many conditions, in particular breast cancer (Warburton et al., 2007).

Unfortunately, physical activity during adolescence does not appear to play a protective role for the risk of breast cancer later in life (Gammon et al., 1998). A recently conducted meta-analysis concluded that physical activity may decrease the risk of prostate cancer, and encouraged men to engage in regular physical activity (Liu et al., 2011). A synthesis of clinical practice guidelines, systematic reviews, meta-analyses, and individual studies suggest that exercise may minimize or prevent adverse physiological effects of cancer and its treatment (Ingram & Visovsky, 2007). A recent *Position Statement on Immune Function and Exercise* (Walsh et al., 2011) offered the following conclusion: "There is consensus that exercise training protects against some types of cancers. Training also enhances aspects of anti-tumour immunity and reduces inflammatory mediators. However, the data linking immunological and inflammatory mechanisms, physical activity, and cancer risk reduction remains tentative."

Preliminary findings in the area of immunosenescence, the natural decline in immune function that occurs with aging, suggest that regular exercise and improved fitness may have potential immune restorative properties and improve "immune risk profile" in the elderly (Simpson & Guy, 2010).

MENTAL HEALTH

People who exercise regularly generally state that they feel better, have increased self-esteem, and have a more positive outlook on life. Not only do they feel better physically, they also they feel better mentally. Epidemiological research with both men and women suggests that physical activity may be associated with reduced symptoms of depression and anxiety and improvements in positive affect and general sense of well-being (USDHHS, 2000). Much of the work in this area has focused on such mental health issues as depression, anxiety, mood, quality of life, cognition, stress, and self-esteem.

Evidence from a review of the literature (prospective studies, randomized controlled trials, and meta-analyses) found that exercise protects against and is an intervention for mild to major depression (Cuijpers, 2009; Donaghy, 2007; Graven et al., 2011; Mead et al., 2009; Nahas & Sheikh, 2011; Rethorst et al., 2009). Research of the National College Health Assessment examined the association between vigorous/moderate or strength-training exercises and mental health in a national sample of college females (Adams et al., 2007). Both vigorous/moderate and strength-training exercises were positively associated with perceived health. Furthermore, both vigorous/moderate and strength-training exercises were negatively associated with several indicators of mental health (e.g., depression, anxiety, and suicidal ideation). Similarly, research examined the association between exercise and mental health and concluded that mental health is modifiable through exercise (Galper et al., 2006; Windle et al., 2010).

The mental health benefits of physical activity, as an intervention, have been summarized elsewhere and include promoting mental health and well-being; preventing and treating mental disorders; and supporting psychosocial rehabilitation (Saxena et al., 2005).

Investigations have focused on populations across the life span, including children, young adults, and older adults. Based on a limited number of small trials, a recently updated Cochrane Review concluded that, when compared to no intervention, exercise reduces anxiety and depression in children and young adults (Larun et al., 2009). A recent Cochrane Review suggests that long-term exercise, of various types, is most likely to benefit mood in adults; however, the magnitude of the effect is indeterminate at this point (Mead et al., 2009). In a recent systematic review of the effect of exercise on cognitive function in older adults, Tseng and colleagues (2011) suggested that there were positive benefits to adopting unimodal, simple exercises for cognitively impaired older adults and a more diversified, multimodal program for healthy older adults. The authors also recommended an exercise regimen of 6 weeks in duration, at least 3 sessions per week lasting 60 minutes each, to increase the likelihood of a positive effect on cognition.

Furthermore, the effect of exercise on individuals with various disorders or diseases, such as schizophrenia, cancer, or other chronic illnesses, has been studied. In a systematic review, Herring and colleagues (2010) concluded that although exercise in sedentary persons with a chronic illness reduces anxiety, training programs lasting as few as 12 weeks and consisting of session of at least 30 minutes resulted in the largest reductions in anxiety. A recently conducted Cochrane Review of the psychological and physical effects of dance and movement therapy on persons afflicted by cancer was unable to arrive at a conclusion because of a dearth of high-quality studies in this area, although there may be a positive effect on quality of life in persons with breast cancer (Bradt et al., 2011). Based on a limited number of small trials, a recently updated Cochrane Review concluded that regular exercise may improve both physical and mental health and well-being in persons with schizophrenia (Gorczynski & Faulkner, 2010).

Various types and modalities of exercise have been employed in studies; an example of one such intervention is tai chi. Tai chi significantly improved both psychological (perceived well-being) and physical (functional capacity, knee extension strength, and flexibility) health over baseline levels (Macfarlane et al., 2005). In a recent systematic review and meta-analysis of the effect of tai chi on psychological well-being, Wang and colleagues (2010) demonstrated an apparent association with reductions in anxiety, depression, mood disturbance, and stress, as well as improvements in self-esteem.

EXERCISE PRESCRIPTION

Literature certainly reflects both the physiological and the psychological benefits that can be experienced with commitment to an active lifestyle. In short, regular physical activity or exercise can help people feel better, look better, and perform better. Unfortunately, as discussed, Americans have failed to embrace the concept and health value of an active lifestyle. Many have been overwhelmed by the misperception that to gain health benefits they must perform vigorous, continual exercise. The result has been discouragement in getting started and poor compliance in staying with it. "No pain, no gain" has been an unfortunate and common refrain (Box 12-8: Quality and Safety Scenario).

People need to be reminded that many of their daily physical activities are actually forms of exercise (Figure 12-4). This approach to physical activity serves as a good foundation to a healthy lifestyle. However, when possible, individuals should also be encouraged to include more formal exercise training in their overall activities to promote optimal cardiorespiratory fitness and significantly improve muscle strength and endurance. The amount of exercise required to achieve these goals is determined by the parameters of an exercise prescription:

F (Frequency)	3 to 5 times a week of aerobic exercise	
	2 to 3 times a week of resistance training	
I (Intensity)	Moderate to vigorous, by heart rate and perceived exertion	
	Able to complete each resistance exercise, 8 to 12 repetitions, without strain	
T (Time)	20 to 60 minutes, plus warm-up and cool-down periods	
	15 to 30 minutes to complete a series of 8 to 10 resistance exercises	
T (Type)	Aerobic (walking, jogging, biking, swimming, rowing, cross-country skiing, elliptical trainer, NordicTrack, StairMaster, aerobics, dancing, skating, or rollerblading)	
	Resistance training (weight machines, free weights, and calisthenics such as push-ups, sit-ups, or pull-ups) (ACSM, 2006)	

Aerobic Exercise

The benefits of aerobic exercise are cumulative; therefore, a frequency of three to five times a week is recommended. Every other day is a good frame of reference and allows for recovery between training sessions, potentially decreasing the chance of overuse injuries. The benefits of exercising more than five times a week are outweighed by the risk of injury, especially with higher-impact activities. When more frequent exercising is a goal, cross-training is recommended. Cross-training means performing different types of exercise on different days of the week or performing different types of exercise within one session. The benefits of cross-training include a decreased risk of musculoskeletal injury, an increased potential for total body conditioning, and improved long-term compliance because variety decreases boredom and eliminates the exercise barrier of limited choices.

The intensity of exercise that results in health and fitness benefits ranges from moderate to vigorous and is comfortable, but challenging (brisk). Intensity is defined by the objective measure of heart rate (HR) and the subjective measure of perceived exertion. The increase in HR during exercise has a strong linear relationship with exercise intensity and aerobic capacity. Resting heart rate (RHR) is the HR measured at rest. Maximum heart rate (MHR) is the rate measured at the highest workload tolerated during exercise. MHR also decreases with age; therefore, a generic formula for determining MHR is 220 minus age. Formulas for determining appropriate exercise HRs have been developed that take RHR and MHR into consideration.

✅ BOX 12-8 QUALITY AND SAFETY SCENARIO

Less Pain, More Gain

In an attempt to encourage increased participation in physical activity, a panel of scientists from the Centers for Disease Control and Prevention and the American College of Sports Medicine came together to review the evidence related to physical activity and to issue a public health message concerning the recommended types and amounts of physical activity. The evidence clearly indicates that the protective effects of exercise can be achieved at more moderate levels of intensity than had been recommended previously. The health and fitness benefits of exercise appear to be related more to the total amount of exercise accomplished (calories expended) rather than to the specific exercise intensity, frequency, and duration. The recommendations are as follows:

- Adults should accumulate 30 minutes or more of moderate-intensity (brisk) physical activity on most (or all) days of the week, for a weekly total of 3 to 4 hours.
- The activity need not be continuous; benefits can be realized with short bouts of activity (a minimum of 10 minutes) over the course of the day.
- This amount of activity will expend about 150 to 200 calories per day (the equivalent of walking 2 miles briskly) or 1000 to 1400 calories per week.

- All types of activity can be applied to the daily total (raking leaves, dancing, or gardening).
- Lower intensity activities should be performed more often, or for longer periods, or both. More vigorous activities should be performed for shorter periods or less frequently.

Because most adults do not meet these standards, they have the most to gain by incorporating a few minutes of increased activity into their day, gradually building up to 30 minutes a day. People who are active on an irregular basis should strive to be more consistent. People who prefer more formal exercise can choose to participate in more vigorous, organized exercise regimens, sports, and recreational activities.

Sedentary individuals gain the most by increasing their activity to the recommended level. However, any person who already meets the standards can derive some additional benefit by becoming more active.

People who do a little bit of exercise are better off than those...who do none and those who do a little more are better off still. (Franklin, 1993, p. 476)

Data from Pate, R. R., Pratt, M., Blair, S. N., Haskell, W. L., Macera, C. A., Bouchard, C. et al. [1995]. Physical activity and public health: A recommendation from the CDC and the ACSM. *Journal of the American Medical Association, 273,* 402-407.

FIGURE 12-4 Physical activity pyramid.

6	No exertion at all
7	
8	Extremely light
9	Very light
10	
11	Light
12	
13	Somewhat hard
14	
15	Hard (heavy)
16	
17	Very hard
18	
19	Extremely hard
20	Maximal exertion

Borg RPE Scale®
© Gunnar Borg, 1970, 1985, 1998.

FIGURE 12-5 Borg RPE Scale®. Copyright © Gunnar Borg, 1970, 1985, 1998. (From Borg, G. [1998]. *Borg's perceived exertion and pain scales.* Champaign, IL: Human Kinetics. For basic information about such factors as scale construction, metric properties, and correct administration, it is necessary to read Borg [1998]. Scales and instructions can be obtained for a minor fee from Dr. G. Borg and his company, Borg Perception, Stockholm, Sweden. E-mail: borgperception@telia.com.)

The **Borg Scale** for rating perceived exertion (RPE) is a psychophysical category scale for the subjective rating of sensations associated with the intensity of physical work (Borg, 1973, 1982) (Figure 12-5). The scale uses ratings based on the individual's overall feeling of exertion and physical fatigue. These ratings correspond well with metabolic responses to exercise, such as HR and oxygen consumption. The strong linear relationship between HR and RPE was originally suggested by Borg and has been verified by subsequent studies. Correlation coefficients from 80% to 90% have been reported consistently using a variety of work tasks and exercise conditions (Borg, 1973, 1982; Skinner et al., 1973). However, perceptions of exertion and the relationship to HR are influenced by both physiological and psychological factors (aches, cramps, pain, fatigue, shortness of breath, anxiety, depression, and introversion or extroversion). Smutok and colleagues (1980) noted that some subjects are more accurate in regulating exercise intensity by RPE than are others and that this variability may be more the result of psychological than physiological factors. Other factors that may alter the strong relationship between HR and RPE are drug-related situations (β-blockers), age, and disease states.

Despite this potential for variability in perception, RPE correlates well with HR clinically, and together they form a complementary means of helping individuals determine a comfortable, beneficial level of exercise intensity. An RPE of 11 to 14

corresponds well with 50% to 85% MHR. Subjective parameters include being slightly short of breath, but not out of breath; being able to talk without difficulty, but unable to sing a song easily; being pleasantly fatigued, but not exhausted; and having mild musculoskeletal discomfort, but no pain.

Attention to RPE helps a person develop a sense of body awareness and an appreciation for the body's response to the stress of activity. Awareness of RPE helps people listen to their bodies and become aware of how it feels to move, where they carry tension, and where they have discomfort. With this increased awareness, individuals can choose how they want to respond, adjusting their exercise practice on a daily basis, making the activity more enjoyable, decreasing the risk of injury, and improving long-term exercise compliance.

The recommendation for the duration of aerobic conditioning exercise is generally 20 to 60 minutes. Less than 20 minutes usually provides minimal benefit. However, for people who are unaccustomed to exercising or for those who are greatly deconditioned, short durations are permissible, gradually increasing to a beneficial, comfortable level as tolerance and confidence improve. Everyone has to start somewhere and doing a little is much better than doing nothing at all.

The benefit of sessions longer than 45 to 60 minutes is again outweighed by the potential for injury. Exercising more than 60 minutes on occasion is certainly not wrong, but a person who increases duration should consider decreasing intensity. Improvements in cardiorespiratory fitness can also be accrued from intermittent bouts of moderate to vigorous exercise (10-minute segments) on a workout day. As discussed, longer bouts of exercise are more beneficial for weight loss. The range of acceptable duration allows for greater flexibility, giving reassurance of benefit to the individual who varies exercise choices daily based on capability, interests, and life demands.

As mentioned, many different choices for mode of aerobic exercise are available. The question is often asked, "What is the best type of aerobic exercise?" The answer is, "the one that the individual is willing to do on a regular basis." Different aerobic exercises have different benefits; they all have their advantages and disadvantages. From a cardiovascular point of view, with relative intensity, frequency, and duration being equal, the benefit is about the same for all modes. Probably the best scenario is cross-training, which results in the most optimal all-around benefits. However, the most important recommendation is that the person starts moving—choosing the person's favorite exercise will increase the likelihood of adhering to an exercise program.

Walking is probably the most accessible and popular form of aerobic exercise. Done briskly, walking provides a good cardiorespiratory challenge in 60% to 80% of the adult population. Walking is also an activity that nearly everyone can do, requires little equipment or cost, can be done almost anywhere, and can be a social or a solitary activity, depending on individual needs. Walking is often the recommended exercise of choice for people who are greatly deconditioned or for those who have physical limitations. Considered a low-impact activity, walking can be easily regulated to accommodate a wide range of fitness levels and motor abilities. Cycling, rowing, and swimming (or water walking or other water aerobics) are non–weight-bearing to low–weight-bearing activities that may be good choices for individuals with physical limitations. Aquatic exercise is a good alternative for individuals with musculoskeletal limitations who need some weight relief with exercise, such as advanced osteoarthritis. Although the buoyancy of the water provides this weight relief, the water also provides resistance to the limbs as they move, encouraging an increase in intensity and conditioning. Individuals should be encouraged to do the types of aerobic exercise that best fit their needs, interests, and lifestyles while providing reasonable benefits.

Warm-Up and Cool-Down Periods

In addition to the endurance phase of exercise, warm-up and cool-down periods should be a regular part of the exercise session. The warm-up period usually lasts 5 to 10 minutes and may include light stretching, calisthenics, or performance of the chosen aerobic activity at a low intensity. This approach prepares both the musculoskeletal and the cardiorespiratory systems for the transition from rest to exercise by increasing blood flow, respiration, body temperature, and muscle flexibility. The warm-up period decreases the risks of injury and heart irregularities.

The cool-down period follows the endurance phase and usually lasts 5 to 10 minutes. This phase allows the body to readjust gradually from the demands of exercise back to baseline. Stretching and slow, rhythmical movement help to increase muscle elasticity, prevent blood pooling and hypotension, and facilitate dissipation of body heat and removal of lactic acid. The result is the prevention of injury, light-headedness, fatigue, and muscle soreness.

Yoga is an excellent example of one form of exercise to use during warm-up and cool-down periods. The word yoga means union or "established in being," which implies a mind-body connection. Simply defined, yoga is mindful stretching. The mind is quiet and awareness is focused on feeling the body as it moves. Movement into and out of yoga postures (called asanas) provides the necessary stimulation of weight-bearing activity to help keep bones strong, provides the movement to increase joint ROM, and stretches and tones muscles. The sun salute (surya namaskar), a series of 12 flexion-extension yoga postures linked together as 1 fluid movement by the breath rhythm, is a wonderful practice to include in the warm-up and cool-down phases of exercise, providing both physiological and mind-body benefits.

Yoga also helps develop an appreciation for the experience of the basic resting state, a mindfulness of how it feels to be relaxed physically and mentally during the activity. In this form, exercise becomes an inner experience: that is, quiet and settled on the inside, dynamic and lively on the outside. The yoga philosophy encourages an appreciation of body sensations, slow stretching, and maintenance of proper posture, all of which help to prevent injury and promote health. There is a growing body of evidence to support the use of yoga to improve range of motion, pain, posture, function, mental health, sleep patterns, disability, and quality of life in select populations (Alfonso et al., 2012; Bussing et al., 2012; Ebnezar et al., 2012; Greendale et al., 2009; Visceglia & Lewis, 2011).

Flexibility

Flexibility is a basic component of physical fitness. Warm-up and cool-down periods provide the opportunity to work on stretching muscles and increasing joint ROM. A safe stretch is one that is gentle and relaxing; a little discomfort may be felt as the muscle stretches, but the discomfort should never reach the point of pain. Stretching mindfully, as in yoga, will ensure a safe stretch. Holding the position for 10 to 20 seconds and repeating the stretch three to five times will encourage optimal flexibility (ACSM, 2006).

Resistance Training

Studies suggest that people who maintain or improve their flexibility and strength are better able to perform daily activities and avoid injury and disability (Pate et al., 1995). Resistance training increases muscle strength and endurance, increases muscle mass, improves metabolic efficiency, maintains or increases bone density, prevents limitations in performance of everyday tasks, decreases the effort required to perform these tasks, and decreases the potential for injury during physical activity.

On the average, after their early twenties people lose about one half a pound of muscle every year through lack of use. This reduction in muscle mass is largely responsible for a decrease in resting metabolic rate, which may translate into weight gain. Resistance training is recommended for the general population because it has a positive effect on many of the degenerative problems associated with the aging process.

Every individual should try to perform activities throughout the day that stimulate muscle strength and endurance. Activities that involve lifting, carrying, or performing repetitive movement against a resistance (vacuuming, raking, shoveling, or baking bread) help preserve lean body mass. If these types of activities are not performed on a regular basis, then the guidelines for resistance training provided in Box 12-4 are suggested. These guidelines are not meant to represent workouts performed by bodybuilders and competitive weight lifters; they are not meant to result in significant muscular hypertrophy. The purpose of weight training from a health perspective is to develop healthy muscles that provide the strength to do daily activities without risk of injury and to stimulate bone health.

The figures in Box 12-4 demonstrate several suggested resistance exercises for upper body strengthening. Resistance training for all major muscle groups is appropriate, but individuals often choose to concentrate on the upper body, because these muscles tend to be neglected in daily activity and other exercise regimens. The ACSM recommends the incorporation of bilateral and unilateral, and single- and multi-joint exercises, including total body exercises (ACSM, 2006). Although many people believe that they need to do three sets of each exercise, excellent results can be attained by doing one set (Hass et al., 2000). A recent meta-analysis of the effect of single versus multiple sets on muscle hypertrophy showed multiple sets to yield a 40% greater improvement in muscle hypertrophy (Krieger, 2010). The ACSM recommends 3 to 5 sets of 8 to 12 repetitions (ACSM, 2006). The weight that is lifted should result in near muscle fatigue at the end of each set (this varies substantially depending on the muscle being trained, the amount of resistance, and the fitness level of the athlete) and should be performed without strain and while maintaining proper form. Once 12 to 15 repetitions can be completed without fatigue, the resistance can be increased (by 5% or less), or the same weight can be used to do an additional set to fatigue. The movements should be performed slowly, preferably coordinated with the breath. Rest intervals vary substantially in the literature; however, a recent review suggested that 3 to 5 minutes allows for hypertrophy and power development and 1 to 3 minutes allows for endurance gains (de Salles, et al., 2009). The ACSM suggests 1 to 3 minutes of rest between sets to develop endurance and 3 to 5 minutes to develop strength and power. Slow, controlled movements result in greater benefits, lower risk of injury, and more appreciation of how the body feels as its muscles are challenged. The recommended frequency depends upon the individual and should be two to three times per week for novice levels, three to four times per week for intermediate levels, and four to five times per week for advanced levels (ACSM, 2006). The exercise variables that comprise the exercise prescription must always be chosen to meet the specific needs and limitations of each individual.

EXERCISE THE SPIRIT: RELAXATION RESPONSE

Exercise should not be considered merely a physical regimen with objective outcomes (calories burned and repetitions completed). Exercise is also a process of challenging the body and the mind to gain a sense of well-being and a feeling of accomplishment, an opportunity to learn about who we really are.

Most people understand the physical benefits of exercise and some people enjoy the challenge of being physically active, but few realize the learning potential inherent in physical activity. Success in embracing a physically active lifestyle may involve a change in focus from the mechanics of exercise to an appreciation for how it feels and what it means to move. Physical activity can be time spent in meditation that fuels both the body and the spirit.

The relaxation response (RR) is an inborn set of physiological changes that offset those of the fight-or-flight (stress) response. When elicited, the RR results in a "letting go" of physical, emotional, and mental tension. The RR is a physiological response inborn in everyone and, although it can sometimes occur without the individual being aware of it, people generally need to develop techniques that help them let go on a more regular basis. Some techniques that are used commonly to elicit the RR include diaphragmatic breathing, meditation, imagery, mindfulness, yoga stretching, and repetitive exercise.

The RR can be combined with exercise to facilitate the release of tension and improve self-awareness and the feeling of well-being. However, a shift in attitude about exercise is also involved, with the focus becoming the process and awareness of movement. Successful elicitation of the RR involves two basic components: a repetitive focus (the breath, a mantra, and the cadence or rhythm of physical activity) and a nonjudgmental attitude (about everyday thoughts and the quality of performance) (Benson & Stuart, 1992). Berger and Owen (1988) have developed exercise characteristics that facilitate stress reduction

and support an exercise environment that allows the successful elicitation of the RR. Activities must:

- Be pleasant and enjoyable.
- Be noncompetitive (competition implies judgment about the self and others).
- Be predictable (elicitation of the RR involves a shift in awareness from the external to the internal environment that will take place only with a sense of safety and reliability).
- Be repetitive and rhythmical (the cadence of activity provides a focus for awareness).
- Facilitate abdominal breathing (watching the breath serves to anchor thoughts in the moment; in combination with cadence, it provides a focused awareness).
- Continue for 20 to 30 minutes at a comfortable intensity on most days of the week (continuity restores a sense of serenity).

All forms of exercise can be used to gain this experience. As discussed, yoga involves mindful stretching with a breathing focus, providing an environment for successful elicitation of the RR. Tai chi is another exercise practice with roots in Eastern philosophy. Known as moving meditation, tai chi combines movement with focused awareness, involving a physical and cognitive focus for moving in choreographed forms that become a meditation.

The quality of body awareness can also be brought into a more traditional exercise practice. Aerobic exercise lends itself well to the elicitation of the RR, because it has rhythmical and repetitive form and because it facilitates abdominal breathing. The practitioner can focus on the breath rhythm, the step cadence of walking or jogging, the pedaling cadence of bicycling, or the stroke cadence of swimming. Mantras can be used to create a positive mindset and to focus the mind in the present moment as the experience unfolds. Resistance training takes on new meaning when coordinated with the breath. Focusing on the muscles and how it feels to move through the ROM enhances the knowledge of what feels good and what does not, providing feedback on accepting physical challenge.

Exercise focus can and should vary on a daily basis depending on need, mood, and intent. Some days it feels right to focus on the more physical aspects of the activity, appreciating the challenge of working harder or longer. Other exercise sessions may be more contemplative, letting creativity run, working through the tension of a lingering stressor, quieting the mind for relaxation, listening to music, or appreciating nature. Focusing on the process rather than the outcomes brings meaning and purpose to the activity and helps achieve something more valuable than mere physical outcomes.

When exercise integrates mind and body, it stops being something that has to be done and instead becomes something desired. Being mindful during physical activity and exercising in the moment increase awareness. With awareness comes choices in the possibilities of self-care. Exercise for fitness of the spirit, walk for the soul, and just let the body do the work. There is a growing body of evidence to support the use of tai chi to improve balance in confidence, pain, mental health, functional mobility, disability, self-efficacy, and quality of life; and to reduce fall risk in select populations (Hall et al., 2011; Huang et al., 2011; Leung et al., 2011; Rand et al., 2011; Wang et al., 2009).

MONITORING THE INNER AND THE OUTER ENVIRONMENT

The primary purpose of exercise is to enhance health. However, because exercise involves stress to the body, the potential to cause or exacerbate health problems is inherent. When a person is not feeling well, the exercise effort should be decreased or stopped until the individual is feeling better. With an infection, a cold, or influenza, the body is under stress and overexertion will only increase that stress and possibly lengthen the healing time. The level of activity should be adjusted to accommodate how the individual feels, slowly progressing to normal workout levels until strength and energy return. This philosophy also holds true for chronic diseases such as arthritis and HIV. During an acute exacerbation, activity should be limited to necessary activities of daily living (ADLs), but on a regular basis staying active is important, adjusting activity levels as tolerated. Exercise can be a useful tool in coping with chronic illness.

Missing an occasional workout will not affect the fitness level; choosing to stop or reduce the amount of exercise when not feeling well is the right choice. However, after missing workouts for 2 weeks, a decline in fitness is inevitable. When starting again, resuming the activity should be slow, gradually working back to the usual level of activity. Inactivity for 3 to 5 months results in the loss of all conditioning benefits gained, and resumption of exercise involves starting over (ACSM, 2006). Being aware of the external exercise environment is also important. Extremes of heat and cold affect performance as the body adjusts to different temperatures and wind conditions. Changing the time of day for exercise (early morning or later evening are better choices for humid days), adjusting fluid intake, and varying the length of warm-up and cool-down periods will improve tolerance for environmental conditions and enhance exercise safety.

Fluid News

Proper hydration is an important component of a good fitness program. Extra fluid is needed to support physiological homeostasis during exercise, especially during hot weather. Drinking a cup of water 15 to 30 minutes before exercise is recommended. If the weather is hot or the indoor exercise area is very warm, then 5 to 12 ounces of fluid should be taken in every 15 or 20 minutes during exercise.

Under certain circumstances, the American College of Sports Medicine recommends consuming beverages containing electrolytes and carbohydrates during exercise over water alone (ACSM et al., 2007). For exercise routines lasting longer than 1 hour, a sports drink with carbohydrates and electrolytes enhances performance and is recommended. This type of liquid provides muscles with energy and helps delay fatigue while meeting fluid needs. Sports drinks containing a 4% to 6% carbohydrate concentration are designed to replace carbohydrates at the proper rate during exercise. They also contain sodium, which promotes fluid retention, enhances flavor, and protects

TABLE 12-1   SPORTS DRINKS THAT HYDRATE AND ENERGIZE

BRAND	CALORIES	CARBOHYDRATE (GRAMS)
All Sport	70	19
Cytomax	80	19
Endura	62	16
Gatorade	50	14
Hydra Fuel	70	17
Isostar	70	16
MET-Rx ORS	75	19
Perform	60	16
Powerade	70	19
Power Surge	80	20
Race Day	63	15
XLR8	62	15

against hyponatremia, which can occur with lengthy exercise sessions. Most sports drinks provide 14 to 20 grams of carbohydrate per 8-ounce serving. The recommended intake is 5 to 12 ounces every 15 to 20 minutes. Which sports drink is the best? Several brands should be tried to determine personal preference in taste, but one should be chosen that contains approximately 50 to 80 calories per 8-ounce serving; any more and the carbohydrate concentration will inhibit fluid absorption. Table 12-1 provides choices for sports drinks that both hydrate and energize.

SPECIAL CONSIDERATIONS

Most adults do not need to consult a physician before starting a moderate-intensity physical activity program. However, men older than 40 years of age and women older than 50 years of age who plan a vigorous program (intensity more than 60% of MHR or Vo$_2$max) or who have either chronic disease or risk factors for chronic disease should consult an appropriate health care provider before starting exercise (Table 12-2 and Box 12-9).

People with CHD or diabetes have special exercise needs. Earlier in this chapter the ways in which exercise and physical activity positively affect primary and secondary prevention in both disease processes were discussed. Limitations in the ability to exercise are related to the severity of the disease and the signs and symptoms of intolerance. For people with CHD and diabetes mellitus (DM), safety with starting a new exercise program requires supervision and guidance from knowledgeable health care providers. Before starting, these individuals should have a medical evaluation, including an exercise tolerance test (ETT), to determine functional capacity and severity of disease.

Coronary Heart Disease

Exercise plays a strong role in rehabilitation after a cardiac event such as myocardial infarction (MI), coronary artery bypass surgery, percutaneous transluminal coronary angioplasty or stent placement, and angina. Increased physical activity appears to benefit individuals from all of these groups. Benefits include the

TABLE 12-2   ACSM RECOMMENDATION FOR MEDICAL EXAMINATION AND EXERCISE TESTING BEFORE BEGINNING AN EXERCISE PROGRAM

	APPARENTLY HEALTHY			INCREASED RISK	
	YOUNGER*	OLDER	NO SYMPTOMS	SYMPTOMS	KNOWN DISEASE[†]
Moderate exercise[‡]	No	No	No	Yes	Yes
Vigorous exercise[§]	No	Yes	Yes	Yes	Yes

From American College of Sports Medicine (ACSM). (2006). *Guidelines for exercise testing and prescription* (7th ed.). Philadelphia: Lippincott Williams & Wilkins.

*Younger implies ≤40 years of age for men, ≤50 years of age for women.

[†]Persons with known cardiac, pulmonary, or metabolic disease.

[‡]Moderate exercise is defined by an intensity of 40% to 60% of Vo_2max, or if the intensity is uncertain, an effort well within the individual's current capacity and that can be comfortably sustained for a prolonged period (60 minutes), slow progression, and generally noncompetitive.

[§]Vigorous exercise is defined by an intensity >60% of Vo_2max, or if the intensity is uncertain, exercise intense enough to represent a substantial cardiorespiratory challenge or result in fatigue within 20 minutes.

BOX 12-9   SYMPTOMS AND SIGNS SUGGESTIVE OF CARDIOPULMONARY DISEASE

- Pain, discomfort (or other anginal equivalent) in the chest, neck, jaw, arm, or other areas that may be ischemic in nature
- Shortness of breath at rest or with mild exertion
- Dizziness or syncope
- Orthopnea or paroxysmal nocturnal dyspnea
- Ankle edema
- Palpitations or tachycardia
- Intermittent claudication
- Known heart murmur
- Unusual fatigue or shortness of breath with usual activities

These symptoms must be interpreted in the clinical context in which they appear, because they are not all specific for cardiopulmonary or metabolic disease.

Data from American College of Sports Medicine. (2006). *Guidelines for exercise testing and prescription* (7th ed.). Philadelphia: Lippincott Williams & Wilkins.

following (Erbs et al., 2006; Heran et al., 2011; Lavie & Milani, 2011; Milani et al., 2011; Oerkild et al., 2011):

- Reduction in total and cardiovascular mortality
- Reduction in hospital admission
- Reduction of symptoms
- Improvement in exercise tolerance and functional capacity
- Increase in the confidence and ability to carry out usual ADLs
- Improvement in psychological well-being and quality of life

Generally, people with CHD demonstrate a reduction in Vo_2max and the ability to do submaximal levels of work. With exercise training, the increase in Vo_2max in persons with CHD averages approximately 20% after 3 months. This improvement in conditioning is the result of both central (cardiac) and peripheral (muscular) changes (ACSM, 2009b). Some of the most significant improvements in exercise tolerance have been noted in individuals with angina. With a decrease in submaximal HR or a decrease in systolic blood pressure (SBP) resulting from conditioning, myocardial oxygen demand is decreased and individuals are able to do a greater amount of work before reaching the anginal threshold. This boost is reflected in an observed increase in rate pressure product (RPP: HR × SBP) at the anginal threshold (ACSM, 2007). An increase in functional capacity allows for progression of exercise tolerance and progression with daily activities and leisure or vocational activities.

Appropriately prescribed and conducted exercise training programs improve exercise tolerance and physical fitness in persons with CHD. Moderate and vigorous regimens are of value, but care must be taken to determine safe exercise parameters for each individual. The parameters of the exercise prescriptions are the same as those for the general population, including frequency, intensity, duration, and mode of exercise.

Aerobic exercise improves cardiorespiratory fitness and functional capacity. Any of the aforementioned aerobic exercises are acceptable for this population, depending on the level of fitness and musculoskeletal limitations. Traditionally, resistance training was not commonly recommended for persons with CHD. The belief was that lifting weights resulted in a disproportionate rise in blood pressure, increased the myocardial oxygen demand, and increased the risk of angina and MI. However, data from several studies indicate that moderate, supervised weight training is feasible, tolerable, and beneficial for individuals with HTN and CHD. Strength training can keep the heart healthy by helping to control body weight, reduce cholesterol levels, and regulate blood glucose levels. Guidelines for determination of appropriate individual training include an aerobic capacity of at least 4 to 5 metabolic equivalents, or METs; an ejection fraction of greater than 30%; and the absence of severe, symptomatic aortic stenosis. However, clinical experience demonstrates that people with more severe disease can use small hand weights to increase muscle tone without risk of cardiovascular compromise.

The exercise intensity for persons who have had a cardiac event but who have not had a symptom-limited exercise tolerance test (ETT) should be kept at a low level based on an elevated heart rate (EHR) of 20 to 30 beats per minute above the resting heart rate (RHR) and a rating of perceived exertion

(RPE) of less than 12. After an ETT has been performed, intensity should then be prescribed based on 50% to 85% maximal heart rate (MHR) and an RPE of 11 to 14, or below the ischemic, anginal, or arrhythmic threshold. Duration and frequency recommendations are similar to those for the general population. People who are the most deconditioned may need to exercise at lower intensities, for short durations, and more frequently throughout the day. Generally, a reasonable goal is three to five times per week for 20 to 40 minutes, plus 5 to 10 minutes each for warm-up and cool-down periods (ACSM, 2007).

Diabetes

Exercise has long been regarded as part of the triad in the management of diabetes in conjunction with diet and medication (insulin or oral medication). In the early 1900s it was determined that exercise lowers the blood glucose concentration of people with diabetes. After the introduction of insulin, studies revealed that exercise can potentiate the hypoglycemic effect of injected insulin. More recently, findings suggest that in individuals who have poor control (i.e., excessive blood glucose levels), exercise may induce a further increase in blood glucose levels, resulting in ketosis. On the average, people with diabetes have a lower MHR, achieve a lower cardiac output at maximal exercise, and have a higher blood pressure during exercise, resulting in lower maximal oxygen consumption. However, these individuals can improve their exercise capacity with training and can experience the benefits related to overall fitness and cardiorespiratory training similar to the benefits gained by people without diabetes.

Apparently, both benefits and risks from exercise exist for people with diabetes. The overall goals regarding physical activity should be to teach individuals to incorporate activity into their daily life, pursue an exercise program if they wish, and develop strategies to avoid the complications of exercise.

As discussed, in addition to diet and weight loss, regular physical activity is an important modality in the prevention and treatment of type 2 diabetes. People with type 2 diabetes should monitor their blood glucose levels and determine their responses to exercise. However, individuals with type 2 diabetes usually can follow the same exercise prescription parameters as those of the general population. Although the same exercise benefits can be achieved by people with type 1 diabetes, the inherent behavior and function of endogenous insulin makes exercising a more difficult proposition for these individuals. The major functions of insulin are to promote glucose uptake into the cells and control metabolic homeostasis during exercise, working in synergy with the counter-regulatory hormones. With exercise, insulin secretion decreases slightly and the concentrations of counter-regulatory hormones increase. This increase stimulates hepatic glucose production, which balances the increased use of glucose by the working muscles, maintaining normoglycemia. However, with injected insulin the plasma insulin concentration does not decrease with exercise, hepatic glucose is not produced as quickly as it is used, and a decrease in blood glucose concentration results. In contrast, people who have poorly controlled diabetes with decreased plasma insulin concentrations already have elevated blood glucose levels, because there is insufficient insulin to assist glucose transport into cells. During exercise the liver is stimulated to produce more glucose, which causes a further elevation in blood glucose levels, worsening the hyperglycemic condition. Ketosis may also result from increased mobilization and incomplete combustion of free fatty acids in muscle cells and accelerated ketone body formation in the liver (Federici & Benedetti, 2006).

Although each person with diabetes should be evaluated and given individual exercise recommendations, the goals of an exercise program are universal:

- Maintain or improve cardiovascular fitness to prevent or minimize long-term cardiovascular complications.
- Improve flexibility that is impaired as muscle collagen becomes glycosylated.
- Improve muscle strength, which may deteriorate as a result of neuropathy.
- Allow people with type 1 diabetes to safely participate in and enjoy physical activities or sports.
- Assist with weight control for people with type 2 diabetes.
- Allow people with diabetes to experience and gain the same benefits and enjoyment from regular exercise as do people without diabetes.

Box 12-10 presents a list of recommendations and precautions for people with diabetes who are interested in regular physical activity and exercise.

BUILDING A RHYTHM OF PHYSICAL ACTIVITY

Participation in regular physical activity increased gradually from the 1960s to the 1980s but seems to have plateaued in recent years. The progress made toward *Healthy People 2020* physical activity goals indicates that most of the population has not embraced a physically active lifestyle (USDHHS, 2010). Although the benefits of physical activity are common to all people, patterns of physical activity vary among population subgroups defined by gender, age, racial background, income, and body fat. The following generalities are true:

- Men are more active than are women.
- Physical activity declines with age.
- Ethnic minorities are less active than are White Americans.
- Higher education and income are associated with more leisure-time activity.
- People who are obese are usually less active than their leaner counterparts.

Adherence and Compliance

Physiological, behavioral, and psychological variables all influence the decision to be physically active. Each person is unique, and success with exercise over the long term comes from recognition of personal motivation or core desire and support from the social environment. Core desire defines the purpose behind putting the effort into developing and maintaining an active lifestyle; it is what motivates the individual to exercise. People should be encouraged to spend some quiet time meditating on why being physically fit is important to them.

BOX 12-10 INNOVATIVE PRACTICE

Recommendations and Precautions for People with Diabetes Who Are Interested in Regular Physical Activity and Exercise

- Notify primary care physician, ophthalmologist, and podiatrist of intent to exercise.
- Monitor blood glucose level before and 20 to 30 minutes after exercise to determine the response to exercise.
- Be sure blood glucose level is less than 300 mg/dL in those with type 1 diabetes or less than 400 mg/dL in those with type 2 diabetes, and urine test results are negative for ketones (if blood glucose level is greater than 240 mg/dL). If blood glucose level is consistently equal to or greater than 250 mg/dL, improved control must be established before continuing exercise.
- If possible, exercise approximately 1 hour after meals when blood glucose level is highest. This plan helps with weight loss, because extra food will not have to be eaten to ward off hypoglycemia. When exercising before meals, a snack may be necessary. (See Table 12-3 for suggestions on food adjustments to maintain blood glucose balance with exercise.)
- Know the action and peak times of insulin dosage and avoid exercising at peak. (Table 12-4 shows the peak action of insulin preparations.)
- Consider adjusting oral medication or insulin dosage to prevent low blood glucose level during exercise. The adjustment will depend on the intensity of the exercise, the duration of the exercise session, and the type of insulin that is used during exercise.
- Be alert for the hypoglycemic lag effect that may occur 12 to 24 hours after vigorous exercise; an extra snack after exercise will help.

- Avoid injecting insulin into a muscle area that will be active during exercise; the pumping action of the muscle may accelerate absorption of the insulin and cause a rapid decrease of blood glucose level.
- Use proper footwear and make frequent foot inspections.
- Avoid high-impact activity when prone to neuropathy in the legs or feet or when there is a history of neuropathy.
- Keep SBP below 180 to 200 mm Hg in the presence of eye or kidney disease.
- Exercising every day is best, but at least 3 to 4 times per week. Start with 10 to 20 minutes and gradually increase to 30 to 40 minutes at 50% to 75% MHR. Continuous aerobic activity helps maintain good blood glucose level control better than intermittent activities. Do not forget the 5-minute to 10-minute warm-up and cool-down periods.
- Avoid high-intensity anaerobic exercise, but low- to moderate-intensity resistance training is acceptable.
- Carry a concentrated form of carbohydrate (sugar packets, glucose tablets, or hard candy) when exercising.
- Wear some form of diabetes identification.
- People with type 2 diabetes need to test blood glucose levels with exercise and potentially adjust oral medications. Consider decreasing medication if blood glucose level is less than 80 mg/dL after exercise. For weight loss, plan the best time to exercise so that snacks can be avoided.

MHR, Maximum heart rate; *SBP*, systolic blood pressure.

TABLE 12-3 FOOD ADJUSTMENTS

DURATION AND INTENSITY	BLOOD GLUCOSE (mg/dl)	SUGGESTED FOOD ADJUSTMENT
<30 min of moderate activity	<100	1 Fruit + 1 bread + 1 meat
Examples: walking 1 mile or bicycling	100-180	1 Bread or 1 fruit
<30 min	>180	May not need snack
30-60 min of moderate activity	<100	1 Fruit + 1 bread + 1 meat
Examples: tennis, swimming, jogging, bicycling, yard work,	100-180	1 Bread or 1 meat
or housework	>180-240	1 Bread or 1 fruit
	>240	May not need snack
60 min of moderate- to high-intensity activity	—	
Examples: competitive sports, strenuous bicycling,		
long-distance running, heavy shoveling		

Modified from Beaser, R. S., & Campbell, A. (2005). *The Joslin guide to diabetes* (2nd ed.). New York: Simon & Schuster.
*If doing strenuous activity or playing sports, consult a physician or exercise physiologist for advice on blood glucose level management. Insulin adjustment may be required in addition to food adjustments (see Table 12-4). Blood glucose level should be tested hourly: 1 bread or 1 fruit per hour unless blood glucose level is ≥180 mg/dL (snack may not be needed for that hour).

TABLE 12-4 PEAK ACTION OF INSULIN PREPARATIONS

RAPID-ACTING	INTERMEDIATE-ACTING	LONG-ACTING
Regular insulin peak action 2-4 hr	Isophane insulin peak action 6-12 hr	Glargine peak action 5-24 hr
Aspart peak action 0.6-0.8 hr	Insulin zinc peak action 8-12 hr	Extended insulin zinc 18-24 hr
Lispro peak action 0.5-1.5 hr		
Glulisine peak action 0.5-1.5 hr		

From Ciccone, C. D. (2007). *Pharmacology in rehabilitation* (4th ed.). Philadelphia: F.A. Davis.

Finding meaning and purpose in an active lifestyle can enhance behavior. Biopsychosocial and spiritual variables need to be considered in promoting physical activity. An individual's biopsychosocial factors and spiritual beliefs affect the behavioral and attitudinal factors that influence the motivation and ability to adhere to an active lifestyle. Generally, however, physical activity is more likely to be initiated and maintained if the individual (NIH, 1998; Pentecost & Taket, 2011):

- Perceives a net benefit
- Chooses an enjoyable activity
- Feels competent doing the activity
- Feels confident in overcoming barriers that may interfere with the activity
- Feels safe doing the activity
- Can access the activity easily on a regular basis
- Perceives no significant negative financial or social cost
- Experiences minimal musculoskeletal discomfort
- Is able to address competing time demands
- Is readily able to fit the activity into the daily schedule
- Balances the use of labor-saving devices with activities that involve physical exertion

Educating the public about physical activity helps to provide guidelines for safe and effective exercise, to reinforce potential benefits, and to alleviate misperceptions that may interfere with the decision to change behavior. However, knowledge about exercise and the intent to exercise do not correlate well with long-term compliance. Confidence in the ability to be physically active—and the confidence that overcoming barriers produces positive benefits that are related to personal goals (self-efficacy)—is strongly related to participation and compliance (Figure 12-6). Exercise self-efficacy is increased when people perform exercise successfully, receive positive feedback about success, view exercise role models, and learn more about the relationships among exercise, health, and body awareness (see the Case Study and Care Plan at the end of this chapter).

Creating a Climate That Supports Exercise

Clearly exercise and fitness need to be social norms. A climate that supports and encourages physical activity should be fostered. Other people and organizations in the individual's social

FIGURE 12-6 Three interacting cognitive processes of Bandura's social-cognitive theory. (Modified from Dzewaltowski, D. A. [1995]. Physical activity determinants: A social-cognitive approach. *Medicine and Science in Sports and Exercise, 26,* 1395-1399.)

environment can influence the adoption and maintenance of physical activity.

Health Care Professionals

People are more likely to increase physical activity if counseled to do so by clinicians. Clinicians inquire about exercise habits, communicate the benefits of increased activity, assist the person in initiating activity, and provide adequate follow-up. Challenging perceived individual barriers to exercise and offering alternative viewpoints can help create new exercise paradigms. Clinicians also serve as role models by demonstrating enthusiasm and the health benefits for being physically active.

Recognizing the stages of behavioral change helps in meeting people at their stage of readiness to change behavior. Providing information on physical activity designed for specific stages of readiness enables people to move from stages of contemplation and preparation into action. An individual in precontemplation is not ready to actively change behavior. This person may respond better to support and information about the benefits of changing behavior rather than being placed in an action environment. The decision to change may come gradually. After a person has made the commitment to change, the action phase lasts about 6 months. Continued follow-up throughout the action phase into maintenance is valuable in helping the individual stay committed until the termination phase is reached and the behavior is secure.

Family and Friends

Social support can be a valuable resource for behavioral change. Significant others or friends can serve as buddies, providing a source of companionship and motivation. These people can offer to share daily responsibilities to make time for exercise (e.g., provide child care). Parents can support their children's activity by having family outings and providing transportation, praise, and encouragement. Joining a fitness club or an exercise group at work provides various forms of stimulation and socialization, which increases the potential for new friendships grounded in an appreciation of the rewards of exercise.

Schools

Schools are one of the most important resources for increasing physical activity. Strategies must be developed to facilitate increased activity in children because it is clear that children are becoming less active and more obese. Schools are providing less opportunity and poorer quality time for physical activity during school hours. All schools should provide opportunities for physical activity that:

- Are appropriate and enjoyable for children of all skill levels and are not limited to competitive sports or physical education classes
- Appeal to girls and boys and to children from diverse backgrounds
- Are offered daily
- Can serve as a foundation for activities throughout life

Schools can also serve as a resource for the community. Expanding operating hours at either end of the school day creates a safe, indoor environment for hall walking.

Communities

Participation in regular physical activity at the community level depends in large part on the availability and proximity of facilities and safe environments. Community government agencies, local health agencies, schools, and places of worship have the potential to provide activity resources to the population at large. Churches seem to be particularly successful in reaching ethnic minorities and older adults. Making neighborhoods safe for outdoor activities can have a major effect on improving activity habits, especially among low socioeconomic and disadvantaged populations, who report lower levels of daily physical activity.

Recognizing that many of the previous recommendations require a financial commitment, government agencies must respond to reports by health agencies and establish public policies that support the importance of physical activity for the general population. Individuals should make a personal commitment to be physically active, but that commitment needs to be supported by a social and political environment that values this type of lifestyle choice.

CASE STUDY

Exercise Self-Efficacy: Sharon G.

Sharon G. is a 53-year-old account executive who is 2 years post-menopause, complains of insomnia, and has chronic low back pain (LBP) and knee pain.

History: Motor vehicle accident (2008), resulting in bone graft to left leg (her left leg is shorter than her right leg). As part of rehabilitation, Sharon started jogging, which was more comfortable than walking with chronic right-sided sacroiliac joint pain. She started running marathons in 2010 and continued until 2011. In 2011 she began to add more variety into exercise and decreased her running, but she still identified herself as being an athlete.

In 2012 Sharon suffered a fall that resulted in chronic LBP, and she was unable to continue aerobic exercise. She began to experience depression and insomnia; exercise had been a significant coping mechanism in the past and now her whole sense of well-being was being affected. As Sharon attempted to rebuild her exercise practice, she would alternate between overexercising, exacerbating symptoms, and then having to stop and recuperate, reinforcing her negative self-image. Magnetic resonance imaging (MRI) studies showed mild arthritis in her knees.

Reflective Questions
1. What are some of her barriers to exercise?
2. How will a regular practice of mindfulness and the RR benefit Sharon's exercise practice?
3. How would she benefit from cross-training?
4. What exercise is she doing that is beneficial for helping to prevent osteoporosis?

LBP, Low back pain; MRI, magnetic resonance imaging.

CARE PLAN

Exercise Self-Efficacy: Sharon G.

NURSING DIAGNOSIS: Altered Sleep Pattern related to low back pain, depression, and recent weight gain

Medications
- Serax (oxazepam) 30 mg, 4 to 6 times a week
- Ginkgo biloba

Defining Characteristics
- Insomnia
- Chronic low back and knee pain
- Depression
- Upset about recent weight gain of 10 lb (61.5 inches, 118 lb); sees ideal body weight as 108 lb

Expected Outcomes
- Walking, treadmill, bicycling, and low-impact aerobics (30 minutes, 3 to 4 times per week)
- Weights 3 to 4 times per week
- Stretching 3 to 4 times per week
- Daily RR
- Build mindfulness into exercise practice

Interventions
- Treadmill and walking daily for 30 minutes
- Weights 2 to 3 times per week
- Yoga and stretching daily

RR, Relaxation response.

SUMMARY

It is important that people incorporate increased activity into their lifestyles on a long-term basis; exercise in the short term is of little overall benefit. Helping individuals gain the knowledge (benefits of exercise and recommended parameters for exercise), skills (self-monitoring), and attitude (core desire) improves compliance. People need to be motivated enough to start, enjoy the activity enough to want to continue, and appreciate the value enough to start again if they lapse. Lapses should be anticipated to avoid the unrealistic sense of total success or total failure. Behavioral change is cyclical rather than linear; success often comes with repeated movement through stages of change and it helps to explore the reasons for the lapse and to view the lapse as a learning experience rather than a failure. The goal is to prevent a relapse that results in a more permanent noncompliance.

The benefits and enjoyment derived from a physically active lifestyle have a significant effect on the quality of life. However, this lifestyle is successful only when it is supported by a degree of self-awareness and self-care. People must realize that they are worth the effort of doing something good for themselves, that they have the right to be happy and healthy, and that exercise can help them achieve that end. By adding a mind-body component to physical activity and not regarding it solely as a physical regimen, people can experience true health rather than mere fitness. A great deal of body exercise is not required; 30 minutes a day can make a significant difference. Success comes with building a rhythm of physical activity into everyday life. The following are some suggestions for a lifestyle approach to exercise:

- Something is better than nothing.
- Attempt small changes over time (gradualism).
- Emphasize moderate intensity.
- Make activity an integral part of life.
- Focus on the process rather than the outcome.
- Clinicians can provide a knowledgeable, supportive, and enthusiastic environment to encourage the change to a healthier, more active way of life.

REFERENCES

Adams, T. B., Moore, M. T., & Dye, J. (2007). The relationship between physical activity and mental health in a national sample of college females. *Women & Health, 45*(1), 69–85.

Alfonso, R. F., Hachul, H., Kozasa, E. H., de Souza, O. D., Goto, V., et al. (2012). Yoga decreases insomnia in postmenopausal women: A randomized clinical trial. *Menopause, 19*(2), 186–193.

Alperson, S. Y., & Berger, V. W. (2011). Opposing systematic reviews: The effects of two quality rating instruments on evidence regarding t'ai chi and bone mineral density in postmenopausal women. *Journal of Alternative and Complementary Medicine, 17,* 389–395.

American Academy of Child and Adolescent Psychiatry. (2004). *Obesity in children and teens, No. 79.* Retrieved April 18, 2005, from www.aacap.org/publications/factsfam/79.htm.

American College of Sports Medicine (ACSM) position stand. (1985-1986). Physical activity and bone health. *Medicine & Science in Sports & Exercise, 36*(11).

American College of Sports Medicine (ACSM). (2006). *ACSM's guidelines for exercise testing and prescription* (7th ed.). Philadelphia: Lippincott Williams & Wilkins.

American College of Sports Medicine (ACSM). (2009a). American College of Sports Medicine position stand. Progression models in resistance training for healthy adults. *Medicine & Science in Sports & Exercise, 41,* 687–708.

American College of Sports Medicine (ACSM). (2009b). *ACSM's exercise management for persons with chronic diseases and disabilities* (3rd ed.). Champaign, IL: Human Kinetics.

American College of Sports Medicine & American Heart Association (ACSM/AHA). (2007). Exercise and acute cardiovascular events: Placing the risks into perspective. *Medicine & Science in Sports & Exercise, 39*(5), 886–897.

American College of Sports Medicine, Sawka, M. R., Burke, L. M., Eicher, E. R., Maughan, R. J., & Stachenfeld, N. S. (2007). American College of Sports Medicine position stand: Exercise and fluid replacement. *Medicine & Science in Sports & Exercise, 39*(2), 377–390.

Anderson, S. L. (2006). Physical therapy for patients with HIV/AIDS. *Cardiopulmonary Physical Therapy Journal, 17*(3), 103–109.

Arne, M., Janson, C., Boman, G., Lindqvist, U., Berne, C., & Emtner, M. (2009). Physical activity and quality of life in subjects with chronic disease: chronic obstructive pulmonary disease compared with rheumatoid arthritis and diabetes mellitus. *Scandinavian Journal of Primary Health Care, 27*(3), 141–147.

Arnold, C. M., & Faulkner, R. A. (2010). The effect of aquatic exercise and education on lowering fall risk in older adults with hip osteoarthritis. *Journal of Aging and Physical Activity, 18,* 245–260.

Baillet, A., Zeboulon, N., Gossec, L., et al. (2010). Efficacy of cardiorespiratory aerobic exercise in rheumatoid arthritis: Meta-analysis of randomized controlled trials. *Arthritis Care & Research, 62*(7), 984–992.

Balistreri, K. S., & Hook, J. V. (2011). Trajectories of overweight among US school children: A focus on social and economic characteristics. *Maternal and Child Health Journal, 15,* 610–619.

Bardi, A. (2007). Can physical activity reduce the risk of breast cancer? *Clinical Nutrition Insight, 33,* 1–3.

Bartels, E. M., Lund, H., Hagen, K. B., Dagfinrud, H., Christensen, R., & Danneskiold-Samsøe, B. (2007). Aquatic exercise for the treatment of knee and hip osteoarthritis. *Cochrane Database of Systematic Reviews* (issue 4).

Bauer, J. M., Kaiser, M. J., & Sieber, C. C. (2008). Sarcopenia in nursing home residents. *Journal of the American Medical Directors Association, 9*(8), 545–551.

Beaser, R. S., & Campbell, A. (2005). *The Joslin guide to diabetes* (2nd ed.). New York: Simon & Schuster.

Belli, T., Ribeiro, L. F., Ackermann, M. A., Baldissera, V., Gobatto, C. A., & Galdino da Silva, R. (2011). Effects of 12-week overground training at ventilatory threshold velocity in type 2 diabetic women. *Diabetes Research and Clinical Practice, 93*(3), 337–343.

Bennell, K. L., & Hinman, R. S. (2011). A review of the clinical evidence for exercise in osteoarthritis of the hip and knee. *Journal of Science and Medicine in Sport, 14,* 4–9.

Benson, H., & Stuart, E. (1992). *The wellness book: The comprehensive guide to maintaining health and treating stress-related illness.* New York: Simon & Schuster.

Berger, B., & Owen, D. (1988). Stress reduction and mood enhancement in four exercise modes: Swimming, body conditioning, hatha yoga, and fencing. *Research Quarterly for Exercise and Sport, 59*(2), 148–159.

Berger, J. S., Brown, D. L., & Becker, R. C. (2008). Low-dose aspirin in patients with stable cardiovascular disease: A meta-analysis. *American Journal of Medicine, 121*(1), 43–49.

Bezalel, T., Carmeli, E., & Katz-Leurer, M. (2010). The effect of a group education programme on pain and function through knowledge acquisition and home-based exercise among patients with knee osteoarthritis: A parallel randomised single-blind clinical trial. *Physiotherapy, 96,* 137–143.

Borer, K. T. (2005). Physical activity in the prevention and amelioration of osteoporosis in women: Interaction of mechanical, hormonal, and dietary factors. *Sports Medicine, 35*(9), 779–830.

Borg, G. A. (1973). Perceived exertion: A note on "history" and methods. *Medicine & Science in Sports & Exercise, 5*(2), 90–93.

Borg, G. A. (1982). Psychophysical bases of perceived exertion. *Medicine & Science in Sports & Exercise, 14*(5), 377–381.

Bradt, J., Goodill, S. W., & Dileo, C. (2011). Dance/movement therapy for improving psychological and physical outcomes in cancer patients. *Cochrane Database of Systematic Review* issue 10.

Braith, R. W., & Stewart, K. J. (2006). Resistance exercise training: Its role in the prevention of cardiovascular disease. *Circulation, 113*(22), 2642–2650.

Brien, S. E., Katzmarzyk, P. T., Craig, C. L., & Gauvin, L. (2007). Physical activity, cardiorespiratory fitness and body mass index as predictors of substantial weight gain and obesity. *Canadian Journal of Public Health, 98*(2), 121–124.

Busch, A. J., Barber, K. A., Overend, T. J., Peloso, P. M., & Schachter, C. L. (2007). Exercise for treating fibromyalgia syndrome. *Cochrane Database of Systematic Review* issue 4.

Busch, A. J., Schachter, C. L., Overend, T. J., Peloso, P. M., & Barber, K. A. (2008). Exercise for fibromyalgia: A systematic review. *Journal of Rheumatology, 35*(6), 1130–1140.

Bussing, A., Ostermann, T., Ludtke, R., & Michalsen, A. (2012). Effects of yoga intervention on pain and pain-associated disability: A meta-analysis. *Journal of Pain, 13*(1), 1–9.

Candow, D. G., Chilibeck, P. D., Abeysekara, S., & Zello, G. A. (2011). Short-term heavy resistance training eliminates age-related deficits in muscle mass and strength in healthy older males. *Journal of Strength and Conditioning Research, 25*(2), 326–333.

Centers for Disease Control and Prevention (CDC). (2008). *Physical activity and good nutrition: Essential elements to prevent chronic diseases and obesity 2008.* Atlanta, GA: U.S. Department of Health and Human Services.

Centers for Disease Control and Prevention (CDC). (2010a). *State indicator report on physical activity, 2010.* Atlanta, GA: U.S. Department of Health and Human Services.

Centers for Disease Control and Prevention (CDC). (2010b). *Vital signs (August).* Atlanta, GA: U.S. Department of Health and Human Services.

Centers for Disease Control and Prevention (CDC). (2011). *Physical activity for everyone: Older adults.* Atlanta, GA: U.S. Department of Health and Human Services.

Chen, S. M., Liu, M. F., Cook, J., Bass, S., & Kai Lo, S. (2009). Sedentary lifestyle as a risk factor for low back pain: A systematic review. *International Archives of Occupational and Environmental Health, 82,* 797–806.

Chodzko-Zajko, W. J., Proctor, D. N., Singh, M. A.F., Minson, C. T., Nigg, C. R., Salem, G. J., et al. (2009). American College of Sports Medicine: Position stand. Exercise and physical activity for older adults. *Medicine & Science in Sports & Exercise, 41*(7), 1510–1530.

Choi, B. K.L., Verbeek, J. H., Tam, W. W.S., & Jiang, J. Y. (2010). Exercises for prevention of recurrences of low-back pain. *Cochrane Database of Systematic Review* issue 1.

Chou, C. H., Hwang, C. L., & Wu, Y. T. (2012). Effect of exercise on physical function, daily living activities, and quality of life in frail older adults: A meta-analysis. *Archives of Physical Medicine and Rehabilitation, 93*(2), 237–244.

Chou, R., & Huffman, L. H. (2007). Nonpharmacologic therapies for acute and chronic low back pain: A review of the evidence for an American Pain Society/American College of Physicians clinical practice guideline. *Annals of Internal Medicine, 147*(1), 492–504.

Chudyk, A., & Patrella, R. J. (2011). Effects of exercise on cardiovascular risk factors in type 2 diabetes. A meta-analysis. *Diabetes Care, 34*(5), 1228–1237.

Cooney, J. K., Law, R., Matschke, V., et al. (2010). Review article: Benefits of exercise in rheumatoid arthritis. *Journal of Aging Research, 13,* 1–14.

Cornelissen, V. A., Arnout, J., Holvoet, P., & Fagard, R. H. (2009). Influence of exercise at lower and higher intensity on blood pressure and cardiovascular risk factors at older age. *Journal of Hypertension, 27*(4), 753–762.

Cowan, D., Radman, H., Lewis, D., & Turpie, I. (2009). A community-based physical maintenance program for frail older adults: The Stay Well program. *Topics in Geriatric Rehabilitation, 25*(4), 355–364.

Cuijpers, P. (2009). Review: Exercise may moderately improve depressive symptoms. *Evidence-Based Mental Health, 12*(3), 77.

de Salles, B. F., Simão, R., Miranda, F., Novaes Jda, S., Lemos, A., & Willardson, J. M. (2009). Rest interval between sets in strength training. *Sports Medicine, 39,* 765–777.

Deshpande, A. D., Harris-Hayes, M., & Schootman, M. (2008). Epidemiology of diabetes and diabetes-related complications. *Physical Therapy, 88*(11), 1254–1264.

Dogra, S. (2011). Better self-perceived health is associated with lower odds of physical inactivity in older adults with chronic disease. *Journal of Aging and Physical Activity, 19*(4), 322–335.

Donaghy, M. E. (2007). Exercise can seriously improve your mental health: Fact or fiction? *Advances in Physiotherapy, 9*(2), 76–88.

Dudgeon, W. D., Phillips, K. D., Bopp, C. M., & Hand, G. A. (2004). Physiological and psychological effects of exercise interventions in HIV disease. *AIDS Patient Care and STDs, 18*(2), 81–98.

Ebnezar, J., Nagarathna, R., Yogitha, B., & Nagendra, H. R. (2012). Effects of integrated approach of Hatha yoga therapy on functional disability, pain, and flexibility in osteoarthritis of the knee joint: A randomized controlled study. *Journal of Alternative and Complementary Medicine, 18*(5), 463–472.

Ehrlich-Jones, L., Lee, J., Semanik, P., et al. (2011). Relationship between beliefs, motivation, and worries about physical activity and physical activity participation in persons with rheumatoid arthritis. *Arthritis Care & Research, 63*(12), 1700–1705.

Elsawy, B., & Higgins, K. E. (2010). Physical activity guidelines for older adults. *American Family Physician, 81*(1), 55–59.

Erbs, S., Linke, A., & Hambrecht, R. (2006). Effects of exercise training on mortality in patients with coronary heart disease. *Coronary Artery Disease, 17,* 219–225.

Escalante, Y., Saavedra, J. M., Garcia-Hermoso, A., & Dominguez, A. M. (2012). Improvement of the lipid profile with exercise in obese children: A systematic review. *Preventive Medicine, 54*(5), 293–301.

Fagard, R. H. (2011). Exercise intensity and blood pressure response to endurance training. *Hypertension, 28*(1), 20–23.

Federici, M. O., & Benedetti, M. M. (2006). Ketone bodies monitoring. *Diabetes Research & Clinical Practice, 74,* S77–S81.

Flegal, K. M., Tabak, C. J., & Ogden, C. L. (2006). Overweight in children: Definitions and interpretations. *Health Education Research, 21*(6), 755–760.

Fillipas, S., Oldmeadow, L. B., Bailey, M. J., & Cherry, C. L. (2006). A six-month, supervised, aerobic and resistance exercise program improves self-efficacy in people with human immunodeficiency virus: A randomized controlled trial. *Australian Journal of Physiotherapy, 52*(3), 185–190.

Fillipas, S., Cherry, C. L., Cicuttini, F., Smirneos, L., & Holland, A. E. (2010). The effects of exercise training on metabolic and morphological outcomes for people living with HIV: A systematic review of randomised controlled trials. *HIV Clinical Trials, 11,* 270–282.

Franklin, B. (1993). *How much exercise is enough? Encyclopedia Britannica.* (pp. 471–476). Los Angeles: Encyclopedia Britannica Inc.

Galantino, M. L., Shepard, K., Krafft, L., Laperriere, A., Ducette, J., Sorbello, A., et al. (2005). The effect of group aerobic exercise and t'ai chi on functional outcomes and quality of life for persons living with acquired immunodeficiency syndrome. *Journal of Alternative and Complementary Medicine, 11*(6), 1085–1092.

Galper, D. I., Trivedi, M. H., Barlow, C. E., Dunn, A. L., & Kampert, J. B. (2006). Inverse association between physical inactivity and mental health in men and women. *Medicine & Science in Sports & Exercise, 38*(1), 173–178.

Gammon, M. D., Schoenberg, J. B., Britton, J. A., Kelsey, J. L., Coates, R. J., Brogan, D., et al. (1998). Recreational physical activity and breast cancer risk among women under age 45 years. *American Journal of Epidemiology, 147*(3), 273–280.

Gleeson, M., Pyne, D. B., Austin, J. P., Francis, J. L., Clancy, R. L., McDonald, W. A., et al. (2002). Epstein-Barr virus reactivation and upper-respiratory illness in elite swimmers. *Medicine & Science in Sports & Exercise, 34*(3), 411–417.

Gorczynski, P., & Faulkner, G. (2010). Exercise therapy for schizophrenia. *Cochrane Database of Systematic Reviews* issue 5.

Graven, C., Brock, K., Hill, K., & Joubert, L. (2011). Are rehabilitation and/or care co-coordination interventions delivered in the community effective in reducing depression, facilitating participation and improving quality of life after stroke? *Disability and Rehabilitation, 33*(17/18), 1501–1520.

Greendale, G. A., Huang, M., Karlamangla, A. S., Seeger, L., & Crawford, S. (2009). Yoga decreases kyphosis in senior women and men with adult-onset hyperkyphosis: Results from a randomized controlled trial. *Journal of the American Geriatrics Society, 57*(9), 1569–1579.

Guadalupe-Grau, A., Fuentes, T., Guerra, B., & Calbet, A. L. (2009). Exercise and bone mass in adults. *Sports Medicine, 39*(6), 439–468.

Guide to Physical Therapist, rev 2nd ed. Alexandria, VA: Americans Physical Therapy Association.

Gulve, E. A. (2008). Exercise and glycemic control in diabetes: Benefits, challenges, and adjustments to pharmacotherapy. *Physical Therapy, 88*(11), 1297–1321.

Hale, L. A., Waters, D., & Herbison, P. (2012). A randomized controlled trial to investigate the effects of water-based exercise to improve falls risk and physical function in older adults with lower-extremity osteoarthritis. *Archives of Physical Medicine and Rehabilitation, 93,* 27–34.

Hall, A. M., Maher, C. G., Lam, P., Ferreira, M., & Latimer, J. (2011). Tai chi exercise for treatment of pain and disability in people with persistent low back pain: A randomized controlled trial. *Arthrtitis Care & Research, 63*(11), 1576–1583.

Hallal, P. C., Victora, C. G., Azevedo, M. R., & Wells, J. C.K. (2006). Adolescent physical activity and health: A systematic review. *Sports Medicine, 36*(12), 1019–1030.

Hamilton, C. J., Swan, V. J., & Jamal, S. A. (2010). The effects of exercise and physical activity participation on bone mass and geometry in postmenopausal women: A systematic review of pQCT studies. *Osteoporosis International, 21,* 11–23.

Han, A., Robinson, V. A., Judd, M. G., Taixiang, W., Wells, G., & Tugwell, P. (2004). Tai chi for treating rheumatoid arthritis. *Cochrane Database of Systematic Review* issue 3.

Hass, C. J., Garzarella, L., de Hoyos, D., & Polloch, M. (2000). Single versus multiple sets in long-term recreational weightlifters. *Medicine & Science in Sports & Exercise, 32*(1), 235–242.

Hayden, J. A., van Tulder, M. W., Malmivaara, A., & Koes, B. W. (2005). Exercise therapy for treatment of non-specific low back pain. *Cochrane Database of Systematic Review* issue 3.

He, M., & Evans, A. (2007). Are parents aware that their children are overweight or obese? *Canadian Family Physician, 53,* 1494–1499.

Hendrick, P., Te Wake, A. M., Tikkisetty, A. S., Wulff, L., Yap, C., & Milosavljevic, S. (2010). The effectiveness of walking as an intervention for low back pain: A systematic review. *European Spine Journal, 19,* 1613–1620.

Heneweer, H., Picavet, H. S., Staes, F., Kiers, H., & Vanhees, L. (2012). Physical fitness, rather than self-reported physical activities, is more strongly associated with low back pain: Evidence from a working population. *European Spine Journal, 21*(7), 1265–1272.

Henwood, T., Keogh, J., & Climstein, M. (2012). Sarcopenia in older adults. *Australian Nursing Journal, 19*(9), 39–40.

Heran, B. S., Chen, J. M., Ebrahim, S., Moxham, T., Oldridge, N., et al. (2011). Exercise-based cardiac rehabilitation for coronary heart disease. *Cochrane Database of Systematic Review* issue 7.

Herring, M. P., O'Connor, P. J., & Dishman, R. K. (2010). The effect of exercise training on anxiety symptoms among patients: A systematic review. *Archives of Internal Medicine, 170,* 321–331.

Hewlett, S., Ambler, N., Almeida, C., et al. (2011). Self-management of fatigue in rheumatoid arthritis: A randomised controlled trial of group cognitive-behavioural therapy. *Annals of the Rheumatic Diseases, 70,* 1060–1067.

Hides, J. A., Jull, G. A., & Richardson, C. A. (2001). Long-term effects of specific stabilizing exercises for first-episode low back pain. *Spine, 26*(11), E243–E248.

Hilde, G., Hagen, K. B., Jamtvedt, G., & Winnem, M. (2007). Advice to stay active as a single treatment for low back pain and sciatica. *Cochrane Database of Systematic Review* issue 6.

Howe, T. E., Shea, B., Dawson, L. J., Downie, F., Murray, A., Ross, C., et al. (2011). Exercise for preventing and treating osteoporosis in postmenopausal women. *Cochrane Database of Systematic Review* issue 7.

Hua, L. P.T., Brown, C. A., Hains, S. J.M., Godwin, M., & Parlow, J. L. (2009). Effects of low-intensity exercise conditioning on blood pressure, and autonomic modulation of heart rate in men and women with hypertension. *Biological Research for Nursing, 11*(2), 129–143.

Huang, J. S., Becerra, K., Oda, T., Walker, E., Xu, R., et al. (2007). Parental ability to discriminate the weight status of children: Results of a survey. *Pediatrics, 120*(1), e112–119.

Huang, T. T., Yang, L. H., & Liu, C. Y. (2011). Reducing the fear of falling among community-dwelling elderly adults through cognitive-behavioural strategies and intense tai chi exercise: A randomized controlled trial. *Journal of Advanced Nursing, 67*(5), 961–971.

Hurley, B., & Armstrong, T. J. (2012). Bisphosphonates vs exercise for the prevention and treatment of osteoporosis. *Journal for Nurse Practitioners, 8*(3), 217–224.

Ingram, C., & Visovsky, C. (2007). Exercise intervention to modify physiologic risk factors in cancer survivors. *Seminars in Oncology Nursing, 23*(4), 275–284.

Irvine, C., & Taylor, N. F. (2009). Progressive resistance exercise improves glycaemic control in people with type 2 diabetes mellitus: A systematic review. *Australian Journal of Physiotherapy, 55*(4), 237–246.

Iwanto, J., Sato, Y., Takeda, T., & Matsumoto, H. (2010). Effectiveness of exercise in the treatment of lumbar spinal stenosis, knee arthritis, and osteoporosis. *Aging Clinical and Experimental Research, 22*(2), 116–122.

Jamtvedt, G., Damm, K. T., Christie, A., Moe, R. H., Haavardsholm, E. A., Holm, I., et al. (2008). Physical therapy interventions for patients with osteoarthritis of the knee: An overview of systematic reviews. *Physical Therapy, 88*(1), 123–136.

Jansen, M. J., Viechtbauer, W., Lenssen, A. F., Hendriks, E. J.M., & de Bie, R. A. (2011). Strength training alone, exercise therapy alone, and exercise therapy with passive manual mobilisation each reduce pain and disability in people with knee osteoarthritis: A systematic review. *Journal of Physiotherapy, 57,* 11–20.

Jones, T. E., Stephenson, K. W., King, J. G., Knight, K. R., Marshall, T. L., & Scott, W. B. (2009). Sarcopenia—mechanism and treatments. *Journal of Geriatric Physical Therapy, 32*(2), 39–45.

Kalyani, R. R., Stein, B., Valiyil, R., Manno, R., Maynard, J. W., & Crews, D. C. (2010). Vitamin D treatment for the preventions of falls in older adults: Systematic review and meta-analysis. *Journal of the American Geriatrics Society, 58,* 1299–1310.

Keller, T. T., Squizzato, A., & Middeldorp, S. (2007). Clopidogrel plus aspirin versus aspirin alone for preventing cardiovascular disease. *Cochrane Database of Systematic Reviews* issue 3.

Kelley, G. A., & Kelley, K. S. (2009). Impact of progressive resistance training on lipids and lipoproteins in adults: A meta-analysis of randomized controlled trials. *Preventive Medicine, 48*(1), 9–19.

Kessenich, C. R. (2007). Nonpharmacological prevention of osteoporotic fractures. *Journal of Clinical Interventions in Aging, 2*(2), 263–266.

Keysor, J. J., & Brembs, A. (2011). Exercise: Necessary but not sufficient for improving function and preventing disability? *Current Opinion in Rheumatology, 23,* 211–218.

Kohrt, W. M., Bloomfield, S. A., Little, K. D., Nelson, M. E., & Yingling, V. R. (2004). American College of Sports Medicine Position stand; physical activity and bone health. *Medicine & Science in Sports & Exercise, 36*(11), 1985-1996.

Koumantakis, G. A., Watson, P. J., & Oldham, J. A. (2005). Trunk muscle stabilization training plus general exercise versus general exercise only: Randomized controlled trial of patients with recurrent low back pain. *Physical Therapy, 85*(3), 209–225.

Krieger, J. W. (2010). Single vs. multiple sets of resistance exercise for muscle hypertrophy: A meta-analysis. *Journal of Strength & Conditioning Research, 24,* 1150–1159.

Kujala, U. M. (2009). Evidence on the effects of exercise therapy in the treatment of chronic disease. *British Journal of Sports Medicine, 43,* 550–555.

Lamina, S. (2010). Effects of continuous and interval training programs in the management of hypertension: A randomized controlled trial. *Journal of Clinical Hypertension, 12*(11), 841–849.

Langdeau, J. B., & Boulet, L. P. (2001). Prevalence and mechanisms of development of asthma and airway hyperresponsiveness in athletes. *Journal of Sports Medicine, 31*(8), 601–616.

Larson-Meyer, D. E., Redman, L., Heilbronn, L. K., & Martin, C. K. (2010). Caloric restriction with or without exercise: The fitness versus fatness debate. *Medicine & Science in Sports & Exercise, 42*(1), 152–159.

Larun, L., Nordheim, L. V., Ekeland, E., Hagen, K. B., & Heian, F. (2009). Exercise in prevention and treatment of anxiety and depression among children and young people. *Cochrane Database of Systematic Review* issue 3.

Lavie, C. J., & Milani, R. V. (2011). Cardiac rehabilitation and exercise training in secondary coronary heart disease prevention. *Progress in Cardiovascular Diseases, 53*(6), 397–403.

Lee, D. J., Meehan, R. T., Robinson, C., Mabry, T. R., & Smith, M. L. (1992). Immune responsiveness and risk of illness in US Air Force Academy cadets during basic cadet training. *Aviation, Space, and Environmental Medicine, 63*(6), 517–523.

Leung, D. P., Chan, C. K., Tsang, H. W., Tsang, W. W., & Jones, A. Y. (2011). Tai chi as an intervention to improve balance and reduce falls in older adults: A systematic and meta-analytical review. *Alternative Therapies in Health and Medicine, 17*(1), 40–48.

Li, J., & Hooker, N. H. (2010). Childhood obesity and schools: Evidence from the National Survey of Children's Health. *Journal of School Health, 80*(2), 96–103.

Lin, Y., Yeh, M., & Huang, L. (2010). Physical activity status and gender differences in community-dwelling older adults with chronic diseases. *Journal of Nursing Research, 18*(2), 88–96.

Lirani-Galvao, A. P.R., & Lazaretti-Castro, M. (2010). Physical approach for prevention and treatment of osteoporosis. *Arquivos Brasileiros de Endocrinologia and Metabologia, 54*(2), 171–178.

Liu, C. K., & Fielding, R. A. (2011). Exercise as an intervention for frailty. *Clinics in Geriatric Medicine, 27*(1), 101–110.

Liu, Y., Hu, F., Li, D., Wang, F., Zhu, L., Chen, W., et al. (2011). Does physical activity reduce the risk of prostate cancer? A systematic review and meta-analysis. *European Urology, 60,* 1029–1044.

Liu-Ambrose, T. Y., Ashe, M. C., & Marra, C. (2010). Independent and inverse association of healthcare utilisation with physical activity in older adults with multiple chronic conditions. *British Journal of Sports Medicine, 44*(14), 1024–1028.

Macfarlane, D. J., Chou, K., & Cheng, W. (2005). The effect of tai chi on the physical and psychological well-being of Chinese older women. *Journal of Exercise Science & Fitness, 3*(2), 87–94.

Mackinnon, L. T. (1992). *Exercise and immunology.* Champaign, IL: Human Kinetics.

Marcus, R. L., Smith, S., Morrell, G., Addison, O., Dibble, L. E., et al. (2008). Comparison of combined aerobic and high-force eccentric resistance exercise with aerobic exercise only for people with type 2 diabetes mellitus. *Physical Therapy, 88*(11), 1345–1354.

Marquard, J. L., Stolee, P., Zaza, C., & Schuehlein, S. (2012). Evaluation of a volunteer-led in-home program for home-bound older adults. *Work, 41*(3), 339–354.

Martin, D. (2011). Physical activity benefits and risks on the gastrointestinal system. *Southern Medical Journal, 104,* 831–837.

Martyn-St James, M., & Carroll, S. (2009). A meta-analysis of impact exercise on postmenopausal bone loss: The case for mixed loading exercise programmes. *British Journal of Sports Medicine, 43*(12), 898–908.

Matthews, C. E., Ockene, I. S., Freedson, P. S., Rosal, M. C., Merriam, P. A., & Hebert, J. R. (2002). Moderate to vigorous physical activity and risk of upper-respiratory tract infection. *Medicine & Science in Sports & Exercise, 34*(8), 1242–1248.

May, S. (2010). Self-management of chronic low back pain and osteoarthritis. *Nature Reviews Rheumatology, 6,* 199–209.

McDermott, A. Y., & Mernitz, H. (2006). Exercise and older patients: Prescribing guidelines. *American Family Physician, 74*(3), 437–444.

McGrath, J. A., O'Malley, M., & Hendrix, T. J. (2010). Group exercise mode and health-related quality of life among healthy adults. *Journal of Advanced Nursing, 67*(3), 491–500.

McKinnis, L. N. (2010). *Fundamentals of orthopedic radiology* (3rd ed.). Philadelphia: F.A. Davis.

Mead, G. E., Morley, W., Campbell, P., Greig, C. A., McMurdo, M., & Lawlor, D. A. (2009). Exercise for depression. *Cochrane Database of Systematic Review* issue 3.

Menschik, D., Ahmed, S., Alexander, M. H., & Blum, R. W. (2008). Adolescent physical activities as predictors of young adult weight. *Archives of Pediatric & Adolescent Medicine, 162*(1), 29–33.

Milani, R. V., Lavie, C. J., Mehra, M. R., & Ventura, H. O. (2011). Impact of exercise training and depression on survival in heart failure due to coronary heart disease. *American Journal of Cardiology, 107,* 64–68.

Moore, L., Harris, C., & Bradlyn, A. (2012). Exploring the relationship between parental concern and the management of childhood obesity. *Maternal and Child Health Journal, 16*(4), 902–908.

Morgan, K. T. (2012). Nutrition, resistance training, and sarcopenia: Their role in successful aging. *Topics in Clinical Nutrition, 27*(2), 114–123.

Nahas, R., & Sheikh, O. (2011). Complementary and alternative medicine for the treatment of major depressive disorder. *Canadian Family Physician, 57*(6), 659–663.

National Institutes of Health. (1998). *Clinical guidelines on the identification, evaluation, and treatment of overweight and obesity in adults.* (Vol. 8, Pub. No. 98–4083), Bethesda, MD: Department of Health and Human Services, National Institutes of Health, National Heart, Lung and Blood Institute.

National Institutes of Health, Osteoporosis and Related Bone Disease—National Resource Center. (2011). *Osteoporosis.* Retrieved July 10, 2012, from www.niams.nih.gov/Health_Info/Bone/Osteoporosis.

National Osteoporosis Foundation. (2011). *Fast facts.* Retrieved July 10, 2012, from www.nof.org/node/40.

National Physical Activity Plan. (2010). Retrieved January 10, 2013, from physical activity.org.

Nieman, D. (1994). Exercise, upper respiratory tract infection, and the immune system. *Medicine & Science in Sports & Exercise, 26*(2), 128–139.

Nieman, D. (2000). Exercise soothes arthritis: Joint effects. *ACSM's Health & Fitness Journal, 4*(3), 20–28.

Nieman, D. C., Johanssen, L. M., Lee, J. W., & Arabatzis, K. (1990). Infectious episodes in runners before and after the Los Angeles Marathon. *Journal of Sports Medicine and Physical Fitness, 30*(3), 316–328.

Nikander, R., Sievanen, H., Heionon, A., Daly, R. M., Uusi-Rasi, K., & Kannus, P. (2010). Targeted exercise against osteoporosis: A systematic review and meta-analysis for optimising bone strength throughout life. *BMC Medicine, 8*(47), 1–16.

Nixon, S., O'Brien, K., Glazier, R. H., & Tynan, A. M. (2005). Aerobic exercise interventions for adults living with HIV/AIDS. *Cochrane Database of Systematic Review* issue 2.

O'Brien, K., Nixon, S., Glazier, R. H., & Tynan, A. M. (2004). Progressive resistive exercise interventions for adults living with HIV/AIDS. *Cochrane Database of Systematic Review* issue 4.

O'Brien, K., Nixon, S., Glazier, R., & Tynan, A. M. (2009). Progressive resistive exercise interventions for adults living with HIV/AIDS. *Cochrane Database of Systematic Review* issue 4.

O'Brien, K., Nixon, S., Tynan, A. M., & Glazier, R. (2010). Aerobic exercise interventions for adults living with HIV/AIDS. *Cochrane Database of Systematic Review* issue 8.

O'Donovan, G., Blazevich, A. J., Boreham, C., Cooper, A. R., Crank, H., et al. (2010). The ABC of physical activity for health: A consensus statement from the British Association for Sport and Exercise Sciences. *Journal of Sports Sciences, 28*(6), 573–591.

Oerkild, B., Frederiksen, M., Hansen, J. F., Simonsen, L., Skovgaard, L. T., & Prescott, E. (2011). Home-based cardiac rehabilitation is as effective as centre-based cardiac rehabilitation among elderly with coronary heart disease: Results from a randomised clinical trial. *Age & Ageing, 40*, 78–85.

Ogden, C. L., Carroll, M. D., Curtin, L. R., McDowell, M. A., Tabak, C. J., & Flegal, K. M. (2006). Prevalence of overweight and obesity in the United States, 1999-2004. *Journal of the American Medical Association, 295*(13), 1549–1555.

Ogden, C. L., Caroll, M. D., Kit, B. K., & Flegal, K. M. (2012). *Prevalence of obesity in the United States, 2009-2010. NCHS data brief, No. 82.* Hyattsville, MD: National Center for Health Statistics.

Oh, R. C., & Lanier, J. B. (2007). Management of hypertriglyceridemia. *American Family Physician, 75*(9), 1365–1371.

Park, Y. H., Song, M., Cho, B. L., Lim, J. Y., Song, W., & Kim, S. H. (2011). The effects of an integrated health education and exercise program in community-dwelling older adults with hypertension: A randomized controlled trial. *Patient Education and Counseling, 82*(1), 133–137.

Pate, R. R., Pratt, M., Blair, S. N., Haskell, W. L., Macera, C. A., Bouchard, C., et al. (1995). Physical activity and public health. A recommendation for the Centers for Disease Control and Prevention and the American College of Sports Medicine. *Journal of the American Medical Association, 273*(5), 402–407.

Pedersen, B. K., & Bruunsgaard, H. (1995). How physical exercise influences the establishment of infections. *Sports Medicine, 19*(6), 393–400.

Pedersen, B., & Ullum, H. (1994). NK cell response to physical activity: Possible mechanisms of action. *Medicine & Science in Sports & Exercise, 26*(2), 140–146.

Pedersen, B., Rohde, T., & Ostrowski, K. (1998). Recovery of the immune system after exercise. *Acta Physiologica Scandinavica, 162*(3), 325–332.

Pejic, R. N., & Lee, D. T. (2006). Hypertriglyceridemia. *Journal of the American Board of Family Medicine, 19*(3), 310–316.

Pentecost, C., & Taket, A. (2011). Understanding exercise uptake and adherence for people with chronic conditions: A new model demonstrating the importance of exercise identity, benefits of attending and support. *Health Education Research, 26*, 908–922.

Perry, S. B., & Downey, P. A. (2012). Fracture risk and prevention: A multidimensional approach. *Physical Therapy, 92*(1), 164–178.

Pescatello, L. S., Franklin, B. A., Fagard, R., Farquhar, W. B., Kelley, G. A., & Ray, C. A. (2004). American College of Sports Medicine position standard. Exercise and hypertension. *Medicine & Science in Sports & Exercise, 36*(3), 533–553.

Peters-Futre, E. M. (1997). Vitamin C, neutrophil function, and upper respiratory tract infection risk in distance runners: The missing link. *Exercise Immunology Review, 3*, 32–52.

Pisters, M. F., Veenhof, C., Schellevis, F. G., et al. (2010). Exercise adherence improving long-term patient outcome in patients with osteoarthritis of the hip and/or knee. *Arthritis Care & Research, 62*(8), 1087–1094.

Polikandrioti, M., & Dokoutsidou, H. (2009). The role of exercise and nutrition in type II diabetes mellitus management. *Health Science Journal, 3*(4), 216–221.

Pyne, D. B., Baker, M. S., Fricker, P. A., McDonald, W. A., Telford, R. D., & Weidemann, M. J. (1995). Effects of an intensive 12-wk training program by elite swimmers on neutrophil oxidative activity. *Medicine & Science in Sports & Exercise, 27*(4), 536–542.

Rand, D., Miller, W. C., Yiu, J., & Eng, J. J. (2011). Interventions for addressing low balance confidence in older adults: A systematic review and meta-analysis. *Age & Aging, 40*(3), 297–306.

Rasmussen-Barr, E., Ang, B., Arvidsson, I., & Nilsson-Wikmar, L. (2009). Graded exercise for recurrent low-back pain: A randomized, controlled trial with 6-, 12-, and 36-month follow-ups. *Spine, 34*, 221–228.

Rethorst, C. D., Wipfli, B. M., & Landers, D. M. (2009). The antidepressive effects of exercise: A meta-analysis of randomized trials. *Sports Medicine, 39*(6), 491–511.

Rixt Zijlstra, G. A., van Haastregt, J. C., Ambergen, T., van Rossum, E., van Eijk, J. T., et al. (2009). Effects of a multicomponent cognitive behavioural group intervention on fear of falling and activity avoidance in community-dwelling older adults: Results of a randomized controlled trial. *Journal of the American Geriatrics Society, 57*(11), 2020–2028.

Roffey, D. M., Wai, E. K., Bishop, P., Kwon, B. K., & Dagenais, S. (2010a). Causal assessment of awkward occupational postures and low back pain: Results of a systematic review. *Spine Journal, 10*(1), 89–99.

Roffey, D. M., Wai, E. K., Bishop, P., Kwon, B. K., & Dagenais, S. (2010b). Causal assessment of occupational sitting and low back pain: Results of a systematic review. *Spine Journal, 10*(3), 252–261.

Roffey, D. M., Wai, E. K., Bishop, P., Kwon, B. K., & Dagenais, S. (2010c). Causal assessment of occupational standing or walking and low back pain: Results of a systematic review. *Spine Journal, 10*(3), 262–272.

Roffey, D. M., Wai, E. K., Bishop, P., Kwon, B. K., & Dagenais, S. (2010d). Causal assessment of occupational pushing or pulling and low back pain: Results of a systematic review. *Spine Journal, 10*(6), 544–553.

Roffey, D. M., Wai, E. K., Bishop, P., Kwon, B. K., & Dagenais, S. (2010e). Causal assessment of workplace manual handling or assisting patients and low back pain: Results of a systematic review. *Spine Journal, 10*(7), 639–651.

Rose, D. J., & Hernandez, D. (2010). The role of exercise in fall prevention for older adults. *Clinics in Geriatric Medicine, 26*(4), 607–631.

Roussel, M., Garnier, S., Lemoine, S., Gaubert, I., Charonnier, L., et al. (2009). Influence of a walking program on the metabolic risk profile of obese postmenopausal women. *Menopause, 16*(3), 566–575.

Sanudo, B., Galiano, D., Carrasco, L., Blagojevic, M., de Hoyo, M., et al. (2010). Aerobic exercise versus combined exercise therapy in women with fibromyalgia syndrome: A randomized controlled trial. *Archives of Physical Medicine & Rehabilitation, 91*(12), 1838–1843.

Sanudo, B., de Hoyo, M., Carrasco, L., Rodriguez-Blanco, C., Oliva-Pascual-Vaca, A., et al. (2012). Effect of whole-body vibration exercise on balance in women with fibromyalgia syndrome: A randomized controlled trial. *Journal of Alternative and Complementary Medicine, 18*(2), 158–164.

Sax, P. E. (2006). Strategies for management and treatment of dyslipidemia in HIV/AIDS. *AIDS Care, 18*(2), 149–157.

Saxena, S., Van Ommeren, M., Tang, K. C., & Armstrong, T. P. (2005). Mental health benefits of physical activity. *Journal of Mental Health, 14*(5), 445–451.

Schamliyan, T. A., Kane, R. L., Wyman, J., & Wilt, T. J. (2008). Systematic review: Randomized, controlled trials of nonsurgical treatments for urinary incontinence in women. *Annals of Internal Medicine, 148*(6), 459–473.

Scharoun-Lee, M., Kaufman, J. S., Popkin, B. M., & Gordon-Larsen, P. (2009). Obesity, race/ethnicity and life course socioeconomic status across the transition from adolescence to adulthood. *Journal of Epdemiology & Community Health, 63*(2), 133–139.

Shaughnessy, M., & Caulfield, B. (2004). A pilot study to investigate the effect of lumbar stabilisation exercise training on functional ability and quality of life in patients with chronic low back pain. *International Journal of Rehabilitation Research, 27*(4), 297–301.

Shaw, K., Gennat, H., O'Rourke, P., & Del Mar, C. (2006). Exercise for overweight or obesity. *Cochrane Database of Systematic Review* issue 4.

Shiri, R., Karppinen, J., Leino-Arjas, P., Solovieva, S., & Viikari-Juntura, E. (2010). The association between obesity and low back pain: A meta-analysis. *American Journal of Epidemiology, 171*, 135–154.

Silva, L. E., Valim, V., Pessanha, A. P.C., Oliviera, L. M., Myamoto, S., Jones, A., et al. (2008). Hydrotherapy versus conventional land-based exercise for the management of patients with osteoarthritis of the knee: A randomized clinical trial. *Physical Therapy, 88*(1), 12–21.

Simpson, R. J., & Guy, K. (2010). Coupling aging immunity with a sedentary lifestyle: Has the damage already been done? A mini-review. *Gerontology, 56*, 449–458.

Skinner, J. S., Hustler, R., Bergsteinova, V., & Buskirk, R. (1973). The validity and reliability of a rating scale of perceived exertion. *Medicine & Science in Sports & Exercise, 5*(2), 94–96.

Slade, S. C., & Keating, J. L. (2007). Unloaded movement facilitation exercise compared to no exercise or alternative therapy on outcomes for people with nonspecific chronic low back pain: A systematic review. *Journal of Manipulative and Physiological Therapeutics, 30*(4), 301–311.

Smith, S. S., Wang, C. H., & Bloomfield, S. A. (2009). *Osteoporosis ACSM's exercise management for persons with chronic diseases and disabilities.* (3rd ed., pp. 270–279). Champaign, IL: Human Kinetics.

Smutok, M., Skrinar, G., & Pandolf, K. (1980). Exercise intensity: Subjective regulation by perceived exertion. *Archives of Physical Medicine & Rehabilitation, 61*(12), 569–574.

Staal, J. B., Hlobil, H., Twisk, J. W., Smid, T., Koke, A. J., & van Mechelen, W. (2004). Graded activity for low back pain in occupational health care: A randomized, controlled trial. *Annals of Internal Medicine, 140*(2), 77–84.

Strasser, B., Siebert, U., & Schobersberger, W. (2010). Resistance training in the treatment of the metabolic syndrome. *Sports Medicine, 40*(5), 397–415.

Tambalis, K., Panagiotakos, D. B., Kavouras, S. A., & Sidossis, L. S. (2009). Responses of blood lipids to aerobic, resistance, and combined aerobic with resistance exercise training: A systematic review of current evidence. *Angiology, 60*(5), 614–832.

Tarnopolsky, M. A. (2008). Nutritional consideration in the aging athlete. *Clinical Journal of Sport Medicine, 18*(6), 531–538.

Terry, L., Sprinz, E., Medeiros, N. B., Oliveira, J., & Ribeiro, J. P. (2006). Exercise training in HIV-1-infected individuals with dyslipidemia and lipodystrophy. *Medicine & Science in Sports & Exercise, 38*(3), 411–417.

Theobald, H. E. (2005). Dietary calcium and health. *Nutrition Bulletin, 30*(3), 237–277.

Tremblay, A., Despres, J. P., & Bouchard, C. (1985). The effects of exercise-training on energy balance and adipose tissue morphology and metabolism. *Sports Medicine, 2*(3), 223–233.

Trudeau, F., Laurencelle, L., & Shephard, R. J. (2004). Tracking of physical activity from childhood to adulthood. *Medicine and Science in Sports and Exercise, 36*(11), 1937–1943.

Tseng, C. N., Gau, B. S., & Lou, M. F. (2011). The effectiveness of exercise on improving cognitive function in older people: A systematic review. *Journal of Nursing Research, 19*, 119–131.

Turcotte, L. P., & Fisher, J. S. (2008). Skeletal muscle insulin resistance: Roles of fatty acid metabolism and exercise. *Physical Therapy, 88*(11), 1279–1296.

Uhlig, T., Fongen, C., Steen, E., Christie, A., & Odegard, S. (2010). Exploring tai chi in rheumatoid arthritis: A quantitative and qualitative study. *BMC Musculoskeletal Disorders, 11*(43), 1–7.

U.S. Department of Health and Human Services. (2008). *2008 Physical Activity Guidelines for Americans.* Washington, DC. Retrieved January 10, 2013, from www.healthgov/pagguidelines/.

U.S. Department of Health and Human Services. (2010). *Healthy People 2020.* Washington, DC: Author. Retrieved from www.healthypeople.gov.

U.S. Department of Health and Human Services. (2000, January). *Healthy People 2010* (Vols. 1 and 2, Conference ed.). Washington, DC: Author.

U.S. Department of Health and Human Services. (2006, December). *Midcourse review. Healthy People 2010.* Washington, DC: Author.

U.S. Census Bureau. (2011, May). *2010 Census shows nation's population is aging.* Washington, DC: Author.

van Middelkoop, M., Rubinstein, S. M., Verhagen, A. P., Ostelo, R. W., Koes, B. W., et al. (2010). Exercise therapy for chronic nonspecific low-back pain. *Best Practice & Research in Clinical Rheumatology, 24,* 193–204.

Visceglia, E., & Lewis, S. (2011). Yoga as an adjunctive treatment for schizophrenia: A randomized, controlled pilot study. *Journal of Alternative & Complementary Medicine, 17*(7), 601–607.

Wai, E. K., Roffey, D. M., Bishop, P., Kwon, B. K., & Dagenais, S. (2010a). Causal assessment of occupational bending or twisting and low back pain: Results of a systematic review. *Spine Journal, 10*(1), 76–88.

Wai, E. K., Roffey, D. M., Bishop, P., Kwon, B. K., & Dagenais, S. (2010b). Causal assessment of occupational lifting and low back pain: Results of a systematic review. *Spine Journal, 10*(6), 554–566.

Wai, E. K., Roffey, D. M., Bishop, P., Kwon, B. K., & Dagenais, S. (2010c). Causal assessment of occupational carrying and low back pain: Results of a systematic review. *Spine Journal, 10*(7), 628–638.

Wallace, J. P., & Ray, S. (2009). Obesity. In *ACSM's exercise management for persons with chronic diseases and disabilities* (3rd ed., pp. 192–200). Champaign, IL: Human Kinetics.

Walrand, S., Guillet, C., Salles, J., Cano, N., & Boirie, Y. (2011). Physiopathological mechanism of sarcopenia. *Clinics in Geriatric Medicine, 27*(3), 365–385.

Walsh, N. P., Gleeson, M., Shephard, R. J., Gleeson, M., Woods, J. A., Bishop, N. C., et al. (2011). Position statement. Part one: Immune function and exercise. *Exercise Immunology Review, 17,* 6–63.

Wang, C., Schmid, C. H., Hibberd, P. L., Kalish, R., Roubenoff, R., et al. (2009). Tai chi is effective in treating knee osteoarthritis: A randomized controlled trial. *Arthritis & Rheumatism: Arthritis Care & Research, 61*(11), 1545–1553.

Wang, C., Bannuru, R., Ramel, J., Kupelnick, B., Scott, T., & Schmid, C. H. (2010). Tai chi on psychological well-being: Systematic review and meta-analysis. *BMC Complementary and Alternative Medicine, 10,* 23. 10.1186/1472-6882-10-23.

Warburton, D. E., Katzmarzyk, P. T., Rhodes, R. E., & Shephard, R. J. (2007). Evidence-informed physical activity guidelines for Canadian adults. *Canadian Journal of Public Health, 98*(Suppl. 2), S16–S68.

Waryasz, G. R., & McDermott, A. Y. (2010). Exercise prescription and the patient with type 2 diabetes: A clinical approach to optimizing patient outcomes. *Journal of American Academy of Nurse Practitioners, 22,* 217–227.

Weltman, N. Y., Saliba, S. A., Barrett, E. J., & Weltman, A. (2009). The use of exercise in the management of type 1 and type 2 diabetes. *Clinics in Sports Medicine, 28*(3), 423–439.

Whitson, H. E., Hastings, S. N., Landerman, L. R., Fillenbaum, G. G., Cohen, H. J., et al. (2011). Back-white disparity in disability: The role of medical conditions. *Journal of the American Geriatrics Society, 59*(5), 844–850.

Windle, G., Hughes, D., Linck, P., Russell, I., & Woods, B. (2010). Is exercise effective in promoting mental well-being in older age? A systematic review. *Aging & Mental Health, 14*(6), 652–669.

Yeh, M. L., Wang, P. C., Lin, J. G., Lin, I. H., & Chen, H. H. (2011). The effect of exercise on body composition in menopausal women: A systematic review and meta-analysis. *Journal of Nursing and Health Care Research, 7*(1), 44.

Yuan, G., Al-Shali, K. Z., & Hegele, R. A. (2007). Hypertriglyceridemia: Its etiology, effects and treatment. *Canadian Medical Association Journal, 176*(8), 1113–1120.

Zehnacker, C. H., & Bemis-Dougherty, A. (2007). Effect of weighted exercises on bone mineral density in post menopausal women without hormone replacement therapy. *Journal of Geriatric Physical Therapy, 30*(2), 79–88.

Zijlstra, G. A.R., van Haastregt, J. C.M., Ambergen, T., van Rossum, E., van Eijk, J. T.M., et al. (2009). Effects of a multicomponent cognitive behavioral group intervention on fear of falling and activity avoidance in community-dwelling older adults: Results of a randomized controlled trial. *Journal of the American Geriatrics Society, 57*(11), 2020–2028.

Zorba, E., Cengiz, T., & Karacabey, K. (2011). Exercise training improves body composition, blood lipid profile and serum insulin levels in obese children. *Journal of Sports Medicine and Physical Fitness, 51*(4), 664–669.

Stress Management

June Andrews Horowitz*

 WEBSITE

http://evolve.elsevier.com/Edelman/
- Study Questions
- Glossary

OBJECTIVES

After completing this chapter, the reader will be able to:
- Analyze concepts of stress, stressor, eustress, and distress.
- Evaluate potential physical, psychological, social, spiritual, and behavioral stressors.
- Analyze the pathophysiology of the stress response and effects on health and illness.
- Examine primary and secondary cognitive appraisals of stress.
- Develop evidence-based stress-management interventions that can be used in clinical practice.
- Explain the nurse's role in stress management and crisis intervention.

KEY TERMS

Active listening
Acupuncture
Affirmation
Anxiety sensitivity
Aromatherapy
Assertive communication
Burnout
Caregiver stress/burden
Cognitive restructuring
Coping
Diabetes
Distress
Empathy
Eustress
Exercise
Expressive writing

Fight-or-flight response
Goal setting
Healthy diet
Healthy pleasures
Humor
Hypnosis
Journal writing
Meridian
Mindfulness
Mini-relaxations
Presence
Primary appraisal
Reflexology
Reiki
Relaxation response
Sandwich generation

Secondary appraisal
Self-awareness
Sleep hygiene
Social support
Sociophysiology
Spillover stress
Spiritual practice
Stress
Stress management
Stress response
Stress warning signs
Stressor
Values clarification
Yoga

*Assistance with this chapter revision was provided by Christy Tran and Danielle Turpin, undergraduate research fellows, Wm. F. Connell School of Nursing, Boston College.

Stress is an excellent paradigm for understanding the relationships among the determinants of health, the leading health indicators, and health outcomes. Stress has been shown to cause or exacerbate many of the leading health problems in the United States today, such as those related to obesity, alcohol and drug abuse, and sexually transmitted diseases (U.S. Department of Health and Human Services [USDHHS], 2011). Consequently, helping individuals, families, and communities to find more effective ways to respond to stress is an important health-promotion goal. The Centers for Disease Control and Prevention (CDC) healthy communities program works to support people in making healthy choices where they live and work (CDC, 2012a).

Stress management has been an effective intervention framework for health promotion, disease prevention, and symptom management. Stress-management strategies such as relaxation and imagery, self-monitoring, goal setting, cognitive restructuring, and problem-solving have long been staples of community health-promotion programs, including Alcoholics Anonymous, SmokEnders, YMCA (Y-USA), and Weight Watchers. These strategies help people to modify health risk behaviors and thereby improve quality of life. However, national health data (CDC, 2012b) indicate the need for continued and expanded use of these modalities across the life span. Although the United States health care system provides excellent, expensive, heroic care, it provides poor quality low-cost health-promotion/preventive care, including stress management. Moreover, to ameliorate many harmful effects of stress, community-level health promotion is essential. Although shifting focus from providing acute care for individuals to enhancing health of communities requires a revolution in our health care delivery systems and outlook, successful community health-promotion initiatives hold promise for the future (Butterfoss, 2009).

The goal of stress management is to improve quality of life by increasing healthy, effective coping, thereby reducing unhealthy consequences of distress. This process produces a dynamic interaction of mind, body, and spirit, which influences physical health and well-being. Stress management is thus an essential tool for expert nursing practice, which recognizes the interface of knowledge on behavior change. The use of critical reasoning to examine multiple factors contributing to symptom development provides a valuable contribution to meeting the goals of *Healthy People 2020*. Stress management can have a significant impact on the following leading health indicators in *Healthy People 2020*: physical activity, obesity, tobacco use, substance abuse, responsible sexual behavior, mental health, injury and violence, environmental quality, immunization, workplace wellness, and access to health care (USDHHS, 2011). (See Chapter 1 for additional discussion of *Healthy People 2020*.) This chapter outlines the psychophysiological aspects of stress, examines strategies shown to mediate its harmful effects, reviews clinical situations in which stress management has been effective, and explores the unique perspective nurses bring that helps individuals identify healthy stress-management strategies.

SOURCES OF STRESS

A stressor is any psychological, social, environmental, physiological, or spiritual stimulus that disrupts homeostasis, thereby requiring change or adaptation (Bartol & Courts, 2009) (Figure 13-1). Stress is a state of threatened homeostasis that triggers an array of adaptive physiological and behavioral responses in an effort to reestablish homeostasis (Kyrou & Tsigos, 2009). These views of stress underscore important ideas: even welcome events, such as a child's wedding, are stressors because they precipitate change, stress is not intrinsically bad or unhealthy, and stress is experienced psychophysiologically. Stress is an essential component of being alive. Stress can be situational or maturational. One's coping strategies and resources will determine the outcomes of each crisis experience.

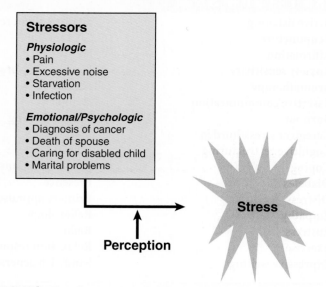

FIGURE 13-1 Stressors can be physiologic or emotional/psychologic. Perception of the stressors will determine whether they cause stress. (Lewis SL, Dirksen SR, Heitkemper MM, et al. (2014). *Medical-surgical nursing: assessment and management of clinical problems,* ed 9, St Louis, 2014, Mosby.)

Individuals encounter a variety of physical, psychological, social, spiritual, and environmental stressors. Stressors range from health and illness experiences, such as childbirth, physical illness, trauma, or blood loss; to activities of daily living, such as caring for children, meeting work deadlines, and cleaning or repairing the house; to less common events, such as taking a critical examination, experiencing the death of a relative, losing possessions in a fire, losing a job, getting a divorce, or getting married. Stressors can be organized into three categories: stressors over which people have no control (extrinsic factors), such as the weather, a traffic jam, or the death of a spouse; stressors that individuals can modify by changing their environment, social interactions, or behaviors; and stressors created or exacerbated (intrinsic factors) by poor time management, procrastination, poor communication, catastrophic negative thinking (expecting the worst), or struggling with self-defeating behaviors. Stress is a person-environment process. The person-environment fit model indicates that the person appraises a situation as taxing or as exceeding his or her resources and endangering well-being (Kahana et al., 2003; Lazarus & Folkman, 1984; Weber, 2011). Stress appraisal is an important concept that helps to explain why two people react in different ways to the same situation. In addition, models of stress have evolved an individualistic perspective to consideration of family and community level stress and coping (Weber, 2011).

Ms. Smith (86 years old) and Ms. Jones (86 years old), both in good health, is a case in point. Both individuals are about to become new residents at an assisted living retirement community in their hometown. Ms. Smith perceives this move as an opportunity to increase the ease of her socializations and activities of daily living, and is looking forward to making new friends and participating in new recreational activities. In contrast, Ms. Jones views this move as abandonment by her family and fears that available resources will be inadequate. Although the event is virtually the same for both Ms. Smith and Ms. Jones, the physiological, psychosocial, and spiritual consequences are personalized because each woman perceives her situation differently. Even though the move to the new environment is the same, each woman has different coping styles and each has different support systems so the experience will differ in its level of stress.

Stress is the physical, psychological, social, or spiritual effect of life's pressures and events. Stress is an interactive process that involves appraisal and response to loss or the threat of loss of the person's homeostasis or well-being at individual, family, and community levels (Weber, 2011). Canadian physiologist Hans Selye first introduced the General Adaptation Syndrome (1950, 1974, 1982), which led the way to continual interest in stress and the effect on the body. Selye reported that, to a certain extent, stress can be challenging and useful, which he identified as eustress. Selye also observed that when stress becomes chronic or excessive, the body is unable to adapt and maintain homeostasis and thus becomes distress. Stress can be both useful and harmful. As stress increases, efficiency and performance also increase, but not endlessly. At a certain point performance and efficiency start to decrease significantly if stress continues unabated. It is important to understand the many causes of stress and the negative physical, psychosocial, and spiritual consequences of distress. Understanding the many-sided sources of stress provides the rationale for a multifaceted approach to its management (Box 13-1: Hot Topics).

Models for understanding human stress are multifaceted and complex. In the past, scientists and clinicians tended to examine and understand stress from their own disciplinary or scientific silos. In other words, understanding stress was typically split into neurobiological and psychosocial camps. However, in recent decades "sociophysiology" has emerged as a multidisciplinary perspective to integrate the "social" and "biological" worlds and answer the following question (Barchas & Barchas, 2011, p. 1): "How do social processes

---

⚠ BOX 13-1   HOT TOPICS

Relationship Between Stress and Development of Breast Cancer and Survivorship

Nurses appreciate the multiple factors in the development of breast cancer and other diseases. Researchers exploring the relationship between stress and breast cancer have demonstrated a relationship among stress (personality traits, stressful life events, and responses to stress), the immune system, genetics, and environmental factors. The physiological influences of stress on breast cancer may be mediated by the immune system. Although women may be unable to prevent stress in their lives, they can learn stress-management strategies. Dealing positively with stress may improve the quality of life for individuals and their families with or at risk for breast cancer.

Growing research evidence supports this understanding of the complex interactions between life stress and breast cancer risk. For example, Kruk (2012) examined the relationship between severe life events and breast cancer risk. The investigator employed case-control examination of 858 Polish invasive breast cancer cases and 1095 controls matched for age and place of residence. Data on life events, sociodemographic characteristics, reproductive factors, family history of breast cancer, current weight and height, and lifestyle habits were collected via a self-administered questionnaire. Unconditional logistic regression analyses with odds ratios with 95% confidence intervals were estimated. After adjustment for potential breast cancer risk factors, women with 4 to 6 individual major life events had 5.33 times higher risk for breast cancer, compared with those in the lowest quartile. Similarly, women with a high lifetime life change score had about 5 times higher risk compared to women with corresponding scores in the lowest range. Several life events (death of a close family member, personal injury or illness, imprisonment/trouble with the law, retirement) were significantly associated with breast cancer risk. Those findings suggest that major life events may have an important etiological role in the development of breast cancer. Surviving breast cancer also poses ongoing challenges to women who experienced breast cancer and their partners (Gregorio et al., 2012).

From Gregorio, S. W., Carpenter, K. M., Dorfman, C. S., Yang, I. L. C., Simonelli, L. F., & Carson III, W. E. (2012). Impact of breast cancer recurrence and cancer-specific stress on spouse health and immune function. *Brain, Behavior, & Immunity, 26(2)*, 228-233; Kruk, J. (March 2012). Self-reported psychological stress and the risk of breast cancer: A case-control study. *Stress, 15(2)*, 162-171; National Cancer Institute. (n.d.). *Psychological stress and cancer: Questions and answers.* Retrieved from www.cancer.gov/cancertopics/factsheet/Risk/stress.

impact the physiology of the organism and how does that altered physiology affect future social behavior?" Thus understanding stress and its management involves attention to the *interactions* of social and biological life at individual and family/communal levels. It follows that stress-management strategies/interventions need to be multifaceted and could be aimed at neurophysiological and interpersonal/social stressors and/or interactions and responses. Establishing empathy by the nurse in understanding stress is beneficial in designing interventions aimed at primary, secondary, and tertiary levels of prevention.

PHYSICAL, PSYCHOLOGICAL, SOCIOBEHAVIORAL, AND SPIRITUAL CONSEQUENCES OF STRESS

Physiological Effects of Stress

An individual's response to stress provides a model to examine changes across biopsychosocial-spiritual domains. In response to a perceived threat (i.e., stressor), the body prepares to meet

the challenge. Perception of threat stimulates a physiological pattern of neuroendocrine activation and behavioral changes mediated by the central nervous system (Figure 13-2) (Bartol & Courts, 2009). In most cases this reaction is an adaptive, short-term, acute response to a stressor. First termed the **fight-or-flight response** (Cannon, 1914) and later called the **stress response** (Selye, 1950, 1974, 1982), the individual's reaction to a real or imagined threat prepares the body for emergency reaction and fosters survival in circumstances of immediate, time-limited threat. The hypothalamus signals the sympathetic nervous system to release epinephrine and norepinephrine, along with other related hormones. A resultant state of arousal is characterized by increased levels of the following: metabolism, pulse rate, blood pressure, respirations, and muscle tension. This physiological arousal proceeds along three main pathways: the musculoskeletal system, the autonomic nervous system, and the psychoneuroendocrine system.

The musculoskeletal system responds by increasing tension and tone. At the same time, the autonomic nervous system, via the sympathetic branch, orchestrates a generalized arousal that includes increases in heart rate, blood pressure, and respiratory

FIGURE 13-2 The stress response. *ACTH,* Adrenocorticotropic hormone; *ANS,* autonomic nervous system; *anti-inflam resp.,* anti-inflammatory response; *BP,* blood pressure; *CRH,* corticotropin-releasing hormone; *epi,* epinephrine; *glu.,* blood glucose level; *HR,* heart rate; *MSS,* musculoskeletal system; *Na ret.,* sodium retention; *norepi,* norepinephrine; *PNE,* pituitary-neuroendocrine system; *RR,* respiratory rate; *SNS,* sympathetic nervous system. (From Wells-Federman, C., Stuart-Shor, E., Deckro, J., Mandle, C. L., Baim, M., & Medich, C. [1995]. The mind/body connection: The psychophysiology of many traditional nursing interventions. *Clinical Nurse Specialist, 9,* 60.)

rate. Additionally, a heightened awareness of the environment is triggered, and blood shifts from the visceral organs to the large muscle groups. Concurrently the psychoneuroendocrine system stimulates the hypothalamic-pituitary-adrenal axis and the secretion of corticosteroids (primarily cortisol) and other neuroendocrine substances into the systemic circulation, increasing blood glucose levels, influencing sodium retention, and, in the acute phase, increasing the anti-inflammatory response.

Study findings (CDC, 2012b) have shown that maladaptive stress can cause or exacerbate disease or symptoms of diseases. Proinflammation associated with stress is emerging as a common pathway in a variety of diseases such as asthma, angina, cardiac arrhythmias, pain, tension headaches, insomnia, and gastrointestinal complaints (Bartol & Courts, 2009). Additionally, stress can produce hyper- or hyporeactivity of hormones regulated by the psychoneuroendocrine system (Bonfiglio et al., 2011).

As mentioned previously, in most cases the stress response is a beneficial adaptive pattern that increases efficiency and quality of performance, but it can prove maladaptive when a stressor continues indefinitely. Maladaptive stress (distress) is an enduring and sometimes self-sustaining cascade of responses that degenerate physical, psychosocial, and spiritual well-being. Not surprisingly, stress and specifically depression have been associated with increased susceptibility to cardiovascular disease, as well as to poor response to its treatment. However, indirect influences of stress and depression on self-care health behaviors might explain these associations. Needless to say, further investigation is needed to demonstrate direct causal links as well as effectiveness of psychological interventions for persons with cardiovascular disease (Whalley et al., 2011).

Psychological Effects of Stress

The psychological effects of stress are best illustrated by its contributory role in negative mood states, including anxiety, depression, hostility, and anger. Exposure to stressful stimuli is associated with elevated cortisol levels and resultant effects on the immune system. Duration, intensity, and timing of a stressor have been shown to affect immune responses in animals. Although systematic studies to explain different patterns of immune response have not yet been conducted with humans, the interactive nature of the mind and immune system is an exciting area of investigation that may contribute to future evidence-based practice (Hou & Baldwin, 2012).

A growing body of clinical research outcomes illustrates the interplay of stress and various health outcomes. For example, research evidence is convincing that individuals with eating disorders experience a high rate of stress, and that appraisal is more important than the nature of any stressful event itself (Courbasson & Jeyarajan, 2011). The relationship between stress and cardiac symptoms also is well documented. Closa and colleagues (2010) demonstrated that for persons awaiting angiography, stress and lack of social support predicted self-reported cardiac symptoms, regardless of actual disease severity. Clinical implications include reducing perceived stress by encouraging reappraisal and support seeking, rather than a ruminative, angry coping style. In conclusion, evidence to date demonstrates a strong association between stress and negative health effects for individuals and their family members.

Sociobehavioral Effects of Stress

In response to stress, individuals often revert to or increase their reliance on less healthy behaviors, such as overeating, excessive use of alcohol or drugs, and smoking. Recognizing that such behaviors are inconsistent with the healthy behaviors needed to cope with stress is easy; however, stopping these behaviors and using health-promoting strategies instead is not. Risky behaviors and traits such as a sedentary lifestyle, obesity, overeating high-fat foods, smoking, substance use, and social isolation have been linked to morbidity and mortality (USDHHS, 2011). Conversely, exercise, healthy diet, smoking cessation, healthy weight maintenance, and social interaction have been identified as leading indicators of health in this country (USDHHS, 2011). Encouraging these health behaviors supports goals of *Healthy People 2020*. However, without understanding how psychosocial factors affect health behaviors, promoting effective self-care is an unrealistic goal (Box 13-2: *Healthy People 2020*).

Spiritual Effects of Stress

Interest in the connection between spirituality and health is significant. Spirituality is defined in many ways but key components typically are that spirituality comprises feelings, thoughts, experiences, and behaviors that arise from a search for meaning and may include interconnectedness with self, others, nature, and a higher force called God, a life-force/higher power, nature, or the transcendent. Spirituality and religion intersect for many, yet they are not synonymous. Many individuals feel spiritual without a formal religious affiliation or practice. In response to stress, people often feel disconnected from life's meaning and purpose; harmful effects on their health and well-being can result. Stressful events can shatter individuals' spiritual center or conversely can move individuals to seek comfort in spirituality or religious practice, beliefs, or community. Encouraging involvement with one's religious/spiritual practices is recommended as a helpful intervention for stress-related problems (Weber, 2011).

The previous section discussed how stress can adversely affect biological, cognitive, emotional, behavioral, and spiritual well-being. This understanding of the psychophysiology of the

---

❤ BOX 13-2 HEALTHY PEOPLE 2020
Health-Related Quality of Life and Well-Being

Health-related quality of life (HRQoL) is a "multi-dimensional concept that includes domains related to physical, mental, emotional and social functioning." HRQoL is a new topic in *Healthy People 2020* and goes beyond "direct measures of population health, life expectancy and causes of death, and focuses on the impact health status has on quality of life. A related concept of HRQoL is well-being, which assesses the positive aspects of a person's life, such as positive emotions and life satisfaction." As explained in this chapter, stress is a challenge to HRQoL Stress management is a key strategy to improving HRQoL.

From Health-related quality of life and well-being, http://healthypeople.gov/2020/topicsobjectives2020/overview.aspx?topicid=19.

BOX 13-3   RESEARCH FOR EVIDENCE-BASED PRACTICE
Impact of Breast Cancer Recurrence and Cancer-Specific Stress on Spouse Health and Immune Function

Spouses of persons with cancer often are primary informal caregivers for their partners. As a group they experience a variety of poor health outcomes. This study examined the relative contributions of cancer recurrence—a cancer-specific stressful event—and the subjective experience of cancer-specific stress in a sample of male spouses of breast cancer survivors. The investigators hypothesized that stress would contribute to poorer physical health and compromised immune function. Given the difficulty of random assignment for this type of study the researchers used a matched-control design, comparing spouses of women with recurrence to a cohort of spouses whose wives were disease-free, but had a history of breast cancer. Spouses of women experiencing a first recurrence were matched to spouses of women with no evidence of disease. Results showed that cancer recurrence status was not a significant predictor of spouses' physical health or immune function; however, among all spouses, cancer-specific stress symptoms were associated with increased physical symptoms and altered T-cell blastogenesis. These findings suggest that health effects for these caregiving spouses were more strongly connected to their subjective experience of cancer as stressful, rather than their partners' current disease status. A practice implication is that exploring spouses' appraisals of the experience should be an essential component of family care when one partner has breast cancer.

Source: Gregorio, S. W., Carpenter, K. M., Dorfman, C. S., Yang, H. C., Simonelli, L. E., & Carson III, W. E. (2012). Impact of breast cancer recurrence and cancer-specific stress on spouse health and immune function. *Brain, Behavior, & Immunity, 26,* 228-233.

mind-body-spirit connection is fundamental to the application of stress management in nursing and provides an obvious rationale for a multifaceted approach. Further support is provided from research endorsing the health-promoting effects of managing stress (Gregorio et al., 2012) (Box 13-3: Research for Evidence-Based Practice).

HEALTH BENEFITS OF MANAGING STRESS

A growing body of evidence underscores the importance of controlling stress to promote health and quality of life for people with a variety of health problems. "The association between stressors and biomarkers specific to physiological systems (i.e., cardiovascular, neuroendocrine, immune, etc.) is an emerging area of interest in biomedical research…with evidence that specific stressors may differentially affect various physiological systems" (Paradies, 2011, p. 11). Thus, interventions that reduce the stress response are an important component of comprehensive disease prevention and management. Psychotherapeutic approaches, such as interpersonal and cognitive-behavioral psychotherapies that focus on perception and management of life stressors, are effective treatments for depression and related mental health disorders (Sadock & Sadock, 2008). These psychotherapies have been incorporated into a range of treatment and secondary prevention programs such as cardiac rehabilitation with great potential for wider adapted use (Menezes et al., 2011). Targeting primary prevention programs is the aim of nurses in assisting with stress reduction before becoming symptomatic.

Promoting a positive attitude and development of skills to cope with stress is foundational to many stress-management interventions. As early as 1982, Kobasa and colleagues made a groundbreaking contribution to understating the stress-illness relationship when they identified characteristics of hardiness. They described individuals with stress-hardy characteristics who, when exercising and accessing social support, were less vulnerable to stress-related symptoms and diseases. The characteristics of stress hardiness are control, challenge, and commitment. For stress-hardy individuals, stress is viewed as a challenge rather than a threat; they feel in control of situations in their lives, and they are committed to rather than alienated from work, home, and family. Hardiness continues to be assessed (recognized) by nurses in assisting individuals and families dealing with crisis and promoting the strengths of survivorship in dealing with new stressors. Another term that is used is resiliency.

Promoting stress management is a key component to disease management and better health outcomes. An example is a pilot study conducted to determine the feasibility of offering the authors' Diabetes Coaching Program (DCP), adapted for African Americans, to a sample of African American adults with type 2 diabetes. The DCP aims to promote resilience, coping, and diabetes empowerment to decrease depression symptoms and influence perceived stress as well as to promote adherence to glucose level monitoring, exercise, and healthy eating. The promising results demonstrated feasibility and potential effectiveness of the DCP to enhance diabetes empowerment, diabetes self-management, and reductions in the progression of obesity, type 2 diabetes, and cardiovascular disease in the African American community (Steinhardt et al., 2009).

Stress management is especially important in situations such as caregiving that extend over long periods of time. Caregiver stress/burden can be described as the appraisal of the experience of caregiving including the taxing nature of behaviors of the recipient of care, role conflict or strain, and physical and mental health effects on the caregiver (McLennon et al., 2011). As the setting for care increasingly is the home and family members take on mounting responsibility for care of loved ones (i.e., children, spouses, or aging parents with chronic conditions), the importance of caring for the caregiver to prevent significant burnout grows. As a result of current trends of delayed parenting and increased life span, the "sandwich generation" of middle-aged adults who are carrying concurrent responsibility for their children and aging parents is at particular risk for severe caregiver burden. Research evidence supports the usefulness of interventions aimed at helping caregivers to find meaning in their activities and role in buffering caregiver stress (McLennon et al., 2011; Quinn et al., 2011). Moreover, the quality of the caregiver–care recipient relationship can affect the caregiver's well-being (Quinn et al., 2009).

In summary, evidence is conclusive that thoughts, feelings, behaviors, beliefs, and biological activity are interrelated.

Perceptions, or the way individuals view situations, can lead to stress and, in turn, adversely affect biological activity, emotions, behavior, and the connection with life meaning and purpose. This interaction among perceptions, stress, and multifaceted effects, in turn, can increase stress and foster a negative stress cycle. The remainder of this chapter presents assessment of stress relating to the physical, psychosocial, and spiritual health and well-being of individuals, and describes application of a variety of strategies shown to help break the negative stress cycle and mitigate its harmful effects across the biological, psychosocial, and spiritual domains.

ASSESSMENT OF STRESS

Assessment of the stress-coping abilities of an individual, family, or community is part of a comprehensive health assessment that includes past and present subjective and objective data. Collecting these data enables the individual and the nurse to determine the status of the person's stress-coping pattern, and actual and potential strengths and weaknesses.

The nurse thoroughly collects data during the history, physical examination, and health patterns assessment (see Chapters 7, 8, and 9). Identifying the stress-coping pattern is especially important. Each individual is the primary data source; no other person can explain accurately the individual's perceptions of the stressors, stress responses, and resources to prevent or alleviate the stress.

Stress is experienced across biological, psychosocial, and spiritual domains; therefore, all perceptions are important to the assessment. Throughout the assessment process, individuals may become aware of information of which they were previously unaware, or they may identify information related to their perceived problems. For example, a man may be aware of the stress of his job but may be unaware that his high blood pressure was caused at least in part by this stress.

Lazarus and Folkman (1984) proposed a theory comprising primary and secondary appraisals of stressful events, situations, or demands and the effectiveness of an individual's coping skills. Primary appraisal of coping includes descriptions of perceived actual and potential positive and negative outcomes. Negative outcomes refer to harm, whereas positive outcomes refer to the challenges resulting from stressors that an individual perceives can be overcome. Examples of negative outcomes are physical injury; disease; loss of a cherished relationship, position, or possession; and death. Positive outcomes include graduation, promotion, and development of important relationships (see the Case Study and Care Plan at the end of this chapter).

Secondary appraisal follows primary appraisal. Secondary appraisal consists of the individual's identification of choices to cope with the actual or potential harm, threat, or challenge. The choices may be internal or external resources and responses. For example, a social resource in coping with the needs of a toddler might be learning strategies in a parent-effectiveness training course. A coping response to the challenges of parenting a toddler might be restructuring the toddler's and parent's schedules to allow for more frequent cycles of activities and rest.

The individual's primary and secondary appraisals of stress provide opportunities to consider the stress experiences in different ways. Resources that had been forgotten may be remembered, or a threat may be newly viewed as a challenge and an opportunity for enhanced development and status. Stress responses are mediated by the appraisal process.

By using measurement instruments with established reliability and validity, nurses can improve assessment of an individual's stress and coping. Tools can help nurses distinguish between diagnoses that have many signs and symptoms in common. For example, disturbances in thinking and feeling processes can be difficult to distinguish and may have confounding clinical pictures. These disturbances can occur separately or simultaneously in the same person. An example of this complexity is the overlapping symptomatology of depression and dementia. The nurse determines whether one health problem is actually the cause of the other in order to develop an effective plan of care (see the Case Study and Care Plan at the end of the chapter).

A wide variety of instruments are available to help nurses assess orientation, attention, cognitive skills and patterns, traits and states of emotions, symptoms of mental health distress and disorders, and overall quality of life. For example, The *Schedule of Recent Experiences* (Holmes, 1981) and the *Impact of Event Scale* (Horowitz et al., 1979) are two well-established instruments used widely in clinical assessment and research to measure stress associated with life changes and events. Burnout, be it work-related or personal, is understood as emotional exhaustion, depersonalization, and a sense of reduced personal accomplishment. The *Maslach Burnout Inventory* (Maslach & Jackson, 1986) is a valid instrument to assess perceptions about work/life balance. Before using any instrument, clinicians and researchers need to check information about its reliability and validity, and training requirements and copyright restrictions (e.g., purchase requirements) that can affect access to its use.

Use of standardized instruments promotes accuracy in developing diagnoses and plans of care, and assists in evaluating the effectiveness of care. For example, a nurse may compare an individual's self-evaluation preintervention scores with postintervention scores and revise the plan of care accordingly. Additionally, nurses may analyze population baseline scores for relevant characteristics and develop programs of research and quality improvements aimed at improving outcomes.

Assessment at the family and community levels also is recommended. Family assessment consists of three major categories: structural, developmental, and functional components of the family (Wright & Leahey, 2009). Environmental factors also contribute to stress so a thorough nursing assessment requires consideration of the community. For example, examining community-level data for unemployment, population density, housing, school quality, crime, suicide incidence, and disease occurrence patterns (i.e., health profiles of the community) as well as availability of various amenities such as green space and access to transportation and healthy foods provides a more complete stress assessment than does individual assessment alone (DeMarco & Segraves, 2011). Moreover, family and community assessment can point to possible stress-reduction interventions such as marshalling available social support or engaging in outdoor activities and exercise.

STRESS-MANAGEMENT INTERVENTIONS

Stress-management strategies are beneficial to people across a broad spectrum of chronological, gender, cultural, and ethnic characteristics. Men and women, young and old, from divergent socioeconomic, cultural, and ethnic backgrounds can benefit from stress-management interventions. Sensitivity to needs and values of individuals and communities, particularly for high-risk groups (vulnerable populations), guides assessment and intervention techniques. The language, belief system, and cultural distinctions of individuals and families in the community guide the choice and adaptation of stress-management strategies. Understanding stress and its management involves attention to the *interactions* of social and biological life at individual and family/communal levels (Barchas & Barchas, 2011); therefore interventions may need to encompass a variety and combination of psychosocial and biological approaches at the primary, secondary, and tertiary levels of prevention. Population-based interventions may be expanded from the individual to the community and to a system- or population-focused practice (Harkness & DeMarco, 2012).

Developing Self-Awareness

Self-awareness is one of the most effective stress-management tools. Self-awareness helps people learn about interactions among mind, body, and spirit; increases a sense of control; and counters self-defeating perceptions. Interventions that promote self-awareness help people make sense of life events and circumstances that may be bewildering or discomforting. Many experiences in life lead to feelings of emptiness and disharmony, because people are unable to connect the experience with thoughts, feelings, actions, and physiological responses. Self-awareness helps individuals recognize stress that they create through negative, exaggerated, unrealistic thinking. This recognition affords an opportunity to change these negative thought patterns, thereby decreasing stress and increasing control. Strategies that increase self-awareness can empower individuals to make new connections and to reframe and reinterpret their experiences in light of their own inner strengths and wisdom.

Techniques for Developing Self-Awareness

Monitoring Stress Warning Signs. The negative stress cycle can be difficult to interrupt. Recognizing warning signs of stress is a necessary first step. Often individuals have long ignored physical, emotional, or behavioral cues or reactions to a stressor that are stress warning signs. A man who suffers from chronic, intermittent backaches and ignores the daily muscle tension caused by poor posture that precedes the backaches provides an example. If he had attended to his early stress warning signs of poor posture and muscle tension, he might have avoided the backache that kept him from exercising and socializing. Becoming aware of these stress warning signs is the first step. Attending to these cues is the next step. After this connection is made, developing skills to reduce negative mood states, unhealthy

behaviors, and physical symptoms becomes much easier. Furthermore, some people misinterpret physiological signs of anxiety (e.g., shortness of breath, racing heartbeat) as indicative of serious physical danger (e.g., suffocation, myocardial infarction). This tendency to misinterpret physical anxiety cues is referred to as anxiety sensitivity, a belief that body sensations associated with anxiety indicate imminent and dangerous outcomes, and is associated with various anxiety disorders and health anxiety. In a study of gender differences in anxiety sensitivity, Thompson and colleagues (2011) found that distraction worked better than sensation focusing on reducing stress for males. By assisting individuals who are prone to anxiety sensitivity to interpret body sensations accurately or to distract from the sensation, nurses can help reduce individuals' misinterpretations, as well as the likelihood of escalation of anxiety symptoms and possibly even development of anxiety disorders.

Nurses teach people to identify their warning signals of stress and to stop, take a few breaths, and break the cycle. Figure 13-3 is a sample form for identifying and recording this information. These signals or cues differ among individuals and can be physical, emotional, behavioral, cognitive, relational, or spiritual. When asked to monitor their responses to a particular event, individuals become more consciously aware of these cues. Although this heightened awareness initially may increase an individual's consciousness of physical pain or emotional discomfort, awareness is a necessary first step in recognizing the negative effects of stress and the relationship of thoughts, feelings, behavior, and biological processes. In addition, nurses and other clinicians have a responsibility to screen for emotional distress to help people recognize and monitor their own physical and mood states. For individuals with health conditions such as coronary artery disease, which is known to have high comorbidity with emotional distress and specifically depression, routine screening should be the standard of care (Menezes et al., 2011).

Try this: ask an individual to identify a stressful experience and the physical or emotional reactions (stress warning signals) to that particular experience. For example, after being instructed to stop, take a breath, and notice the physical and emotional response to a stressful situation, one woman related the following:

> On my way to work yesterday, I sat in a huge traffic jam. I noticed that my heart was racing, my breathing had changed, and my hands were gripping the steering wheel. I felt angry and frustrated because I was going to be late for work.

Although these responses seem quite obvious, most people are unaware of the effects of stress on their minds and bodies. In the preceding example, the building of the woman's stress may continue to escalate at work, influencing her interactions with coworkers. Once individuals become aware of these effects, they may be able to release tension more easily, countering the negative effects of stress and increasing a sense of control. Techniques that help to reduce negative effects of stress include using distraction by purposefully shifting focus to pleasant thoughts or engaging in a diversion activity, and using a relaxation response technique, as described in the following section.

Physical Symptoms

_____ Headaches
_____ Indigestion
_____ Stomachaches
_____ Sweaty palms
_____ Sleep difficulties
_____ Dizziness

_____ Back pain
_____ Tight neck and shoulders
_____ Racing heart
_____ Restlessness
_____ Tiredness
_____ Ringing in ears

Behavioral Symptoms

_____ Excess smoking
_____ Bossiness
_____ Compulsive gum chewing
_____ Attitude critical of others

_____ Grinding of teeth at night
_____ Overuse of alcohol
_____ Compulsive eating
_____ Inability to get things done

Emotional Symptoms

_____ Crying
_____ Nervousness and anxiety
_____ Boredom (no meaning to things)
_____ Edginess (ready to explode)
_____ Feeling powerless to change things

_____ Overwhelming sense of pressure
_____ Anger
_____ Loneliness
_____ Unhappiness for no reason
_____ Easily upset

Cognitive Symptoms

_____ Trouble thinking clearly
_____ Lack of creativity
_____ Memory loss
_____ Forgetfulness

_____ Inability to make decisions
_____ Thoughts of running away
_____ Constant worry
_____ Loss of sense of humor

Spiritual Symptoms

_____ Emptiness
_____ Loss of meaning
_____ Doubt
_____ Unforgiving
_____ Martyrdom
_____ Looking for magic
_____ Loss of direction
_____ Cynicism
_____ Apathy
_____ Needing to "prove" self

Relational Symptoms

_____ Isolation
_____ Intolerance
_____ Resentment
_____ Loneliness
_____ Lashing out
_____ Hiding
_____ Clamming up
_____ Lowered sex drive
_____ Nagging
_____ Distrust
_____ Lack of intimacy
_____ Using people

FIGURE 13-3 Stress warning signals. (From _Medical symptom reduction clinic patient notebook._ [n.d.]. Boston: The Benson-Henry Institute for Mind Body Medicine of Massachusetts General Hospital, Harvard Medical School.)

**Learning and Practicing a Relaxation Response Technique.** Eliciting the relaxation response is another technique to help people develop awareness and counter the negative effects of stress. Relaxation response techniques oppose the stress response by reducing sympathetic arousal (Benson, 1975). The immediate physiological effects of relaxation are decreases in heart rate, blood pressure, respiratory rate, and muscle tension.

The long-term physiological effect is a decrease in central nervous system arousal with a concomitant decrease in musculoskeletal system, autonomic nervous system, and psychoneuroendocrine system arousal. To the extent that stress causes or exacerbates a symptom, eliciting the relaxation response can break this stress-symptom cycle. In addition to these physiological changes, psychological changes such as improved mood and behavioral changes, including a reduction in risky behaviors, can occur. The relaxation response can counteract stress-related disease processes, particularly processes associated with immunological, cardiovascular, and neurodegenerative disorders (Walsh, 2011).

The relaxation response is an innate physiological response (Benson, 1975); therefore, a number of techniques that involve mental focusing can be used. Details on these techniques and guidelines for clinical applications can be found in Chapter 14. All of these techniques have two basic components:

- The repetition of a word, sound, phrase, prayer, image, or physical activity
- The passive disregard of everyday thoughts when they occur

Electronic recordings (e.g., DVDs, CDs, MP3 players) can be used to help guide this process of focusing, especially during the initial learning phase.

Nurses often can introduce individuals to the immediate calming effects of the relaxation response in less than 5 minutes. One effective way is to have the person make a fist and notice what happens to the breathing pattern. Most people have a tendency to hold their breath while tensing a body part. Now ask the person to take a few deep diaphragmatic breaths while making a fist. Most people will notice that the tension is much harder to maintain while taking a deep breath. This awareness helps to recognize the relationship between breath and tension. Lamaze techniques for helping mothers manage pain during delivery are based on this connection between breathing and relaxation. Most people hold their breath when they perceive a threat (stress), feel anxious, or become angry. By stopping and taking a few deep breaths when they become aware of physical changes (holding the breath or clenching the jaw) or emotional changes (feeling anxious or angry), individuals can elicit the relaxation response, reduce sympathetic arousal, calm negative mood states, and gain a sense of control. Yoga and deep breathing can assist with mindfulness (i.e., awareness of perception) and promote relaxation.

Using Mini-Relaxations. Mini-relaxations can be taught quickly and used throughout the day to help develop awareness and to counter the negative effects of stress on the mind, body, and spirit. Individuals can be taught to monitor minor stress warning signs (jaw and shoulder tension) and to use a mini-relaxation exercise to keep these initial symptoms of stress from developing into an incapacitating tension headache. A mini-relaxation exercise can be anything from a few conscious, deep diaphragmatic breaths to several minutes of sitting quietly (Box 13-4: Quality and Safety Scenario).

Alternative and Complementary Therapies. A variety of alternative and complementary therapies can prevent and reduce harmful effects of stress (Snyder & Lindquist, 2010). These therapies include acupuncture, hypnosis, aromatherapy, reflexology, Reiki, and chiropractic and herbal therapies. These approaches have developed outside the mainstream of traditional Western medicine; however, developing evidence of efficacy has promoted growing acceptance of some of these approaches. People increasingly are using alternative and complementary practices as self-help measures, and research to study their effects has exploded in recent years (Dossey et al., 2009). Nurses can help individuals evaluate the safety and efficacy of various alternative and complementary therapies. In particular, herbal remedies require cautious use because they can have harmful, as well as beneficial, effects, and they sometimes interfere with other treatments and medications. Among the alternative therapies available, there is strong evidence of effectiveness of acupuncture and hypnosis, and they are becoming widely accepted within mainstream health care.

Acupuncture is an ancient Chinese technique used to reduce pain and to prevent and manage various disorders by placement

---

☑ BOX 13-4 QUALITY AND SAFETY SCENARIO

A Stress-Management Strategy for Nurses

Develop the skill of personal presence. Presence is the gift of self through availability and attention to needs. Presence means "being there" for another person. To be available to others in this way, first practice the skill of being present with yourself. One effective way of developing this skill is through mindfulness, which is the ability to focus attention on what you are experiencing from moment to moment. Mindfulness encompasses the abilities of slowing down and bringing your full attention (thoughts, feelings, and body sensations) to the action in which you are engaged at the moment. The practice can be particularly useful in allowing yourself to extend the benefits of eliciting the relaxation response in more areas of your daily life.

The following are some ideas for practicing personal presence (mindfulness):

- When you awaken each morning, bring your full attention to your breathing. Allow your awareness to expand gradually into the room and then slowly begin to listen to the sounds of the outdoors.

- On your way to work, focus on how you walk, drive, or ride the transit. Take some deep diaphragmatic breaths and relax your body as you travel.
- Take a moment to attend to your breath, relax your body, and focus your mind before entering a care recipient's room.
- As you eat a meal, carefully examine it through all of your senses—the sight, smell, touch, taste, and the sound of each bite. Mindfully enjoy this new experience.
- Recurring events of the day can become cues for a mini-relaxation (the ringing telephone; auscultating a heartbeat; answering a call light, before, during, and after rounds or report).
- Make the transition home from work mindful. Leave thoughts and worries of work at work and be conscious of your home environment each day.

Once again, focus on your breathing and become completely aware of your surroundings as you go to sleep. Practice mindfully letting go of today and tomorrow as you allow your mind and body to get some much needed rest.

Modified from The Benson-Henry Institute for Mind Body Medicine of Massachusetts General Hospital. (n.d.). *Stress.* Retrieved from www.massgeneral.org/bhi/basics/whatisMBM.aspx.

of fine needles at specific meridian points on the body. Acupuncture is not a self-help approach, so seeking treatment from an experienced acupuncturist is required. The Western scientific community cannot explain why acupuncture works but acknowledges its effectiveness. Even the World Health Organization has listed illnesses that can be managed with acupuncture (Killeen, 2009), and some health insurance plans provide reimbursement for acupuncture treatments.

Hypnosis comes from a Greek word meaning sleep. Hypnosis narrows consciousness and elicits relaxation, inertia, and passivity, like sleep, yet awareness is never lost completely and the hypnotized person can respond (Brann et al., 2011). The exact mechanisms through which hypnosis works are not known, although perhaps its ability to induce deep relaxation and its possible action in shifting brain activity from the "analytical" left side to the "nonanalytical" right side might be explanatory. Nevertheless, its effectiveness in managing a variety of conditions, notably smoking and anxiety-related problems, and managing pain is well recognized. Trained therapists provide hypnotherapy to manage stress and various mental health problems, including phobias, addictions, and posttraumatic stress disorder. Self-hypnosis, a form of deep relaxation similar to relaxation techniques described in this chapter, can be a useful stress-reduction tool. Self-help guides provide safe and easy-to-follow guidelines. One note of caution is warranted: hypnosis is not recommended for people with organic brain disorders, psychotic disorders, or other severe mental disorders.

Reiki (pronounced ray-kee) is made up of two Japanese words: *Rei,* or universal spirit (sometimes thought of as a supreme being), and *ki*. Thus, the word Reiki means universal life energy. Reiki is a therapy that uses energy fields with the intent to affect health. To transmit ki, believed to be a life-force energy, the Reiki practitioner places hands on or near the person receiving treatment. In the United States, Reiki is designated as a form of complementary and alternative medicine (CAM) (National Center for Complementary and Alternative Medicine, n.d.; Snyder, & Lindquist, 2010).

Expressive Writing. Transforming thoughts and emotions related to stressful experiences into written language has demonstrated positive effects on health (North et al., 2011). In its therapeutic meaning, expressive writing involves telling a "story" about traumatic, emotionally charged, or stressful events and personal reactions. Journal writing—more specifically, self-confessional writing—is a form of expressive writing that typically is done via entries in a journal over time that describe unfolding personal responses to life events. Expressive writing is useful in disclosing and processing emotions, and in measurably improving physical and mental health.

Expressive writing, including journaling, can help people reflect on stressful events and their reactions to these events. Such reflection is an opportunity to reform perceptions and to consider alternative ways to manage stress. Individuals may find resolutions to conflicts that work uniquely for them. These resolutions then may increase a sense of control and mediate negative consequences of stress. This self-reflective process shares elements of cognitive-behavioral therapy—an intervention effective in reducing harmful effects of stress.

Nurses can advise people to get a special notebook for a journal and write about a stressful event for 15 minutes a day, in a setting in which they will not be interrupted. From a health perspective, people will be more effective when making themselves the only audience. The nurse should warn that the individual may feel sad or depressed immediately after the writing session, but these feelings usually dissipate within an hour. Nonetheless, exploring deep thoughts and feelings on paper is not a panacea. When an individual is coping with death, divorce, or some other major stressor, feeling better instantly after writing cannot be expected. A person can, however, develop a clearer understanding of feelings and of the situation through journal writing. In other words, journal writing helps people objectify experiences, identify the influence of stress on symptoms, and develop insights into more effective problem-solving. Some individuals may recognize the need for psychotherapeutic support through journal writing, and an appropriate referral can then be made.

Nutrition: Healthy Diet

Countering negative effects of stress requires caring for physical health and well-being. The mind and body are connected; therefore, paying attention to one while ignoring the other does not promote overall health. The body requires rest, a healthy diet of balanced food choices, and exercise. Over the last few decades, nutrition has moved to the forefront as a major component of health promotion, disease prevention, and symptom management. Food is now viewed as a positive influence on health, physical performance, and state of mind, rather than simply a fuel needed to prevent disease and sustain life. Adaptive eating is characterized by balanced eating patterns and caloric intake as well as appropriate body weight for height. Nutrition is an important component of early intervention strategies to improve physical, cognitive, emotional, social, and spiritual functioning (Luck, 2009).

However, the American lifestyle has made practicing healthy eating habits increasingly difficult. Americans frequently replace nutritionally balanced meals with readily available high-fat, high-calorie food (United States Department of Agriculture [USDA], 2012). One of the frustrations that nurses experience is trying to help children and adults develop healthy eating habits. This effort takes planning and correctly choosing a variety of foods, and eating a diet low in fat, saturated fat, and cholesterol, with plenty of vegetables, fruits, and grain products. The current U.S. dietary guidelines (USDA, 2012) are based on the following two overarching concepts: focus on caloric balance over time to achieve and maintain a healthy weight; focus on consuming nutrient-dense foods and beverages. Daily food choices should be made from the five food groups. Key recommendations also highlight the importance of calorie control and physical activity. A detailed discussion of the health benefits of balanced nutrition and guidelines throughout the life span can be found in Chapter 11.

Encouraging healthier dietary choices helps people to recognize that control over their health and well-being is possible. This knowledge, in turn, helps counter the negative effects of stress and lower the stress-disinhibition effect that can influence poor dietary choices. Nurses encourage people to monitor their daily dietary patterns to gain awareness of how they use food in times of stress. Tools like food diaries (24-hour recall) help people to monitor the amount and quality of what they eat and drink and to set realistic goals. An example of an online free program is www.myfitnesspal.com, which combines nutrition tips and a way to monitor exercise in a journal format (MyFitnessPal, 2012).

Physical Activity

Combining a healthy diet with a regular exercise routine has many health benefits and can positively affect quality of life. For example, one of the most effective ways to lose weight and improve self-esteem is to combine exercise with nutritious eating. Exercise (physical activity that improves strength, flexibility, and conditioning) and balanced nutrition serve as protective factors against several major chronic diseases. Regular physical activity decreases the risk of death from heart disease, lowers the risk of developing diabetes, and is associated with a decreased risk of colon cancer (United States Department of Health and Human Services [USDHHS], 2011). Exercise helps prevent high blood pressure and helps lower blood pressure in people with elevated levels. Regular physical activity, even at moderate levels, is associated with lower death rates for adults of any age. Psychological well-being is enhanced and the risk of developing depression can be reduced; regular physical activity appears to reduce symptoms of depression and anxiety and to improve mood.

Additionally, children and adolescents need weight-bearing exercise for normal skeletal development, and young adults need this type of exercise to achieve and maintain peak bone mass (USDHHS, 2011). Regular physical activity also increases the ability of older people, and those with certain chronic, disabling conditions, to perform activities of daily living. Nevertheless, high stress could increase injury risk for athletes, and injured athletes may experience greater stress than noninjured peers when they are sidelined from competition. Chapter 12 provides a comprehensive discussion of the benefits of exercise and clinical application throughout the life span.

Regular physical activity helps people adopt a more active lifestyle as they begin to feel better physically and emotionally, thereby breaking the negative stress cycle (Figure 13-4). Positive effects can be obtained with exercise of only moderate intensity. For example, a brisk walk of 30 to 60 minutes, 3 to 5 times a week, promotes fitness and decreases risk of disease. Being physically active on a daily basis is extremely important; therefore, nurses can help individuals increase physical activity by suggesting a variety of activities in which they might engage each day (Box 13-5). An exercise diary can generate a baseline for usual activity to set realistic goals and monitor progress. By simply changing a few daily routines, individuals can gain enormous physical, psychosocial, and spiritual rewards that promote health and break the negative stress cycle.

Sleep Hygiene

Health and the ability to meet life's many demands and manage stress effectively require proper rest. Many people suffer

FIGURE 13-4 Regular physical activity helps adopt a more active lifestyle.

BOX 13-5 HELPING INDIVIDUALS INCREASE PHYSICAL ACTIVITY

Nurses can suggest ways for individuals to increase physical activity throughout the day, including:

- Have fun and play active games with children.
- Engage in a sport.
- Find a friend with whom to walk or jog.
- Take a class in yoga or tai chi.
- Get and walk a dog.
- Garden on the weekends.
- Walk or bicycle to school or work.
- Take the stairs, never the elevator.
- Park the car at the farthest point in the parking lot at work, school, or when shopping.

By simply changing a few daily routines, a person can gain enormous physical, psychosocial, and spiritual rewards that promote health and break the negative stress cycle.

---

from sleep deprivation and sleep disorders (e.g., sleep apnea) that can cause or exacerbate conditions such as depression and fatigue and contribute to poor concentration and ineffective problem-solving. Insomnia can be induced by stress or other cognitive-behavioral factors, such as unrealistic expectations, inappropriate scheduling of sleep, trying too hard to sleep, consuming caffeine, getting inadequate exercise, and a number of other factors including illness, alcohol use, or drug use (Stuart, 2009b). Determining the extent to which sleep disturbance is the result of behavior or stress-related issues is a necessary assessment. Overcoming sleep disturbances cannot be done quickly. Changing these behaviors requires patience and persistence. Once factors associated with sleep disturbance are identified, nurses can help individuals improve their sleep patterns by counseling them to follow several sleep hygiene or behavior guidelines (keeping a sleep diary, having a regular sleep-wake cycle, and making prudent dietary changes). Referral for appropriate evaluation of possible disorders such as sleep apnea also is a necessary nursing intervention. Assisting people to make healthy behavior changes in their sleep habits provides another opportunity for people to increase self-regulation, confidence,

---

BOX 13-6 SLEEP HYGIENE STRATEGIES

Nurses find the following suggestions to be helpful for individuals with sleep disturbance resulting from behavioral or stress-related issues:

- Keep a sleep diary, which helps determine sleep patterns more accurately, assess progress, and reinforce behavior change.
- Challenge irrational beliefs.
- Reduce consumption of alcohol and caffeine. (Chapter 11 gives some tips.)
- Avoid use of sleeping pills.
- Have a regular sleep-wake schedule, even on the weekends.
- If unable to fall asleep within 20 to 30 minutes or if waking up and unable to fall back to sleep within that time, get out of bed and do something until groggy and sleepy again.

- Focus on relaxation, not sleep. Use a relaxation tape, and practice diaphragmatic breathing. Limit naps during the day to less than 45 minutes. Longer naps reset the biological clock and disturb nighttime sleep.
- Exercise within 3 to 6 hours of bedtime. Exercise improves sleep by producing a significant rise in body temperature, followed by a compensatory drop a few hours later, making it easier to fall asleep and stay asleep. Furthermore, because exercise is a physical stressor, the brain compensates by increasing the amount of deep sleep.
- Take a hot bath 2 hours before bedtime. The temperature drop after the bath helps to induce sleep.
- Sleep in a cool room. Individuals grow sleepier and become less active when body temperature falls.

Modified from Stuart, G. W. (2009b). Psychophysiological responses and somatoform and sleep disorders. In G. W. Stuart & M. T. Laraia (Eds.), *Principles and practice of psychiatric nursing* (9th ed., pp. 241-253). St Louis: Mosby.

---

and control, thereby reducing stress and improving quality of life. Box 13-6 presents several sleep hygiene strategies.

Cognitive-Behavioral Restructuring

Many stressful situations can be created or exacerbated by negative, exaggerated, catastrophic thinking. Cognitive-behavioral therapy (CBT) is a conceptually based short-term intervention to modify this thinking and related behaviors, and thereby reduce stress. In the context of therapy, cognitive-behavioral restructuring is a technique or series of strategies that help people evaluate their thoughts, challenge them, and replace them with more rational cognitive and behavioral responses (Beck, 1976, 1979; Clark & Beck, 2012). Although advanced training is needed to provide CBT, nurses can safely and effectively use basic strategies. A helpful resource for nurses is the Beck Institute for Cognitive Behaviour Therapy (Beck Institute for Cognitive Behaviour Therapy, 2012).

Appraisal, or the way in which a situation is viewed, can be a major cause of stress, making CBT especially suited for stress management. When situations are viewed in a negative, distorted, or illogical manner, such perceptions can adversely affect emotions, behaviors, beliefs, and physiological parameters. Cognitive-behavioral restructuring teaches people to recognize that negative thinking often causes emotional distress and associated behaviors. This recognition, in turn, alters problematic thinking and behavior, reduces the negative consequences of stress, and enhances health (Stuart, 2009a; Stuart & Wells-Federman, 2009).

Cognitive-behavioral restructuring does not gloss over or deny misfortune, suffering, or negative feelings. Many circumstances exist in peoples' lives for which it is appropriate to feel sad, anxious, angry, or depressed. More accurately, cognitive-behavioral restructuring is a technique that helps some people become unstuck from these moods so that they can experience a broader range of feelings and try out new behaviors (Stuart, 2009a). In this structured method, individuals are asked to consider their cognitive appraisal of a situation and how this assessment affects feelings, behaviors, and physiological processes. Reframing, or cognitive reappraisal, educates individuals in monitoring thoughts and replacing those that are negative and irrational with those that are more realistic and helpful. Adding behaviors that are consistent with reframed thinking follows.

For example, a woman may have had plans to meet a friend for lunch on a day she woke up with a migraine headache. She might begin to think such thoughts as "This always happens to me when I have plans," "This headache will never go away," "I shouldn't have to deal with this," or "My day is ruined." The result of this negative, irrational self-talk is disappointment, frustration, and anger. This emotional arousal will, in turn, increase muscle tension and a variety of other stress-related symptoms, which may exacerbate the headache. To help individuals develop the skill of cognitive-behavioral restructuring, nurses can teach them to examine a stressful situation using the four-step innovative practice CBT approach highlighted in Box 13-7.

In the previous example, the woman may reflect that "I am having a migraine headache and I hate that it is on a day that I had made plans, but I will take my medication, listen to my relaxation tapes, and rest. I'll call my friend and see if we can change our plans. Perhaps she can come over to visit me for tea this afternoon if I feel better." Although it is understandable that anyone would be disappointed and upset over this situation, applying the four-step cognitive restructuring technique can help identify healthy choices and gain a sense of control.

Based on the work of pioneers such as Aaron Beck (1976, 1979) and Albert Ellis (Ellis, 1962; Ellis & Dryden, 1987), cognitive therapy has emerged during the past 5 decades as a treatment designed to alter dysfunctional beliefs and thoughts associated with depression, anxiety disorders, and other emotional problems (Clark & Beck, 2012). Over time, theorists, clinical researchers, and clinicians recognized the effectiveness of this approach for many persons, as well as the value of linking helpful alterations in thinking to complementary behavioral changes. As a result, CBT emerged. CBT is an efficacious treatment approach for many stress-related and mental health disorders. For example, researchers have shown that CBT is effective, alone or with other therapies or medication, in alleviating postpartum depression (Grote et al., 2009). Evidence provides strong support for use of cognitive-behavioral restructuring as a stress-management

BOX 13-7 **INNOVATIVE PRACTICE**

The Four Step Approach to Cognitive Restructuring Enhanced with Technology

To help individuals develop the skill of cognitive restructuring, nurses can teach them to examine a stressful situation using the following four-step approach:

1. *Stop* (break the cycle of escalating, negative thoughts).
2. *Breathe deeply* (elicit the relaxation response and release tension).
3. *Reflect* (ask, "What is going on here? What am I thinking? Is the thought true? Is the thought helpful? Am I jumping to conclusions or magnifying the situation?").
4. *Choose* a more realistic, rational response. Try out the alternative response in a future situation.

Alternative Approach

Teaching/coaching can be done face-to-face or can be provided via technology (e.g., a website and/or smart phone application that shows the above steps with feedback interface). Via technology, feedback can be given via text or e-mail messages to correct negative thoughts and to provide suggestions and positive reinforcement for steps 2 to 4 when success is reported. Phone and/or face-to-face interaction can augment contact via technology when possible. Tracking successful cognitive restructuring via online entry can provide useful outcome data. As Internet and smart phone penetration increase and costs decrease, use of such technological interventions will increasingly be cost-effective ways to reach more individuals and can be applied across a range of technological platforms (e.g., computers, smart phones, and tablets). Reminder generic affirmations also can be added via text messaging at very-low cost to encourage practice of the steps.

Four Step Approach, modified from Clark, D. A., & Beck, A. T. (2012). *The anxiety and worry workbook: The cognitive behavioral solution.* New York: Guilford Press; Stuart, G. W. (2009b). Psychophysiological responses and somatoform and sleep disorders. In G. W. Stuart & M. T. Laraia (Eds.), *Principles and practice of psychiatric nursing* (9th ed., p. 241). St Louis: Mosby.

approach. Box 13-8: Diversity Awareness presents relevant information related to the effects of racial/ethnic discrimination on cognitive appraisals of interactions as threatening and harmful resulting in increased overall stress burden.

Affirmations

Affirmations can be an effective stress-management and cognitive-behavioral restructuring skill, because they are a method of countering self-defeating negative thoughts and attitudes in addition to being helpful in addressing spiritual needs. An affirmation is a positive thought, in the form of a short phrase or saying, which has meaning for the individual. By reinforcing new ways of thinking or behaving in the present moment, affirmations are statements that people can use to reaffirm new intentions and to clarify goals.

Nurses coach individuals to create an affirmation as a way of developing a more helpful, realistic belief system. For example, thoughts such as "I can't handle this" and "My day is ruined" can be countered with "I can handle this" and "I know ways to increase my comfort." Repeating an affirmation often throughout the day, perhaps after eliciting the relaxation response or as part of a breathing exercise, can become second nature and can help to enhance self-esteem and reduce stress.

 BOX 13-8 **DIVERSITY AWARENESS**

Social Stressors Can Lead to Discrimination for Vulnerable Populations

Health is perceived through one's spiritual beliefs, holistic practice, and bio-medical perspectives. Nurses understand cultural sensitivity when providing care and the importance of clear communication in multicultural care. Greater concern for health literacy and improved coordination with support organizations are needed. Barriers such as discrimination and geopolitical tension may affect the ability to cope through frustration and may influence health care outcomes. *Healthy People 2020* identifies the need to close the gap and supports health equity by addressing chronic disease and infant mortality rates. For example, social stressors have been linked to increased depressive symptoms among antepartum African American women (Dailey et al., 2011). Thus, in addition to the need for universal symptom screening, it is essential that nurses develop and test interventions to ameliorate effects of social stressors such as discrimination for vulnerable populations.

Social Support

Having supportive family, friends, and coworkers is for many individuals an important contributor to effective coping and stress hardiness (Kobasa et al., 1982). Many people believe that confiding in others and talking out problems can be a helpful way to get good advice or uncritical support. Social support comprises a network of close family, friends, coworkers, and professionals. Social support literature notes that both the number of supports and the quality of the relationships are important (van Woerden et al., 2011).

Research outcomes demonstrate the protective health effects of social support. However, influences may vary by type or source of support. For example, van Woerden and colleagues (2011) examined the effects of social support from personal, professional, and community networks and other factors in relation to self-rated health using a cross-sectional postal and Web-based survey with a random sample of 10,000 households in Wandsworth, London. Results demonstrated that social support from family or friends, at work, and by civic participation was associated with a lower likelihood of poor self-rated health, but that social support from neighbors was associated with a higher likelihood of reporting poor health. The outcomes suggest that most of the health effects of social support are complementary. Nonetheless, the finding that the health effects of family social support were insignificant after controlling for the other social support variables suggests that it can be compensated by support from other sources. Sociodemographic variables (e.g., gender, age, being married, being employed, and owning a home) were also associated with better self-rated health. The principal message is that a variety of sources of social support may promote health and that nurses should ask individuals about all types of social support in order to help them cultivate and use support from many sources. In addition, substituting support from a different source when it is lacking from one usual source such as family can be a helpful strategy.

Nursing interventions are aimed to facilitate social support to promote effective coping and reduce stress. Using information available in their local communities or through national organizations, nurses suggest support groups (see Chapter 8), website chat rooms, social networking sites, educational classes, and exercise facilities, to name a few. Individuals and their families are often referred to volunteer organizations such as the American Lung Association, American Heart Association, American Cancer Society, and the Arthritis Foundation for resources related to specific health-promotion/maintenance needs that also may provide social support opportunities.

Assertive Communication

Effective communication is an important stress-management skill. An important coping and problem-solving skill, communication, can be adversely affected by exaggerated negative thoughts and deeply held negative beliefs and assumptions (Stuart, 2009a). (See Chapter 4 for additional discussion of communication.) People who have difficulty with communication usually have one or all of the following problems:

- Disparity between what they say (statement) and what they want (intent)
- Confusion about or resistance to stating clearly how they feel, what they want, or what they need (lack of assertiveness), with either a tendency to deny their own feelings (passiveness) or indifference toward the feelings of others (aggressiveness)
- Difficulty listening to others

The importance of matching the statement with intention is illustrated by the following example:

As Timothy is leaving for his basketball game on a Saturday afternoon, his mother tells him, "Remember to be home early tonight." When Timothy arrives home at 9:00 pm, his mother, who is waiting at the front door, yells, "Where were you? Is this your idea of early? You know your father and I had plans tonight. We were counting on you. You think only of yourself. This always happens. You'll never change. You'll always be irresponsible and selfish."

The first guideline for effective communication is that people need to be clear about what they want and what they need (intent) in statements to others. Although it would be wonderful if a son or daughter, spouse, friend, or others were great mind readers, assuming that people automatically know what is meant does little to help with communication. Nurses help individuals match statements with intentions. This process requires that individuals recognize distorted, exaggerated thoughts and emotions and take responsibility for their part of the conversation. Communicating effectively is a learned art and skill.

Reviewing the previous example, if the mother's intention was to have her son home before 8:00 PM, then her statement needed to indicate this. She could have said, "I hope you enjoy the game, but remember your father and I are going out tonight. We need to have you home before 8:00 PM to take care of your sister." It is important that the person understands that the other person in the conversation is not obligated to respond as one would wish. However, a request can be much clearer when the statement reflects the intent.

The next guideline for effective communication is to be assertive. Assertive communication, in most cases, is the most effective way to communicate. An assertive statement is nonjudgmental, expresses feelings and opinions, and reaffirms perceived rights. The general format of an assertive statement is: *I feel* [emotion], *when you* [the behavior], *because* [explanation].

The formula requires that all three elements be included. Cognitive restructuring, as described earlier, facilitates assertive communication because it requires individuals to identify their thoughts and feelings. In the previous example, Timothy's mother could:

- *Stop* (breaking the cycle of escalating, negative thoughts)
- *Breathe deeply* (releasing physical tension; promoting relaxation)
- *Reflect:*
  - How do I feel emotionally? (e.g., frustrated)
  - What are my automatic thoughts? ("If he cared about us, then he would have been home on time. He's always selfish and irresponsible. He's never going to change.")
- *Choose:*
  - A more realistic, helpful way of thinking ("He's not always selfish and irresponsible. Even though it feels like he doesn't care about us when he does this, I know he cares.")

Becoming aware of her automatic thoughts and feelings would help Timothy's mother plan an assertive statement when Timothy comes home. She could then say, "I feel frustrated [emotion] when you are late [behavior], because I expected you would be home in time to care for your sister while your father and I went out, or that you would have called if you were going to be late [explanation]." This statement both makes her feelings clear and explains why she feels this way, which in turn provides a better opportunity to work on problem-solving. When people cannot verbalize both their feelings and their needs, others are forced to figure out what they are. When others fail to do so correctly, individuals may feel victimized and blame the others for not understanding. Nurses help people recognize that they have a right and a responsibility to speak up and to do so in an assertive manner. The nurse helps individuals in matching their emotion with the explanation (frustration equals unmet expectation). It is important to remind them that this way of communicating may feel awkward and uncomfortable at first. Practicing this technique many times will be required before communication improves. Role play can be a useful technique to practice. Other people need time to become accustomed to the changes. Effective communication takes both practice and patience with everyone involved.

Empathy

Empathy is an effective stress-management intervention because it assists with communication. Empathy is the ability to consider another person's perspective and to communicate this understanding back to that person. Empathy guides individuals to become better listeners.

Empathy can be facilitated through the technique of active listening. Active listening requires conscious, empathic, nonjudgmental awareness. Listening also helps clarify the issues involved and can deescalate many emotional exchanges. The use of focus groups can assist the nurse in understanding concerns, such as a parent group concerned about nutrition choices in the lunch room. For example, during a situation in which a parent announces, "I'm fed up with the food selection in the cafeteria" the response may be important to resolving the issues without promoting further miscommunications and increasing problems. Rather than being caught by a defensive, emotional reaction, individuals can learn to communicate empathetically using the four-step approach:

- *Stop* (breaking the cycle of escalating, negative thoughts)
- *Breathe deeply* (releasing physical tension; promoting relaxation)
- *Reflect:*
  - How do I feel emotionally? (hurt, angry)
  - What are my automatic thoughts? ("How could [person] say that? It's not my fault. I have things to do. [Person] always accuses me. This is never going to change.")
  - What are the thoughts and emotions being expressed by the other person?
  - The practice of asking this question will provide a different view. The individual can then begin to plan a response.
- *Choose:*
  - "My feelings are hurt, but I don't have to react defensively."
  - "I'm going to try to understand [person's] perspective using this phrase: 'You sound____about____' and listen to [person's] response."

By using this phrase, an individual can gain awareness from another person's perspective (Rogers, 1951). Continuing with the scenario, the response might be, "You sound upset about the choice of food available..." Possible responses to this empathetic statement might include, "It's not just about that. Everything went wrong today and this was just one more thing when my child complains about lunch," or, "You're right. I hate having to pay for food that my child will not eat."

When one uses active listening, the other person often feels heard. An opportunity to clarify any misunderstanding becomes available. This exercise may help reduce emotional arousal, defensive behavior, and conflict. Active listening allows the individual to buy time and to get a better perspective on what the other person is thinking and feeling. Individuals can then make a choice as to how they want to respond. They may choose to use assertive communication or to step away from the interaction. Active listening promotes empathic, objective, and nonjudgmental communication. Nurses recommend use of stress-management skills that include active listening techniques to facilitate effective communication, which, in turn, reduces conflict and stress.

Healthy Pleasures

Engaging in **healthy pleasures** (activities that bring feelings of peace, joy, and happiness) is, for most individuals, an important part of life. However, for individuals who are feeling overwhelmed with daily hassles of work/life balance, illness, or loss, this practice may have been lost. Individuals may feel that they do not deserve to have pleasure or that they are waiting for happiness until they feel better, until the stressors are resolved or until they go away. This belief makes breaking the stress cycle even more challenging; however, rewards motivate behavior (Stuart, 2009a). By asking people to pursue a healthy and pleasurable activity every week, motivating them to become more

involved in their lives and break this cycle is often easier. The activity can be simple and it need not cost money. For example, people often find pleasure in enjoying nature, spending time with a friend, reading a book, or watching a movie. Hobbies are purposeful leisure activities that can balance hectic, stressful lives. A hobby should be chosen from interest and/or talent. Many hobbies have added benefits of increasing activity (e.g., gardening) or promoting social engagement (e.g., a book club or chorus). Nurses advise individuals to make leisure activities a regular part of the week as a purposeful and conscious plan to break the stress cycle.

Spiritual Practice

In response to stress, people can feel disconnected from life's meaning and purpose, which in turn affects spiritual health and well-being. Meeting spiritual needs may be facilitated by **spiritual practice** or activities that help people find meaning, purpose, and connection. For example, individuals may choose to elicit the relaxation response through prayer. This focused, relaxed state of mind might help them develop a spiritual perspective that can engender a shift in values and beliefs to help cope with a stressor they cannot change, such as chronic illness or loss of a loved one. Expression of anger or confusion in the face of difficulties, trauma, or tragedy also can provide a therapeutic outlet, but conversely may engender spiritual or religious doubt, or a sense of alienation from one's beliefs. Nurses suggest a referral to a chaplain or clergy member, provide spiritual music or art work, recommend spiritual reading material, and provide personal **presence** (see Box 13-4).

Nurses propose activities that provide a sense of meaning and purpose. Keeping a journal can be an important strategy to help individuals focus on aspects of life that are more positive and that become clouded from view when feeling overwhelmed by stress. Finding ways of helping others (tutoring children, reading to the blind, or visiting an older adult) can have a positive influence on spiritual health and well-being. Altruism, generosity, kindness, and service to others are more than moral virtues. These attributes not only help to make the world a better place but also help people find meaning and purpose in life. Religious and existential well-being has provided some defense against depression for people living with chronic and life-threatening conditions. Older, chronically ill, and homebound people can be encouraged to produce written or oral histories that can be a legacy or, when able, to contact others needing care or to make telephone calls to raise funds for a favorite charity. In addition, nurses and other health care professionals can assist individuals and families to describe and clarify their personal religious and spiritual perspectives, especially in light of evolving practices/meaning structures and high rates of interfaith marriages/partnerships (Walsh, 2011). Spirituality and religious affiliation cannot be equated. Additionally, being part of a "faith community" may provide an important source of social support for many people. Within faith communities nurses (also known as "parish" nurses) act as facilitators, educators, and referrers to individuals and families in promoting holistic care. Nurses can encourage individuals to search for a community that is comfortable, accepting, and supportive.

Clarifying Values and Beliefs

To manage stress and develop a balanced lifestyle, people must recognize the things and values that are important to them, reflect on where they are in life, evaluate what needs to be changed, and generate an action plan for that change (Keegan, 2009) (see Chapter 4). This process is known as values clarification. The first step is to identify what is important, meaningful, and valuable so as to assess whether actions are consistent with beliefs. What people believe and value guides their actions by

endorsing certain behaviors and changing others. When people assess their values and beliefs, they employ the ability to make their own choices rather than relying on beliefs and values dictated to them by others.

One method nurses use to help people identify what they value and, ultimately, to help them clarify the relationship between their beliefs and actions is to ask them to identify what is important or meaningful to them. The form in Figure 13-5 is an example of questions used in the Medical Symptom

---

"What Is Important and Meaningful to You in Life?"

In each of the following areas, what do you want for yourself, today, next week, a year from now?

Under each of the following categories, please ask yourself these important questions.

Professional, educational, and intellectual
Today _____
Next week _____
A year from now _____

Relationships
Today _____
Next week _____
A year from now _____

Creative things
Today _____
Next week _____
A year from now _____

Spiritual
Today _____
Next week _____
A year from now _____

Volunteer and altruistic
Today _____
Next week _____
A year from now _____

Health
Today _____
Next week _____
A year from now _____

Fun and play
Today _____
Next week _____
A year from now _____

Material objects
Today _____
Next week _____
A year from now _____

FIGURE 13-5 What is important and meaningful to you in life? (From *Medical symptom reduction program patient notebook*. [n.d.]. Boston: The Benson-Henry Institute for Mind Body Medicine of Massachusetts General Hospital, Harvard Medical School.)

Reduction Program at The Benson-Henry Institute for Mind Body Medicine of Massachusetts General Hospital (n.d.) in Boston. Individuals are asked to identify what is important and meaningful to them in eight domains. Nurses change the domains to reflect more accurately the values and beliefs of the individuals they are counseling. After reviewing the results, individuals may find that they have not been doing certain things that are important to them (becoming more physically active, eating a healthier diet, volunteering, or spending time with their children). When people detect inconsistencies between their values and their actual living habits, they can begin to develop a working plan for correcting these inconsistencies. This process enables them to make conscious choices and to have more control (Figure 13-5).

Setting Realistic Goals

Developing an action plan for change to work toward a more balanced health-promoting lifestyle that is consistent with a person's values and beliefs is an important stress-management strategy. Setting realistic, attainable goals facilitates this exercise. Goal setting is a dynamic process that involves both the individual and the nurse. Goals should be specific, concrete, measurable, and achievable. Nurses facilitate this process by respecting the individual's input and using a values clarification exercise (such as the one mentioned) to facilitate a more complete database to guide individuals to identify and prioritize problems to be addressed, and set mutually agreed on long-term and short-term goals. Nurses encourage individuals to challenge themselves when their behaviors are not consistent with what they identified as important and meaningful to them. For example, when an overweight man with hypertension and high cholesterol levels continues to smoke and eat high-fat foods, nurses help him to look at these behaviors relative to what is meaningful to him, such as his family. The cost and benefit are usually clear and the responsibility for the change is with the individual, not the nurse. Nurses ask the following questions to help individuals clarify long-term goals:

- What is important to you?
- What would you like to change about your life?
- What can you do to start that change?
- When will you take that action?
- How will you measure success?
- How will you maintain the desired change?
- How can I help you to reach your goal?

Setting realistic, attainable goals helps to create a sense of confidence and achievement and to build enthusiasm to set future goals. This process, in turn, increases a sense of control and mitigates the negative effects of stress.

Humor

Humor is an enjoyable and effective antidote to stress for many people. Humor can have health-promoting properties (Stuart, 2009c; Wooten, 2009). When acting as a stress reducer, humor produces laughter. Laughter creates predictable physiological changes in the body. Similar to how it behaves with other forms of exercise, the body responds in two stages: (1) an arousal phase with an increase in physiological parameters, and (2) a

> **BOX 13-9   HUMOR STRATEGIES FOR STRESS REDUCTION***
>
> Nurses help individuals use humor for health promotion and stress reduction in a variety of ways, including:
> - Keeping a humor journal: looking for the unintentional amusing remark, watching for funny things young children say or do, and looking in the newspaper for humorous grammatical errors or an inappropriate choice of words and writing them in a journal
> - Looking on the Internet for humorous resources
> - Creating a scrapbook of humorous cartoons, pictures, stickers, poems, and songs
> - Reading a cartoon or joke in the newspaper every day and sharing it with a friend
> - Watching funny movies or reruns of old television programs
> - Finding and spending time with funny, light-hearted people
>
> *For more information about using humor to reduce stress, see Box 6-4, p.143.

resolution phase, during which these parameters return to resting values or lower values (Wooten, 2009).

Humor can open different perspectives on problems and facilitate objectivity, which increases a sense of self-protection and control. Finding humor in a stressful situation can help people to reframe perceptions of the event. Some hospital staffs are using laughter libraries, humor rooms, comedy carts that can be wheeled into an individual's hospital room, and clowns to bring laughter and joy to the bedside. Humor has potential as an accessible, enjoyable, and inexpensive stress-reduction strategy that can offer people new perspectives on their world and themselves. Nevertheless, recognizing that humor can mask conflict or be hurtful is critically important in judging when and how to use it in clinical and work setting encounters (Box 13-9).

EFFECTIVE COPING

When people believe that they can cope effectively, the harmful effects of stress can be minimized. The stressful situation is perceived as a challenge rather than a threat. This often elusive difference has vital mind, body, and spirit effects. When people believe that their lives are more balanced and under control, they are productive, but not driven; are aroused, but not anxious; and may even be physically or mentally tired, but not exhausted.

Effective coping helps people face great adversity (such as illness) and recognize the opportunity that the situation often presents. First and foremost, individuals must recognize that coping is the ability to find a balance between acceptance and action, between letting go and taking control. Many stress-management strategies help individuals distinguish these differences by providing a format for observing or objectifying their experiences. Other strategies such as exercise and balanced nutrition help individuals promote physical health and well-being to counter the harmful effects of stress.

Nurses help individuals improve effective coping by guiding them in the art of choosing the right strategy at the right time. In doing so, people gain a sense of control that minimizes or buffers harmful effects of stress. Nurses use the interventions described in this chapter to assist individuals to manage extrinsic and intrinsic stressors.

When individuals cannot control or influence the situation (extrinsic stressors), nurses advise them to do the following:

- Take care of physical health and well-being: exercise; eat healthy, balanced meals; and practice sleep hygiene.
- Accept: learn to accept that some situations or people cannot be changed or avoided. Forgiveness and letting go of resentment are often a part of acceptance.
- Use distraction: distraction involves putting a worry aside, when necessary, until the situation can be dealt with directly. This prioritizing is quite different from procrastinating or denial, because it is a necessary delay rather than avoidance.
- Reduce emotional arousal: practice mini-relaxations, listen to a relaxation recording, use the four-step cognitive-behavioral restructuring technique, exercise, seek social support, pray, meditate, use humor and affirmations, write in a journal, or engage in a healthy pleasure.

When individuals can alter or influence the situation, or when they are contributing to or creating the stress (intrinsic stressors), nurses advise them to do the following:

- Take care of physical health and well-being: exercise; eat healthy, balanced meals; and practice sleep hygiene.

- Reduce emotional arousal: practice mini-relaxations, listen to music or a relaxation DVD or CD, engage in exercise, seek social support, pray, meditate, use humor and affirmations, write in a journal, engage in a healthy pleasure, and/or use the four-step cognitive-behavioral restructuring strategy:
  - *Stop* (breaking the cycle of escalating, negative thoughts)
  - *Breathe deeply* (eliciting the relaxation response and releasing tension)
  - *Reflect* (asking, "What is going on here? What am I thinking? Is the thought true? Is the thought helpful? Am I jumping to conclusions or magnifying the situation?")
  - *Choose* a more realistic, rational response and related behavioral reaction.
  - *Problem-solve:*
    - Clarify values, beliefs, and expectations.
    - Gather information.
    - Seek advice, support, assistance, or information.
    - Use assertive communication and empathy.
    - Set realistic goals, design action strategies, and determine the best steps to handle the problem.
    - Take action.

See the Care Plan for John R. for an example of a plan for effective coping.

CASE STUDY

Health Assessment: John R.

John R., a 29-year-old man separated from his wife, walked into the health maintenance organization (HMO) stating he had a severe sore throat, could not eat, had not worked for a day, and was feeling "awful." He wanted to see the doctor and get a prescription for an antibiotic. The medical record revealed two episodes within the last 9 months of complaints of a sore throat, culture of organism, and antibiotic treatment. The separation from his wife occurred 1 year ago. He had not had a physical in 2 years. During the assessment interview, the nurse gathered the following information: John R. appeared tired; he presented his problem in short, terse statements; he was irritable about the clinic's slow service; and he expressed a need to get back to work. Within the last 3 weeks, he had been required to work overtime because he faced deadline penalties, and his boss said that John R.'s promotion, due in 2 months, depended on his performance now. The company is struggling and layoffs may be pending. John R. said that, in general, things were fine. His wife was

apparently happy without him and he was too busy to care or to think about that relationship. He made one remark about his boss, "What do you do with a nervous boss?" He described his diet as fast food "taken on the run." He said he gets about 6 hours of sleep per night and awakens one to two times near morning. He has infrequent contact with family members, who live in the area. In accordance with the clinical protocol for the health center, the nurse collects a throat culture.

Reflective Questions

1. As John R.'s nurse, how would you comprehensively assess his health?
2. What are several different diagnoses and possible individual, family, etiological factors to consider?
3. What work-related health issues may be a concern?
4. What other issues may impact the community where John R. is employed?

CARE PLAN

Plan for Effective Coping: John R.

* NURSING DIAGNOSIS: Ineffective Coping related to increased stress at work and limited coping strategies

Defining Characteristics to Assess
- Physiological disturbances
- Abuse of alcohol or drugs
- Participation in potentially dangerous activities
- Engaging in lifestyle with risk to health
- Impairment of social role functioning:
  - Nonproductive lifestyle
  - Failure to function in usual social roles
  - Nonperformance of activities of daily living

- Inappropriate behaviors in social situations
- Self-absorption
- Lack of concern for or detachment from usual social supports
- Poor morale:
  - Unhappiness
  - Lack of future orientation
  - Hopelessness
  - Unacceptable quality of life
  - Pessimism
- Defensive patterns:
  - Inflexibility
  - Hypervigilance

Continued

◎ CARE PLAN

Plan for Effective Coping: John R.—cont'd

- Avoidance
- Inertia
- Refusal or rejection of help

Expected Outcomes

John R. will:
- Report increased information on and consequences to himself of stressors experienced.
- Practice the relaxation response for 20 to 30 minutes every day through prayer or contemplation; use multiple mini-relaxations throughout each day.
- Report increasing weekly exercise or activity and healthy changes in nutrition and sleep or rest patterns.
- Develop effective coping and problem-solving abilities to manage stress, beginning with the stress at work.

- Evaluate result of throat culture and consult with primary care provider if positive and antibiotic is indicated.

Interventions
- Promote an attitude of openness to new information.
- Enroll him in a cognitive-behavioral group program to learn stress-management strategies and health promotion.
- Monitor his daily practice of relaxation response.
- Monitor his changes in exercise or activity, nutrition, sleep or rest patterns, and mood.
- Guide him to develop two coping strategies through cognitive-behavioral restructuring.
- Schedule a follow-up appointment or telephone check-in to monitor well-being.

*NANDA Nursing Diagnoses—Definitions and Classification 2012-2014, Herdman T.H. (ED). Copyright © 2012, 1994-2012 NANDA International. Used by arrangement with John Wiley & Sons Limited. In order to make safe and effective judgements using the NANDA-I nursing diagnoses it is essential that nurses refer to the definitions and defining characteristics of the diagnoses listed in this work.

SUMMARY

Health and the ability to cope effectively with the many demands of work/life balance require management of stress. Combining careful assessment and choice of strategies, thoughtful and honest feedback, and continued support, nurses assist people to cope more effectively with the innumerable actual and potential stressors they may encounter. Research to discern the interplay of physiological, psychological, social, and spiritual responses to stress has yielded important knowledge for practice. However, uncovering the intricate workings of the brain within the context of human stress and coping experiences is a daunting and critical challenge for today's health researchers.

Stress-management strategies provide an opportunity for individuals to acquire the necessary skills to cope more successfully and become confident in self-management. Such awareness enables the individual to challenge and change perceptions, decrease stress reactivity, improve self-management skills, and minimize the harmful consequences of stress. This process positively influences health promotion, disease prevention, and symptom management. Understanding influences of stress on health and illness is essential to all nursing practice.

REFERENCES

Barchas, P. R., & Barchas, J. D. (2011). Sociophysiology 25 years ago: Early perspectives of an emerging discipline now as part of neuroscience. *Annals of the New York Academy of Sciences, 1231,* 1–16.

Bartol, G. M., & Courts, N. F. (2009). The psychophysiology of body mind healing. In B. Dossey, C. Guzetta, & L. Keegan (Eds.), *Holistic nursing: A handbook for practice* (5th ed., pp. 601–613). Sudbury, MA: Jones & Bartlett. doi:10.1111/j. 1749-6632.2011.06135.x.

Beck, A. T. (1976). *Cognitive therapy and the emotional disorders.* New York: International Universities Press.

Beck, A. T. (1979). *Cognitive therapy of depression.* New York: Guilford Press.

Beck Institute for Cognitive Behaviour Therapy. (2012). Retrieved from www.beckinstitute.org/.

Benson, H. (1975). *The relaxation response.* New York: William Morrow & Co.

Bonfiglio, J., Inda, C., Refojo, D., Holsboer, F., Arzt, E., & Silberstein, S. (2011). The corticotropin-releasing hormone network and the hypothalamic-pituitary-adrenal axis: Molecular and cellular mechanisms involved. *Neuroendocrinology, 94*(1), 12–20. doi: 10.1159/000328226.

Brann, L., Owens, J., & Williamson, A. (2011). *The handbook of contemporary clinical hypnosis [electronic resource]: Theory and practice.* Chichester, West Sussex, UK: John Wiley & Sons. Retrieved from http://nccam.nih.gov/health/whatiscam/.

Butterfoss, F. D. (2009). Evaluating partnerships to prevent and manage chronic disease. *Public Health, Practice, and Policy, 6*(2), A64.

Cannon, W. (1914). The emergency function of the adrenal medulla in pain and the major emotions. *American Journal of Physiology, 33,* 356–372.

Centers for Disease Control and Prevention (CDC). (2012a). *The guide to community preventive services: The community guide; what works to promote health.* Retrieved from http://www.thecommunity guide.org/index.html.

Centers for Disease Control and Prevention (CDC). (2012b). *National prevention strategy: America's plan for better health and wellness.* Retrieved from www.cdc.gov/Features/PreventionStrategy/.

Clark, D. A., & Beck, A. T. (2012). *The anxiety and worry workbook: The cognitive behavioral solution.* New York: Guilford Press.

Closa, L. T., Nouwen, A., Sheffield, D., Jaumdally, R., & Lip, G. Y. (2010). Anger rumination, social support, and cardiac symptoms in patients undergoing angiography. *British Journal of Health Psychology, 15,* 841–857. ISSN: 1359-107X. PMID: 20205981.

Courbasson, C., & Jeyarajan, J. (2011). Individuals with eating disorders and stress. In A. P. Barnes & J. E. Montefuscio (Eds.), *Role of stress in psychological disorders* (pp. 99–111). New York: Nova Science Publishers.

Dailey, D. E., Dawn, E., & Humphreys, J. C. (2011). Social stressors associated with antepartum depressive symptoms in low-income African American women. *Public Health Nursing, 28,* 203–212. ISSN: 0737-1209. PMID: 21535105.

DeMarco, R., & Segraves, M. M. (2011). Community assessment. In G. Harkness & R. DeMarco (Eds.), *Community and public health nursing: Evidence for practice* (pp. 175–191). Philadelphia: Lippincott Williams & Wilkins.

Dossey, B., Keegan, L., & Guzetta, C. (2009). *Holistic nursing: A handbook for practice* (5th ed.). Sudbury, MA: Jones & Bartlett.

Ellis, A. (1962). *Reason and emotion in psychotherapy.* New York: L. Stuart.

Ellis, A., & Dryden, W. (1987). *The practice of rational emotive therapy (RET).* New York: Springer.

Gregorio, S. W., Carpenter, K. M., Dorfman, C. S., Yang, H. C., Simonelli, L. E., & Carson, W. E. III (2012). Impact of breast cancer recurrence and cancer-specific stress on spouse health and immune function. *Brain, Behavior, & Immunity, 26,* 228–233.

Grote, N. K., Swartz, H. A., Geibel, S. L., Zuckoff, A., Houck, P. R., & Frank, E. (2009). A randomized controlled trial of culturally relevant, brief interpersonal psychotherapy for perinatal depression. *Psychiatric Services, 60,* 313–321. ISSN: 1075-2730. PMID: 19252043. CINAHL AN: 201022075.

Harkness, G., & DeMarco, R. (Eds.). (2012). *Community and public health nursing: Evidence for practice.* Philadelphia: Lippincott Williams & Wilkins.

Healthy People 2020. (2012). Retrieved from http://healthypeople. gov/2020/topicsobjectives2020/overview.aspx?topicid=19.

Holmes, T. H. (1981). *The schedule of recent experiences.* Seattle: University of Washington Press.

Horowitz, M., Wilner, N., & Alvarez, W. (1979). Impact of event scale: A measure of subjective stress. *Psychosomatic Medicine, 41*(3), 209–218.

Hou, R., & Baldwin, D. (2012). A neuroimmunological perspective on anxiety disorders. *Human Psychopharmacology, 27*(1), 6–14. doi: 10.1002/hup.1259.

Kahana, E., Lovegreen, L., & Kahana, M. (2003). Person, environment, and person-environment fit as influences on residential satisfaction of elders. *Environment and Behavior, 35,* 434–435.

Keegan, L. (2009). The art of holistic nursing and the human health experience. In B. Dossey, C. Guzetta & L. Keegan (Eds.), *Holistic nursing: A handbook for practice* (5th ed., pp. 101–110). Sudbury, MA: Jones & Bartlett.

Killeen, T. K. (2009). Complementary and alternative therapies. In G. W. Stuart & M. T. Laraia (Eds.), *Principles and practice of psychiatric nursing* (9th ed., pp. 549–556). St Louis: Mosby.

Kobasa, S. C., Maddi, S. R., & Kahn, S. (1982). Hardiness and health: A prospective study. *Journal of Personality and Social Psychology, 42,* 391–404.

Kruk, J. (2012). Self-reported psychological stress and the risk of breast cancer: A case-control study. *Stress, 15,* 162–171.

Kyrou, I., & Tsigos, C. (2009). Stress hormones: Physiological stress and regulation of metabolism. *Current Opinion in Pharmacology, 9*(6), 787–793. doi: 10.1016/j.coph.2009.08.007.

Lazarus, R., & Folkman, S. (1984). *Stress, appraisal, and coping.* New York: Springer.

Luck, S. (2009). Nutrition. In B. Dossey, C. Guzetta & L. Keegan (Eds.), *Holistic nursing: A handbook for practice* (5th ed., pp. 209–222). Sudbury, MA: Jones & Bartlett.

Maslach, C., & Jackson, S. E. (1986). *Burnout inventory.* (Manual research edition, 2nd ed.). Palo Alto, CA: Consulting Psychologists Press.

McLennon, S. M., Habermann, B., & Rice, M. (2011). Finding meaning as a mediator of burden on the health of caregivers of spouses with dementia. *Aging & Mental Health, 15,* 522–530. doi: 10.1080/13607863.2010.543656.

Menezes, A. R., Lavie, C. J., Milani, R. V., O'Keefe, J., & Lavie, T. J. (2011). Psychological risk factors and cardiovascular disease: Is it all in your head? *Postgraduate Medicine, 123,* 165–176. ISSN: 0032-5481. PMID: 21904099.

MyFitnessPal. (2012). *Free calorie counter.* Retrieved from www.my fitnesspal.com/.

National Cancer Institute. (n.d.). *Psychological stress and cancer: Questions and answers.* Retrieved from www.cancer.gov/cancertopics/ factsheet/Risk/stress.

National Center for Complementary and Alternative Medicine. (n.d.). Retrieved from http://nccam.nih.gov/.

North, R. J., Pai, A. V., Hixon, J. G., & Holahan, C. J. (2011). Finding happiness in negative emotions: An experimental test of a novel expressive writing paradigm. *Journal of Positive Psychology, 6,* 192–203. ISSN: 1743-9760.

Paradies, Y. (2011). A theoretical review of psychosocial stress and health. In A. B. Barnes & J. E. Montefuscio (Eds.), *Role of stress in psychological disorders* (pp. 1–19). New York: Nova Science Publishers.

Quinn, C., Clare, L., & Woods, B. (2009). The impact of the quality of relationship on the experiences and wellbeing of caregivers of people with dementia: A systematic review. *Aging & Mental Health, 13,* 143–154.

Quinn, C., Clare, V., & Woods, R. T. (2011). The impact of motivation and meanings on the wellbeing of caregivers of people with dementia. *International Psychogeriatrics, 22,* 43–55.

Rogers, C. (1951). *Client-centered therapy.* Boston: Houghton Mifflin.

Sadock, B. S., & Sadock, V. A. (2008). *Kaplan & Sadock's concise textbook of clinical psychiatry* (3rd ed.). Philadelphia: Wolters Kluwer/ Lippincott Williams & Wilkins.

Selye, H. (1950). *Stress.* Montreal: Acta Inc.

Selye, H. (1974). *Stress without distress.* Philadelphia: J. B. Lippincott Co.

Selye, H. (1982). History and present status of the stress concept. In L. Goldberger & S. Breznitz (Eds.), *Handbook of stress: Theoretical and clinical aspects* (pp. 7–17). New York: Free Press.

Snyder, M., & Lindquist, R. (Eds.), (2010). *Complementary/alternative therapies in nursing* (6th ed.). New York: Springer.

Steinhardt, M. A., Mamerow, M. M., Brown, S. A., & Jolly, C. A. (2009). A resilience intervention in African American adults with type 2 diabetes: A pilot study of efficacy. *Diabetes Educator, 35,* 274–284. ISSN: 0145-7217. PMID: 19204102.

Stuart, E., & Wells-Federman, C. L. (2009). Cognitive therapy. In B. Dossey, L. Keegan & C. Guzzetta (Eds.), *Holistic nursing: A handbook for practice* (5th ed., pp. 171–175). Sudbury, MA: Jones & Bartlett.

Stuart, G. W. (2009a). Cognitive and behaviour change interventions. In G. W. Stuart & M. T. Laraia (Eds.), *Principles and practice of psychiatric nursing* (9th ed., pp. 559–570). St Louis: Mosby.

Stuart, G. W. (2009b). Psychophysiological responses and somatoform and sleep disorders. In G. W. Stuart & M. T. Laraia (Eds.), *Principles and practice of psychiatric nursing* (9th ed., pp. 241–253). St Louis: Mosby.

Stuart, G. W. (2009c). Therapeutic nurse-patient relationship. In G. W. Stuart & M. T. Laraia (Eds.), *Principles and practice of psychiatric nursing* (9th ed., pp. 13–42). St Louis: Mosby.

The Benson-Henry Institute for Mind Body Medicine of Massachusetts General Hospital. (n.d.). *Stress.* Retrieved from www.mass general.org/bhi/basics/whatisMBM.aspx.

Thompson, T., Keogh, E., & French, C. C. (2011). Sensory focusing versus distraction and pain: Moderating effects of anxiety sensitivity in males and females. *Journal of Pain, 12,* 849–858. ISSN: 1526-5900. PMID: 21481646.

United States Department of Agriculture. (2012). *Dietary guidelines for Americans.* Retrieved from www.cnpp.usda.gov/dietaryguide lines.htm.

United States Department of Health and Human Services (USDHHS). (2011). *Healthy People 2020.* Retrieved from www.healthypeople. gov/2020/topicsobjectives2020/default.aspx.

van Woerden, H. C., Poortinga, W., Bronstering, K., Garrib, A., & Hegazi, A. (2011). The relationship of different sources of social support and civic participation with self-rated health. *Journal of Public Mental Health, 10*, 126–139. ISSN: 1746-5729.

Walsh, A. (2011). The relaxation response: A strategy to address stress. *International Journal of Athletic Therapy & Training, 16*(2), 20–23.

Weber, J. G. (2011). *Individual and family stress and crises.* Thousand Oaks, CA: Sage Publications.

Wells-Federman, C., Stuart-Shor, E., Deckro, J., Mandle, C. L., Baim, M., & Medich, C. (1995). The mind/body connection: The psychophysiology of many traditional nursing interventions. *Clinical Nurse Specialist, 9*, 60.

Whalley, B., Rees, K., Davies, P., Bennett, P., Ebrahim, S., Liu, Z., et al. (2011). Psychological interventions for coronary heart disease. *Cochrane Database of Systematic Reviews* (8), CD002902–CD002902. doi: 10.1002/14651858.CD002902.pub3.

Wooten, P. (2009). Humor, laughter, and play: Maintaining balance in a serious world. In B. Dossey, L. Keegan, & C. Guzzetta (Eds.), *Holistic nursing: A handbook for practice* (5th ed., pp. 239–249). Sudbury, MA: Jones & Bartlett.

Wright, L. M., & Leahey, M. (2009). *Nurses & families: A guide to family assessment and intervention* (5th ed.). Philadelphia: F.A. Davis.

Complementary and Alternative Strategies

*Elizabeth Kudzma and Jennifer Brunton**

 WEBSITE

OBJECTIVES

After completing this chapter, the reader will be able to:
- Compare holistic, allopathic, and complementary and alternative health modalities.
- Describe the nursing role in complementary health therapies.
- Explain the origin and practice of selected holistic health strategies.

- Identify complementary and alternative medicine (CAM) resources and guidelines.
- Discuss complementary and alternative medicine (CAM) safety and effectiveness.

KEY TERMS

Acupressure	Cranial and cranio-sacral therapies	Meridians
Acupuncture	Curandero	Moxibustion
Affordable Care Act	Dance therapy	Music therapy
Allopathic medicine	Distant healing	National Center for Complementary
Alternative therapy	Energy work	and Alternative Medicine (NCCAM)
American Holistic Nurses Association	Hatha yoga	National Prevention Strategy
(AHNA)	Healing touch (HT)	Naturopathy
Aromatherapy	Health	Nutritional counseling
Art therapy	Herbal therapy	Physical therapy
Asana	Holism	Polarity therapy
Attunement	Homeopathy	Prana
Ayurvedic medicine	Hydrotherapy	Prayer
Biofeedback	Hypnotherapy	Presence
Centering	Imagery	Probiotics
Chakras	Integrative therapy	Qi
Chi	Jin Shin Jyutsu	Qi gong
Chiropractic medicine	Kundalini	Reflexology
Complementary and alternative medi-	Massage	Reiki
cine (CAM)	Meditation	Shiatsu
Complementary therapy	Melatonin	Spinal or bone manipulation

*Thanks to Suzy Harrington for her contribution of this chapter in previous editions.

Tai chi
Therapeutic touch (TT)
Touch therapies

Traditional Chinese medicine (TCM)
Wellness

Whole medical systems
Yoga

 THINK ABOUT IT

Mrs. C. is 62 years old. She has been experiencing osteoarthritis of the knees for the last 5 years. As a younger person, 30 to 40 years ago, she was extremely active; she was a cross-country runner and played a lot of tennis. She is not overweight and occasionally uses a knee brace. She still wishes to play tennis and enjoys walking; however, the knee pain is becoming more problematic. On the worst days, she takes two 500-mg tablets of the nonsteroidal antiinflammatory drug Tylenol. Mrs. C. understands this is a chronic condition. She does not want to take a drug stronger than Tylenol, although she is considering corticosteroid and hyaluronic acid (viscosupplementation) injections. Also in the future, arthroscopy or knee replacement surgery may be indicated; however, she hopes this is in the distant future. The local hospital offers wellness classes that describe alternative and complementary therapies for knee osteoarthritis, including therapeutic touch (TT), healing touch (HT), dietary supplements (glucosamine and chondroitin), and acupuncture. She understands that these complementary therapies may help relieve chronic pain, particularly of musculoskeletal

origin. After looking at sites on the Internet, Mrs. C. has outlined these next-step questions:

- *What is the difference between therapeutic touch and healing touch therapy?*
- *What occurs in a usual visit for acupuncture or a therapeutic or healing touch session?*
- *How do these therapies work? Do energy therapies have a well-described theoretical framework?*
- *What is the best understanding of the biological and physiological mechanisms for these therapies?*
- *What is the best understanding of the safety status of these therapies?*
- *Is either therapy more effective than the other?*
- *Would Mrs. C.'s use be considered complementary, alternative, or integrative?*
- *What does study evidence say about the efficacy of these therapies?*

Sources: Coakley, A. M., & Barron, A. (2012). Energy therapies in oncology nursing. *Seminars in Oncology Nursing, 28*(1), 55-63; Fazzino, D. L., Quinn Griffin, M. T., McNulty, R., & Fitzpatrick, J. (2010). Energy healing and pain: A review of the literature. *Holistic Nursing Practice, 24*(2), 79-88; NCCAM, http://nccam.nih.gov/research/results/spotlight/060210.htm.

HOLISTIC VERSUS ALLOPATHIC

The American Nurses Association recognizes holistic nursing as an official nursing specialty with its own defined scope and standards of practice. The American Holistic Nurses Association (AHNA) defines holistic nursing as "all nursing that has healing the whole person as its goal and integrates complementary and alternative medicine (CAM) approaches into clinical practice." According to the AHNA, a holistic nurse:

- Is a legally licensed nurse who takes a mind-body-spirit-emotion approach to the practice of nursing
- Serves as a bridge between conventional healing and complementary and alternative healing practices, and is trained in both health care models
- Works in a variety of settings—from hospitals to universities to private practice
- May specialize in one or more modalities (or methods of healing), such as acupuncture, chiropractic, or energetic healing (AHNA, 2012a)

Although many of the CAM modalities require specialty-trained practitioners, all nurses can incorporate a holistic mind-body-spirit-emotion approach into their everyday practice (Lundy & Janes, 2009). Whole health is comprised of five dimensions—physical, spiritual, emotional, intellectual, and social; other sources add environmental as a sixth element. To be truly healthy, all the dimensions must be healthy. Western or allopathic medicine traditionally supports the physical dimension, and most often promotes curative interventions rather than preventive modalities.

What Is the Difference Between Holism and Allopathy?

Health care and delivery in the United States, or allopathic medicine, focuses on identifying diseases and conditions by a physician or other midlevel provider (for example, nurse practitioner), and using drugs and surgery to treat bacteria and other ailments (Dosch, 2012; Mork, 2012). Consumers are often dissatisfied with conventional health care and feel that, within the conventional model, they are viewed as machines or as components of an assembly line. Too often in modern health care practice an individual seeking care is identified by the disease or condition causing the ailment. For example, a person seeking care may be called a diabetic or an asthmatic. Many consumers are seeking alternative styles of health care that focus on seeing care recipients as whole people, increasing well-being, and giving consumers greater control over self-care. Behind the idea of holism is the understanding that people are not just physical bodies; people have emotional, spiritual, and relationship aspects involved with well-being that combine within the physical body to make a whole person (Angner, 2008). Holism entails a focus on proactive, healthy living and considers not only prevention but also the root cause of the illness. This movement in the healing arts reflects the theory of holism and recognizes that all aspects of the person must be considered when planning and delivering care (Brown, 2011).

The field is broad and constantly changing, but an authoritative and governmental source, the National Institutes of Health's National Center for Complementary and Alternative Medicine (NCCAM), defines CAM as "a group of diverse medical and health care systems, practices, and products that are not generally considered part of conventional medicine or Western allopathic medicine and the traditional medical providers in the United States health care system" (NCCAM, 2012a). NCCAM has separate definitions of complementary, alternative, and integrative. It defines complementary therapy as the use of CAM in conjunction with and as a complement to allopathic traditional medicine. Alternative therapy uses CAM in place of traditional medicine. Integrative therapy is the scientific, evidence-based use of combined CAM and traditional medicine with an emphasis on safety and effectiveness (NCCAM, 2012b).

Wellness

The World Health Organization and holistic health practitioners begin classically from the same place when they believe "Health is a state of complete physical, mental and social well-being and not merely the absence of disease or infirmity" (WHO, 1948). Mosby (2009) defines wellness as "a dynamic state of health in which an individual progresses toward a higher level of functioning, achieving an optimum balance between internal and external environments." Wellness provides a sense of empowerment to persons seeking care. Smith and colleagues (2006) summarized the WHO glossary terms by noting that wellness allows an optimal state of health in individuals and groups. It allows the fullest potential of an individual in many dimensions (physical, psychological, social, spiritual, economic) and the fulfillment of role expectations (family, community, religious, occupational). Another source (Corporate Wellness, 2012) reports the following:

> Wellness is an active process of becoming aware of and making choices toward a more successful existence.
> Process means that improvement is always possible.
> Aware means that we are continuously seeking more information about how we can improve.
> Choices mean that we consider a variety of options and select those in our best interest.
> Success is determined by individuals to be their collection of life accomplishments (Corporate Wellness, 2012)

Working toward health and wellness is an ongoing process that includes self-knowledge and self-care. When disease occurs, holistic practitioners seek to support the person's natural healing systems, to consider the whole person, and to consider the environment (both physical and mental) surrounding the person. Many of the interventions used in holistic health care practice are backed by centuries of tradition, but they are often considered complementary or alternative practices and are not currently incorporated into most conventional health care practices (Dossey & Keegan, 2013).

Moving Mainstream

Alternative and complementary practices are moving into mainstream medical practice. A 2007 National Health Interview Survey (NHIS) (Barnes, Bloom, & Nahin, 2008) identified that approximately 38% of adults use CAM modalities and 83 million adults spent $33.9 billion out-of-pocket on CAM. CAM costs are 11.2% of total out-of-pocket expenditures on health care. The $14.8 billion spent on nonvitamin, nonmineral, natural products is equivalent to approximately one third of total out-of-pocket spending on prescription drugs ($47.6 billion), and the $11.9 billion spent on CAM practitioner visits is equivalent to approximately one fourth of total out-of-pocket spending on physician visits ($49.6 billion) (NCCAM, 2012c; see http://nccam.nih.gov/research/results/spotlight/123108.htm).

A holistic approach to health care not only prevents, assesses, and treats disease but also promotes wellness (Lundy & Janes, 2009). Using holistic modalities can also help meet the goals of *Healthy People 2020*. This includes increasing quality and years of life, improving nutrition, increasing physical activity, and decreasing illegal substance abuse and harassment throughout the life span (see Box 14-1: *Healthy People 2020*).

Clinical Practice Guidelines

Clinical practice guidelines for CAM modalities exist to identify and describe evidence-based recommended courses of intervention (NCCAM, 2012d) (Box 14-2: Quality and Safety Scenario). Ideally, CAM and allopathy are not divergent but can effectively be used simultaneously with each other. See Box 14-3 for a list of NIH NCCAM clinical practice guidelines to provide best evidence-based practice support.

Uses in Practice

Many medical and nursing schools are adding courses on alternative/complementary therapies to their curricula (Snyder & Lindquist, 2009). *Dr. Dean Ornish's Program for Reversing Heart Disease,* which originally incorporated a strict low-fat diet, yoga or other mild exercise, and meditation/relaxation (BlueCross BlueShield Association, 2012; Ornish, 1995), is now available in many areas of the country. Dr. Ornish was one of the first to acknowledge that comprehensive lifestyle changes could reverse cardiac disease even without drugs or surgery. Medicare now includes coverage for his programming (Ornish, 2012, *Preventive Medicine Research Institute*, www.pmri.org/dean_ornish.html).

Alternative/complementary therapies can also be used as an adjunct to conventional medical care (Robin, 2010; Rost, 2009). Rapidly increasing numbers of physician practices, managed care groups, insurers, and hospitals are including holistic health practices (Northrup, 2010; Weil, 2000, 2011). The Cancer Center at St. John Hospital in Detroit, Michigan, has a clinic that also offers qi gong, tai chi, yoga classes, hypnotherapy, and guided imagery (Van Elslander Cancer Center, 2012). With a vision "to promote health and healing of body, mind, and spirit," the Woodwinds Health Campus located in Woodbury, Minnesota, offers complementary therapies including the use of essential oils, energy-based therapies, imagery, music, acupuncture, acupressure, and massage (Woodwinds Health Campus, 2010). The Veterans Affairs Hospital in Salt Lake City, Utah, offers 13 complementary therapies (herbal and nutritional supplement education, acupuncture, hypnosis, qi gong, meditation, yoga, and prayer) as an adjunct to conventional health care (Smeeding & Osguthorpe, 2005). Franklin Memorial Hospital, in western Maine, offers Reiki services to inpatients (Kendall, 2007). The Birchtree Center in western Massachusetts offers professional holistic development classes for nurses that can help them prepare for Holistic Nursing Certification (HNC) (Birchtree Center, 2012, www.birchtreecenter.com/prof_dev.html). This integration of

From U.S. Department of Health and Human Services (USDHHS). (2011). *Healthy People 2020.* Retrieved July 10, 2012, from www.healthypeople.gov/2020/about/default.aspx.

BOX 14-1 HEALTHY PEOPLE 2020

Selected National Health and Wellness Objectives

- (Developmental) Increase the proportion of insured persons with coverage for clinical preventive services.
- (Developmental) Increase the proportion of persons who receive appropriate evidence-based clinical preventive services.
- Increase the proportion of adolescents who have had a wellness checkup in the past 12 months.
- Increase the proportion of schools with a school breakfast program.
- Reduce the proportion of adolescents who have been offered, sold, or given an illegal drug on school property.
- Increase the proportion of adolescents whose parents consider them to be safe at school.
- (Developmental) Increase the proportion of middle and high schools that prohibit harassment based on a student's sexual orientation or gender identity.
- Increase the proportion of elementary, middle, and senior high schools that provide comprehensive school health education to prevent health problems in the following areas: unintentional injury; violence; suicide; tobacco use and addiction; alcohol or other drug use; unintended pregnancy, HIV/AIDS, and STD infection; unhealthy dietary patterns; and inadequate physical activity.
- Increase the proportion of elementary, middle, and senior high schools that provide school health education to promote personal health and wellness in the following areas: hand washing or hand hygiene; oral health; growth and development; sun safety and skin cancer prevention; benefits of rest and sleep; ways to prevent vision and hearing loss; and the importance of health screenings and check-ups.
- Increase the proportion of college and university students who receive information from their institution on each of the priority health risk behavior areas

(all priority areas; unintentional injury; violence; suicide; tobacco use and addiction; alcohol and other drug use; unintended pregnancy, HIV/AIDS, and STD infection; unhealthy dietary patterns; and inadequate physical activity).

- (Developmental) Increase the proportion of worksites that offer an employee health-promotion program to their employees.
- Increase the proportion of persons who report that their health care providers always involved them in decisions about their health care as much as they wanted.
- (Developmental) Increase the proportion of patients whose doctor recommends personalized health information resources to help them manage their health.
- Increase the proportion of adults who meet current federal physical activity guidelines for aerobic physical activity and for muscle-strengthening activity.
- Increase the proportion of adolescents who meet current federal physical activity guidelines for aerobic physical activity and for muscle-strengthening activity.
- Increase the proportion of physician office visits that include counseling or education related to physical activity.
- Health-Related Quality of Life and Well-Being is a new topic area for *Healthy People 2020.* Health-related quality of life (HRQoL) is a multidimensional concept that includes domains related to physical, mental, emotional, and social functioning. It goes beyond direct measures of population health, life expectancy, and causes of death, and focuses on the impact health status has on quality of life. A related concept of HRQoL is well-being, which assesses the positive aspects of a person's life, such as positive emotions and life satisfaction.

BOX 14-2 QUALITY AND SAFETY SCENARIO

How Should Complementary and Alternative Medicine (CAM) Be Evaluated?

Those who use therapeutic touch (TT) believe strongly that it is an effective intervention because they have seen it work. Despite an impressive body of research, the efficacy of TT continues to be questioned. Much of the research on TT has attempted to test efficacy using a randomized controlled clinical trial (RCT) study design to conform to current scientific paradigms concerning the acceptability of research evidence. Appreciation for the value of energy therapies including TT probably lies beyond strict application of statistical design and the use of randomized controlled trials (Coakley & Barron, 2012).

Many complementary and alternative therapies, including TT, are tailored specifically to the individual and produce personalized treatment plans that are nonstandardized; these applications may not fit requirements of a RCT design. A TT treatment is dictated by the needs of the individual and is finished when the practitioner believes that it is finished, not within a rigid time limit imposed by a study protocol. A TT practitioner cannot participate in a blind trial, because

client touch, centering, assessment, and intentionality are integral to the practice. TT may also be particularly useful in certain subsets of persons seeking care, for example, in managing the pain and anxiety associated with cancer treatment (Coakley & Barron, 2012). Additionally, healers may be unable to perform identically from day to day, and psychological and physical changes within the healer may affect the ability to heal. Herman and colleagues (2006) suggest using health services research designs, which include pragmatic trials rather than RCTs, to study alternative/complementary therapies.

- What standards of proof should the nurse require before adopting an alternative/complementary therapy in clinical practice?
- Have all (or even some) of the alternative/complementary therapies commonly used by nurses today been subjected to these standards?
- Have all (or even most) of the standard therapies commonly used by nurses and medicine today been subjected to these standards?

Sources: Coakley, A. B., & Barron, A. (2012). Energy therapies in oncology nursing. *Seminars in Oncology Nursing, 28*(1), 55-63; Faculty of Harvard Medical School & Natural Standard. (2008). *Complementary and alternative medicine: Therapeutic touch.* Retrieved July 10, 2012, from www.intelihealth.com/IH/ihtIH/WSIHW000/8513/34968/358873.html?d=dmtContent; Herman, P. M., D'Huyvetter, K. D., & Mohler, M. J. (2006). Are health services research methods a match for CAM? *Alternative Therapies in Health and Medicine, 12*(3), 78-83.

holistic practices with standard allopathic medicine (Mork, 2012) serves to introduce more people to complementary therapies and may give these practices more robust credibility, especially with those who currently question their value (Box 14-4: Hot Topics).

Healthy People 2020

Holistic interventions are used to promote wellness and are used to meet the *Healthy People 2020* vision of improving the health of Americans and helping them live long and

BOX 14-3 COMPLEMENTARY AND ALTERNATIVE MEDICINE (CAM) CLINICAL PRACTICE GUIDELINES (CPGS): FEATURED GUIDELINES

Allergy and Immunology
- Diagnosis and Management of Food Allergy (*Journal of Allergy and Clinical Immunology*)
- Guidelines for the Diagnosis and Management of Asthma (*NHLBI*)

Cardiology
- Soy and Cardiovascular Health (*Circulation*)

Family Medicine
- Clinical Use of Dietary Supplements and Nutraceuticals (*Endocrine Practice*)
- Dietary Reference Intakes for Calcium and Vitamin D (*Institute of Medicine of the National Academies*)
- Herbs and Supplements in Managed Care (*The Permanente Journal*)
- Evaluation and Management of Chronic Insomnia in Adults (*Sleep*)
- Psychological and Behavioral Treatment of Insomnia (*Sleep*)

Gastroenterology
- Probiotics and Children (*Journal of Pediatric Gastroenterology and Nutrition*)

Neurology
- Alternative Therapies for Parkinson's Disease (*Neurology*)
- Migraine Headaches in Children and Adolescents (*Journal of Pediatric Health Care*)

Oncology
- Exercise Guidelines for Cancer Survivors (*Medicine & Science in Sports & Exercise*)
- Integrative Oncology: Complementary Therapies and Botanicals (*Society for Integrative Oncology*)
- Integrative Oncology in Lung Cancer (*Chest*)

Pain Management
- Chiropractic Management of Fibromyalgia (*Council on Chiropractic Guidelines and Practice Parameters*)
- Chronic Pain Management (*Anesthesiology*)
- Diagnosis and Treatment of Low-Back Pain (*Annals of Internal Medicine*)
- Management of Fibromyalgia Syndrome in Adults (*University of Texas, School of Nursing*)
- Osteopathic Manipulative Treatment for Low-Back Pain (*Journal of the American Osteopathic Association*)
- Pain Management Task Force Final Report (*Office of The Army Surgeon General*)

Pediatrics
- Migraine Headaches in Children and Adolescents (*Journal of Pediatric Health Care*)
- Probiotics and Children (*Journal of Pediatric Gastroenterology and Nutrition*)
- The Use of Complementary and Alternative Therapies in the Treatment of Fragile X Syndrome (*The Fragile X Clinical and Research Consortium*)

Psychiatry and Mental Health
- Management of Traumatic Stress Disorder and Acute Stress Reaction (*VA/DoD*)
- Posttraumatic Stress Disorder—Associated Nightmares (*Journal of Clinical Sleep Medicine*)

Rheumatology
- Osteoarthritis of the Hip and Knee (*Osteoarthritis Cartilage*)
- Osteoarthritis of the Knee (*The Journal of the American Academy of Orthopaedic Surgeons*)

Women's Health
- Botanicals for Menopausal Symptoms (*Obstetrics and Gynecology*)

From NCCAM. (2012d). *Clinical practice guidelines.* Retrieved July 8, 2012, from http://nccam.nih.gov/health/providers/clinicalpractice.htm.

BOX 14-4 HOT TOPICS

When Traditional Medicine and Complementary and Alternative Medicine (CAM) Collide

As a recent immigrant to the United States, Mary M. was excited for the birth of her first child and wanted to have a natural experience and deliver at home with the support of a doula (trained but not medically licensed labor coach), as she herself was born. Her pregnancy is low risk. What questions should Mary expect from her obstetrician and how can she prepare for the meeting? To her surprise, her obstetrician denies her request without discussion. What role does culture and spirituality play? As a nurse, how would you respectfully advocate to the obstetrician for Mary? Would information about nurse midwives be helpful for Mary? Are there state/governmental regulations limiting home deliveries? What about a birthing center, if one is available? What might be several recommendations for collaborative practice and integration of complementary and alternative modalities?

healthy lives. Although none of the objectives are specific to CAM, it is inherently integrated throughout, as many CAM modalities support the mission and its overarching goals. Examples are increasing physical activity and flexibility in all age groups, decreasing pain, and reducing substance

abuse (U.S. Department of Health and Human Services [USDHHS], 2011).

Affordable Care Act and National Prevention Strategy

The Affordable Care Act is very broad, but it supports CAM and states that health care workforce plans shall include licensed CAM disciplines (Weeks, 2010). Complementary and alternative medicine practitioners and integrative practices are mentioned in several areas, including workforce planning; patient-centered medical homes; wellness, prevention, and health-promotion services; comparative effectiveness research; and birthing services.

The National Prevention Strategy, released in June 2011 as a result of the Affordable Care Act (National Prevention Council, 2011), has the following four strategic directions:
- Healthy and Safe Community Environments: Create, sustain, and recognize communities that promote health and wellness through prevention.
- Clinical and Community Preventive Services: Ensure that prevention-focused health care and community prevention efforts are available, integrated, and mutually reinforcing.
- Empowered People: Support people in making healthy choices.

- Elimination of Health Disparities: Eliminate disparities, improving the quality of life for all Americans.

The second direction has a holistic objective: "Enhance coordination and integration of clinical, behavioral, and complementary health strategies." Inclusion of CAM into future research and evaluation and integration into care are mentioned several times throughout the document (National Prevention Council, National Prevention Strategy, 2011, www.health care.gov/prevention/nphpphc/strategy/report.pdf).

HOLISTIC NURSING

Holistic practices are moving into mainstream health care practice; therefore, nurses must understand the interventions that constitute holistic practice in order to discuss these practices with individuals who are using them to facilitate integrative care. Nurses who understand holistic practices may make referrals to alternative/complementary practitioners. Nurses also find that holistic interventions such as energy work, bodywork, aromatherapy, prayer, meditation, massage, imagery, music therapy, and the movement arts of yoga, tai chi, and qi gong provide a useful adjunct to current nursing theory (Current Nursing, 2011) and practice.

The American Holistic Nurses Association (AHNA) defines holistic nursing as nursing practice that heals the whole person. It is a "specialty practice that draws on nursing knowledge, theories, expertise and intuition to guide nurses in becoming therapeutic partners with people in their care. This practice recognizes the totality of the human being—the interconnectedness of body, mind, emotion, spirit, social/cultural, relationship, context, and environment" by integrating complementary and alternative modalities (CAM) into clinical practice to broaden and enrich nursing treatment of physiological, psychological, and spiritual needs. Florence Nightingale is thought to be one of the first holistic nurses because she believed in care of the person, focusing on unity, wellness, and the interrelationship of human beings with their environment. Holistic therapy is considered an "attitude, a philosophy, a way of being" although some holistic nurses specialize in one or more modalities (AHNA, 2012b, www.ahna.org/AboutUs/WhatisHolistic Nursing/tabid/1165/Default.aspx; Dossey & Keegan, 2013).

The American Holistic Nurses Association "advances the profession of holistic nursing by providing continuing education in holistic nursing, helping to improve the health care workplace through the incorporation of the concepts of holistic nursing, educating professionals and the public about holistic nursing and integrative health care, and promoting research and scholarship in the field of holistic nursing" (AHNA, 2012a, www .ahna.org/AboutUs/MissionStatement/tabid/1931/Default. aspx). The AHNA website offers a variety of resources including a directory of holistic practitioners based on modality and location, descriptions of healing modalities (AHNA, 2012d), and guidance on starting a holistic private practice.

INTERVENTIONS

The National Institutes of Health National Center for Complementary and Alternative Medicine (NCCAM) divides CAM modalities into several loose domains and an additional "whole medical system category" that incorporates all domains. The domains are not formally defined but include biologically based or natural products' practices, mind and body medicine, manipulative body-based practices, and an "other" category to include movement therapies and the manipulation of energy fields. Because each modality has its own identified guidance for purpose, efficacy, and safety, this section will not be specific, but will briefly define many of the modalities and highlight a few of the more common ones. In addition, inclusion in one domain versus another is not exclusive, because many could belong to several categories.

Whole Medical Systems

Whole medical systems are complete systems of theories and practices that have evolved culturally over time, and because they are different from Western allopathic medicine, they are considered CAM. Examples include traditional healers, medicine men, indigenous healers, and witch doctors. The 2007 NHIS (Barnes, Bloom, & Nahin, 2008) found that 0.4% of adults and 1.1% of children had consulted a traditional healer (usage varied for the seven specific types of healers identified in the survey). The 2007 NHIS asked about the use of Ayurveda, homeopathy, and naturopathy. Although relatively few respondents said they had used Ayurveda or naturopathy, homeopathy ranked tenth in usage among adults (1.8%) and fifth among children (1.3%).

Ayurvedic Medicine

Ayurvedic medicine originated in India and has evolved over thousands of years as one of the world's oldest medical systems. It integrates CAM modalities such as herbs, massage, and special diets to balance the body, mind, and spirit while preventing illness and promoting wellness. Basic premises include the beliefs that all living and nonliving things in the universe are joined together and good health is achieved when one's mind and body are in harmony (NCCAM, 2012h). Two ancient books, over 2000 years old and written in Sanskrit, are considered the heart of the practice and identify eight branches of ayurvedic medicine: internal medicine; surgery; treatment of head and neck disease; gynecology/obstetrics; pediatrics; toxicology; care of the elderly and rejuvenation; and sexual vitality. Treatment practices include eliminating impurities, decreasing symptoms, increasing resistance to disease, and reducing worry and increasing harmony. Nearly 80% of the Indian population continues to utilize ayurvedic medicine.

Traditional Chinese Medicine

Traditional Chinese medicine (TCM) evolved over thousands of years in China and includes herbs, acupuncture, and other CAM treatments. The theoretical framework includes the complementary yet opposing yin and yang life forces, and the balance and harmony of the vital energy, or life force (qi), circulating through the body's meridian pathways. TCM describes the organs and tissues in the body through corresponding elements of fire, earth, metal, water, and wood. It also uses eight principles to analyze symptoms and categorize conditions, including cold/heat, interior/exterior, excess/deficiency, and yin/yang (NCCAM, 2012e, http://nccam.nih.gov/health/whatiscam/chinesemed.htm).

Naturopathy

Naturopathy evolves from a medical system in nineteenth century Europe guided by the healing power of nature (Lazarides,

2010). Underlying principles are first do no harm, physician as teacher, treat the whole person, prevention, healing power of nature, and treat the cause (Stengler, 2010). Practitioners do not use prescription drugs, injections, x-rays, or surgery, but instead implement a variety of CAM modalities, emphasizing adopting a healthy lifestyle, strengthening and cleansing the body, and using noninvasive treatments (NCCAM, 2012f: nccam.nih.gov/health/naturopathy).

Homeopathy

Homeopathy treats the whole person and believes that symptoms are a body's effort to rid itself of disease. Treatment stimulates the body's healing ability through the administration of small amounts of dilute substances that cause illness or symptoms. It is based on three basic principles: like cures like; the more a remedy is diluted, the greater the potency; and illness is specific to the individual. Treatment is based on the whole person, rather than on the symptoms (Wardle, 2011).

Biologically Based Practices/Natural Products

Biological or natural products are the oldest form of CAM, making up the foundation of our modern pharmacology approach. Medicinal herbs were found in the personal effects of a mummified prehistoric man in the Italian Alps (NCCAM, 2012a). Botanical remedies were inventoried in great detail in the Middle Ages. The 2007 NHIS (Barnes, Bloom, & Nahin, 2012a) found that nearly 20% of American adults use natural products as CAM. This area of CAM includes nutritional counseling, herbs, vitamins, minerals, probiotics, and aromatherapy. According to NCCAM, daily multivitamins and calcium supplements are not thought of as CAMs.

Nutritional counseling uses diet and supplementation therapeutically as the primary or adjunctive treatment for illness, as well as for maintaining good health (Balch, 2010). Examples are promotion of foods high in iron to treat anemia and caloric restrictions for promotion of weight loss. Dietitians and nutritionists suggest a variety of techniques such as food pairing and macrobiotics for optimal healing and for preventive health (Gardner et al., 2007).

Herbal therapy is the use of herbs or their chemical properties to treat specific conditions or to enhance the function of various body systems, such as boosting the immune system, treating allergies, or preventing a cold. Herbal medicines may act on the body like prescription drugs and may affect how the body reacts to other medications; therefore it is important to research dosage and efficacy and to remind care recipients to share information regarding use of all supplements and herbs with their health care provider to facilitate coordinated and safe care (Snyder & Lindquist, 2009). A recent systematic review reported that most herbal medicinal products were not linked to drug interactions with serious consequences, but the scarcity of data in this area does not allow for definite conclusions (Posadzki, Watson & Ernst, 2012) (Table 14-1).

Probiotics are live microorganisms found in the human digestive tract, such as "friendly bacteria." They are taken to enhance the digestive system either as a supplement or in natural forms, such as yogurt or other fermented foods.

TABLE 14-1 HERBS: THEN AND NOW*

HERBS AS MEDICINE

DRUG NAME	PLANT/TREE
Digitalis (heart drug)	Foxglove plant
Paclitaxel (cancer drug)	Pacific yew tree
Aspirin	Willow tree
Quinine (malaria drug)	Cinchona tree
Morphine	Opium poppy
Galantamine (Alzheimer's drug)	Daffodil bulbus
Vincristine (cancer drug)	Rosy periwinkle
Reserpine (blood pressure drug)	Indian snakeroot plant

From National Center for Complementary and Alternative Medicine (NCCAM, 2012g). *Herbs at a glance* (pp. 2-3). Retrieved July 12, 2012, from http://nccam.nih.gov/sites/nccam.nih.gov/files/herbs/NIH_Herbs_at_a_Glance.pdf.

*What are herbs? An herb (also called a botanical) is a plant or plant part used for its scent, flavor, and/or therapeutic properties. An herbal supplement is a type of dietary supplement that contains herbs, either alone or in mixtures.

TABLE 14-2 STUDIES DEVELOPED BY NURSES USING AROMATHERAPY WITH POSITIVE RESULTS

SYMPTOM	OILS
Wound	Chamomile and lavender
Pressure ulcer/MRSA	Tea tree and aloe vera gel
Postoperative nausea	Ginger
Nausea	Peppermint
Agitation	French lavender
Agitation	Not specified
Agitation	Bergamot
Agitation	Ylang ylang, sweet marjoram, and bergamot
Pre-phlebotomy	*Piper nigrum*
Terminal agitation	Lavender, sandalwood, and frankincense
Terminal agitation	Lavender
Terminal agitation	Frankincense

Summarized from Buckle, J. (2007). Literature review: Should nursing take aromatherapy more seriously? *British Journal of Nursing, 16*(2), 116-120.
MRSA, Methicillin-resistant *Staphylococcus aureus.*

Hydrotherapy is the use of water, ice, steam, and hot and cold temperatures to maintain and restore health. Treatments include full body immersion, steam baths, saunas, spas, and the application of hot and/or cold compresses.

Aromatherapy uses aromatic plant materials and the essential oils of plants to treat physical imbalances (Buckle, 2003), as well as to achieve psychological and spiritual well-being through inhalation, external application, or ingestion. The essential oils have pharmacological, physiological, and psychological effects on the human body. The use of aromatherapy, like many CAMs, without professional clinical training is strongly discouraged. Individuals must have this training to know the specific warnings and contraindications for each oil, as well as to understand how to handle the oils (Lee et al., 2012) (Table 14-2).

Manipulative and Body-Based Practices

Manipulative and body-based practices focus on the manipulation of bones and joints, soft tissues, and circulatory and lymphatic systems. According to the 2007 NHIS (Barnes, Bloom, & Nahin, 2008), these ranked in the top 10 CAM therapies. Categories include spinal or bone manipulation and massage.

Spinal or Bone Manipulation

Spinal or bone manipulation is the application of controlled force on a bone or joint and is performed by chiropractors, physical therapists, osteopathic physicians, and some conventional medical doctors. Spinal manipulation was recorded in ancient Greece and became foundational to chiropractic and osteopathic medicine in the late nineteenth century.

Chiropractic medicine focuses on manipulation of the spine and joints, focusing on spinal alignment for optimal nervous system functioning. Chiropractors often integrate other CAMs such as massage, nutrition, and specialized kinesiology into their practice.

Cranial and cranio-sacral therapies also focus on a natural configuration of the skeletal system, focusing on the skull and the cranio-sacral system for the treatment of body imbalances. Cranio-sacral therapy originated in osteopathy and focuses on the bones of the cranium, spine, and sacrum, using gentle pressure to restore free movement of cerebrospinal fluid, allowing for normal functioning.

Physical therapy integrates a variety of modalities including massage, manipulation, heat and cold, movement, and electrical impulses to treat the body after damage or injury, reduce swelling, relieve pain, and restore function and range of motion (ROM) to the body.

Massage

Massage incorporates different techniques in the manipulation of muscles and soft tissues of the body, such as stroking, kneading, pulling, or pinching the skin for pain relief, in order to increase circulation, to facilitate healing, and to reduce stress and increase relaxation (Fritz, 2008). It is one of the oldest therapies and has references in writing in ancient China, Japan, India, Egypt, Greece, and Rome. Even Hippocrates mentions it in his writings. Different types of therapies have different techniques and purposes such as Bowenwork therapy, Feldenkrais method, lymphatic therapy, neuromuscular therapy, Rolfing structural integration, and trigger point therapy.

Mind-Body Medicine

Mind and body practices focus on the interactions between the brain, the body, and behavior, using the mind to affect the body and the body to affect the mind. Categories include meditation, imagery, and body movement. This concept dates back 2000 years to traditional Chinese and ayurvedic medicine practices. Hippocrates noted that treatment relied upon attitude, environmental influences, and natural remedies. Deep breathing, meditation, yoga, guided imagery, and progressive relaxation were in the top CAM therapies according to the 2007 NHIS (Barnes, Bloom, & Nahin, 2008).

Meditation

Meditation is a focused attention to increase relaxation, quiet the mind, and reduce stress. Although it is often a part of many religious cultures, it is not necessarily a religious activity and can be practiced while being still or while being active, such as during walking. Like massage, different types have a variety of purposes and techniques. Breath meditation is the simplest because it can be done anywhere and can evoke the relaxation response (Box 14-5). It can be taught and is useful for anyone who is having a "bad day." Centering focuses on a sacred word. Mindfulness meditation is a way of paying attention or being mindful of a variety of topics such as thoughts, actions, or the environment. Walking meditation is a form of mindfulness because the individual is mindful of the interaction of the inner body, the external body, and the environment with each step.

Imagery

Imagery is "a gentle but powerful technique that focuses and directs the imagination" in order to, among other things, promote a sense of well-being and to help people relax (www.health journeys.com/what_is_guided_imagery.asp). During imagery practice, images are presented verbally but are designed to evoke all the senses, causing the person to focus attention on the image and thus relax as if they are actually there. For example, if the person's special place is a beach, the practitioner might ask the individual to hear the water softly lapping at the shore, to see the white sand (senses of hearing and sight), and to feel the warm sun falling softly on the skin (sense of touch) as the smell of orange blossoms drifts through the air (sense of smell) (Kwekkeboom et al., 2008).

Hypnotherapy is a form of guided relaxation and focused attention of the unconscious mind. It is used for memory recall and for behavior changes such as discontinuing the use of tobacco products.

Biofeedback is a relaxation technique concentrating on vital functions such heart rate, breathing rate, and blood pressure. This visualization identifies which actions can change the rates and is used for stress and an irregular heart rate. Neurolinguistic

---

BOX 14-5 TEACHING THE TECHNIQUE OF BREATH MEDITATION

- You may stand, sit, or lie quietly as you begin to focus on your breath.
- Inhale and feel the air come into your nostrils, move down your throat, and into your lungs. Do not try to control the breath. Just observe it.
- Exhale and feel the air move up from your lungs and into your throat. Feel the warmth of the exhaled air in your nostrils.
- Breathe. Feel the air move in and out. Concentrate on the breath. Do not try to control the breath. Just observe it.
- Continue watching the breath for 5 to 10 minutes. As other thoughts come into focus, notice them and let them go. Focus again on the breath.
- As you become comfortable with breath meditation, you may easily add simple imagery to this technique.
- As you inhale, imagine breathing in peace or love or wellness.
- As you exhale, imagine breathing out pain or sorrow or grief.
- As you inhale, breathe in whatever it is that you need.
- As you exhale, breathe out whatever you wish to be free of in your life.

programming (NLP) changes behavior by changing patterns of thinking and speaking.

Movement Therapy

Movement therapies use movement and bodywork to promote physical, mental, emotional, and spiritual well-being. The movement arts such as qi gong, tai chi, and yoga are helpful for body, mind, and spirit, and, though technically not energy work, do manipulate life energies.

Qi gong (pronounced chee gung) is part of traditional Chinese medicine, combining relaxed movements with a meditative aspect and controlled breathing to move qi energy through the energy channels and increase vital energy.

Tai chi (pronounced tie chee) began as a Chinese martial art and combines physical movement, breath control, and meditation in a dancelike sequence of poses based on the movements of animals. One pose flows into the next in a slow, relaxed, gentle, unbroken rhythm, bringing an awareness of the moment-to-moment state of the body and producing a meditative state.

Yoga also uses postures, controlled breathing, and meditation (Besant, 2011; Iyengar, 2008). It comes from the Hindu tradition, originated as a form of spiritual practice, and aids in flexibility, agility, balance, and relaxation. The postures have names such as proud warrior, waterfall, runner's pose, downward-facing dog, mountain pose, and eagle pose. Many types and branches of yoga exist. Karma yoga is the yoga of right action and good works; bhakti yoga is the yoga of devotional practices; raja yoga is the yoga of meditative practices; jnana yoga is the yoga of the study of spiritual texts; mantra yoga is the yoga of repetition of a sacred phrase; laya yoga is the yoga of blending self with the Supreme (Sivananda, 2005).

Hatha yoga, the yoga of physical practice of various postures called asanas and of breath control, is most familiar to Western cultures. Hatha yoga also includes breathing exercises known as pranayama. Prana means vital energy and is synonymous with breath (Iyengar, 2008). Control of the breath helps the yogi control the mind and keep it focused on the present moment or the Supreme Being, or both. Breath control also helps move the subtle energy (prana or kundalini) through channels in the body (nadis) to nourish the body organs and the spirit (Iyengar, 2008).

Dance therapy is another movement-based mind-body modality, using dance to allow the body and mind to move freely in response to the music. Dependent on the person and the mood desired, all forms of music can be used.

Energy Work

People are animate beings with energy, a life force present in all living and nonliving elements of the universe. This energy is the animating force that flows through the body and extends beyond the body to interact with the energy in the environment (Pierce, 2007). The human energy field may be detected, assessed, and manipulated by an energy practitioner. Certain types of body energy are well-known. Electrical energy in the body is reflected in diagnostic studies including electrocardiographic and electroencephalographic tracings.

People can be affected by the energy of their environments, including the energy of other people. For example, anxiety is contagious and moves readily and quickly from person to person. There are medical uses for energy that comes from the environment. The energy of radiation is used to shrink tumors; sound energy, in the form of ultrasound waves, is used to break kidney stones. Music, a form of sound energy, can be relaxing or stimulating and has been used to decrease pain, depression, and disability (Siedliecki & Good, 2006). Light energy is useful in treating seasonal affective disorder and melatonin, a naturally occurring herb, may alter the sleep-wake cycle (Lam et al., 2006; Srinivasan et al., 2006). Color, another form of light energy, may have an effect on emotions and behaviors. Lasers, focused light energy, are used in many types of surgery and to treat other disorders (Frech & Adler, 2007; Kujawa et al., 2004).

"Some CAM practices involve manipulation of various energy fields to affect health. Such fields may be characterized as veritable (measurable) or putative (yet to be measured). Practices based on veritable forms of energy include those involving electromagnetic fields (e.g., magnet therapy and light therapy). Practices based on putative energy fields (also called biofields) generally reflect the concept that human beings are infused with subtle forms of energy; qi gong, Reiki, and healing touch are examples of such practices." (NCCAM, 2012b, http://nccam.nih.gov/health/whatiscam)

Other energies can affect healing. Many cultures believe that an energy flows through the body that nourishes organs and promotes optimal functioning. Chinese call this energy chi (or qi), Japanese call it ki, and East Indians call it prana. Some conceive of this energy in the form of chakras, or energy centers. In the West, this energy is often called subtle energy, life energy, or universal energy. Most of the detailed information on this energy system originally came from ancient practices and texts, including descriptions by people who have the exceptional ability to see the energy as it affects people. Personal experience may reveal the subtle energy in the body, as demonstrated by the exercise in Box 14-6.

BOX 14-6 FEEL YOUR OWN ENERGY

This exercise will help you feel your own energy, or chi.

- Sit quietly, back straight, feet touching the floor.
- Place your hands in your lap.
- Take a few deep breaths. Become quiet and still.
- Breathe slowly in and out for a few minutes.
- Slowly raise your hands in front of you, palms facing, hands about 15 inches apart. Cup your fingers as though you are holding a basketball between your hands.
- Concentrate on the space between your hands. What is there? Can you feel anything?
- Slowly bring your palms closer together, focusing on the space between your hands.
- Can you feel warmth? Does it feel spongy? Can you move your hands around a shape?
- What you are feeling is the energy coming from the energy centers in your hands. Focus on the energy. Try to increase the sensation of fullness in the space between your hands.
- If you do not feel anything right away, bring your hands back out to 15 inches apart and slowly move your hands together again. Try no more than 3 times each time you attempt the exercise.

BOX 14-7 RESEARCH FOR EVIDENCE-BASED PRACTICE

Assessment of Fragile Families and Well-Being, Father Incarceration, and Child Development

The *Fragile Families and Child Wellbeing Study* follows a cohort of nearly 5000 children born between 1998 and 2000 in U.S. cities. Approximately 75% of these children were born to unmarried parents, who are at greater risk of family disintegration and living in poverty.

American men have high rates of incarceration and there are high rates of fatherhood among these men. Data from the *Fragile Families and Child Wellbeing Study* were used to study the relationships between paternal incarceration and developmental progress of approximately 3000 urban children. Cross-sectional and longitudinal regression models were used that controlled not only the fathers' basic demographics and a complex set of potential cofounders but also several measures of preincarceration child and family development.

The study found "significant increases in aggressive behaviors and attention problems among children whose fathers are incarcerated" (p. 49). These effects were stronger than with other forms of father absence and were stronger for children who lived with fathers before the prison absence. These effects were thought to involve family stresses beyond those of usual father/child separation. Psychological well-being was also decreased because these men are at greater risk for experiencing adverse health conditions (e.g., depression), which may reduce their involvement with their children. These findings suggest that children of incarcerated fathers, especially those who previously lived in the home, may require extra support from caretakers, teachers, and health care providers, especially screenings for health-promotion strategies by school nurses and pediatric nurse practitioners. Fragile fathers and families should be an important population to encourage participation in wellness programs to mitigate upset and stress and improve the well-being of their children.

Sources: Geller, A., Cooper, C. E., Garfinkel, I., Schwartz-Soicher, O., & Mincy, R. B. (2012). Beyond absenteeism: Father incarceration and child development. *Demography, 49*(1), 49-76; *Fragile families and child wellbeing study.* (2012). Retrieved July 11, 2012, from www.fragilefamilies.princeton.edu/index.asp.

BOX 14-8 DIVERSITY AWARENESS

Hot and Cold Diseases

Hispanic culture considers disease causation as an imbalance between hot and cold. Specific diseases are classified by their causation, and the treatments (food, home remedies, and medications) used to ameliorate disease are generally temperature opposites; for example, a cold treatment is used for a hot disease. Some hot diseases are constipation, diarrhea, fever, pregnancy, ulcers, and rashes. Examples of cold diseases include arthritis, a cold, indigestion, menstrual cramps, stomachaches, and muscle spasms.

Hispanic use of complementary and alternative therapies is substantial; these therapies are often used to support chronic conditions. Diabetes is a hot disease. Hypertension, which is considered to be caused by anger, fear, nervousness, and thick blood, is a hot disease. It is treated by the cold treatments of lemon juice and various teas. Asthma is a cold disease, treated by traditional herbal mixtures and by massage. Home treatments traditionally complement traditional therapies and include cactus, aloe vera, and bitter gourd. If home treatments, which are generally initiated by an influential female in the home, are not successful, family and friends are consulted for advice. A spiritual leader (curanderismo) may also be consulted to perform a healing ritual for an especially recalcitrant problem. If this treatment fails to resolve the problem, an allopathic physician may be consulted.

Because there is potential for drug interactions between allopathic medicines and the traditional medicines of the Hispanic population, it is especially important that allopathic providers understand the home treatments that this population is using. One way to ease the assessment of the use of home treatments is with an open mind and with acceptance of folk practices.

Sources: Dayer-Berenson, L. (2010). *Cultural competencies for nursing.* Sudbury, MA: Jones & Bartlett Learning; Tabur, M. M., Crowe, T. K., & Torres, E. (2009). A review of curanderismo and healing practices among Mexicans and Mexican Americans. *Occupational Therapy International, 16*(1), 82-88; Ortiz, B. I., Shields, K. M., Clauson, K. A., & Clay, P. G. (2007). Complementary and alternative medicine use among Hispanics in the United States. *Annals of Pharmacotherapy, 41*, 994-1004.

Any illness, stress, emotional upset, or spiritual distress can affect the flow of life energy. For example, in fragile families, the energy flow that normally contributes to well-being can become blocked, unbalanced, or chaotic (Box 14-7: Research for Evidence-Based Practice). These disruptions in the flow of life energy can cause or exacerbate illness in the physical body and can increase emotional and spiritual distress. The basic goal behind the various modalities of energy work is to release blockages to energy flow, stimulate deficient life energy, and rebalance life energy.

Energy healing takes place in many cultures. There are other types of healing and healers. Shamanism has existed in many parts of the world for centuries. As the population of Hispanic Americans increases in the United States, the curandero (healer) of Mexican, Central American, and South American cultures, who often treats diseases with heat and cold, is becoming more familiar. Faith healers are associated with many different religions (Box 14-8: Diversity Awareness).

Acupuncture

Acupuncture manipulates life energy (chi or qi) by stimulating precisely mapped points on the skin surface. The points overlie the channels, called meridians, through which chi travels. The channels are named for the organs they affect, such as the lung meridian, heart meridian, and kidney meridian. Acupuncture may be used to diagnose disharmony; the points become tender to palpation in the presence of a disturbance in energy flow. The acupuncture points act as valves in the meridian system. When the points are stimulated, acupuncture acts as a treatment modality to correct disturbances in flow. When stimulated, the valve may open to release blocked or excess chi or close to allow chi to collect if chi is deficient. Stimulation of the points may be accomplished in several ways: by inserting fine needles into the points, by electro-stimulation, by laser, by light stimulation, and by burning herbs on or over the points to increase point stimulation, a technique called moxibustion. Acupuncture is one of the oldest healing practices in the world.

Acupressure and Reflexology

Acupressure stimulates meridian points with pressing, knuckling, rubbing, squeezing, and stretching movements. The technique is taught in some massage schools because it is often used along with massage to move and balance the body's energies. Shiatsu uses a sequence of rhythmic pressure on acupressure meridians. Reflexology is another method of moving energy by

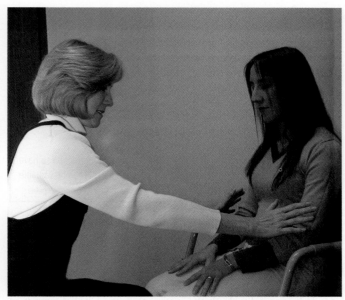

FIGURE 14-1 The assessment phase of therapeutic touch. The practitioner is attempting to sense disturbances or imbalances in the person's energy field.

using hand pressure. Rather than application of pressure to acupuncture points, the reflexologist applies pressure to mapped points on the feet or hands, or both. Pressure is applied with the thumbs, pressing deeply into the point to release tension and stimulate circulation of blood, lymph, and energy. Reflexology is more than massage because practitioners believe that the points correspond to the organs of the body and that stimulating the points will stimulate the organs (Reflexology Association of America, 2012; see www.reflexology-usa.org/articles/definitions_of_reflexology.html).

Touch Therapies

In touch therapies such as therapeutic touch, healing touch, Reiki, pranic healing, qi gong healing, and polarity therapy, among others, practitioners use their hands to direct life energies drawn from the environment to the individual in an effort to restore balance and harmony within the human energy system (www.intelihealth.com/IH/ihtIH/WSIHW000/8513/34968/358873.html?d=dmtContent). During these therapies, the hands can be placed directly on the person's body (contact) or at a distance from the body (no contact).

Therapeutic touch (TT) was conceptualized by nursing theorist Martha Rogers. She felt humans were composed of energy fields that interacted with the energy fields of their environments (Wright, 2007). TT practice comprises three essential elements. The first element is centering by the practitioner. Centering is a process of becoming calm, present in the moment, and connected with the individual being treated, allowing the practitioner to give the person undivided attention. The centered practitioner is able to let go of personal feelings and emotions and is more open to inner perceptions (Krieger, 1998). The practitioner remains centered throughout the treatment. During assessment, the second element, the practitioner's hands move over the individual's body at a height of about 3 inches

above the skin in an attempt to sense disturbances or imbalances in the person's energy field (Figure 14-1).

Assessment is performed before treatment begins and continues throughout treatment. Krieger (1993) describes the treatment techniques, the third element of TT practice. These techniques consist of methods to change the patterns in the human energy field (unruffling), to direct energy to the person to replenish depleted energy (modulation), and to balance or redistribute the individual's energies (modulation). Healing touch (HT) is similar to TT but adds full-body techniques for moving energy and disorder-specific energetic interventions to the modulation phase of TT (Hover-Kramer, 2011).

Reiki comes from Japanese tradition and requires training by a Reiki master. In addition to teaching the hand placements and symbolic gestures used in Reiki, the master attunes the student. Attunement opens the energy channel, enabling the student to bring universal energy through the body and to the recipient (Assefi et al., 2008; Baldwin et al., 2010). Therapeutic touch theory and clinical interventions are probably the most cited in the literature. Even though the energy therapies—TT, HT, and Reiki—have had sufficient attention in the nursing literature and contribute to satisfaction of care recipients in meaningful ways, there is a need for more research with larger samples that compare the various practices and modalities (Coakley & Barron, 2012; Fazzino et al., 2010).

Jin Shin Jyutsu uses fingertips pressed to specific healing point combinations to balance energy along specific pathways. Polarity therapy is a combination of energy work, caring intention, movement exercises, and dietary regimens and is aimed at clearing energy blockages and building health (American Polarity Therapy Association, 2012). Many use magnets or magnet therapy to control magnetic fields around many body systems to aid in healing and in the functioning of the systems. Color therapy integrates the nervous system and the body with the use of electronic instrumentation and color receptivity. Eye movement desensitization and reprocessing (EMDR) focuses on using alternative stimuli, either eye movement or sound, to reprogram traumatic stress responses.

Other Energy Modalities

Although the basis for many religious faiths, simple prayer focuses on the subtle energy life force known by different names. Prayer has different meanings to different people. A prayer may be a request for divine intervention, a type of meditation (centering prayer), or a form of intentionality that is useful in healing (Chopra, 2010, 2012). People pray for themselves, and they pray for others (Mao et al., 2007).

Praying for others may be a form of distant healing. Although the results of recent research on distant healing have not shown significant results, many who practice energy work believe that their efforts are effective over long distances. One method of participating in distance healing is the healing circle. The members of the healing circle join hands. Each member sends healing energy to his or her neighbor on the right until the energy is flowing around the circle. When the energy is flowing readily, each member of the group focuses the energy on one group member, who acts to send the energy to someone they know in need of

TABLE 14-3	BEING THERE VERSUS BEING WITH

THE NURSE WHO IS BEING THERE	THE NURSE WHO
Is attentive	Is available with whole self
Is task oriented	Enters the person's world
Does the right thing	Becomes vulnerable
Fulfills a role	Is present as a whole person
Assists with coping	Alleviates suffering
Provides security	Enables growth

BOX 14-9	WELLNESS QUIZ

- Do you wake up with enthusiasm for the day ahead?
- Do you have the high energy you need to do what you want?
- Do you laugh easily and often, especially at yourself?
- Do you confidently find solutions for the challenges in your life?
- Do you feel valued and appreciated?
- Do you appreciate others and let them know it?
- Do you have a circle of warm, caring friends?
- Do the choices you make every day get you what you want?

If you answered "no" to any of these questions, congratulations! You have identified areas in your life that you may want to change. This can be valuable information.

From Caton, S. (Ed.). (© 2003). *Wellness from within: The first step.* Anaheim, CA: American Holistic Health Association. Retrieved July 8, 2012, from http://ahha.org/ahhastep.htm.

healing. Each member of the circle may, in turn, receive energy from the group and send it to an individual in need of healing.

Music therapy is the use of specific kinds of music (or sounds) to produce desired changes in behaviors, emotions, and physiological processes. Music influences the limbic system, the area of the brain involved with emotions and feelings. Various types of music may be used therapeutically, and some music is composed specifically for therapeutic effect (Aigen, 2005). This music is called designer music, which may include sound frequencies that alter brainwave frequencies to achieve a particular brain state or emotion. When using music as therapy, the music choice should be tailored to the individual. People's musical tastes vary widely; the music that some find relaxing may be grating to others (Karkou & Sanderson, 2006). Music may also improve sleep quality in older adults (Hui-Ling & Marion, 2006).

Nursing Presence

The way people interact with one another can cause pain or promote healing and is determined by a person's **presence.** A classic study by Halldorsdottir (1991) examined individuals' perceptions of their interactions with nurses. Subjects maintained that nurse interactions followed a continuum from life-destroying to life-sustaining to life-giving. Individuals perceived life-giving nurses as a healing force; they were perceived as "being present with," rather than simply being there for, the individuals.

As described by Fredriksson (1999), "being there" would normally be considered acceptable nursing behavior (Table 14-3). However, the individuals in the Halldorsdottir (1991) study demonstrate that nurses can be much more than acceptable; the nurse's presence can actually contribute to healing. In examining the differences in "being there" and "being with," Fredriksson (1999) found that when nurses are "being with" subjects, the nurses' attention was focused rather than merely attentive, their touch was caring rather than task oriented, and nurses did not merely hear, they listened.

When using presence as a holistic intervention and establishing a whole person–to–whole person relationship, the nurse becomes vulnerable to the pain of the individual. Nurses may choose to avoid this pain by walking away, maintaining a professional distance, and being too busy with other tasks to be fully present. The key to overcoming these barriers to using presence in nursing practice is self-knowledge and self-care (Finfgeld-Connett, 2008; Hendren, 2010; McMahon & Christopher, 2011).

Holistic health involves knowing the physical self, the emotional self, the mental self, and the spiritual self; seeking a comfortable

balance among these aspects of being; and knowing what changes need to be made to achieve this balance (AHNA, 2012c). This knowledge is vital to both the nurse attempting holistic practice and the individual interested in pursuing holistic health.

The *Wellness Quiz* can assist both nurses and individuals in the exploration of self that begins the process of self-care (Box 14-9). An example of a more detailed assessment instrument, a personal health workbook is presented in **Website Resource 14A.**

Self-exploration is valuable to the nurse who wants to use presence in his or her practice because presence requires authenticity (Anderson, 2007). The more that is known about oneself, the more there is of oneself to offer to another, and "the only thing you ever have to offer to another human being, ever, is your own state of being" (Dass, 1976, p. 6).

When self-knowledge is gained, one or more of the holistic health strategies mentioned in this chapter can be useful in helping people achieve optimal wellness. In addition to the strategies mentioned, many other holistic interventions can be helpful. These strategies include homeopathy, **art therapy,** flower essences, crystals, and additional forms of bodywork and movement therapies. Every person is a whole, unique being; therefore, each person needs to explore the possible strategies and decide which modalities are the best methods to achieve an improved state of wellness.

People beginning this self-exploration and the practice of holistic health strategies may find that the practice changes their lives. Both using presence and giving the gift of self enhance personal growth in the giver by helping the giver find meaning in the relationship (Covington, 2005) (Box 14-10: Innovative Practice).

SAFETY AND EFFECTIVENESS

Most CAM therapies lack a strong scientific evidence base, as many have not been studied with rigorous, well-designed clinical trials. NIH is sponsoring research to fill the knowledge gap and build this foundation for safety, efficacy, and suitability for specific conditions.

The U.S. Food and Drug Administration (FDA) regulates dietary supplements, but the regulations are less strict than those for prescription or over-the-counter medications. For example, safety and efficacy do not have to be proved before marketed, although, once on the market, it does monitor label claims and inserts.

BOX 14-10 INNOVATIVE PRACTICE
Reconnecting Nurses Emotionally and Spiritually

Repar and Patton (2007) report on a program to assist nurses to "reconnect emotionally and spiritually with themselves, their clients, and fellow health-care workers" (p. 182). Nursing has become a more difficult career with compassion fatigue and increasing clinical demands leading to nurse burnout. Heavy caseloads, limited control over the work environment and schedule, rotating hours, and health systems in transition contribute to the problem. A program at the University of New Mexico Hospitals was developed called Arts-in-Medicine (AIM).

This program offers a 10-minute chair massage and allows nurses time to make art and to relax and be introspective during 1½-hour sessions during the workday on the units where they work. Each unit is visited by artists, massage therapists, and movement therapists approximately twice a semester. In addition, three longer sessions called Afternoon Delights (p. 184) help nurses relax and learn to practice self-care.

Sources: Repar, P. A., & Patton, D. (2007). Stress reduction for nurses through Arts-in-Medicine at the University of New Mexico Hospitals. *Holistic Nursing Practice, 21*(4), 182-186. Available at http://artsinmedicine.unm.edu/ArticleStressNurses.pdf; Irving, J. A., Dobkin, P. L., & Park, J. (2009). Cultivating mindfulness in health care professionals: A review of empirical studies of mindfulness-based stress reduction. *Complementary Therapies in Clinical Practice, 15,* 61-66.

Most CAM providers are not credentialed in a standardized national system, so credentialing regulations and standards vary nationally (NCCAM, 2012i). Some require training, testing, and continuing education, but most do not. Many practitioners belong to professional organizations that establish requirements for their profession (Box 14-11).

Although generally safe when used properly, the following are some CAM safety precautions:

- Carefully select CAM practitioners with appropriate training and experience.
- Take time to research and understand the treatment and ensure it is appropriate for the individual and the purpose.
- Be aware of scams.
- Treatment may not be covered by insurance.

BOX 14-11 MORE WEBSITE INFORMATION

- The NCCAM website at http://nccam.nih.gov/health/ and http://nccam.nih.gov/health/whatiscam/#informed provides further guidance on how to be an informed consumer, how to obtain information for the health care professional, and how to find and select a CAM practitioner.
- The NCCAM Clearinghouse (nccam.nih.gov) provides information on CAM and NCCAM, including publications and searches of federal databases of scientific and medical literature. The Clearinghouse does not provide medical advice, treatment recommendations, or referrals to practitioners. The Office of Dietary Supplements (ODS) seeks to strengthen knowledge and understanding of dietary supplements by evaluating scientific information, supporting research, sharing research results, and educating the public. Its resources include publications (such as *Dietary Supplements: What You Need to Know*), fact sheets on a variety of specific supplement ingredients (such as vitamin D and black cohosh), and the *PubMed Dietary Supplement Subset* (ods.od.nih.gov).
- PubMed® is a service of the National Library of Medicine (NLM); PubMed contains publication information and (in most cases) brief summaries of articles from scientific and medical journals (see www.ncbi.nlm.nih.gov/sites/entrez).
- NIH National Library of Medicine's MedlinePlus provides resources that help answer health questions. MedlinePlus brings together authoritative information from the National Institutes of Health as well as other government agencies and health-related organizations (see www.medlineplus.gov).

From NCCAM. (2012a). *What is complementary and alternative medicine?* Retrieved July 8, 2012, from http://nccam.nih.gov/health/whatiscam/.

- Quality is not always regulated for dietary supplements, and, like all "medicines," they may have side effects or react dangerously with other medications and supplements. In addition, they may not have been tested on children or pregnant women, so check labels with care.
- Some energy treatments may have side effects and cause inflammation that can affect other conditions and may not have been tested on children or pregnant women.
- Always inform both the allopathic and the holistic practitioner about the care and treatment received by other health care practitioners.

CASE STUDY
Use of Therapeutic Touch: George P.

George P., an 82-year-old White man, came to the clinic reporting neck pain and stiffness of approximately 4 months' duration. He was previously treated with ibuprofen (Motrin), acetaminophen, and oxycodone (Percocet) as well as with physical therapy. At the time of the initial clinic visit, Mr. P. was still taking Motrin but had stopped taking Percocet because the pain "isn't bad enough to take drugs [narcotics]." He rated his neck pain as 5 on a scale of 1 to 10. Neck range of motion (ROM) had improved, but it still caused problems for him when driving. Mr. P. lives next to a very busy street and did not feel that he could turn his neck well enough to see the traffic coming. He was afraid to pull out into the street. His daughter had driven him to the clinic. She said, "Pop is still in pain. He has little interest in doing anything. He walks like an old man and he can't work in his garden because of the pain." The goal of treatment for George P. is pain relief and increased ROM.

Reflective Questions
1. What holistic health strategies might be used to relieve George's pain and to help him increase his ROM?

2. After the treatment goals are reached, what holistic health strategies would you recommend to assist George P. in maintaining and improving his health?

Therapeutic touch (TT) was offered to George P. Although he was skeptical that this treatment would be effective, he agreed to treatment to please his daughter. Increased heat was noted in the neck and shoulder areas. A 30-minute TT treatment was performed, with special attention given to the neck and shoulder area. Immediately following the TT treatment, Mr. P. rated his pain as 0 on a scale of 1 to 10 and reported that he "couldn't remember when he'd been so relaxed"; and the excess heat had dissipated. Mr. P. was also given some simple yoga exercises for the neck and advised to perform the exercises twice a day, five gentle repetitions each time. Mr. P. was seen in the clinic a total of eight times for TT and was given increasingly difficult yoga stretches for the neck and shoulders. His pain rating at the end of treatment remained at 0 on the 1 to 10 scale. He had stopped taking Motrin, saying, "I don't need it anymore." His neck ROM had improved, and he was driving and working in his garden again. He continues his yoga stretches and has started performing daily qi gong exercises.

Use of Therapeutic Touch: George P.

*NURSING DIAGNOSIS: Disturbed Energy Field Disturbance related to slowing or blocking of energy flow secondary to repetitive motion injury

Defining Characteristics
- Perceptions of changes in patterns of energy flow, such as:
  - Temperature change: warmth, coolness
  - Visual changes: image, color
  - Disruption of the field: vacant, hole, spike, bulge
  - Movement: wave, spike, tingling, dense, flowing
  - Sounds: tone, words

Related Factors
- Pathophysiological: illness, injury
- Treatment-related: immobility, perioperative experience, labor and delivery
- Situational: pain, fear, anxiety, grieving
- Maturational: age-related developmental difficulties or crises

Expected Outcomes
- The person will report increased sense of relaxation.
- The person will report decreased anxiety and tension.
- The person will demonstrate evidence of physical relaxation (e.g., decreased blood pressure, pulse, respiratory rate, and muscle tension).
- The person will report an increased sense of well-being.

Interventions
- Provide privacy if possible.
- Explain energy therapy (therapeutic touch, Reiki, healing touch) and obtain permission to treat.
- Position the person comfortably.
- Become quiet and still (centered) and bring the focus to the person.
- Assess (scan) the energy field for openness and flow.
- Clear the exterior energy field by combing through the field from head to toe (unruffling).
- Move the palms of the hands toward the person, 2 to 4 inches over the person's body, from head to feet in a smooth, light movement.
- Sense the cues to energy imbalance (i.e., warmth, coolness, tightness, heaviness, tingling, emptiness).
- Focus on perceived areas of imbalance to repattern the energy flow.
- Reassess and smooth the exterior energy field, ensuring that the energy flow is open in the feet.
- Gently stop the treatment and provide the person time to rest.
- Encourage the person to discuss the experience.

Modified from Carpenito, L. J. (2009). *Nursing diagnosis: Application to clinical practice* (13th ed.). Philadelphia: Lippincott.
**NANDA Nursing Diagnoses—Definitions and Classification 2012-2014*, Herdman T.H. (ED). Copyright © 2012, 1994-2012 NANDA International. Used by arrangement with John Wiley & Sons Limited. In order to make safe and effective judgments using the NANDA-I nursing diagnoses it is essential that nurses refer to the definitions and defining characteristics of the diagnoses listed in this work.

SUMMARY

Holistic health strategies are designed to view the individual as a biopsychosocial-spiritual whole being. Many holistic health strategies have been practiced in other cultures for many years; some began as religious practices. As these practices moved to the West, the health-promoting nature of these therapies came to the forefront and the emphasis on religion waned. Many of these strategies can be used to help nurses and those they serve reach the *Healthy People 2020* goals. A body of research already exists supporting the use of these therapies and more research is being performed. Although the studies to date have been unsuccessful in providing definitive evidence that would persuade some health care practitioners of the utility of the practices, many individuals—including holistic health practitioners—are convinced that these practices help promote and maintain health.

Every person is a unique, individual being; therefore, some exploration of self, the various strategies, and the practitioner will be necessary before determining which strategy is the right fit for the individual. The right-fit strategy will increase both physical and mental well-being. **Website Resource 14B** presents a summary list of definitions of many holistic strategies. Nurses need to understand holistic health strategies because individuals are using them in increasing numbers. Nurses who begin to practice holistic interventions may find them a useful and exciting adjunct to their nursing practice.

REFERENCES

Aigen, K. (2005). *Music-centered music therapy*. Gilsum, NH: Barcelona.

American Holistic Nurses Association (AHNA). (2012a). *About us.* Retrieved July 8, 2012, from www.ahna.org/AboutUs/MissionStatement/tabid/1931/Default.aspx.

American Holistic Nurses Association (AHNA). (2012b). *What is holistic nursing?* Retrieved July 8, 2012, from www.ahna.org/AboutUs/WhatisHolisticNursing/tabid/1165/Default.aspx.

American Holistic Nurses Association (AHNA). (2012c). *Fact sheet: What is holistic nursing?* Retrieved July 6, 2012, from www.ahna.org/Home/NewsRoom/FactSheetHolisticNursing/tabid/1239/Default.aspx.

American Holistic Nurses Association (AHNA). (2012d). *Description of healing modalities.* Retrieved July 8, 2012, from www.ahna.org/Home/ForConsumers/HolisticModalities/tabid/1921/Default.aspx.

American Polarity Therapy Association. (2012). *About polarity therapy.* Retrieved July 10, 2012, from www.polaritytherapy.org/polarity/index.html.

Anderson, J. H. (2007). The impact of using nursing presence in a community heart failure program. *Journal of Cardiovascular Nursing, 22*(2), 89–94.

Angner, E. (2008). The philosophical foundation of subjective measure of well-being. *Capabilities and Happiness*, 286–298.

Anspaugh, D. (2010). *Wellness: Concepts and applications.* New York: McGraw-Hill.

Assefi, N., Bogart, A., Goldberg, J., & Buchwald, D. (2008). Reiki for the treatment of fibromyalgia: A randomized controlled trial. *Journal of Complementary and Alternative Medicine, 14*(9), 1115–1122.

Balch, P. A. (2010). *Prescription for nutritional healing: A practical A-to-Z reference to drug-free remedies using vitamins, minerals, herbs and food supplements* (5th ed.). New York: Avery Trade.

Baldwin, A. L., Vitale, A., Brownell, E., Scicinski, J., Kearns, M., & Rand, W. (2010). The touchstone process: An ongoing critical evaluation of reiki in the scientific literature. *Holistic Nursing Practice, 24*(5), 260–276.

Barnes, p., Bloom, B., & Nahin, R. (2008). Complementary and alternative medicine use among adults and children: United States, 2007. *National Health Statistics Reports, 24*, 1–24.

Besant, A. (2011). *Introduction to yoga.* CreateSpace Publishing.

Birchtree Center. (2012). *Professional development for nurses: Preparation for certification in holistic nursing (HNC).* Retrieved July 10, 2012, from www.birchtreecenter.com/prof_dev.html.

BlueCross BlueShield Association. (2012). *Dr. Dean Ornish's program for reversing heart disease.* Retrieved July 10, 2012, from www.blueadvocacy.org/plans/program/dr_dean_ornish_program_for_reversing_heart_disease.

Brown, L. (2011). *Two systems of medicine.* Retrieved July 7, 2012, from www.holistic.com/holistic/learning.nsf/ed8732a8bed2f2a4872569060015ca74/6d6ad242c4e75c9c87256b8f00021919!OpenDocument.

Buckle, J. (2003). *Clinical aromatherapy: Essential oils in practice* (2nd ed.). New York: Churchill Livingstone.

Buckle, J. (2007). Literature review: Should nursing take aromatherapy more seriously? *British Journal of Nursing, 16*(2), 116–120.

Carpenito, L. J. (2009). *Nursing diagnosis: Application to clinical practice* (13th ed.). Philadelphia: Lippincott.

Caton, S. (Ed.), (2003). *Wellness from within: The first step.* Anaheim, CA: American Holistic Health Association. Retrieved November 13, 2011, from http://ahha.org/ahhastep.htm.

Chopra, D. (2010). *Reinventing the body, resurrecting the soul: How to create a new you.* New York: Three Rivers Press.

Chopra, D. (2012). *Spiritual solutions: Answers to life's greatest challenges.* Easton, PA: Harmony Press.

Coakley, A. M., & Barron, A. (2012). Energy therapies in oncology nursing. *Seminars in Oncology Nursing, 28*(1), 55–63.

Corporate Wellness. (2012). *Definition of wellness.* Retrieved July 8, 2012, from www.definitionofwellness.com/.

Covington, H. (2005). Caring presence: Providing a safe space for patients. *Holistic Nursing Practice, 19*(4), 169–172.

Current Nursing. (2011). *Nursing theories.* Retrieved November 29, 2012, from http://currentnursing.com/nursing_theory/nursing_theorists.html.

Das, R. (1967). *The only dance there is.* New York: Jason Aronson.

Dayer-Berenson, L. (2010). *Cultural competencies for nursing.* Sudbury, MA: Jones & Bartlett Learning.

Dosch, L. (2012). *Allopathic medicine vs. holistic health.* Retrieved July 10, 2012, from www.ehow.com/about_5434926_allopathic-medicine-vs-holistic-health.html#ixzz1Zpsg8C5P.

Dossey, B. M., & Keegan, L. (2013). *Holistic nursing: A handbook for practice* (6th ed.). Sudbury, MA: Jones & Bartlett Learning.

Faculty of Harvard Medical School & Natural Standard. (2008). *Complementary and alternative medicine: Therapeutic touch.* Retrieved July 10, 2012, from www.intelihealth.com/IH/ihtIH/WSIHW000/8513/34968/358873.html?d=dmtContent.

Fazzino, D. L., Quinn Griffin, M. T., McNulty, R., & Fitzpatrick, J. (2010). Energy healing and pain: A review of the literature. *Holistic Nursing Practice, 24*(2), 79–88.

Finfgeld-Connett, D. (2008). Concept synthesis of the art of nursing. *Journal of Advanced Nursing, 62*, 381–388. 10.1111/j.1744-618X.2008.00090.x. From www.equip.org/PDF/DN105.pdf.

Frech, E. J., & Adler, D. G. (2007). Endoscopic therapy for malignant bowel obstruction. *Journal of Supportive Oncology, 5*(7), 303–310.

Fredriksson, L. (1999). Modes of relating in a caring conversation: A research synthesis on presence, touch and listening. *Journal of Advanced Nursing, 30*(5), 1167–1176.

Fritz, S. (2008). *Mosby's fundamentals of therapeutic massage* (4th ed.). St Louis: Mosby.

Gardner, C. D., Kiazand, A., Alhassan, S., et al. (2007). Comparison of the Atkins, Zone, Ornish, and LEARN diets for change in weight and related risk factors among overweight premenopausal women. *Journal of the American Medical Association, 297*(9), 969–977.

Halldorsdottir, S. (1991). Five basic modes of being with another. In D. A. Gaut & M. M. Leininger (Eds.), *Caring: The compassionate healer* (NLN Pub. No. 15-2401, pp. 37–49). New York: National League for Nursing Press.

Hendren, R. (2010, May 11). Nurses find simple ways to improve satisfaction. *Media Health Leader.* Retrieved from www.healthleadersmedia.com/content/NRS-250810/Nurses-Find-Simple-Ways-to-Improve-Satisfaction##.

Herman, P. M., D'Huyvetter, K., & Mohler, M. J. (2006). Are health services research methods a match for CAM? *Alternative Therapies in Health and Medicine, 12*(3), 78–83.

Hover-Kramer, D. (2011). *Creating healthy relationships: Professional standards for energy therapy practitioners.* Fulton, CA: Energy Psychology Press.

Hui-Ling, L., & Marion, G. (2006). Music improves sleep quality in older adults. *Journal of Advanced Nursing, 53*(1), 134–144.

Irving, J. A., Dobkin, P. L., & Park, J. (2009). Cultivating mindfulness in health care professionals: A review of empirical studies of mindfulness-based stress reduction. *Complementary Therapies in Clinical Practice, 15*, 61–66.

Iyengar, B. K. S. (2008). *Iyengar yoga: The path to holistic health.* London: Dorling Kindersley Publishers, Ltd.

Karkou, V., & Sanderson, P. (2006). *Arts therapies: A research-based map of the field.* Edinburgh: Elsevier.

Kendall, M. (2007). Ancient wisdom, modern care. *Advance for Nurses, 13*, 24.

Krieger, D. (1993). *Accepting your power to heal: The personal practice of therapeutic touch.* Santa Fe, NM: Bear & Company.

Krieger, D. (1998). Healing with therapeutic touch (interview). *Alternative Therapies in Health and Medicine, 4*(1), 87–92.

Kujawa, J., Talar, J., Gworys, K., Gworys, P., Pieszynski, I., & Janiszewski, M. (2004). The analgesic effectiveness of laser therapy in patients with gonarthrosis: An evaluation. *Ortopedia, Traumatologie, Rehavilitacja, 6*(3), 356–366.

Kwekkeboom, K. L., Hau, H., Wanta, B., & Bumpus, M. (2008). Patients' perceptions of the effectiveness of guided imagery and progressive muscle relaxation interventions used for cancer pain. *Complementary Therapies in Clinical Practice, 14*, 185–194.

Lam, R. W., Levitt, A. J., Levitan, R. D., Enns, M. W., Morehouse, R., Michalak, E. E., et al. (2006). The Can-SAD study: A randomized controlled trial of the effectiveness of light therapy and fluoxetine in patients with winter seasonal affective disorder. *American Journal of Psychiatry, 163*(5), 805–812.

Lazarides, L. (2010). *A textbook of modern naturopathy.* London: Waterfall.

Lee, M. S., Choi, J., Posadzki, P., & Ernst, E. (2012). Aromatherapy for health care: An overview of the systematic reviews. *Maturitas, 71*(3), 257–260.

Lundy, K., & Janes, S. (2009). *Community health nursing: Caring for the public's health.* Burlington, MA: Jones & Bartlett Learning.

Mao, J. J., Farrar, J. T., Xie, S. X., Bowman, M. A., & Armstrong, K. (2007). Use of complementary and alternative medicine and prayer among a national sample of cancer survivors compared to other populations without cancer. *Complementary Therapies in Medicine, 15*(1), 21–29.

McMahon, M. A., & Christopher, K. A. (2011). Toward a mid-range theory of nursing presence. *Nursing Forum, 46*, 71–82. doi: 10.1111/j.1744-6198.2011.00215.x.

Mork, R. (2012). *Holistic versus allopathic medicine.* Retrieved July 10, 2012, from www.life123.com/health/alternative-medicine/naturopathy/holistic-versus-allopathic-medicine.shtml.

Mosby. (2009). *Mosby's medical dictionary* (8th ed.). St Louis: Elsevier.

National Center for Complementary and Alternative Medicine (NCCAM). (2012a). *What is complementary and alternative medicine?* Retrieved July 10, 2012, from http://nccam.nih.gov/health/whatiscam/.

National Center for Complementary and Alternative Medicine (NCCAM). (2012b). *CAM basics: What is complementary and alternative medicine?* Retrieved July 6, 2012, from http://nccam.nih.gov/health/whatiscam/.

National Center for Complementary and Alternative Medicine (NCCAM). (2012c). *The use of complementary and alternative medicine in the United States: Cost data.* Retrieved July 19, 2012, from http://nccam.nih.gov/news/camstats/costs/costdatafs.htm.

National Center for Complementary and Alternative Medicine (NCCAM). (2012d). *Clinical practice guidelines.* Retrieved July 10, 2012, from http://nccam.nih.gov/health/providers/clinicalpractice.htm.

National Center for Complementary and Alternative Medicine (NCCAM). (2012e). *Traditional Chinese medicine: An introduction.* Retrieved July 19, 2012, from http://nccam.nih.gov/health/whatiscam/chinesemed.htm.

National Center for Complementary and Alternative Medicine (NCCAM). (2012f). *Naturopathy: An introduction.* Retrieved July 10, 2012, from http://nccam.nih.gov/health/naturopathy/naturopathyintro.htm.

National Center for Complementary and Alternative Medicine (NCCAM). (2012g). *Herbs at a glance.* Retrieved July 10, 2012, from http://nccam.nih.gov/health/herbsataglance.htm.

National Center for Complementary and Alternative Medicine (NCCAM). (2012h). *Ayurvedic medicine: An introduction.* Retrieved July 10, 2012, from http://nccam.nih.gov/health/ayurveda/introduction.htm.

National Center for Complementary and Alternative Medicine (NCCAM). (2012i). *How to find a CAM practitioner.* Retrieved July 10, 2012, from http://nccam.nih.gov/health/howtofind.htm.

National Prevention Council, National Prevention Strategy. (2011). *Office of the Surgeon General.* Washington, DC. Retrieved July 10, 2012, from www.healthcare.gov/prevention/nphpphc/strategy/index.html.

Northrup, C. (2010). *Women's bodies, women's wisdom (revised edition): Creating physical and emotional health and healing.* New York: Bantam.

Ornish, D. (1995). *Dr. Dean Ornish's program for reversing heart disease.* New York: Ballantine.

Ornish, D. (2012). *Preventive Medicine Research Institute.* Retrieved July 8, 2012, from www.pmri.org/dean_ornish.html.

Pierce, B. (2007). The use of biofield therapies in cancer care. *Clinical Journal of Oncology Nursing, 11*(2), 253–258.

Posadzki, P., Watson, L., & Ernst, E. (2012). Contamination and adulteration of herbal medicinal products (HMPs): An overview of systemic reviews. *European Journal of Clinical Pharmacology.* July 29 [Epub ahead of print]. Retrieved on November 29, 2012, from www.ncbi.nlm.nih.gov/pubmed/22843016.

Reflexology Association of America. (2012). See www.reflexology-usa.org/articles/definitions_of_reflexology.html.

Repar, P. A., & Patton, D. (2007). Stress reduction for nurses through Arts-In-Medicine at the University of New Mexico Hospitals. *Holistic Nursing Practice, 21*(4), 182–186.

Robin, M. (2010). *Wellness on a shoestring: Seven habits for a healthy life.* Missouri: Unity House.

Rost, A. (2009). *Natural healing wisdom and know-how: Useful practices, recipes and formulas for a lifetime of health.* New York: Black Dog and Leventhal Publishers.

Siedliecki, S. L., & Good, M. (2006). Effect of music on power, pain, depression and disability. *Journal of Advanced Nursing, 54*(5), 553–562.

Sivananda, S. S. (2005). *Practice of yoga* (8th ed.). Shivanandanagar, India: The Divine Life Society.

Smeeding, S., & Osguthorpe, S. (2005). The development of an integrative healthcare model in the Salt Lake City Veterans Affairs Healthcare System. *Alternative Therapies in Health and Medicine, 11*(6), 46–51.

Smith, B., Tang, K., & Nutbeam, D. (2006). WHO health promotion glossary: New terms. *Health Promotion International, 21*(4), 340–345.

Snyder, M., & Lindquist, R. (2009). *Complementary/alternative therapies in nursing* (6th ed.). New York: Springer.

Srinivasan, V., Smits, M., Spence, W., Lowe, A. D., Kayumov, L., Pandi-Perumal, S. R., et al. (2006). Melatonin in mood disorders. *World Journal of Biological Psychiatry, 7*(3), 138–151.

Stengler, M. (2010). *The natural physician's healing therapies: Proven remedies medical doctors don't know.* New Jersey: Prentice Hall Press.

Tabur, M. M., Crowe, T. K., & Torres, E. (2009). A review of curanderismo and healing practices among Mexicans and Mexican Americans. *Occupational Therapy International, 16*(1), 82–88.

United States Department of Health and Human Services (USDHHS). (2011). *Healthy People 2020.* Retrieved July 10, 2012, from www.healthypeople.gov/2020/about/default.aspx.

Van Elslander Cancer Center. (2012). *Services.* Retrieved July 12, 2012, from www.stjohn.org/VanElslander.

Wardle, J. (2011). *Clinical naturopathy: An evidence-based guide to practice.* Elsevier: Churchill Livingstone.

Weeks, J. (2010). *The Integrator blog: News, reports, opinion and networking for the business, education, policy and practice of integrative medicine, CAM, and integrated health care.* Retrieved November 30, 2012, from http://theintegratorblog.com/site/index.php?option=com_content&task=view&id=658&Itemid=189.

Weil, A. (2000). *Spontaneous healing: How to discover and embrace your body's natural ability to maintain and heal itself.* New York: Ballantine Books.

Weil, A. (2011). *Spontaneous happiness.* Boston: Little, Brown.

Woodwinds Health Campus. (2010). *Healing arts therapy.* Retrieved July 10, 2012, from www.healtheast.org/woodwinds/healing-arts.html.

World Health Organization (WHO). (1948). Preamble to the Constitution of the World Health Organization as adopted by the International Health Conference, New York, 19 June–22 July 1946; signed on 22 July 1946 by the representatives of 61 States (Official Records of the World Health Organization, No. 2, p. 100) and entered into force on 7 April 1948. Retrieved July 7, 2012, from www.who.int/about/definition/en/print.html.

Wright, B. W. (2007). The evolution of Rogers' science of unitary human beings: 21st century reflections. *Nursing Science Quarterly, 20*(1), 64–67.

CHAPTER

15

Overview of Growth and Development Framework

Tawna Cooksey-James

WEBSITE

http://evolve.elsevier.com/Edelman/
- Study Questions
- Glossary

OBJECTIVES

After completing this chapter, the reader will be able to:
- Explain the importance of growth and development as a framework for assessing and promoting health.
- Define the terms growth, development, and maturation.
- Discuss factors that influence growth in an individual.
- Describe Erikson's theory of psychosocial development.
- Contrast Piaget's and Vygotsky's theories of cognitive development.
- Compare Kohlberg's and Gilligan's theories of moral development.
- Evaluate a person's growth and development and determine normal and abnormal areas.

KEY TERMS

Cephalocaudal
Denver Developmental Screening Test
Development
Developmental patterns
Differentiation
Erikson's theory of psychosocial development

Gilligan's theory of moral development
Growth
Growth charts
Growth patterns
Kohlberg's theory of moral development
Learning

Maturation
Piaget's theory of cognitive development
Proximodistal
Scaffolding
Vygotsky's theory of cognitive development
Zone of proximal development

? THINK ABOUT IT

Vaccine Issues and Controversies

A 4½-year-old child begins to scream as the nurse approaches with her "kindergarten shots." The mother tries to comfort her child, as she turns anxiously to the nurse and states, "I've heard vaccinations can be dangerous. No wonder she's frightened. Are they really necessary?"
- What influence might the mother's anxiety have on the child's behavior?
- What approaches and information can the nurse have for the mother?
- What approaches can the nurse take to gain the child's cooperation?

Unit 4 introduces growth and development as a framework for health assessment and promotion throughout the life span. Understanding human growth and development facilitates nursing assessment of health knowledge and behavior. Further, health education is more effective when the nurse acknowledges and incorporates growth and developmental needs as well as the individual's prior understanding of and beliefs about health and health-related concepts.

Health promotion during growth and development would not be complete without the inclusion of *Healthy People 2020.*

TABLE 15-1   GROWTH AND DEVELOPMENT

Overview of Developmental Periods

PERIOD	AGE	CHARACTERISTICS
Infant	Birth to 12 months	Fully dependent on others for basic needs
		Ends as infant begins to explore environment, walks alone, and develops basic communication skills
Toddler	12 months to 3 years	Motor development progresses significantly
		Child achieves a degree of physical and emotional autonomy while maintaining a close identity with the primary family unit
Preschool child	3 to 6 years	Child has increased interest and involvement with peers and may have social interactions with many people
School-age child	6 to 10 years	Marked by entrance into elementary school; interests turn away from family toward peers
Adolescent	11 to 18 years	Period of transition, adjustment, and personal exploration; ends when adolescent demonstrates readiness to assume full adult responsibilities of financial, emotional, and social independence
Young adult	18 to 35 years	Establishing an occupation or career, finding and learning how to live with a partner, and starting and rearing a family
Middle adult	35 to 65 years	Being established in a marriage, an occupation or career, and a community; may continue to be a time of transition; adjusts to physiological changes of middle age
Older adult	More than 65 years	May be a time of continued involvement in work and active socializing; adjusts to decreased physical strength and health; retirement; reduced income; decreasing independence; and deaths of spouses, friends, and self

Throughout Unit 4, specific topics and objectives from *Healthy People 2020* will be examined in chapters appropriate to the age and individual developmental level in the life span under discussion. Although these objectives will serve as guides for the promotion of health care at each level, the topic "access to health services" crosses all levels and the entire life span. The first four objectives that increase access to health services for all people and families including increase the proportion of persons with health insurance; increasing the proportion of insured persons with coverage for clinical preventive services; increasing the proportion of persons with a usual primary care provider; and increasing the number of practicing primary care providers, including nurse practitioners (*Healthy People*, 2020). Without access to health services, health promotion cannot occur and a person has difficulty achieving and maintaining health. With passage of the Affordable Care Act by President Obama on March 23, 2010, increased access to health services by all persons may be obtained (U.S. Department of Health and Human Services [USDHHS], 2012).

This chapter focuses on the study of health promotion at individual developmental levels by exploring basic concepts of growth and development as well as providing an overview of representative theories of development. Each of the following nine chapters provides health assessment and promotion strategies appropriate for selected age groups across the life span. The age groups described are prenatal; infant; toddler; preschool child; school-age child; adolescent; and young, middle, and older adult (Table 15-1).

OVERVIEW OF GROWTH AND DEVELOPMENT

Understanding of growth and development has continued to expand with advances in science. Today we find ourselves at the intersection of the genomic era and the age of technology. We are only just beginning to appreciate the long-term impact of early interactions on later health and health-related behavior.

Individuals continue to evolve throughout the life span, and developmental transitions occur beyond childhood and adolescence, extending into the young, middle, and older adult

years. Today, aging adults are receiving increased attention as the average life expectancy increases and adults older than 85 become the fastest growing age group, providing new challenges for health assessment and promotion.

Growth

Growth refers to a quantifiable change in structure. In the body, this change means an increase in the number and/or size of the cells, resulting in an increase in the size and weight of the whole, or any of its parts. During childhood, physical changes in height, weight, and head circumference, or growth parameters, are measured and charted regularly. While growth refers to these obvious changes to the whole individual, it also refers to the increases (and as we age, decreases) in the size of specific organs and systems. The health history and physical assessment of an individual should include all body systems, but should emphasize systems undergoing the most change. Table 15-2 outlines growth as it takes place throughout the body systems and life span. The growth of some systems, such as the skeletal and muscular systems, is influenced by gender, whereas the growth of others, such as the nervous and respiratory systems, is independent of gender. Growth changes that take place in young, middle-aged, and older adults should be noted. People who think of growth only as it applies to infants, children, and adolescents are missing important changes from conception and throughout adulthood.

Influences on an individual's potential for growth include genetic factors, prenatal and postnatal exposures, nutrition, and environmental factors (see the Case Study and Care Plan at the end of this chapter). Other influences include emotional health as well as traditional cultural practices that influence childrearing, lifestyle, and health care practices (Box 15-1: Diversity Awareness). Although growth potential is primarily determined by individual genetics, health and environmental exposures influence the attainment of that potential. The timing of exposure to environmental hazards may determine to a great extent the amount and kind of effects of these influences. For example, if a pregnant mother is exposed to the rubella virus, the developing fetus is much more vulnerable than either the mother

Text continued on p. 343

TABLE 15-2 GROWTH AND DEVELOPMENT

Flowchart Showing Directions of Growth Changes Throughout Life Cycle*

OVERVIEW OF DEVELOPMENTAL CHANGES	PRENATAL →	INFANCY →	CHILDHOOD →	PUBERTY AND ADOLESCENCE →	ADULTHOOD → MIDDLE AGE → OLD AGE
Heart and Circulatory System					
Action of heart and circulatory system is under control of autonomic nervous system	Heart formed and begins to beat about third week	Heart grows somewhat more slowly than rest of body (weight doubled by 1 yr, body weight tripled) Grows steadily during childhood With birth, considerable change in paths and relative volumes of blood flow, reflected in loss of certain fetal structures and changes in heart and major vessels	Heart grows somewhat more slowly than rest of body	At puberty, heart takes part in rapid growth, reaching mature size with rest of body	Heart weight remains relatively constant after age 25 (only organ other than prostate that does not decrease in weight with age) Cardiac output decreases 30-40% between ages 25 and 65 Capacity to increase rate and strength of beat during physical work is diminished Cardiac strength lessens with age, whereas expenditure of energy is more than in youth
Throughout life cardiac rate is responsive to organ needs and emotional states (fear, anxiety, tension, depression)	Heart rate high, ≈150 beats/min		Heart rate falls steadily throughout childhood		After maturity, women have slightly higher pulse rate than men, 65 beats/min (girls' temperature remains stationary, higher than boys'); men maintain same pulse rate in maturity (slightly lower body temperature than women)
		130 beats/min	70-80 beats/min	60 beats/min in adolescence, rate differs with gender	
			Heart rate more variable during childhood—regular Not until middle childhood does peripheral blood picture become same as adult		
Urinary System					
Parallels growth as a whole	Young fetus is about 90% water	Newborn is about 70% water	Composition of urine in healthy child (after age 2 yr) changes very little as child matures; thus renal function and urinalysis can be used as monitor of well-being		Adult is about 58% water
Proportion of body water and solids follows pattern related to growth—tendency for human organism to dry out as life progresses	Urinary system begins in first month	Urinary system does not complete full development until end of first year			Glomerular filtration rate decreases about 47% from age 20 to 90
Function of kidneys, with other organ systems, is to help in regulation of internal environment of body		All renal units immature at birth; thus fluid and electrolyte imbalance occurs readily Kidney function adequate at birth if not subjected to undue stress			
Digestive System					
As a whole, grows as total body grows, although evidence suggests that various parts of gastrointestinal system undergo separate periods of growth, maturity, and senescence	Before birth nutrients are supplied through placental circulation; digestion and absorption do not occur in GI tract	Stomach size increases rapidly in first months, then grows steadily throughout childhood			All actions of GI tract (food intake, digestion, absorption, elimination) not only respond to physiological needs but from birth to old age also are sensitive to tensions and anxiety

Continued

TABLE 15-2 GROWTH AND DEVELOPMENT

Flowchart Showing Directions of Growth Changes Throughout Life Cycle—cont'd

OVERVIEW OF DEVELOPMENTAL CHANGES	PRENATAL →	INFANCY →	CHILDHOOD →	PUBERTY AND ADOLESCENCE →	ADULTHOOD →	MIDDLE AGE →	OLD AGE
Digestive System, cont'd				Spurt of growth at puberty			
	Salivary glands small at birth	Digestive apparatus immature at birth (food passes through rapidly, reverse peristalsis common) Acidity of gastric juices varies over life span; low during infancy, rises during childhood, plateaus about age 10, rises during puberty Free gastric acid (HCl) more marked in boys Increase rapidly during first 3 mo; reach relative adult proportions by age 2			Data suggest generalized atrophy of entire GI tract with advancing age Nutritional needs vary according to individual variation—decreasing metabolism → enzyme production—↓ HCl ↓ — stomach volume—tone of large intestine may become impaired until decrease with senescence (also diminished taste)		
Special Senses Most are well developed at birth, although their association with higher centers comes about gradually during early life and diminishes with advancing age	Begin very early in embryonic development—3-6 wk	Sense of touch is developed first, then hearing and vision Vision: infant can perceive simple differences in shape but not complex patterns (greater proportion of total growth before birth); various dimensions of vision develop at various ages, eye muscles function at mature level first year, fusion begins 9 mo until 6 yr; refractive power changes over life cycle—hyperopia increases until eyeball reaches adult size (≈8 yr), then reverses trend toward emmetropia; postpubertal years—toward myopia until 30 yr when myopia decreases and hyperopia increases					
Adipose Tissue Although adipose tissue varies greatly among individuals, overall lifetime pattern exists Fat accumulation varies greatly with body build and constitution Relationship between caloric intake, amount of exercise, and utilization or accumulation of fat is not yet fully understood but is basis of much interrelated research	Accumulates rapidly before birth; peaks at seventh gestational month Premature infant may look wrinkled and scrawny because of lack of adipose tissue	Increases rapidly during first 6 mo	Decreases from first to seventh yr in both genders	Then begins to increase slowly to puberty Fat begins to accumulate slowly and continues uninterrupted in girls, producing feminine curves, and accounts for much of weight gain	Some girls become slim after full maturation; many maintain about same amount of adipose tissue as at puberty	Typically both genders tend to gain weight in 50s and 60s but do not maintain same body contours of earlier years at same weight (increased deposit on abdomen and hips)	Usually fat stores are lost after seventh decade in both genders Sharpness in contours, increasingly prominent bony landmarks
	Gender differences are not noted in body shape of prepubescent children			Deposition of fat differs in body—amount decreases sharply at time of maximal growth spurt (increased weight caused by increase in muscle mass and bones)	After full maturation, fat accumulation begins →		

Lymphoid Tissue

Lymphoid tissue is scattered widely throughout body and includes lymph nodes, tonsils, adenoids, thymus, spleen, and lymphocytes of blood; follows unique pattern of growth, rapid in infancy and begins to atrophy at puberty

Begins during last month of uterine life—cross placenta at levels equal to mother's and remain for several months after delivery

Grows most rapidly during infancy and childhood, reaching maximal size a few years before puberty; parallels development of immunity

Thus increased incidence of disease with increasing age of child

Then atrophies and is smaller in volume at full maturity than during childhood

Thymus so small that it is difficult to locate in older people

Respiratory System

Growth parallels that of total body growth

Respiratory apparatus is a highly organized system of organs under nervous and hormonal regulation, which functions in coordination with rest of body

Gender difference in gas exchange becomes apparent during puberty

Before birth, air sacs do not contain air; oxygen supplied through maternal circulation

When umbilical cord is cut, infant must use own breathing apparatus—breathing irregular at first both in rate and in depth—fast in infancy and gradually slowing through childhood until maturity is reached

No gender difference in respiratory rate at any time of life

Respiratory exchange gradually becomes more efficient as life advances. Actual volume of air inhaled with each breath increases as lung size expands with general body growth. Vital capacity and maximal breathing capacity rise gradually in both genders, increasing more in boys during puberty; adult men have more efficient respiratory exchange, are capable of greater feats of muscular exertion without exhaustion than women.

Basal metabolic rate declines (rate higher in men than in women)

Skeletal System

Bone growth passes through successive stages of development from connective tissue to cartilage to osseous tissue; completion of calcification indicates end of growing period and is thus a useful measure of growth rate and physiological maturity

Most growth ceases during adolescence

Follows cephalocaudal law of development

70% of head growth before birth; bones of hands and wrist laid down in cartilage

After first year, legs fastest growing, 66% of total increase in height; longer puberty is delayed, greater the leg length

Trunk fastest growing, 60% of total increase

Reserved during growth spurt

Length of trunk and depth of chest reach peak growth

Maximal height in early 20s to 30s

Then gradual decline until onset of senescence

Thinning of vertebral disks beginning in middle years; most rapid in last decade

Continued

TABLE 15-2 GROWTH AND DEVELOPMENT

Flowchart Showing Directions of Growth Changes Throughout Life Cycle—cont'd

OVERVIEW OF DEVELOPMENTAL CHANGES	PRENATAL→	INFANCY→	CHILDHOOD→	PUBERTY AND ADOLESCENCE→	ADULTHOOD→	MIDDLE AGE→ OLD AGE
Skeletal System, cont'd		At birth, shafts of metacarpals are ossified (and visible by radiography); carpal bones begin to ossify	Growth of both genders nearly even until onset of puberty in girls first (≈10 yr); Boys begin ≈2 yr later, but markedly greater; Peak in height comes before peak in weight			Spinal column shortens (osteoporosis) with thinning vertebrae—shortening of trunk with long extremities—reversal of growth proportions in infancy
Muscle System Number of striated muscle fibers is roughly the same in all human beings. Tremendous difference in size, not only from fetus to adult but also among adults, is caused by ability of individual muscle fibers to increase in size	Muscle formation begins early, assuming final shape by end of second month	Increases rapidly during infancy but slowly during childhood	Growth in both genders is same in childhood	With onset of puberty, muscle strength is greater in boys (when muscle growth is stimulated by testosterone) Greatest increase begins in puberty; muscle size precedes muscle strength in boys Increase in muscle size means increasing strength in children; increase in skill is more intimately related to maturation of nervous system	Muscle mass continues to increase gradually—maximal strength in early adulthood—then declines slightly—according to use and genetic constitution; Will increase in bulk and strength as used until onset of senescence	Atrophy and loss of muscle tone
Nervous System Growth and maturation of central and peripheral nervous systems (brain, cord, peripheral nerves, many sense organs) reflected by changing size of head	Growth very rapid during intrauterine development; head grows at greater rate than rest of body	Has all the brain cells in first year, which will continue to increase in size; number and complexity of axons, dendrites, and synapses will continue to increase All neural tissues grow rapidly during infancy and early childhood		(No neural growth spurt at puberty)	Function continues with use	Depletion of fully functioning brain cells, whether they are lost, shrink, or lose connections; Decrease in myelin sheath, impulses decrease; slowed down speed of action and reaction

System / General Description	Birth / Fetal	Childhood	Puberty / Adolescence	Adulthood	Older Adult / Aging
	Segmented spinal nerves are mature, fully myelinated, and functioning at term (e.g., knee jerk), but acquisition of myelin in cortex, and cord is closely correlated with observed behavior (myelination of this tract follows cephalocaudal, proximodistal law)				
	Brain grows rapidly after birth, reaching 90% of total size by age 2	By middle childhood almost reaches adult size	Then slow increase to full maturity		Brain weight decreases with age
	Equipment for sense of taste and smell present at birth and perhaps most acute at that time				Taste less acute, less discriminatory with advancing age
					Structural changes in CNS result in impaired perception

Reproductive System

System / General Description	Birth / Fetal	Childhood	Puberty / Adolescence	Adulthood	Older Adult / Aging
Organs of reproductive system show little increase during early life but rapid development just before and coincident with puberty	Genital organs form during uterine life; uterus undergoes growth spurt before birth (hormonal stimulation from mother)	Quiescent during childhood →	Maturation at puberty (menstruation) →		Involution after menopause
Maturation and fulfillment of reproductive functions of maturity (in female) are followed by involution in later years	Female sex organs well formed but not functioning at birth (but have full quota of sensory nerves)	Regained size by age 10 to 11 →	Adult size at puberty →		Begins to atrophy with advancing age
	Uterus undergoes involution to half its birth weight				
	In male—testes, as with ovaries, remain dormant and small, not even growing in proportion to rest of body (with sensory nerves)		Until puberty, interstitial cells of Leydig reappear and secrete testosterone, so testes and penis continue to increase in size; pubic hair appears		
	Mammary glands develop in both genders during fetal life	Nonsecretory during childhood until puberty→	Development rapid →	Enlarge during pregnancy, developing alveoli →	Atrophy with advanced age
	Enlargement of breasts at birth (both genders) →			Maximum increase with pregnancy →	
	Sex hormones: until puberty girls and boys produce male hormones (androgens) and female hormones (chiefly estrogens) in small and roughly equal amounts				

Integumentary System

System / General Description	Birth / Fetal	Childhood	Puberty / Adolescence	Adulthood	Older Adult / Aging
Includes skin and its appendages and adnexa (nails, hair, sebaceous glands, eccrine and apocrine sweat glands)	Hair, skin, and sebaceous glands fully formed in utero	Matures slowly until puberty (children prone to rashes)	Rapid spurt in maturation of skin and all its structures		Changes in skin most obvious sign of aging (exposure and environmental conditions)
Although all skin is similar, this organ shows considerable variability in different parts of body (and from individual to individual) and varies greatly during life span	Lanugo begins to decrease before birth and continues regression few weeks postnatally →		Replaced by body hair, less extensive distribution; marked difference in type and distribution of hair at puberty →		Regenerative and growth power decreases and skin loses elasticity

Continued

TABLE 15-2   GROWTH AND DEVELOPMENT

Flowchart Showing Directions of Growth Changes Throughout Life Cycle—cont'd

OVERVIEW OF DEVELOPMENTAL CHANGES	PRENATAL →	INFANCY →	CHILDHOOD →	PUBERTY AND ADOLESCENCE →	ADULTHOOD →	MIDDLE AGE →	OLD AGE
Integumentary System, cont'd	Activity of sebaceous glands decreases after birth →			Increases rapidly at puberty (more prone to acne)			
Endocrine System Consists of number of glandular structures scattered throughout body Although small in size, their hormones influence all growth and development of whole organism	Immaturity of entire endocrine system puts infant at disadvantage if required to adjust to wide fluctuations in concentration of water, electrolytes, glucose, amino acids. All are interrelated, but each organ develops at own rate: • Thyroid—increases from midfetal life to maturity; slightly larger in boys than girls; growth spurt at adolescence • Adrenals—after birth decrease in size and continue throughout first year, increase again during childhood (but smaller than birth); spurt at puberty, reaching maturity with rest of body; greater increase in male gonads and testes and female ovaries (endocrine glands as well as reproductive organs), follow genital type of growth pattern • Hypophysis, or pituitary gland—produces or stimulates hormones that influence growth • Parathyroid—produces hormones that maintain homeostasis of calcium and phosphorus • Islets of Langerhans—dispersed throughout pancreas; produce insulin and glucagon					With age, decline occurs in all endocrine gland functions	

*This chart indicates only general trends and directions of growth and development; it is not all-inclusive. No distinct ages, absolute values, or ranges of normal variations are intended in this flowchart. Modified from the format originally developed in Sutterly, D. C., & Donneley, G. F. (1973). *Perspectives in human development: Nursing throughout the life cycle.* Philadelphia: J. B. Lippincott. Modified from Papalia, D. E., & Feldman, R. D. (2011). *Experience human development* (12th ed.). New York: McGraw Hill.
CNS, Central nervous system; *GI,* gastrointestinal.

BOX 15-1 DIVERSITY AWARENESS

Childhood Lead Poisoning in Hispanic Children

While the U.S. has made tremendous progress in eliminating some of the more significant sources of lead (lead paint was banned in 1978; the use of leaded gasoline was phased out during the early 1990s), lead poisoning remains a significant threat to today's children. Chronic low-level lead exposure results in learning disabilities, impaired growth, poor eye-hand coordination, antisocial behavior, dental decay, and hearing loss. The National Safety Council (NSC) emphasizes that, while lead exposure continues to affect large numbers of children, lead poisoning is a totally preventable disease. During the past two decades, public health and provider efforts have resulted in a 90% decline in the overall number of children affected. However, the risk for children of Hispanic families has remained steady.

In 1997 the Centers for Disease Control and Prevention (CDC, 1997) issued new guidelines for blood lead screening. Children were to be screened if they met any of the following criteria:

- Receives services from public assistance programs for the poor
- Lives in an area where more than 27% of the housing was built before 1950
- Parent or guardian answers yes to any of the following:
  - Does your child live in or regularly visit a house that was built before 1950?
  - Does your child live in or regularly visit a house that was built before 1978 with recent or ongoing renovations or remodeling?
  - Does your child have a sibling or playmate who has or did have lead poisoning?

These screening questions primarily target those children whose exposure is through lead-based paint. However, this is not the primary source of lead exposure for the majority of children in Hispanic families. Food and culturally defined health practices bring additional risk to this population. Foods packaged or canned outside the United States, especially in Mexico or South America; foods cooked, stored, eaten, or drunk using ceramic containers or pottery made outside the United States, especially in Mexico or South America; Mexican or South American raisins, and wrapped Mexican candies (specifically tamarind fruit candies and lollipops), all increase lead exposure (MMWR, 2009).

Empacho, a common Hispanic term for stomach or intestinal upset or obstruction, is often treated with a folk remedy that coincidentally is 70% to 90% lead. It is known by many names, including *Alarcon, Azarcon, Coral, Greta, Liga, Maria Luisa,* and *Rueda*. Another common Hispanic folk remedy containing lead is *Pay looah*.

Further, an often-overlooked risk is the use of warm, hot, or boiled tap water from contaminated pipes. Many Hispanics feel that heating the water rids it of contaminants, although any heat mobilizes the lead and makes it easier to absorb. This is also true of pottery that is heated by cooking in it, placing heated fluids in it, or heating it in the microwave. While typical instruction pamphlets teach that tap water should be run for a full minute before it is consumed, it fails to state that the water consumed should come from the cold tap if it is to be consumed.

When screening for lead poisoning in Hispanic children, the nurse remembers to include questions about the use of folk remedies, pottery, imported foods and candies, as well as the use of boiled or hot tap water. In addition, the nurse should include dietary education that encourages decreasing fat intake, because lead is retained in fat, and increasing vitamin C, calcium, and iron intake, all of which reduce the amount of lead in the body.

For more information about the health effects of lead on children, how to identify children with elevated lead levels, or obtain a lead dust test kit, visit the following websites:

- National Safety Council (NSC)
  www.nsc.org/resources/issues/lead.aspx
- Centers for Disease Control and Prevention: General Lead Information
  www.cdc.gov/nceh/lead/faq/about.htm
- Environmental Protection Agency: Protect Your Child From Lead Poisoning
  www.epa.gov/lead
- Environmental Protection Agency: Eliminating Child Lead Poisoning
  http://yosemite.epa.gov/OCHP/OCHPWEB.nsf/content/leadhaz.htm/$file/leadhaz.pdf
- Mayo Clinic: Lead Poisoning
  www.mayoclinic.com/health/lead-poisoning/FL00068

or an older child, especially during the first trimester when all organs systems are in a stage of rapid growth and development. Teens who fracture a limb at the bone's growth plate are also more affected than older teens and young adults who have completed their growth spurt.

Growth Patterns

Expected **growth patterns** exist for all people. Growth is not steady throughout life. The periods of extremely rapid growth—prenatal, infancy, and adolescence—are contrasted with slower rates of growth during the toddler, preschool, and school-age periods. Infants typically double their birth weight by 6 months of age and triple their birth weight by 1 year of age. The well-known "growth spurt" in height typically occurs early in adolescence for girls and later in adolescence for boys.

Different parts of the body increase in size at different rates. For example, during early life the head is the fastest growing section, followed by the trunk, and then the arms and legs. Newborns' heads account for one quarter of their overall length, as opposed to adults' heads that account for one ninth of their overall height. The growth changes in proportion of body parts from infancy to adulthood are demonstrated in Figure 15-1.

Growth Charts

Growth is one of the most important indications of a child's overall health and well-being. Accurate growth assessment depends on precise measurement of growth parameters using proper equipment, correct and consistent techniques, careful plotting of measurements, and thoughtful interpretation of the data (Falkenstern & Bauer, 2009).

Based on input from an expert panel, the Centers for Disease Control and Prevention (CDC) recommended that health practitioners within the United States use the 2006 World Health Organization (WHO) international **growth charts** for children from birth to 24 months, and continue to use the revised 2000 CDC growth charts (including the body mass index [BMI] and the 3rd and 97th percentiles) for children ages 2 to 20 years. This recommendation was based on the fact that WHO growth charts were compiled from healthy breastfed infants living in optimal conditions and achieving the greatest potential of growth possible, which was recognized as the desired standard against which to compare the growth of all other infants (CDC, 2010). In creating the WHO growth charts, researchers gathered data from six countries (Brazil, Ghana, India, Norway, Oman, and the United States) using longitudinal and cross-sectional methods

FIGURE 15-1 Changes in body proportions from birth to adulthood. (Based on a figure from Crouch, J. E., & McClintic, J. R. [1976]. *Human anatomy and physiology* [2nd ed.]. New York: John Wiley & Sons. Done with permission from John Wiley and Sons, 2012.)

BOX 15-2   RESEARCH FOR EVIDENCE-BASED PRACTICE

Comparing the New Growth Charts: Prediction of Future Obesity?

Because the CDC and WHO growth charts use the same indicators for growth, they have undergone comparative studies to indicate differences when using each chart in order to respond to the need for public health prevention efforts addressing the increasing prevalence of childhood obesity (Mei & Grummer-Strawn, 2011).

From the beginning, it was recommended that when using the WHO growth charts to screen for abnormal or unhealthy growth that the 3rd and 97th percentiles were used instead of the 5th and 95th percentiles, respectively. Health practitioners needed to be aware that fewer children would be identified as underweight since slower growth among breastfed infants is normal within the first 6 months.

In early comparative studies, aware that lower growth was expected, Goodell and colleagues (2009) concluded that rapid weight gain during the first year of life predicted obesity in 2 to 3 year olds. Maalouf-Manasseh and colleagues (2011) also concluded that gaining weight more rapidly in the first year than that indicated by the WHO growth charts may be an early indication of later obesity.

However, in their comparative studies, Ziegler and Nelson (2012) observed that the weight percentiles of the WHO growth charts were higher in the first 6 months and lower between 6 and 24 months when compared to the CDC

percentiles for the same age ranges. Their conclusion was explained not only by appreciating that breastfed infants grow somewhat slower than formula-fed infants but also by realizing the attrition rate of low weight gaining breastfed infants that occurred when compiling data for the WHO growth charts.

Therefore, while the WHO growth charts may be used for national and international observations of malnutrition, it is imperative that additional data be obtained before the WHO standards can be applied for local public health interventions. The low weight of the WHO growth charts should not be used to misclassify a child as overweight or obese with the use of corrective interventions (Ziegler & Nelson, 2012).

Although the new WHO growth charts furnish health care providers and researchers with an improved tool to assess and track the growth of children from newborns to 24 months of age, care must be taken not to misinterpret the results of the individual child. As indicated by the evidence presented, it is too early to use the WHO growth chart as the magic bullet of early identification and intervention of future obesity in children during the first year of life. However, continued investigation holds many implications in the future planning of health care efforts against the obesity epidemic.

(Mei & Grummer-Strawn, 2011). The outstanding strength of the WHO growth charts is that they are globally representative (Ziegler & Nelson, 2012). Both the CDC and the WHO growth charts describe weight-for-age, length (or stature)-for-age, weight-for-length, and BMI-for-age, and include the 5th and 95th and the 3rd and 97th percentiles (CDC, 2010). The WHO and the CDC growth charts for each gender with instructions for use can be viewed and downloaded from the CDC website: www.cdc.gov/growthcharts/.

When assessing growth data for use in the growth charts, it is important to remember that a single measurement taken at one point in time, although helpful in providing a baseline, does not allow for the best assessment of a child's growth. Serial measurements, plotted on a growth chart over time, best reflect a child's pattern of growth. Slowed growth, plateaus, or decreases

in height, weight, and head circumference (CDC, 2009), as well as rapid increases, raise questions for health care providers about the adequacy of a child's nutritional intake, syndromes or disease states, neglect, or emotional problems (Falkenstern & Bauer, 2009). See Box 15-2: Research for Evidence-Based Practice on the use of the new growth charts and preschool children.

Concept of Development

Development refers to gradual change and expansion of ability and advance in skill from a lower to a more-advanced complexity. In contrast to growth, which is a quantitative or precisely measurable change, development is a qualitative change. Qualitative changes are more challenging to describe, because they cannot be measured in precise units. Development has best been conceptualized as a process that can be assessed because it follows certain sequencing or patterns, although the timing of this advancement is individual.

Developmental Patterns

All individuals follow similar **developmental patterns,** with one stage of development building on and leading to the next. Early development proceeds as follows:

Pattern of Development:
- **Cephalocaudal** = head to toe
- **Proximodistal** = midline to periphery
- **Differentiation** follows a pattern: simple to complex, and general to specific

Examples of Patterns of Development:
- Cephalocaudal: Infants gain neck and head control before controlling the movements of the extremities.
- Proximodistal: Infants' central nervous systems develop before peripheral nervous systems.
- Differentiation: Infants use a whole-hand grasp before learning the finer control of the pincer grasp, and they coo or babble before they speak.

Although the sequence of development is predictable, the exact timing of the sequencing is individual. Individuals develop at their own rate, on their own schedule. For example, infants creep and crawl before they walk and their primary teeth erupt in a predictable sequence, but each will walk and develop primary teeth on an individual schedule. However, there are guidelines or parameters that assist parents and health care providers in assessing whether children are progressing in an acceptable developmental sequence within a reasonable time frame. Areas of assessment usually focus on personal and social, gross and fine motor, and language development. The **Denver Developmental Screening Test,** which was revised in 1992 (now known as Denver II), is a screening tool that assists health care providers in monitoring children's development in each of these areas from birth to 6 years of age. The Denver II is presented in **Website Resource 17A.**

Social expectations can influence developmental tasks with expectations that an individual achieve certain landmarks during each period of development. However, the age at which a child is expected to master certain developmental tasks is determined partly by cultural expectations. Some cultures are comfortable with breastfeeding their children well into childhood, whereas others expect the transition to self-feeding with a cup much earlier. When assessing a child's abilities, nurses are aware that a child who has never been given the opportunity to learn or master a skill may be developmentally capable, but fails when tested. For example, a child who is capable of learning colors or numbers can do so only if taught, just as the child who was breastfed well into childhood, never having been offered a cup, may well be developmentally capable of drinking from a cup but probably will fail at early attempts.

Development is closely interrelated with the concepts of both learning and maturation. **Learning** is the process of gaining specific knowledge or skills that result from exposure, experience, education, and evaluation. **Maturation** is an increase in competence and adaptability that reflects changes in the complexity of a structure that makes it possible for that structure to

BOX 15-3 QUALITY AND SAFETY SCENARIO

Anticipatory Guidance

The nurse is often in a position to provide anticipatory guidance to parents, which involves teaching parents ways to handle a situation before it becomes an issue or problem. Knowledge of normal growth and development provides a foundation for this teaching. For example, the toddler period is one of intense exploration of the environment, when locomotion is the major gross motor skill acquired. The nurse, knowing the number one cause of death in toddlers is accidents, provides the following teaching to the parents of a child who is entering the toddler period:
- Always use a federally approved car restraint and check for proper installation and placement.
- Supervise child closely near any source of water, including buckets, bathtubs, toilets, and especially swimming pools.
- Turn pot handles toward the back of the stove and use the back burners whenever possible.
- Place all toxic substances in a locked cabinet and have the poison control contact number easily accessible. Avoid the use of syrup of ipecac unless advised by a poison control representative to do so.
- Move a toddler from the crib to a bed.
- Provide barriers on open windows.
- Decrease the water heater temperature to avoid scald burns from tap water.
- Avoid foods that pose a choking hazard such as nuts, hard candies, raisins, fresh carrots, whole grapes, chewing gum, hot dogs, and fish with bones.
- Guard against running into the street when walking and playing outside.

begin to function or to function at a higher level. Maturation of a structure, system, or individual refers to the emergence of the genetic potential of that structure, system, or individual. Learning cannot occur unless the individual is mature enough to understand and control behavior. Children can be toilet trained only when their bodies have matured to the point of developing internal and external sphincter control. Earlier attempts will be frustrating for both child and parent.

Growth and development are complex, interrelated processes that are influenced by and, in turn, influence the health of an individual. The nurse who understands this relationship is aware of the need for age-specific health assessment and promotion strategies (Box 15-3: Quality and Safety Scenario).

THEORIES OF DEVELOPMENT

Specific aspects of development of the person have been studied for centuries. Many theories of development are used in the study of individuals throughout the life span; the nurse may wish to refer to a text on developmental psychology to become familiar with some of these theories. In this unit, five theories are introduced to gain a holistic view of the progression of individual development throughout the life span. These theories were originally developed by Erikson, Piaget, Vygotsky, Kohlberg, and Gilligan.

Psychosocial Development: Erikson's Theory

Erik Erikson described the development of identity of the self through successive stages that unfold throughout the life span

TABLE 15-3 GROWTH AND DEVELOPMENT

Erikson's Eight Stages of Human Development

AGE GROUP	PSYCHOSOCIAL STAGE	LASTING OUTCOMES
1. Infancy	Basic trust versus basic mistrust	Faith and hope
2. Toddler stage	Autonomy versus shame and doubt	Self-control and willpower
3. Preschool stage	Initiative versus guilt	Direction and purpose
4. School age	Industry versus inferiority	Method and competence
5. Adolescence	Identity versus role confusion	Devotion and fidelity
6. Young adulthood	Intimacy versus isolation	Affiliation and love
7. Middle adult-hood	Generativity versus stagnation	Production and care
8. Older adulthood	Ego integrity versus despair	Renunciation and wisdom

Modified from Erikson, E. H. (1995). *Childhood and society* (35th anniversary ed.). New York: Norton; Erikson, E. H., & Erikson, J. M. (1998). *The life cycle completed.* New York: Norton.

(Erikson, 1968, 1995; Erikson & Erikson, 1998). Although he studied with Freud and supported the psychosexual theory of development, Erikson's theory of psychosocial development is based on the need of each person to develop a sense of trust in self and others and a sense of personal worth. Erikson described a healthy personality in positive terms, not merely through the absence of disease.

Psychosocial development is based on critical stages, each requiring resolution of a conflict between two opposing forces (e.g., intimacy versus isolation). Each stage depends on the preceding stage, which must be accomplished successfully for the person to proceed. Erikson's use of a psychosocial framework acknowledges the influence of other people and the environment but maintains that it is ultimately the individual who must master each of the conflicts. Although each of the conflicts is predominant at a certain stage in life, it is important to recognize that all of the conflicts exist in each person, to some extent, at all times and that a conflict, once resolved, may emerge again in appropriate situations. These stages are summarized in Table 15-3 and discussed more fully in the chapters on each developmental age group. See the Case Study at the end of this chapter about an infant girl and how hospitalization could affect her stage of psychosocial development.

Cognitive Development

Another aspect of development is cognitive development. Jean Piaget, a Swiss psychologist, also trained in biology and philosophy, is well-known for his theory of cognitive development. He viewed children as biological organisms interacting with their environment, and his theory contends that cognitive development reflects children's attempts to make sense of their worlds. Piaget developed his cognitive theory by observing his

own children (Piaget, 1950). Hence, the major criticism of his work is that he underestimated children's capabilities and gave little or no consideration for cultural differences. Lev Vygotsky, a Russian contemporary, was also trained in both the physical sciences and psychology. He presented his theory of cognitive development stating that a child's development could not be separated from the social and cultural context in which it occurs. He also credited children with more innate ability to learn and emphasized the importance of language (Vygotsky, 1986). Both Piaget and Vygotsky are presented in more detail in the following sections.

Cognitive Development: Piaget's Theory

Jean Piaget's theory of cognitive development is concerned primarily with structure rather than content, with how the mind works rather than with what it does. Piaget uses the word scheme to describe a pattern of action or thought. A scheme is used to take in or assimilate new experiences or may be modified or accommodated by new experiences. Each person is striving to maintain a balance, or equilibrium, between assimilation and accommodation (Phillips, 1975; Piaget, 1950).

Piaget described the stages of cognitive development throughout the developmental years. Through a natural unfolding of ability, the child acquires sequentially predictable cognitive abilities. Given adequate environmental stimuli and an intact neurological system, the child gradually matures toward full ability to conceptualize. Piaget's theory of cognitive development encompasses the time from birth to approximately 15 years of age. Each of the four distinct stages is summarized in Table 15-4 and discussed more fully in the specific chapters on each developmental age. Piaget suggests that quantitative, but no further qualitative, changes in cognitive function take place after about age 15.

Cognitive Development: Vygotsky's Theory

One of the significant differences between the cognitive theories of Piaget and Vygotsky is that Piaget believed that development preceded learning. Piaget proposed that a level of cognitive development must be reached *before* learning could take place. Vygotsky thought that by viewing development and learning in this way, that adults would teach to the lowest ability, aiming instruction at those mental functions or intellectual operations that had already matured in the child (Wink & Putney, 2001). In contrast, Vygotsky proposed that learning precedes development. He states that learning pulls development, which is in stark contrast to Piaget, who felt children were not capable of learning something until they were developmentally ready.

Vygotsky argued that, while learning may be similar among children at certain times or phases of development, it is not identical in all children because of their differing social and cultural experiences (Vygotsky, 1978). He felt Piaget overemphasized the intellectual and biological universality of developmental stages. Vygotsky was more interested in the cultural and social influences on learning and development as well as how individual children actively internalize what they learn from others. For Vygotsky, development begins as an interpersonal process of "meaning making" and then becomes an individualized

TABLE 15-4 GROWTH AND DEVELOPMENT

Piaget's Stages of Cognitive Development

STAGE	AGE	CHARACTERISTICS
Sensorimotor	Birth to 2 years	Begins with a predominance and reliance on reflexes that permit the body to learn
		Reflexes decrease and voluntary acts develop
		Imitation predominates
		Thought is dominated by physical manipulation of objects and events
		Develops the concept of object permanence and the ability to form mental representations
Preoperational	2 to 7 years	Advancing use of language and movement
		Development of egocentric, animistic, and magical thinking
		Uses representational thought to interpret and learn, not in terms of general properties, but in terms of the relationship or use to them
		No cause-and-effect reasoning
		Thought is dominated by the senses—what is seen, heard, or experienced
Concrete operations	7 to 11 years	Mental reasoning processes assume logical approaches to solving concrete problems, including cause and effect
		Collecting; mastering facts
		Can consider other points of view
		Thought influenced by social contacts
		Language is perfected
Formal operations	11 to 15 years	True logical thought and manipulation of abstract concepts emerge
		Morality established

Modified from Schuster, C. S., & Ashburn, S. S. (1992). *The process of human development: A holistic life span approach* (2nd ed.). Boston: Lippincott; Piaget, J., & Inhelder, B. (2000). *The psychology of the child.* New York: Basic Books; Piaget, J. (1959). *Language and thought of the child.* New York: Routledge.

BOX 15-4 INNOVATIVE PRACTICE

How to Raise a Genius

It is clear that the American Academy of Pediatrics (AAP) recommendation of *no screen time (television/video/computer/phone) for children younger than 2 years* has not been widely heeded and continues to have negative effects on the cognitive development of young children. While limited viewing of age-appropriate, educational television may be beneficial to children of preschool age, television has a unique effect on children younger than age 2 that has been associated with poorer cognitive development (Kirkorian et al., 2008).

One study found that 94 children younger than age 2 years were exposed to an average of 12 hours of screen time in a typical week and that 34% of their parents were not able to correctly identify the expert recommendation for television watching for children younger than 2 years (Funk et al., 2009). Recent studies have associated television watching with decreased language development. A study of 329 children ranging in age from 2 to 48 months found that even audible television that decreased the child's exposure to discernible adult speech led

to decreased child vocalizations and delayed speech development (Christakis et al., 2009). Similar research results found that television viewing by itself was significantly negative for the child younger than 2 years of age, but that these negative results were fully mediated by the inclusion of two-sided adult-child conversations (Zimmerman et al., 2009). Previous studies reported that infants and toddlers learn faster and better when they are able to interact with adults, rather than just watch and listen. Children who interacted with their parents through reading or games showed an increase in language skills.

- How can nurses teach parents the recommendation for television viewing for children younger than age 2 years?
- How can nurses use the results of this study when teaching parents that face-to-face interaction and two-way conversations with their children promote development more than watching TV or videos?

process of "making sense." There are no predetermined levels of development; rather, experience is in the front—leading and expanding development in unlimited ways.

Although **Vygotsky's theory of cognitive development** is less known to health care professionals, educators have embraced his theory, especially what he refers to as the zone of proximal development. The **zone of proximal development** is the distance between the actual and potential developmental level (Wink & Putney, 2002). In this zone, children are pulled toward new learning through their interaction with others and the environment. The guidance given by others in this zone is referred to as **scaffolding.** According to Vygotsky, all people need to understand not only the way in which an

individual learns and develops but also the social, cultural, and political context in which that learning and development takes place. This difference has the potential for profound impact on how the nurse approaches teaching and learning (Box 15-4).

Moral Development: Kohlberg's Theory

One aspect of cognitive development is the development of moral thinking and judgment. Lawrence **Kohlberg's theory of moral development** is based on interviews that focused on hypothetical moral dilemmas such as: Should a man steal an expensive drug that would save his dying wife? From these interviews, Kohlberg developed his theory, which is outlined

TABLE 15-5 **GROWTH AND DEVELOPMENT**

TABLE 15-5 **GROWTH AND DEVELOPMENT**

Kohlberg's Stages of Moral Development

STAGE	GOAL
Preconventional	Avoiding punishment
	Gaining reward
Conventional	Gaining approval
	Avoiding disapproval
Postconventional	Agreeing upon rights
	Establishing personal moral standards
	Achieving justice

Compiled from Kohlberg, L. (1981). *The philosophy of moral development* (Vol. 1). San Francisco: Harper & Row.

in Table 15-5 (Kohlberg, 1969, 1981). The three stages of moral development—preconventional, conventional, and postconventional—are based on Piaget's theory of cognitive development and emphasize ethics of justice. Progression through the successive stages of moral development generally takes place during the school-age, adolescent, and young-adult years. Beyond the young-adult years, stabilization or increased consistency of thought and perhaps an increased correlation between moral judgment and moral action occur (Kohlberg, 1981).

Moral Development: Gilligan's Theory

Carol **Gilligan's theory of moral development** (Gilligan, 1982; Gilligan et al., 1988) suggests that there is a different process of moral development in women in society. While a doctoral student, Gilligan did research with Lawrence Kohlberg at Harvard University. She discovered that Kohlberg's original research was conducted using only men and that women often scored lower in Kohlberg's subsequent investigations. She asserted that women were not inferior in their moral development, just different. In developing her own research with female subjects, she proposed her own theory of moral development, which, like Kohlberg's, has three stages (Table 15-6). However, Gilligan concluded that the transitions between stages are based on changes in one's sense of self rather than on changes in cognitive development, as Kohlberg proposed. She also reported that women think more in terms of caring and relationships than men do, who are more inclined to think in terms of rules and justice.

TABLE 15-6 **GROWTH AND DEVELOPMENT**

Gilligan's Stages of Moral Development (for Women)

STAGE	CHARACTERISTICS	GOAL
Preconventional	What is practical to others and best for self, realizing connection to others	Individual survival
Conventional	Sacrifices wants and needs to fulfill others' wants and needs	Self-sacrifice is goodness
Postconventional	Moral equal of self and others	Principle of nonviolence, do not hurt self or others

Compiled from Gilligan, C. (1982). *In a different voice: Psychological theory and women's development.* Cambridge, MA: Harvard University Press; Gilligan, C., Ward, J. V., & Taylor, J. M. (Eds.). (1988). *Mapping the moral domain: A contribution of women's thinking to psychology and education.* Cambridge, MA: Harvard University Press.

CASE STUDY

Birth of a Disabled/Chronically Ill Child: Avery

Avery is a 33-year-old female pregnant with her third child; her other two children are ages 5 and 10 years. At 26 weeks' gestation, Avery is hospitalized for contractions. Despite pharmacological attempts to stop labor, Avery's labor continues to the active phase. Avery and her partner just learned that a baby born this prematurely may have many problems, including cerebral palsy. As the perinatologist leaves the room, Avery turns to the nurse and starts to cry.

Reflective Questions

1. What is the nurse's role when the parents learn a child has a chronic disease and/or disability?
2. What can the nurse anticipate for these new parents during the labor? At the birth of the baby? In the first 2 weeks after birth? Over the baby's first year of life? Over the first 5 years?
3. How will this child's growth, development, and goals for health promotion be affected? How about those of the parents? What about those of the siblings?
4. What factors might contribute to Avery's development of chronic sorrow?
5. If Avery becomes depressed, how might this affect the growth and development of the new baby? What effect might this have on her relationship with her partner? What effect might her depression have on her other children?
6. What will be the impact of this child's disabilities on the siblings?
7. How might the nurse intervene to lessen the effects of chronic sorrow?

CARE PLAN

Birth of a Disabled/Chronically Ill Child: Avery

*NURSING DIAGNOSIS: Chronic Sorrow (parental) related to missed opportunities and unending caregiving for a new child

Definition

Cyclical, recurring, and potentially progressive pattern of pervasive sadness experienced (by a parent, caregiver, individual with chronic illness or disability) in response to continual loss, throughout the trajectory of an illness or disability

Defining Characteristics

- Parental expression of disparity between preconceived notions of parenting and reality
- Parental expression of an ongoing or recurrent sense of sadness or loss
- Parental expressions of negative feelings (e.g., anger, depression, disappointment, emptiness, frustration, self-blame, helplessness, hopelessness, loneliness, overwhelmed) that are often triggered by health care crises or conflict with expected social norms for child or family

◎ **CARE PLAN**

Birth of a Disabled/Chronically Ill Child: Avery—cont'd

Related Factors
- Change in family structure
- Change in parental role expectation
- Parental coping styles
- Goal: Assist family unit to attain, maintain, or regain optimal health

Expected Outcomes
- Grief resolution: *Adjustment to actual or impending loss.* For example: Parents verbalize reality of loss, progress through stages of grief, decreasing preoccupation with loss, verbalize acceptance of loss and resolve feelings about loss.
- Hope: *Optimism that is personally satisfying and life-supporting.* For example: Parents express inner peace, expectation of a positive future.
- Psychosocial adjustment: *Adaptive psychosocial response of an individual to a significant life change.* For example: Parents set realistic goals, maintain productivity, verbalize optimism about present, use effective coping strategies, report feeling socially engaged.

Nursing Interventions
- Grief work facilitation: *Helping another cope with painful feelings of actual or perceived responsibility.* For example: Listen to expression of grief, encourage identification of fears, assist in identifying needed modifications in lifestyle.
- Hope inspiration: *Enhancing the belief in one's capacity to initiate and sustain actions.* For example: Help identify areas of hope in their lives, demonstrate hope by recognizing the disability or illness as only one facet of the child, provide parents opportunities to be involved with support groups, especially with other parents of children who are disabled/chronically ill who have transcended.

- Coping enhancement: *Assisting a person to adapt to perceived stressors, changes, or threats that interfere with meeting life demands and roles.* For example: Provide an atmosphere of acceptance, seek to understand each parent's perspective of the situation, appraise and discuss alternate responses to situation, foster constructive outlets for negative feelings, assist the parents to identify positive strategies to deal with limitations and manage necessary lifestyle changes.
- Resiliency promotion: *Assisting individual, families, and communities in development, use, and strengthening of protective factors to be used in coping with environmental and societal stressors.* For example: Encourage positive health-seeking behavior, facilitate development and use of neighborhood resources.

References

Bulechek, G. M., Butcher, H. K., Dochterman, J. M., & Wagner, C. (Eds.). (2012). *Nursing interventions classification (NIC)* (6th ed.). St. Louis: Mosby.

Johnson, M., Moorhead, S., Bulechek, G., & Butcher, H. (2011). *NANDA, NOC, and NIC linkages* (3rd ed.). St Louis: Mosby.

Kao, B., Plante, W., & Lobato, D. (2009). The use of the impact on sibling scale with families of children with chronic illness and developmental disability. *Child: Care, Health and Development, 35*(4), 505–509.

Masterson, M. K. (2010). *Chronic sorrow in mothers of adult children with cerebral palsy: An exploratory study.* Doctoral Dissertation (UMI AA13408137): Kansas State University.

Moorhead, S., Johnson, M., Maas, M., & Swanson, E. (Eds.), (2012). *Nursing outcomes classification (NOC)* (5th ed.). St. Louis: Mosby.

Patrick-Ott, A., & Ladd, L. D. (2010). The blending of Boss's concept of ambiguous loss and Olshansky's concept of chronic sorrow: A case study of a family with a child who has significant disabilities. *Journal of Creativity in Mental Health, 5,* 74–86.

NANDA Nursing Diagnoses—Definitions and Classification 2012-2014, Herdman T.H. (ED). Copyright © 2012, 1994-2012 NANDA International. Used by arrangement with John Wiley & Sons Limited. In order to make safe and effective judgments using the NANDA-I nursing diagnoses it is essential that nurses refer to the definitions and defining characteristics of the diagnoses listed in this work.

SUMMARY

Individuals make many choices that affect their health each day, and a number of factors influence how these choices are made. The stage of growth and development, as well as the context in which learning takes place, influences how individuals experience different situations and realize the choices available. Knowing theories of the concepts of human growth and development, nurses have a clear understanding of the challenges an individual is likely to encounter as well as the skills the individual is likely to have and/or need for successful growth and development, and maturation throughout the life span. Theories provide nurses with frameworks for health assessment, promotion, and intervention.

REFERENCES

Centers for Disease Control and Prevention (CDC). (2009). Children with elevated blood lead levels related to home renovation, repair, and painting activities—New York State, 2006-2007. *Morbidity and Mortality Weekly Report (MMWR), 58*(03), 55–58.

Centers for Disease Control and Prevention (CDC). (2010). Use of World Health Organization and CDC growth charts for children aged 0–59 months in the United States. *Morbidity and Mortality Weekly Report (MMWR), 59*(rr09), 1–15.

Centers for Disease Control and Prevention (CDC). (2011a). CDC health disparities and inequalities report—United States, 2011. *Morbidity and Mortality Weekly Report (MMWR), 60*(Suppl), 1–116.

Centers for Disease Control and Prevention (CDC). (2011b). Lead poisoning of a child associated with use of a Cambodian amulet—New York City, 2009. *Morbidity and Mortality Weekly Report (MMWR), 60*(3), 69–71.

Centers for Disease Control and Prevention (CDC). (2011c). Ten great public health achievements—United States, 2001—2010. *Morbidity and Mortality Weekly Report (MMWR), 60*(19), 619–623.

Centers for Disease Control and Prevention (CDC). (2012). *Prevention tips.* Retrieved July 1, 2012, from www.cdc.gov/nceh/lead/tips.htm.

Christakis, D. A., Gilkerson, J., Richards, J. A., Zimmerman, F. J., Garrison, M. M., Xu, D., et al. (2009). Audible television and decreased adult words, infant vocalizations, and conversational turns. *Archives of Pediatric and Adolescent Medicine, 163*(6), 554–558.

Erikson, E. H. (1968). *Identity, youth, and crisis.* New York: Norton.

Erikson, E. H. (1995). *Childhood and society* (35th anniversary ed.). New York: Norton.

Erikson, E. H., & Erikson, J. M. (1998). *The life cycle completed.* New York: Norton.

Falkenstern, S. K., & Bauer, L. A. (2009). Helping kids grow. *Nurse Practitioner, 34*(3), 30–38.

Funk, J. B., Brouwer, J., Curtiss, K., & McBroom, E. (2009). Parents of pre-schoolers: Expert media recommendations and ratings knowledge, media-effects beliefs, and monitoring practices. *Pediatrics, 123*(3), 981–988.

Gilligan, C. (1982). *In a different voice: Psychological theory and women's development.* Cambridge, MA: Harvard University Press.

Gilligan, C., Ward, J. V., & Taylor, J. M. (Eds.), (1988). *Mapping the moral domain: A contribution of women's thinking to psychology theory and education.* Cambridge, MA: Harvard University Press.

Goodell, L. S., Wakefield, D. B., & Ferris, A. M. (2009). Rapid weight gain during the first year of life predicts obesity in 2-3 year olds from a low-income, minority population. *Journal of Community Health, 34,* 370–375.

Kirkorian, H. L., Wartella, E. A., & Anderson, D. R. (Spring 2008). Media and young children's learning. *Future of Children, 18*(1), 39–61.

Kohlberg, L. (1969). Continuities and discontinuities in childhood and adult moral development. *Human Development, 12,* 93–120.

Kohlberg, L. (1981). *The philosophy of moral development (Vol. 1).* San Francisco, CA: Harper & Row.

Maalouf-Manasseh, Z., Metallinos-Katsaras, E., & Dewey, K. G. (2011). Obesity in preschool children is more prevalent and identified at a younger age when WHO growth charts are used compared with CDC charts. *Journal of Nutrition, 141,* 1154–1158.

Mei, Z., & Grummer-Strawn, L. M. (2011). Comparison of changes in growth percentiles of U.S. children on CDC 2000 growth charts with corresponding changes on WHO 2006 growth charts. *Clinical Pediatrics, 50*(5), 402–407.

Phillips, J. L. (1975). *The origins of intellect: Piaget's theory* (2nd ed.). San Francisco, CA: W.H. Freeman.

Piaget, J. (1950). *The psychology of intelligence.* London, England: Routledge and Kegan Paul.

U.S. Department of Health and Human Services (USDHHS). (2012). *What's changing and when.* Retrieved July 1, 2012, from www.healthcare.gov/law/timeline.

United States Department of Health and Human Services (USDHHS). (2011). *Healthy People 2020.* Retrieved December 1, 2012, from www.healthypeople.gov/2020/about/default.aspx.

Vygotsky, L. S. (1978). *Mind in society: The development of higher psychological processes.* Cambridge, MA: Harvard University Press.

Vygotsky, L. S. (1986). *Thought and language.* Cambridge, MA: MIT Press.

Wink, J., & Putney, L. (2002). *A vision of Vygotsky.* Boston, MA: Allyn & Bacon.

Ziegler, E. E., & Nelson, S. E. (2012). The WHO growth standards: Strengths and limitations. *Current Opinion Clinical Nutrition Metabolic Care, 15*(3), 298–302.

Zimmerman, F. J., Gilkerson, J., Richards, J. A., Christakis, D. A., Xu, D., Gray, S., et al. (2009). Teaching by listening: The importance of adult-child conversations to language development. *Pediatrics, 124*(1), 342–349.

⊖volve WEBSITE

http://evolve.elsevier.com/Edelman/
- Study Questions
- Glossary
- Website Resources
  16A: Summary of Fetal Growth and Development During Pregnancy
  16B: Systematic Adaptation of the Fetus to Extrauterine Life
  16C: Effects of Teratogens on Embryo and Fetus
  16D: Physical and Diagnostic Tools Used During Pregnancy
  16E: Prenatal Assessment Guide

OBJECTIVES

After completing this chapter, the reader will be able to:
- Differentiate fetal development and the newborn transition to extrauterine life.
- Analyze changes in the maternal system during pregnancy based on their influences on pregnancy adaptation.
- Interpret the role of the nurse in promoting the physical, mental, and spiritual health of the childbearing family.
- Compare fetal problems caused by maternal drinking, smoking, drug use, and viral exposure during pregnancy.
- Outline the nursing role during labor and birth with a focus on the physical, emotional, spiritual, and educational needs of the woman giving birth and her family.
- Analyze the influence of factors such as ethnicity, legislative priorities, and the sociopolitical context of the health care delivery system on prenatal and childbirth care and the needs of families.

KEY TERMS

Acquired immunodeficiency syndrome (AIDS)	Colostrum	Fourth stage of labor
Amniocentesis	Conception	Fundus
Amniotic membranes	Congenital defect	Gestation
Anemia of pregnancy	Cytomegalovirus (CMV)	Gestational hypertension
Apgar scoring system	Dilation	Gonococcus (GC)
Bacterial vaginosis	Down syndrome	Group B *Streptococcus*
Bradycardia	Embryo	Hepatitis B (HBV)
Candida albicans	Endometrium	Herpes simplex
Cervical effacement	Estrogen	Human chorionic gonadotropin
Chlamydia	Fertilization	Human immunodeficiency virus (HIV)
Chloasma	Fetal alcohol spectrum disorder (FASD)	Hydramnios
Chorionic membranes	Fetal heart monitor	Infant mortality rate (IMR)
Chorionic villi	Fetus	Infertility
	First stage of labor	Labor

? THINK ABOUT IT

First Pregnancy Labor

Laura, currently 41 weeks into her first pregnancy, is admitted at 2:00 AM to St. Jude's Medical Center with uterine contractions occurring every 8 minutes since midnight. Her cervix is dilated to 2 cm and is 80% effaced, and her station is –3. Her husband is out of town on a business trip, and Laura's neighbor has accompanied her to the hospital. Although Laura attended Lamaze classes with her husband, she is anxious about the labor. She says to the nurse, "My back is about to break, I have so much bottom pressure, and I wanted to go natural, without medication and all this high-technology stuff, including the monitor."

- Based on your knowledge of ethical and legal principles of care, how would you as a caregiver appropriately respond to Laura's needs with labor and delivery?
- What factors in Laura's database would support the use of the fetal heart monitor? What factors would not support use of the monitor?
- What political, legal, ethical, and other factors might be relevant to the widespread use of monitors in American maternity units today?
- How does the use of fetal heart rate monitoring fit into a health-promotion approach to labor and delivery?

The process of conception, pregnancy, and birth involves a complex interaction of many factors, including the physiological and psychological changes in the woman and family and the development of a fetus into a viable newborn. The focus of this chapter is on the pregnant woman, her family, and the developing fetus; discussing one without the others is impossible. The nurse must consider all three entities when seeking to promote a healthy pregnancy and healthy family system after birth.

BIOLOGY AND GENETICS

The physical changes during pregnancy include natural processes involving fertilization of the egg by the sperm, implantation of the fertilized egg into the uterus, embryonic or fetal growth and development, placental development and function, and maternal changes related to the pregnancy process.

Duration of Pregnancy

Pregnancy begins with the union of a sperm and egg, a process called fertilization. Under normal healthy circumstances, a full-term pregnancy lasts approximately 9 solar months, 10 lunar months, or 40 weeks. An accurate estimated date of delivery is determined by using Nägele's rule. This is done by adding 7 days to the date of the first day of the last normal menstrual period and subtracting 3 months. A usual pregnancy consists of 9 months, divided into three equal periods called trimesters. Oftentimes these trimesters form the basis for discussion of expected fetal and maternal changes during pregnancy.

Fertilization

The union of sperm and egg requires several crucial factors, many of which are not fully understood. When a sperm cell penetrates an egg in the ampulla of the fallopian tube, the beginning of a human being (called a zygote) results. Additional division of zygotic cells results in more differentiated structures that eventually produce an embryo and subsequently a fetus.

An absence of one or more critical factors may cause infertility (failure of the couple to become pregnant despite usual sexual activity over 1 year's time). For example, both a sperm cell and an egg cell must be mature and in the fallopian tube for approximately 5 hours for union of sperm and egg to occur (the process of conception). The sperm must be of uniform size, be normally formed, possess high motility, and have an ability to secrete enzymes that dissolve the membrane surrounding the egg. Cellular changes within the egg prevent other sperm from entering the ovum after the sperm penetrates it (Mattson & Smith, 2011). The woman attempting pregnancy must have a certain basal body temperature and fallopian tubes free of adhesions or obstructions. A woman will likely conceive within 24 hours after ovulation.

Implantation

Transplantation of the fertilized egg in the uterine cavity after its trip through the fallopian tube requires approximately 6 days (Coad & Dunstall, 2011). Once the zygote reaches the uterus, it stays there for up to 5 days, receiving nutrition from the endometrium, the inner lining of the uterus (Tortora & Derrickson, 2011). The process of fertilization and implantation triggers the production of large amounts of the hormone progesterone, which stimulates the formation of endometrial cells known as the decidua. The decidua provides nutrition for the embryo, a term that defines the growing conceptus up to 8 weeks of age.

Fetal Growth and Development

Much is known about the stages of physical development in each structural system of the embryo. However, metabolic functions, particularly those relevant to the endocrine and neurological systems, are less well-defined. Appropriate fetal development depends on these events occurring in a specified period and order during each trimester of pregnancy. If this does not occur, an abnormality in structure or function (a **congenital defect**) may result. This defect may be noted at birth, did not occur at conception (called a genetic defect), but most likely resulted from some disruption that occurred after conception and during fetal development. **Website Resource 16A** presents a summary of fetal growth and development.

Placental Development and Function

After implantation of the zygote, the **placenta** develops through an integration of embryonic and decidual cells. The **chorionic membranes** and **amniotic membranes,** which surround the fetus throughout **gestation,** also begin to form. The amniotic fluid, manufactured by the amniotic membrane, supports the developing fetus and protects it from injury.

The basic structure of the placenta allows maternal-fetal blood exchange to nourish the fetus and allow excretion of fetal waste products. Throughout most of gestation, increasing placental development allows maternal blood to flow through the intervillous spaces and fetal circulation to flow through the **chorionic villi** (Cunningham et al., 2010a). The unique structure of the placenta permits the exchange of certain molecules but prevents fetal and maternal blood supplies from mixing for most of the pregnancy. Substances with larger and heavier molecules (such as heparin or insulin) normally do not pass through the placenta to the fetus, but lighter molecules (such as anesthetic gases, oxygen, carbon dioxide, and electrolytes) readily cross the placenta. Because of the difficulty involved in predicting exactly which substances will cross the placenta, the nurse needs to encourage pregnant women and those contemplating pregnancy to avoid any substance that might cause harm to the fetus.

The fetus, which continues to gain strength and maturity during the later weeks of gestation, generally rests its head in the lower maternal pelvis by the end of pregnancy (Figure 16-1). The membranes protect the fetus from infection and act as a container for the amniotic fluid. As birth begins, the membranes may rupture, causing the loss of amniotic fluid and stronger uterine contractions, reflective of the **labor** process. If the membranes rupture more than 24 hours before birth, uterine infection and potential fetal harm may result.

As gestation nears completion, placental function gradually decreases, which may serve as a stimulus for the onset of labor. When pregnancy continues beyond 42 weeks, or 2 weeks beyond the calculated due date, placental function decreases even more, posing concerns about the well-being of the fetus (Polin et al., 2011).

The discussion of fetal development provides only a brief glimpse about the prenatal period. Maternal changes and culmination of the prenatal period, labor, and birth are also important to address.

FIGURE 16-1 Diagrammatic representation of relationship of fetus, placenta, membranes, and uterus during gestation. (From Lowdermilk, D., Perry, S., Cashion, K., & Alden, K.R. [2012]. *Maternity and women's health care* [10th ed.]. St. Louis: Elsevier Mosby.)

Maternal Changes

A woman experiences various physiological effects based on a combination of hormonal and mechanical changes during pregnancy. Hormonal influences tend to increase as the pregnancy progresses. The mechanical (hemodynamic) changes reach a peak in the seventh or eighth month and then gradually decline as the pregnancy nears completion (Cunningham et al., 2010b). Clinical symptoms will manifest during this peak stress time.

Signs of Pregnancy

A woman may assume that she is pregnant because she has skipped her menstrual period or experiences nausea and vomiting, changes in breast sensations and size, or increased urinary frequency (presumptive signs of pregnancy). If she suspects she is pregnant, the woman should undergo a pregnancy test. If performed too early, a home pregnancy test may produce a false-negative result attributable to a low level of **human chorionic gonadotropin (hCG).** This hormone, produced by the placenta and found in a pregnant woman's urine and blood, triggers a positive pregnancy result. These tests have a high degree of accuracy (97%) if the instructions are followed exactly. As the pregnancy progresses, the woman may experience **presumptive signs of pregnancy,** which are subjectively experienced; **probable signs of pregnancy,** which are objectively observed by the health care provider; and **positive signs of pregnancy,** which are positive signs that verify that a pregnancy exists (Box 16-1). During the first trimester of pregnancy, using sophisticated testing with **ultrasound,** health care providers can determine fetal presence and placental adequacy early in pregnancy. This technology, using high-frequency sound waves that bounce off the fetus and are interpreted by a computer, allows visualization of the fetus and gestational structures throughout pregnancy (Norwitz & Schorge, 2010).

Adaptive Changes of Other Systems

In addition to pregnancy-related changes in the reproductive system, adaptive changes in other body systems occur. The urinary system undergoes dramatic changes during gestation as follows:

- A 50% increase in glomerular filtration rate (GFR) occurs related to the influences of **estrogen** and progesterone.
- Ureters increase in diameter by 25% secondary to progesterone influence.

BOX 16-1 SIGNS OF PREGNANCY AND TIME OF OCCURRENCE

Presumptive
- Breast changes (e.g., tenderness) (3-4 weeks)
- Fatigue (12 weeks)
- Urinary frequency (6-12 weeks)
- Nausea and vomiting (4-14 weeks)
- Amenorrhea (4th week)
- Quickening (16-20 weeks)

Probable
- Enlargement of the uterus (12-14 weeks)
- Softening of the uterine isthmus (Hegar's sign) (6th-12th week)
- Bluish or cyanotic color of cervix and upper vagina (Chadwick's sign) (6th-8th week)
- Softening of the cervix (Goodell's sign) (5th week)
- Ballottement of the fetus (16th-28th week)
- Positive test for hCG in the maternal urine or blood serum (4th-12th week)
- Changes in skin pigmentation (chloasma and linea nigra) (2nd half of pregnancy)

Positive
- Detection of fetal heart tones by auscultation, ultrasonography, or a Doppler (8-17 weeks)
- Palpation of fetal body parts using Leopold maneuvers (19-22 weeks)
- Fetal movements visible and detected by examiner (late pregnancy)
- Radiological or ultrasonographic demonstration of fetal parts (6-16 weeks)

hCG, Human chorionic gonadotropin.

- Urinary output increases about 80% related to the total body water increase.
- Bladder capacity increases to about 1500 mL to accommodate extra fluids.

The cardiovascular system changes also beginning early in pregnancy as follows:

- Cardiac output increases up to 50% to meet the demands of pregnancy.
- Total blood volume increases up to 45% during pregnancy. Physiological anemia of pregnancy may result because of a greater increase in the volume of plasma compared with the volume of red blood cells.
- Heart rate increases by 10 beats/min to compensate for the increase in blood volume.

Respiratory system changes include the following:

- Tidal volume (volume of air inspired) increases by 30% to 40% to increase the effectiveness of air exchange. Total oxygen consumption increases about 20%.
- The diaphragm is displaced upward secondary to the enlarging uterus and causes shortness of breath during the last trimester.

Increased elasticity and softening of connective tissue of the musculoskeletal system cause the following changes during pregnancy:

- The joints relax, especially the pelvic joints that support the pregnancy and create pliability at the time of birth.
- Lumbar and dorsal curves of the spine increase late in pregnancy and contribute to low back pain and the waddle of pregnancy.
- Separation of the symphysis pubis occurs secondary to influence of relaxin hormone.

Changes in the integumentary system occur, which may include the following:

- Hormones and stretching of the connective tissue of the abdomen attributable to an enlarging uterus lead to stretch marks (**striae gravidarum**).
- A narrow, brownish line (**linea nigra**) divides the abdomen, running from the umbilicus to the symphysis pubis. The linea nigra fades after the pregnancy ends.
- An increase in pigmentation caused by melanocyte-stimulating hormone causes darkened areas on the face termed the mask of pregnancy (**chloasma**).

The gastrointestinal (GI) system undergoes dramatic changes during pregnancy, such as the following:

- The enlarging and space-occupying uterus cramps the intestinal region, causing a slowing of both peristalsis and emptying time of the stomach.
- Relaxin causes a decrease in gastric motility leading to constipation.
- Frequent "heartburn" results from reflux of stomach contents into the esophagus secondary to upward displacement of the stomach and a relaxed gastroesophageal sphincter (Gilbert, 2011; Heffner & Schust, 2010; Stables & Rankin, 2011).

Reproductive System

Effects on the reproductive system include changes in the uterus, breasts, vagina, vulva, and ovaries. The prepregnant uterus is approximately the size of a closed fist. The uterus at term has the capacity to contain a 3.2 to 4-5-kg (7 to 10 lb) infant and the placenta. As the uterus enlarges, the **fundus** (the upper uterine segment) moves higher in the abdomen (Figure 16-2). The breasts begin enlarging early in the pregnancy, and in late pregnancy they may secrete small amounts of **colostrum,** a precursor of mature breast milk. The vagina and vulva receive a greater blood supply and appear darker (cyanotic) as a result. Some women will notice an increase in vaginal secretions and experience a whitish discharge (Mattson & Smith, 2011).

Hormones such as hCG and estrogen, secreted by the placenta and the fetus, create an optimal intrauterine environment for the fetus and stimulate many changes in the pregnant woman's body. The developing fetus contributes to the provision of an adequate environment for its own growth and nourishment, despite the possibility of creating discomforts for the pregnant woman.

Preconception Care of Women

The rates of adverse birth outcomes (preterm and low birth weight, infant deaths, and birth defects) and maternal pregnancy complications in the United States are all higher than goals targeted in *Healthy People 2020*. Given the adverse trends seen in preterm birth rates and related infant death rates, a comprehensive public health research agenda that investigates the social, genetic, and biomedical factors contributing to these adverse outcomes was convened by the Centers for Disease Control and Prevention (CDC). The *3rd National Summit on Preconception Health and HealthCare* met in the summer of 2011 and set the following objectives:

- Advance opportunities to improve preconception health that are supported by provisions of the Affordable Care Act (ACA).

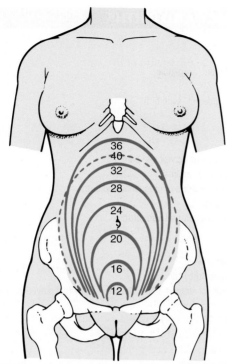

FIGURE 16-2 Upper level of enlarging uterus by weeks of normal gestation with a single fetus. (From Seidel, H. M., Ball, J. W., Dains, J. E., & Benedict, G. W. [2011]. *Mosby's guide to physical assessment* [7th ed.]. St Louis: Mosby.)

- Promote use of the evidence base for preconception care.
- Showcase the ideas, innovation, and expertise that have emerged from the field over the past 5 years.

The key points introduced included that preconception health is a gateway for broader conversations about women's wellness; that health practices and policies with an individual focus have finite success; and that researchers have been advocating for broadening the spectrum of improving health using life course for more than a decade (CDC, 2011a).

Preconception care offers an effective and efficient means to reduce complications of pregnancy for both the mother and her newborn. Women should be made aware that certain preconception interventions may improve not only the outcomes of pregnancy but also the overall health of the woman as well. The following interventions may be included:
- Folic acid supplementation to reduce the risk for neural tube defects by two thirds
- Rubella vaccination to reduce the risk of severe congenital defects
- Diabetes management to reduce risk of birth defects threefold
- Hypothyroidism management to promote healthy fetal neurological development
- Hepatitis B vaccination for at-risk women to prevent chronic liver disease
- Human immunodeficiency virus/acquired immunodeficiency syndrome (HIV/AIDS) screening and treatment to prevent transmission to fetus

- Screening and treatment for sexually transmitted infections (STIs) to reduce ectopic pregnancy and/or fetal anomalies
- Oral antiepileptic medication management to minimize birth defect potential
- Cessation of acne treatment with isotretinoin (Accutane) to prevent defects
- Smoking cessation counseling to reduce negative perinatal outcomes
- Screening and treating of depression to reduce the risk of postpartum depression
- Elimination of alcohol use to prevent fetal alcohol spectrum disorders
- Obesity control to reduce risks of cerebrovascular disease (CVD), diabetes, or surgical births (CDC, 2011e)

As a group, nurses are challenged to effectively translate the concept of preconception care to all women in their practice setting. By informing women that existing health conditions and medications can affect pregnancy outcomes, nurses can provide a positive environment for the woman's future pregnancy and improve overall health practices.

Normal Discomforts

Changes in the woman's body during pregnancy support a nursing diagnosis of *Alteration in comfort with relevant interventions* for most women. Women may feel a sense of relief that other pregnant women have these concerns and that interventions exist to increase their comfort at various points during gestation. Particularly for those experiencing a first pregnancy, the nurse serves as a valuable support person to help expectant couples adjust to the challenges and discomforts of pregnancy, a goal for the earlier-stated diagnosis.

Teaching the Woman about Changes to Expect in the Body During Pregnancy

In addition to serving as a caregiver, advocate, and support person, the nurse serves as a teacher throughout the pregnancy care process. Active teaching responsive to an individual's concerns about pregnancy may occur in the clinic, physician's office, or other care environments. Nursing interventions should address recommended professional practice guidelines for education during the prenatal period to prevent complications for the family. For example, the nurse may offer textbooks, pamphlets, videotapes, and referrals to websites and other media to increase a couple's knowledge of fetal, maternal, and family changes during gestation and then encourage and answer any questions based on the material. Going beyond one-to-one teaching, the nurse may also refer couples to early pregnancy and Lamaze childbirth preparation classes to enlarge their social support network and increase knowledge about labor and delivery. Throughout the care process, the nurse is sensitive to the cultural and ethnic beliefs and behaviors of the individual or family. By incorporating knowledge of these beliefs and behaviors, the nurse protects the pregnant woman and her baby by providing individualized care addressing the childbearing rituals held by various cultural groups (Table 16-1). A summary of perinatal care guidelines is provided in Table 16-2.

TABLE 16-1   CULTURAL VALUES RELATED TO PREGNANCY AND BIRTH*

Group	Values
Filipino	Structured prenatal care for those who can afford it Pregnancy normal event with family focused on pregnant woman's needs Pregnant woman encouraged to eat well, sleep often, and not to work out of home Sexual intercourse taboo during last 2 weeks of pregnancy Pregnant woman encouraged to eat fresh eggs close to delivery to help baby "slide out" with birth Woman very modest about body needs and care during pregnancy Father passive with birth process; pregnant woman active participant with birth Breastfeeding encouraged until child is a toddler
American Indian	In many tribes women are expected to seek prenatal care with pregnancy; some tribes accept late care Dialogue with women in tribal community important to maximize pregnancy and birth process Meditation, self-control practice, and indigenous plants (herbal teas) used for discomforts of pregnancy and birth Pregnant woman stoic about birth process; father present but not active participant Female kin present to support woman in labor; breastfeeding and bottle feeding encouraged after birth Father may avoid hunting immediately after birth or until infant's cord detaches
Arab American	Pregnancy normal event; may not access prenatal care because of that belief Much family support given to pregnant woman to allow maximal rest and minimal work Present orientation: little preparation for birth, fears labor pains but responds once they come Expressive with labor but not active with control of pain; relies on family members for support; father not active, may feel powerless with birth process Very modest about care, especially with opposite-gender health care provider Prefer bottle feeding; colostrum believed to harm baby
Blacks	Most access prenatal care after first trimester or seek care earlier with problems Female kin provide most of support with pregnancy and birth; male support less visible Open expression of pregnancy and birth discomfort; active participant in birth process May self-medicate with cultural remedies for pregnancy complaints May avoid being in photographs because of fear of stillbirth May crave certain foods: chicken, greens, clay, starch, or dirt (pica) If of Muslim faith, may wish to have head covered during labor and birth process Breastfeed if given information on the benefits of this method
Mexican American	Often face barriers to prenatal care because of lack of insurance, fear of health care system, lack of transportation to clinic May consider prenatal care not necessary because childbirth is normal life event Education and acculturation influence prenatal care access Pregnancy considered to follow marriage; family supports respect and assistance to pregnant woman Pregnant woman does not smoke, work, drink alcohol, or use drugs; pregnancy a time to rest, walk, eat well, sleep, drink chamomile tea, and avoid cold air Grandmother may move into the home close to delivery time to help and provide folk remedies after birth Modest about care and needs; same-gender health care provider encouraged Generally walks during labor to enhance birth; wants family for support; woman active and father delegates support to female members of family Generally breastfeeds for up to 1 year
Vietnamese	Generally early prenatal care unless immigrant status, then depend on family for care Encouraged to eat healthy foods, get rest, avoid strenuous activity during last trimester Focus on keeping pregnant woman warm, encouraging salt water for oral care, and maintaining good hygiene Sexual intercourse taboo with pregnancy Father present but not active with pregnancy Birth a time of hot and cold imbalance; mother "suffers in silence," may moan or grunt; mother depends on female relatives for support and guidance Mother breastfeeds for up to 1 year; avoids cold foods for this period

Compiled from Spector, R. E. (2008). *Cultural diversity in health & illness* (7th ed., pp. 101-137). Upper Saddle River, NJ: Pearson/Prentice Hall; Purnell, L. D. (2009). *Guide to culturally competent health care.* Philadelphia: F.A. Davis; Haas, A. (2011). Cultural diversity in childbirth education. *Midwifery Today with International Midwife, 97,* 39; Lewallen, L. (2011). The importance of culture in childbearing. *Journal of Obstetric, Gynecologic, and Neonatal Nursing, 40*(1), 4-8; Callister, L. (2011). Global and cultural perinatal nursing research: Improving clinical practice. *Journal of Perinatal & Neonatal Nursing, 25*(2), 139-143; Bowers, P. (2011). Cultural perspectives in childbearing. *Nursing Spectrum.* [Online]. Retrieved from http://ce.nurse.com/ce263-60/cultural-perspectives-in-childbearing/.
*General ideas about beliefs and behaviors of each of these cultural groups have been given with no intent to stereotype all persons who represent these groups' beliefs or behaviors. It is hoped that this information will provide direction to the nurse who will continue to assess each individual to render care that meets each person's traditional values in a biomedical model of health care in the United States today.

TABLE 16-2   PERINATAL CARE GUIDELINES

FIRST TRIMESTER	SECOND TRIMESTER	THIRD TRIMESTER	LABOR STAGES	POSTPARTUM
Complete assessment to identify risk factors	Assess adaptation to pregnancy and fetal well-being	Review physiological changes	Admission to birthing facility	Complete a head-to-toe physical assessment: Breasts Uterus Bladder Bowels Lochia Emotional status Circulatory status Episiotomy
Awareness of subtle or overt physical, sexual, or emotional abuse	Update heath history	Monitor changes related to pregnancy	*First stage:* Complete maternal/fetal assessments Determine labor progress Assist with comfort measures Monitor fetal heart rate Support family in their efforts Praise efforts	Assess for postpartum blues/depression
Assess physical and psychosocial progress in adaptation to pregnancy	Continue to recognize cultural influences	Assess expectant family's readiness for labor, birth, and parenting role	*Second stage:* Offer encouragement Assist with pushing efforts Document activities	Encourage bonding and attachment
Inquire about physical changes and discomforts; explain causes and identify appropriate relief measures	Encourage informed decision-making and positive health care practices	Review finalized birth plan	*Third stage:* Provide care as needed Document time of placental delivery Administer meds as ordered	Demonstrate breastfeeding techniques
Provide anticipatory guidance appropriate for her individual needs • Educational needs: Hazards during pregnancy • Use of drugs, alcohol, and smoking Seat belts, high-risk behaviors Warning/danger signs to report Nutrition and weight management Sexuality	Review potential risk factors and when to report Ensure community referrals/resources as needed Educational needs: Oral hygiene Nutritional needs Safety issues in workplace Discomforts of pregnancy Relief of common discomforts of pregnancy Prepared childbirth classes	Identify community resources available to family Explain any diagnostic tests ordered Meet educational needs: needs for newborn care Monitoring fetal movements Strategies to cope with discomforts Promote family safety Including partner in process Childbirth preparation	*Fourth stage:* Monitor vital signs; fundus, assess bladder status Encourage parental-infant interaction Monitor newborn's well-being Provide perineal care, food, fluids Provide family support	Provide anticipatory guidance needed for this family Educational needs: Nutrition Fatigue Childcare Immunizations Sexuality Family planning Breast engorgement Family adaptation Follow-up care needed Danger signs to report Sibling readiness for new member Self-care activities

Total Weight Gain

Total weight gain during pregnancy reflects not only the growth of the baby and placenta, but also the growth of the uterus and breasts, the storage of maternal fat, and the increased amounts of blood and other body fluids. It has been nearly 2 decades since guidelines for how much weight a woman should gain during pregnancy were issued by the Institute of Medicine (IOM). More research has been conducted on the effects of weight gain in pregnancy on the health of both mother and baby. The IOM released new weight gain guidelines in 2009 that are based on revised body mass index (BMI) categories and now have a recommendation for obese women. To meet

the recommendations of the report, women need to gain within the weight gain ranges for their BMI category. Achieving the recommended gain will require individualized attention and support from a woman's care providers as well as her family and community.

The new IOM guidelines reflect changing U.S. demographics, particularly the surge in the number of women who are overweight or obese. Healthy women at a normal weight for their height (BMI of 18.5 to 24.9) should gain 25 to 35 pounds during pregnancy, the new guidelines state. Underweight women (BMI less than 18.5) should gain more, 28 to 40 pounds, and overweight women (BMI of 25 to 29.9) should gain less, 15 to

25 pounds. Obese women (BMI greater than 30) should limit their gain to 11 to 20 pounds (IOM, 2011).

Obesity is a public health concern worldwide, arising from multifaceted and complex causes that relate to individual choice and lifestyle, and the influences of wider society. In addition to a long-standing focus on both childhood and adult **obesity**, there has been more recent concern relating to maternal **obesity**. Infants of obese mothers are more likely to be born prematurely, to be stillborn, or to die in the first 28 days of life. In addition, they are more likely to be born with a congenital abnormality (Heslehurst, 2011). Despite the serious health implications of obesity in pregnancy, the current level of awareness of such risks among childbearing women is limited (Keely et al., 2011).

Ideally, all women with a BMI >30 should be provided with accurate and accessible information about the risks associated with obesity in pregnancy at a preconception visit. Weight-loss interventions would be most appropriately employed before pregnancy, but if that is not possible, nurses need to recognize the need for opportunistic health promotion aimed at disseminating information about the risks of obesity in pregnancy to overweight and obese women of childbearing age. Most women are highly motivated to have healthy infants and this could be a key factor in health-promotion discussions that inform women of the risks of obesity in pregnancy and promote healthy lifestyle choices and weight-loss strategies preconceptually and between pregnancies.

Labor and Birth

Pregnancy culminates with labor and giving birth. The process of giving birth elicits a significant emotional response from the delivering family. A description of the events of a usual labor and birthing process must occur to establish a background for considering the physiological changes in the mother and the infant.

Several theories offer explanations for the cause of labor. Many factors likely interact, including uterine distention, mechanical irritation, progesterone deprivation, placental aging and hormones, and posterior pituitary activity. Labor usually begins around 40 weeks of gestation, suggesting that hormonal control similar to that regulating the menstrual cycles also contributes to its onset (Cunningham et al., 2010c).

Labor may be divided conveniently into the following four distinct stages:

- **Dilation stage**—lasts from the onset of true labor contractions to complete dilation of the cervix. It is divided into three phases: latent (0- to 3-cm dilation); active (4- to 7-cm dilation); and transition (8- to 10-cm dilation)
- **Pushing stage**—lasts from complete dilation (10 cm) of the cervix to birth
- **Placental stage**—lasts from the time of birth of the newborn to delivery of the placenta and membranes, which can range from 2 to 15 minutes
- **Recovery stage**—defined as the first 4 hours after childbirth where physiological and psychological adjustments begin to occur

The first stage of labor starts with regular timing of uterine contractions and ends with complete dilation (opening) and cervical effacement (thinning of the cervix). Signs of beginning

BOX 16-2 SIGNS OF BEGINNING LABOR

- Bloody show or loss of the mucous plug that seals cervical canal during pregnancy
- Regular uterine contractions
- Contractions increasing in intensity, duration, and frequency
- Palpable hardening of the uterus during contractions
- Pain in the lower back radiating to the front of the abdomen

labor include those listed in Box 16-2. The cervix, the lower portion of the uterus, must dilate from a closed position (0 cm) to a totally open position (10 cm, or 4 inches, in diameter). During the first stage, the cervix must also completely efface or shorten from a length of 1 to 2 inches to a barely palpable (paper-thin) thickness. For most women, painless Braxton-Hicks contractions throughout pregnancy cause some cervical dilation and thinning, or at least cervical softening, before the onset of active labor.

During the **first stage of labor,** the presenting part of the fetus begins to press on the cervix, lower uterine segment, and nerve endings around the cervix and vagina. Women's responses to this process vary; pain thresholds and cultural perceptions of and responses to pain differ among laboring women (see Table 16-1). The fundus, the active contractile part of the uterus, becomes thicker as labor progresses, retracts the lower uterine segment and cervix, and helps push the fetus toward the cervix and eventually through the vagina for birth (Cohen & Friedman, 2011). Stage one lasts an average of 8 to 12 hours for women experiencing a first birth and somewhat less for women having a second or additional child. Based on a laboring woman's needs, various pain medications, nonpharmacological measures, Lamaze breathing, and other distractive techniques may alleviate the discomfort associated with first-stage labor. Periodic vaginal examinations by the nurse or other health care provider indicate a laboring woman's cervical dilation and effacement and descent of the fetus into the birth canal (a concept called **station**). In a full-term pregnancy, loss of the amniotic membrane usually increases pressure of the fetal head against the cervix, making dilation and effacement more efficient, and tends to augment the labor process.

During the **second stage of labor,** the fetus descends through the lower birth canal toward the woman's perineum. The upper uterine segment greatly thickens, and the abdominal muscles assist in the descent and expulsion of the fetus. Women who have attended childbirth classes often are better prepared to actively push the baby through the pelvis and perineum during contractions. Cultural practices may support pushing from a squatting or upright position and not in a supine one. Nurses must acknowledge that the maternity health care system has a unique culture that may clash with the cultures of many of our care recipients. For many women, an overwhelming urge to bear down during uterine contractions occurs at this time. The fetal head accommodates to the mother's pelvis and vaginal structure and, finally, the head becomes flush with the vaginal opening on the woman's perineum. The woman at this point actively pushes to expel the newborn.

The **third stage of labor** begins after the birth of the newborn and lasts until placental expulsion. Placental separation usually takes place within 5 to 30 minutes after completion of the second stage. After delivery of the placenta the health care provider examines the placenta to determine that all placental tissue is intact and to detect any abnormalities that could affect the infant's condition and adaptation to extrauterine life.

The **fourth stage of labor** generally consists of the first 2 hours after childbirth, during which the mother faces the greatest risk of postpartum hemorrhage. An expected blood loss of 250 to 500 mL may cause the mother to experience a moderate decline in blood pressure (Cohen & Friedman, 2011). She may also experience an increase in pulse rate (**tachycardia**) to compensate for blood loss during the early postpartum period. The Care Plan at the end of this chapter addresses the nurse's role in managing the **stages of labor**.

Overview of Care

Professional members of the health care team play an important role in labor and delivery, but a woman's family or significant other (i.e., husband, partner, friend, family) also inherently contributes to her care during labor and birth, particularly in certain cultures (see Table 16-1). Many practitioners suggest that the expectations and beliefs of a birthing couple have a great effect on how the woman fulfills the mothering role. Therefore the nurse needs to collaborate with the people who care for the pregnant woman to meet that family's needs during pregnancy, labor, and delivery.

The importance of the nurse's knowledge, caregiving, and support cannot be underestimated during the first stage of labor. Active emotional and physical nursing support decreases the length of many women's labors, use of analgesics and anesthetics, and number of operative deliveries and may help women reach their birthing goals (Association of Women's Health, Obstetrical, and Neonatal Nursing [AWHONN], 2010). Provided that they are accepted by a woman's culture, independent nursing interventions to increase comfort (e.g., giving backrubs or massages, offering ice or warm fluids by mouth, assisting with ambulation and position changes, and providing a clean and dry environment) may help the laboring woman cope with the challenges of labor. Many women will request medication to diminish the pain of labor and birth, and the nurse may need to review options for medication with each woman or couple. During the first stage the mother must not bear down, because this may cause cervical swelling; often, active nursing support and distractive techniques, such as breathing and visual refocus, can prevent pushing before the second stage of labor. A woman may depend on the nurse to model breathing techniques to relieve labor discomfort. The nurse may need to explain usual interventions during this stage of labor, including the use of a **fetal heart monitor** (a machine that detects and records fetal heart rate and activity during labor), intravenous fluids, digital blood pressure machine, and urinary catheter. Open and clear communication among the health care providers and laboring woman and her significant others, particularly during frequent and difficult uterine contractions, will improve coping before the pushing stage begins.

During the second stage of labor, the woman needs reassurance and support for her pushing efforts. Constant reinforcement and education by the nurse about labor progress, fetal heart monitor tracings, and other interventions will give the mother and her support system the guidance needed to give birth to the infant. Throughout labor the nurse considers the specific cultural and ethnic needs to support nursing assessment and positive responses to labor by the childbearing family.

Active nursing support during the third and fourth stages of labor includes observing for excessive vaginal bleeding after the placenta is expelled, assisting the woman in breastfeeding her new baby, monitoring vital signs, and implementing uterine massage if the uterus becomes boggy or fails to contract over the placental site. Emotional support during assessments and delivery of information to explain the rationale for assessments are also important nursing roles supported by professional practice standards.

Throughout the entire labor and birth process, the nurse makes careful observations of the laboring woman and fetus so that she can detect early any difficulties with the progress of labor or with maternal or fetal health. Problems may include unusual fetal or uterine activity, presence of **meconium** (fetal stool) in the amniotic fluid, fetal tachycardia (heart rate greater than 160 beats per minute) or fetal **bradycardia** (heart rate less than 110 beats per minute) in a full-term infant, and fetal heart rate decreases with uterine activity during labor (Mattson & Smith, 2011). These events must be reported immediately to the health care provider, with a complete oral and electronic description of the event. The nurse must be aware that abnormal fetal and maternal signs and patterns may be related to factors such as maternal diabetes or hypertension; type, timing, or dosage of labor medications; uterine contraction pattern; maternal or fetal infections; maternal anemia; preeclampsia; presence and character of amniotic fluid; bleeding in the pregnant woman or fetus; or early gestational age of the infant (Gilbert, 2011).

Our major role as nurses is to provide safe and evidence-based care to promote optimal birth outcomes for all women. Nurses need to remember there is more than one way to provide this care. Nurses are educated to assess every woman as an individual and to plan care with mutual goal setting for the best outcomes. By assisting all persons seeking care from diverse cultures and by adopting our practices as much as possible to embrace the cultural traditions of others, we will enhance the childbearing experience and promote the health of women, newborns, and families.

CHANGES DURING TRANSITION FROM FETUS TO NEWBORN

Most newborns experience a smooth transition from intrauterine to extrauterine life. When difficulty occurs, however, the newborn's viability depends on the nurse's understanding of the fine balance of chemical, physiological, and anatomical changes that occurs as it makes the transition to postnatal life (Katz et al., 2011). **Website Resource 16B** presents details about the adaptation of the fetus to extrauterine life.

TABLE 16-3 APGAR SCORING

SIGN	SCORE		
	0	1	2
HEART RATE	ABSENT	SLOW (<100)	>100
Respiratory effort	Absent	Weak cry, hypoventilation	Good strong cry
Muscle tone	Flaccid, limp	Some flexion of extremities	Active motion, extremities well flexed
Reflex irritability	No response	Grimace	Cry
Color	Blue, pale	Body pink, extremities blue	Completely pink

From Cohen, W.R., & Friedman, E.A. (2011). *Labor and delivery care: A practical guide.* Malden, MA: Wiley-Blackwell; Norwitz, E. R., & Schorge, J. O. (2010). *Obstetrics and gynecology at a glance* (3rd ed.). Malden, MA: Blackwell Publishing.

Nursing Interventions

Nursing activities during this adaptation process include assessment and interventions aimed at specific protection of the infant and prevention of complications. Cold stress should be avoided by keeping the newborn dry and warmly wrapped and by avoiding environments that cause heat loss. Overall, the nurse should minimally disturb, but maximally observe and document, the newborn's behavior during reactive periods.

Apgar Score

Assessment of the newborn after the first few hours of life is essentially the same as assessment of the young infant (see Chapter 17). One technique, specific to timing after birth, is the Apgar scoring system. This scoring historically has been used to provide a simple clinical measure to evaluate the newborn's general condition at birth. The Apgar score, made at 1 minute and 5 minutes of age, may be repeated again at 10 minutes of age until the infant's condition has stabilized. A total score is calculated by adding the values allotted to the categories noted in Table 16-3. The highest possible score is 10. A score of 8 to 10 indicates that the baby is adapting well. The Apgar score does not predict the neurological development of an infant, but may relate to the infant's risk of illness or death during the first year of life, which is important information for parents of an infant with a low Apgar score (Wong & MacLennan, 2011).

Gender

Gender differences occur in fetal growth. Generally boys grow faster than girls in the third trimester, and at birth boys are slightly heavier, are longer, and have a larger head circumference than girls (Bao & Swaab, 2011). Although more boys are conceived, they tend to be aborted spontaneously more often than girl embryos; the two X chromosomes possessed by female embryos may protect them from the early hazards of pregnancy. After birth, boys continue to have a lower survival rate than do girls (Coch et al., 2010).

Race and Culture

Race may affect the health of the fetus in several ways. For example, in the United States, non-Whites (mainly Blacks) have more fraternal twin pregnancies than Whites (Cunningham et al., 2010d). Because their organs are less mature, twin fetuses face an increased risk for **premature delivery** as a result of gestational factors in the mother. Currently the United States is forty-ninth in the world ranking for infant mortality rate (IMR), with a rate of 6.06 (Central Intelligence Agency [CIA], 2011). This rate, which reflects the number of infants who die before the end of their first year of life and is the leading indicator of a nation's health, reflects the higher IMRs and low-birth-weight outcomes of Blacks, American Indians, and other ethnic minority populations in the United States. This rate illustrates the complex sociopolitical issues that produce birth outcomes in this country and those needing attention to improve the IMR (CDC, 2011b; CIA, 2011; MacDorman & Matthews, 2011; U.S. Department of Health and Human Services [USDHHS], 2010).

Race is also a factor in the frequency of certain genetic and congenital malformations (Box 16-3: Hot Topics). For example, more Native American, Latino, or Asian descent babies have cleft palates (an opening in the oral palate) than do Black babies (Mayo Clinic, 2011). Black babies have higher rates of sickle cell anemia (abnormally shaped red blood cells) than White babies. Interestingly, the total number of malformations tends to be about the same in all races that have been studied (Whites, Blacks, Hispanics, and Asians) (March of Dimes, 2011).

A woman's ethnic background may also influence the health of her fetus based on a link to socioeconomic status. For increasing numbers of homeless pregnant women, income may support family survival needs, but not prenatal care. Minority group pregnant women may have fewer economic resources to obtain a nutritious diet or early and consistent high-quality prenatal care. These outcomes may relate to access to health care factors or cultural beliefs that do not support recommended foods or prenatal care (Box 16-4: *Healthy People 2020*).

Genetics

Genetic influences affect the survival and later well-being of the child through several known mechanisms. Down syndrome (trisomy 21) remains the most recognized and most commonly occurring example of an extra chromosome. Extra chromosomes, deleted chromosomes, or translocations usually cause multiple malformations incompatible with life, causing early loss of the fetus via spontaneous abortion. Single malformations in an otherwise normal fetus (e.g., clubfoot, cleft palate, or neural tube defect) probably result from a combined effect of many genes (March of Dimes, 2011). These defects, found at birth, may be surgically corrected or managed during the child's life. Invasive techniques of amniocentesis, chorionic villus sampling, and chromosome analysis have expanded genetic counseling options and interventions for women facing possible fetal genetic defects. The nurse works with other members of the health care team to inform these women and couples of genetic and high-risk screening resources when family history or other factors indicate that a fetal genetic defect may be likely.

⚠ BOX 16-3   HOT TOPICS
Genetic Testing May Lead to Ethical Dilemmas

Prenatal genetic testing provides important opportunities for assessment of genetic risk and diagnosis. However, some genetic tests do not identify all of the possible gene mutations that can cause a particular condition, or they have limited predictive value. Because some genetic tests may not provide all the information that families may want, the test may subsequently require difficult decisions without providing full information. As an example, a cystic fibrosis carrier testing can identify couples who are both carriers. When the cystic fibrosis mutations are identified in the parents, prenatal diagnosis can be performed to determine whether a fetus has inherited a cystic fibrosis gene mutation from each parent. Knowing that a fetus has inherited two cystic fibrosis mutations, however, does not, at this time, predict the severity of the disease in the infant. For couples in this situation, the ethical dilemma involves the decision to continue or to end a pregnancy without having knowledge of the severity of the disorder.

Should the Information Be Obtained if No Treatment or Intervention Exists?

Genetic testing can lead to specific treatments or interventions for some conditions but not for others. This is the case with some disorders that can be detected in expanded newborn screening. When phenylketonuria (PKU) is identified, dietary intervention allows individuals with this condition to lead healthy and productive lives. Currently, however, not all conditions can be adequately treated. Genetic testing for some conditions for which there are no treatments might have the potential to cause psychological harm, stigmatization, and discrimination. Genetic testing for Huntington's disease (HD), a progressive motor and cognitive disorder with onset in midlife, is one example. There are no effective treatments or preventive measures currently available. Thus, choosing to have genetic testing for HD is highly personal, and it is recommended that individuals consider extensive pretest counseling. These tests may lead to decisions that cannot be reversed and are based on a woman's best guess as to what would be the best course of action for her and her family. The dilemma that occurs then is whether a newborn should be tested for disorders that we cannot treat.

Ethical decision-making models/frameworks are valuable tools that can assist nurses in addressing ethical dilemmas. Principles of autonomy, informed consent, privacy/confidentiality, beneficence, nonmaleficence, and justice are applicable to use in the ethics involved in genetic testing. These principles should be sensitive to human needs, should be responsive to contextual considerations, and should emphasize the uniqueness of each situation.

1. What might be the nurse's role in assisting the family in their decision-making process?
2. What assurances can be made regarding privacy and confidentiality of the genetic information to prevent future employment or health insurance discrimination?
3. What resources are available to nurses to keep current on prenatal genetic testing?

♥ BOX 16-4   HEALTHY PEOPLE 2020
Selected National Health-Promotion and Disease-Prevention Objectives for the Prenatal Period

- Reduce the rate of fetal deaths at 20 or more weeks of gestation to no more than 5.6 fetal deaths per 1000 live births. (Baseline: 6.2 per 1000 live births in 2005)
- Reduce the rate of fetal and infant deaths during the perinatal period (28 weeks of gestation to 7 days after birth) to no more than 5.9 perinatal deaths per 1000 live births. (Baseline: 6.6 per 1000 live births in 2005)
- Reduce the rate of neonatal deaths (within the first 28 days of life) to 4.1 neonatal deaths per 1000 live births. (Baseline: 4.5 per 1000 live births in 2006)
- Reduce the rate of maternal mortality to 11.4 maternal deaths per 100,000 live births. (Baseline: 12.7 per 100,000 live births in 2007)
- Reduce the rate of maternal illness and complications due to pregnancy (complications during hospitalized labor and birth) to 28%. (Baseline: 31.1% of pregnant females suffered complications during hospitalized labor and delivery in 2007)
- Reduce the rate of cesarean births among low-risk (full-term, singleton, vertex presentation) women to 23.9%. (Baseline: 26.5% of low-risk females giving birth for the first time had a cesarean birth in 2007)
- Reduce the rate of low-birth-weight (LBW) newborns to 7.8%. (Baseline: 8.2% of live births were low birth weight in 2007)
- Reduce the rate of very-low-birth-weight (VLBW) newborns to 1.3%. (Baseline: 1.5% of live births were very-low-birth-weight in 2007)
- Reduce the rate of total preterm births to 11.4%. (Baseline: 12.7% of live births were preterm in 2007)
- Reduce the rate of late preterm births or live births at 34 to 36 weeks of gestation to 8.1%. (Baseline: 9.0% of live births were late preterm or occurred at 34 to 36 weeks of gestation in 2007)
- Increase the proportion of pregnant women who receive early and adequate prenatal care to 77.6%. (Baseline: 70.5% of pregnant females received early and adequate prenatal care in 2007)
- Increase abstinence from alcohol, cigarettes, and illicit drugs among pregnant women to 98.3% (alcohol), 98.6% (cigarette smoking), and 100% (illicit drugs). (Baselines: *alcohol,* 89.4% of pregnant females aged 15 to 44 years reported abstaining from alcohol in the past 30 days in 2007 to 2008; *cigarette smoking,* 89.6% of females delivering a live birth reported abstaining from smoking cigarettes during pregnancy in 2007; and *illicit drugs,* 94.9% of pregnant females aged 15 to 44 years reported abstaining from illicit drugs in the past 30 days in 2007 to 2008)
- Increase the proportion of women of childbirth potential with intake of at least 400 mcg of folic acid from fortified foods or dietary supplements to 26.2%. (Baseline: 23.8% of nonpregnant females aged 15 to 44 years reported a usual daily total intake of at least 400 mcg of folic acid from fortified foods or dietary supplements in 2003 to 2006)
- Increase the proportion of women delivering a live birth who received preconception care services and practiced key recommended preconception health behaviors to following values: took prenatal vitamins (33.1%); did not smoke cigarettes before pregnancy (85.4%); did not drink alcohol before pregnancy (56.4%); and maintained a healthy weight before pregnancy (53.4%). (Baselines: 30.1% of females delivering a recent live birth took multivitamins/folic acid every day in the month before pregnancy as reported in 2007; 77.6% of females delivering a recent live birth did not smoke in the 3 months before pregnancy as reported in 2007; 51.3% of females delivering a recent live birth did not drink alcohol in the 3 months before pregnancy as reported in 2007; and 48.5% of females delivering a recent live birth had a normal weight [i.e., a BMI of 18.5 to 24.9] before pregnancy as reported in 2007)

From U.S. Department of Health and Human Services (USDHHS). (2010). *Healthy People 2020.* [Online] Available at www.healthypeople.gov/2020/topicsobjectives2020/objectiveslist.aspx?topicId=26.

BOX 16-5 ASSESSMENT FOR PREGNANCY ACCORDING TO GORDON'S FUNCTIONAL HEALTH PATTERNS

Health perception–health management pattern: Aware of or participates in management of pregnancy, or both; expects an uncomplicated pregnancy based on woman's or significant other's active involvement in her own care; able to state complications of pregnancy that mandate physician notification; engages in health-promotion behaviors specific to pregnancy.

Nutritional-metabolic pattern: Follows diet changes of pregnancy as recommended by nurse; has appropriate weight for height and has gained adequate weight for gestational age of pregnancy; eats three meals a day and two snacks (afternoon and evening), focusing on increased amounts of vegetables and fruits; drinks healthy fluids including at least 8 glasses of water per day; has elastic skin turgor.

Elimination pattern: Experiences occasional constipation from progesterone influence of GI peristalsis relaxation, usually corrected by increased fluids, nightly walking, and more diet roughage; voids 7 to 10 times a day, depending on amount of fluids consumed; no known hemorrhoids or difficulty in elimination; voiding without excess frequency, urgency, or burning; understands signs of UTI.

Activity-exercise pattern: Walks 3 times a week for 20 minutes without complaints of unusual fatigue or soreness; active at home with housework and at work teaching primary school; swam 2 times a week before pregnancy and move to current residence.

Sleep-rest pattern: Generally sleeps 7 to 8 hours a night; has increased total daily sleep somewhat with fatigue of pregnancy—naps for 1 hour on weekends and 30 minutes after work; sleeps on side and with two pillows for comfort; uses no sleep aids; generally able to relax and initiate sleep without difficulty; occasionally has headache at end of workday and takes acetaminophen (Tylenol) for relief or listens to soft music after work to enhance relaxation.

Cognitive-perceptual pattern: Realizes the need to decrease work activity and increase rest periods as she nears end of pregnancy; answers questions in appropriate tone and words during pregnancy visits; has intact memory (alert and remote); reads about pregnancy and early parenthood to prepare for the birth.

Self-perception–self-concept pattern: States she is excited about pregnancy after a year of trying to conceive; well groomed, wears maternity clothes because "I want to"; believes she looks "nice" due to pregnancy.

Roles-relationships pattern: Lives with husband of 3 years; visits extended family, 60 miles away, every month; shares family roles with husband, accepts this balance; has many friends who support her pregnancy; perceives extensive employee and employer support with pregnancy and time off after delivery.

Sexuality-reproductive pattern: States, "I have a satisfying love life and enjoy my husband"; before pregnancy, engaged in sexual intercourse 4 to 5 times a week with desire to become pregnant; with pregnancy and fatigue, has intercourse generally 2 to 3 times a week, with pattern acceptable to both partners; no known STIs in past or present.

Coping-stress tolerance pattern: Concerned about fatigue affecting performance as primary school teacher; walks 3 times a week for 20 minutes to "center myself and feel good"; smiles often, good sense of humor; supportive family excited about her pregnancy.

Values-beliefs pattern: Protestant religion; prays daily and gains strength from religion.

Other data:
- Medication history:
  Prenatal vitamin (Materna), 1 tablet each morning
  Ferrous sulfate, 1 tablet each morning
  Acetaminophen (Tylenol) 650 mg for occasional headaches
- Physical examination:
  5 feet, 4 inches tall
  Weight 140 lb (at 14 weeks of pregnancy; weight gain of 5 lb with pregnancy)
  29 years of age
  PERRLA
  TPR 98.2-76-16
  BP 114/78 mm Hg right arm (sitting, left arm)
  Peripheral pulses equal, strong bilaterally
  Skin warm, dry, elastic turgor; mucous membranes intact, moist; alert, oriented ×3

Modified from Peterson, R. (2012). *Clinical companion for fundamentals of nursing* (8th ed.). St. Louis: Mosby; Gordon, M. (2010). *Manual of nursing diagnosis* (12th ed.). Sudbury, MA: Jones & Bartlett Learning.
BP, Blood pressure; *GI,* gastrointestinal; *PERRLA,* pupils equally round and reactive to light and accommodation; *STIs,* sexually transmitted infections; *TPR,* temperature, pulse, respirations; *UTI,* urinary tract infection.

GORDON'S FUNCTIONAL HEALTH PATTERNS

Box 16-5 provides an example of a pregnancy assessment using Gordon's functional health patterns (2010).

Health Perception–Health Management Pattern

Based on her culture and life experience, a woman may view pregnancy as an illness, as a completely natural and healthy state, or as a combination of the two. This perception will influence her view of her changing body, her attitude toward the usual discomforts of pregnancy such as fatigue or backache, her choice of health-oriented or illness-oriented care, and her decision to seek prenatal care. The woman who sees herself as healthy and pregnancy as a normal part of her life most likely will seek a health care provider with a similar outlook. Another woman with the same perception may seek help from a socially approved group, as defined by her culture, and avoid standard Western medicine during pregnancy (e.g., Roma [gypsies]). Generally, women with a positive view of pregnancy will continue active participation in their respective social circles and careers. However, the woman who sees her pregnancy as a time of illness may use this as a reason to withdraw from her work and social obligations.

A woman's acceptance of her pregnancy influences her health management practices and choices. The woman who denies or has strong negative feelings about her pregnancy may fail to eat properly, get enough rest and exercise, breastfeed, or seek prenatal care. A woman may deny a pregnancy because she never intended to become pregnant despite having sexual intercourse without birth control. Approximately 50% of American pregnancies are unintended, particularly among adolescents, women older than age 40, women with low income, and women who lack access, cultural acceptance, education, experience sexual violence, and lack financial resources to purchase or use contraception (Monea & Thomas, 2011; USDHHS, 2010).

These women, faced with an unplanned or a closely spaced pregnancy, may expose a fetus to alcohol, tobacco, and **sexually transmitted infections (STIs)**, abuse a child who was never wanted, or fail to obtain follow-up care for a high-risk child (i.e., experienced complications from childbirth) (USDHHS, 2010; U.S. Preventive Services Task Force [USPSTF], 2011a).

The nurse who works with a pregnant population is sensitive to a wide range of views expressed by these women and works with each to effectively manage their pregnancies. For example, Hispanic women are less likely to receive early prenatal care based on a belief that pregnancy is not an illness. The nurse targets interventions that focus on this group's needs and beliefs while adhering to professional practice standards that will improve their outcomes.

Nutritional-Metabolic Pattern

Massive amounts of literature support the importance of optimal nutrition during pregnancy for maternal and fetal well-being. Maternal malnutrition before and during pregnancy may exert a teratogenic effect on the fetus. A **teratogen** is an agent that causes either a functional or a structural disability in the organism based on exposure to that agent (Merriam-Webster, 2012). Teratogens principally affect the central nervous system (CNS) of the fetus, leading to impaired intelligence and performance later in life. They are discussed more in the Environmental Processes section later in the chapter.

Various factors influence the quality of nutrition needed for positive fetal development and birth outcome. Fetal development suffers in cases of adolescent pregnancy or in pregnancies of older women who experience poor nutrition between and during several pregnancies. Maternal nutritional deficiencies during one's own fetal, infant, and childhood periods also contribute to the development of structural and physiological disadvantages to supporting a growing fetus. For example, women who are severely underweight before pregnancy often experience higher rates of low-birth-weight infants and preterm labor than do women of appropriate prepregnant weight (Cunningham et al., 2010e). Inherited maternal stature and pelvic development may influence pregnancy and efficiency of labor and delivery. A lack of income to buy healthy food may also exist, and sometimes cultural values related to food intake influence the quality of nutrition during pregnancy.

To meet increased metabolic, energy, and structural needs for pregnancy, most nutritionists recommend that a pregnant woman increase her intake by approximately 300 calories each day (USDHHS, 2010). This results in a total weight gain of about 25 to 35 pounds (Figure 16-3). If at the end of 20 weeks of gestation the woman has not gained at least 10 pounds, she risks delivering an ill infant suffering from intrauterine growth restriction (IUGR). These risks also exist when a woman continues to gain insufficient weight throughout the pregnancy or in a woman who was underweight or overweight before pregnancy. Although the rate of gain and the total gain during pregnancy vary among women, a correlation exists between an erratic pattern of weight gain or a too-rapid weight gain and a lack of fetal well-being (Debruyne et al., 2012). The nurse advises the pregnant woman to eat a well-balanced diet.

FIGURE 16-3 Many practitioners recommend a weight gain of 25 to 30 pounds for women within a normal weight range before conception.

A well-balanced diet for a pregnant woman parallels that needed by all human beings, with increases of certain components as recommended by the Food and Nutrition Board of the National Academy of Science (Institute of Medicine [IOM], 2011; USDHHS, 2010). The nurse recommends that the entire family eat a healthy diet. The nurse encourages the pregnant woman to drink 8 to 10 glasses of water per day to develop amniotic fluid and prevent urinary tract infections often seen with pregnancy. The nurse may also need to encourage the woman to modify her diet to include more fiber and roughage to avoid constipation during pregnancy (Table 16-4).

Protein requirements during pregnancy increase to about 70 grams (g) per day, or a daily increase of 25 g above normal (Dudek, 2010). This ensures an adequate supply of amino acids for fetal growth and development, blood volume expansion, and maternal tissue growth. Other protein sources, such as cheese, cream soups, puddings, tofu, and yogurt, may be better tolerated by some women and by those from cultures (Hispanic) that do not drink milk. Animal protein and less expensive legume sources provide protein and, if combined with other healthy food sources, provide high-quality meals (e.g., tuna and rice, peanut butter, and whole-wheat bread). Protein foods cost more than other foods. Therefore the nurse may need to teach pregnant couples about economical ways to meet protein needs for fetal development.

Mineral intake must also increase during pregnancy. Increased protein intake usually provides the extra needed essential minerals, particularly phosphorus and calcium. The rapid deposit of calcium in fetal bones and teeth during the third trimester of pregnancy requires adequate maternal calcium stores from early pregnancy and continued calcium intake to prevent maternal bone demineralization. Other calcium sources include green, leafy vegetables and calcium-fortified foods, sources more acceptable to cultures with a history of lactose intolerance (African, Mexican, and some European groups).

A woman who eats a well-balanced diet should gain sufficient vitamins and minerals for maternal and fetal needs during pregnancy. However, most health care providers recommend that the pregnant woman include 30 mg of elemental iron daily

TABLE 16-4 NUTRITIONAL NEEDS FOR PREGNANT AND LACTATING WOMEN

NUTRIENT	PREGNANCY	LACTATION	SOURCES	COMMENTS
Calories	+300	+500	Eat a variety from all food groups	Begin to increase calories in second and third trimesters
Protein	70 g	70 g	Lean meat, fish, eggs, poultry, milk, and dairy products	Supports fetal growth and development; formation of placenta and amniotic fluid; and expanded blood volume
Calcium	1000 mg/day	1000 mg/day	Milk, cheese, dark green leafy vegetables, nuts, and dried fruit	Women with low calcium intake require calcium supplements with vitamin D
Iron	27 mg/day	9 mg/day	Lean meats, dark green leafy vegetables, eggs, whole grain, dried fruit, and shellfish	Provides iron for fetal liver storage, which sustains infant for first 4 to 6 months of life
Folic acid	600 mcg	500 mcg	Fresh green leafy vegetables, liver, peanuts, whole-grain breads, and cereals	All women of childbearing age should take 400 mcg of folic acid daily to prevent neural tube defects in first trimester
Fats	30% of daily calories	30% of daily calories	Low-fat dairy products and lean cuts of meat	Provides a valuable source of energy for the body during pregnancy
Carbohydrates (CHOs)	7-11 servings daily	7-11 servings daily	Dairy products, fruits, vegetables, whole-grain cereals, and breads	Provides fiber necessary for proper bowel functioning. CHO intake needs to be sufficient to prevent ketoacidosis from protein use for energy

From Thompson, J., & Manore, M. (2012). *Nutrition: An applied approach* (3rd ed.). San Francisco, CA: Benjamin Cummings.

to benefit both mother and fetus, particularly during the last trimester. Anemia of pregnancy is a global health problem affecting nearly half of all pregnant women worldwide. High fetal demands for iron render iron deficiency the most common cause of anemia of pregnancy. In certain geographical populations, human pathogens such as hookworm, malarial parasite, and human immunodeficiency virus (HIV) are important factors in anemia of pregnancy. The hemoglobinopathies—sickle cell disease and thalassemia—represent diverse causes of anemia of pregnancy, requiring specialized care. Iron deficiency anemia is common among pregnant women, and anemia contributes to hemorrhage, postpartum infection, and preterm birth. Anemia occurs more often among pregnant adolescent, Black, and older White women (Lee & Okam, 2011).

In recent years, a number of studies have been performed to evaluate the possible health benefits of an increased intake of folic acid. However, the only well-documented benefit emerging from randomized controlled trials, nonrandomized intervention trials, and observational studies is the risk reduction of neural tube defects (NTDs). NTDs are congenital malformations that include anencephaly, encephalocele, and spina bifida caused by the failure of fusion of the neural tube that normally closes between the 22nd and 28th days since conception (on an average of 40 to 42 days after the first day of the last menstrual period). The occurrence of NTDs varies among the population between 0.8 and 3 per 1000 births, and it is estimated that 324,000 pregnancies are affected every year worldwide. Increased consumption of folic acid can decrease NTD risk to 0.6 per 1000 births (Mastroiacovo & Leoncini, 2011). To decrease NTD risk, it is recommended that all women capable of becoming pregnant should consume more folic acid. The goal is that every woman could start her pregnancy with an optimal folate status. Evidence-based research thus supports that women planning pregnancy and those in their first trimester take 0.4 mg (400 micrograms [mcg]) of folic acid in a daily

multivitamin supplement to prevent neural tube defects and anemia. This is particularly important for women with multiple gestations who experience a greater risk of anemia. However, research has shown that only 25% of women of childbearing age consume this amount of folic acid, which is critical for early fetal development (USDHHS, 2010).

Fats and carbohydrates must supply the caloric requirements during pregnancy. Although increased protein intake provides more calories, the body-building requirements of pregnancy and fetal growth demand most of the added protein. Fats and carbohydrates remain the most important sources of energy and essential vitamins and minerals. Supplemental vitamins and minerals, although not known to cause maternal or fetal harm if taken in reasonable dosages, probably cost the pregnant woman more to meet the nutritional needs of pregnancy than does a well-balanced diet.

The practice of pica, a psychobehavorial disorder characterized by the ingestion of nonfood substances such as dirt, clay, starch, and ice, may negatively influence the quality of a pregnant woman's nutrition during pregnancy. Pica in humans can be classified by the type of ingested substance. The three main substances consumed by pregnant women are soil or clay (geophagia), ice (pagophagia), and laundry or corn starch (amylophagia). Other pica cravings include burnt matches, stones, charcoal, mothballs, soap, sand, plaster, coffee grounds, baking soda, paint chips, and glue (Njiru et al., 2011). Common in rural pregnant Black women, this practice may contribute to iron deficiency anemia and interfere with nutrient absorption, particularly among women of lower economic status. Other potential complications may include lead poisoning, fecal impaction, parasitic infections, prematurity, perinatal mortality, low-birth-weight infants, and anemia in the infant (Dudek, 2010). Pica is often practiced by African American women, usually in the rural southern United States. It is thought to occur as a result of an iron deficiency that leads to the craving and/or a carryover from behaviors practiced in Africa (Mattson & Smith, 2011). The nurse completes a nutritional assessment on any pregnant woman. The nurse identifies instances of pica and suggests a culturally sensitive diet that will better meet the needs of the woman and her developing fetus. It is essential that the nurse remain nonjudgmental but stress the importance of an adequate diet, folic acid, and iron supplements, and the dangers of pica.

The best time to teach a woman about prenatal nutrition is before she becomes pregnant. Most women do not seek prenatal care until they suspect pregnancy. Therefore the nurse often delivers information about optimal nutrition to the pregnant woman after critical fetal development has already begun. If all school children received nutrition information as part of their kindergarten through twelfth grade curriculum (a primary prevention approach), women might have better overall personal nutrition established through lifestyle practices of individuals and families that would support high-quality prenatal nutrition later in their lives. Without such a primary prevention approach, secondary prevention intervention during pregnancy occurs through laboratory monitoring of iron levels, assessment of the woman's feelings of well-being, determination of the woman's actual intake of essential nutrients, and assessment of her pattern and total weight gain during the pregnancy. Many pregnant women work outside the home and may be among the increasing numbers of American families who spend 40% of their food budgets on food eaten outside the home (USDHHS, 2010). The nurse alerts the pregnant woman and her family to the documented high amounts of cholesterol, calories, sodium, and fat and low amounts of iron and calcium that these foods contain so as to improve nutritional intake during pregnancy.

In June 2011, the United States Department of Agriculture (USDA) unveiled a new food icon, *MyPlate,* which replaces *MyPyramid* as the government's primary food group symbol. *MyPlate* is meant to serve as a simple guide to help consumers choose healthful foods. In order to build a "healthy plate," *MyPlate* suggests that consumers choose fruits, vegetables, whole grains, low-fat dairy products, and lean protein foods to get essential nutrients without excess calories. Strategies for creating such a plate include filling half of your plate with fruits and vegetables; using whole grains for at least half of your daily grains consumed (e.g., 100% whole-grain cereals, breads, and pasta); switching from whole milk to skim or 1% milk; and choosing a variety of protein sources (e.g., seafood, small portions of lean meat and poultry, and beans). It also recommends that women should avoid shark, swordfish, king mackerel, or tilefish when they are pregnant or breastfeeding. These fish contain high levels of mercury and should be avoided. In summary, the pregnant woman needs to follow the *USDA Daily Food Plans for Moms* as follows:

- Fruits and vegetables—7 or more servings daily (3 servings of fruit and 4 of vegetables)
- Whole-grains or enriched breads/cereals—6 to 9 servings daily
- Dairy products—3 to 4 servings of low-fat or nonfat milk, yogurt, or cheese daily

- Meat and beans—3 servings daily (one serving = 2 ounces) (USDA, 2011).

See Chapter 11 for more information on nutrition including *MyPlate.*

Elimination Pattern

Fetus

The fetus accomplishes all essential elimination functions through the placenta. Carbon dioxide, water, urea, and other waste products pass through the placenta, to be eliminated by the mother's body. By the end of the first trimester, the fetus swallows, makes respiratory movements, and urinates. However, these abilities become truly functional only after birth.

Pregnant Woman

The pregnant woman experiences changes in her elimination pattern because of the enlarging uterus and hormonal influences. These changes (urinary frequency during the first and third trimesters, constipation, and hemorrhoids) cause normal, minor discomforts. Anticipatory guidance by the nurse helps the pregnant woman cope with these changes and prevent complications of pregnancy. For example, teaching the pregnant woman commonsense measures (Box 16-6: Innovative Practice) may prevent urinary tract infections (UTIs), typically a problem that is more common during pregnancy. With a known correlation between UTIs and premature labor, a focus on preventing and managing these infections must occur during pregnancy.

Activity-Exercise Pattern

Fetus

Early spontaneous movements of the fetus may be reflexive, stimulated by passive uterine movement. Ultrasonographic observation of fetal movement shows repetitive movements early in pregnancy; at about 16 weeks, the pregnant woman feels these movements, termed **quickening.** By the end of the second trimester, fetal movement occurs less frequently because of lack of space in the uterus. The woman and her partner look forward to the regular daily cycle of movements, indicators of fetal well-being. An absence of or dramatic increase in fetal movements for more than 8 hours may indicate fetal distress. The nurse routinely teaches a pregnant woman to count the number of fetal movements each day typically starting at 28 weeks' gestation and report any changes in fetal activity to the health care provider.

Pregnant Woman

The physical changes during pregnancy and the rigors of labor and delivery require that a pregnant woman be in the best physical condition of her life. Fortunately many pregnant women view pregnancy as a normal, natural state, and they often participate actively in physical activities or sports enjoyed before pregnancy. Generally a woman should avoid high-risk sports, such as sky diving and high-altitude climbing, because these could cause trauma to the fetus from low oxygen pressure or a maternal fall. Nurses encourage each woman to choose activities based on her interests,

Evidence-Based Practice for Preventing Urinary Tract Infections and Promoting Genitourinary Health

- Increase fluid intake to approximately 8 to 10 glasses per day; plain water is best to flush the body's systems of potential toxins; drink a glass of water before sexual intercourse to allow urinary output afterward to prevent UTIs.
- Avoid bladder irritants such as caffeine products, alcohol, artificial sweeteners, spicy foods, and carbonated beverages.
- Make urination a regular habit; avoid waiting to urinate until bladder is full.
- Urinate before and after sexual intercourse to cleanse the urethra and empty the bladder.
- Be aware that vigorous or frequent intercourse may contribute to increased risk of UTIs.
- Maintain consistently good perineal hygiene, including wiping from front to back after urination and defecation.
- Take all prescription medications given for UTIs, even when the symptoms of the infection have been alleviated.
- Drink cranberry juice to acidify the urine or take cranberry pills; these products may relieve some of the symptoms of a UTI. Cranberry *(Vaccinium macrocarpon)* has demonstrated antiinflammatory, antiadhesive, and antioxidant properties.
- Seek health care advice for a vaginal infection, which may contribute to development of a UTI.
- Nurses need to be aware that most UTIs are caused by *Escherichia coli* and the majority of women may be asymptomatic. Obtaining a urine specimen and culture is needed with any degree of suspicion of a UTI.
- Approximately half of UTIs in pregnancy occur in women with preexisting asymptomatic bacteriuria, and these UTIs have poor outcomes, including preterm rupture of membranes, preterm birth, neonatal infection, preeclampsia, maternal anemia, amnionitis, and maternal septic shock (O'Dell, 2011).
- The nurse should assess for increased risk of developing a UTI: congenital or structural abnormalities of the genitourinary system, previous surgery to the genitourinary system; pregnancy; previous UTIs; high intake of carbonated beverages; and poor intake of water.

UTI, Urinary tract infection.

comfort, and good judgment. When a sport or activity causes exhaustion or pain, it should be modified or discontinued. Later in pregnancy the woman should be encouraged to choose safe physical activities because of changes in her center of gravity attributable to the enlarging uterus and in the musculoskeletal system.

The woman with a sedentary lifestyle before pregnancy should slowly increase her activity level during pregnancy. A daily swim or 30-minute walk provides a good introduction to a regular exercise program. Regular exercise contributes to joint flexibility, improved cardiovascular and gastrointestinal fitness, uterine tone for an efficient labor, fewer pregnancy discomforts, weight control and a lower risk for diabetes, and overall feelings of well-being in the pregnant woman (USDHHS, 2010). For the self-directed woman, prenatal classes or a consumer-oriented book of prenatal exercises will facilitate an adequate exercise program. For most women, group exercise with other pregnant women is more enjoyable than exercising alone. The benefits of physical activity in the general population are established and research suggests regular physical activity following childbirth is linked with improved health outcomes. However,

many women do not resume prepregnancy exercise levels. The nurse encourages women to enter a structured diet and exercise program sponsored by the birthing hospital to help women lose weight after childbirth (Gaston & Gammage, 2011).

In an uncomplicated pregnancy, a couple may continue their usual sexual activity. However, threatened abortion or history of abortion in the first trimester, early rupture of membranes, and other complications may call for restrictions on sexual intercourse or orgasm.

Sleep-Rest Pattern

Fetus

Electroencephalographic studies have shown four cyclical states of activity in the fetus: complete wakefulness, drowsy wakefulness, rapid eye movement sleep, and quiet sleep. Evidence suggests that a diurnal (day-night) pattern exists during the fetal period. Sleep is required for somatic and brain growth and development. Sleep-wake patterns change with central nervous system maturation. In one research study, the median relative percentage time spent in a quiet state was 26%. The median duration of time spent in a quiet state was 15.7 minutes within a 1-hour recording. Both quiet states and active states were established in 84% of the fetuses studied (Suwanrath & Suntharasai, 2010). Infant development entails increasing amounts of quiet sleep as well as increasing periods of quiet alertness. Both states require remarkable neural organization; thus sleep-wake patterns are an excellent window to the infant's neurological status.

Pregnant Woman

Fatigue reflects the significant physical and emotional changes occurring in the pregnant woman. The nurse counsels a woman that fatigue usually subsides by the fourth month but may return later in pregnancy. Rest breaks during the day and 8 hours of sleep each night help prevent fatigue and increase the pregnant woman's comfort. The nurse encourages each pregnant woman to rest when her body signals it is tired because of the rapidly growing fetus and the woman's needs for physical renewal. This encouragement must be directed particularly toward working women, who may need a physician's note for their employer that validates the need for rest during the workday.

Many pregnant women do not sleep well because they need to urinate several times a night during the first and third trimesters. In addition, some women experience positional discomfort in late pregnancy that prevents effective sleep and, therefore, increases their fatigue. Fatigue may influence a woman's evaluation of her role as a pregnant woman, her body changes, and her cultural beliefs related to her ability to succeed in pregnancy. The nurse helps the woman express her thoughts and feelings and find ways to support better sleep and rest patterns (e.g., sleeping upright in a chair at night for easier breathing).

Cognitive-Perceptual Pattern

Fetus

During the prenatal period, although motor functions lag behind, all fetal sensory systems function or nearly function.

FIGURE 16-4 The pregnant woman enjoys time with family while pregnant.

These systems include vision, hearing, taste, smell, touch, and proprioceptive and vestibular senses (Polin et al., 2011). The fetus with all senses intact does experience the discomfort of pregnancy and the pain of labor contractions. The visual system matures relatively late in gestation, especially compared with the tactile, olfactory, and auditory systems. Although capable of seeing by 30 weeks of age, the fetus has little opportunity to use this ability in utero because of the absence of light (Del Giudice, 2011). After approximately 25 weeks, pregnant women note that their babies respond to a loud, sudden noise. Some pregnant women and their partners offer sensory stimulation to the fetus by singing or rubbing the woman's abdomen. This parental behavior may assist in the bonding process between parent and baby. Thus the nurse may wish to include this kind of information in prenatal teaching sessions.

Pregnant Woman

Physical and psychological processes remain closely intertwined as pregnancy progresses. Psychological stresses and normal emotional growth affect the physical status of the pregnancy, interactions of the family members, and the eventual relationship between mother and infant. When considering the emotional aspects of pregnancy, the nurse recognizes that the woman's personality, environment, physical state, family, and sociocultural and spiritual background affect the ways in which she handles the psychological changes (Figure 16-4).

Two major categories of psychological influences are normal psychological growth required of parents to emotionally and physically prepare them for parenthood; and internal or external stressors on the pregnant woman that decrease her ability to provide the best environment for the developing fetus. The pregnant woman undergoes many cognitive changes that ultimately result in her psychological readiness for motherhood.

Emotional Changes. Hormonal and other physical changes assist the woman in the psychological work of pregnancy. Progesterone level increases affect the woman's general mood, causing her to be more introverted and passive. These mood changes help her to focus her energy on the growing child and

her own growth and development. In addition to hormonal changes, the presence, growth, and movements of the fetus become more a part of the woman's experiential self. According to Rubin (1984), the classic researcher on maternal-infant bonding, the pregnant woman receives immediate sensations of touch, motion, and weight from the fetus that she can share only partially with others. These support a maternal feeling of separateness and uniqueness that causes the woman to turn inward. She frequently worries that the shift in energy away from the world toward herself and her child may cause her to lose contact, drift away from valued relationships, and lose feelings of competence in her areas of achievement. She spends time analyzing her experiences and their possible influence on her effectiveness as a future parent. She constantly studies the qualities of human relationships and shows increased sensitivity and perceptiveness to many people. To others, the woman may seem overly sensitive and analytical during pregnancy (Rubin, 1967, 1984).

Although a woman's mood varies based on a variety of factors and at different times during the pregnancy, many women experience wide mood swings, emotional lability, irritability, and changes in sexual desire. Physical discomforts, hormonal changes, feelings about altered body image, cultural considerations, work and relationship adjustments, and demanding cognitive maturational processes may also cause these emotional changes.

Rubin's classic work stimulated nurses to look beyond the physiological and pathological aspects of childbearing to the intricate process of becoming a mother, and to identify areas for providing help. Current research identifies two simultaneous processes in the transition to motherhood: engagement and growth and transformation. Engagement is making a commitment and being engrossed in mothering through active involvement in the child's care. At the same time, the woman's engagement leads to the woman's growth and transition as she becomes a mother (Miller, 2011).

Current descriptions for the stages in the process of establishing a maternal identity in becoming a mother include the following:
- Commitment, attachment, and preparation for the pregnancy
- Acquaintance, learning, and physical restoration during the first 6 weeks after birth
- Moving toward a new normal from 2 weeks to 4 months

Stressors Influencing Development. The mother's age, fears related to a previous fetal loss, feelings about the pregnancy, life situation and culture, degree of stress, the presence of other children, loss of control at times, unintended pregnancy, and the influence of loved ones may serve as stressors that influence the ways in which she completes the developmental tasks of motherhood. Women with unwanted pregnancies have multiple risk factors and would benefit from targeted interventions (Maxson & Miranda, 2011). A young pregnant woman facing the additional developmental task of adolescence may have difficulty incorporating the pregnant body or the role of mother into her still undefined self-image. Cognitively, she may still be unable to make plans for the baby or even accept the pregnancy until she feels the baby move. Anticipatory guidance is critical when an adolescent faces overlapping developmental challenges of age and pregnancy.

On the other hand, a pregnant woman older than 35 years may feel more isolated by her situation than does the pregnant woman in her twenties. Frequently established in career and family, the older pregnant woman needs to learn to balance her growth and development in these valued areas with her new sense of self. Fears related to being considered at high risk because of age may increase her anxiety and ambivalence about the pregnancy, even if she was previously infertile. As a first-time mother, she may worry about managing the physical demands of labor and delivery, sleeplessness of motherhood, chances of having an abnormal child, and the need to juggle conflicting life responsibilities and relationships.

A woman with other children moves through the developmental tasks differently than does a woman who is pregnant for the first time. Even with a desired pregnancy, the woman may worry about incorporating the new infant into her relationships and managing the time needed for a new baby. She may have fears and anxieties about labor and delivery because of a previous negative experience. She may be much more aware of the problems involved with caring for a new infant and may not be excited about another pregnancy experience that demands a redefinition of motherhood or additional childrearing expenses.

Developmental Tasks

Rubin (1967, 1977, 1984) describes four major developmental tasks that a woman seeks to accomplish as she learns to become a mother. These include ensuring safe passage through pregnancy and childbirth, ensuring acceptance of the child by significant people in her family, binding to her unknown child, and learning to give of self. According to Rubin, all four tasks must be confronted simultaneously, but each task assumes greater priority at certain times than do other tasks. Each woman works through these tasks based on her unique style, cultural values, and life priorities. At the end of pregnancy, however, all tasks must be integrated to create a presentation, similar to a tapestry (Rubin, 1984).

Ensuring Safe Passage

- The woman engages in a variety of prenatal care options appropriate to her culture and life experience. For example, pregnant Cambodian women rely on older same-culture women to give prenatal care and advice and rely little on prenatal classes or visits. Some Hispanic American women, based on their view that pregnancy is a healthy, natural experience, may not seek prenatal care but seek a strong matriarchal support system for a positive outcome.
- The woman becomes more protective of herself and the fetus by avoiding crowds, revolving doors, small spaces, and people believed to place the mother at risk. She tires of being pregnant but fears the effect of delivery on her safety and that of her child (Rubin, 1972, 1984). Although sharing fears and desires with her partner, family, or health care provider helps, only the safe delivery

of a normal child can fully free a pregnant woman from her fears to meet this developmental task (Rubin, 1972, 1977).

Ensuring Acceptance of the Child

- The woman must believe that her child will be accepted into her family based on her definition of family. According to Rubin (1984), the partner's receptivity to the child is particularly important, and many women fantasize about the gender of their child based on a partner's preference.
- The woman frequently judges her partner's degree of receptivity to the infant by the amount of love and attention that she, herself, receives from him during her pregnancy.
- She may desire support from other women, rather than her partner, based on her life experience, values, and cultural background.

Binding into Her Unknown Child

- This task is the most complex cognitive process for the pregnant woman (Rubin, 1984). To accomplish this task, the woman must integrate the fetus as an integral part of herself but also as a separate being. Completion of this task occurs with birth of the baby.
- Initially, the woman fantasizes about the baby through associative images: when she eats an egg, she thinks of the baby. Fantasies in the second and third trimesters relate more specifically to what the child will be like; the woman may imagine the baby in little girl or little boy clothes.
- During the eighth month, the woman begins nesting activity by preparing the nursery and thinking increasingly of the baby as an external reality in her home.

Learning to Give of Herself

- Although the actual mothering activity occurs after birth, the learning process to become a mother begins during pregnancy.
- The woman begins the task by examining what she will gain and lose by becoming a mother.
- She then explores the meaning of giving by examining how others give to her and to others and how she has given to others in the past (Rubin, 1984).
- Gifts for herself and the baby represent meaningful manifestations of her own and others' acceptance of her motherhood and her ability to give to her child and develop her identity as mother (Rubin, 1967, 1972).

Self-Perception–Self-Concept Pattern

To develop a maternal identity, the woman must first accept the pregnant body image. Initially she may show ambivalence based on her need to "fit" the pregnancy with her perception of self. She may dislike the physical changes of pregnancy or gladly "show off" her pregnant body to others. During the second trimester, however, the woman frequently begins to feel more positive about her changing womanly image as she feels the baby move, and increased amounts of estrogen and progesterone enhance her sense of vitality, inner peace, and acceptance. Her body begins to look pregnant, and generally others respond positively to this change (Rubin, 1972).

By the third trimester, however, the woman frequently tires of the pregnancy. Her sense of awkward moments supersedes feelings of well-being. She may experience uncomfortable, sleepless nights, the constant need to urinate, Braxton-Hicks contractions, and other discomforts. Some women experience infant movement or mild contractions as pleasurable, sensual sensations, whereas others find them extremely uncomfortable. By pregnancy's end, these women yearn to have their former body boundaries back, to hold the baby in their arms, or to have someone else carry the baby.

After birth, the woman gradually sees the infant more and more as a separate individual, dependent on her care. The mother starts to bond with her baby based on her self-perception. If she feels good about herself, she will show love toward the infant; when she feels ugly or unlovable, she may make uncomplimentary remarks about the infant's appearance (Rubin, 1984).

Maternal Role

The pregnant woman's personality, maturity level, and psychological development influence her readiness to assume the role of mother. The way in which society in general and her culture in particular perceive motherhood and the role of women, as well as the way in which her own views mesh with these perceptions, will affect the ease of the transition. The family situation, the availability of peer role models, and the relationship with her mother are also significant. Internalization of the mother role occurs only after the birth, when the woman interacts with the infant in a reciprocal relationship (Rubin, 1977).

Nursing Interventions

The woman may feel overwhelmed by her feelings and thoughts during pregnancy. Although others acknowledge her physical changes, only she experiences the psychological changes of excitement, ambivalence, or confusion associated with being pregnant.

During prenatal assessment, the nurse should address expected cognitive changes and self-image issues with each pregnant woman and respond nonjudgmentally to concerns expressed in this area. In one-to-one sessions or group prenatal classes, women and their partners should be encouraged to discuss their ideas and feelings related to the emotional and relationship changes expected during pregnancy, because these changes influence the future intimate relationship.

Education and practice on the maternal role and being a mother is an effective intervention in increasing self-confidence in caring and maternal identity. During their transition to motherhood, pregnant women want attentive, proactive, professional psychosocial support from nurses. They expect nurses to oversee the transition period and to be capable of supporting them in dealing with changes in pregnancy and in preparing for birth and motherhood.

Roles-Relationships Pattern

The pregnant family changes throughout the pregnancy and postpartum period as each family member explores and responds to new roles and relationships. A pregnant woman without a partner may feel isolated during pregnancy and depend on family or friends as she adjusts to her situation. Cultural beliefs and traditions may produce stresses during pregnancy, change roles and relationships, or provide emotional and physical support to the pregnant family as it prepares for the baby.

The partner of the pregnant woman faces many new situations that influence that person's parental development. The pregnant woman may seem to be a different person to others because of her emotional response to the pregnancy, introspection, fantasies, need for more rest, and changes in sexual drive. The partner may feel a rivalry with the fetus and baby, because the mother is devoting increasing amounts of time to the baby. He may resent the attention that she receives during the pregnancy and the additional demands that she may make on his time. He may experience more financial pressure because of baby expenses and his partner's need to stop working on a short-term or long-term basis. These perceptions may lead him to batter or otherwise abuse his partner, possibly causing poor pregnancy and newborn outcomes (Box 16-7: Quality and Safety Scenario). The nurse assesses each pregnant woman for abuse and intervenes appropriately to protect the safety and health of the family during gestation.

The male partner may be concerned about his ability to fulfill the father role and support his wife or significant other. His fathering role models may be limited because of a lack of contact with his own father or because he spends time with men who are not actively parenting. He may never have held a baby before and may worry that he might drop or harm his own child. If his partner experiences pregnancy complications, he may feel guilty about causing the pregnancy. Table 16-5 gives a more complete list of both the father's and the mother's emotional responses to a first pregnancy. The nurse must work with the pregnant family to help them adapt to a first pregnancy, because this one affects how they will cope with subsequent pregnancies.

Children in the family also experience role changes during and after the pregnancy. The very young child, unaware of the concept of a new baby before the infant arrives, may experience a changed relationship with his pregnant mother. She may have less time to play, be more irritable from fatigue, or limit or stop active play late in pregnancy because of increased awkwardness and concern about her safety. After the baby arrives, the child may be kept away from both baby and mother by well-meaning friends and relatives, have to share parents with others, or may want to breastfeed from the mother as the baby does. When permitted to see the newborn, the child may be admonished to "be careful" or "don't touch the baby." Thus a young child may not accept the baby with open arms.

The older child understands the newborn's significance more clearly but still experiences apprehensions about the effects of the baby on the family. Older children may have been told that they will become a big brother or sister, but does this mean they will lose toys and time with parents, and have to give up a private bedroom? Older children may worry about their mother, who seems more tired, less available, and perhaps even sick at times. Her enlarging abdomen may appear frightening. With help from the nurse, parents can make

BOX 16-7 **QUALITY AND SAFETY SCENARIO**

Birth Outcomes in Abused Pregnant Women

Nurses and other providers who deliver health care to women must address the issue of abuse of the pregnant woman by an intimate partner. Intimate partner violence is a significant public health problem with negative physical and psychological outcomes. It has been associated with increased levels of sexually transmitted infections, preterm labor, low-birth-weight infants, anxiety, substance abuse behaviors, and postpartum depression (Brownridge et al., 2011). Consider the following research study and the questions that follow to understand the issue further.

Several studies have attempted to identify risk factors associated with experiencing violence during pregnancy. However, all of these previous studies compared women who were abused during pregnancy to nonabused pregnant women. To further the understanding of risk factors for experiencing violence during pregnancy, it may be useful to investigate factors that differentiate female victims of intimate partner violence (IPV) who were and were not victimized during pregnancy. This will allow us to shed light on unique aspects of pregnancy violence. In addition, the current study examines risk factors using a nationally representative sample. The **risk factors** identified included *young age, less than a high school education, unemployment of mother and/or father,* and *violence in the family of origin; unmarried status* increased the risk of violence during pregnancy, but also the relative risk was even greater if the women separated or divorced while pregnant; *paternal uncertainty* and accusations of infidelity have been associated with an increased risk of violence among pregnant women. Male partners may develop paternal assurance tactics, such as the use of violence to establish control, to combat paternal uncertainty and increase the probability that the children he raises are his own and there is no infidelity on the part of the woman. *Patriarchal domination* has also been linked to an increased risk of violence against women. Pregnancy may symbolize a time when the woman assumes more control over her own body and may represent a degree of independence from her male partner; violence against the pregnant partner may represent a male partner's attempt to reassert control. Many women who are abused during pregnancy have reported that their partners attempt to

socially isolate them from family, friends, and other social support systems. The majority of women reporting physical violence during pregnancy are also victims of *verbal abuse* and psychological aggression. In fact, psychological abuse may be the predominant form of abuse during pregnancy in some cultures. And women who had a *partner with a drinking problem* were more than 3 times as likely to be abused during pregnancy compared to women whose partner did not have a drinking problem.

The **health outcomes** of violence against pregnant women include being *kicked, punched, thrown down stairs, threatened with knives, choked, scalded, pushed out of moving cars,* and *having objects thrown* at them. A number of violence-related injuries also include *cuts, bruises, fractures, concussions, dental injuries, stab wounds, vaginal bleeding,* and *persistent headaches*. Mental health issues include *depression, stress, distress, fearfulness, anxiousness,* and feelings of *isolation*.

Nursing Implications

Overall, this study indicates a need for nurses to screen for high-risk factors prenatally, to be aware of the health risks secondary to violence, and to tailor nursing interventions supportive of pregnant women facing abuse. Nurses need to be aware of the issues surrounding pregnancy violence and have the ability to provide pregnant women with the resources and information necessary to ensure their safety.

Questions

• How do the current health care system and the sociopolitical context of care in this country contribute to the high numbers of pregnant women facing abuse from their intimate partners?

• What kind of interventions do you believe would be effective for these abused women?

• How should U.S. health care policy ethically and legislatively address the problem of intimate partner abuse during pregnancy?

Data from Brownridge, D. A., Taillieu, T. L., Tyler, K. A., Tiwari, A., Ko Ling, C., & Santos, S. C. (2011). Pregnancy and intimate partner violence: Risk factors, severity, and health effects. *Violence Against Women, 17*(7), 858-881.

pregnancy an exciting time of learning and growing for the family (Box 16-8). Chapter 18 also discusses the sibling relationship in greater detail.

In extended families, expectant grandparents also experience changes during the pregnancy of their daughter or daughter-in-law. The maternal grandmother, seeing her daughter assume the mother role, may now view her daughter as a rival, because they are both mothers. The grandparents may be reminded of their own aging, resenting when their advice about pregnancy and parenting goes unheeded. A positive outcome of a pregnancy may be a new closeness between woman and mother if the daughter turns to her mother to seek advice and share feelings. The nurse may encourage expectant parents to use pregnancy as a transition time for their own parents, which can enhance extended family cohesion in the future.

During pregnancy and after birth, each family member begins to establish an emotional attachment to the imagined or real new baby. Research shows that when the mother has a strong support system to develop deep feelings of attachment to the fetus, she will most likely attach to the baby after birth. Therefore the nurse assesses the support system of each

pregnant woman and implements primary and secondary interventions to increase family bonding with a new baby.

Sexuality-Reproductive Pattern

The pregnant woman's body image and merging of this body image with her definition of femininity greatly influence her feelings about her sexuality. For a previously infertile couple, achieving pregnancy may be a blessed event, despite the need for technology that affects a woman's concept of self and femininity and a man's concept of self and masculinity. The reflections of others, particularly those of a pregnant woman's husband, partner, or friend, help a woman to accept changes in her body, leading to better adjustment in their sexual relations.

On the other hand, women may experience different sexual feelings during pregnancy. Some women experience an increase in desire, but many worry about intercourse during pregnancy, fearing that it will cause miscarriage, infection, or an early birth. Other women may suffer from nausea during pregnancy or simply lack sexual interest. Physical discomfort, fatigue, and awkwardness as well as fear of membrane rupture, infection, or harm to the fetus may also diminish the woman's

TABLE 16-5   POSSIBLE RESPONSES TO FIRST PREGNANCY

PHASE OF PREGNANCY	FATHER'S RESPONSE	MOTHER'S RESPONSE
First trimester	Fear of losing wife or child	Loss of interest in coitus
	Self-doubt as a future father	Possible less sexual effectiveness
	May develop new hobby outside of partner as way of distancing self	Sleepiness and chronic fatigue
		Nausea
		Increased dependence
		Feels ambivalent toward reality of pregnancy
		Anxious about process of labor and prospect of caring for a child
		Worries about miscarriage
		Becomes aware of physical changes in her body
		May develop a closer relationship with her mother with a common experience of motherhood
Second trimester	Increased respect	Solemnity, hilarity, and playfulness about fetal movements
	Awe as quickening comes	Talks about and with fetus
	Names for fetus coined	Increased eroticism
	May give partner extra attention she desires	Expects partner to demonstrate interest in caring for her and baby
		Feels movement and thinks of child as an individual
Third trimester	Fear of coitus hurting fetus	Abstinence (often recommended by physician)
	Abstinence difficult	Sleepiness
	Envy or pride, or both, at wife's creativity	Backache
	Worry about birth	Abdominal discomfort
	Keen awareness of male-female differences	Sexual isolation
	May show a greater level of tenderness and protectiveness	Heightened sense of femininity
		Assembles items needed for care of infant and selects possible names
Postpartum	Eagerness to resume marital relations	Pain and fear of harm from too early coitus
	Concern over endangering wife's recovery	Low eroticism
	Sense of triumph in becoming a father	Concern about effect on husband of continued abstinence
	Tenderness toward wife and baby	Sense of completion as a mother
Pregnancy as a whole	Increased romanticism	Increased romanticism
	Increased nurturance	Increased optimism
	Increased family life participation	Family roles replacing marital emphases
	Financial stress	Fear of miscarriage or problems with baby
	Concern about lack of skills in baby care	Pride of accomplishment
		Emotional stress, feeling overloaded

Sources: Dunkel Schetter, C. (2011). Psychological science on pregnancy: Stress processes, biopsychosocial models, and emerging research issues. *Annual Review of Psychology, 62,* 531-558; Yu, M., McElory, J. A., Bullock, L. C., & Everett, K. D. (2011). Unique perspectives of women and their partners using the Prenatal Psychosocial Profile Scale. *Journal of Advanced Nursing, 67*(8), 1767-1778.

BOX 16-8   NURSING STRATEGIES TO HELP PARENTS PREPARE SIBLINGS FOR THE NEONATE

- Explain the pregnancy and birth appropriate to the child's age.
- Answer all the child's questions.
- Use relevant literature to educate the child about the coming baby.
- Encourage discussion and questions by talking about the new baby during relaxed family times rather than during busy, rushed times.
- Have the child participate in decisions, such as choosing a name, clothes, and toys for baby.
- When sibling classes are available as part of the childbirth education process, encourage parents and child to attend.
- Suggest that the child go with the mother during clinic or office visits.
- Allow and discuss negative comments about the pregnancy or baby.
- Encourage child to make drawings or give small gifts to the baby when it is born.

interest in sexual relations. Sexual dissatisfaction of the couple may result from restrictions in sexual positions, pain on penetration, increased vaginal discharge, breast tenderness, or the other physical discomforts of pregnancy such as fatigue and heartburn. In some cases the enlarging uterus will require the couple to modify positions for intercourse, particularly during the latter part of pregnancy. The couple's feelings about the woman's changing body may alter their sexual relationship. The nurse's first step in primary prevention intervention in this area is to support the couple's needs and to relate, in a sensitive fashion, accurate information that facilitates couple intimacy during pregnancy.

Some women experience a decreased desire for sexual intercourse but an increased desire for holding, touching, and other signs of physical affection from their husbands or partners. The nurse encourages the couple to explore other activities for mutual sexual satisfaction.

In summary, the nurse can use the following guidelines concerning sexual activity:

- Sex is generally considered safe in pregnancy.
- Abstinence should be recommended only for women who are at risk for preterm labor, or antepartum hemorrhage because of placenta previa.
- There is little evidence to show that sex at term may help induce labor, but this practice is considered safe in women with low-risk pregnancies (Jones et al., 2011).
- The resumption of intercourse postpartum should be dictated by a woman's level of comfort.

Coping-Stress Tolerance Pattern

Physical and psychological adaptations of the woman to pregnancy affect her perception of stressors and her ability to cope with all aspects of her life. Even normal discomforts of pregnancy may be stressful for a woman, mandating her to modify her usual routine to cope more effectively. Anxiety tends to be high during the first trimester as the woman adapts to pregnancy and anticipated life changes. During the second trimester, the woman feels less anxious, but anxiety returns during the third trimester with impending labor and delivery. Throughout pregnancy women may demonstrate their anxieties through psychosomatic complaints and behaviors, such as nausea and vomiting after the first trimester, excessive eating, food cravings, sleeplessness, and fainting. Realistically, every pregnant woman probably experiences some degree of stress. However, many women have considerable stress or ongoing stress, such as poverty, marital difficulties, or unsatisfactory living or working conditions, that influences their coping abilities.

A pregnant woman's anxieties may be reflected in her dreams and fantasies. Many pregnant women report dreams about their babies being deformed or dead, themselves dying, or a family member being injured. Many women at the end of their pregnancies express fears about body mutilation with delivery. Other women may manifest their anxiety by smoking, drinking, or using drugs (legal or illegal), all of which can harm the fetus. Prenatal depression and/or anxiety has been associated with excessive activity and growth delays in the fetus as well as prematurity, low birthweight, disorganized sleep, and less responsiveness to stimulation in the neonate. Infants of depressed/anxious mothers have difficult temperaments, and later in development attentional, emotional, and behavioral problems have been noted during childhood and adolescence, as well as chronic illnesses in adulthood (Field, 2011). The nurse must direct a pregnant woman who is not coping well to relevant resources for assistance. The nurse must also assess each woman's progress in taking on the mothering role as the pregnancy nears term. This information can be shared with the postpartum nursing staff to encourage discussion in this important area.

The nurse encourages the pregnant woman to use tension-relieving strategies such as listening to soft music, using humor, crying, sleeping, talking to a friend, meditating, exercising, and fantasizing during times of stress. These strategies are safe for the fetus and provide relief from many normal tensions and anxieties during pregnancy and afterward. Overall, the nurse plays a key role by responding nonjudgmentally and promoting the coping of women during pregnancy.

Values-Beliefs Pattern

Although pregnancy has been described as the fulfillment of the deepest and most powerful wish of a woman, this fulfillment often coincides with a woman's fear of losing part of herself. She gives up some relationships and pleasures to assume other anticipated satisfactions. She may find that she values friendships with other mothers now, whereas before pregnancy her friendships focused on work or school colleagues. She may discover, much to her husband's confusion, that she values different qualities in him than she did before anticipating birth. Her husband may also experience a shift in his values.

Pregnant women and their partners may experience changes in their spiritual values. For women with strong spiritual needs related to their cultural backgrounds, spiritual interventions will help them integrate various dimensions of their lives, develop the ability to parent successfully, and find meaning in the changes and goals of pregnancy. Seen as a mystical event or miracle, conception may lead to an increased faith in God or a favorite saint. Nonreligious couples may start to attend church after the baby's birth, because they want religion to be part of their child's life. Religious beliefs may influence a woman's decision to undergo certain tests or procedures, such as amniocentesis or abortion. Some women may feel forced to reproduce because their religious or cultural mores forbid contraception or encourage large families. In these groups, each pregnancy may be seen as another unwanted, but unavoidable, burden or may be valued because more children signify a stronger family.

ENVIRONMENTAL PROCESSES

Physical Agents

A healthy infant is the outcome of most pregnancies. However, genetic abnormalities and environmental hazards may cause fetal harm, spontaneous abortion (natural loss of conceptive products), or minor or serious congenital defects. Diagnostic methods that identify an early pregnancy or a fetal loss may assist couples in practicing healthy decisions to prevent loss or congenital abnormalities. Cunningham and colleagues (2010f) note that congenital defects affect 3% to 4% of all live births and contribute to infant mortality rates by causing structural or functional disability incompatible with life. Real-time ultrasonography identifies approximately 85% of fetal anomalies by 36 weeks of gestation (Gilbert, 2011). This knowledge, gained before giving birth, permits expectant couples and the health care delivery team to access resources for improving the baby's life or support family grieving if the baby is not expected to live. With progress made in diagnostic tools and the Human Genome Project, some couples may be able to prevent fetal defects or manage them during pregnancy to improve the quality of their baby's life after birth (see the Case Study at the end of this chapter). Unfortunately, even when no genetic or congenital defects exist, the fetus may still be injured during the process of labor and delivery and face a lesser quality of life.

Teratogens are environmental agents that cause spontaneous abortions or congenital defects. Unlike genetic abnormalities, which occur only at conception, environmental agents may affect the developing infant at any point during gestation. Fetal organs have critical periods of development and if affected at that time by a teratogen, the infant may have a defect in that organ system. **Website Resource 16C** depicts the effects of teratogens on the embryo and fetus. Teratogens normally do not cause a congenital defect during the first 14 days after conception. However, the embryo may be lost later during early gestation (a spontaneous abortion). Therefore, as a primary prevention strategy, any woman contemplating or attempting pregnancy should be counseled to avoid teratogens that might cause fetal loss or damage.

Physical Factors and Diagnostic Tools

Modern diagnostic tools, such as ultrasonography, amniocentesis, chorionic villus sampling, and alpha-fetoprotein screening have been used to identify a number of fetal problems. Many of these tools are presented in **Website Resource 16D**. Certain risk factors, such as family history, maternal and paternal age, maternal illness, or previous fetal abnormalities, may indicate the need for these diagnostic tools during a woman's pregnancy. These tools commonly identify problems related to abnormal size or rate of fetal growth, chromosomal abnormalities, neural tube defects, and fetal lung immaturity. The nurse, in consultation with the health care team, must participate in providing informed consent to women before these diagnostic tools are utilized.

Biological Agents

Biological processes in the fetal environment, which include infections and other health problems of the mother, may affect fetal growth and development. A pregnant woman who acquires an asymptomatic viral infection may not seek health care because she believes that the fetus will not be harmed. However, viral agents may cause fetal damage early in pregnancy. The woman with a health problem, such as diabetes, may also cause fetal damage if she fails to adhere to her health care provider's directives.

When the nurse discusses with pregnant couples the effects of biological processes on the fetus, she must emphasize that the timing of the maternal infection or illness is critical to predicting fetal defects. Maternal infections during the first trimester of pregnancy may cause severe fetal defects or death, depending on the organism. Infections later in pregnancy may also seriously affect the fetus, but less often. Unfortunately, pregnancy renders many women more susceptible to viral illness, supporting an argument for all women of childbearing age to be fully immunized. Many vaccines (measles, mumps, rubella, and polio) cannot be given during pregnancy because of potential risk to the fetus, but others present no risk (tetanus and diphtheria). A TORCH (**t**oxoplasmosis, **o**ther agents, **r**ubella, **c**ytomegalovirus, **h**erpes simplex) screen may be done to detect the presence of five teratogenic perinatal infections: toxoplasmosis, hepatitis B, rubella, cytomegalovirus, and herpes simplex (Table 16-6).

Toxoplasmosis

Toxoplasmosis is caused by a protozoan that infects people through consumption of undercooked meat, handling of cat feces, and exposure to infected soil in countries outside the United States (Friars, 2007). An infected pregnant woman may have

TABLE 16-6 TORCH PERINATAL INFECTIONS

INFECTION	AGENT	SOURCE	FETAL-NEONATAL RISKS	COMMENTS
Toxoplasmosis	Protozoan *Toxoplasma gondii*	Raw or undercooked meat; unpasteurized goat's milk; feces of infected cats	IUGR, hydrocephaly, seizures, neurological and cognitive effects, chorioretinitis, intracranial calcifications	Instruct mother to not eat undercooked or raw meat; avoid exposure to cat litter
Other/hepatitis B	Hepadnavirus	Blood or blood products; sexually transmitted via body fluids	Generally asymptomatic, but majority become chronically infected	Newborn should receive HBIG within 12 hours after birth and HepB vaccine postpartum
Rubella	Rubella virus	Direct or indirect contact with droplets of infected person	CNS defects, developmental delay, deafness, cataracts, IUGR, microcephaly, cardiac defects, glaucoma	Screen all pregnant women with rubella antibody titers
Cytomegalovirus	Herpesvirus	Transmitted by droplet infection from person to person	Microcephaly, IUGR, CNS abnormalities, deafness, blindness, jaundice, GI defects, seizures	Prevention of maternal primary infection in early pregnancy; stress good personal hygiene
Herpes simplex	HSV-1 and -2	Sexually transmitted infection to mother; fetus contacts it during birth from genital lesions	Intense herpetic lesions on eyes, mouth, and skin; keratitis; conjunctivitis	Practice safer sex; careful handwashing; surgical birth if active lesions

Compiled from Gilbert, E. S. (2011). *Manual of high risk pregnancy* (5th ed.). St. Louis: Mosby Elsevier; Mattson, S., & Smith, J.E. (2011). *Core curriculum for maternal-newborn nursing* (4th ed.). St. Louis: Saunders Elsevier; Fantasia, H., Fontenot, H. B., Sutherland, M., & Harris, A. L. (2011). Sexually transmitted infections in women. *Nursing for Women's Health, 15*(1), 46-58; Shet, A. (2011). Congenital and perinatal infections: Throwing new light with an old TORCH. *Indian Journal of Pediatrics, 78*(1), 88-95.
CNS, Central nervous system; *GI,* gastrointestinal; *HBIG,* hepatitis B immune globulin; *HepB,* hepatitis B; *HSV,* herpes simplex virus; *IUGR,* intrauterine growth restriction.

flulike symptoms or mild to severe upper respiratory symptoms believed to be unrelated to an infection. Vertical transmission from an infected pregnant woman to the fetus predominantly occurs when infection is acquired for the first time during pregnancy. Overall, about one third of infected pregnant women give birth to an infant with toxoplasmosis, and the risk of vertical transmission rises sharply with gestational age at maternal infection. However, fetuses infected during an early pregnancy period are much more likely to show clinical signs of infection, such as chorioretinitis or intracranial calcification (Tamaruet et al., 2011). About 60% of maternal infections acquired during the third trimester will result in fetal infection, which might manifest as skin rashes, enlarged lymph nodes and liver, inflammation of the heart, pneumonia, jaundice, or severe central nervous system damage after birth or years later (Greener, 2011). Nurses can offer some simple hygiene suggestions that reduce the risk of infection. For example, humans can acquire *toxoplasmosis* from eating undercooked or raw meat (especially lamb and pork), from being exposed to contaminated soil or water, or from consuming uncooked vegetables. Clearly, nurses should advise pregnant women to cook meat thoroughly and wash and scrub vegetables well, especially those eaten raw. Pregnant women should use good hand-washing technique, avoid eating raw meat, wear gloves when gardening, and avoid handling cats or cleaning cat litter boxes to avoid exposure to *Toxoplasma*.

Syphilis

An infected mother transfers syphilis, an STI that is caused by a protozoan, to her fetus. The causative organism, *Treponema pallidum,* can be transferred across the placenta and can infect the developing fetus as early as 6 weeks of gestation. The risk of vertical transmission and infection in the newborn is directly related to the stage of maternal syphilis during pregnancy; transmission occurs more frequently during primary or secondary syphilis in the mother than during latent stages of the disease. Although preventable and treatable, the number of congenital and neonatal syphilis cases has increased over the last several years (CDC, 2011c). Maternal risk factors for acquiring syphilis include homelessness, human immunodeficiency virus (HIV) positive status, single marital status, and a history of STIs. Maternal syphilis has been associated with complications such as hydramnios, spontaneous abortion, and preterm births. Fetal complications such as fetal syphilis, fetal hydrops, prematurity, fetal distress, and stillbirth also occur. Neonatal complications can include congenital syphilis, seizures, neonatal death, and late sequelae (Follett & Clarke, 2011). The infant may be born with localized mucocutaneous lesions, nasal congestion, anemia, and generalized septicemia, but may appear healthy at birth only to have symptoms appear later. Routine testing of high-risk women for syphilis at the first prenatal visit and during the third trimester and antibiotic treatment (crystalline penicillin G) for affected women and their partners have reduced the number of infants with congenital syphilis (Shet, 2011).

Rubella

Despite the broad use of the measles, mumps, and rubella vaccine, or MMR, and the resulting immunity to rubella, approximately 20% of women reach their childbearing period without immunity to this disease (USDHHS, 2010). The risk of vertical transmission from a nonimmune mother with primary rubella infection in the first trimester of pregnancy is considerably high at 80% to 90%. Beyond the first 12 weeks of gestation, fetal organogenesis is nearly complete, and deafness may be the only consequence in the infected infant (Shet, 2011). The symptoms of rubella may cause the mother to think she has a minor viral infection, but rubella during the first trimester may cause improper fetal development of the ears, eyes, and heart and deafness. No treatment exists for an infected fetus; however, a pregnant woman may receive the vaccine to protect future pregnancies if she has no history of rubella infection. After giving birth, new mothers often receive the vaccine before being discharged with a recommendation to avoid pregnancy for at least 3 months to prevent fetal harm from the vaccine.

Cytomegalovirus

Cytomegalovirus (CMV) is a leading cause of congenital infections and long-term neurodevelopmental disabilities among children. It is the most common infection that can cause serious fetal complications. CMV infects an estimated 1% to 2% of all infants born in the United States. Most mothers infected with CMV have mild, often nonspecific symptoms, but their infants may experience hearing loss, blindness, enlarged liver and spleen, seizures, intracranial calcifications, and neurodevelopmental disabilities (Nigro & Adler, 2011). Unfortunately, no means exist to prevent or manage this viral infection. Perhaps an immunization similar to that for rubella will be developed in the future. Until vaccines and nontoxic antiviral agents are available, hygienic measures are important as prophylaxis.

Herpes Simplex Virus

Herpes simplex virus infections remain extremely common today, with many people unaware that they have the disease. Herpes simplex may cause spontaneous abortion or fetal neurological damage. Infants infected at birth may show localized or generalized disease with symptoms of vesicular skin lesions, microcephaly, hydrocephalus, chorioretinitis, conjunctivitis, seizures, respiratory distress, or gastrointestinal bleeding. These symptoms may cause newborn death. An infant delivered vaginally by a woman with active genital herpes has a 40% to 60% chance of being infected (CDC, 2011d), supporting a decision for a cesarean birth for any women with active vaginal or perineal herpes lesions. Risk factors for the transmission of herpes from mother to newborn have been detailed. The pregnant woman who acquires genital herpes as a primary infection in the latter half of pregnancy, rather than before pregnancy, is at greatest risk of transmitting this virus to her newborn. This is true for both herpes simplex virus type-1 and type-2 (Gardella & Brown, 2011). Generally acyclovir (Zovirax) is not recommended during pregnancy for treatment of viral lesions. The nurse educates the infected woman about comfort measures at this time, including ways to keep the lesions dry and application of comfort measures to reduce the pain of the lesions (Li, 2011).

Chlamydia, Gonococcus, Group B *Streptococcus*, Bacterial Vaginosis, and *Candida albicans*

Infections caused by these bacteria and yeast (*Candida albicans*) may occur in the woman's vagina or cervix, infecting the infant during a vaginal birth. Chlamydia, the most common bacterial STI, appears most often among poor women with little access to care. Although few symptoms are seen, infection may cause preterm labor, premature rupture of membranes, low-birth-weight infants, or newborn conjunctivitis or pneumonia. Routine treatment of the newborn's eyes after birth with erythromycin destroys the organisms. Maternal gonococcus (GC) infection can be transmitted to the newborn from the mother's genital tract at the time of birth and can cause ophthalmia neonatorum, systemic neonatal infection, maternal endometritis, or pelvic infection. The risk of transmission from an infected mother to her infant is nearly 50% (Allstaff & Wilson, 2011). Newborn infants often receive erythromycin ointment in the eyes to prevent GC infection. Screening at 36 to 37 weeks of pregnancy for group B *Streptococcus* infection has been recommended, because this infection causes preterm rupture of the amniotic membranes, premature labor, fetal respiratory distress syndrome, fetal septicemia, and meningitis (Gilbert, 2011). Bacterial vaginosis may also cause premature labor (U.S. Preventive Services Task Force, 2011b). *Candida albicans*, the cause of a common vaginal fungal infection, may also cause an oral infection called thrush in the newborn. Routine assessment of pregnant women, and occasionally their sexual partners (GC), for these bacterial and yeast infections must occur during pregnancy so that treatment can occur and prevent fetal infection at the time of birth.

Human Immunodeficiency Virus (HIV)

Acquired Immunodeficiency Syndrome. The U.S. Public Health Service and the U.S. Preventive Services Task Force recommend that all pregnant women in the United States be tested for HIV infection, ideally at the first prenatal visit (USPSTF, 2011c). Any woman in a high-risk group (e.g., intravenous drug users, women who have bisexual partners or multiple sexual contacts, women with a history of STIs, women who exchange sex for money or drugs, or Black or Hispanic women living in poverty) should be tested for antibodies to HIV. For the HIV-positive woman or one who engages in high-risk sexual practices, counseling must occur before conception. Counseling should include both the direct effect of the virus on pregnancy and the effect of pregnancy on HIV disease progression. Although unclear, it appears that HIV infection becomes worse during pregnancy because of a woman's altered immune status. Some early pregnancy discomforts, such as fatigue, anorexia, and weight loss, may mask the early symptoms of HIV infection and thus postpone a definitive diagnosis.

Infants born to HIV-positive women have an infection rate of up to 25% (CDC, 2011f). Affected infants may not be seropositive for HIV for many months after birth and then later develop the disease. Recent use of zidovudine (AZT) protocol treatments throughout pregnancy has improved the prognosis of an HIV-positive woman and has decreased viral transmission to the fetus, although the drug remains expensive and may be inaccessible for women who do not receive prenatal care.

The pregnant woman who has acquired immunodeficiency syndrome (AIDS) or who is HIV positive should be carefully monitored by a health care team for opportunistic infections that occur frequently. The nurse can be instrumental in helping this woman coordinate her contacts with care providers, answering her questions, and working as a member of the team to provide optimal care for the woman and her child. Frequently the pregnant woman with AIDS does not seek care, based on fears of being reported for her disease. Involving the woman in continuous prenatal care decreases her risk of preterm rupture of membranes, problems with fetal growth, postpartum infection, drug and alcohol abuse, and difficulty in addressing sociocultural barriers to a better life (Wilson, 2011).

Although important in decreasing the transmission of any disease, astute preventive measures are mandatory for nurses who are exposed to HIV-infected body fluids, such as blood, amniotic fluid, and vaginal secretions (universal precautions should be followed). All health care providers must follow hospital and birth center policies regarding the use of gloves and gowns and the disposal of needles and other potentially contaminated equipment to prevent the transmission of this disease in particular.

Hepatitis B

Hepatitis B virus (HBV) infection remains a significant concern during pregnancy, because it affects the maternal liver and has a high fetal transmission rate (60%) if present during the third trimester. High-risk groups for HBV infection include women from Asia, Pacific Islands, and sub-Saharan Africa, as well as health care workers, intravenous drug users, and women with multiple sex partners (CDC, 2011g). Based on the large number of infected women who fail to show symptoms until liver damage has occurred, all pregnant women early in pregnancy and those at risk should be screened routinely for this virus (U.S. Preventive Services Task Force, 2011d). HBV immunization (three injections over a period of 6 months) may be given before or during pregnancy to a mother who is seronegative (CDC, 2011h). According to Gilbert (2011), most women harboring the virus transmit it through the placenta to the fetus or through contaminated urine, feces, saliva, or vaginal fluids during birth. Many women carrying the virus deliver prematurely, and some infants may have acute hepatitis or later develop liver cancer.

Other Health Concerns

Pregnant women may also develop any of the infections of nonpregnant women. For example, pregnant women frequently experience upper respiratory tract and gastrointestinal tract infections, adding to the discomforts of pregnancy. However, there is no evidence the viruses causing these infections have a teratogenic effect on the fetus.

Fever frequently occurs with illness. A high, prolonged fever (hyperthermia) in a pregnant woman may harm the fetus, especially during the first trimester. Some literature indicates that high fever is associated with miscarriages, stillbirths, and premature deliveries. Whether the high fever or an underlying illness causing the fever has created the problem must be determined.

Some reports have also correlated prolonged use of a sauna or hot tub, causing hyperthermia, with birth defects such as microcephaly, anencephaly, and hypotonia. Until health care providers understand this issue better, the nurse should advise pregnant women to avoid prolonged sauna or hot tub use and spending time with people who are ill or carrying disease. When a pregnant woman develops a high fever, she should be advised to contact her health care provider immediately.

Pregnant mothers may have other health problems that influence their physiological processes and thus harm the developing fetus. Black women experience twice the rate of hypertension and diabetes mellitus as do White women. These higher rates may account for the three to four times higher maternal mortality rate seen among pregnant Black women as compared with White women (CDC, 2011i).

Diabetes. Diabetes may exist before or during pregnancy, affecting both mother and fetus. Pregnancy increases the need for maternal insulin to balance the woman's blood glucose level. Currently the American College of Obstetricians and Gynecologists (ACOG) recommends that all pregnant women complete a glucose tolerance test at 28 weeks of gestation to identify abnormal blood glucose utilization and the need for additional monitoring. Complications from diabetes during pregnancy include polyhydramnios (excessive amniotic fluid volume), acidosis, increased rate of infection, vascular complications, and increased risk of pregnancy-induced hypertension. Because of an increased incidence of intrauterine death after 36 weeks of gestation attributable to an aging placenta, close monitoring in the last month is essential. Neonatal complications from diabetes include hypoglycemia, respiratory distress syndrome, hyperbilirubinemia, and hypocalcemia. Infants of mothers with diabetes also have a higher incidence of congenital anomalies, such as a heart lesion or meningocele (Gilbert, 2011). The diabetic pregnant woman needs close health care team supervision and ongoing health teaching, including diet and exercise management, in order to control her disease effectively.

Heart Disease and Hypertension. Heart disease and hypertension are the two serious maternal cardiovascular problems during pregnancy. Rheumatic heart disease, a common problem, contributes to congestive heart failure, threatening the lives of both mother and fetus. The fetus may require premature delivery. Chronic hypertension, seen more frequently in first-time mothers older than age 35, increases the chance of stillbirths, premature delivery, and development of **gestational hypertension**, which increase both maternal and infant mortality rates. Mothers with these problems must be monitored closely throughout pregnancy to prevent complications (Czeizel & Bánhidy, 2011).

Rh Blood Group Incompatibility. Rh blood group incompatibility sometimes affects fetal development. This problem usually occurs when the mother has Rh-negative red blood cells and the fetus has Rh-positive red blood cells, inherited from a father who has Rh-positive blood. Rh incompatibility affects 10% to 15% of White women, 5% of Black women, but few Asian women (Rubarth, 2011). In this disorder, maternal antibodies develop, cross the placental membranes, and destroy the Rh-positive red blood cells of the fetus. Based on the severity of

the response, the infant may develop varying levels of hyperbilirubinemia after birth or may die in utero from the anemia of erythroblastosis fetalis (hemolytic disease of the newborn).

All women should be assessed for blood type, Rh factor, and antibody development to Rh-positive cells at their first prenatal care visit and again at 24 to 28 weeks of pregnancy unless the father of the baby is Rh negative (USPSTF, 2011e). Rh incompatibility between a mother and future fetus may be prevented by administering $Rh_o(D)$ immune globulin (RhoGAM) to an Rh-negative mother at 28 weeks of gestation and within 72 hours after birth. The immunization prevents the mother's sensitization to fetal Rh-negative cells by inactivating fetal red blood cells in the mother before she can develop an antibody response. The ideal injection time is after the mother's first delivery of an Rh-positive infant, miscarriage, or therapeutic abortion. The incompatibility generally does not occur during the first pregnancy, and the immunization prevents problems with later pregnancies.

Chemical Agents

Drugs ingested by the mother may be teratogens to the fetus. The tragic experience with the tranquilizer drug thalidomide, which caused limb deformities during the early 1960s, led to a recommendation that medications should be avoided during pregnancy unless absolutely necessary (Box 16-9: Research for Evidence-Based Practice). The fact remains, however, that during the most critical early weeks of fetal development and growth, when many women do not know they are pregnant, ingested drugs may seriously affect the fetus. Based on fetal gestational age and drug metabolism, drugs may alter the placenta itself or directly affect development and growth of the fetus. The drugs that most commonly cause congenital defects are prescription medications, over-the-counter (OTC) drugs, street drugs, nicotine (cigarettes), caffeine, and alcohol. The U.S. Food and Drug Administration has labeled some of these drugs with an "X"; this means that scientific studies have shown negative fetal effects when pregnant women take them.

Prescription Medications

Women frequently become pregnant while taking medications for illnesses diagnosed before pregnancy, such as hypertension, or they may receive medication to treat an illness acquired during pregnancy, such as a urinary tract infection (UTI). Some of the more common drugs that have been studied for fetal effects include antibiotics and anticonvulsants.

Most short-term and usual-dose antibiotics do not cause fetal harm. The tetracyclines are categorized as pregnancy category D (positive evidence of human fetal risk) because they combine with calcium ions and are deposited in deciduous teeth (causing discoloration) and bones (inhibiting bone growth and causing deformities) (King & Brucker, 2009). Primary teeth seem most affected, but when the antibiotic is given near the time of delivery the permanent teeth may be damaged also.

On the basis of our current state of knowledge, the vast majority of antibiotics do not cause serious harm to the unborn child if used properly and at the appropriate doses during pregnancy. The treatment with an antibiotic that is contraindicated

---

BOX 16-9   RESEARCH FOR EVIDENCE-BASED PRACTICE

Substance Use in Pregnancy

Objective: To improve awareness and knowledge of problematic substance use in pregnancy and to provide evidence-based recommendations for the management of this challenging clinical issue for all health care providers.

Options: This guideline reviews the use of screening tools, general approach to care, and recommendations for clinical management of problematic substance use in pregnancy.

Outcomes: Evidence-based recommendations for screening and management of problematic substance use during pregnancy and lactation.

Evidence: Medline, PubMed, CINAHL, and The Cochrane Library were searched for articles published from 1950 using the following key words: substance-related disorders, mass screening, pregnancy complications, pregnancy, prenatal care, cocaine, cannabis, methadone, opioid, tobacco, nicotine, solvents, hallucinogens, and amphetamines. Results were initially restricted to systematic reviews and randomized controlled trials/controlled clinical trials. A subsequent search for observational studies was also conducted because there are few RCTs in this field of study. Articles were restricted to human studies published in English.

Recommendations

- All pregnant women and women of childbearing age should be screened periodically for alcohol, tobacco, and prescription and illicit drug use.
- When testing for substance use is clinically indicated, urine drug screening is the preferred method. Informed consent should be obtained from the woman before maternal drug toxicology testing is ordered.
- Policies and legal requirements with respect to drug testing of newborns may vary by jurisdiction, and caregivers should be familiar with the regulations in their region.

- Health care providers should employ a flexible approach to the care of women who have substance use problems, and they should encourage the use of all available community resources.
- Women should be counseled about the risks of periconception, antepartum, and postpartum drug use.
- Smoking cessation counseling should be considered as a first-line intervention for pregnant smokers. Nicotine replacement therapy and/or pharmacotherapy can be considered if counseling is not successful.
- Methadone maintenance treatment should be a standard of care for opioid-dependent women during pregnancy. Other slow-release opioid preparations may be considered if methadone is not available.
- Opioid detoxification should be reserved for selected women because of the high risk of relapse to opioids.
- Opiate-dependent women should be informed that neonates exposed to heroin, prescription opioids, methadone, or buprenorphine during pregnancy are monitored closely for symptoms and signs of neonatal withdrawal (neonatal abstinence syndrome).
- The risks and benefits of breastfeeding should be weighed on an individual basis because methadone maintenance therapy is not a contraindication to breastfeeding.

Nursing implications: Using these guidelines, nurses can assist in helping pregnant women improve access to health care, and assistance with appropriate addiction care leads to reduced health care costs and decreased maternal and neonatal morbidity and mortality.

Source: Wong, S., Ordean, A., & Kahan, M. (2011). Substance use in pregnancy. *Journal of Obstetrics & Gynaecology Canada, 33*(4), 367-384.

---

does not justify termination of pregnancy. However, ultimately no medicine, including antibiotics, can be described as absolutely safe (Mylonas, 2011).

The prevalence of antiepileptic drug use in pregnant women is very low. Although their main indication is epilepsy, antiepileptic drugs are increasingly being used in the treatment of bipolar mood disorders, migraine, and neuropathic pain syndrome, which means their prevalence will increase in the future (Mølgaard-Nielsen & Hviid, 2011). The effects of anticonvulsants on the fetus have been documented thoroughly. Women with seizure disorders have carried infants to term while being treated with hydantoin, barbiturates, and other antiseizure medications. Infants born to mothers taking hydantoin (Dilantin) may have fetal hydantoin syndrome, reflected in microcephaly, retardation, cleft lip and palate, and congenital heart disease. Barbiturates, such as phenobarbital, may cause newborn addiction. Women with seizure disorders should discuss their medication requirements with their physicians before becoming pregnant and have close health care team monitoring throughout pregnancy.

Over-the-Counter Drugs

Pregnant women frequently choose to treat minor illnesses with OTC drugs. Research on acetylsalicylic acid (aspirin) and acetaminophen (Tylenol) indicates that both medications are safe in recommended dosages. However, aspirin alters platelet function and may cause maternal and newborn bleeding if taken close to delivery. Acetaminophen can be toxic to the liver. Certain ingredients in common cold remedies have been associated with fetal irritability (Briggs et al., 2011). Ibuprofen has been known to prolong labor based on its antiprostaglandin effect. Any drug may harm a fetus, so all drugs should be avoided during pregnancy unless prescribed by the health care provider.

The nurse includes information on the known and probable effects of medications on the fetus in prenatal teaching of couples. Discussion of herbal treatments is included, because little research exists on their effects and interactions with over-the-counter and prescribed medications. The nurse recognizes that many cultural groups use these nontraditional agents, because they believe that they will effectively manage pregnancy-related concerns. The nurse may need to encourage an individual to reconsider the use of herbs when evidence exists that these may harm the fetus or mother.

Drug Abuse

Given the prevalence of drug use and abuse in our society, it is imperative that nurses be able to recognize, manage, and refer as appropriate substance abuse problems for their care recipients. Substance abuse during pregnancy poses significant risk because all substances consumed by the mother pass freely through the placenta, and thus the fetus as well as the mother experiences substance use, abuse, and addiction. All pregnant women and women of childbearing age should be screened periodically for alcohol, tobacco, and prescription and illicit drug use.

Maternal use of narcotics, tranquilizers, cocaine, amphetamines, marijuana, and other drugs may cause serious health problems to both the mother and the unborn child. These drugs represent an enormous cost to society by causing increased risks of low-birth-weight infants and preterm infants as well as deficits in child development if the mother ingests them during pregnancy (National Institute on Drug Abuse [NIDA], 2011).

Narcotics. Chronic narcotic use during pregnancy is increasing in prevalence. Signs of narcotic withdrawal in the newborn include tremors, irritability, hyperactivity, vomiting, diarrhea, sweating, poor feeding, and possibly convulsions. No evidence suggests withdrawal in infants whose mothers used cocaine or amphetamines, although there is an increased risk for preterm births, neonatal irritability, placental abruption, premature rupture of membranes, and fetal distress (Gilbert, 2011). Frequent maternal marijuana use during pregnancy may cause fetal immunological problems, but evidence conflicts with an unclear impact. Current research has shown that some infants born to women who used marijuana during their pregnancies display altered responses to visual stimuli, increased tremulousness, and a high-pitched cry, which could indicate problems with neurological development (NIDA, 2011). To avoid these problems, nurses must recognize women who abuse drugs and assist them in seeking appropriate help. This task may be difficult because drug abusers often try to hide their habit, fear being reported to the police, and may be unable to change their lifestyle without extensive intervention.

Alcohol. Many women in today's society drink alcohol regularly. However, alcohol crosses the placenta and may cause fetal death early in pregnancy. Fetal exposure to alcohol throughout pregnancy may cause fetal alcohol syndrome (FAS) or fetal alcohol spectrum disorder (FASD), a collection of symptoms including IUGR, increased risk of facial anomalies, structural brain abnormalities, mental health problems, attention-deficit/hyperactivity disorder (ADHD), and retardation. It is clinically proven that alcohol consumption during all stages of pregnancy puts the fetus at risk of being born with lifelong alcohol-related brain damage (Fleisher, 2011). Recent studies report symptoms of fetal alcohol disorder in children whose mothers may have consumed just a couple of drinks a day at certain stages of pregnancy. Another study confirmed that fetal alcohol syndrome is not the only problem connected with drinking during pregnancy: It is also a risk factor for early alcohol abuse and dependence in the child (Herrick et al., 2011; Warren et al., 2011). Numerous studies have shown that no safe level of alcohol use exists during pregnancy; therefore, alcohol should be avoided during this time and when attempting conception. The consequences of prenatal alcohol exposure are often grave, inhibiting both physical and intellectual development, societal acceptance, and adult success. The evidence is clear—alcohol can be more damaging to the developing fetus than heroin, cocaine, or any other drug, producing by far the most serious neurobehavioral effects in the fetus. Nurses need to stress this finding to make all women aware to avoid alcohol during their pregnancy.

Nicotine. In the United States, it is estimated that about 16% of pregnant women smoke during their pregnancies. Carbon monoxide and nicotine from tobacco smoke may interfere with the oxygen supply to the fetus. Nicotine also readily crosses the placenta, and concentrations in the fetus can be as much as 15% higher than maternal levels. Nicotine concentrates in fetal blood, amniotic fluid, and breast milk. Combined, these factors can have severe consequences for the fetuses and infants of mothers who smoke (NIDA, 2011). The USPSTF recommends that clinicians ask all pregnant women about tobacco use and provide augmented, pregnancy-tailored counseling framework for engaging women in smoking cessation discussions:

- Ask about tobacco use.
- Advise to quit through clear, personalized messages.
- Assess willingness to quit.
- Assist to quit.
- Arrange follow-up and support.

Evidence indicates that maternal smoking causes increased rates of spontaneous abortion and ectopic pregnancy, decreased fertility, intrauterine growth restriction (IUGR), increased numbers of low-birth-weight or preterm infants, placental abnormalities, vaginal bleeding, congenital anomalies, perinatal mortality, and premature rupture of the membranes. The best advice for pregnant mothers or women considering pregnancy is ceasing all use of tobacco products, decreasing smoking if one is a heavy smoker, and avoiding places where smoking occurs. The nurse needs to understand the context of smoking in a woman's life and the complexity of her choice to quit smoking in order to propose solutions to decrease fetal exposure to nicotine (Box 16-10: Research for Evidence-Based Practice).

Caffeine. Coffee, cocoa, tea, cola, and chocolate contain caffeine, another addictive drug. Gene mutations have been found in laboratory animals exposed to moderate amounts of caffeine; however, these defects have not been found in human beings. One study found a weak association between excess caffeine intake (more than 300 mg or more than 3 cups of coffee per day) during pregnancy with a slight increase in birth defects, but not statistically significant (Browne et al., 2011). Until additional research clarifies the relationship between caffeine intake and fetal effects, nurses should teach pregnant women to avoid excess caffeine intake.

Chemical Substances

The influence of chemicals on human development remains unclear. Some natural substances found to be teratogenic in animals, but not necessarily in human beings, include insect and bacterial toxins, insecticides, herbicides, and fungicides, including dichlorodiphenyltrichloroethane, or DDT. Recent studies involving pregnant women who eat fish with high mercury levels (shark, swordfish, king mackerel, canned tuna, or tilefish) support evidence that mercury negatively affects fetal development, particularly brain development, and may be associated with preterm labor (Lando & Zhang, 2011). Women can safely eat up to 12 ounces of cooked fish weekly. Some studies report stillbirths, abortions, preterm births, and mental retardation in fetuses exposed to lead. This area needs more study, particularly

BOX 16-10   RESEARCH FOR EVIDENCE-BASED PRACTICE
Nicotine Replacement Therapy in Pregnancy

Maternal tobacco smoking during pregnancy is the most significant preventable cause of poor health outcomes for women and their babies, with morbidity resulting from placental abruption, miscarriage, stillbirth, prematurity, low birth weight, neonatal or sudden infant death, and asthma. Frequently, clinicians use nicotine replacement therapy (NRT) in attempts to help pregnant smokers stop smoking. However, although NRT is an effective smoking cessation treatment for nonpregnant smokers, its efficacy and safety in pregnancy have not been demonstrated adequately.

The **purpose** of this study was to determine the efficacy and safety of nicotine replacement therapy (NRT) with or without behavioral support when used to support smoking cessation in pregnancy.

Design, setting, and participants: In a systematic review of randomized controlled trials (RCTs) in which NRT was used with or without behavioral support to promote smoking cessation, trials providing unequal behavioral support to different trial groups were excluded. Included were randomized controlled trials (RCTs) with designs that permitted independent effects of any type of NRT (e.g., patch, gum) for smoking cessation to be isolated. A total of five trials was identified that met criteria, giving a total of five included trials that enrolled a total of 695 pregnant smokers.

Findings: There is currently insufficient evidence to demonstrate that NRT, used by pregnant women for smoking cessation, is either effective or safe. Although birth outcomes were generally better among those infants born to women who had used NRT, none of these observed differences reached statistical significance. By ensuring that the only difference between the arms of included trials was the provision of NRT to all participants, we have isolated the independent effects of NRT that are of most importance to clinicians. Clinical guidelines assume that when pregnant women are heavily dependent upon nicotine, using NRT will be less harmful to them and their babies than continued smoking; however, these findings have not produced evidence for this assumption. Additional studies are needed to determine the safety and efficiency of NRT.

Nursing implications: In the absence of evidence for either the effectiveness or the safety of NRT use in pregnancy, perhaps nurses should emphasize the importance of using proven, behavioral strategies to promote smoking cessation in pregnancy to ensure optimal outcomes.

Data from Coleman, T., Chamberlain, C., Cooper, S., & Leonardi-Bee, J. (2011). Efficacy and safety of nicotine replacement therapy for smoking cessation in pregnancy: Systematic review and meta-analysis. *Addiction, 106*(1), 52-61.

with more women working in traditional male workplaces where there are environmental contaminants. Nurses assess and provide women in their first trimester with information on environmental agents that are potentially damaging throughout gestation and counsel them on ways to avoid exposure.

Medications Given During Childbirth

The final time that the fetus encounters drugs through the mother is during the birthing process. Many women desire medications for labor discomforts, and usually only medications deemed safe and monitored closely during labor and birth have been used (e.g., epidural anesthetics, opiate agonists in small doses). Some analgesic drugs administered during labor can cause neonatal sedation and respiratory depression and can influence the rate and quality of the infant's adaptation to extrauterine life. Studies of visual attentiveness and sucking behavior, as well as neurological tests and electroencephalography, suggest that fetal depressant effects may last as long as days after birth.

Mechanical Forces

The amniotic fluid reservoir protects the fetus during pregnancy and during mild to moderate trauma to the mother's abdomen. However, major trauma to the mother's abdomen, such as that sustained in a severe car accident, may cause maternal bleeding, preterm labor, and other concerns. The nurse instructs the pregnant woman in the proper way to wear both a lap belt and shoulder harness to protect her and her fetus while driving. All women in the second and third trimesters should be encouraged to seek medical care following an accident believed to influence the health of mother or fetus.

The uterus, another mechanical force, also influences the fetus. Near the end of pregnancy, the fetus outgrows the uterus and becomes molded by it, particularly in cases of multiple pregnancy. Some children have congenitally dislocated hips from uterine pressure and fetal position in utero. Most deformities return to normal either naturally or with repositioning after birth. Fetal malposition cannot be prevented; therefore, the neonate is assessed for problems and support is provided to the parents about the newborn's appearance.

The actual labor and birth process represents the final mechanical force. Few newborns experience injury during this process, and those who do usually recover with limited effect. It is difficult to predict and prevent traumas during birth, such as when delivery of an infant who is larger than expected requires vacuum extraction, which may injure the child. In these cases, based on health care team assessment, the mother may undergo cesarean section to protect herself and the baby.

Radiation

Scientific evidence indicates that exposure to x-rays, especially early in pregnancy, may cause chromosomal changes, spontaneous abortion, mental retardation, microcephaly, fetal loss, or malignancy later in life (Wiesel et al., 2011). The fetus is most sensitive to radiation effects between 8 and 15 weeks of pregnancy and thus should be spared any radiation exposure during that period (Shaw et al., 2011). Literature supports a greater incidence of leukemia in children of women exposed to x-rays during pregnancy compared with children whose mothers were not exposed. Unless the benefits of radiographic information clearly outweigh the risks of exposing the fetus to x-rays, these examinations should not be performed during gestation. If radiography is deemed necessary, wearing a lead apron, using as low a radiation dose as possible, and following other recommendations made by the National Council on Radiation Protection and Measurements should be used to protect the developing fetus.

DETERMINANTS OF HEALTH

Social Factors and Environment

Community and Work

Many more women now work outside the home, either in careers or in jobs needed for family economic survival. As each woman considers or experiences pregnancy, she will need to ask herself questions that will optimize her pregnancy outcome. These questions include the following: Is my work strenuous or possibly dangerous to my baby because of exposure to toxic substances? Do I need to work for long periods, influencing my need for rest? Will workplace stressors influence my coping with pregnancy and my family needs?

A safe workplace environment (one that does not involve exposure to hazardous substances or organisms and provides adequate breaks for worker rest and body movement) will allow a pregnant woman to work until her baby is due, unless her health becomes impaired. The nurse helps each woman assess the safety of her workplace and suggest ways to decrease hazards in that setting. These hazards include exposure to viruses, fungi, industrial products (hydrocarbons or pesticides), smoke, radiation emitted by medical diagnostic equipment, air pollutants, and asbestos and possibility for workplace violence, mental and physical stress, and even noise pollution. The nurse encourages the pregnant worker to consider workplace ergonomics, addressing how the current work space will meet her changing physical needs.

Some employers in this country have been designated creators of "family friendly" work environments, because they have willingly made accommodations to support breastfeeding and pregnant workers and families. These accommodations allow women to prioritize their pregnancy and family needs. Evidence indicates that such approaches reduce pregnancy complications and increase work productivity. Although few in number, family friendly employers offer health-promotion programs focusing on healthy nutrition, stress management, and exercise for employees, who experience better health outcomes.

As a rule, however, too few employers support flexible work schedules for prenatal care visits, rest periods for pregnant workers, or removal of vending machines to support optimal nutrition for pregnant working class women. Some working women, regardless of status, believe that once they announce their pregnancy, they will face workplace pressure to stop working or change positions in the company based on their gestational needs. Based on experience, some employers fear that their pregnant employees will overuse sick time or seek a reduced workload.

In a recent study of pregnancy within the workplace, two factors were identified that may be challenging. In many workplaces, pressures on women to 'ignore' pregnancy and to 'push on' through sickness and exhaustion may relate to certain workplace cultures referred to as 'male norms'. The partiality for 'male norms' could be seen as creating problems for these pregnant women, who feel obliged to downplay their 'inherent femaleness' by minimizing their pregnancy in order to fit in with workplace notions of reliability and presence.

Secondly, health advice on pregnancy might also be difficult to implement within women's workplaces because of underlying assumptions, reflected in health advice, that women's care is most appropriately performed in the home. It is significant that health guidance on pregnancy carework makes little reference to place, and offers slender guidance on how pregnancy carework might be implemented at work. Common sense suggests that instructions about napping during the day and using ice packs to relieve hemorrhoids would be entirely inappropriate within most workplaces, whatever the occupation of the pregnant woman (Gatrell, 2011).

The pregnant woman must deal with these situations by being factual and assertive about her ability to continue working. National law dictates that it is illegal to discriminate against a woman because she is pregnant. If a woman believes that she has been treated unfairly because of her pregnancy, she may pursue the issue legally or become active in local women's rights organizations to gain support. However, when a woman leaves a job that did not support her pregnancy, she often gives up accrued leave time or takes a lower salary at another job. These outcomes influence her choices during pregnancy and early parenting.

Workplaces vary greatly in allowing leave time during and after pregnancy. Federal legislation, the Family and Medical Leave Act, obligates employers of at least 50 people to provide up to 12 weeks of paid leave for new parents or women who have medical problems during pregnancy. Ideally a woman who desires children should explore the issue of leave during a job interview, but many women fail to do this until they are already pregnant. A woman often requires written verification from her physician if she needs a leave of absence from her job attributable to pregnancy complications. Although she may wish to return to work shortly after giving birth, the woman is counseled to allow sufficient time to regain her strength and adapt to parenting. The nurse may help the couple make reasonable decisions related to locating resources for child care, exploring "shared-time" with other new mothers or part-time employees (for example, middle-age adults caring for their older parents), or finding ways of balancing work and family needs.

Culture and Ethnicity

Cultural groups have unique ideas and beliefs related to pregnancy, childbirth, and childbearing that must be understood by the nurse in order to render individualized care to each pregnant woman. As part of the assessment, the nurse determines the cultural attachment of a woman by asking the following question: Does she think that some or most of the childbearing ideas of her culture are old fashioned, but does she feel obligated to follow these ideas, at least superficially, because of family pressure? In this situation, the nurse may need to be a confidant for the woman who needs to vent her frustrations about cultural restrictions.

Nonconscious stereotyping and prejudice contribute to racial and ethnic disparities in health care. Contemporary training in cultural competence is insufficient to reduce these problems because even educated, culturally sensitive nurses can activate and use their biases without being aware they are doing so. Research in social psychology shows that over time stereotypes and **prejudices** become invisible to those who rely on them. Automatic categorization of an individual as a member of a social group can unconsciously trigger the thoughts (stereotypes) and feelings (**prejudices**) associated with that group. This implies that, when activated, implicit negative attitudes and stereotypes shape how nurses evaluate and interact with minority groups. This makes minority group care recipients uncomfortable and discourages them from seeking or complying with treatment (Stone & Moskowitz, 2011).

Nurses need to be very cognizant of their stereotyping and prejudices and "park them at the door-stop" before interacting with minority women. Have nurses ever thought about why pregnant women do not seek prenatal care or do not return for follow-up care once they have encountered a negative reception? If nurses would reverse roles with minority women and just imagine how it feels to encounter negative attitudes when needing health care, perhaps biased attitudes would change dramatically (Nelson & Henriksen Hellyer, 2011).

Nurses need an awareness of how culture, tradition, and acculturation may affect the women for whom they provide care, as this is the first step toward understanding diverse cultural behavior. The next step is for nurses to be aware of the three 'levels' of culture when offering health advice and planning healthcare for various diverse groups:

- The *primary* level of culture refers to rules that are known by all and obeyed by all and may be almost unconsciously performed by women (e.g., health, healing and health-belief systems, or how illness, diseases, and their causes are perceived by that specific culture).
- The *secondary* level is the underlying rules and guidelines known by the group but not generally relayed to outsiders. This may include taboos and rituals relating to behavior, which may be followed depending on the individual.
- A *tertiary* level is visible to the outsider, such as traditional dress, foods, and religious ceremonies (Esegbona-Adeigbe, 2011).

Intercultural caring by nurses is complex. However, nurses need to have a positive attitude and demonstrate acceptance of different cultures. This can be achieved by nurses taking the stance of respecting, listening, and understanding diversity, as well as acknowledging any barriers such as culture. Nursing support may assist the individual in adjusting both her needs and those of the culture she represents to experience a satisfactory pregnancy.

The nurse has an obligation to read about and seek information on cultures encountered in practice and to become active in community organizations that represent cultures whose members get prenatal care from the nurse. Above all, the nurse must be open to a variety of viewpoints, judging them not against personal beliefs, but rather in relation to the general concept of health promotion and today's goal to provide culturally competent care to a variety of cultural groups (Box 16-11: Diversity Awareness box).

Levels of Policy Making and Health

Both legislative actions and social movements influence childbearing. In some countries, such as China, the government decrees the number of children a couple may have and imposes economic or social sanctions to enforce these restrictions.

BOX 16-11 DIVERSITY AWARENESS

Nursing Roles in Providing Culturally Competent Care

In recent years, a greater emphasis has been placed on nurses recognizing and appreciating **diversity** in order to acquire cultural competency. Cultural knowledge is the most important construct of cultural competence for nurses, being crucial for the accurate appreciation of a care recipient's worldview. Delivery of culturally competent care implies that a nurse acknowledges and acts on the unique history that a pregnant woman and family bring to a health care interaction. The nurse supports culturally competent care by:

- Recognizing that cultural diversity exists and affects the process and outcome of health care
- Respecting people as unique individuals who, by their differences from the majority, bring a broadened definition of appropriate health care
- Using data gained from a cultural assessment for completion of a care plan
- Encouraging cultural behavior that protects the biopsychosocial, spiritual, and safety needs of the individual
- Gaining insight into the nurse's own beliefs and values about people who may be different or have different needs than the majority or those of the nurse's own culture; understanding how these beliefs and values influence the outcomes of health care delivery with childbearing families
- Recognizing the values of the health care system reflected in the customs and practices of birthing facilities and responding to these facilities based on one's value system
- Providing interpreters to improve communication between the individual and health care providers
- Becoming literate in languages, customs, and cultural practices of people commonly seen in the health care environment

---

Although Americans may have as many children as they desire, various coalitions lobby strongly for families. The recent Family and Medical Leave Act validates the federal government's commitment to prioritizing family issues by giving new parents time off from work during the early months of parenthood, while supporting these individuals' professional work goals and needs.

The U.S. government remains concerned about the health of pregnant women and ways to decrease fetal and infant morbidity and mortality. Historically, states have used federal monies from Medicaid and Title V maternal and child health block programs to provide services for pregnant women and children. Many countries provide universal access to prenatal care, but in the United States low-income women rely on Medicaid, a joint federal-state program, to cover most of the cost of prenatal care. With constraints on state and federal budgets, many of which fund community prenatal clinics, concerns have been expressed about whether sufficient money will exist for funding women and children's care programs. Local health departments may offer free or low-cost prenatal care for women who are pregnant, but again, the extent of services depends on state government or local allocation of funds. Despite this free or low-cost care, more than 49 million Americans overall lack health insurance and, therefore, face barriers that affect their easy access to prenatal care (Carrillo et al., 2011; USDHHS, 2010). Many ethnically diverse populations, and in particular Hispanic groups, lack insurance and a level of education that increases their understanding of health-related information for family health promotion. Educating women during the childbearing cycle is particularly important to increase the chances of families obtaining and understanding health-promotion information for healthier behaviors (USDHHS, 2010).

With the nurse's help in data collection, consumers should be encouraged to express their views and opinions on pregnancy and parenting topics to their elected governmental representatives. This expression indeed works; many states recently legislated hospital stays of at least 48 hours for women with vaginal deliveries and even longer stays for women with cesarean deliveries. These laws evolved from public concern over premature discharges of new mothers as part of managed care insurance directives. Longer stays help health care providers identify potential problems in the mother or the baby before discharge, such as difficulty breastfeeding. Continued legislative work on insurance reform may improve family planning services so that couples can plan pregnancies to better meet their sociocultural and financial goals and needs (USDHHS, 2010). Insurance reform, driven by legislative change, may also improve health care coverage for underinsured individuals who lack a consistent source of prenatal care or report difficulties in receiving care because of communication, structural, or personal barriers within their insurance system (Broussard et al., 2011).

Economics

When the pregnant woman begins prenatal care, personal financial resources influence the kind of care she receives, the need to remain employed during or after a pregnancy, the acceptance of her pregnancy, the nutritional status of the woman, and other choices. The expenses of planning and experiencing a pregnancy may determine whether the woman or her family faces a financial crisis. The nurse needs to understand the financial history and priorities of the couple, because this information will affect access to and use of prenatal care.

The nurse inquires in a sensitive fashion about a woman's or couple's finances to make appropriate referral to resources for care (e.g., Title V or Medicaid programs). Until recently, Medicaid provided no adolescent family planning services, a situation that may have influenced high rates of pregnancy in some sectors of this country (USDHHS, 2010). Many low-income women qualify for the U.S. Department of Agriculture's supplemental feeding program for Women, Infants, and Children (WIC). This program provides essential foods such as milk, cheese, and eggs to pregnant and lactating women. During prenatal visits, the nurse may help a woman or family plan a budget for food and other essential requirements based on individual family needs, cultural values, need for a healthy diet during pregnancy, and income level. Local food banks and second-hand clothing and baby supply stores may provide needed items for these families. Occasionally women may access free transportation and child care at the prenatal clinic if the nurse provides information about this program.

Health Services/Delivery System

Options for care during pregnancy range from medical-based care by an obstetrician or general practitioner to more health-promotion–focused care by a nurse practitioner or midwife.

Geographical availability of options, finances, previous experience, partner's preference, cultural or social acceptability of certain options, and preexisting or newly recognized risk factors will influence a woman's choice of care. Based on her culture and the belief that pregnancy is not an illness, a woman may not seek Western medical prenatal care, but rather may rely on individuals of her culture to provide care until the actual labor, when she will go to a hospital.

Unless complications arise a woman generally chooses where she will labor and give birth and the extent of labor and birthing process intervention. The movement toward home birth that began during the early 1970s continues to meet some consumer needs for a more family-oriented, natural, health-focused experience. However, most couples choose a hospital birth setting because of availability of emergency equipment and personnel in case of complications. Some insurance companies will reimburse only births done in hospitals and in birth centers or birthing rooms attached to a hospital. The nurse helps expectant couples become aware of the care and birthing alternatives to make an informed choice for a positive labor and birth experience. Women who lack resources to access the health care delivery system and teaching by the nurse during regular prenatal visits generally are less able to make informed decisions that affect their childbearing experiences.

Many expectant couples also make an informed choice about the actual process of labor and birth by developing a birth plan—those components of care and intervention that the couple desires for the birth experience. A pregnant woman and her partner may choose natural childbirth or a method of analgesia or anesthesia. The nurse helps the pregnant woman and her partner choose the most appropriate method by providing information about options and encouraging questions about each option. Collaboration between the nurse and woman or couple in meeting their birth plan goals is important, because research shows that women remember their labor and birthing experiences for a long time. A positively viewed birth experience may support a couple's involvement as active health care consumers, thus facilitating their future health of their family.

The nurse may encourage the pregnant couple or woman to attend prenatal classes. These provide valuable information and preparation for birth for many couples. The International Childbirth Education Association, the American Society for Psychoprophylaxis in Obstetrics (ASPO), and many local groups offer a variety of classes for the expectant couple. These classes may include information on early pregnancy, Lamaze-ASPO or Bradley methods, cesarean birth, breastfeeding, infant cardiopulmonary resuscitation, and parenting. Sibling classes for the newborn and involvement of children in the birth experience may also increase sibling bonding.

NURSING APPLICATION

Teaching the pregnant woman and her partner during the prenatal period is the most important role of the nurse. Even the woman who has previously given birth or who has a high degree of education may need or want information from the health care team that will assist her family to adapt effectively to changes of pregnancy to support a healthy birth outcome.

To provide appropriate teaching, the nurse performs a comprehensive assessment that involves the entire family, such as that presented in **Website Resource 16E.** Assessment, the first step in the nursing process, allows the nurse to determine maternal and fetal physical and psychological risks, the woman's informational base for pregnancy and birth, and cultural and family needs. Assessment should also include physical, spiritual, emotional, and sociocultural inspection and recognition of abuse. Battering increases during pregnancy and may be detected by physical, emotional, behavioral, and history assessment of the woman. Pregnant women at high risk for abuse include adolescents, those with low incomes, and those with a history of alcohol or drug abuse, as well as a partner with a similar history (American College of Obstetricians and Gynecologists [ACOG], 2011; U.S. Preventive Services Task Force, 2011a). In cases of suspected abuse, the nurse, in consultation with other members of the health care team, provides support and resources for the woman to make an informed decision about protecting herself and her fetus during pregnancy. The nurse may also want to refer the person to a professional counselor for a brief counseling outreach intervention or abuse shelter for personal safety (Brownridge et al., 2011).

As discussed in this chapter, assessment may also be made by using Gordon's (2010) functional health patterns, a common conceptual framework for clinical assessment (see Box 16-5). Data used in the assessment process will likely be collected during the prenatal visit and may change based on life occurrences of the pregnant woman. A woman may be defined as high risk during her pregnancy if she experiences heavy bleeding, premature labor, elevated blood pressure, or extreme anxiety; if there is fetal distress; or if the woman shows unexpected behavior or symptoms. After noting these high-risk conditions, the nurse should refer the pregnant woman to an obstetrical specialist or other resources for pregnant women and their families (see the Case Study below).

After a complete assessment during each prenatal visit, the nurse develops a teaching plan for the individual. Throughout the prenatal course, the nurse collaborates with the woman and her partner to assess their learning and support needs. For

example, literature on bottle feeding or breastfeeding may be provided to help a woman decide on a method, and books, videos, and websites may help couples understand more about birth and, therefore, feel that they have more control during labor and in meeting their birthing goals. If the woman plans to attend group prenatal classes, the nurse should coordinate her teaching content and process with those expected in the classes, thereby preventing undue repetition. The nurse teaching prenatal classes should provide a list of topics to participants in the class to share with their health care providers. A woman may be knowledgeable in some areas, and the nurse can use this knowledge as a foundation for further individualized teaching. Box 16-12 covers relevant topics to be covered by the nurse during prenatal care interactions with pregnant women. These topical areas relate to nursing interventions discussed earlier in this chapter. Basic handouts detailing information such as danger signs will provide information that a woman can post at home should she experience unexpected complications of her pregnancy.

BOX 16-12 TOPICS FOR PRENATAL CARE TEACHING

1. Rationale for and interpretation of physical findings and laboratory results
2. Value of keeping appointments
3. Danger signs that should be reported
4. Breast care to prepare for lactation
5. Breastfeeding versus bottle feeding
6. Exercise and rest
7. Fetal growth and development
8. Physical and psychological changes during pregnancy and relief measures
9. Effects of smoking, drinking, and drugs on the fetus
10. Nutrition
11. Work and play
12. Body mechanics
13. Personal hygiene
14. Sex during pregnancy
15. Preparation for labor and birth
16. Superstitions and old wives' tales
17. Signs of impending labor
18. Supplies and preparations for the baby
19. Partner's and siblings' responses

CASE STUDY

Active Labor: Susan Wong

Mrs. Wong, a first-time mother, is admitted to the birthing suite in early labor after spontaneous rupture of membranes (SROM) at home. She is at 38 weeks of gestation with a history of abnormal alpha-fetoprotein levels at 16 weeks of pregnancy. She was scheduled for ultrasonography to visualize the fetus to rule out an open spinal defect or Down syndrome, but never followed through. Mrs. Wong and her husband disagreed about what to do (keep or terminate the pregnancy) if the ultrasonography indicated a spinal problem, so they felt they did not want this information.

Reflective Questions

1. As the nurse, what priority data would you collect from this couple to help define relevant interventions to meet their needs?

2. How can you help this couple if they experience a negative outcome in the birthing suite? What are your personal views on terminating or continuing a pregnancy with a risk for a potential anomaly? What factors may influence your views?

3. With the influence of the recent Human Genome Project and the possibility of predicting open spinal defects earlier in pregnancy, how will maternity care change in the future?

Prediction of Human Disease

An organism's complete set of DNA is called its genome. Virtually every single cell in the body contains a complete copy of the approximately 3 billion DNA base pairs, or letters, that make up the human genome. The Human Genome

Continued

CASE STUDY

Active Labor: Susan Wong—cont'd

Project (completed in 2003), conducted by the National Human Genome Research Institute, produced a very high–quality version of the human genome sequence that is freely available in public databases. Researchers have been able to use DNA sequencing to search for genetic variations and/or mutations that may play a role in the development or progression of a range of diseases. Clearly, there are implications and ethical considerations for the health sciences here. Along with the important information uncovered by the Human Genome Project, a great controversy arose. Even though blood tests are now available for the detection of various fatal diseases such as Huntington's disease, cystic fibrosis, and colon cancer, many people would rather live with uncertainty than know they have an incurable life-threatening disease. Sadly, the tests, which have been developed, are to detect the disease and not cure it.

Another consideration is the use of genetic information by existing and prospective employers. Imagine a situation where employment preference is given to those who can demonstrate they are 'genetically free' of future diseases that might limit their capacity to work. Still, three major unsolved problems in perinatal and neonatal health include: (1) preterm birth; (2) the neonatal consequences of vaginal versus cesarean birth; and (3) neonatal gastrointestinal disease, specifically necrotizing enterocolitis. Hopefully within the near future, the Human Genome Project's research will be able to address all three to improve pregnancy outcomes.

In just a decade, the Human Genome Project has sparked an explosion of information that has proved useful to basic and clinical scientists. We must remain cautious as to how and when this new information and technology is used in the future to ensure it is for the betterment of mankind.

Sources: Gregory, K. E. (2011). Microbiome aspects of perinatal and neonatal health. *Journal of Perinatal & Neonatal Nursing, 25*(2), 158-162; Kuehn, B. (2011). Scientists see promise and challenges in translating genomics to the clinic. *Journal of the American Medical Association, 305*(13), 1285-1286.

◎ CARE PLAN

Nursing Management for Stages of Labor: Susan Wong

*NURSING DIAGNOSIS: Ineffective Coping related to active labor status

Defining Characteristics
- Initiation of labor at 2:00 AM with SROM
- First-time mother who did not attend childbirth classes
- Supportive spouse
- Current gestational age of 38 weeks
- Contraction pattern defined as moderate intensity, frequency every 2 minutes, 60 seconds in duration
- After 6 hours of labor, 4 cm dilated, 100% effaced, and stage: active phase
- Moaning, moving around in bed, and stating, "I can't take this much longer; it hurts too much!"

Related Factors
- Prenatal history of abnormal alpha-fetoprotein levels at 16 weeks
- Prenatal care since 12 weeks pregnant
- History of depression in college
- Works as engineer with large manufacturing firm
- Gravida 1, para 0
- Recent resident of city, moved from East Coast approximately 4 months ago
- 25 years of age, Asian family history, married 1 year

Expected Outcomes
- Mother will state level of pain to be less than 4 on a scale of 1 to 10 during labor.

- Mother will successfully use visual imagery techniques, massage, and slow deep breathing for relaxation during labor.
- Mother will state early in labor at least three ways to cope effectively with pain and will implement these strategies as relevant.
- Fetus will demonstrate an expected FHR pattern and will experience no compromise during labor.
- Mother and family will verbalize needs during labor and delivery to health care team.

Interventions
- Assess level of labor discomfort every 20 to 30 minutes and as needed according to pain scale rating of 1 to 10.
- Implement and document nursing interventions (backrubs, heat and cold applications, position changes, back pressure and massage, and Jacuzzi therapy, among others) to relieve labor discomforts.
- Assess cultural beliefs with labor and delivery management and implement interventions as needed to meet practice standards.
- Provide teaching about labor and delivery progress and breathing, visual imagery, and massage techniques that may decrease labor discomfort.
- Provide verbal and nonverbal reassurance during labor.
- Teach about fetal response during labor and rationale for nursing interventions to support fetal health, such as use of left side position to increase placental blood flow.
- Throughout labor, answer any questions from mother and family members about needs and responses to labor process.
- Involve family members as much as possible during labor and as requested by mother to improve her ability to cope.

*NANDA Nursing Diagnoses—Definitions and Classification 2012-2014, Herdman T.H. (ED). Copyright © 2012, 1994-2012 NANDA International. Used by arrangement with John Wiley & Sons Limited. In order to make safe and effective judgments using the NANDA-I nursing diagnoses it is essential that nurses refer to the definitions and defining characteristics of the diagnoses listed in this work. *Retired NANDA Nursing Diagnosis. FHR*, Fetal heart rate; *SROM*, spontaneous rupture of membranes.

SUMMARY

Dramatic changes occur during pregnancy; a new life forms and develops and the expectant family members (mother, father, siblings, and other close members) experience major changes in their roles and relationships with each other. Although all fetal development processes, changes in pregnant women's bodies, and role transitions among family members share common elements, each family uniquely experiences pregnancy because of life experience and personal values. The focus is the entire family, although the nurse most often deals directly with the pregnant woman. The nurse provides valuable resources and information that the family may use to meet its specific needs. The overall nursing goal involves assisting each family to have a healthy pregnancy and birth outcome, to lay the foundation for satisfactory parenting and family life.

REFERENCES

Allstaff, S., & Wilson, J. (2011). Sexually transmitted infections in pregnancy. *Pulse, 71*(24), 24–25.

American College of Obstetricians and Gynecologists (ACOG). (2011). *Violence against women.* [Online] Retrieved from www.acog.org/departments/dept_notice.cfm?recno=17&bulletin=186#repro.

Association of Women's Health, Obstetrical, & Neonatal Nursing (AWHONN). (2010). *Achieving constant quality care: Using research to guide clinical practice* (2nd ed.). Washington, DC: Author.

Bao, A., & Swaab, D. (2011). Sexual differentiation of the human brain: Relation to gender identity, sexual orientation and neuropsychiatric disorders. *Frontiers in Neuroendocrinology, 32*(2), 214–226.

Briggs, G. G., Freeman, R. K., & Yaffe, S. J. (2011). *Drugs in pregnancy and lactation* (9th ed.). Philadelphia: Lippincott Williams & Wilkins.

Broussard, D., Sappenfield, W., Fussman, C., Kroelinger, C., & Grigorescu, V. (2011). Core state preconception health indicators: A voluntary, multi-state selection process. *Maternal & Child Health Journal, 15*(2), 158–168. doi: 10.1007/s10995-010-0575-x.

Browne, M., Hoyt, A., Feldkamp, M., Rasmussen, S., Marshall, E., Druschel, C., et al. (2011). Maternal caffeine intake and risk of selected birth defects in the National Birth Defects Prevention Study. *Birth Defects Research. Part A, Clinical and Molecular Teratology, 91*(2), 93–101.

Brownridge, D. A., Taillieu, T. L., Tyler, K. A., Tiwari, A., Ko Ling, C., & Santos, S. C. (2011). Pregnancy and intimate partner violence: Risk factors, severity, and health effects. *Violence Against Women, 17*(7), 858–881. doi: 10.1177/1077801211412547.

Carrillo, J., Carrillo, V. A., Perez, H. R., Salas-Lopez, D., Natale-Pereira, A., & Byron, A. T. (2011). Defining and targeting health care access barriers. *Journal of Health Care for the Poor & Underserved, 22*(2), 562–575.

Centers for Disease Control and Prevention (CDC). (2011a). *3rd National Summit on preconception health and health care.* Available at www.beforeandbeyond.org/?page=summit-abstracts.

Centers for Disease Control and Prevention (CDC). (2011b). CDC health disparities and inequalities report, United States, 2011. *MMWR, 60*(Suppl), 49–50.

Centers for Disease Control and Prevention (CDC). (2011c). *Syphilis—CDC fact sheet.* [Online] Retrieved from www.cdc.gov/std/syphilis/stdfact-syphilis.htm.

Centers for Disease Control and Prevention (CDC). (2011d). *Genital herpes—fact sheet.* [Online] Retrieved from www.cdc.gov/std/herpes/stdfact-herpes.htm.

Centers for Disease Control and Prevention (CDC). (2011e). *Guidelines for preconception care of women.* [Online] Retrieved from www.cdc.gov/ncbddd/preconception/QandA.htm#3.

Centers for Disease Control and Prevention (CDC). (2011f). *HIV among women.* [Online] Retrieved from www.cdc.gov/hiv/topics/women/index.htm.

Centers for Disease Control and Prevention (CDC). (2011g). *Hepatitis B fact sheet.* [Online] Retrieved from www.cdc.gov/hepatitis/HBV/HBVfaq.htm#overview.

Centers for Disease Control and Prevention (CDC). (2011h). *Hepatitis B vaccination.* [Online] Retrieved from www.cdc.gov/vaccines/vpd-vac/hepb/default.htm.

Centers for Disease Control and Prevention (CDC). (2011i). *Preventing and managing chronic disease to improve the health of women and infants.* [Online] Retrieved from www.cdc.gov/reproductivehealth/womensrh/ChronicDiseaseandReproductiveHealth.htm.

Central Intelligence Agency (CIA). (2011). Country comparison: Infant mortality rate. *The World factbook.* [Online] Retrieved from www.cia.gov/library/publications/the-world-factbook/rankorder/2091rank.html.

Coad, J., & Dunstall, M. (2011). *Anatomy & physiology for midwives* (3rd ed.). Chennai, India: Elsevier Churchill Livingstone.

Coch, D., Dawson, G., & Fischer, K. W. (2010). *Human behavior, learning, and developing the brain.* New York: Guilford Publications.

Cohen, W. R., & Friedman, E. A. (2011). *Labor and delivery care: A practical guide.* Malden, MA: Wiley-Blackwell.

Cunningham, F. G., Gant, N. F., Leveno, K. J., Gilstrap, L. C., Hauth, J. C., & Wenstrom, K. D. (2010a). Implantation, embryogenesis, and placental development. In *Williams obstetrics* (23rd ed., Chapter 3, pp. 39–90). New York: McGraw-Hill.

Cunningham, F. G., Gant, N. F., Leveno, K. J., Gilstrap, L. C., Hauth, J. C., & Wenstrom, K. D. (2010b). Maternal physiology. In *Williams obstetrics* (23rd ed., Chapter 5, pp. 121–150). New York: McGraw-Hill.

Cunningham, F. G., Gant, N. F., Leveno, K. J., Gilstrap, L. C., Hauth, J. C., & Wenstrom, K. D. (2010c). Prenatal care. In *Williams obstetrics* (23rd ed., Chapter 8, pp. 201–230). New York: McGraw-Hill.

Cunningham, F. G., Gant, N. F., Leveno, K. J., Gilstrap, L. C., Hauth, J. C., & Wenstrom, K. D. (2010d). Prenatal diagnosis and fetal therapy. In *Williams obstetrics* (23rd ed., Chapter 13, pp. 313–340). New York: McGraw-Hill.

Cunningham, F. G., Gant, N. F., Leveno, K. J., Gilstrap, L. C., Hauth, J. C., & Wenstrom, K. D. (2010e). Antepartum assessment. In *Williams obstetrics* (23rd ed., Chapter 15, pp. 373–388). New York: McGraw-Hill.

Cunningham, F. G., Gant, N. F., Leveno, K. J., Gilstrap, L. C., Hauth, J. C., & Wenstrom, K. D. (2010f). Genetics. In *Williams obstetrics* (23rd ed., Chapter 12, pp. 285–312). New York: McGraw-Hill.

Czeizel, A. E., & Bánhidy, F. (2011). Chronic hypertension in pregnancy. *Current Opinion in Obstetrics & Gynecology, 23*(2), 76–81.

Debruyne, L., Whitney, E. N., & Pinna, K. (2012). *Nutrition and diet therapy* (8th ed.). Boston: Wadsworth.

Del Giudice, M. (2011). Alone in the dark? Modeling the conditions for visual experience in human fetuses. *Developmental Psychobiology, 53*(2), 214–219. doi:10.1002/dev.20506.

Dudek, S. G. (2010). *Nutritional essentials for nursing practice* (6th ed.). Philadelphia: Lippincott Williams & Wilkins.

Esegbona-Adeigbe, S. (2011). Acquiring cultural competency in caring for black African women. *British Journal of Midwifery, 19*(8), 489–496.

Field, T. (2011). Prenatal depression effects on early development: A review. *Infant Behavior & Development, 34*(1), 1–14.

Fleisher, S. (2011). Alcohol and pregnancy: Advising women not to take risks. *British Journal of Midwifery, 19*(6), 396–397.

Follett, T., & Clarke, D. (2011). Resurgence of congenital syphilis: Diagnosis and treatment. *Neonatal Network, 30*(5), 320–328.

Friars, C. (2007). Toxoplasmosis and pregnancy. *Practicing Midwife, 10*(4), 20–21.

Gardella, C., & Brown, Z. (2011). Prevention of neonatal herpes. *BJOG: An International Journal of Obstetrics and Gynecology, 118*(2), 187–192.

Gaston, A., & Gammage, K. L. (2011). The effectiveness of a health-based message on pregnant women's intentions to exercise postpartum. *Journal of Reproductive & Infant Psychology, 29*(2), 162–169. doi:10.1080/02646838.2010.541230.

Gatrell, C. (2011). Putting pregnancy in its place: Conceiving pregnancy as carework in the workplace. *Health & Place, 17*(2), 395–402.

Gilbert, E. S. (2011). *Manual of high risk pregnancy and delivery* (5th ed.). St. Louis: Mosby.

Greener, M. (2011). The tragedy of congenital abnormalities. *Nurse Prescribing, 9*(3), 117–121.

Gregory, K. E. (2011). Microbiome aspects of perinatal and neonatal health. *Journal of Perinatal & Neonatal Nursing, 25*(2), 158–162.

Gordon, M. (2010). *Manual of nursing diagnosis* (12th ed.). Sudbury, MA: Jones & Bartlett Learning.

Heffner, L. J., & Schust, D. J. (2010). *The reproductive system at a glance* (3rd ed.). Oxford, UK: Wiley-Blackwell.

Herrick, K., Hudson, L., & Burd, L. (2011). The elephant in the cradle: Fetal alcohol spectrum disorders. *Zero to Three, 31*(3), 44–50.

Heslehurst, N. (2011). Identifying 'at risk' women and the impact of maternal obesity on National Health Service maternity services. *Proceedings of the Nutrition Society, 70*(4), 439–449.

Hill, L. (2011). Adjusting to motherhood. *Community Practitioner, 84*(5), 40–41.

Institute of Medicine (IOM). (2011). *Weight gain during pregnancy: Reexamining the guidelines.* Retrieved from www.iom.edu/Reports/2009/Weight-Gain-During-Pregnancy-Reexamining-the-Guidelines.aspx.

Jones, C., Chan, C., & Farine, D. (2011). Sex in pregnancy. *Canadian Medical Association Journal, 183*(7), 815–818.

Katz, C., Bentur, L., & Elias, N. (2011). Clinical implication of lung fluid balance in the perinatal period. *Journal of Perinatology, 31*(4), 230–235.

Keely, A., Gunning, M., & Denison, F. (2011). Maternal obesity in pregnancy: Women's understanding of risks. *British Journal of Midwifery, 19*(6), 364–369.

King, T. L., & Brucker, M. C. (2009). *Pharmacology for women.* Sudbury, MA: Jones & Bartlett Learning.

Kuehn, B. (2011). Scientists see promise and challenges in translating genomics to the clinic. *Journal of the American Medical Association, 305*(13), 1285–1286.

Lando, A., & Zhang, Y. (2011). Awareness and knowledge of methylmercury in fish in the United States. *Environmental Research, 111*(3), 442–450.

Lee, A., & Okam, M. (2011). Anemia in pregnancy. *Hematology/Oncology Clinics of North America, 25,* 241–259.

Li, D. (2011). Does antiviral medication for treating herpes simplex during pregnancy increase the risk of birth defects in offspring? *Evidence-Based Medicine, 16*(1), 30.

MacDorman, M. F., & Mathews, T. J. (2011). *Understanding racial and ethnic disparities in U.S. infant mortality rates.* NCHS Data Brief No. 74, Hyattsville, MD: U.S. Department of Health and Human Services, CDC, National Center for Health Statistics.

March of Dimes. (2011). *Genetic birth defects. March of Dimes fact sheets.* [Online] Retrieved from www.marchofdimes.com/birth defects_cleftpalate.html.

Mastroiacovo, P., & Leoncini, E. (2011). More folic acid, the five questions: Why, who, when, how much, and how. *Biofactors, 37*(4), 272–279. doi:10.1002/biof.172.

Mattson, S., & Smith, J. E. (2011). *Core curriculum for maternal-newborn nursing* (4th ed.). St. Louis: Saunders Elsevier.

Maxson, P., & Miranda, M. (2011). Pregnancy intention, demographic differences, and psychosocial health. *Journal of Women's Health, 20*(8), 1215–1223.

Mayo Clinic. (2011). *Cleft lip and cleft palate. Mayo Clinic Health Library.* [Online] Retrieved from www.mayoclinic.com/health/cleft-palate/DS00738/DSECTION=risk-factors.

Merriam-Webster. (2012). *Merriam-Webster's Medical Dictionary.* Springfield, MA: Merriam-Webster, Incorporated.

Miller, T. (2011). Transition to first-time motherhood. *Practising Midwife, 14*(2), 12–15.

Mølgaard-Nielsen, D., & Hviid, A. (2011). Newer-generation antiepileptic drugs and the risk of major birth defects. *Journal of the American Medical Association, 305*(19), 1996–2002.

Monea, E., & Thomas, A. (2011). Unintended pregnancy and taxpayer spending. *Perspectives on Sexual & Reproductive Health, 43*(2), 88–93. doi: 10.1363/4308811.

Mylonas, I. (2011). Antibiotic chemotherapy during pregnancy and lactation period: Aspects for consideration. *Archives of Gynecology & Obstetrics, 283*(1), 7–18.

National Institute on Drug Abuse (NIDA). (2011). *Pregnancy and substance abuse.* [Online] Retrieved from http://health.nih.gov/topic/PregnancyandSubstanceAbuse.

Nelson, J., & Henriksen Hellyer, J. M. (2011). The patient's responsibility. *American Journal of Nursing, 111*(2), 11.

Nigro, G., & Adler, S. (2011). Cytomegalovirus infections during pregnancy. *Current Opinion in Obstetrics & Gynecology, 23*(2), 123–128.

Njiru, H., Elchalal, U., & Paltiel, O. (2011). Geophagy during pregnancy in Africa: A literature review. *Obstetrical & Gynecological Survey, 66*(7), 452–459.

Norwitz, E. R., & Schorge, J. O. (2010). *Obstetrics and gynecology at a glance* (3rd ed.). Malden, MA: Blackwell Publishing.

O'Dell, K. (2011). Pharmacologic management of asymptomatic bacteriuria and urinary tract infections in women. *Journal of Midwifery & Women's Health, 56*(3), 248–265.

Polin, R. A., Fox, W. W., & Abman, S. H. (2011). *Fetal & neonatal physiology* (4th ed.). St Louis: Saunders Elsevier.

Rubarth, L. (2011). Blood types and ABO incompatibility. *Neonatal Network, 30*(1), 50–53.

Rubin, R. (1967). Attainment of the maternal role. Part I. Processes. *Nursing Research, 16,* 237–245.

Rubin, R. (1972). Fantasy and object constancy in maternal relationships. *Maternal and Child Nursing Journal, 1*(2), 101–111.

Rubin, R. (1977). Bonding in the postpartum period. *Maternal and Child Nursing Journal, 6,* 67–75.

Rubin, R. (1984). *Maternal identity and the maternal experience.* New York: Springer.

Shaw, P., Duncan, A., Vouyouka, A., & Ozsvath, K. (2011). Radiation exposure and pregnancy. *Journal of Vascular Surgery: Official Publication, The Society for Vascular Surgery [and] International Society for Cardiovascular Surgery, North American Chapter, 53*(Suppl. 1), 28S–34S.

Shet, A. (2011). Congenital and perinatal infections: Throwing new light with an old TORCH. *Indian Journal of Pediatrics, 78*(1), 88–95.

Stables, D., & Rankin, J. (2011). *Physiology in childbearing with anatomy and related biosciences* (3rd ed.). London, UK: Ballière Tindall Elsevier.

Stone, J., & Moskowitz, G. (2011). Non-conscious bias in medical decision making: What can be done to reduce it? *Medical Education, 45*(8), 768–776. doi: 10.1111/j.1365-2923.2011.04026.x.

Suwanrath, C., & Suntharasai, T. (2010). Sleep-wake cycles in normal fetuses. *Archives of Gynecology & Obstetrics, 281*(3), 449–454.

Tamaru, S., Kikuchi, A., Takagi, K., Wakamatsu, M., Horikoshi, T., & Ogiso, Y. (2011). Fetal therapy of severe symptomatic toxoplasmosis using azithromycin. *Journal of Obstetrics & Gynaecology Research, 37*(7), 953–957. doi: 10.1111/j.1447-0756.2010.01459.x.

Tortora, G. J., & Derrickson, B. H. (2011). *Principles of anatomy and physiology* (13th ed.). Malden, MA: John Wiley & Sons.

United States Department of Agriculture (USDA). (2011). *Daily food plan for moms.* [Online] Retrieved from www.choosemyplate.gov/mypyramidmoms/pyramidmoms_plan.aspx.

U.S. Department of Health and Human Services (USDHHS). (2010). *Healthy People 2020.* Washington, DC: U.S. Government Printing Office. [Online] Retrieved at www.cdc.gov/nchs/healthy_people/hp2020.htm.

U.S. Preventive Services Task Force (USPSTF). (2011a). *Screening for family and intimate partner violence.* [Online] Retrieved from www.uspreventiveservicestaskforce.org/uspstf/uspsfamv.htm# summary.

U.S. Preventive Services Task Force (USPSTF). (2011b). *Screening for bacterial vaginosis in pregnancy to prevent preterm delivery.* [Online] Retrieved from www.uspreventiveservicestaskforce.org/uspstf/uspsbvag.htm.

U.S. Preventive Services Task Force (USPSTF). (2011c). *Screening for HIV.* [Online] Retrieved from www.uspreventiveservicestaskforce.org/uspstf05/hiv/hivrs.htm.

U.S. Preventive Services Task Force (USPSTF). (2011d). *Screening for hepatitis B virus infection in pregnancy.* [Online] Retrieved from www.uspreventiveservicestaskforce.org/uspstf/uspshepbpg.htm.

U.S. Preventive Services Task Force (USPSTF). (2011e). *Screening for Rh (D) incompatibility.* [Online] Retrieved from www.ahrq.gov/clinic/pocketgd1011/gcp10s2e.htm.

Warren, K. R., Hewitt, B. G., & Thomas, J. D. (2011). Fetal alcohol spectrum disorders: Research challenges and opportunities. *Alcohol Research & Health, 34*(1), 4–14.

Wiesel, A., Spix, C., Mergenthaler, A., & Queisser-Luft, A. (2011). Maternal occupational exposure to ionizing radiation and birth defects. *Radiation and Environmental Biophysics, 50*(2), 325–328.

Wilson, S. (2011). HIV and pregnancy: Past, present and future. *HIV Nursing, 11*(1), 9–11.

Wong, L., & MacLennan, A. (2011). Gathering the evidence: Cord gases and placental histology for births with low Apgar scores. *The Australian & New Zealand Journal of Obstetrics & Gynecology, 51*(1), 17–21. doi: 10.1111/j.1479-828X.2010.01275.x.

Infant

Susan Scott Ricci

evolve WEBSITE

http://evolve.elsevier.com/Edelman/
- Study Questions
- Glossary

- Website Resources
  17A: Growth Chart for Girls, Birth to 36 Months
  17B: Growth Chart for Boys, Birth to 36 Months
  17C: Recommended Immunization Schedule for Persons Aged 0 Through 6

OBJECTIVES

After completing this chapter, the reader will be able to:
- Evaluate the infant's health status and give examples of basic growth and developmental principles.
- Analyze the developmental tasks for the infant and the behavior indicating that these tasks are being met.
- Explain the immunization schedule and other safety and health-promotion measures to a parent.
- Detect common parental concerns about infants and describe a model for parent education to allay these concerns.
- Examine accidents that occur during infancy and recommend appropriate counseling for accident prevention and safety.
- Differentiate ways in which nurses can be active in promoting major policies and influencing legislation concerning health.
- Outline governmental strategies to meet the goals of improving infant health.

KEY TERMS

Active immunization
Birth defect
Body mass index (BMI)
Child abuse
Denver Developmental Screening Test
Failure-to-thrive syndrome

Growth
Growth index
Oral stage of development
Passive immunization
Paternal engrossment
Reflexes

Sensorimotor period
Sickle cell anemia
Sudden infant death syndrome (SIDS)
Tay-Sachs disease
Trust versus mistrust
Weaning

💡 THINK ABOUT IT

Car Safety Seats

Infants are at particular risk from automobile accidents. The proper use of occupant protection systems (infant car safety seats with seat belts) can reduce the risk of death and injury significantly. Although many public service campaigns encourage parents to restrain their infants while riding in automobiles (and all states have laws requiring some type of passenger safety restraint for infants), some parents neglect or remain unaware of the importance of providing safety for their vulnerable infants.

Nurses must have up-to-date knowledge about car occupant protection systems and their proper use to help parents find new products and obtain the most current information available. Parents often rely on the salesperson of the infant car seat for their information about protection systems and the proper use of car seats. However, informational brochures and media campaigns fall short because they usually fail to provide explanations or demonstrations. As a result, parents may misinterpret the information that they receive.

- What type of program might you develop to reach and inform parents about the importance of car seat safety?
- In what settings might such a program be implemented?
- How would you modify your teaching plan to meet the needs of illiterate parents?
- How would you modify your program to ensure that parents who come from cultural backgrounds different than your own would respond well to the information?

♥ BOX 17-1   HEALTHY PEOPLE 2020

Selected National Health-Promotion and Disease-Prevention Objectives for Infants

- Reduce the rate of all infant deaths (within 1 year). Target: 6.0 infant deaths per 1000 live births (Baseline: 6.7 infant deaths per 1000 live births within first year of life in 2006)
- Reduce the rate of neonatal deaths (within the first 28 days of life). Target: 4.1 neonatal deaths per 1000 live births (Baseline: 4.5 neonatal deaths per 1000 live births occurred within the first 28 days of life in 2006)
- Reduce the rate of infant deaths related to birth defects (all birth defects). Target: 1.3 infant deaths per 1000 live births (Baseline: 1.4 infant deaths per 1000 live births were attributed to birth defects (all birth defects) in 2006)
- Reduce the rate of infant deaths from sudden infant death syndrome (SIDS). Target: 0.50 infant deaths per 1000 live births (Baseline: 0.55 infant deaths per 1000 live births were attributed to sudden infant death syndrome in 2006)
- Reduce the 1-year mortality rate for infants with Down syndrome. Target: 43.7 deaths within the first year of life per 1000 infants with Down syndrome (Baseline: 48.6 deaths within the first year of life per 1000 infants diagnosed with Down syndrome occurred from 2005 to 2006)
- Increase the proportion of infants who are put to sleep on their backs. Target: 75.9% (Baseline: 69.0% of infants were put to sleep on their backs in 2007)
- Increase the proportion of infants who are breastfed. Target: 81.9% (Baseline: 74.0% of infants born in 2006 were ever breastfed as reported from 2007 to 2009)

From U.S. Department of Health and Human Services (USDHHS). (2010). *Healthy People 2020.* [Online] Available at www.healthypeople.gov/2020/topicsobjectives2020/objectiveslist.aspx?topicId=26.

Providing a safe and sound source of attachment and interaction is paramount to healthy infant development. Caregiving and mothering activities are the primary ingredients of an infant's preparation for life and ultimate independence. Nurses play a vital role in influencing this positive interaction through health promotion and education.

This chapter focuses on the infant and family during the infant's developmental period of 1 to 18 months. Because the infant is completely dependent, this chapter addresses the infant's parents and significant others as sources of health-promotion activities. The relationship initiated at birth between parents and infant is the basis for the interdependence that is required for proper psychological and physical infant development. Health care professionals must focus on parent education as a means of fostering healthy, satisfying relationships within the family unit, and promoting the development of healthy future generations.

The principles of normal growth and development are used as a structural framework for this chapter. Understanding these principles helps the nurse identify deviations from the norm and institute appropriate health-promoting interventions.

To promote and maintain health during infancy, a balance between the infant's internal and external environmental forces must be established; any disruption places the infant at risk. Several processes that greatly influence this balance are identified, and appropriate interventions are outlined to assist the nurse in promoting a healthy infant population (American Academy of Pediatrics, 2011a; Hockenberry & Wilson, 2010) (Box 17-1: *Healthy People 2020*).

BIOLOGY AND GENETICS

Human development begins when a single sperm penetrates a mature ovum. The changes that follow are undeniable and wondrous. During this early period of growth and development the infant depends completely on others, primarily the parents, to meet all personal needs (Box 17-2). To assist the parents in their understanding of their infant's needs and progress, the nurse must know what behaviors to expect at certain age levels. These developmental landmarks serve as a basis for anticipatory guidance (Table 17-1). Parents are aware of age-appropriate behavior to anticipate and facilitate these developmental landmarks. This knowledge, along with the nurse's anticipatory guidance, can also promote closer family relationships. In addition to the growth landmarks, the infant must accomplish developmental tasks to form a healthy personality.

Developmental Tasks

Every infant faces developmental tasks and must accomplish them individually. Different practices in various societies affect the perception and resolution of the tasks, but all must be faced (Pillitteri, 2010).

The infant's first and most basic task is survival, which includes the physical tasks of breathing, sucking, eating, digesting, eliminating, and sleeping. Because many of these tasks involve the infant's mouth, this stage of life often is referred to

BOX 17-2 GROWTH AND DEVELOPMENT

During Infancy

One Month
- Follows and fixes on bright object with eyes when it moves within field of vision
- Still has head lag when pulled to sitting position
- Displays tonic neck, grasp, and Moro reflexes
- Turns head when prone, but unable to support
- Displays sucking and rooting reflexes
- Holds hands in fists
- Makes small, throaty sounds
- Gains 5 to 7 ounces weekly for 6 months
- Grows 1 inch monthly for 6 months
- Cries when hungry or uncomfortable
- Lifts head momentarily when prone

Two Months
- Has closed posterior fontanel
- Listens actively to sounds
- Lifts head almost 45 degrees off table when prone
- Follows moving object with eyes
- Recognizes familiar faces
- Pays attention to speaking voice
- Assumes less flexed position when prone
- Vocalizes; distinct from crying
- Turns from side to back
- Begins to have social smile

Three Months
- Visually inspects object and stares at own hand with apparent fascination when either appears in field of vision
- Has longer periods of wakefulness without crying
- Laughs aloud and shows pleasure in vocalization
- Holds head erect and steady; raises chest, usually supported on forearms
- Smiles in response to mother's face
- Begins prelanguage vocalizations (coos, babbles, and chuckles)
- Carries hand or object to mouth at will
- Actively holds rattle, but will not reach for it
- Turns eyes to object placed in field of vision

Four Months
- Begins drooling, indicated by appearance of saliva; does not know how to swallow it
- Holds head steady when in sitting position
- Recognizes familiar objects
- Shows almost no head lag when pulled to sitting position
- Rolls from back to side and from abdomen to back
- Inspects and plays with hands; pulls clothing or blanket over face in play
- Begins eye-hand coordination
- Chews and bites
- Enjoys social interaction
- Demands attention by fussing
- Reaches out to people
- Is aware and interested in new environment
- Grasps object with two hands
- Squeals

Five Months
- Reaches persistently; grasps with entire hand
- Plays with toes

- Smiles at mirror image
- Begins to postpone gratification
- Shows signs of tooth eruption
- Sleeps through night without food
- Weighs twice the birth weight
- Sits with slight support
- Vocalizes displeasure when desired object is taken away
- Is able to discriminate strangers from family
- Makes cooing noises
- Squeals with delight
- Looks for object that has fallen
- Rolls from back to stomach or vice versa

Six Months
- Gains approximately 3 to 5 ounces weekly during the second 6 months
- Grows approximately 1 inch monthly for 6 months
- Is able to lift cup by handle
- Begins to hitch in locomotion
- Sits in high chair with straight back
- Begins to imitate sounds
- Vocalizes to toys and mirror image
- Babbles with one-syllable sounds: "ma, ma, da, da"
- Has definite likes and dislikes
- Likes to be picked up
- Plays peek-a-boo
- Makes "guh" and "bah" sounds

Seven Months
- Has eruption of upper central incisors
- Bears weight when held in standing position
- Sits, leaning forward on both hands
- Fixates on one very small object
- Produces vowel sounds: "ba-ba" and "da-da"
- Shows fear of strangers
- Displays emotional instability by easy and quick changes from crying to laughing
- Repeats activities that are enjoyed
- Bangs objects together
- Approaches toy and grasps it with one hand
- Imitates simple acts

Eight Months
- Feeds self with finger foods
- Sits well alone
- Stretches out arms to be picked up
- Greets strangers with bashful behavior
- Begins to show regular patterns in bladder and bowel elimination
- Responds to "no"
- Makes consonant sounds: t, d, and w
- Dislikes dressing and diaper change
- Releases object at will
- Shows nervousness with strangers
- Pulls toy toward self

Nine Months
- Creeps and crawls (backward at first)
- Shows good coordination and sits alone
- Responds to adult anger; cries when scolded

📊 BOX 17-2 GROWTH AND DEVELOPMENT

During Infancy—cont'd

- Explores object by sucking, chewing, and biting it
- Responds to simple verbal requests
- Drinks from cup or glass with assistance
- Pulls self to standing position
- Begins to show fears of going to bed and being left alone
- Imitates waving "bye-bye"
- Releases object with flexed wrist
- Repeats facial expressions of adults
- Uses thumb and index finger in pincer grasp

10 Months
- Sits by falling down
- Says "da-da" and "ma-ma"
- Understands "bye-bye"
- Looks at and follows pictures in book
- Crawls and cruises about well
- Pays attention to own name
- Picks up objects fairly well
- Extends toy to another person without releasing
- Pulls self to standing position and stands while holding onto solid object

11 Months
- Is able to push toys and place several objects in container
- Attempts to walk without assistance
- Begins to hold spoon
- Stands erect with help of person's hand
- May have eruption of lower lateral incisors
- Holds crayon to mark on paper
- Imitates definite speech sounds
- Reacts to restrictions with frustration

12 Months
- Loses Babinski's sign
- Develops evident hand dominance
- Weighs triple the birth weight
- Has equal circumference of head and chest
- Walks with help
- Knows own name

- Has slow vocabulary growth because of increased interest in walking
- Develops lumbar curve
- Uses spoon in feeding, but often puts it upside down in mouth
- Drops object deliberately for it to be picked up
- Shakes head for "no"
- Plays pat-a-cake
- Recovers balance when falling over
- Tries to follow when being read to
- Does things to attract attention
- Imitates vocalization lead

15 Months
- Creeps up stairs
- Uses "da-da" and "ma-ma" labels for correct parents
- Tolerates some separation
- Drinks from cup well, but rotates spoon
- Asks for object by pointing
- Plays interactive games such as peek-a-boo and pat-a-cake
- Expresses emotions; has temper tantrums
- Walks without help

18 Months
- Has closed anterior fontanel
- Has long trunk, short and bowed legs, and protruding abdomen
- Walks up stairs with help
- Turns pages of book
- Has short attention span
- Begins to test limits
- Has bowel movements at appropriate time when placed on potty
- Indicates wet pants
- Gets into everything
- Fills and handles spoon without rotating it, but spills frequently
- Runs clumsily and falls often
- Is extremely curious
- Places object in hole or slot
- Becomes communicative, social being
- Imitates behavior of parents, such as mimicking household chores

---

as the oral stage of development, reflecting the primary importance of the mouth as the center of pleasure. More developmental tasks that must be accomplished during infancy are listed in Box 17-3.

To assist the infant's parents in encouraging achievement of these tasks, the nurse discusses the importance of stimulation and environmental interactions. Many neurological structures are far from completely developed at birth (Coch et al., 2010). To continue growing, the brain depends not only on internal, embryological, and maturational forces, but also on external stimulation. This external stimulation appears to influence the internal, anatomical, and maturational processes by means of at least three different mechanisms (Kail & Cavanaugh, 2012):

- Stimulation favors progressive complex branching of dendrites (the connection between nerve cells).
- Stimulation increases the degree of vascularization of certain anatomical structures of the brain, such as the centers associated with vision.
- Stimulation increases the process of myelination, which is closely related to the rate of development of a variety of functions. Myelin coats the brain and nerve tissue, which then becomes activated.

When counseling parents, the nurse stresses the importance of a variety of stimuli within the infant's environment. A variety of auditory and visual stimuli should be available, such as colorful mobiles, radio, spoken voice, and toys, to assist the infant in achieving developmental tasks. The sense of touch is an extremely important stimulus, bringing the infant in tune with caregivers in different environments, making it a reality. Ensuring that appropriate sensory stimuli are available is vital to the infant's growth and developmental progression (Kail & Cavanaugh, 2012).

Concepts of Infant Development

The study of how a helpless infant grows and develops into a fully functioning, independent adult has fascinated many

TABLE 17-1 PARENTING TASKS FOR DEVELOPMENTAL LANDMARKS IN INFANCY

AGE (MONTHS)	LANDMARK	PARENTING TASK
1	Lifts head when prone	Place infant in prone position and dangle colorful object above head
2	Has social smile	Promote by talking to infant and allowing opportunity to smile
4	Squeals	Encourage and praise for doing
5	Rolls from back to front	Place infant in protected area (crib or playpen) and encourage to move by placing toy out of reach
8 to 9	Uses pincer grasp to feed self	Make finger foods available
10	Pulls self to standing position	Provide safe environment; place chair or object of appropriate height within reach
11 to 12	Initiates vocalization	Talk to infant frequently and include in family gatherings
12 to 15	Walks	Encourage and provide clutter-free, safe walkway; praise for attempts
15	Drinks from cup	Supply cup with appropriate drink; do not scold for clumsiness in handling cups or spills
18	Mimics household chores	Give rags to help with chores, dusting, allow to fold clothes, and so on

BOX 17-3 GROWTH AND DEVELOPMENT
Developmental Tasks Accomplished in Infancy

- Achieves physiological equilibrium after birth
- Establishes self as a dependent person, but separate from others
- Becomes aware of animate versus inanimate and familiar versus unfamiliar and develops rudimentary social interaction
- Develops a feeling of affection for others and the desire for affection from others
- Manages the changing body and learns new motor skills, develops equilibrium, begins eye-hand coordination, and establishes rest-activity rhythm
- Learns to understand and control the physical world through exploration
- Develops a beginning symbol system, conceptual abilities, and preverbal communication
- Directs emotional expression to indicate needs and wishes

From Steinberg, L., Bornstein, M. H., Vandell, D. L., & Rook, K. S. (2011). *Lifespan development: Infancy through adulthood.* Belmont, CA: Wadsworth, Cengage Learning.

researchers. Their theories describe the development of human behavior as overlapping stages that occur in somewhat predictable patterns in an individual's life (Meyerhoff, 2010). Because these developmental theories are presented in Chapter 15, only their specific application to the infant is discussed here.

Psychosocial Development

Erikson's psychosocial developmental theory is concerned primarily with a series of tasks or crises that each individual must resolve before encountering the next one. The central task

during infancy is the development of a sense of trust versus mistrust. Establishing this basic trust or mistrust determines the manner in which the infant approaches all future stages of growth. The infant first develops a sense of trust in the mother (or other caretaker) and then in other significant people. Trust influences the infant's future relationships, allowing for deeper commitment and intimacy. To develop trust the infant requires maximal gratification and minimal frustration to experience a healthy balance between inner needs and outer satisfaction. If the mother or caretaker is consistently responsive to the infant, meeting physical and psychological needs, the infant will likely learn to trust his or her caretaker; view the world as a safe place; and grow up to be secure, self-reliant, trusting, cooperative, and helpful towards others.

Prompt, skillful, and consistent response to the infant's needs helps foster security and trust because it enables the infant to predict what will happen within the environment. When unpredictability and disorganized routines exist, the infant will develop fear, anger, and insecurity, which eventually lead to mistrust. The infant can demonstrate desire by crying but depends on the sensitivity and willingness of others to provide relief. If the most important people fail to do this, the infant has little foundation on which to build faith in others or self in adulthood.

Cognitive Development

Piaget's cognitive developmental theory focuses on intellectual changes that occur in a sequential manner as a result of continual interaction between the infant and the environment (Berk, 2012). Piaget's sensorimotor period (up to age 18 months) describes the time during which infants develop the coordination to master activities that allow them to interact with the environment. During this period the infant solves problems using sensory systems and motor activity rather than symbolic processes, which develop later.

Research has shown that fetuses are able to distinguish light from dark and that sight is present at birth. Rod cells in the retina of the eyes, which are responsible for light perception, are functional at birth although the retina (the organ of visual perception) is not fully developed until approximately 4 months of age. However, the infant can perceive color and shape. Infants are startled by loud noises and are soothed by soft voices, indicating that their sense of hearing is functioning. Their hearing can also be tested with audio equipment at birth. Babies cry when pricked with a diaper pin and fuss when too hot or too cold; therefore, the senses of pain and temperature are operative also. Touching, stroking, and rocking typically comfort a fussing infant. Infants will also react to odors and tastes.

In addition to perceiving stimulation, the newborn is capable of reflexive behavior. Reflexes are responses that normally are exhibited after particular types of new stimulation (Woods, 2011). Because the response occurs after the stimulus, reflexes are unlearned. Some infant reflexes, such as rooting and sucking, have survival value. The rooting reflex, activated by lightly stroking the angle of the lips or cheek, helps the infant locate the food source. The infant will turn toward the side that is being stroked and will open the lips to suck. The sucking reflex

TABLE 17-2 GROWTH AND DEVELOPMENT

Piaget's Five Stages of Infant Development

STAGE	DESCRIPTION
Stage 1: birth to 1 month	Modification of reflexes Practices and perfects reflexes present at birth Sucking reflex becomes more refined and voluntary
Stage 2: 1 to 4 months	Primary circular reactions Repeats behavior that previously led to an interesting event Only the infant's own body involved in activities
Stage 3: 4 to 10 months	Secondary circular reactions begin Repetitions involve events or objects in the external world Appears to perform actions with a purpose Hand-eye coordination
Stage 4: 10 to 12 months	Coordination of secondary reactions Combines two or more previously acquired strategies to obtain a goal
Stage 5: 12 to 18 months	Tertiary circular reactions Uses active experimentation to achieve previously unattainable goals Infant purposely varies movements to observe results

is initiated when an object is placed in the infant's mouth. Together, these reflexes ensure that the infant can obtain food. Infants also have reflexes that result in grasping, yawning, hiccoughing, coughing, and sneezing.

Armed with these reflexes and sensory capabilities, the infant is ready to begin interacting with the environment (seeing, hearing, touching, tasting, and smelling) to acquire valuable information.

The infant progresses in various ways between birth and age 18 months, with early capabilities changing and becoming intentional. Piaget outlines five stages within the sensorimotor period that describe the infant's development, from the early reflexive behavior to differentiation between self and environment (Table 17-2).

The infant in the sensorimotor period uses behavioral strategies to manipulate objects, to learn some of their properties, and to reach goals by combining several behaviors. The infant's behavior is tied to the concrete and the immediate; schemes can be applied only to objects that can be perceived directly.

Knowledge of child developmental theories is extremely valuable to the nurse during interactions with infants. Understanding the infant's level of cognitive thought and emotional and social development helps the nurse decipher a child's communications more meaningfully and interpret behaviors and the processes that motivate the child more accurately. This knowledge can be incorporated in the anticipatory guidance offered to the parents. The nurse stresses that a variety of sensory and motor stimuli fosters learning within the infant's environment.

Denver Developmental Screening Test

The **Denver Developmental Screening Test (DDST)** is one of several standardized tools that screen for developmental problems in children from birth to 6 years of age. Three purposes have been identified for administering the Denver II: screening

apparently healthy infants for developmental problems; validating intuitive concerns about an infant's development with an objective test; and monitoring high-risk children for developmental problems.

Four areas of development are screened: personal-social; fine motor–adaptive; language; and gross motor. Unique features of the Denver II are its recent and sophisticated standardization and its inclusion of norms for various subgroups based on place of residence, ethnicity, and mother's level of education. The Denver II includes four test behavior descriptors to rate the infant's behavior, reflecting the administrator's subjective impression of the infant's overall behavior. Behavioral ratings are established for compliance with the examiner's requests for alertness and interest in the surroundings, fearfulness, and attention span.

The nurse tells the parents before the test that the DDST is not an intelligence test but, rather, a test of the child's developmental level. By adding the number of accomplished and unaccomplished items on the test form, the screener estimates the child's developmental level. By referring to guidelines on the instruction sheet, the child is scored P (passed) or F (failed) on each item. The DDST can be administered with minimal materials and time and, ideally, should be administered to an infant at approximately 3 or 4 months of age, again at 10 months, and again at 3 years (Coch et al., 2010).

Another infant developmental and social-emotional screening tool is the Ages and Stages Questionnaire (ASQ). It takes parents about 15 minutes to administer the test, which is then scored by the health care professional. The ASQ can be used for infants 1 month old to children up to age 66 months. The ASQ consists of 21 questionnaires with each questionnaire having approximately 30 questions. It is available in both English and Spanish languages.

Still another infant assessment tool is the Infant Developmental Inventory (IDI) that tracks developmental skills in five areas: social, self-help, gross motor, fine motor, and language. Monthly developmental milestones on the chart help parents obtain a more comprehensive picture of how infants develop. Parents can also report any questions or concerns about their infant's health, development, or behavior. Health care providers may further assess the infant's development by observing behaviors and recording them on the chart, in which case the baby's progress will be scored "typical," "borderline," or "delayed" in each developmental area. The Infant Developmental Inventory can be used up to 18 months of age.

The infant's growth index—height and weight measurements plotted on a standard growth chart to assess for normal progression—is also important. Physical growth (height and weight) is a valid health status indicator that should be measured during each routine office or clinic visit. During the first year of life, growth is rapid. An infant who is growing properly is at low risk for developing a chronic disease (Puckett & Black, 2010).

The nurse plots the infant's length and weight measurements against exact chronological age on growth grids. In 2000 the National Center for Health Statistics published growth grids that have been standardized to the present growth charts for female and male infants from birth to age 36 months. These growth charts are presented in **Website Resources 17A** and **17B.** Body mass index (BMI) is a feature of the new pediatric growth charts recently released by the Centers for Disease Control and Prevention (CDC). The CDC recommends that health care providers use the World Health Organization (WHO) growth standards to monitor growth for infants and children from birth to 2 years of age in the United States and use the CDC growth charts for U.S. children age 2 years and older (CDC, 2011a). Growth charts are not intended to be used as a sole diagnostic instrument. Instead, growth charts are tools that contribute to forming an overall clinical impression for the child being measured (Parsons et al., 2011).

With the addition of body mass index to the charts, the CDC significantly increased the usefulness of this tool as a warning signal for potential obesity as early as 2 years of age. Parents have an opportunity to change their children's eating habits before a weight problem develops. The revised pediatric growth charts more accurately reflect the cultural and racial diversity currently found in the United States and can track children and young people through age 20. The growth charts indicate data that children are heavier today than in the past, but height has remained virtually unchanged.

An infant's growth index, as determined by length and weight, is only one factor in assessing health status. Differences in growth curves can influence the diagnosis of under- and overnutrition, and the interpretation of adequate growth following nutritional intervention. The nurse has an overall understanding of growth and developmental principles to counsel parents regarding their infant's progress.

Gender

The infant's gender is determined at the moment of fertilization. Immediately after delivery, the parents usually ask, "Is it a girl or a boy?" The answer has far-reaching implications for many family units. Gender is one of the many important factors that influence parents' way of relating to the infant.

Studies have revealed many biological and behavioral differences between male and female infants. Boys are, on average, larger and have proportionately more muscle mass at birth. Girls are generally smaller but physiologically more mature at birth and are less vulnerable to stress. Boys show more motor activity, whereas girls display a greater response to tactile stimulation and pain (Polan & Taylor, 2010). As the infant develops, further differences are noted. By 6 months, girls respond to visual stimulation with longer attention spans and are more socially responsive than are boys; girls also tend to sit up, walk, and crawl earlier than do boys. Girls also learn to communicate with language at an earlier age, whereas male infants use their whole bodies in communicating (Coch et al., 2010).

The gender of the infant, a major concern of many expectant parents, may well influence parental relationships and expectations. The infant's gender can evoke disappointment; in some cases, a woman may feel disappointed in a girl because she knows that her husband wanted a boy. Today, the trend is to want one child of each gender. Because of the availability in America of better forms of contraception and economic factors

such as the expense of raising children, most couples are having fewer children today when compared with the 1950s. The importance and stress of producing the "right-sex" infant is evident. Being the "wrong sex" can, combined with other factors, place an infant at risk for child abuse. The parents may find fault with and place blame on the infant for not meeting this expectation (Olson et al., 2011).

Health intervention focuses on the identification of high-risk families and the promotion of positive relationships between infants and parents. The nurse promotes the good health, appearance, and developmental potential of the infant. Increasing the parents' feelings of adequacy and self-esteem will promote their acceptance and care of the infant. Most importantly, follow-up care for these families is a high priority to ensure that adequate support and help are available.

Race

Race refers to the classification of human beings into groups based on particular physical characteristics, such as skin pigmentation, head form, and stature, attributable to a common inheritance. Caucasoid, mongoloid, and negroid are the three racial types generally recognized (Dorland, 2012). A range of physical variation exists among people of different races with regard to growth rate, dentition, body structure, blood groups, and susceptibility to certain diseases as well as a great many other variables.

In assessing an infant, the nurse not only collects data but also compares the data with established norms, such as a standardized growth chart. When the norms chosen are not appropriate for the individual (for example, an Asian infant's growth is assessed based on norms for White children), the assessment will not be accurate. The nurse who works with families from a variety of racial groups has an understanding of each background and how it relates to health and health care. To facilitate nursing care for a family from a racial group different from that of the health care provider, effective communication must be established. This communication will help foster an understanding of the other's point of view and frame of reference. Each family member is viewed as an individual, as well as a family unit. There is no stereotyping of families within a racial or ethnic group. Despite common language, color, or historical background, not all members of a particular racial group are alike. This diversity presents, without doubt, considerable challenges for nurses who work with families with infants (Schwartz & Scott, 2011). Universal norms by which to measure one's growth and skill capacity do not exist. The nurse recognizes the differences and intervenes appropriately. The orientation of health maintenance and disease prevention is basic to good health practices, regardless of racial makeup. This concept is the main focus of all health care. (Refer to Chapter 2 for further details.)

Genetics

The desired and expected outcome of any pregnancy is the birth of a healthy, perfect baby. Parents experience disappointment when they discover that their baby has been born with a defect. A birth defect is an abnormality of structure, function, or metabolism as a result of a genetic or environmental influence on the fetus, often a combination of both. Couples may refrain from having another child because they have had one with a serious birth defect and do not want to risk another. In these situations, genetic counseling provides information that is needed to understand a hereditary disorder and its associated risks. The main goal of counseling is to explain **birth defects** to affected families and to allow prospective parents to make informed decisions about childbearing.

Using the basic laws governing heredity and knowing the frequency of specific birth defects in the population, the genetic counselor can often predict the probability of recurrence of a given abnormality in the same family. An important aspect of primary prevention is identifying families at increased risk and referring them for counseling (R. Lewis, 2011). Aspects to be reviewed in the initial interview include the following:

- *Maternal age.* The risk of having a child with Down syndrome increases significantly for the woman older than 35 years of age. In this syndrome, three chromosomes appear in the 21 chromosome group (trisomy 21). Characteristic features of Down syndrome include upward-slanting eyes; small, malformed ears; large, protruding tongue; broad hands and feet; and some degree of mental retardation.
- *Ethnic background.* Several genetic disorders occur with higher frequency in certain groups. Anyone can be a carrier of Tay-Sachs, but the disease is most common among the Ashkenazi Jewish population. About 1 in every 27 members of the Ashkenazi Jewish population carries the Tay-Sachs gene (Sheth, 2012). Abnormal deposits of lipids (fats) in the cells of the cerebral cortex, spleen, liver, and lymph nodes are characteristic of Tay-Sachs disease. An autosomal recessive gene transmits it. Blacks have a much greater chance of carrying the sickle cell trait than does the general population. Sickle cell anemia is an autosomal recessive condition that occurs in 1 out of every 500 Black births and causes severe hemolytic anemia crises. One in 12 African Americans has the sickle cell trait (CDC, 2011b).
- *Family history.* Certain diseases, such as Huntington's chorea, hemophilia, or mental retardation, are often hereditary. Huntington's chorea (an autosomal dominant disease involving the brain) is characterized by deterioration of intellectual functions and involuntary movements of the limbs, face, and trunk. Once symptoms are manifested, a steady deterioration leads to death in about twenty years. Hemophilia is a sex-linked recessive coagulation disorder caused by a functional deficiency of a clotting factor; it leads to prolonged bleeding. Hemophilia passes from an unaffected carrier mother to her male offspring. It affects 1 in 5000 male births. About 400 babies are born with hemophilia each year in the United States (CDC, 2011c).
  - *Reproductive history.* Spontaneous abortions, stillbirths, and previous live-born children with birth defects or slow development may indicate an increased risk.
  - *Maternal disease.* Several maternal disorders are associated with a higher frequency of birth defects, including diabetes mellitus, seizure disorder, mental retardation, and phenylketonuria. Prenatal diagnosis offers the couple

the option of aborting a fetus that is affected with certain genetic disorders. For many people, however, this option is unacceptable. Chapter 16 discusses the various tests used for prenatal diagnosis.

The nurse's role throughout the genetic counseling process is to provide the vital link between the counseling team and the high-risk couple. The nurse is involved in case finding, referral, and family education. As a result of the new and expanding technology devoted to genetic and genomic research, a growing number of genetic tests are available for the screening, diagnosis, and treatment of rare and common diseases. All nurses will need to become knowledgeable about the basics of genetics and genomics and their applications to clinical care so that they can provide quality health care that is appropriate to their setting, population, geographical location, access, and coverage. This knowledge will allow nurses to provide appropriate information to care recipients regarding genetic tests that are part of their own health care (Lea et al., 2011).

GORDON'S FUNCTIONAL HEALTH PATTERNS

Health Perception–Health Management Pattern

Health promotion is aimed at assisting the infant and family to change behavior to produce better physical and emotional health in adulthood. The old saying "an ounce of prevention is worth a pound of cure" has great merit and if considered, and acted on, this can be very effective in promoting an individual's health. To reach this goal, the nurse encourages childrearing practices that promote normal growth and development, fosters attitudes and values compatible with health, and teaches appropriate use of health services (Whitehead, 2011). The nurse promotes the infant's health through the parents, who determine the care practices for the dependent infant.

Health is largely a subjective judgment. Each person's perception of health is related to physical and mental capabilities, self-concept, relationships with others and the environment, and personal goals and values (Jarvis, 2012). With this understanding, the nurse uses every opportunity to convey confidence in the parents' health perception–health management pattern and to improve their ability to implement behaviors that promote the infant's health. When parents learn and adopt behaviors that improve their own health, they are more likely to ensure that the health needs of their infant are met. Parental modeling increases the chances that good health practices will be retained throughout the child's life.

The goals of nursing practice with infants and their families are to promote individual motivation for health, to assist the family to identify health needs, and to develop problem-solving skills using the family's own resources. To meet these goals, the nurse identifies the family's perception of good or bad health practices, which greatly influences participation in health-promoting activities. Age, gender, educational level, cultural orientation, financial status, and occupation combine to influence health perception. When parents believe that the infant is more susceptible to a health problem if promotional behavior is not enacted, they become more motivated to adopt the behavior.

The nurse's task helps the parents recognize their infant's susceptibility and the potential consequences when healthy practices are not instituted. The nurse works within the family's health perception framework to become acquainted with the characteristics that influence the infant's health. Unless caregivers meet their own personal needs, they will be unable to meet their infant's developmental needs. The empowerment and growth of mothers is a key element to facilitate the successful development of their infants (Harkness & DeMarco, 2011). The nurse supports the parents, strengthening their parental confidence and self-esteem, providing information on meeting their infant's needs, and reinforcing their health perception–health management pattern.

Nutritional-Metabolic Pattern

One of the most important aspects of health promotion in the infant is nutritional status. Many opinions have been expressed about the infant's nutritional needs. As research in this area continues, recommendations and opinions will change; however, some basic facts about nutrition remain fairly consistent. Infant nutritional requirements are based on what is considered necessary to support life, provide for growth, and maintain health.

Essential Nutrients

Water, proteins, fats, carbohydrates, vitamins, and minerals are the essential nutrients in any diet. Because the first year of life is a period of rapid growth, nutritional needs during this period are especially important and always changing. Water is vital to survival. A person can live for several weeks without food but can survive only a few days without water. Because the infant's body weight is approximately 75% water, the baby must consume large amounts of fluid to maintain water balance. Water requirements average from 125 to 150 mL/kg of body weight per day during the first 6 months of life and from 120 to 135 mL/kg per day during the second 6 months (DeBruyne et al., 2012). The sources of water are fluids (primarily milk) and food; most strained foods are 75% to 85% water. Most infant diets meet the basic water requirement.

The infant must also consume sufficient high-quality protein to facilitate growth and development. Recommended protein requirements are 9 grams (g) per day during the first 6 months and 10 g per day during the second 6 months. No more than 20% of an infant's daily energy requirement should come from protein because they are not able to process and excrete the excess nitrogen from higher protein diets (Thompson & Manore, 2012).

Carbohydrates should supply 30% to 60% of the energy intake during infancy. Approximately 37% of the calories in human milk and 40% to 50% of the calories in commercial formulas are derived from lactose or other carbohydrates. The recommended intake of carbohydrates is set at 60 g per day for infants up to 6 months of age and 95 g per day for infants 7 to 12 months old (Dudek, 2010).

A minimum of 3.8 g/kcal and a maximum of 6 g/kcal of fat (40% to 50% of calories) are recommended for infants (Thompson & Manore, 2012). This quantity is present in human milk and in all formulas prepared for infants. Significantly lower intakes, such as in skim milk feedings, can result in an inadequate energy intake.

Vitamins are essential nutrients in the infant's diet that regulate metabolism and allow more efficient use of carbohydrates, fats, and proteins within the body. Although most infants receive adequate vitamin intake through formula, breast milk, and food, recent research has raised a concern about a vitamin D deficiency in infants who receive only breast milk. Vitamin D deficiency is actually quite common among U.S. infants. The Institute of Medicine (IOM) recently revised the recommended dietary allowances (RDAs) for vitamin D. According to the IOM, nutritional rickets is on the rise in the United States among American children with certain risk factors: dark-skinned infants, infants breastfed for long periods without receiving any vitamin supplementation, and infants with decreased exposure to sunlight. The IOM recommends that this population needs vitamin D supplementation of 400 international units/day to be initiated within the first 2 months of life and that this supplementation needs to be continued throughout the time the infant is breastfeeding (Institute of Medicine, 2011).

Minerals are found in relatively small amounts in the infant's body but are vital elements in body structure and control of certain body functions. Mineral intake for infants appears to be adequate, except for iron and fluoride.

The full-term infant is born with stores of iron adequate to meet needs for hemoglobin production for approximately 4 to 6 months. After this time, body stores may need to be replenished. Although iron in human milk is bioavailable, both breastfed and formula-fed infants should receive an additional source of iron by 6 months of age. Iron-fortified formula and cereals are the most commonly used food sources.

Fluoride, concentrated in the bones and teeth, helps reduce dental caries. Although fluoride is important for strong tooth development, it is not recommended during the first 6 months of life. Supplementation is necessary only when the diet contains insufficient fluoridated water.

A review of these requirements shows that milk (breast or formula) meets most of the infant's nutritional needs when consumed in adequate amounts, plus vitamin D supplementation for the high-risk infants. No data support the theory that solid foods are needed to meet these nutritional needs, at least during the first 6 months of life.

Food Additives

In addition to their questionable nutritional value, additives in commercial baby food can negatively influence an infant's health status. The purposes of food additives vary, including adding nutritional value; preserving or extending shelf life; facilitating preparation; improving flavor, color, and texture; and keeping flavors and textures consistent (WHO, 2011).

Commercially prepared baby foods are generally safe, nutritious, and high quality. In response to consumer demand, baby food manufacturers have removed much of the added salt and sugar that their products once contained and have eliminated most food additives.

BOX 17-4 RESEARCH FOR EVIDENCE-BASED PRACTICE

The WIC Program: An Economic Analysis of Breastfeeding and Infant Formula

The Special Supplemental Nutrition Program for Women, Infants, and Children (WIC) has provided free infant formula while simultaneously attempting to promote breastfeeding. The cost structure was analyzed of WIC food packages in relation to breastfeeding.

Methods: The analysis provides 2010 estimates for the cost and utilization of each of the WIC food packages for pairs of infants and their mothers. New food packages were introduced in all states by 2009 and were intended to promote breastfeeding. The analysis accounts for the composition of the new food packages, although utilization projections predate the implementation of those packages, so current rates of breastfeeding may be understated.

Results: The projections suggest that just fewer than 74% of infant participants are estimated to receive food packages associated with exclusive formula use. Relative to food packages for mother-infant pairs who exclusively breastfeed, the exclusive formula packages are around 25% more expensive for infants in the first 6 months of life but 64% less expensive during the second 6 months.

Conclusions: Simulations suggest that the achievement of the *Healthy People 2020* breastfeeding targets among WIC participants would have a minimal effect on food package costs. Simulations for extreme cases (e.g., all fully breastfeeding for 1 year) suggest that food package costs could be reduced by 18% if all WIC mother-infant pairs engaged in exclusive breastfeeding for the first 6 months, followed by exclusive formula use in the next 6 months. A 38% reduction could be achieved if all mother-infant pairs received the partial breastfeeding packages.

Nursing implications: Perhaps a mixed message is being sent to new mothers when they receive both infant formula coupons (supplemental nutrition assistance program [SNAP] food stamps) and breastfeeding encouragement through WIC. Although the WIC message is partial to breastfeeding practices, the infant formula is still made available to all mothers. Nurses employed in postpartum units as well in community clinics can offer help to mothers attempting to establish breastfeeding by encouraging participation in a 'breastfeeding hot line' whereby new mothers can contact nurses for assistance and support in challenging times. Hopefully, by being able to follow-up with breastfeeding mothers who may need additional support during their learning process, nurses can reduce the temptation for mothers to utilize the WIC coupons for purchasing infant formula.

From Drago, R. (2011). The WIC program: An economic analysis of breastfeeding and infant formula. *Breastfeeding Medicine, 6,* 281-286.

Nutrition problems include undernutrition, in which infants do not receive an adequate supply of an essential nutrient, and overnutrition, in which they receive more of a certain nutrient than is needed for healthy growth and development (Dudek, 2010). For infants in the United States, both of these problems are present. A parent who wants the infant to have family foods rather than commercial baby food can blenderize a small portion of the table food at each meal. This choice necessitates cooking without salt or sugar, which is the practice of baby food manufacturers. Making baby food is easy and economical. Written resources are available for parents who are interested in more details about home food preparation for infants.

Parents should be encouraged to read baby food labels carefully. Nurses can obtain lists of baby foods and their ingredients from the manufacturers. The best overall recommendation that nurses make to parents is to provide their infants with a well-balanced diet and avoid excesses.

Breastfeeding

Research throughout the years has demonstrated unequivocally that exclusive breastfeeding is the preferred method of infant feeding for the first 6 months of life and should be continued for at least the first year of life and beyond for as long as mutually desired by mother and child (American Academy of Pediatrics [AAP], 2011a). Breast milk is often called the perfect food for the infant and for the mother, because of its composition and because it does not have to be purchased, cooked, or stored. Both the American Dietetic Association and the AAP have released position statements in support of breastfeeding. This has influenced a number of health-promotion strategies in the United States. In *Healthy People 2020,* objectives MICH 21 through MICH 24 address breastfeeding. In all objectives the target is to increase these activities by 10% by 2020 (U.S. Department of Health and Human Services [USDHHS], 2010) (Box 17-4: Research for

BOX 17-5 BABY-FRIENDLY HOSPITAL INITIATIVE BREASTFEEDING GUIDELINES

- Have a written breastfeeding policy that is communicated routinely to all health care staff.
- Train all health care staff in the skills necessary to implement this policy.
- Inform all pregnant women about the benefits and management of breastfeeding.
- Help the mother initiate breastfeeding within 30 minutes after birth.
- Show mothers how to breastfeed and how to maintain lactation even when they are separated from their infants.
- Give newborn infants no food or drink other than breast milk unless medically indicated.
- Practice rooming-in; allow mothers and infants to remain together 24 hours a day.
- Encourage breastfeeding on demand.
- Do not give pacifiers to breastfeeding infants.
- Foster the establishment of breastfeeding support groups and refer mothers to these groups when discharged from the hospital or clinic.

From World Health Organization and United Nations Children's Fund. (2009). *Baby-friendly hospital initiative.* [Online] Retrieved from www.who.int/nutrition/publications/infantfeeding/9789241594950/en/index.html.

Evidence-Based Practice). If the nation is to meet the Surgeon General's goal by the year 2010, efforts to promote breastfeeding must be strengthened in hospitals, health maintenance organizations, private health care offices, and public health clinics.

WHO, the United Nations Children's Fund (UNICEF), and the *Healthy People 2010 Midcourse Review* (2006) have adopted the *Baby-Friendly Hospital Initiative* in an attempt to establish a global effort to increase breastfeeding. To become a baby-friendly health care facility, the 10 steps to successful breastfeeding must be implemented, as shown in Box 17-5.

BOX 17-6	ADVANTAGES OF BREASTFEEDING

Breast Milk
- Has the correct balance of all essential nutrients for infants
- Is full of immunological agents to protect against disease
- Is easier to digest than is formula
- Contains antiinflammatory properties
- Promotes growth of *Lactobacillus bifidus*
  - Reduces risk of childhood obesity, ear infections and diabetes
  - Reduces risk of asthma and respiratory viruses

Breastfeeding
- Is cheaper and more convenient than formula
- Provides a unique bonding experience for both infant and mother
- Assists in the process of uterine involution for the mother
- Decreases postpartum vaginal bleeding
- Decreases costs for public health programs (e.g., WIC)
- Decreases SIDS rate, overweight, and obesity in adulthood
- Decreases environmental burden for disposal of formula cans and bottles
- Promotes weight reduction for new mother

BOX 17-7	SOLID FOOD INTRODUCTION SEQUENCE

- Cereals, particularly rice because of nonallergenic property
- Fruits such as peaches, pears, and applesauce
- Vegetables, with yellow vegetables (squash and carrots) given before green vegetables (peas or beans)
- Strained meats, such as nonallergenic lamb or veal

Research shows that women's decisions of whether to breast-feed are influenced by information they receive from their health care providers. Low levels of actual or perceived professional support and lack of knowledge, support, and measures needed to cope with breastfeeding difficulties are found to be associated with formula-use decisions (Brown et al., 2011). Because of the important role in the mother's choice of infant feeding, nurses can be instrumental in working toward the national goal to increase breastfeeding by educating all women about the advantages of the practice (Box 17-6). Community nurses who are caring for breastfeeding mothers stress the following tips to increase the duration of this activity:

- Drink 1 quart of fluids daily to produce a sufficient quantity of breast milk.
- Consume 300 to 400 kcal/day above prepregnancy energy intake to avoid excessive weight loss (Samour & King, 2012).
- Learn the appropriate interventions for engorged breasts, sore nipples, plugged ducts, infection, and leaking nipples.
- Learn about the use of breast pumps and milk storage.
- Join breastfeeding support groups for continued help within the community.
- Learn about the effects of drugs, environmental pollutants, alcohol, and nicotine on breast milk.

Introduction of Solid Foods

Timing of the first introduction of solid food during infancy may have potential effects on lifelong health. No scientific evidence is available on the best time to introduce solid foods during infancy. At approximately 4 to 6 months of age, the infant is usually physiologically and developmentally ready to have solid foods, either commercial or home-prepared. The AAP (2011b) recommends that waiting until the child is 6 months of age to introduce solid food decreases the tendency to develop food allergies and reduce the risk of childhood obesity. The introduction of various foods was recommended to supply a more appealing, diversified diet for the infant; supply energy, iron, and vitamins; and provide needed trace elements (AAP, 2011b). The decision to start solid foods at 4 to 6 months of age is based more on neuromuscular and developmental readiness of the infant than on any hard scientific data, but research does validate the lowered risk of developing food allergies if solid foods are not introduced until 6 months of age (Kuo et al., 2011).

All infants develop according to their own schedules, and some are ready to start eating solid foods earlier than other infants. The addition of foods should be governed by an infant's nutritional needs and readiness to handle different forms of foods (Rapley, 2011). The order of food introduction and the specific amounts to be given are based on tradition rather than on scientific fact. No scientific studies have been performed to determine whether there is a specific order of infant food introduction necessary or amounts needed for optimal development. The sequence of solids typically recommended by the AAP is cereal, fruits, vegetables, and meats. The typical sequence in which foods are introduced is shown in Box 17-7. A few tips to assist the parents in making the introduction of solid foods a smooth transition are listed in Box 17-8.

Recommendations for food introduction by age and sequence are shown in Table 17-3.

Weaning

Weaning is a gradual, caring process that introduces the infant to a cup, which replaces the bottle or breast. Weaning should be started when the infant is ready. Developmentally, the infant can usually learn to use a cup by age 5 to 6 months; however, many children continue to nurse after they start using a cup. The infantile extrusion reflex needs to be absent. This reflex is present in very young infants and involves the tongue pushing out any material in the mouth not associated with sucking. The safety advantages of this are obvious, but weaning cannot be commenced until the infant has matured sufficiently for the reflex to be absent. In addition, weaning should not be started until the infant can sit only slightly supported and turn away his/her head to indicate food refusal. The AAP recommends breastfeeding for at least the first year of life. WHO and UNICEF suggest that the health benefits of breast milk are important throughout the second and third years of life and should be continued. However, because breast milk is very low in iron content (0.3 to 0.5 mg/L), there has been concern about the possible impact of this advice on the development of anemia, a condition that if left untreated could cause irreversible developmental delays (Ntouva et al., 2011). Weaning should be started at this age by periodically offering sips of water or juice. Initially the infant may not be eager to accept these offers but should

BOX 17-8 TIPS FOR INTRODUCING SOLID FOODS

Assess the infant's readiness to consume solid foods first:
- The infant can sit up (with support) and can hold her/his head and neck up well.
- The infant's birth weight has doubled.
- The infant is interested in what you are eating and may even try to grab food from your plate.
- The infant can keep food in her/his mouth rather than letting it dribble out.
- The infant shows signs of being hungry by wanting to nurse more often.

If readiness is validated, then begin with the following:
- The infant's first solid foods should be smooth and runny. Gradually, the infant will be ready to accept a slightly rougher texture.
- Puréed foods are used until the infant has teeth; chopped foods are used when the infant can chew.
- Introduce only one new food at a time and in small amounts for a period of 5 to 7 days. When the new food is not tolerated or the infant is allergic to it, the new food can be identified quickly and discontinued.
- The infant must learn how to handle solid foods. Because infants use sucking movements, part of the food is ejected from the mouth. With time and practice, the infant learns how to take solid food from a spoon.
- Do not mix solid foods together; the infant should learn to appreciate different tastes and textures.
- Always feed the infant in an upright position; do not feed the infant solids from the bottle.
- Until 1 year of age, feed the infant milk before solid foods.
- Look at, smile at, and talk to the infant during feeding.
- Do not give honey to infants less than 12 months of age because of the risk of infant botulism.*
- Respect the infant's likes and dislikes; rejected foods may be reintroduced later.
- Avoid peanuts and peanut butter because of the potential for severe allergic reactions.

*Honey has been credited throughout the centuries with therapeutic and medicinal uses. However, honey should not be given to infants under 1 year of age. Honey is a known source of bacterial spores that produce a toxin that can cause infant botulism. This rare, but serious, form of food poisoning affects the nervous system of infants and can result in death. Researchers also suspect a link between infant botulism and some cases of SIDS, because breathing is affected in the most severe stages of food poisoning. Botulism spores are quite common, found in dust, soil, and uncooked food. Honey is the only food implicated in infant botulism. Because honey is not essential for the nutrition of infants, parents and caregivers should be reminded not to feed it to infants younger than 1 year. Honey should never be added to baby food or placed on the nipple of a pacifier.

TABLE 17-3 FIRST FOODS FOR THE INFANT

AGE (MONTHS)	ADDITION
4 to 6	Iron-fortified rice cereal, followed by other cereals
5 to 7	Strained vegetables and fruits and their juices
6 to 8	Protein foods (cheese, meat, fish, chicken, and yogurt)
9	Finely chopped meat, toast, teething crackers
10 to 12	Whole egg, whole milk (allergies less likely now)

into organic acids that demineralize the teeth until they decay. By not using the bottle as a pacifier, parents can prevent this condition.

Some additional tips for counseling parents are as follows:
- Keep a calm, relaxed attitude throughout the weaning process.
- Do not force an infant to use a cup; it is more detrimental to wean sooner than later.
- Introduce the cup for one feeding per day and progress until the breast or bottle is surrendered.
- Put only purified tap water into the bottle, and give the infant juice and milk from a cup.
- Remember that infants enjoy the accomplishment of using a cup; it is one of their first steps toward independence.

Anticipatory Guidance

The infant progresses from a diet of milk alone to a diet of milk and solid foods within a short period. Understanding the infant's nutritional needs and developmental capabilities, the nurse can guide the parents in meeting them and in the process foster healthy family-infant relationships. The health-promotion activity used in meeting proper infant nutrition focuses on parent education and positive reinforcement of parenting abilities.

Elimination Pattern

The infant develops an elimination pattern by the second week of life, usually associated with the frequency and amount of feedings. Both breastfed and bottle-fed infants progress to a pattern of fewer stools per day after the first few months of life.

A breastfed infant's stools have an orange-yellow color and a soft, even consistency, with a slightly sour but clean smell, dissimilar to stools passed later in life. A bottle-fed infant's stools are harder and smellier and resemble those of an infant eating solid food. The breastfed infant has many daily stools during the first and second months of life, progressing to one stool per day or even one stool every 4 to 5 days in the later months before solid foods are introduced. The bottle-fed infant has two to four stools per day during the first month, tapering to one a day or even fewer at the end of infancy (Polan & Taylor, 2010).

For the first year of life, an infant cannot control the bowels. Bowel evacuation remains under involuntary, reflexive control until myelination of the spinal cord is complete, usually by 14 to 18 months of age (Kliegman et al., 2011). Nurses advise overanxious parents to delay toilet training until the infant is developmentally ready. The stress in American culture on daily bowel movements makes many mothers concerned about their

become accustomed to this new experience fairly quickly (Box 17-9: Quality and Safety Scenario).

Some infants accept the cup readily; other infants are extremely reluctant to give up the bottle, especially the bedtime bottle. Allowing infants to sleep with propped bottles can lead to aspiration if the milk flows too rapidly or the infant becomes too sleepy to coordinate sucking and swallowing. Another potential problem is baby-bottle tooth decay, of all upper teeth and some of the lower posterior teeth, from direct contact with sugar, syrup, honey-sweetened water, or fruit juice. When the infant falls asleep and stops sucking on the bottle, the sugary solution pools around the infant's teeth and remains there for long periods. The carbohydrate in the solution is fermented

---

☑ **BOX 17-9   QUALITY AND SAFETY SCENARIO**

How to Hold Your Infant for Feedings

- Sit or lie down comfortably with your back supported.
- Make sure the infant has one arm on either side of your breast as you pull him/her close.
- Use firm pillows or folded blankets under the infant as a means of support during the feeding. As the infant gets older, the extra support will likely be unnecessary.
- Support the infant's back and shoulders firmly.
  - Do not push on the back of the infant's head.
  - Correct positioning enables good attachment.
  - The infant should be at a 90-degree angle, with his/her nose meeting the mother's nipple.
- After the infant's mouth is open wide, pull him/her quickly to your breast.

Three Common Breastfeeding Positions
Football
- Hold the infant's back and shoulders in the palm of your hand.
- Tuck the infant up under your arm, keeping the infant's ear, shoulder, and hip in a straight line.
- Support the breast. After the infant's mouth is open wide, pull him/her quickly to you.
- Continue to hold your breast until the baby feeds easily.

Lying Down
- Lie on your side with a pillow at your back and lay the infant such that you are facing each other.
- To begin, prop yourself up on your elbow and support your breast with that hand.
- Pull the infant close to you, lining up his/her mouth with your nipple.
- After the infant is feeding well, lie back down. Hold your breast with the opposite hand.
- Cradle the infant in the arm closest to the breast with his/her head in the crook of your arm.

- Have the infant's body facing you, tummy to tummy.
- Use your opposite hand to support the breast.

Across the Lap
- Lay your infant on firm pillows across your lap.
- Turn the infant, facing you.
- Reach across your lap to support the infant's back and shoulders with the palm of your hand.
- Support your breast from underneath to guide it into his/her mouth.

Breastfeeding Is Going Well When...
- Your infant is feeding approximately 8 times in 24 hours for 30 to 40 minutes at each feeding. Some infants need to eat more frequently until they learn to breastfeed efficiently. Other infants gain weight although they feed less often.
- At least one breast softens well at each feeding.
- You feel a tug, but not pain, when he/she sucks.
- The infant's arms and shoulders are relaxed during the feeding.
- The infant has bursts of 10 or more sucks and swallows at the beginning of each feeding.
- As your breast softens; the infant slows down to two to three sucks and swallows at a time.
- Your infant is content when you finish breastfeeding.
- By the time the infant is 4 days old, you should see at least six wet diapers and two bowel movements every 24 hours.
- Signs that a good attachment has been made are:
  - The infant's nose is free from the breast.
  - The infant's chin is firmly pressed against the breast.
  - The infant has round cheeks.
  - If any areola is visible, it should be more above the top lip versus the bottom lip.

Adapted from Surtees, A., & Kelleher, D. (2011). Maternity focus: Techniques to support breastfeeding. *British Journal of Healthcare Assistants,* *5*(3), 134-136; Hughes, G. (2011). How to...help with positioning and attachment. *Midwives, 14*(4), 26.

---

infant's elimination patterns. The breastfed infant may go for several days without having a bowel movement, which usually is not a problem. When the infant's behavior and feeding and sleeping patterns are normal, no elimination problem exists. A breastfed infant rarely becomes constipated when consuming adequate amounts of breast milk. Usually the nurse only has to reassure the parents and discuss normal elimination patterns. Urination increases as fluid intake increases. An infant who voids 6 to 12 times a day during the first few months of life is usually healthy and well hydrated. Voiding is involuntary until sometime during the second year of life, when bladder sensation develops. Irregular patterns of voiding characterize the remaining period of infancy.

Anticipatory Guidance

Anticipatory guidance and health promotion concerning elimination patterns of the infant consist of parental teaching and reassurance, with special emphasis on good hygienic practices. Reassuring the parents about the infant's inability to control elimination is important so that their expectations are realistic.

Activity-Exercise Pattern

Physical activity and exercise contribute to development and coordination throughout the life span; infants receive their exercise through play. Initially infants engage in play with themselves with their hands or feet, by responding to various sounds, and by rolling and getting into various positions. By manipulating objects and achieving pleasurable sensations, infants learn about themselves and the objects in the environment.

Activity Through Play

Although the word play suggests physical activity, the infant's first play is actually an exercise of the senses. The infant's first toys are visual. Through play, infants learn to hone their senses, to exercise their physical abilities, and to relate to other people. Most of the infant's play is solitary and repetitious. As each discovery is made, self-confidence and pride in the achievement are reinforced (as is the skill) through repetition.

As the infant enters the second half of the first year and becomes mobile, the family should provide the infant with increasing opportunities for spontaneous play and exploration. A planned play period in a safe environment should be

FIGURE 17-1 The mother provides an infant with comfort by her closeness.

established. The infant should have unrestrictive clothing so that movement can be free and unhampered. The caregiver should not interfere directly with the play but should be attentive to the infant's needs.

An important nursing role is assisting parents to promote play, stressing the importance of providing opportunities that are appropriate for the infant's age. Buying expensive toys is unnecessary; common household items, such as pots, pans, lids, and spoons, provide excellent objects for play purposes.

Activity Through Stimulation

Parental stimulation of the infant is an important developmental technique; the infant needs stimulation to learn about the world. This activity does not require expensive objects, but rather involves experiences in sight, sound, and touch that are free and can be provided by any parent (Figure 17-1). Examples of stimulating experiences for infants include the following:

- Having lullabies sung to them
- Listening to tape recordings of a heartbeat
- Seeing colorful mobiles in crib
- Being rocked in a rocking chair
- Having a familiar face smiling close by
- Having space to wander when developmentally ready
- Looking at themselves in mirrors
- Listening to music

Anticipatory Guidance

Knowledge of developmental landmarks allows the nurse to guide parents in proper play and stimulation for infants. Handing a 15-month-old child a ball and placing the child in a fenced-in back yard to play is not enough. These activities must provide interpersonal contact, activity, and exercise. Activity and exercise through stimulation and play are extremely important for adequate and healthy development (Berk, 2012).

Sleep-Rest Pattern

The amount of sleep that infants need is closely related to their rate of growth. Initially infants sleep approximately 80% of the time, as demanded by their rapid growth. As growth begins

TABLE 17-4 GROWTH AND DEVELOPMENT

Normal Sleep Patterns for Infants

AGE (MONTHS)	HOURS IN 24-HOUR PERIOD
2 to 3	Low: 10 Average: 16½ High: 23
3 to 4	Low: 8 to 10 nightly High: 11 to 12 nightly (2 or 3 naps daily)
6 to 12	11 to 12 nightly (2 or 3 naps daily)
12 to 18	8 to 12 nightly (1 or 2 naps daily)

to slow toward the middle of the first year of life, less sleep is needed. The 12-month-old infant sleeps only 12 of 24 hours, a pattern that remains essentially unchanged through the second year (St. James-Roberts, 2012). To assist parents in understanding normal sleep and rest patterns, the nurse stresses that no set schedule exists (Table 17-4).

Anticipatory Guidance

Health-promotion activities can also help the parents determine the individual needs of their infant. The nurse stresses that longer sleep patterns are signs of maturation and that sleep and rest are recognized as having a significant influence on the infant's growth and development. Sleep problems are highly prevalent in early childhood. Frequently, parents seek professional help when they suspect their child suffers from a sleep problem. The nurse may offer the parents helpful comments for promoting infant sleep patterns, such as the following:

- Provide a quiet room for the infant that is separate from the parents' room.
- Learn behavioral clues that signal that the infant is going to sleep and is not interacting socially.
- Learn to become sensitive to sleep cycles and rest periods that the infant is establishing and base care accordingly.
- Attempt to schedule feeding times during wakeful rather than drowsy periods.
- Learn that certain cycles are intrinsic to infants and that each infant is unique.
- Perform rituals for the infant, such as rocking or reading a bedtime story, to provide comfort and security and let the infant know the expected behavior.

If parents express a sleep concern, the nurse assesses their reactions, considers their definition of the concern, assesses the sleep environment, and observes the infant's own unique sleep patterns. Only then can the nurse's health-promotion approach be individualized to assist the family in caring for the infant.

Sudden Infant Death Syndrome

Sudden infant death syndrome (SIDS) is defined as the sudden death of an infant under 1 year old that is unexpected and unexplained after a thorough postmortem examination. SIDS is the only cause of death derived by exclusion of other causes. Despite declines in prevalence during the past 2 decades, SIDS continues to be one of the leading causes of infant mortality

BOX 17-10   SAFE TO SLEEP PUBLIC EDUCATION CAMPAIGN

The Safe to Sleep campaign—formerly known as the Back to Sleep campaign—aims to educate parents, caregivers, and health care providers about ways to reduce the risk for sudden infant death syndrome (SIDS) and other sleep-related causes of infant death.

Safe to Sleep is an expansion of the original Back to Sleep campaign, which started in 1994. Back to Sleep was named for its recommendation to place healthy babies on their backs to sleep, the most effective action that parents and caregivers can take to reduce the risk of SIDS. Since that campaign started, the percentage of infants placed on their backs to sleep has increased dramatically, and the overall SIDS rates have declined by more than 50 percent.

The expanded Safe to Sleep campaign builds on the success and reach of the Back to Sleep campaign. In addition to strategies for reducing the risk of SIDS, Safe to Sleep also describes actions that parents and caregivers can take to reduce the risk of other sleep-related causes of infant death, such as suffocation.

Safe to Sleep campaign collaborators include the *Eunice Kennedy Shriver* National Institute of Child Health and Human Development (NICHD); the Maternal and Child Health Bureau of the Health Resources and Services Administration (HRSA); the Centers for Disease Control and Prevention (CDC), Division of Reproductive Health; the American Academy of Pediatrics (AAP); the American College of Obstetricians and Gynecologists (ACOG); First Candle; and the Association of SIDS and Infant Mortality Programs (ASIP).

The safe sleep strategies outlined in Safe to Sleep materials and publications are based on recommendations defined by the AAP Task Force on SIDS. The Task

Force released expanded guidelines in October 2011. More information about these recommendations is available at the NICHD/NIH website.

Based on the AAP Task Force recommendations, parents and caregivers can make changes to their babies' sleep environment to make it safer and to reduce the risk for SIDS and other sleep-related causes of infant death.

Courtesy Thinkstock.

Modified from National Institute of Child Health and Human Development, *Safe to Sleep Public Education Campaign.* (2013). Retrieved from www.nichd.nih.gov/sids/Pages/sids.aspx.

in the post-neonatal period. SIDS is a complex, multifactorial disorder, the cause of which is still not fully understood. Behavioral risk factors identified in epidemiological studies include prone and side sleeping positions, preterm birth and/or infant low birth weight, smoke exposure, soft bedding, bed sharing, not breastfeeding, and overheating (Yikilkan et al., 2011) (Box 17-10). These factors may also be associated with sleep disorders in infants, principally with bedtime problems, abnormal night awakenings, and arrhythmic sleep. Although SIDS affects infants from all social strata, lower socioeconomic status, younger maternal age, inadequate prenatal care, and lower maternal education level are consistently associated with SIDS. The incidence of SIDS has varied over time and among nations. Sudden **infant death syndrome (SIDS)** is the third leading cause of infant mortality in the United States and the leading cause of death among infants 28 to 364 days of age (Miller et al., 2011). By definition, the cause of SIDS is not known.

Although the *Back to Sleep* program by the AAP has resulted in a lower number of infant deaths from SIDS, there have been identified consequences to the supine sleeping position, including deformational plagiocephaly (defined as having an abnormally flat head shape, as a complication of supine sleeping) and delayed gross motor delays. Plagiocephaly occurs when external forces are applied to the molding skull of an infant and cause it to become misshaped, usually with asymmetrical head shape, misaligned ears, and facial asymmetry. Infants who sleep on their backs do not have the opportunity

to lift their heads or use muscles that they would use while in the prone position. Babies who are least exposed to "tummy time" tend to be slower in achieving major milestones such as rolling over, sitting up, crawling, and pulling up to stand (Eron et al., 2011).

The primary intervention to decrease the risk of plagiocephaly is "tummy time." Parents should be instructed to allow supervised tummy time while the infant is awake and cautioned about the amount of time their infant spends in a car seat. Delayed gross motor development can be prevented by reducing the amount of time the infant spends in the supine position. Tummy time is the key intervention in preventing gross motor delays in infants. This prone position provides the infants with increased physical challenges and gives them a chance to begin developing head control by strengthening neck muscles. Nurses should educate the parents to introduce prone positioning in short periods several times a day. As infants get stronger, they will use arm muscles to lift themselves and aid them to reach for toys or other objects. This strengthening is essential in assisting them in rolling over, crawling, pulling up to stand, and developing fine motor development including coordination and sensory processing.

Objective MICH 1.8 from *Healthy People 2020* (USDHHS, 2010) is to reduce infant deaths from sudden infant death syndrome (SIDS) from 0.55 infant deaths per 1000 live births to 0.50 infant deaths per 1000 live births. Objective MICH 1.9, to reduce infant deaths from SIDS and other causes (including

SIDS, unknown causes, accidental suffocation, and strangulation in bed), was to improve from 0.93 infant deaths per 1000 live births in 2006 to 0.84 infant deaths per 1000 live births by 2020. Both objectives advocate a 10% reduction in infant deaths.

When an infant dies suddenly, unexpectedly, and for no apparent reason, a family crisis occurs. The parents are devastated and completely unprepared for the shock, reacting with intense guilt, blaming themselves and each other, and agonizing over the part they may have played in the infant's death. Because many unanswered questions remain, these feelings are universal. Parents think there is something they could have done to prevent the tragedy. In most cases, nothing could have been done. Too frequently, the first sign that something was wrong is death. The nurse is in an excellent position to help the family through this crisis. Dealing with the family's grief is very difficult. Many families find strength in their faith to help them through this difficult time. Other family members and close friends can assist the family in their grieving process. Many receive solace and support from talking to other parents who have lost an infant to SIDS. Several parent groups are available from local chapters of the SIDS Foundation; the nurse can refer them to their local chapter.

The nurse's main supportive role for families coping with SIDS is listening and offering compassionate guidance through the weeks and months that follow. The nurse encourages parents to talk about their infant. Too soon, family and friends expect the surviving family to "get over it." A parent, however, is never able to "get over it"; it is only put in perspective and not so near the surface. Nurses need to actively participate in helping parents through their grieving process and remember a standard time frame is not applicable (McGrath, 2011).

Nursing assessment of the infant at risk for SIDS includes observing the infant for apneic episodes. Usually, however, nursing assessment occurs after death and consists of support and providing appropriate resources for the family. Nursing diagnoses for sudden infant death might include the following:
- Spiritual distress related to coping with death
- Ineffective family coping related to the loss of an infant
- Dysfunctional grieving related to the parents' inability to cope

Nurses also discuss with the family feelings about caring for future children. Life can appear out of control and parents may believe that they cannot care for another infant. These feelings must be resolved before another pregnancy is contemplated. When dealing with the families of SIDS victims, nurses can feel uncomfortable and helpless. As health professionals, they might speak in terms of easing the pain or alleviating the guilt of these families, but many times simple nonverbal human contact is sufficient to express concern and understanding.

Cognitive-Perceptual Pattern

Cognition is the process by which an individual recognizes, accumulates, and organizes the knowledge of the environment, beginning with the perception or recognition of an event within that environment. Cognitive development is concurrent with biological, adaptive, and psychosocial achievement. The infant's biological and cognitive developmental patterns

TABLE 17-5 GROWTH AND DEVELOPMENT
Visual Development During Infancy

AGE	BEHAVIOR THAT INDICATES VISION
1 to 3 months	Fixes gaze on object 12 to 24 inches away
	Takes interest in bright colors and faces
	Follows objects in field of vision
3 to 6 months	Begins to show interest in hands
	Follows in range of 90 degrees
	Recognizes familiar objects
	Able to see full color by now
6 to 9 months	Visual scanning becomes more integrated
	Capable of organized depth perception
	Begins to perceive distances accurately
	Both eyes should focus equally now
9 to 12 months	Able to look for concealed items
	Converges on objects in close proximity
	Peripheral vision is well developed
	Judges distance well
12 to 18 months	Eye-hand coordination develops
	Depth perception more refined
	Ability to identify forms and shapes

(Piaget's sensorimotor period) were discussed earlier in this chapter. The focus of this section is on the infant's sensory and language development and the importance of stimulation to both developmental areas. From birth, infants possess sensory capabilities; all sensory organs are well developed and functioning. As the infant is cared for and handled, the special senses become organized neurologically into a pattern of behavior that will greatly influence subsequent development.

Vision

The infant's initial visual impressions are unfocused, bizarre, unfamiliar, and meaningless. Because everything is new and only somewhat significant, visual stimuli must be moving, bright, or flashing to capture the infant's attention. The infant's eyes are well developed at birth, but the muscles that attach the eyes to their sockets are weak. This weakness may be stressful to parents, because the infant's eyes do not appear to function simultaneously. Parents can be assured that most infants coordinate their eye movements by the age of 3 months; by 6 months this function is mature. Table 17-5 summarizes visual developmental milestones.

Hearing

After the amniotic fluid drains from the middle ear several days after birth, the infant's hearing becomes acute. Hearing is one of the better-developed senses in the infant; the fetus can even hear in utero and responds to loud sounds (Figure 17-2). The newborn can distinguish sound frequencies and turns toward a voice or another sound. The infant may be familiar with the mother's voice early in life. Sounds gradually gain significance and meaning when they are associated with caregivers, food, and pleasure.

The ability to listen and discriminate among sounds is an important task during infancy. The closer the infant is to the sound, the more easily the sound can be discriminated. The groundwork for verbal ability begins to develop long before

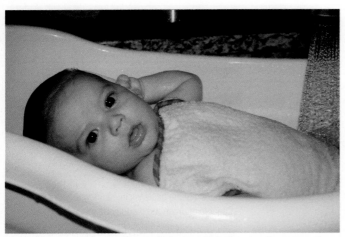

FIGURE 17-2 Babies respond to startling, loud noises, confirming their sense of hearing.

TABLE 17-6 GROWTH AND DEVELOPMENT

Normal Development of Hearing

AGE	BEHAVIOR THAT INDICATES HEARING
1 to 3 months	Is startled by loud noises
	Stops activity when spoken to
3 to 6 months	Turns eyes and head toward sound
	Responds to mother's voice
	Imitates own noises: "ooh" and "ba-ba"
6 to 9 months	Responds to own name
	Looks toward sounds
	Recognizes familiar sounds
9 to 12 months	Points to familiar objects or people
	Imitates simple words and sounds
	Locates a sound in any direction
12 to 18 months	Follows simple spoken directions
	Distinguishes between sounds
	Spoken words are well on their way

words appear, and many believe that infants whose mothers talk to them tend to speak earlier than infants who are not exposed to these sounds (Crandell et al., 2011). Table 17-6 summarizes the infant's auditory development.

Smell

The ability to smell is fully developed at birth. The infant has many receptors in the nose, but it lacks the cilia that line the inside of the adult's nose. As a result, the infant has a keen sense of smell, because odors reach the receptor cells easily. Within 2 weeks after birth, an infant can differentiate the odor of the mother's milk from other sources of milk, an ability developed when the infant is held closely (Puckett & Black, 2010). At this time the infant begins associating the parents with their body odors, a perception that is important to infant-parent bonding.

Taste

The sense of taste is present at birth and salivation begins at approximately 3 months of age. The four primary sensations

are sour, salty, sweet, and bitter. The taste buds for sweet tastes are more abundant during early life than they are in later life, which may account for the preference for sweets that is characteristic of infants and children.

Touch and Motion

Tactile sensation is well developed at birth, particularly on the lips and tongue. Perceptions of motion and touch are perhaps the most important of all senses. Rocking and other motions are sensations of equilibrium picked up by the middle ear. Skin-to-skin touching should be performed regularly; evidence shows that touch helps relieve the unspent tensions that infants develop and accelerates neuromuscular development (Puckett & Black, 2010). Infants respond with pleasure to rocking and other motions and to tactile sensations of warmth, closeness, and cuddling.

Language Development

Language development, an important aspect of the infant's cognitive and perceptual pattern, is affected by development of the intellect, maturation of the central nervous system, development of the organs of speech, and exposure to human verbalization.

As in other areas of development, language acquisition follows a definite sequence. During the first 2 months, most of the infant's sounds are vowels and are made primarily in the front part of the mouth (Coch et al., 2010). Crying is the major means of communication during this period. Cooing sounds are heard at approximately 2 to 3 months, usually in response to an adult's voice. By 6 months, babbling sounds are heard, and by 9 to 10 months, the infant forms two-syllable sounds. By 12 months, words such as "ma-ma," "bye-bye," and "da-da" are emerging. From 15 to 18 months, an expressive jargon with rhythmic intonations develops, but words are recognized only rarely. The infant uses jargon along with pointing to express wishes.

Anticipatory Guidance

The nurse's knowledge and understanding of an infant's cognitive and perceptual behavior facilitates interaction with infants and serves as a guide in parental counseling. The main focus centers on stimulation, because each of the infant's senses is receptive to environmental stimulation. This activity helps the infant learn from the environment. When an infant is exposed to appropriate sensory stimulation, greater curiosity, improved mental capabilities, accelerated neuromuscular growth, enhanced gastrointestinal functioning quicker weight gain, more rapid language development, and pleasing mother-infant interactions are likely to occur (Cohen, 2012).

Parents are the primary providers of pleasurable and stimulating experiences for the infant. The nurse assists them by offering suggestions about suitable stimuli for each sensory modality.

Self-Perception–Self-Concept Pattern

Self-perception has a pervasive influence on all aspects of life. Self-concept consists of a set of attitudes regarding what each person thinks, believes, and feels about the self. These attitudes form a personal self-belief that is an abstraction referred as "me." Many researchers believe that the infant determines self-existence by first noting that actions such as crying or smiling have an effect on others, which depends on receiving feedback (Berk, 2012). Studies confirm that infants can identify themselves and therefore form a self-concept. Infants at 4 months of age were found to be particularly fascinated with their images in mirrors and smiled more at themselves than they did at pictures of other infants (Puckett & Black, 2010).

As the infant continues to grow and mature, many circumstances combine to influence self-concept. How others relate to the infant's body and the messages that the infant receives from the body lead to knowledge of a physical self. The ability to use the body to influence others can lead the psychological self to conclude that someone cares about the infant (Coch et al., 2010).

The infant's development of body image is gradual. At birth the infant has diffuse feelings of hunger, pain, anger, and comfort, but no body image. Initially, the infant knows only the self and regards the external world as an extension of the self. Only when infants begin to experience the environment through sensory modalities are they able to distinguish their bodies from animate and inanimate objects.

Nursing Suggestions

The nurse plays a vital role in assisting parents to foster the development of a positive self-concept and a good body image in their infant. The nurse first identifies personal self-concept and how it influences individuals (Rochat, 2011). The nurse stresses that the way in which parents treat the infant influences the infant's self-concept. Basically, infants and young children incorporate their parents' interactions with them (good or bad) into their own view of self. Parents must understand that their infant's self-concept is an important, continuing event. What the infant knows and later believes about the self will affect all interactions with others, and by influencing what the infant will later attempt, the self-concept may have broad effects on the development of new skills. The mental state or the idea of "me" is that part of the self that makes reference to itself. This mental state develops over the first 2 years of life and is a function of both brain maturation processes as well as socialization (M. Lewis, 2011).

Roles-Relationships Pattern

Researchers have explored extensively the effect of early bonding between parents and their infants, emphasizing that this initial attraction sets the stage for the later development of love and affiliation. The bonding process has many other implications for the infant's future development as well (Oppenheim & Goldsmith, 2011).

Attachment and Bonding

The parent-infant relationship does not begin with the birth of the infant; many aspects have been molded by the life experiences of the parents long before they reached parenthood. The kind of mothering that a woman received as an infant and the concept of mother that she developed as she grew represent early effects that can influence the mother-infant relationship. The mother's overall self-concept will affect her ability to relate to her infant, as will her relationship with the infant's father.

The establishment of this emotional bond between the mother and her infant is known as attachment. This emotional bond is considered crucial for the optimal physical and emotional development of the infant. Maternal behaviors such as how the mother holds, feeds, and looks at the infant demonstrate the process of attachment. Attachment is developed by proximity and interaction with the infant. Positive feedback between the caregiver and the infant through social, verbal, and nonverbal responses facilitates the attachment process (Hawkins, 2010).

Various theories have attempted to explain the basis for attachment behavior. Freudian psychoanalytical theory emphasizes that the bond between child and mother develops as a result of the mother's fulfillment of the infant's innate desire to socialize and the physical requirements for survival. Social learning theory contributes the principles of reinforcement to the attachment process; as the mother meets the infant's needs, discomfort is reduced or removed. The infant associates the pleasurable feeling of being satisfied with the mother, who becomes a significant other in the infant's life. The bonding process is the basis for the mother-infant relationship, which, in turn, forms the basis for the interdependence that is necessary for the infant's psychological and physical development. All infants are born with the building blocks that develop into attachment behaviors and thus all infants have the ability to form an attachment relationship with their primary caregiver (Underwood & Rosen, 2011).

In their early studies on attachment, Klaus and colleagues (2000) formulated the following seven crucial principles:

- A sensitive period appears to exist during the first minutes and hours after birth, when it seems necessary for the mother and father to have close contact with their infant for later development to be optimal.
- Species-specific responses to the infant appear to exist in the human mother and father when the infant is first given to them.
- The attachment process seems to be structured such that the parents become attached to one infant at a time or in the case of a multiple birth to each infant simultaneously.
- For attachment to occur appropriately, the infant must respond to the mother and father by some signal, such as body or eye movements. This principle has been called the "you can't love a dishrag" phenomenon.
- Individuals who witness the birth process become strongly attached to the infant.
- Some adults find it difficult to go through the processes of attachment and detachment simultaneously. Becoming attached to an infant, while still mourning the loss or threatened loss of another person, is difficult for parents.
- Some early events may have long-lasting effects. For example, anxiety over an infant with a transient disorder in the child's early days may result in long-term concerns or behavior that will have implications for future development.

✹ BOX 17-11 INNOVATIVE PRACTICE
*The Touchpoints Model**

The birth of a baby is a life-changing event for a couple and family. Although most infants develop through predictable yet individual patterns of development, parents, especially first-time parents, are usually unaware of these patterns or have difficulty assessing their infant's progress and problems. All of these processes can be stressful for the parents, the entire family, and the infant.

The Touchpoints Model Program at Children's Hospital in Boston, Massachusetts, delivers a training model for practitioners, emphasizing the building of supportive alliances between parents and professionals around key points in the development of young children. The model is an outgrowth of Dr. T. Berry Brazelton's book *Touchpoints* (2006) and research at Children's Hospital in Boston. The Touchpoints model provides a form of outreach through which multidisciplinary practitioners can engage parents around important, predictable phases of their baby's development. The Touchpoints model stresses preventive health through development of relationships between parents and providers; acknowledges that developing and maintaining relationships is critical to appreciating cultural, religious, and societal family dynamics; and encourages the practitioner to focus on strengths in individuals and families. Touchpoints is not a stand-alone model; it is intended to be integrated into ongoing pediatric, early childhood, and family intervention programs.

Contact Information
The Touchpoints Project
Child Development Unit
Children's Hospital
1295 Boylston Street
Boston, MA 02215

*Touchpoints has gone on-line. Parents and professionals can get advice and information from Dr. Brazelton at Brazelton, T. B. (2011). *Brazelton Touchpoints Center*. [Online] Available at www.touchpoints.org; Lester, B. M., & Lester, J. D. (2010). *Nurturing children and families: Building on the legacy of T. Berry Brazelton*. Chichester: Wiley-Blackwell Publishers (Newer clinical applications).

Just as the infant's behavior influences attachment, it also continues to influence the evolving maternal-paternal-infant relationship as the infant develops. Studies have shown that if the process of attachment is encumbered, later problems are more likely to occur, such as child abuse, failure-to-thrive syndrome, and behavior problems. Failure-to-thrive is a physical sign that an infant is receiving inadequate nutrition for optimal growth and development (Jaffe, 2011).

Many factors are present when a relationship is being established and maintained. Most people enter a relationship with unrealistic expectations. Parents are no exception—they are going to be wise, patient, and devoted, and they will nurture their infant. Because the parents' self-esteem is associated closely with their infant's interactions and accomplishments, when parents' self-esteem is low, disappointment, anger, and a disturbance in the relationship with their infant can occur. In some instances this disturbed parent-infant relationship is short-lived and nothing harmful develops. When a disturbed parent-infant relationship continues, however, the infant is at risk for abuse and behavior problems (Box 17-11: Innovative Practice).

The process of bonding is also important for fathers. Recently, a process called paternal engrossment has been used to describe the behavior pattern of fathers when they interact with their infants. The following are the major characteristics of engrossment: visual awareness of the infant; tactile awareness, often expressed in a desire to hold the infant; awareness of distinct characteristics, with emphasis on the features that resemble the father; perception of the infant as perfect; development of a strong feeling of attraction to the infant that leads to intense focusing of attention; a feeling of extreme elation; and a sense of deep self-esteem and satisfaction (Berk, 2012).

Child Abuse

Child abuse has occurred throughout history, yet its prevalence is difficult to estimate, partly because, like an iceberg, it is mostly hidden. Family traditionally has been considered a safe place for its members, but many infants are at risk for maltreatment. Infant and child abuse has always been a part of human history. Acceptable behavior toward infants is largely a learned phenomenon; the art of parenting is not instinctively acquired, as many people believe. Abusing parents are seldom "monsters"; they are merely individuals ineffectively coping with the demands of parenthood, for which there is little or no preparation, as well as other life stressors.

The scope of child abuse is extensive: estimates indicate that more than 3 million infants and children in the United States are victims of abuse annually, which means 1 in 20 children are physically abused each year. Infants from birth to 1 year of age are the most vulnerable victims of abuse and neglect at the rate of 20.6 per 1000 children (AAP, 2011c). Children under 4 years of age are the most frequent victims. Women are more frequent abusers than are men, because they are the primary caregivers. Men abuse more severely and commit sexual abuse more frequently. Child abuse does not discriminate; it occurs in families of every race, creed, and socioeconomic class.

The child-abuse syndrome is a clinical condition in infants who have suffered serious active or passive abuse at the hands of their parents or other caregivers. Physical trauma is not the only facet, but it is the most overt indicator of a dysfunctional family unit and a disturbed parent-infant relationship (AAP, 2011c).

Active manifestations of abuse include the following:
- Brain injuries, subdural hematomas, and skull fractures
- Soft-tissue injuries, such as bruises, lacerations, or burns
- Fractures of the long bones and ribs; multiple fractures in various stages of healing
- Sexual abuse manifested by genital tissue injury; sexually transmitted infections

Passive manifestations of abuse include the following:
- Poor nutrition, failure to thrive, and severe malnutrition
- Poor physical condition: neglected safeguards against disease, poor skin condition, and lack of medical attention
- Emotional neglect: rejection, indifference, and deprivation of love
- Moral neglect: allowing the infant or child to remain in an immoral atmosphere

Abusing parents often have common patterns of behavior. As children, their own parents may have abused them. In this way, child abuse is cycled from generation to generation. The development of the maternal role on which the infant depends for health, progress, and survival begins during the mother's early childhood. Unless she received love and proper mothering, she will have difficulty with a relationship that entails the complete dependency of another person. She may find the relationship with her own infant to be unrewarding, threatening, and frustrating. Feelings of inadequacy and guilt in the mother and father roles compound the problems.

Abusing parents are often socially isolated and have few people to whom they can turn during times of crisis; they also cannot support one another emotionally. These parents may view the infant as the person who can provide the love, support, and nurturing that is lacking in their own lives. When the infant does not fulfill their expectations, the risk of abuse becomes acute (Denton et al., 2011).

The abused infant or child is frequently singled out as someone who is different. This infant may be chronically ill, may have been premature, may be hyperactive, may have been the product of a difficult and complicated pregnancy, or may have an obvious anomaly. Early bonding disturbances (inadequacies in feeding, holding, and caring for the infant) are characteristic signals.

The long-term effects of child abuse are profound. The victims lack basic trust (a major task of infancy) and confidence and self-worth. These deficits follow the victims into adulthood and parenthood, and the vicious cycle continues. One of the discouraging findings is that infants and children who were abused frequently grow up to be abusing parents (AAP, 2011c).

Across the United States great interest has been generated in attempts to identify parents in the prenatal and perinatal periods that have significant potential for child abuse. Nurses play a critical role in recognizing infants who have been intentionally harmed, because they are often the first to begin taking a history on the infant. Nurses work collaboratively with community agencies to provide follow-up care for the infant in danger of continued abuse. Nurses take appropriate action if they suspect an infant is at risk. Some of the biggest challenges of child protection come from our own internal reluctance to act, but doing nothing is not an option. The following measures have been undertaken to help prevent child abuse:

- Predictive questionnaires to be given to parents on postpartum units
- Recognition of parents who have difficulty relating to their infants through body language clues or verbalizations
- Closer follow-up during the postpartum period by the public health nurse
- Crisis hot lines made available to parents in distress

Before focusing on nursing interventions (Box 17-12), the nurse makes several observations to assist in identifying a high-risk infant by answering the following questions:

- Does the mother hold the infant close and establish eye contact?
- Does the mother speak negatively about the infant?
- Does the mother intensely dislike the duties of motherhood, such as diapering, feeding, and so on?
- Does the mother expect too much of the infant at a particular stage of development?

BOX 17-12 NURSING INTERVENTIONS TO PREVENT ABUSE OF INFANTS

- Promote and facilitate early parent-infant bonding.
- Promote a trusting relationship.
- Provide more frequent office visits and be available by phone.
- Provide infant care instructions to enhance mothering ability.
- Provide for community health person to make home visits.

- Does the mother focus her attention on the infant rather than on her husband?
- Does the mother have a good support system available?
- Does the mother act overly concerned about the infant's gender?

Most communities are seeking ways in which child abuse can be prevented through educational efforts, improved agency coordination, and development of new collaborative efforts and services for parents and infants. Laws for reporting abuse have been enacted in every state. Reporting all cases of suspected abuse and neglect is mandatory. Everyone must assist in this endeavor to prevent continued abuse. It takes a community effort to address the problem.

Homelessness

Along with food, health, and personal safety, probably no greater basic need for human beings exists than shelter. The loss of shelter is detrimental to the health and well-being of all people. Homelessness in the United States is a national disgrace. Most estimates place the number of homeless people at 4 million. Two percent of all children are homeless (NHCHC, 2011).

To say that the well-being of the next generation is being jeopardized by homelessness is not an exaggeration. Homelessness devastates every aspect of a child's life, causing damage with long-term implications that remain unknown. Homelessness endangers a child's health throughout childhood. Homeless infants are often exposed to unsafe and unsanitary conditions in shelters in which infectious diseases thrive. These dangers are combined with a lack of access to regular health care; common childhood ailments such as ear infections become extremely serious and sometimes life-threatening illnesses before they are treated.

Ear infections are among the most common health problems encountered in children. For a bacterial infection, a course of antibiotics usually relieves the condition. Rarely are long-term complications encountered. For the homeless infant, however, the story is different. Families are cut off from their regular clinics and providers. The struggle for basic life needs is intense. The poverty, isolation, and disorientation of prolonged homelessness can be complicated by drug or alcohol abuse, provoked, at least in part, by situational despair. The fundamental ability of a family to function is hampered or paralyzed.

For the homeless family, the fever caused by an infant's acute ear infection may not have the highest priority. Availability, accessibility, and affordability of health care are serious concerns. As a result, the infection may never be treated, and the problem becomes prolonged (the infection evolves to a chronic state). Hearing and language development can be impaired.

These children simply do not receive routine, reliable health care. They remain at high risk for many health problems. Their health problems remain undiagnosed and undertreated, if they receive attention at all. Complications and secondary problems abound. Infants are born onto the streets without cribs and are rarely held. They may find refuge in an overcrowded shelter one night, and the next night their shelter is a doorway hidden in an alley; the following night home is an abandoned car. From the beginning of life these infants encounter an unbeatable cycle of nowhere to go, no place to call home, and no safe sanctuary, only the feeling of aloneness and unpredictability (Gillard, 2012).

The pioneering work of Erik Erikson has defined the necessary stages of human development. Each level of maturation must be mastered sequentially, but to do so takes a secure environment, opportunities to succeed, and emotional support. The hidden tragedy for homeless children is the stifling development of their personal growth. Homelessness can be eliminated. The key factors are increased affordable housing, increased income for low-income families, and strengthened service and support for families at risk of homelessness. Families at risk of homelessness for solely economic reasons can often be helped with short-term loans and grants. Community-based programs can help identify these families before they lose their homes.

Efforts are increasingly made to link the homeless with all available programs and services, such as the Special Supplemental Nutrition Program for Women, Infants, and Children (WIC), food stamps, Head Start, and housing subsidies. These programs should continue to provide assistance after the family is resettled in permanent housing. These families will need more comprehensive services with special problems such as domestic violence, mental illness, and substance abuse.

Because of the multitude of needs, a partnership that provides a variety of resources must be developed. Nurses can take a leadership position in helping the homeless achieve a sense of security and adequate health care. By involvement in community health care for the homeless and provision of compassionate care, nurses can give the homeless a clear signal of hope and concern about their plight. Drawing attention to this social problem by speaking to community groups to obtain their support is another way that nurses can help. Volunteering time in community shelters and organizing health care days through the local health department is another way to address the problem.

Nurses can become active in raising the nation's conscience and helping to call attention to this national disgrace. Housing and support services must be provided to assist the homeless in regaining a foothold in society. With the right support services and health care, many homeless people can be stabilized and reintegrated into the community. These families with infants are not "throwaways," but people who have fallen on hard times need to be offered a variety of helping hands. Through this help, the nation's health can improve. Ending homelessness is everyone's responsibility and it will only be possible if we address the underlying causes such as poverty, social inequity, intimate partner violence, health insurance costs, and family breakdown. (See the Case Study and Care Plan at the end of this chapter.)

Sexuality-Reproductive Pattern

An infant's identity begins at birth, when the gendered child is identified and caretakers behave a certain way toward the infant because of its gender. The infant's sexuality gives direction to its physical, emotional, social, and intellectual responses throughout life. Infants have a great oral sensitivity, enjoy skin-to-skin contact, and explore their own bodies for pleasure during the first year of life. A healthy, accepting attitude by caretakers is important in an infant's evolving sexual development.

Coping-Stress Tolerance Pattern

The term *stress* implies intense reaction to an experience and changes in usual behavior. Stress is a normal phenomenon that occurs throughout the life span, as, for example, when an individual experiences a developmental or situational crisis.

Developmental Crisis

Developmental crises are turning points or periods of great change. Most stressors that an infant experiences are a necessary part of growth and development. For example, learning new skills creates stress. The infant who is unable to move forward while learning to crawl experiences stress. The infant expresses this stress by crying for help. Other stressors are more psychosocial in nature, such as being left with a babysitter or in an unfamiliar place.

Situational Crisis

Situational crises are not anticipated easily and do not occur necessarily as part of the normal growth and development process. One major situational crisis during infancy is separation from the significant other. The following three distinct phases are evident in the reaction to separation (Puckett & Black, 2010):

- *Protest.* Infant cries loudly, screams for the mother, and refuses attention of the substitute caregiver.
- *Despair.* Infant stops crying and becomes less active, withdraws, and becomes apathetic.
- *Withdrawal.* Infant takes an interest in surroundings but tends to ignore or reject the mother when she returns, because she failed to meet the infant's needs.

Initially, with no time framework and no understanding of waiting, the infant has little ability to cope with stress. As maturity and a sense of security provided by the caregiver increase, the infant begins to wait a short time to have needs met without protest. An infant who experiences stress reacts by crying, the main tool of communication. The infant gradually learns to tolerate greater stress with time.

Nursing Interventions

Nursing interventions that assist the infant and family in stressful situations are listed in Box 17-13. By allaying anxiety in the infant's caregiver, the nurse facilitates coping behaviors in the infant. The stressful situation and the problem-solving activities can be turned into growth-producing experiences for the family, with coping capacities strengthened for the future.

BOX 17-13 NURSING INTERVENTIONS TO ASSIST IN STRESSFUL SITUATIONS DURING INFANCY

- Attempt to meet the infant's needs promptly.
- Allow favorite toy or item of security to be present during stressful experiences.
- Allow familiar caregiver to be present to calm the infant.
- Attempt to keep the number of strangers interacting with the infant to a minimum.
- Attempt to provide a warm and accepting environment for the infant.
- Allow freedom of expression (crying) to reduce tension in the infant.
- Identify the infant's established daily routine and try to follow through with it.
- Reinforce the infant's need for expression.
- Establish a trusting relationship with the infant.
- Provide opportunity for play so the infant can vent fears.
- Provide emotional support for the parents so they can, in turn, give support to their infant.

Values-Beliefs Pattern

A value is a standard or principle that reflects a person's judgment on what is important in life. When people communicate, they send both the content message of the spoken words and the unspoken message of who they are and what they believe. Values are pervasive and important and give a focus to both individuals and groups within a particular culture. Because values are attitudes learned especially from significant others within the environment, the parents' values-beliefs pattern greatly influences the care and development of the infant.

Nursing Interventions

By understanding and respecting the parents' value system, the nurse works within their framework of values in the counseling situation. The nurse communicates personal values to the family. To work successfully within a different value system, the nurse incorporates the following attitudes concerning the values-beliefs pattern into the nursing process (Clark, 2009):

- Believe in the ultimate worth of the infant and the family, regardless of their behavior or situation.
- Grant families the freedom to make their own informed choices and to experience the responsibilities and consequences of their decisions.
- Use knowledge of the family's value system in specific ways to reward and reinforce positive health practices.
- Value the growth potential inherent in developmental and situational crisis situations.
- Recognize your own value system and its influence on your behavior.
- Work with families without applying your personal value system in judging their behavior.
- Broaden your value system by accepting lifestyles different from your own.

The nurse influences the behavior of the parents, who have the greatest influence on their infant's values-beliefs pattern. The nurse accomplishes this task by modeling (living congruently with professed values), acting as a consultant by sharing pertinent information with parents, and modifying one's own values. Nurses can anticipate a family crisis of values and can help to promote positive coping and effective use of social supports (Gardner et al., 2011).

Modeling can be a potent influence on another individual's behavior. In the counseling situation, the family looks to the nurse for guidance and assistance in promoting healthy childrearing practices. The methods by which the nurse interacts with the infant, listens to the parents' concerns, and demonstrates respect for the family unit are influencing factors in changing behavior.

Second, the nurse acts as a consultant to influence values. Advice on childrearing practices is overwhelming to parents; everyone has opinions. The nurse listens before giving advice to determine whether parents will accept the advice and to allow parents to decide whether the advice can be useful. Repeated attempts to convert parents to the nurse's value system can make them defensive and resistant to the advice.

Third, by expressing values and attitudes, but remaining open to other approaches, the nurse influences the values-beliefs pattern. Parents can realize that they are free to change and are not bound to values that others outside their value system express (Gardner et al., 2011). Communication skills can more effectively promote the health of the infant and family.

ENVIRONMENTAL PROCESSES

Physical Agents

This section discusses various factors within the environment that can affect the infant's health status. The entire realm of accident prevention and safety promotion is applicable here.

According to the Centers for Disease Control and Prevention (CDC), unintentional injuries, including motor vehicle traffic crashes, falls, poisonings, suffocations, drownings, and fires/burns, are the number one cause of death for people ages 1 to 44 and the fifth-leading cause of death for all ages. Beyond the emotional damage that accompanies such tragedies, the American Public Health Association (APHA) reports that unintentional injuries cost the country more than $69 billion per year (12% of total health care spending) (APHA, 2011).

One of the overall goals for the Quality and Safety Education for Nurses (QSEN) project is to meet the challenge of preparing future nurses who will have the knowledge, skills, and attitudes necessary to continuously improve the quality and safety of the health care systems within which they work. One of their competencies promotes safety within the environment.

Some areas applicable to this competency of safety for infants would be the use of flame-retardant sleepwear and knowledge of measures to promote crib safety and toy safety.

Infant sleepwear made for sizes 9 months and smaller can be flame resistant or non–flame resistant. Flame-resistant clothing usually is labeled as such and is either a synthetic fiber or treated cotton. Parents should be advised to select flame-resistant sleepwear for their infant, and follow the laundry instructions carefully to maintain this property. Sleepwear in sizes larger than 9 months is required to be either flame resistant or snug fitting.

Snug-fitting clothing that conforms to the body has less opportunity to ignite when exposed to a flame than loose-fitting clothing. Smaller sizes are not required to be snug fitting, because a smaller infant is less likely to be mobile enough to expose himself/herself to a fire hazard.

All new cribs are required to meet strict safety standards; however, if parents accept a secondhand crib, they need to be advised to check the following:

- The slats should be no farther than 2⅜ inches apart. Wider slats could allow an infant's head to become trapped between them.
- Check for any decorations or projections that could snag an infant's clothes. Avoid cribs with decorative cutouts in the headboard or footboard.
- Some older cribs were painted with lead-based paint, which could poison an infant who mouths or chews the wood. If unsure, strip the old paint and repaint it with new lead-free enamel.
- Check all the screws and bolts that hold the crib together; make sure none are missing and all are tight. Avoid cribs with drop side rails. If a drop side rail detaches or becomes loose, an infant may become trapped between the mattress and railing.
- The crib mattress should be firm and should fit very snugly, with no room for the baby to become trapped between the mattress and the crib. Do not cover the mattress with plastic or a quilt, which can suffocate a baby.

Never put an infant to sleep on a waterbed, pillow, quilt, beanbag chair, or sofa. All of these surfaces increase the chance that a baby could suffocate or get his/her head or another part of his/her body trapped in the furniture.

Do not put pillows or stuffed animals in an infant's crib, because they can cause suffocation. Crib quilt bumpers also pose a risk for suffocation and should not be used. When your infant learns to sit, lower the mattress so he/she cannot fall out of the crib. Remove mobiles, and make sure draperies and window blind cords are well out of his/her reach.

Anticipatory guidance to promote infant toy safety would include instructions for parents purchasing new toys to follow the age guidelines on the packaging. Infant toys should have no tiny parts that pose choking hazards, and nothing on the toy should be sharp or detachable. Infants explore objects with their mouths, so anything they pick up should be too big to swallow. The more chewable and unbreakable a toy is, the safer it will be.

Accidents are always unexpected and, in retrospect, usually could have been prevented. Unintentional injuries are the leading cause of death for children in the United States and globally. Research shows that every 1½ minutes an infant is seen in the emergency department for an unintentional injury (APHA, 2011). Adults take for granted that they are living in a world designed by adults for adults. They must remind themselves constantly that infants also live in this complex world and that they learn at a remarkable rate, primarily by exploring and playing in the environment. These experiences render them extremely vulnerable to accidents, a major problem and a challenging field for preventive measures.

FIGURE 17-3 Accident prevention for infants in their car seats includes the use of safety belts.

Accidents occur in many situations: in the home, outside, on the playground, and in automobiles. The use of safety belts prevents infant injury (Figure 17-3). Most accidents, however, occur in the home. Their number and seriousness are closely linked to the infant's developmental stage. Accidents tend to increase with the mobility of the infant, but even a 2 month old can wiggle or fall from a high place. Keeping the environment free from hazards and ensuring caregiver supervision are crucial for this age group.

Nurses have the opportunity to help parents and caregivers anticipate and understand the common hazards of early life and provide specific guidance for accident prevention.

Unintentional Injuries

Falls. Falls are most common after 4 months of age, when the infant has learned to roll over, but they can occur at any age. Falls involving infants happen more often in the home environment, on stairs, from furniture, and out of windows. The best advice is never to place an infant unattended on a raised surface that has no type of guardrails. When in doubt, the safest place is the floor (Smithson et al., 2011). Safety tips to assist parents in preventing falls are listed in Box 17-14.

Burns. In the United States, burns are the third leading cause of unintentional injury death in children ages 1 to 14 years, accounting for more than 600 deaths per year in children from birth to 19 years of age (Bowman et al., 2011).

Burns are the most frequent and frightening of all accidents during infancy. The majority of fire deaths occur in the home and most victims die from smoke or toxic gases and not from the burns (Bowman et al., 2011). Because nearly all burns are preventable, the attendant caregiver can experience severe guilt.

Fire from matches or other sources, hot liquids, ultraviolet light from the sun, electricity or electrical outlets, and heating elements such as radiators, registers, and floor heaters can all cause burns. Box 17-15 lists safety tips to assist parents in preventing burns.

Swallowing/Choking on Foreign Objects. Any small object that an infant puts in the mouth has the potential to be swallowed and choked on. More than 65% of deaths from

BOX 17-14   SAFETY TIPS TO PREVENT FALLS

- Keep sides up and firmly secured when the infant is in the crib.
- Place the infant seat on a stable surface, preferably the floor. The infant should be strapped in securely.
- Check high chairs, strollers, and carriages for safety, and restrain the infant who is active.
- All windows above the first floor should be locked and have operable window guards.
- Clean up food or liquid spills immediately from the floor.
- Remember that polished floors are hazardous, especially when throw rugs are present.
- Close off stairways with doors or properly installed gates, at the top and bottom.
- To prevent falls, set the crib mattress at the lowest adjustment level after the infant can pull up and stand.
- Place furniture away from windows and anchor pieces to the wall.
- Avoid the use of baby walkers.
- Never leave an infant alone on a bed, changing table, or piece of furniture.
- Avoid bringing strollers onto escalators.

Data from Newman, A. (2011). *The ultimate guide to babyproofing your home and general baby safety.* Hamburg, Germany: Axel Publishing and New York Department of Health, Bureau of Injury Prevention (2009), http://www.health.state.ny.us/prevention/injury prevention/

BOX 17-15   BURN PREVENTION GUIDELINES

- Keep the infant out of the sun when ultraviolet rays are strongest, generally from 10 AM to 3 PM.
- Sunscreen, clothing with long sleeves, pant legs, and a brimmed hat are essential to prevent sun overexposure.
- Remember that fireplaces can be a serious hazard. Fine-mesh screens attached to a frame are safer than freestanding screens. Never leave an infant alone in a room where a fire is burning; make sure the fire is extinguished before going to bed.
- Avoid bathing the infant in a sink or adult tub near hot water faucets. Test the bath water temperatures before placing the infant in it; keep one hand on the infant at all times during the bath.
- Be sure that all infant's clothing is made of nonflammable materials.
- Avoid handling hot liquids near the infant.
- Turn the handles of cooking utensils toward the back of the stove.
- Keep all electrical cords taut, especially those for coffee pots; keep cords out of the infant's sight.
- Cover electrical outlets with protective plastic caps.
- Place a barrier in front of any heat-producing element, especially floor heaters.
- Keep all matches and lighters out of the infant's reach.
- Teach the older infant the meaning of hot.
- Close oven doors when the oven is in use or when cooling.
- If you must smoke, keep the heat of cigarettes or cigars away from the infant.
- Install smoke detectors on every level of the home and in every sleeping area.

BOX 17-16   NURSING INTERVENTIONS TO REDUCE CHOKING HAZARDS FOR INFANTS

- Keep small objects out of an infant's reach.
- Avoid propping bottles and making large holes in nipples to prevent aspiration of formula into the infant's lungs.
- Discourage the use of powder on infants to reduce the risk of pneumonia from inhaling zinc stearate.
- Burp the infant thoroughly before placing in the crib; place infant in side-lying position.
- Older children should not give food to the infant, who may choke on it. An adult should be near to supervise children around infants.
- Adults should not set a bad example by putting pins or other objects in their mouths; older infants like to mimic adults.
- Inspect toys for loose, removable parts that could end up in the infant's mouth.

hot dogs, paper clips, nuts, corn, buttons, popcorn, chips, apple with peel, and parts of broken toys are frequently swallowed. Many objects can fit into this category and into the infant's mouth. The carelessness of a caregiver, relative, friend, or babysitter in leaving small objects available and within reach, or giving toys unsuited to the infant's stage of development, frequently causes these accidents.

When choking occurs, the adult should place the infant across the adult's knees and deliver 5 back blows (slaps) followed by 5 chest thrusts repeatedly until the object is expelled or the infant becomes unresponsive. Abdominal thrusts are not recommended for infants because thrusts in the abdominal area could potentially damage the relatively large and unprotected liver (American Heart Association, 2011). Cardiopulmonary resuscitation (CPR) should be performed if the infant becomes unresponsive. The American Heart Association does not recommend using under-the-diaphragm abdominal thrusts for choking infants younger than age 1 year.

Prevention of swallowing foreign objects is the best treatment. Some safety measures for parents and caregivers of infants are listed in Box 17-16.

The entire balance of safety for infants depends on allowing them plenty of opportunity to explore and play within the environment while protecting them from harmful agents. According to the AAP, the greatest threat to the health of infants is not illness but injuries, many of which can be prevented. The nurse informs the infant's parents, babysitters, family friends, and day care workers about the need to childproof their environments when an infant is present. The nurse can explain ways to promote the safety of these varied environments (Box 17-17).

Biological Agents

The fetus is partially protected from some biological agents in the environment by the placental barrier and the mother's defense system. After birth, however, the infant is thrust into an environment that is filled with infectious, disease-causing agents. These bacterial or viral organisms can be found in food, cribs, the air, pets, the parents, and the siblings—literally everywhere. Even the healthiest environment harbors disease-causing

foreign-body aspiration occur in infants. Liquids are the most common cause of choking in infants, whereas balloons, small objects, and foods are the most common causes of foreign-body airway obstruction in children (APHA, 2011). Parents should be advised that objects such as safety pins, peanuts, beads, coins,

BOX 17-17 HOME CHILDPROOFING TIPS

- Remove any heavy, sharp, or breakable objects from tables and low shelves.
- Bolt bookcases to the wall and remove heavy books to prevent falls.
- Test floor and table lamps to make sure they cannot be pulled over.
- Disconnect unused appliances and wrap up cords.
- Secure all other cords to prevent appliances from being pulled down.
- Safely discard unused and unneeded medicines.
- Avoid referring to medicines as candy.
- Store potentially toxic substances out of sight and reach.
- Close reachable outlets with safety covers.
- Tie drapery and blind cords out of the infant's reach.
- Choose stair gates with openings too small for an infant's head and child-resistant fasteners such as pressure bars.
- Avoid accordion or expandable gates with openings that can trap an infant's head.
- Install smoke detectors and check the batteries at least once a month.
- Use sturdy screens in front of fireplaces.
- Place crib, playpen, and high chair well away from heaters, fans, and electrical outlets.
- Install childproof latches on drawers and cupboards. Store all cleaning compounds and detergents in a high, locked cupboard.
- Buy all medicines in bottles with childproof lids and keep them in their original labeled containers for identification in case of accidental ingestion.
- Install lids on garbage pails and never leave any harmful materials in them, such as sharp can lids or spoiled food.
- Check the floor regularly for objects small enough to be swallowed.
- Cut blind cords into two pieces.

agents. Although the infant cannot escape exposure to these pathogens without being completely isolated, immunizations are given to assist the infant's defense against some communicable diseases.

Acquired Immunodeficiency Syndrome

Acquired immunodeficiency syndrome (AIDS) is spread by contact with the human immunodeficiency virus (HIV) through blood and body secretions. The virus attacks the T cell lymphocytes, affecting formation of TH4 (T helper or T inducer) cells, which direct the immune response. The infant with HIV infection is unable to resist normal infections. Transmission of HIV from mother to infant is the most likely cause of childhood HIV. Transmission can occur during pregnancy, at delivery, or during breastfeeding (Read & Newell, 2011) (see Chapter 16). There is no immunization against HIV infections currently, but frequently preventive options are offered to mothers, and babies are usually delivered by cesarean birth. Antiretroviral drugs reduce viral replication and can decrease mother-to-child transmission of HIV either by lowering plasma viral load in pregnant women or by providing postexposure prophylaxis in their newborns. In developed countries, highly active antiretroviral therapy (HAART), which usually comprises three drugs, has reduced the mother-to-child transmission rates to around 1% to 2%, but HAART is not always available in developing countries (Siegfried et al., 2011a).

Because infants can retain maternal antibodies for HIV infection for as long as 18 months, the diagnosis of HIV infection in an at-risk infant (one whose mother is infected) is extremely difficult. In the last few years, investigators have demonstrated the utility of highly accurate blood tests in diagnosing HIV infection in infants 6 months of age and younger. Standard assay has limited utility in diagnosing HIV reactivity among infants until the age of 18 months, by which time many HIV-infected infants expire. The test for diagnosing infants and children younger than 18 months is DNA polymerase chain reaction (DNA-PCR) either by a dried blood spot or by a whole blood sample (Jain et al., 2011). Although signs and symptoms of illness can occur at any time, they usually begin during the first year of life. In infants the symptoms of the disease include failure-to-thrive, oral candidiasis, recurrent bacterial infections, persistent pulmonary infiltrates, chronic diarrhea, and delays in reaching important milestones in motor skills and mental development such as crawling, walking, and speaking. Early recognition and triaging of infants suspected of having HIV infection provide an opportunity for early diagnosis and treatment, which could prevent the adverse impact of rapidly progressive HIV disease (Jeena et al., 2011).

In response to the urgent need to reduce the number of new HIV infections globally, the WHO and the UNAIDS (Joint United Nations Program on HIV/AIDS) funded research to determine whether male circumcision should be recommended for the prevention of HIV infection (WHO and UNAIDS, 2011). Based on the research findings presented, experts recommended that male circumcision be recognized as an important intervention to reduce the risk of heterosexually acquired HIV infection in men. There is strong evidence that medical male circumcision reduces the acquisition of HIV in heterosexual men by between 38% and 66% over 24 months. Incidence of adverse events is very low, indicating that male circumcision, when conducted under these conditions, is a safe procedure. Inclusion of male circumcision into current HIV prevention measure guidelines is warranted, with further research required to assess the feasibility, desirability, and cost-effectiveness of implementing the procedure (Siegfried et al., 2011b). Parents must weigh their decision to circumcise their male infant based on their own values, religious backgrounds, and culture in light of this new information.

Nursing assessment focuses on a careful and complete history of the infant and mother, signs and symptoms of the disease, growth and development history, and psychosocial concerns. Parents are assessed carefully to determine their level of anxiety; knowledge of the disease process, including prognosis, treatment, and transmission; and awareness of resources, support systems, coping strategies, and the infant's needs.

No other disease causes as much public awareness and panic as does AIDS. Part of this behavior is ignorance. Nurses play a major role in educating the public about the disease process, its mode of transmission, and most of all, preventive measures. Preventive education should begin with young children. Most school health programs include information on AIDS. School nurses can contribute to the success of these programs, as can nurses working in prenatal clinics, to spread the importance of prevention. Nurses in all settings can engage in research related to AIDS to gather further clarification of this fatal disease.

Although the infant is not an active participant in the spread of HIV, parents should understand the means by which the virus is transmitted and not allow their infant to become a passive participant because of their own high-risk behaviors.

Immunization

Disease prevention by immunization is a public health priority in *Healthy People 2020* and society as a whole. Progress continues toward the goal of protecting children from serious disease through immunizations. The most recent schedule recommends the rotavirus vaccine (Rota) in a three-dose schedule at ages 2, 4, and 6 months. The influenza vaccine is now recommended as an annual vaccine for all children ages 6 to 59 months. In addition, varicella vaccines should be administered at age 12 to 15 months, and a newly recommended second dose should be administered at age 4 to 6 years (CDC, 2011d). For current year immunizations see http://www.cdc.gov/vaccines/recs/schedules/child-schedule.htm#hcp.

The two types of immunization are active and passive. In **active immunization,** all or part of a disease-causing microorganism or a modified product of that microorganism is injected into the body to make the immune system react defensively. This substance is generally a toxin of the disease organism; depending on the virulence and certain other characteristics of the organism, it is used in the vaccine in a live, killed, or attenuated form (Clem, 2011). The attenuated form is alive, but its virulence has been reduced significantly by treatment with laboratory procedures that use, for example, heat or chemicals, which reduces the potency of microorganisms. Examples of active immunization include diphtheria, tetanus, and acellular pertussis (DTaP); inactivated polio vaccine (IPV); and measles, mumps, and rubella (MMR). Active immunity is relatively long lasting, waning over several years if at all.

Passive immunization is accomplished by injecting blood from an actively immunized person or animal. After an individual has been exposed to a disease, a passive immunization is given to prevent the disease from developing. Passive immunizations provide a short immunity, usually 1 to 6 weeks, which will protect the person until the danger of contracting the disease is passed. Passive immunization also helps reduce the severity of the disease when it is contracted. Because of the short duration, active immunization is still needed to remain permanently immune. Passive immunity occurs naturally in newborns when maternal antibodies are passed through the placenta or in breast milk.

The Committee on Infectious Diseases of the AAP and the CDC (2011d) recommends immunization schedules that are revised periodically as new information arises. Table 17-7 lists the current recommendations for healthy infants. More detailed immunization information is provided in **Website Resource 17C.**

Immunization provides one of the most cost-effective means of preventing infection in infants. Immunizations not only help protect those receiving the vaccinations from developing potentially serious diseases but also help protect entire communities by preventing and reducing the spread of infectious agents. Immunization is additionally important because

AGE (MONTHS)	IMMUNIZATION
Birth	HepB-1
1 month	HepB-2
2 months	DTaP-1 + Hib-1 + PCV + Polio + RV
4 months	DTaP-2, Hib-2 + Polio + PCV-2 + RV
6 months	HepB-3 + DTaP-3 + Hib-3 + Polio + PCV-3 + RV influenza (yearly)
12 to 15 months	Hib-4 + MMR + PCV + HepA + varicella
15 to 18 months	DTaP-4

TABLE 17-7 RECOMMENDED IMMUNIZATION SCHEDULE FOR INFANTS

Modified from Centers for Disease Control and Prevention. (2012). *Recommended immunization schedules for persons aged 0-6 years—United States, 2012.* [Online] Retrieved from www.cdc.gov/vaccines/recs/schedules/child-schedule.htm.
*DTaP, Diphtheria, tetanus, acellular pertussis vaccine; HepA, hepatitis A vaccine; HepB, hepatitis B vaccine; Hib, Haemophilus influenzae type b conjugate vaccine; MMR, measles, mumps, rubella vaccine; PCV, pneumococcal vaccine; Polio, polio vaccine; RV, protects against infections caused by rotavirus.

currently available antibiotics cannot destroy viruses; therefore, immunization offers the only means of control. Nurses have a special responsibility to keep informed of the recommendations and document all vaccinations given. Emphasis must be placed on educating parents about the importance of immunization. Children need a series of vaccinations, starting at birth, to be fully protected against 12 potentially serious diseases. To motivate parents to have their infants immunized, the nurse can work toward increasing health education to achieve greater health maintenance knowledge, send reminders for upcoming visits and needed immunizations, vigorously advocate for all infants to receive comprehensive health care, including immunizations, provide health services that make immunizations feasible and available, develop a close relationship with the family, and continue surveillance of the immunization status of every infant in the health care system.

Chemical Agents

Drugs

Despite advances such as childproof caps on medications, childproof packaging, increased educational efforts, and increased awareness of commonly ingested substances, deaths attributable to unintentional poisonings still occur. Unintentional poisonings are an unfortunate and usually preventable cause of death and disability in infants and children. The very nature of a young child predisposes the child to explore the surrounding environment. As children grow and learn to become independent, they are compelled to investigate new and interesting items, places, and objects, such as medications. On the basis of calls to the U.S. poison control centers, each year more than 1 million children less than 5 years of age experience potentially toxic ingestions (Gutierrez et al., 2011).

Aspirin is the medicine most commonly ingested, with acetaminophen and vitamins close behind. Ibuprofen and other aspirin substitutes are becoming increasingly popular with parents as antipyretics. Vitamins can be harmful; however, many vitamins contain iron, making them potentially lethal. Infants are frequently attracted to vitamins because of their appealing colors, scents, and flavors, especially children's vitamins.

Recent changes in packaging and limits on the number of tablets contained in each bottle have reduced deaths resulting from overdose. Drug manufacturers are using childproof caps increasingly as a safety measure. Despite a concerted effort by manufacturers, childproof bottle caps vary in effectiveness (Clark, 2009). Frequently the safety caps are adultproof, although children can readily open them.

This accessibility points to the dangers of medications, regardless of the bottle. All medications still must be secured in a safe place when infants are in the home or visiting other homes. Some additional guidelines to help prevent accidents involving drugs include the following:

- Use a prescription drug only for the purpose and the person for whom it is intended. Do not use medication prescribed for someone else for a similar condition in the infant.
- Discard unused drugs by taking them to dump into trash on toxic dump days; many infants have been poisoned by eating tablets found in the trash at home.
- Request safety caps on all prescription drugs.
- Keep all medicines under lock and key.
- Have the telephone number of the nearest poison control center readily available.

The main points to be emphasized in giving parents guidance in accident prevention are to eliminate specific environmental hazards, such as drugs, from exploring infants, and to supervise infants while they play, gradually replacing supervision with safety training (Irving, 2011).

Plants

Houseplants are another source of poison. Most people fail to think of houseplants as potentially poisonous, because people do not consider eating them. However, infants test almost everything by putting it in their mouths, and a number of plants can be deadly when eaten. As a result, plants are one of the leading sources of poisoning of infants, and amateur foragers frequently learn the hard way that not everything that looks good can be eaten. Most plants, however, have an unpleasant taste and therefore are consumed only in small amounts. Effects of unintentional poisonings are typically dose dependent; therefore, as children age and their sense of taste becomes more defined, the risk of large-dose unintentional poisonings decreases because they are better able to discriminate the unpleasant taste.

Household plants are frequently placed on the floor, where the leaves or flowers are easy to pull off and taste. The best intervention for plant poisoning is prevention, which, in this case, means previous knowledge. Table 17-8 identifies several common household and garden plants that are poisonous. The nurse must know which plants are harmful when ingested and must inform parents of the potential dangers to infants.

The most prominent groups of plants involved in exposures are those containing oxalates, and the most common symptom is gastroenteritis. The top 12 identified plants (in descending order) nationally were *Spathiphyllum* species (peace lilly), *Philodendron* species (philodendron), *Euphorbia pulcherrima* (poinsettia), *Ilex* species (holly), *Phytolacca americana* (pokeweed), *Toxicodendron radicans* (poison ivy), *Capsicum* (pepper), *Ficus*

TABLE 17-8   POISONOUS PARTS OF COMMON HOUSE AND GARDEN PLANTS

PLANT	TOXIC PART	SYMPTOMS
Apple	Seeds	Release cyanide when ingested in large quantities; can be fatal
Azalea	All parts	Nausea, vomiting, dyspnea, paralysis; can be fatal
Buttercup	All parts	Inflammation around mouth, stomach pains, vomiting, diarrhea, and convulsions
Castor bean	Seeds	Burning of mouth and throat, excessive thirst, and convulsions; one or two seeds are near the lethal dose for adults
Croton species	Plant juice	Gastroenteritis
Daffodil	Bulb	Nausea, vomiting, and diarrhea; can be fatal
Dieffenbachia	All parts	Intensive burning and irritation of the mouth and tongue; death can occur when base of tongue swells enough to occlude air passages
English holly	Berries	Nausea, vomiting, diarrhea, central nervous system depression; can be fatal
English ivy	Leaves and berries	Dyspnea, vomiting, diarrhea, coma, and death
Hyacinth	Bulb	Nausea, vomiting, and diarrhea; can be fatal
Iris	Underground stems	Digestive upset
Jasmine	All parts	Hallucinations, elevated temperature, tachycardia, and paralysis
Lily of the valley	All parts	Arrhythmia, mental confusion, weakness, shock, and death
Mistletoe	Berries	Acute stomach and intestinal irritations with diarrhea; can be fatal
Oak tree	Acorns	Kidney failure, gastritis
Oleander	All parts	Digestive upset, bloody diarrhea, respiratory depression, cardiac arrhythmia, blurred vision, coma, and death
Philodendron	All parts	Burning of lips, mouth, and tongue; swelling of tongue; dyspnea; kidney failure; death
Poinsettia	Leaves	Severe irritation to mouth, throat, and stomach; can be fatal
Potato	All green parts	Cardiac depression; can be fatal
Tomato	Green parts	Cardiac depression; can be fatal
Violet	Seeds	Taken in quantity, cathartic effects can be serious to infant
Yew	Foliage, seeds, bark	Nausea, vomiting, diarrhea, dyspnea, and dilated pupils; death is sudden

(rubber tree, weeping fig), *Crassula argentea* (jade plant), *Dieffenbachia* (dumb cane), *Epipremnum aureum* (pothos), and *Schlumbergera bridgesii* (Christmas cactus) (Petersen, 2011).

The National Clearinghouse for Poison Control Centers lists plants as the third most commonly ingested poison, after aspirin and household cleaning agents. Safety education is stressed at all well-baby visits beginning in the first 6 months of life. Prevention of plant poisoning and other accidents depends on a reciprocal relationship between protection and education that must be related to age. Keep all poisonous substances, medicines, cleaning agents, health and beauty aids, paints, and plants locked in a safe place out of an infant's sight and reach. Never store poisonous substances in containers other than original ones (for example, empty jars or soda bottles). Safe behavior is a learned behavior, gradually acquired in a progressive process with increasing age.

When parents are being taught, anticipatory guidance should include ways to prevent ingestions, the phone number for the nationwide poison control center (1-800-222-1222), early recognition of common signs and symptoms of poisoning, and the importance of never giving remedies before the poison control center is contacted. It is also important to discuss with parents and caregivers the importance of storing these medications out of the reach of infants and children, using safety locks on cabinets, and keeping purses (or any other places of storage of these medications) out of the reach of infants and children who are at risk for unintentional poisoning. When parents are provided anticipatory guidance, particular emphasis must be placed on the prevention of unintentional poisonings. Guidance should be given on the basis of developmental age rather than chronological age (Wilkerson et al., 2011).

As nurses, part of our role is that of education. Talking with parents outside the health care arena would be a great start. Girl Scout meetings, meetings of parent-teacher associations, church gatherings, day care centers, and other community-based activities can provide a forum for teaching and learning, and such training sessions could also provide an opportunity for questions to be answered.

Box 17-18 lists specific safety measures for parents to prevent plant poisoning for infants (Henslow, 2011; Krenzelok & Mrvos, 2011; Petersen, 2011).

BOX 17-18 NURSING INTERVENTIONS TO PREVENT PLANT POISONING IN INFANTS

- Keep plants out of reach of infants and young children.
- Never eat any part of a plant except the parts that are grown or sold as food.
- Keep jewelry made from unknown seeds or beans away from exploring infants.
- Learn to identify poisonous plants around your house and garden.
- Do not use unknown plants as medicines or teas.
- Pay close attention to infants at play inside and outside.
- Seek help whenever anyone chews or swallows a poisonous plant.
- Be aware that infants are more susceptible than are adults to the effects of poisonous plants.
- Keep the poison control center telephone number handy (800-222-1222).

Toxins

Infants are at particular risk from toxic factors in the environment; as dependent, developing organisms, they are inherently vulnerable. Generally the exposure of infants to potential toxins is quite different from that of adults because of differences in physical environment, activities, and diet. Daily activities of infants, such as proximity to the floor or carpet inside the home and the lawn or soil outside, hand-to-mouth behaviors, and smaller body size and composition, place them at great risk for environmental toxins. Infants are exposed to a host of environmental pollutants on a regular basis. These exposures occur through all possible environmental media: air, water, soil, and food. Infants have a unique exposure pattern and unique vulnerabilities. For example, some studies identify that the infant's oral habits and unique diet (ingesting more fruits, vegetables, and water than do adults) magnify their exposure to certain agents. Finally, because infants have a longer life span, toxins that have a long latency or cumulative toxicity (such as certain carcinogens) pose a greater risk to them than to adults (Yu et al., 2011).

Some pesticides that are used to control insects that feed on cereal grains, fruits, and vegetables are notorious for their slow accumulation in human tissue. Produce washes are available now to rid vegetables and fruits of these potential toxins. Over sufficient time, exposure to relatively small amounts of pesticides can result in the buildup of toxic quantities and lead to chronic disease in humans.

Lead is another environmental toxin that has no known physiological role in the human body. Although lead is essentially a contaminant, most people absorb a certain amount through exposure to lead-based paint in older homes, contaminated soil, household dust, drinking water, lead crystal, and lead-glazed pottery. Before 1950, lead-based paint was used on the inside and outside of most homes. It was used to make several colors including white, and was known to dry to a hard, durable surface. In 1977 federal regulations banned lead from paint for general use. However, homes built before 1977 are likely to contain lead-based paint. Numerous toys made in China have been recalled and deemed unsafe because they contain lead-based paint. Studies have revealed a high lead content in dust, dirt, and soil. Lead in the air comes primarily from automobile emissions (National Institute of Environmental Health Sciences [NIEHS], 2011a). Absorption of lead is closely related to particle size. Airborne lead of small particle size is readily absorbed through the lungs, whereas larger particles fall to the ground. Lead affects practically all systems within the body. At high levels, lead can cause convulsions, coma, and even death. Lower levels of lead can adversely affect the brain, central nervous system, blood cells, and kidneys.

Infants are vulnerable to lead exposure for several reasons. In proportion to their weight, infants inhale more air and more lead than do adults. Additionally, infants breathe closer to the ground, where a higher concentration of lead is located. Their dust-raising play and habit of putting their hands in their mouths add to their lead consumption; they also have a greater rate of gastrointestinal absorption of lead and other chemicals than do adults. Both exercise and blockage of the nasal passages increase mouth breathing, and the mouth is a far less capable filter than the nose. Mouth breathing, coupled with their greater frequency of respiratory tract infections, exposes infants to a greater amount of environmental toxins. The growing prevalence of asthma is also evidence of environmental exposure to lead and other pollutants. Approximately 7 million children have asthma. Statistics show that asthma rates have doubled in the last decade and death rates from asthma have increased in recent years. The reality is that we do not know why asthma is becoming more prevalent, but air pollution is a contributing factor (NIEHS, 2011b).

Human potential and development are clearly important natural resources, and a growing body of evidence now links increased lead exposure to impaired intellectual performance and potential. Clinical lead poisoning affects many children, but it is preventable; excess lead in the infant's environment is made by, and should be eliminated by, human beings. Childhood lead exposure has been linked to numerous health problems including learning disorders, attention deficit disorder, and hearing loss. Researchers suspect that there is no threshold of exposure to lead for many of these adverse outcomes, especially as a neurotoxicant (Wedeen, 2011). Progress has been made in reducing blood lead levels in infants and young children. But still today, more than 300,000 American children remain at risk for lead exposure. Many infants and young children live in poverty and old rented dwellings, which can lead to or exacerbate effects of lead exposure. The following factors have contributed to the reduction of blood lead levels (U.S. Department of Health and Human Services [USDHHS], 2010):

- Decline in lead used in gasoline
- Decline in manufactured food and soft drink cans containing lead solder
- Ban on leaded paint for residential (indoor) use
- Established standard for lead exposure in industry
- Ban on lead-containing solder in household plumbing
- Implementation of lead poisoning prevention programs
- Ban of toys manufactured in China containing lead-based paint

Parents need education regarding measures that can reduce their infant's exposure to lead:

- Keep areas in which the infant plays as dust free and clean as possible.
- Do not remove lead paint yourself.
- Do not bring dust into the home.
- If work or a hobby involves lead, change clothes and bathe before entering the environment of infants (e.g., day care centers).
- Do not burn painted wood in fireplace.
- Eat a balanced diet rich in calcium, iron, and vitamin C.

Infants do not necessarily escape noxious chemicals when they are indoors. The levels of contaminants that cause air pollution are approximately the same indoors as they are outdoors, with perhaps higher indoor concentrations of carbon monoxide, nitrogen dioxide, and various hydrocarbons from tobacco smoke; poorly ventilated heating and cooking equipment; and aerosol sprays. There are radon checks and carbon dioxide detectors that can be used to assess the presence of these contaminants. Many consequences of exposure to air pollution may not be observed during infancy, but can surface in problems that affect both physical and mental well-being over a lifetime.

Among the acute illnesses of infancy, respiratory disease is ranked first, representing between 50% and 75% of all childhood diseases (NIEHS, 2011c). In addition to the inconvenience and incapacity induced by respiratory diseases, medical costs are high. Dirty air aggravates and, in some cases, causes nearly all respiratory problems. Infants with chronic respiratory disease can become adults with respiratory problems.

Water pollution can cause gastrointestinal disturbances in the infant. Parents and health care providers are quick to blame food, teething, or a virus for simple diarrhea, when the underlying cause may come from the kitchen tap. Numerous strong chemicals are used today to purify drinking water. These chemicals can irritate the delicate lining of the gastrointestinal tract and cause disturbances. Nurses encourage parents to boil all water for 20 minutes before they give it to their infant to help eliminate any potential problem.

Table 17-9 lists major pollutants and their health effects.

Motor Vehicles

This section refers to the effects of motion or action of forces on the infant; the focus here is on motor vehicle accidents.

TABLE 17-9   MAJOR POLLUTANTS AND THEIR HEALTH EFFECTS

POLLUTANTS	MAJOR SOURCES	EFFECTS
Carbon monoxide	Vehicle exhaust	Replaces oxygen in red blood cells; causes dizziness, coma, or death
Lead	Antiknock agents in some gasoline, old paint chips, metal pieces, pottery, and soil	Accumulates in bones and soft tissues; affects blood-forming organs, kidneys, and central nervous system
Nitrogen dioxide	Industrial wastes, vehicle exhaust	Causes structural and chemical changes in lungs; lowers resistance against URIs
Radon	Earth and rock beneath homes, well water, and building materials	Lung cancer
Ozone	Formed when hydrocarbons and nitrogen dioxide react	Produces smog; irritates mucous membranes, causing coughing, choking, and impaired lung function; contributes to asthma and bronchitis
Sulfur dioxide	Burning coal and oil, industrial processes	Increases colds, coughs, and asthma; contributes to acid rain
Passive smoking	Tobacco products	Causes high incidence of URIs, pneumonia, bronchitis, and asthma; linked to cancer

From the Environmental Protection Agency (EPA). (2011). *Air quality*. [Online] Retrieved from www.epa.gov/iaq/.
URI, Upper respiratory infection.

Automobiles present a danger to people of all ages, but especially to infants. Usually an infant is injured because of improper restraint inside the automobile. Many parents have been misled by thinking that it is better to be thrown clear of an accident than it is to be restrained. Many also think that it is safer to hold an infant on the lap in the front seat rather than to have the infant restrained in the back seat. On the contrary, these practices increase the probability of a fatality. A free-moving child not only distracts the driver but also positions the child in a more vulnerable position for being thrown.

Adult seat belts are unsuitable for infants or children younger than 4 years of age, because their pelvic structure is small; the AAP recommends that safety seats for infants be used (USDHHS, 2010). The American Academy of Pediatrics released a new policy statement that provides four evidence-based recommendations for best practices in the choice of a child restraint system to optimize safety in passenger vehicles for children from birth through adolescence: rear-facing car safety seats for most infants up to 2 years of age; forward-facing car safety seats for most children through 4 years of age; belt-positioning booster seats for most children through 8 years of age; and lap-and-shoulder seat belts for all who have outgrown booster seats. In addition, a fifth evidence-based recommendation is for all children younger than 13 years to ride in the rear seats of vehicles (AAP, 2011d). All children should be in the back seat because of the potential danger posed by air bags. Infant safety in motor vehicles depends entirely on the responsible adults.

Each year infants die from heat stroke after being left unattended in motor vehicles. More than half of the deaths are children younger than 2 years of age. Research has found that on days when ambient temperatures exceeded 86° F, the internal temperatures of a vehicle quickly reaches above 120° to 140° F (Iannelli, 2011). At those temperatures, children are at great risk (http://pediatrics.about.com/od/summersafety/a/heat_illness.htm), which can lead to a high fever, dehydration, seizures, stroke, and death.

Even at relatively cool ambient temperatures, the temperature can rise inside the vehicle to more than 100° F, which places the infant at risk for hyperthermia. Vehicles heat up rapidly, with the majority of the temperature rise occurring within the first 15 to 30 minutes. Leaving the windows opened slightly does not significantly slow the heating process or decrease the maximal temperature attained (Null, 2011).

Nurses can take the lead in increasing public awareness and improving parental education regarding heat rise in motor vehicles. The take home message here is to never leave an infant alone in a motor vehicle. Make "look before you leave" a routine whenever you get out of the car.

The nurse can also suggest the automobile safety precautions listed in Box 17-19.

Much of automobile safety is common sense, but the nurse must cover all areas in anticipatory preventive teaching. The importance of automobile safety cannot be overemphasized.

Radiation

In its broadest sense, radiation means the transfer of electromagnetic waves or energy through space (Yu et al., 2011). Radiation of all types presents a potential hazard in the infant's environment. The risk level depends on the amount of radiation and the length of exposure and on the particular tissues involved. The infant's rapidly growing and immature cells are especially vulnerable.

The infant is exposed to two basic categories of radiation: natural background radiation, which comes from cosmic rays and radioactive material existing naturally in the soil, water, and air; and human-made radiation, which includes x-rays and radiation from nuclear power plants, microwave ovens, and other electronic devices found in the home (USDHHS, 2010). Infants have a developing immune response. As their immune system develops, immunity occurs in response to external factors such as the environment. Their exposure to ultraviolet radiation alters development of the immune system, leading to long-term implications for suppression of immunity in adulthood (McGee et al., 2011).

Cancer

Most people think of cancer as a disease of adults. Cancer, however, is the leading cause of death from disease in children more than 1 year of age. On average, 1 to 2 children develop the disease each year for every 10,000 children in the United States. The most common cancers found from infancy to age 5 years are Wilms' tumor, retinoblastoma, acute lymphocytic leukemia, neuroblastoma, and rhabdomyosarcoma (National Cancer Institute [NCI], 2011).

Nursing interventions to identify risk factors include taking a careful history, which usually reveals a slow progression of symptoms (e.g., cat's eye reflex, strabismus, painful red eye, and blindness). For example, the nurse who suspects retinoblastoma should ask questions such as the following to identify risk factors:

- Are tumors of the eyes common in your family?
- If so, can you identify which relatives had this and what was done for these tumors?

BOX 17-19 AUTOMOBILE SAFETY PRECAUTIONS

- Be a good role model. Make sure you always wear your seat belt.
- Never leave a child unattended in a parked car or around cars.
- Never hold a child in the lap in the front seat.
- Always use an infant car seat that is properly installed by following the manufacturer's instructions.
- Keep car doors and windows locked.
- Use safety restraints for passengers and driver.
- Do not be distracted by an infant while driving.
- Continue to use car seats as directed by the manufacturer; then use seat belts.
- Never place an infant in a rear-facing car safety seat in the front seat of a vehicle that has a passenger airbag.
- Make sure the seat belt is routed through the correct belt path for adult seat belts.
- Always lock your car and secure the keys so that children cannot access keys.
- Install a trunk release mechanism, so that children will not be trapped in the trunk.
- Take the child out of the car seat first, and then worry about getting other items (e.g., groceries) out of the car.

- Have you noticed your child having any eye problems, such as crossed or lazy eyes, or difficulty seeing?
- Have you noticed any changes in your child's eyes?

Nurses with physical assessment skills can perform screening and ophthalmoscopic examinations on high-risk infants and children. These eye tests include checking for the following:

- Visual acuity, which can be determined by the fixation test, used to screen vision in infants and children 6 months to 5 years of age
- Red reflex, which appears whitish in the infant with retinoblastoma (the cat's eye reflex, the most common presenting sign of this cancer)
- Lid lag, which is found in exophthalmos

Nurses play a major role in cancer detection, treatment, and prevention through their astute assessment skills, interview techniques, and community education to increase awareness of this disease to parents.

DETERMINANTS OF HEALTH

Social Factors and Environment

Community and Work

As infants grow and develop, their boundaries extend beyond the home environment. Many mothers and fathers of infants return to the work force, placing them in community day care centers.

Today few young families can escape financial burdens. The two-income and single-mother families are ways of life and the trend will continue. With more than half of all American mothers working outside the home, the need for child care service is growing. This situation is usually an emotional issue for families; the separation process can be traumatic for both infant and parent.

Findings from social science research regarding the effects of day care on an infant's development and health can be summarized as follows: little evidence suggests that day care permanently enhances or slows intellectual development; day care can be used, even from earliest infancy, without damaging the mother-infant relationship; and day care can lead to a slight increase in minor illnesses, but excluding ill infants from the center is not an effective means of reducing the spread of illness (Beijers et al., 2011).

The question of how old an infant should be before being placed in day care is frequently asked of health professionals. Many experts believe that a mother and infant should have 4 to 6 months together before the mother returns to work. Brazelton and Sparrow (2006) make a good case for the mother and infant transitioning through four stages of attachment together before the mother returns to work.

- In the first stage, which takes 10 to 14 days, the infant learns to be attentive to the mother, and the mother learns cues from the infant about being both ready for and tired of attentiveness.
- The second stage, which lasts 8 weeks, is a stage of playful interaction, when the mother learns how to recognize the infant's nonverbal cues and helps the infant maintain the alert state.
- The third stage, from the tenth week to the fourth month, is when the mother and infant learn to play games together.

BOX 17-20 PROSPECTIVE DAY CARE FACILITY QUESTIONS

- Is the center licensed by the state?
- Is the day care facility open all year?
- How many children are present at the center?
- What is the age range of children at the center?
- What is the teacher-to-child ratio? (For infants, 1:3 is recommended.)
- Describe the day care program.
- What meals are served?
- What is the cost?
- Are there openings?
- What are the qualifications of caregivers?
- Are the caregivers happy and interacting with the infant?
- Are infants content?
- Are parents welcome to drop in?

- During the fourth stage, which occurs in the fourth month, infants rapidly learn about themselves and their world. Brazelton suggests that a mother, when possible, should spend the first 4 months with her new infant.

A nationwide survey of family day care found that nearly 50% of all infants in day care centers in the United States are cared for in one of three types of arrangements (Clark, 2009):

- Private homes that provide informal day care to infants of relatives, friends, and neighbors
- Regulated independent care licensed by state agencies
- Regulated, sponsored care provided by licensed workers operating as part of home networks under umbrella agencies

The nurse has a vital role in assisting families with infants who need day care. Many factors are reviewed when a family is looking for an appropriate day care program; the nurse can counsel and guide the family in its search. The means by which the nurse counsels and guides the family in selecting a day care center are as follows:

- Promote awareness of the three types of day care available in their local communities.
- Counsel parents on questions to ask employees of a prospective day care facility (AAP, 2011e) (Box 17-20).
- Help parents learn ways to cope with the separation behaviors manifested by their infant:
  - Remain calm in the situation.
  - Attempt to reduce the number of adults who interact with the infant and always introduce them.
  - Encourage the parents to bring an infant's special cuddly toy from home to the day care facility to promote security.
  - Listen to the parent's understanding of the separation and expected behaviors.
  - Reassure parents that it takes time for the infant to make the transition from parent to another caregiver and vice versa.
  - Emphasize that at certain developmental levels stranger anxiety may be heightened (8 months), and separation behaviors of crying and clinging may be repeated.
  - Work toward promoting a good relationship among parents, infant, and caregiver by providing opportunities for open discussions of concerns.

Culture and Ethnicity

Culture defines how health care information is received, how rights and protections are exercised, what is considered to be a health problem, how symptoms and concerns about the problem are expressed, who should provide treatment for the problem, and what type of treatment should be given. In short, culture is the lens through which one views the world, affecting everything that an individual and their family perceives and does.

The developing infant is subject to the influences of culture from the moment of conception. Partly because of the long dependency period, the family environment is the setting within which the infant experiences overall cultural attitudes. The lives of infants tend to be more under the direct control of parents or other caregivers than the lives of older children, who often are actively involved in selecting their own environments through contacts with peers, teachers, and other adults. The special demands of infancy require extensive and specific caregiving routines across cultures. The parents' perceptions of illness, wellness, roles, childrearing practices, religious values, language, and health practices are all modeled for the infant. In short, culture helps form the infant's view of the world (Giger & Davidhizar, 2012).

The family's ethnicity includes ideas about health, illness, food preferences, moral codes, and family life that persist across generations and survive even the upheaval of coming to a new country. All cultural groups confront repeated challenges as they transfer their families from familiar to unfamiliar surroundings. Infants are exposed to an appropriate mode of behavior that is in accordance with their family's cultural standards. By observing and imitating family members, infants take cues for behavior. These perceptions are then incorporated into their own self-concepts (Puckett & Black, 2010).

In attempting to foster trust with diverse populations, nurses need to help women and their families feel comfortable enough to engage in a dialogue and share information. One approach is being careful not to prejudge as foolish or ill-conceived specific cultural practices and beliefs about health care. For example, a perinatal nurse describes a practice common in Hispanic culture in which an infant who has a sunken fontanel is held upside down by the feet to "fill" the hole. Instead of deeming such a practice foolish and scoffing at it, the nurse should let the families know that a more effective practice is to also "give the infant lots of water, or human milk, or formula, … [and] make sure that the infant gets lots of liquids" (Swota & Hester, 2011). With such an approach, families are not embarrassed to let nurses know about their traditional cultural practices. This will help bridge the gap and build trust in their relationship.

To assess and plan appropriate interventions for different ethnic groups, nurses must be aware of their own cultural backgrounds. An important consideration is to examine all customs and values in relative terms, seeing none as either good or bad (Box 17-21). Change is inevitable in family life, whether it is resisted or welcomed. An important function of the nurse is to help families monitor the rate of change that is acceptable to various members and reach a consensus.

Culturally competent nursing interventions have been shown to improve outcomes in those seeking care. Research

BOX 17-21 FACTORS THAT FACILITATE MULTICULTURAL HEALTH CARE BY NURSES

- Self-exploration of values and beliefs concerning other cultures and their beliefs
- Knowledge of the historical experience, recent and long-term, of ethnic groups that live in the community
- Demographic data that include family size, socioeconomic status, and future expectations that are characteristic of diverse ethnic groups
- Understanding and sensitivity to cultural health care practices different from own
- Recognition of folk beliefs and cultural attitudes toward health and illness
- Awareness of the nature of problems encountered by ethnic group members when they enter the health care system, including fear and distrust of health care professionals, language barriers, and discrimination by caregivers

From Giger, J. N., & Davidhizar, R. E. (2012). *Transcultural nursing: Assessment and intervention* (6th ed.). Philadelphia: Elsevier; Andrews, M. M., & Boyle, J. S. (2011). *Transcultural concepts in nursing care* (6th ed.). Philadelphia: Lippincott Williams & Wilkins.

has identified several strategies that nurses can use that improve communication and reduce stress for culturally diverse populations: answering questions carefully, teaching by demonstration, and "taking time to explain in simple English." In addition, if women felt that the staff truly cared for their infant, this facilitated communication across multiple barriers because they "felt safe to ask questions" or express needs (Wiebe & Young, 2011). Thus, nurses who are mindful of the specific views of a culture respect the boundaries of the particular cultural perceptions, beliefs, and practices. Culturally competent nurses have achieved efficacy in communication skills and incorporate health care practices and beliefs of a particular culture in health care plans. Furthermore, respect for the individual's cultural values is viewed as essential if the nurse is to successfully help the family achieve a state of health and wellness.

The nurse identifies the power structure within a given cultural group. This knowledge may help dictate which family member to approach with the health teaching. Although the nurse might assume it would be the infant's mother, this may not necessarily be the case. Among some Native American tribes, the grandmother, not the parents, has the authority over the grandchildren. In many Latino cultural groups, the infant's father, not the mother, makes decisions about the infant's welfare (Andrews & Boyle, 2011). The nurse assesses the cultural groups' practices and beliefs before planning interventions. Improving the quality and safety of nursing care for culturally diverse women globally should be the primary goal of all perinatal nurses. Approaches to infant care practices vary among cultural groups (Box 17-22: Diversity Awareness).

Language

Language is an important medium for understanding and working together. The nurse may avoid or tend to mumble a person's name when it is foreign; people hesitate to express themselves when the material is unfamiliar. The nurse must consider how

BOX 17-22 DIVERSITY AWARENESS BOX

Quick Guide for Cross-Cultural Nursing Care

The dominant American attitudes about infants and approaches to infant care have undergone many changes in the past several years. With the increased numbers of women in the work force, fathers are becoming more involved in infant care and day care for infants is increasing. Although children are valued, and raising children within the nuclear family remains a priority, an increasing number of American women are focusing on careers, delaying childbirth, and limiting family size.

Members of some cultures view childbearing and childrearing differently. The birth of a child is crucial for many Hispanic, Navajo, Black, Middle Eastern, and Mormon women, whose social role and status are attained through reproduction within the marital relationship. Preference for a male child exists among families of many cultures, particularly Middle Eastern and Asian (Giger & Davidhizar, 2012).

In the dominant American culture, an infant frequently is wrapped warmly in blankets, placed in an infant seat or stroller, and put to sleep in a crib in a room separate from the parents. Mothers of other cultures may choose to carry or wrap their infants differently; women from some cultures carry their infants with them at all times and sleep with them. Southeast Asian infants may be carried in a hip sling or a blanket carrier. Native American infants often are carried in a cradleboard (a wooden frame into which an infant is bundled and tied). The cradleboard is properly blessed before it is used and can be carried, attached to the mother's back, hung from a tree, or propped up to keep the infant comfortable, safe, and secure (Andrews & Boyle, 2011).

Cultural beliefs and practices are continually evolving and changing. Nurses acknowledge and explore their meanings with all the families with which they meet. Nurses work actively to reduce the experience of culture shock for ethnic minority families, remembering that American medical beliefs and practices may appear strange to others. All behavior must be evaluated from within the context of the family and their cultural background and experience.

Nurses must facilitate health-promoting attitudes and practices and show empathic concern and respect for individuals of all cultural backgrounds. By incorporating the assessment of cultural beliefs and practices into the individual's plan of care, nurses can demonstrate respect and take a step forward in developing culturally appropriate patterns of caring.

In American culture the number of women choosing to breastfeed has steadily increased in recent years. Many factors are involved in the decision-making process. Nurses who care for families of newborns are aware of the multiplicity of factors influencing feeding choice and encourage and support parents in their decisions to promote health of newborns.

The family is the primary health care provider for the infant. The family determines health promotion of the family including when an infant is ill. Many cultural groups choose between the traditional or folk beliefs that they believe to be appropriate to them and Western medical treatment. The Vietnamese use both. For example, to decrease an infant's fever, a basil leaf is tied to the wrist with a piece of cheesecloth. For colic, a silver coin is dipped in wine and rubbed or scratched on the infant's back. Nurses are cautious in imposing their own values, beliefs, and attitudes on others. Rather than judging people, the nurse ascertains how each family's values and beliefs influence health outcomes.

The nurse remembers that all behaviors must be evaluated from within the context of the family's cultural background and experiences. Nurses who strive to foster health-promoting attitudes and behaviors begin at the most basic level: empathic concern and respect for the individual. By incorporating the assessment of cultural beliefs and practices into the infant's plan of care, nurses demonstrate respect, reduce alienation, and take a step toward developing culturally appropriate patterns of health promotion. Respecting another's language and religion is extremely important.

---

the individual who speaks a different language feels about being unable to express thoughts and feelings or to understand what is being said. Both parties may play the avoidance game.

The nurse takes steps to remove communication barriers, including the following:

- Using a professional interpreter to help in the communication process
- Using pictorial flash cards in the individual's native language to assist in explaining instructions
- Sending a health care worker to an educational center or school to learn the basics of the language to help in the interpreting process in the health care facility

Even a person who speaks the nurse's language may not understand and comprehend instructions given by the nurse. The negative impact of poor communication is huge, resulting in poor health outcomes, health disparities, and high health care costs. The importance of good health communication is relevant to all populations seeking care, including those from culturally and linguistically diverse backgrounds (Hasselkus, 2011).

Religion

In this pluralistic and democratic society, Americans are confronting the ethical and religious values that impinge on health care services. Interestingly, some providers believe that religion plays no role in individuals' health care practices; therefore, they eschew people's religious or ethical concerns and deal mainly with the physical or psychological problems at hand. However, the individual's religious and ethical concerns are generally the major source for human values when evaluating health care services.

Religious beliefs can become risk factors when they affect decisions concerning treatment. An example may be the parents who refuse a blood transfusion, surgery, or other medically indicated treatment required to save their infant's life. A court order is needed in many instances to treat these infants. The decision is the parents' responsibility, based on their customs and beliefs, and should be respected. Deciding not to offer an opinion may be extremely difficult, but usually the opinion is unwanted. Religion is often a powerful force, and when the nurse causes conflict and interferes, a gap can be formed. This gap may force the parents to seek nonprofessional health care to help them with their health-related and religious ideas about birth, death, stress, birth control, and other matters. To work successfully with an individual, the person's religious background should be investigated and understood thoroughly. Most nurses recognize that attending to the spiritual needs of families enhances the overall quality of their nursing care and the satisfaction of their care recipients.

Levels of Policy Making and Health

Legislation

Health and well-being have become generally accepted rights of everyone, without regard to race, gender, age, economic or social status, or creed. The federal government has pledged to promote the general welfare of the United States in the belief that it belongs to everyone.

To fulfill this pledge, several goals were established. One of these concerns is infant health. The goal, as described by the U.S. Department of Health and Human Services (2010), is to "Improve the health and well-being of women, infants, children and families."

The infant mortality rate has been on a steady decline since the turn of the century, a result of better infant nutrition; improved technology; improved housing; and improved prenatal, obstetrical, and pediatric care (USDHHS, 2010). To meet the goal of improving infant health, major health problems in this age group must be reduced. A major hazard for infants is low birth weight. To address this problem, factors that increase the risk of low birth weight in infants must be identified (Box 17-23).

Many of these factors can be prevented, or risks can be identified early and managed to prevent low-birth-weight infants. The major focus for prevention is prenatal care for all women.

Another major threat to infant survival is congenital disorders, such as malformations of the brain and spine (e.g., microcephaly and myelomeningocele), congenital heart defects (e.g., ventricular septal defects), and combinations of malformations, such as Down syndrome or Tay-Sachs disease. Although some congenital abnormalities cannot be prevented, others can be detected by performing prenatal screening and promoting research to determine their etiology.

Other factors identified by the U.S. Department of Health and Human Services (2010) and *Healthy People 2020* that contribute to the high infant mortality rate are injuries at birth, SIDS, accidents, respiratory distress syndrome, and inadequate parenting.

The federal government's plans to attain the goal of healthy infants are the following:

- Promote family planning services such that all pregnancies are planned and all infants are wanted.
- Provide pregnancy and infant care services through Maternity and Infant Care (MIC) projects to high-risk populations. The WIC program improves the nutritional status of both mother and infant.
- Encourage educational efforts by schools, health providers, and the media to promote prenatal care.
- Promote massive immunization efforts such that each infant is protected from communicable disease.

Nursing's Role. Nurses have important roles in promoting change in response to a continually expanding knowledge base, consumer health care needs, and governmental legislation. By actively participating in groups involved with health planning, the nurse helps make governmental policy more responsive to infants' health care needs.

The nurse's role in the development of health care policies has the following three stages: identifying resources for the community to meet its specific needs; planning for resources

BOX 17-23 LOW-BIRTH-WEIGHT RISK FACTORS

Maternal Factors
- Low socioeconomic status
- No prenatal care
- Preeclampsia and eclampsia
- Hypertension
- Chronic renal disease
- Advanced diabetes
- Malnutrition
- Cigarette smoking (10 per day or more)
- Drug addiction
- Maternal age (younger than 15 or older than 35)
- Alcohol abuse
- Marital status

Fetal Factors
- Multiple gestation (twins)
- Congenital malformation
- Chromosomal abnormality
- Chronic intrauterine infection
- Placental insufficiency

not available to the community; and coordinating the resources available to the community to promote better use of them.

The nurse can become a member of a health planning council, a concerned citizen's group, or an advisory group to a local legislator or to a state health department grant task force. In this capacity, the nurse's responsibility is to inform the other committee members. Because nurses have firsthand experience with many community needs, they are in a good position to speak out and inform others.

The nurse within the community also has several resources available to assist when a need is identified to promote the infant's health, including resources on the federal level (U.S. Department of Health and Human Services), state level (public health department), local level (MIC clinics and well-baby clinics), and community groups (Parents Anonymous, hot lines, La Leche League, March of Dimes, and SIDS groups).

Coordinating for resources, the nurse actively participates in assessing the availability of services within the community and makes recommendations to consolidate or expand existing services. Increasing public awareness of community resources, their services, and existing needs is the basis of the nurse's role in developing policy.

Economics

Even in this society of considerable affluence, many people live below the poverty level. Poor families tend to be characterized as lacking education, having high unemployment rates, being large in size with female heads of household, residing in crowded living areas, and lacking adequate bathroom facilities (U.S. Census Bureau, 2010). According to the latest U.S. Census Bureau report (2010), there were more than 43 million people living in poverty in 2009. For children 18 years or younger, the poverty rate was approximately 21%. Poverty rose among all ethnic groups, but even more so for Blacks and Hispanics.

Virtually every major health problem is found more frequently in segments of the population with low income than in high-income groups. The infant mortality rates in low-income families remain significantly higher than those in high-income families, despite an overall decrease in infant mortality rate nationally (Glasco, 2011; USDHHS, 2010).

Studies have demonstrated that parents with low incomes are often unaware of their infant's developmental needs; they frequently are faced with many environmental and social stresses that demand their time, energy, and other resources (Lareau, 2011). Many parents have so many unfulfilled needs of their own that they cannot meet their infants' needs. Poverty has contributed to the increase in the homeless population, with the fastest growing segments being families with children, currently at 23%. One in 50 children is homeless, and half of these children are under age 5 years. Children who are born into poverty are at risk for an array of negative outcomes that can extend into adulthood. There is substantial evidence that supports the association of poverty with lower educational and cognitive outcomes. These children are also at risk for behavioral and emotional problems (Van Allen & Sterling, 2011).

In many cases, infants from families in poverty have delayed language development. With limited educational and life experiences, their parents are often unable to be ideal models for language development. Infants learn early language sounds from their parents, but their attempts at language must be reinforced.

Armed with the knowledge of how economics can affect the infant's growth, development, and health status, the nurse, before deciding interventions, assesses the family situation by performing the following tasks:

- Establish a relationship with the family to obtain pertinent information.
- Evaluate the home environment in which the infant interacts.
- Elicit the parents' health perceptions about their own health and that of the infant.
- Complete a thorough physical examination of the infant to identify any problem areas.
- Identify community resources that are available to the low-income family.

Nurses should also collaborate with other health care providers to assist families to identify resources to address their economic needs and improve health outcomes. One key role for nurses is to empower families to effectively engage and negotiate the health care system through advocacy.

Health Services/Delivery System

The U.S. health care delivery system is diverse and large; many different sectors merge to provide infant care. Within this enormous, multidisciplinary system, the nurse is an advocate who facilitates the family's passage through the many facets of care. Table 17-10 lists a suggested schedule for health-promotion infant care.

The value of health promotion and preventive health care has been validated; it is cost-effective and is here to stay. As nurses' roles continue to expand within the various parts of the health care system, their duty is to keep pace with the needs, concerns, and available strategies (Clark, 2009; Stanhope & Lancaster,

2012). Because many conditions that cause morbidity or mortality in infants are preventable when health-promotion practices are employed, nurses have the mission of working within the health care system to promote infant health (USDHHS, 2010).

NURSING APPLICATION

The primary role of the nurse in promoting the health of an infant is to provide the family with education during the most critical developmental period. Initial health-promotion efforts should focus on the nutritional needs of the infant during the first 18 months of life. Basic principles of biological growth and development set the stage for appropriate developmental tasks and psychological growth in the coming months.

The nurse promotes the health of the infant through his or her interactions with the parents since the infant is dependent upon them for care. The nurse is in a position to encourage practices in the home that create the most optimal conditions for normal growth and development. An important starting point for the nurse is to teach new parents about the nutritional value of breastfeeding and to encourage those efforts. Professional support and education play a vital role in increasing the rates of breastfeeding women.

Following a routine immunization and well-child health visit schedule is another aspect of health promotion of the infant. Nurses play a role in this task by educating parents about the importance of immunization. In addition, nurses should remain informed about the immunization recommendations and assist the family in maintaining documentation of vaccines administered. If cost or access to care is a factor, families can be referred to free or low-cost vaccination clinics.

Injuries and accidents are a major concern for the infant population. Accident prevention and safety are topics that should be addressed by the nurse when working with families. Although it is difficult to address the many ways in which an infant can be injured, nurses should be prepared to educate about the most common hazards. Some of the educational topics that can be addressed include fall and burn prevention, choking hazards, unintentional poisonings, environmental hazards, and automobile safety. Also, a significant source of illness in infants and children is associated with infectious diseases from either a bacterial or a viral source. Particularly in younger infants, parents should be taught about the importance of frequent handwashing, avoidance of sick contacts, and signs and symptoms of illness that require immediate medical attention.

The health-promotion goals of the nurse working with infants are met through the family. The nurse must ascertain the health perceptions and motivation of the family including their use of good or bad health practices. The family must be motivated to provide good health practices for the infant. As the nurse plans health-promotion activities for families of infants, it is imperative that factors influencing health perception are identified. The ability of the nurse to provide a supportive relationship with the parents is a key element in facilitating successful infant development. The nurse working with this population has a unique opportunity to influence the health status of both the infant and the family for years to come.

TABLE 17-10   SUGGESTED SCHEDULE FOR HEALTH-PROMOTION INFANT CARE

AGE (MONTHS)	PROMOTIONAL ACTIVITY	AGE (MONTHS)	PROMOTIONAL ACTIVITY
1	Complete physical assessment: PKU test Immunizations: HepB-2 **Parent discussion includes:** Basic infant needs: to be touched, held, fondled, rocked, and talked to Appropriate toy: colorful mobile Nutrition: formula or breast milk		Use of finger foods Playing games with infant: pat-a-cake, peek-a-boo, waving bye-bye, and shaking hands Appropriate toys: blocks, stack toys, and jack-in-the-box Fear of strangers
2	Complete physical assessment Immunizations: DTaP-1, Hib-1, Polio, and PCV-1, RV-1 **Parent discussion includes:** Placing infant in prone position to allow lifting of head Need of infant to be exposed to a variety of stimuli within environment Need of infant for change of scenery Colic and other common problems	12	Complete physical assessment Immunizations: MMR; PCV; Hib; Varicella and HepA Laboratory work: CBC **Parent discussion includes:** Accident prevention Getting into things Infant's need to touch and investigate environment, with supervision Parent's need to read, show pictures, and repeat body parts to infant Infant's need for limited independence Sleeping patterns
4	Complete physical assessment Immunizations: DTaP-2, Hib-2, Polio-2, PCV-2, RV-2 **Parent discussion includes:** Stimulation of infant Providing a mirror in which the infant can see reflection Being talked to and played with Appropriate toy: rattle		Appropriate toys: sets of measuring cups, nesting toys, pots and pans, and wooden spoons
6	Complete physical assessment Immunizations: DTaP-3, Hib-3, HepB-3, Polio-3, PCV-3, RV-3, and flu vaccine Laboratory work: hematocrit level **Parent discussion includes:** Accident prevention Teething and use of cool rings Allowing infant to crawl to explore environment Stranger anxiety	15	Complete physical assessment Immunizations: DTaP **Parent discussion includes:** Negativism as normal aspect of development Age of curiosity in infant Toys appropriate for age: push-pull toys and ball Accident prevention Elimination patterns Discipline: stress positive aspects of behavior, when possible
9	Complete physical assessment **Parent discussion includes:** Accident prevention Dental caries prevention: cleaning teeth with gauze daily Infant's need for space to crawl about Use cup if weaning	18	Complete physical assessment Immunizations: HepA-2 **Parent discussion includes:** Accident prevention Begin toilet training, if child is ready Encourage vocalization Socialization with other small children Importance of reading to child Setting limits on behavior Coping mechanisms of parents

CBC, Complete blood count; *DTaP,* diphtheria, tetanus, acellular pertussis vaccine; *HepB,* hepatitis B vaccine; *Hib, Haemophilus influenzae* type B conjugate vaccine; *MMR,* measles, mumps, rubella vaccine; *PCV,* pneumococcal vaccine; *Polio,* polio vaccine; *RV,* rotavirus.

CASE STUDY

Homelessness: Homeless Minority Infants

As a community health nurse in an inner-city health center, you are increasingly aware that the homeless population in your city appears to be the forgotten aggregate. Your community health center provides primary care to a culturally diverse and indigent population. As a nurse, you believe that the homeless population within your city has numerous health needs. Beyond the basic requirements, many homeless people have mental and substance abuse problems, a deficiency in life skills, and poor family support, and most of all lack access to child health services.

The homeless population has all of the usual health problems you would expect in the general population in addition to other problems resulting from their homeless lifestyle. Although there are several glaring concerns, you plan to focus your attention first on securing immunizations for the homeless infants and, secondly, to obtain formula for them.

Reflective Questions

1. In planning health services for this special population, what facts do you need to know?
2. What barriers to accessing health care for minority infants confront the homeless family?
3. How can you overcome some of the barriers in developing your plan for health care?

Discussion

1. In planning health services for this special population, what facts do you need to know? The following are some of the first questions that should be asked:
   - How many homeless minority infants are in this aggregate?
   - Where are they?
   - How can they access health care in the city?

Homelessness: Homeless Minority Infants—cont'd

To answer these questions, it might be prudent to collaborate and partner with other health and social service agencies, local hospitals, and the state health and human services agency. Collaboration and partnering can bring in additional resources and reduce duplication and gaps in services.

2. What barriers to accessing health care for infants confront the homeless family?
   - Lack of transportation
   - Lack of trust in the medical establishment
   - Judgmental care on the part of health care providers and nurses
   - No health insurance to cover medical visits
   - Preventive care, such as immunizations, not a priority when you are hungry
   - No money to get prescriptions filled
   - Waiting until condition is serious before seeking treatment

3. How can you overcome some of the barriers in developing your plan for health care?
   - Provide health care in the city shelters for use by homeless minority families.
   - Set up a mobile health care team and visit the shelters to provide care.
   - Offer free immunizations for all family members.
   - Establish educational sessions within the shelters to provide information.
   - Stress the importance of preventive measures to reduce illness in infants.
   - Obtain free formula from companies or hospitals to give to homeless infants.
   - Work closely with other health care interests within the community.

CARE PLAN

Homelessness: Homeless Minority Infants

Homelessness is a community dilemma and an example of an economic problem that places infants at risk. Families are the fastest growing group of homeless people. Homeless families do not have health insurance; infants within these families are more likely to lack immunizations, proper nutrition, a safe environment, and a stable family situation. The community health nurse in this chapter's Case Study wants to address two aspects of homeless infants: (1) immunizations and (2) nutrition.

*NURSING DIAGNOSIS: Ineffective Health Maintenance related to nonadherence to appropriate immunization schedule as manifested by increased incidence of communicable diseases

Defining Characteristics
- History of lack of health-seeking behavior by caregiver
- Lack of financial or other resources
- Reported or observed impairment of personal support systems
- Lack of knowledge regarding health-promotion practices
- Inability to access health care
- Limited basic personal resources

Related Factors
- Ineffective family coping
- Perceptual-cognitive impairment
- Lack of material resources
- Ineffective individual coping

Expected Outcomes
Caretaker of infant will:
- Begin health-seeking behavior on behalf of the minority infant.
- Increase health-promotion and health-maintenance knowledge.
- Gain access to available health care resources.
- Participate in life change to improve health status; meet goals for health care maintenance.

Nursing Interventions
- Assess caretaker's feelings, values, and personal situation.
- Assess for family patterns, economic issues, and cultural patterns that influence compliance.
- Assist caretaker and minority family to access health care resources available to them.
- Refer caretaker and family to community agencies to address social and economic issues.
- Educate caretaker and family on the importance of immunizations and disease prevention.
- Provide for follow-up care to increase chance of health status change taking place.

*NURSING DIAGNOSIS: Risk for Imbalanced Nutrition—Less than Body Requirements related factors and socioeconomic factors as manifested by low height and weight measurements for chronological age on growth chart

Defining Characteristics
- Pale conjunctival and mucous membranes
- Poor muscle development
- Inadequate food intake to maintain body weight
- Weight loss, fatigue, frequent irritable, fussy, crying behavior
- Growth and development milestones not met
- Frequent illnesses suggesting depressed immunity

Related Factors
- Inability to obtain adequate food or fluid or both to nourish body because of socioeconomic factors

Expected Outcomes
Infant will demonstrate the following:
- Progressive weight gains toward desired goal
- Weight within normal range for height and weight
- Minority infant consuming adequate nourishment
- Infant free of signs of malnutrition

Nursing Interventions
- Assess healthy body weight for age and height.
- Observe minority infant's ability to consume food and fluids.
- Monitor food and fluid intake weekly.
- Access nutritional resources for the caretaker or family.
- Refer to appropriate community agencies to meet needs.
- Assist the caretaker or family to identify area needing change that will make the greatest contribution to improve nutrition.
- Implement instructional dialogue that is appropriate for their level.
- Provide for follow-up care to assist them in changing their health status.

References: Ackley, B. J, Ladwig G. B. (2011). *Nursing diagnosis handbook: An evidence-based guide to planning care* (9th ed). St. Louis: Elsevier; Moyet, L. J. (2009). *Nursing diagnosis: Application to clinical practice* (13th ed.). Philadelphia: Lippincott Williams & Wilkins.
*NANDA Nursing Diagnoses—Definitions and Classification 2012-2014, Herdman T.H. (ED). Copyright © 2012, 1994-2012 NANDA International. Used by arrangement with John Wiley & Sons Limited. In order to make safe and effective judgments using the NANDA-I nursing diagnoses it is essential that nurses refer to the definitions and defining characteristics of the diagnoses listed in this work.

BOX 17-24   HOT TOPICS

Traveling with Infants

Overseas travel is increasing. Taking infants on a long trip to a foreign country can be a positive experience; however, the importance of careful planning and realistic expectations should not be underestimated. Although package holidays, especially to established tourist resorts, generally offer families a protected environment, they do not give complete immunity from travel-related illnesses or accidents.

The most frequently reported infant travel problems are diarrhea, malaria, and accidents. Often, parents focus on vaccine-related concerns during their pretravel consultation. Although no trip can ever be guaranteed as risk-free, awareness of issues and careful planning facilitate safer travel. Without being alarmist, nurses need to provide realistic, consistent advice. The following are some key points to include:

- Parents should be advised not to take infants to regions where malaria may be transmitted because infants with malaria have a high death rate.

- If parents decide to take their infant to malarial areas, they must be advised about appropriate antimalarial drugs and bite avoidance measures.
- International travel should preferably be delayed until initial routine childhood vaccinations have been completed (usually by the age of 4 months).
- Infants are more susceptible to serious consequences of diarrhea. Good food and water hygiene is crucial, and, whenever possible, breastfeeding is best.
- Appropriate pediatric medical care can be limited or nonexistent in some geographical regions.

Questions

- What specific insect bite avoidance behaviors should parents be informed of by the nurse?
- Which infant immunizations need to be completed before traveling overseas?
- What information about availability of health care needs to be explored before traveling?

SUMMARY

Society is changing, as are people's needs and ideas. Families today want more information and knowledge, and they demand that health care professionals be more responsive to their needs. Their demand has been a catalyst for the nurse's expanded health care role and responsibility for health promotion.

Health-promotion and disease-prevention practices that are applicable during infancy can be used in the nurse's expanded role. A four-pronged approach is stressed:

- Giving anticipatory guidance to the family unit as the infant grows and develops
- Teaching and counseling to ensure the infant's optimal development
- Being a family advocate to ensure the safety and development of the family unit
- Screening to identify infants at risk of developing a condition via history gathering, physical exam, observation of parent-child interaction, and laboratory testing

Anticipating potential health problems during infancy and effectively intervening to avert these problems are nursing processes that promote health. Early detection and reduction of risk factors avoid many health problems, such as abuse. By anticipating problems and helping families to avoid them, the nurse promotes health maintenance.

Using the infant's normal growth and development, psychosocial tasks, common health problems, and health maintenance strategies, the nurse makes an assessment of the infant, the family, and the infant's developmental status to provide anticipatory guidance.

By teaching (Box 17-24: Hot Topics), an essential component of the nursing process, the nurse transmits knowledge to families to ensure continuity of care and long-term health maintenance. By counseling, the nurse listens to the identified problem, helps the family to recognize the real issues, and allows the family to make its own decisions regarding health care.

Because the infant is in no position to advocate effectively, the nurse assumes this role. The ultimate goal of nursing intervention in maintaining the infant's health is future self-care. As the infant grows and matures, well-established family health maintenance habits can only enhance the lives of healthy future generations. The nurse is challenged to join this effort of investment in the future.

REFERENCES

American Academy of Pediatrics (AAP). (2011a). *Breastfeeding: Best for baby and mother.* [Online] Retrieved from www.aap.org/breastfeeding/files/pdf/Winter2011Newsletter.pdf.

American Academy of Pediatrics (AAP). (2011b). *Switching to solid foods.* [Online] Retrieved from www.healthychildren.org/english/ages-stages/baby/feeding-nutrition/pages/Switching-To-Solid-Foods.aspx.

American Academy of Pediatrics (AAP). (2011c). *Child abuse and neglect.* [Online] Retrieved from www.aap.org/sections/childabuseneglect/.

American Academy of Pediatrics (AAP). (2011d). *AAP updates recommendation on car seats.* [Online] Retrieved from www.aap.org/advocacy/releases/carseat2011.htm.

American Academy of Pediatrics (AAP). (2011e). *Choosing a child care center.* [Online] Retrieved from www.healthychildren.org/English/family-life/work-play/pages/Choosing-a-Childcare-Center.aspx?

American Heart Association (AHA). (2011). *American Heart Association guidelines for cardiopulmonary resuscitation and emergency cardiovascular care of pediatric and neonatal patients: Pediatric basic life support.* [Online] Retrieved from www.heart.org.

American Public Health Association (APHA). (2011). *National Public Health Week calls attention to injury prevention.* [Online] Retrieved from www.jhsph.edu/publichealthnews/articles/2011/public_health_week_2011.html.

Andrews, M. M., & Boyle, J. S. (2011). *Transcultural concepts in nursing care* (6th ed.). Philadelphia: Lippincott Williams & Wilkins.

Beijers, R., Jansen, J., Riksen-Walraven, M., & de Weerth, C. (2011). Nonparental care and infant health: Do number of hours and number of concurrent arrangements matter? *Early Human Development, 87*(1), 9–15.

Berk, L. E. (2012). *Infants and children: Prenatal through middle childhood* (7th ed.). Boston: Allyn & Bacon/Longman Publishers.

Bowman, S., Aitken, M., Maham, S., & Sharar, S. (2011). Trends in hospitalizations associated with pediatric burns. *Injury Prevention: Journal of the International Society for Child and Adolescent Injury Prevention, 17*(3), 166–170.

Brazelton, T. B., & Sparrow, J. A. (2006). *Touchpoints: Your child's emotional and behavioral development* (2nd ed.). Cambridge, MA: Perseus/Da Capo Press.

Brown, A., Raynor, P., & Lee, M. (2011). Healthcare professionals' and mothers' perceptions of factors that influence decisions to breastfeed or formula feed infants: A comparative study. *Journal of Advanced Nursing, 67*(9), 1993–2003.

Centers for Disease Control and Prevention (CDC). (2011a). *Growth charts.* [Online] Retrieved from www.cdc.gov/growthcharts/.

Centers for Disease Control and Prevention (CDC). (2011b). *Sickle cell trait.* [Online] Retrieved from www.cdc.gov/ncbddd/sicklecell/traits.html.

Centers for Disease Control and Prevention (CDC). (2011c). *Hemophilia.* [Online] Retrieved from www.cdc.gov/Features/HemophiliaDay/.

Centers for Disease Control and Prevention (CDC). (2011d). *Recommended immunization schedules for persons aged 0-18 years—United States, 2011.* Retrieved from www.cdc.gov/vaccines/recs/schedules/child-schedule.htm#hcp.

Clark, M. J. (2009). *Community health nursing: Advocacy for population health* (5th ed.). Upper Saddle River, NJ: Pearson Prentice Hall.

Clem, A. (2011). Fundamentals of vaccine immunology. *Journal of Global Infectious Diseases, 3*(1), 73–78.

Coch, D., Dawson, G., & Fischer, K. W. (2010). *Human behavior, learning, and the developing brain: Typical development.* New York: Guilford Publications.

Cohen, D. (2012). *How the child's mind develops* (2nd ed.). Oxford, UK: Taylor & Francis.

Crandell, T., Crandell, C., & Zanden, J. V. (2011). *Human development* (10th ed.). Boston, MA: McGraw-Hill.

DeBruyne, L., Whitney, E. N., & Pinna, K. (2012). *Nutrition and diet therapy* (8th ed.). Belmont, CA: Wadsworth Publishers.

Denton, J., Newton, A., & Vandeven, A. (2011). Update on child maltreatment: Toward refining the evidence base. *Current Opinion in Pediatrics, 23*(2), 240–248.

Dorland, W. A.N. (2012). *Dorland's illustrated medical dictionary* (32nd ed.). Philadelphia: Elsevier Health Sciences.

Dudek, S. G. (2010). *Nutritional essentials for nursing practice* (6th ed.). Philadelphia: Lippincott Williams & Wilkins.

Eron, N. B., Dygert, K. M., Squillace, C., Webster, N. J., Andrianos, A., Crockett, E. G., et al. (2011). The physician's role in reducing SIDS. *Health Promotion Practice, 12*(3), 370–378. doi:10.1177/1524839909341033.

Gardner, S. L., Carter, B. S., Enzman-Hines, M., & Hernandez, J. A. (2011). *Merenstein & Gardner's handbook of neonatal intensive care* (7th ed.). St. Louis: Mosby Elsevier.

Giger, J. N., & Davidhizar, R. E. (2012). *Transcultural nursing: Assessment and intervention* (6th ed.). St. Louis: Mosby Elsevier.

Gillard, A. (2012). *Homelessness.* Belmont, CA: Gale Cengage Learning.

Glasco, D. (2011). *Children in poverty.* Richmond, VA: Kindom Publishing Group.

Gutierrez, J., Negrón, J., & García-Fragoso, L. (2011). Parental practices for prevention of home poisoning in children 1-6 years of age. *Journal of Community Health, 36*(5), 845–848.

Harkness, G. A., & DeMarco, R. (2011). *Community health and public health nursing: Evidence for practice.* Philadelphia: Lippincott Williams & Wilkins.

Hasselkus, A. (2011). Health communication: Implications for diverse populations. *Perspectives on Communication Disorders & Sciences in Culturally & Linguistically Diverse (CLD) Populations, 18*(1), 12–19.

Hawkins, S. (2010). The midwife's role in facilitating maternal-infant bonding and attachment. *MIDIRS Midwifery Digest, 20*(3), 355–360.

Henslow, G. (2011). *Poisonous plants in field and garden.* Charleston, SC: Nabu Press.

Hockenberry, M. J., & Wilson, D. (2010). *Wong's nursing care of infants and children* (9th ed.). St. Louis: Mosby.

Iannelli, V. (2011). *Kids in hot cars alert.* [Online] Retrieved from http://pediatrics.about.com/od/safety/a/05_hot_cars.htm.

Institute of Medicine (IOM). (2011). *Dietary supplement fact sheet: Vitamin D.* [Online] Retrieved from http://ods.od.nih.gov/factsheets/vitamind.

Irving, L. (2011). Preventing unintentional injuries in children and young people under 15. *Community Practitioner: The Journal of the Community Practitioners' & Health Visitors' Association, 84*(3), 36–38.

Jaffe, A. (2011). Failure to thrive: Current clinical concepts. *Pediatrics in Review/American Academy of Pediatrics,* 100–107.

Jain, K., Mahajan, R., Shevkani, M., & Kumar, P. (2011). Early infant diagnosis: A new tool of HIV diagnosis in children. *Indian Journal of Community Medicine, 36*(2), 139–142.

Jarvis, C. (2012). *Physical examination and health assessment* (6th ed.). St. Louis: Elsevier.

Jeena, P., Reichert, K., Adhikari, M., Popat, M., Carlin, J., Weber, M., et al. (2011). Clinical manifestations and outcome in HIV-infected young infants presenting with acute illness in Durban, South Africa. *Annals of Tropical Pediatrics, 31*(1), 15–26.

Kail, R. V., & Cavanaugh, J. C. (2012). *Human development: A life-span view* (6th ed.). Florence, KY: Cengage Learning.

Klaus, M. H., Kennell, J. H., & Klaus, P. H. (2000). *Bonding: Building the foundations of secure attachment and independence.* New York: Perseus Book Group.

Kliegman, R. M., Stanton, B., St. Geme, J., Schor, N., & Behrman, R. E. (2011). *Nelson textbook of pediatrics* (19th ed.). St. Louis: Elsevier.

Krenzelok, E. P., & Mrvos, R. (2011). Friends and foes in the plant world: A profile of plant ingestions and fatalities. *Clinical Toxicology (15563650), 49*(3), 142–149.

Kuo, A., Inkelas, M., Slusser, W., Maidenberg, M., & Halfon, N. (2011). Introduction of solid food to young infants. *Maternal and Child Health Journal, 15*(8), 1185–1194.

Lareau, A. (2011). *Unequal childhood: Class, race and family life* (2nd ed.). Berkley, CA: University of California Press.

Lea, D., Skirton, H., Read, C. Y., & Williams, J. K. (2011). Implications for educating the next generation of nurses on genetics and genomics in the 21st century. *Journal of Nursing Scholarship, 43*(1), 3–12.

Lewis, M. (2011). The origins and uses of self-awareness or the mental representation of me. *Consciousness and Cognition, 20*(1), 120–129.

Lewis, R. (2011). *Human genetics: Concepts and applications* (10th ed.). Boston: McGraw-Hill.

McGee, H., Malley, R., Muller, H., & Woods, G. (2011). Neonatal exposure to UVR alters skin immune system development, and suppresses immunity in adulthood. *Immunology & Cell Biology, 89*(7), 767–776. doi:10.1038/icb.2010.170.

McGrath, J. (2011). Neonatal nurses: What about their grief and loss? *Journal of Perinatal & Neonatal Nursing, 25*(1), 8–9.

Meyerhoff, M. (2010). *A parent's guide to the mind of the infant and toddler.* Tallahassee, FL: William Gladden Foundation Press.

Miller, L. C., Johnson, A., Duggan, L., & Behm, M. (2011). Consequences of the "Back to Sleep" program in infants. *Journal of Pediatric Nursing, 26*(4), 364–368.

National Cancer Institute (NCI). (2011). *Childhood cancers.* [Online] Retrieved from www.cancer.gov/cancertopics/factsheet/Sites-Types/childhood.

National Health Care for the Homeless Council [NHCHC]. (2011). *Children, Youth and Homlessness.* Retrieved from http://www.nhchc.org/wp-content/uploads/2011/09/Children2011.pdf.

National Institute of Environmental Health Sciences (NIEHS). (2011a). *Lead.* [Online] Retrieved from www.niehs.nih.gov/health/topics/agents/lead/.

National Institute of Environmental Health Sciences (NIEHS). (2011b). *Asthma.* [Online] Retrieved from www.niehs.nih.gov/health/topics/conditions/asthma/.

National Institute of Environmental Health Sciences (NIEHS). (2011c). *Air pollution and respiratory disease.* [Online] Retrieved from www.niehs.nih.gov/health/impacts/respiratory/.

Ntouva, A. A., Rogers, I. I., MacAdam, A. A., & Emmett, P. P. (2011). Weaning practices and iron status of exclusively breast fed infants. *Journal of Human Nutrition & Dietetics, 24*(3), 297–298.

Null, J. (2011). *Hyperthermia deaths of children in vehicles.* [Online] Retrieved from http://ggweather.com/heat/.

Olson, D. H., DeFrain, J. D., & Skogrand, L. (2011). *Marriages and families: Intimacy, diversity and strengths* (7th ed.). Boston: McGraw-Hill.

Oppenheim, D., & Goldsmith, D. E. (2011). *Attachment theory in clinical work with children: Bridging the gap between research and practice.* New York: Guilford Publications.

Parsons, H., George, M., & Innis, S. (2011). Growth assessment in clinical practice: Whose growth curve? *Current Gastroenterology Reports, 13*(3), 286–292.

Petersen, D. D. (2011). Common plant toxicology: A comparison of national and Southwest Ohio data trends on plant poisonings in the 21st century. *Toxicology & Applied Pharmacology, 254*(2), 148–153.

Pillitteri, A. (2010). *Maternal and child health nursing: Care of the childbearing and childrearing family* (6th ed.). Philadelphia: Lippincott Williams & Wilkins.

Polan, E., & Taylor, D. (2010). *Journey across the lifespan: Human development and health promotion* (4th ed.). Philadelphia: F.A. Davis.

Puckett, M. B., & Black, J. K. (2010). *Understanding infant development.* St. Paul, MN: Redleaf Press.

Rapley, G. (2011). Baby-led weaning: Transitioning to solid foods at the baby's own pace. *Community Practitioner, 84*(6), 20–23.

Read, J. S., & Newell, M. (2011). Efficacy and safety of cesarean delivery for prevention of mother-to-child transmission of HIV-1. *Cochrane Database of Systematic Reviews* CD005479. doi: CD005479 10.1002/14651858.

Rochat, P. (2011). The self as phenotype. *Consciousness and cognition, 20*(1), 109–119.

Samour, P. Q., & King, K. (2012). *Pediatric nutrition* (4th ed.). Sudbury, MA: Jones & Bartlett Learning.

Schwartz, M. A., & Scott, B. M. (2011). *Marriages and families: Diversity and change* (6th ed.). Paramus, NJ: Pearson.

Sheth, K. (2012). Tay-Sachs disease. *PubMed Health.* [Online] Available at www.ncbi.nlm.nih.gov/pubmedhealth/PMH0002390/.

Siegfried, N., van der Merwe, L., Brocklehurst, P., & Sint, T. T. (2011a). Antiretrovirals for reducing the risk of mother-to-child transmission of HIV infection. *Cochrane Database of Systematic Reviews 7*: CD003510. doi: 10.1002/14651858. CD003510.pub3.

Siegfried, N., Muller, M., Deeks, J. J., & Volmink, J. (2011b). Male circumcision for prevention of heterosexual acquisition of HIV in men. *Cochrane Database of Systematic Reviews 2011,* (2): CD003362. doi: 10.1002/14651858.CD003362.pub2.

Smithson, J., Garside, R., & Pearson, M. (2011). Barriers to, and facilitators of, the prevention of unintentional injury in children in the home: A systematic review and synthesis of qualitative research. *Injury Prevention: Journal of the International Society for Child and Adolescent Injury Prevention, 17*(2), 119–126.

St. James-Roberts, I. (2012). *The origins, prevention and treatment of infant crying and sleeping problems: An evidence-based guide to preventing and managing problems for healthcare professionals and families they support.* Oxford, UK: Taylor & Francis.

Stanhope, M., & Lancaster, J. (2012). *Public health nursing: Population-centered health care in the community* (8th ed.). St. Louis: Mosby.

Swota, A., & Hester, D. (2011). Ethics for the pediatrician: Providing culturally effective health care. *Pediatrics in Review, 32*(3), 39–43.

Thompson, J., & Manore, M. (2012). *Nutrition: An applied approach* (3rd ed.). San Francisco, CA: Benjamin Cummings.

Underwood, M. K., & Rosen, L. H. (2011). *Social development: Relationships in infancy, childhood, and adolescence.* New York: The Guilford Press.

U.S. Census Bureau. (2010). *Characteristics of the population below the poverty level.* Washington, DC: U.S. Government Printing Office.

U.S. Department of Health and Human Services (USDHHS). (2006). *Healthy People 2010 midcourse review.* Washington, DC: U.S. Government Printing Office.

U.S. Department of Health and Human Services (USDHHS). (2010). *Healthy People 2020.* [Online] Retrieved from www.healthypeople.gov/2020/topicsobjectives2020/objectiveslist.aspx?topicId=26.

Van Allen, K., & Sterling, Y. M. (2011). Pediatric nurses address children and the economy: Part 1. The impact of poverty on children and families. *Journal of Pediatric Nursing, 26*(4), 369–372.

Wedeen, R. P. (2011). Lead poisoning: The evolving definition. *International Journal of Occupational & Environmental Medicine, 2*(1), 1–3.

Whitehead, D. (2011). Before the cradle and beyond the grave: A lifespan/settings-based framework for health promotion. *Journal of Clinical Nursing, 20*(15/16), 2183–2194.

Wiebe, A., & Young, B. (2011). Parent perspectives from a neonatal intensive care unit: A missing piece of the culturally congruent care puzzle. *Journal of Transcultural Nursing, 22*(1), 77–82. doi: 10.1177/1043659609360850.

Wilkerson, R., Northington, L., & Fisher, W. (2011). Ingestion of toxic substances by infants and children. *Critical Care Nurse, 25*(4), 35–44.

Woods, D. (2011). *Primary newborn care.* Cape Town, South Africa: EBW Healthcare.

World Health Organization (WHO). (2011). Evaluation of certain food additive and contaminants. *World Health Organization Technical Report Series* (960), 1.

World Health Organization (WHO) and Joint United Nations Program on HIV/AIDS (UNAIDS). (2011). *New data on male circumcision and HIV prevention: Policy and programme implications.* Retrieved from http://data.unaids.org/publReport/2007/mc_recommendations_en.pdf.

Yikilkan, H., Ünalan, P., Cakir, E., Ersu, R., Cifcili, S., Akman, M., et al. (2011). Sudden infant death syndrome: How much mothers and health professionals know. *Pediatrics International, 53*(1), 24–28. doi: 10.1111/j.1442-200X.2010.03202.x.

Yu, M., Tsunoda, H., & Tsunoda, M. (2011). *Environmental toxicology: Biological and health effects of pollutants* (3rd ed.). London, England: CRC Press.

18

Toddler

Tawna Cooksey-James, Ali Salman, and Yi-Hui Lee

evolve WEBSITE

http://evolve.elsevier.com/Edelman/
- Study Questions
- Glossary

OBJECTIVES

After completing this chapter, the reader will be able to:
- Describe the physical growth, developmental, and maturational changes that occur during the toddler period.
- List the recommended health-promotion and disease-prevention visits for the toddler with the appropriate topics for anticipatory guidance for their parents.
- Compare and contrast developmentally appropriate approaches to toddlers at different ages.
- Analyze the factors that contribute to the heightened vulnerability of toddlers to injury and abuse.
- Develop a plan to reach *Healthy People 2020* target objectives specific for toddlers.

KEY TERMS

Amblyopia	Masturbation	Strabismus
Autism spectrum disorders	Night terrors	Styes
Autonomy	Object permanence	Temperament
CDC growth charts	Otitis media	Toilet training
Child abuse	Parallel play	Visual-reinforcement audiometry
Conditioned-play audiometry	Preoperational stage	World Health Organization (WHO)
Doubt	Rituals	growth charts
Egocentrism	Sensorimotor stage	
Lumbar lordosis	Shame	

❓ THINK ABOUT IT

Refraining the Terrible Two's

A young mother tells the nurse that she is convinced her 22-month-old child, who used to be the sweetest child around, has entered what must be the terrible two's. She reports that her child's favorite words include "mine" and "no," with "no" being the response to every request the mother makes. In addition, the child is becoming increasingly stubborn and just threw her first public temper tantrum. The mother says that she is tired of saying and hearing "no" and turns to the nurse for help.

- How does the nurse explain the relationship between the child's stage of psychosocial development and meaning behind the child's behaviors?
- What suggestions can the nurse give to the mother to respond sensitively to her child's evolving need for independence while balancing her own need to provide for and protect her child?

Having spent their first year of life getting to know and trust their parents and other child care providers and their immediate environments, toddlers' increasing mobility now allows them to begin to expand their worlds, bringing excitement and challenges to both themselves and their parents. Toddlers are ready to develop a sense of self and separate from their parents, and understanding and respecting this evolving independence is a common parental challenge. Their behaviors can be frustrating, but the toddlers' delight in their own emerging competence and achievements can bring a sense of joy and accomplishment to everyone around them (Warren et al., 2008).

Nurses explain to parents and other primary care providers the many physical and developmental changes that occur in toddlers and describe how these changes contribute to their vulnerability to injury and overall health as well as to the health and vulnerability of the family unit. Unfortunately, the recommended schedule for health-promotion and disease-prevention visits for this age group advocates fewer contacts than during infancy. Parents may begin to fall into a pattern of illness care, missing the continued opportunity to receive anticipatory guidance and health-promotion information until they are required by preschool or school prerequisites. The nurse plays an integral role in encouraging health-promotion efforts and behaviors (Hagan et al., 2008; Hockenberry & Wilson, 2011).

BIOLOGY AND GENETICS

The toddler period begins at 12 to 18 months and extends to 3 years of age. The overall growth rate slows significantly, and the increasingly active toddler begins the process of shedding baby fat and straightening his or her posture. Toddlers have a protuberant abdomen, accentuated by a lumbar lordosis, and a characteristic gait, in which their feet are planted wide apart and appear flat because of an extra fat pad in the instep for stability.

A slow, steady growth in height of 2 to 4 inches per year and in weight of 4 to 6 pounds per year occurs during toddlerhood and remains steady until puberty. Birth weight usually quadruples by 2½ years of age, and the toddler's height at age 2 years is approximately 50% of the final adult height (Hockenberry & Wilson, 2011). Use growth charts to determine the parameters within which an individual toddler's growth lies for head circumference, height, and weight. The Centers for Disease Control and Prevention (CDC) recommends that health care providers use the 2006 World Health Organization (WHO) growth charts to monitor growth for infants and children up to 2 years of age in the United States, and then use the 2000 revised CDC growth charts for U.S. children ages 2 to 20 years (CDC, 2010b; Grummer-Strawn et al., 2010). The toddler's height may be measured in a recumbent position for length, as in infancy, or in a standing position for stature. When using the CDC growth charts for toddler's ages 2 years and older, measure the height in a standing position to obtain the toddler's stature and then use the appropriate chart based on stature.

The nurse continues to measure head circumference throughout the toddler period. The anterior fontanel usually closes by 18 months, the skull begins to thicken, and by 24 months it is 80% of its adult size (Hockenberry & Wilson, 2011).

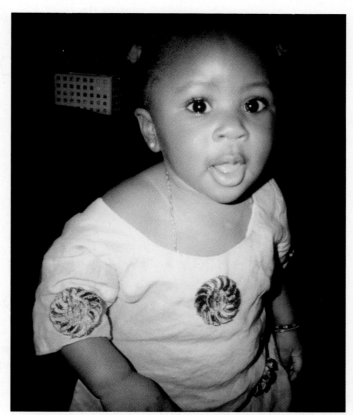

FIGURE 18-1 Toddler demonstrates mouth breathing.

The kidneys are well differentiated by the toddler years, and specific gravity and other urine findings are similar to those of adults. The daily excretion of urine for the 2-year-old child is 500 to 600 mL, increasing to 750 mL for the 3 year old. Toddlers empty their bladders less frequently than infants and begin to develop voluntary control of urination. However, full bladder control comes later and begins after 18 to 24 months when the toddler first becomes physiologically able to control the bladder.

The toddler's gastrointestinal tract also reaches functional maturity, although it continues to grow into adulthood. The toddler tends to need meals and snacks more frequently than an older child or adult. Most toddlers develop sufficient voluntary control of internal and external anal sphincters to accomplish successful bowel training. Bowel control usually occurs before urinary control.

Lung capacity continues to increase as the toddler grows, and the respiratory rate decreases from a mean of 30 breaths per minute at 1 year of age to 25 breaths per minute at 3 years. The diameter of the toddler's upper respiratory tract is small when compared with that of an older child or adult and may lead to mouth breathing when the nose is obstructed with mucus (Figure 18-1). This small diameter, coupled with the toddler's exploratory nature and lack of judgment in deciding what to place in the mouth, can result in accidental airway obstruction, which demands emergency action.

The proximal anatomy of the ear, eustachian tube, and nasal pharynx continue to resemble those of the infant more closely than those of the adult, continuing the risk for otitis media.

Maxillary (upper) teeth

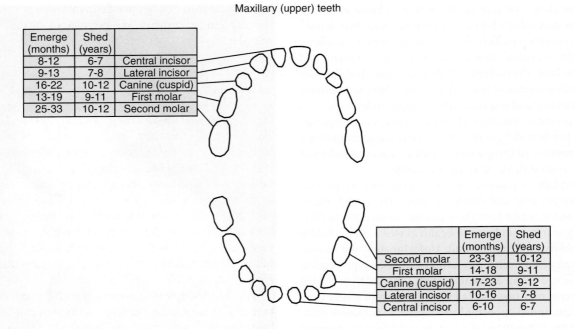

Emerge (months)	Shed (years)	
8-12	6-7	Central incisor
9-13	7-8	Lateral incisor
16-22	10-12	Canine (cuspid)
13-19	9-11	First molar
25-33	10-12	Second molar

	Emerge (months)	Shed (years)
Second molar	23-31	10-12
First molar	14-18	9-11
Canine (cuspid)	17-23	9-12
Lateral incisor	10-16	7-8
Central incisor	6-10	6-7

Mandibular (lower) teeth

FIGURE 18-2 Eruption (and shedding) of primary teeth.

The tonsils and adenoids remain proportionately large during the toddler years (Seidel et al., 2011).

With the exception of reproductive functions, most endocrine organs become functionally mature during the toddler and preschool years, although function continues at a minimum. The production of glucagon and insulin can be limited or labile, producing variations in blood glucose levels throughout early childhood. The production of cortisol, aldosterone, and deoxycorticosterone by the adrenal cortex remains somewhat limited, but they appear to function effectively in protecting the young child from the hazards of fluid and electrolyte imbalance well-known in infancy. Secretion of epinephrine and norepinephrine from the adrenal medulla increases sufficiently to perform homeostatic functions of the autonomic nervous system and to mediate certain aspects of increased emotional components of behavior. Regulation of growth during early childhood remains one of the most important functions of the endocrine system.

Changes in the circulatory system include a decrease in heart rate, an increase in blood pressure, and a change in vascular resistance in response to growth in the size of various blood vessel lumens. The toddler's heart rate ranges from 80 to 120 beats per minute and the mean blood pressure is 90/56 mm Hg. Getting the toddler to sit still for a blood pressure reading can be difficult, but it is worth the effort to obtain several baseline readings for future reference.

The capillary beds gradually increase their capacity to respond to heat and cold in the environment, providing the toddler with more effective thermoregulation. Toddlers can also begin to take voluntary measures to relieve the discomfort of heat or cold. For example, the older toddler can put on clothing or move to warmer or cooler areas, assisting physiological efforts to maintain a constant internal thermal environment.

The immune response continues to mature. As toddlers expand their worlds through play groups and day care centers, exposure to new and different organisms is greatly increased. They may experience a period during which they appear to succumb to many minor respiratory tract and gastrointestinal tract infections. As immunity begins to develop against the organisms in their new environments, their resistance similarly increases.

Passive immunity to communicable disease acquired through transfer of maternal antibodies during fetal life has disappeared, and active immunity through the initial immunization series is usually completed by the age of 18 months. The next scheduled immunizations do not occur until age 4 to 6 years, before entering kindergarten. If a toddler is behind in the initial immunization series, a separate schedule is available that gives catch-up schedules and minimal intervals between doses (CDC, 2011). For updated CDC immunization schedules refer to the CDC website at www.cdc.gov/vaccines/schedules/.

All 20 primary or deciduous teeth erupt by the end of toddlerhood (Figure 18-2). Timing of these eruptions can vary widely, but a variation in the sequence alerts the nurse to inquire about early trauma to the mouth or familial traits for nonsequential tooth eruption. Other important aspects of dental care at this age are included in health teaching and are listed in Box 18-1.

A mature swallowing pattern, using the tongue rather than the cheeks, has not yet developed, and toddlers continue to be at risk for choking. Toddlers who are mouth, rather than nose, breathers because of ongoing respiratory illness or allergies may have an underdeveloped palatal arch. With normal breathing, the tongue rests on and naturally widens the palate; however, when the child is forced to breathe through the mouth, the tongue rests in the lower jaw, not on the palate. This resultant narrowing of the palatal arch predisposes these toddlers for dental crowding when the permanent teeth erupt.

BOX 18-1   NURSING INTERVENTIONS TO PROMOTE DENTAL HEALTH CARE FOR TODDLERS

Brushing

- When teeth are present, begin to use a soft-bristled brush. The finger-wrapped gauze method used during infancy is no longer adequate because teeth are too close together to reach all tooth surfaces.
- Introduce only a moist toothbrush at first. After the toddler has accepted the toothbrush, begin using toothpaste. A pea-size amount is adequate. If the child does not like the taste of the toothpaste, use plain water.
- Toothpaste should contain supplemental fluoride if not in water supply.
- Toddlers do not have the motor coordination to brush their own teeth. They may enjoy imitating parents and put the toothbrush in their mouths, but an adult should be responsible for the actual brushing.
- Brush daily; for many toddlers, this practice becomes part of the bedtime routine. When the child appears too tired to cooperate in the evening, the parent should choose some other time of day when this important task will not be so difficult.

Foods

- Limit foods high in sugar because they contribute to dental caries.
- When the young toddler still drinks from a bottle, only plain water should be given. Milk and juices should be offered by cup. If milk or juice is given in a bottle, it should never be done at naptime or bedtime.

Visits to the Dentist

- The first visit to the dentist should occur during the toddler years. Many dentists suggest an introduction-orientation, inspection-consultation type of visit when the child is approximately 18 to 24 months of age. This type of visit provides an early, enjoyable introduction to professional dental health promotion and care.
- Once molars are present, arrangements with the dentist need to be done to have dental sealants.

U.S. Preventive Services Task Force. (July 2010). Retrieved from www.uspreventiveservicestaskforce.org.

An increase in the size and strength of muscle fibers continues. During this period, as during infancy, the use of muscle tissues is the primary stimulus for increased size and strength for gross and later fine motor movement. Myelination of the corticospinal tract is functionally sufficient to support most movement, but achievement of full control does not occur until much later in life. Throughout early childhood, voluntary motor movement is often accompanied by involuntary movements on the opposite side of the body. This mirroring of action is more pronounced in children who suffer some damage to the central nervous system, but the mechanisms by which this occurs are unknown. The toddler generally does not show complete dominance of one side of the body and may still switch hands when eating, throwing a ball, or engaging in other-handed activities.

Genetics are passed from each parent to their child and great similarities may show between the generations. Most genetic syndromes and disease entities are diagnosed either during the prenatal period or during infancy. However, some genetic syndromes and diseases are not detected until the toddler years or even later. The most common initial sign is a change in growth pattern or developmental delays. Developmental delays are often not diagnosed during infancy because the subtle language, motor, or cognitive deficiencies do not interfere with the expected performance and behavior of the infant as they do with the more actively developing toddler.

GORDON'S FUNCTIONAL HEALTH PATTERNS

Health Perception–Health Management Pattern

Toddlers may eventually learn that being sick means feeling bad or having to stay in bed, but they have little, if any, understanding of the meaning of health. They may perform requested health-promotion activities, such as brushing teeth, but they may simply brush their teeth as part of their bedtime ritual and not because they know this activity will prevent dental caries. Toddlers depend on their parents for health management, and their overall health will be greatly influenced by their parents' health perceptions and health management priorities (Box 18-2: *Healthy People 2020*).

Toddlers identify with parents, caregivers, and other important role models, internalizing a wide range of lifestyle attributes. Parents' and caregivers' health perceptions and health behaviors should model the perceptions and behaviors desired for health promotion. Toddlers whose parents eat a variety of foods are more likely to try new foods. Such modeling increases the chances that good practices will be retained throughout the toddler's life. The nurse's task is to help parents strengthen their confidence and self-esteem as parents and provide them with the information needed to anticipate and meet the developmental needs of their toddler as they develop as a family.

Nutritional-Metabolic Pattern

The American Academy of Pediatrics (AAP, 2012) recommends breastfeeding for 1 year or longer as preferred between a mother and a child. Adequate iron intake must be ensured as the toddler changes from breast milk or iron-fortified formula and cereal to whole cow's milk, which is low in iron. Whole cow's milk also interferes with the absorption of iron from other food sources. A toddler who continues to ingest whole milk from a bottle tends to drink up to 32 ounces per day. This practice blunts the child's appetite at mealtimes and can lead to an exclusion of foods that contain iron in the diet (American Academy of Pediatrics, Healthy Children, 2012a), requiring iron from fortified foods or supplements. The use of a bottle with milk or juice, especially at bedtime, has also been associated with dental caries (baby bottle tooth decay) because of the high sugar content. If parents want to give a bottle at bedtime, it should contain only water.

Fruit juice and other drinks are often overconsumed because they taste good, because they are conveniently packaged and easily carried around by the toddler, and because they are viewed as nutritious. However, the American Academy of Pediatrics, Healthy Children (2012b) cautions parents to use only 100% juice that is pasteurized, that children 1 to 6 years of age have two fruit servings each day, only one of which should be juice, and that fresh fruit should be encouraged. They further state that 4 to 6 ounces (oz) (120 to 180 mL) of fruit juice equals one fruit serving. Fruit juice has no nutritional advantage over

❤ BOX 18-2   **HEALTHY PEOPLE 2020**

Selected Health-Promotion and Disease-Prevention Objectives for Toddlers

- Increase age-appropriate vehicle restraint system use in children ages 1 to 3 years to 79% from baseline of 72% for children ages 1 to 3 years restrained in front-facing child safety seats in 2008.
- Reduce unintentional injury and death among children ages 1 to 4 years from 2000 to 2005 levels, especially the three leading causes of death/100,000 for this age group: (1) drowning-related deaths of 27%, (2) pedestrian-related deaths of 15%, and (3) fire- and burn-related deaths of 14%.
- Increase the proportion of young children screened for an autism spectrum disorder (ASD) and other developmental delays by 24 months of age from 2007 baseline level of 19.5% of children ages 10 to 36 months to 21.5%.
- Reduce iron deficiency among young children ages 1 to 2 years in 2005 to 2008 from 15.9% to 14.3%, and children ages 3 to 4 years in 2005 to 2008 from 5.3% to 4.3%.
- Eliminate elevated blood lead levels in children ages 1 to 5 years (baseline was 0.9% of children ages 1 to 5 years had 1.5 mcg/dL average blood lead levels in 2005 to 2008).
- Reduce exposure to selected environmental toxins as measured by blood and urine concentrations of the substances or their metabolites in children ages 1 year and older in 2003 to 2004, especially reduce (1) cadmium, (2) mercury, and (3) lead levels.

- Reduce the number of antibiotics prescribed for young children. Reduce the number of courses of antibiotics for ear infections for young children under age 5 years; especially reduce antibiotics prescribed for ear infections in 2007 from 47% to 35%.
- Achieve and maintain effective vaccination coverage levels for universally recommended vaccines among young children ages 19 to 35 months from 2008 levels, especially (1) 4 doses of DTaP from 85% to 90%; (2) 3 doses of Hib from 57% to 90%; (3) 4 doses of pneumococcal conjugate vaccine (PCV) from 80% to 90%; (4) 2 doses of hepatitis A vaccine from 40% to 60%; (5) a birth dose of hepatitis B vaccine from 2006 and 2008 levels from 51% to 85%; and (6) 2 or more doses of rotavirus vaccine from 2009 level from 38% to 80%.
- Increase the proportion of children ages 19 to 35 months in 2008 who receive the recommended doses of DTaP, polio, MMR, Hib, hepatitis B, varicella, and PCV vaccines from 68% to 80%.
- Reduce invasive pneumococcal infections among children under 5 years of age in 2008: (1) new invasive pneumococcal infections (from 20.3 to 12 cases/100,000), and (2) invasive penicillin-resistant pneumococcal infections (from 4.3 to 3 cases/100,000).

From *Healthy People 2020: Midcourse review.* (2010). Office of Disease Prevention & Health Promotion (ODPHP) of the Office of Public Health, U.S. Department of Health and Human Services. Retrieved from http://odphp.osophs.dhhs.gov/pubs/; Borse, N. N., Gilchrist, J., Dellinger, A. M., Rudd, R. A., Ballesteros, M. F., & Sleet, D. A. (2008). *CDC Childhood Injury Report: Patterns of unintentional injuries among 0 to 19 year olds in the United States, 2000–2006.* Atlanta, GA: National Center for Injury Prevention and Control, Centers for Disease Control and Prevention. Retrieved from www.cdc.gov/safechild/images/CDC-childhoodinjury.pdf.

whole fruit and in fact lacks the fiber contained in whole fruit (AAP, Healthy Children, 2012c).

A decrease in the growth rate during toddlerhood results in a decrease in appetite. Parents need to be reminded of this if they begin to worry about their toddler's nutritional intake. Keeping a daily record over a 3- to 5-day period presents a better picture of a child's intake and is a useful teaching tool for this age group.

Toddlers often use mealtime as an occasion to assert individuality and control as well as exploration (Figure 18-3). Families will vary in their expectations of eating behavior and mealtime routines. The nurse's best guide for parents of toddlers is to remind them that parents are in charge of what food is offered, when it is offered, and where (Box 18-3: Research for Evidence-Based Practice). Box 18-4 lists some nursing interventions to promote healthy eating in toddlers. However, it is up to the toddler to decide the amount to actually eat. Periodically, a toddler may even refuse a meal altogether. Parents need to be encouraged to offer healthy, age-appropriate food choices. Toddlers will eat them, as long as they do not fill up on empty calories from juice and high-carbohydrate snacks that are often given to children "so they eat something." Further, parents should not focus too much attention on food intake or punish children for refusing food. Toddlers may learn how easily parents can be controlled by their behavior around food intake and may then continue the behavior for the attention alone.

Maintaining a record of food intake over time, the nurse can demonstrate the adequacy of the nutrients that the toddler is already receiving during mealtimes and help parents develop a plan to offer more of the essential foods during meals (Holt et al., 2011). Children with inadequate nutrition are predisposed to impaired immune systems, leading to infections and delayed healing and recovery. They also are predisposed to depletion of muscle mass, leading to diminished functional capacity. In addition, although inadequately understood, nutrients and neurotropic factors interact with one another for brain and behavioral development (More, 2008; Rosales & Zeisel, 2008).

The family who has a vegetarian or vegan diet may need some assistance from the nurse or a dietitian. Vegetarian and vegan diets vary widely, so it is important to assess precisely the foods that are eaten, the foods that have been eliminated from the diet, and the supplements that are used.

Elimination Pattern

Toilet training is often a major parental concern during toddlerhood. The nurse anticipates this developmental stressor and initiates discussion with the parents to determine their understanding of the child's signs of developmental readiness and their attitude and commitment to establishing a toileting pattern for their toddler. Emotional and physiological readiness for toilet training rarely develops before 18 months of age. Parents who begin before their child is ready usually experience frustration.

Nursing Interventions

By suggesting the sequence in Box 18-5: Quality and Safety Scenario, the nurse assists parents with toilet training. The parent

10 tips
Nutrition Education Series

kid-friendly veggies and fruits

10 tips for making healthy foods more fun for children

ChooseMyPlate.gov

Encourage children to eat vegetables and fruits by making it fun. Provide healthy ingredients and let kids help with preparation, based on their age and skills. Kids may try foods they avoided in the past if they helped make them.

1 smoothie creations
Blend fat-free or low-fat yogurt or milk with fruit pieces and crushed ice. Use fresh, frozen, canned, and even overripe fruits. Try bananas, berries, peaches, and/or pineapple. If you freeze the fruit first, you can even skip the ice!

2 delicious dippers
Kids love to dip their foods. Whip up a quick dip for veggies with yogurt and seasonings such as herbs or garlic. Serve with raw vegetables like broccoli, carrots, or cauliflower. Fruit chunks go great with a yogurt and cinnamon or vanilla dip.

3 caterpillar kabobs
Assemble chunks of melon, apple, orange, and pear on skewers for a fruity kabob. For a raw veggie version, use vegetables like zucchini, cucumber, squash, sweet peppers, or tomatoes.

4 personalized pizzas
Set up a pizza-making station in the kitchen. Use whole-wheat English muffins, bagels, or pita bread as the crust. Have tomato sauce, low-fat cheese, and cut-up vegetables or fruits for toppings. Let kids choose their own favorites. Then pop the pizzas into the oven to warm.

5 fruity peanut butterfly
Start with carrot sticks or celery for the body. Attach wings made of thinly sliced apples with peanut butter and decorate with halved grapes or dried fruit.

6 frosty fruits
Frozen treats are bound to be popular in the warm months. Just put fresh fruits such as melon chunks in the freezer (rinse first). Make "popsicles" by inserting sticks into peeled bananas and freezing.

7 bugs on a log
Use celery, cucumber, or carrot sticks as the log and add peanut butter. Top with dried fruit such as raisins, cranberries, or cherries, depending on what bugs you want!

8 homemade trail mix
Skip the pre-made trail mix and make your own. Use your favorite nuts and dried fruits, such as unsalted peanuts, cashews, walnuts, or sunflower seeds mixed with dried apples, pineapple, cherries, apricots, or raisins. Add whole-grain cereals to the mix, too.

9 potato person
Decorate half a baked potato. Use sliced cherry tomatoes, peas, and low-fat cheese on the potato to make a funny face.

10 put kids in charge
Ask your child to name new veggie or fruit creations. Let them arrange raw veggies or fruits into a fun shape or design.

USDA United States Department of Agriculture Center for Nutrition Policy and Promotion

DG TipSheet No. 11
June 2011
USDA is an equal opportunity provider and employer.

Go to www.ChooseMyPlate.gov for more information.

FIGURE 18-3 Tips for making healthy foods more fun for children. (From United States Department of Agriculture, Center for Nutrition Policy and Promotion. [2011]. Available at http://www.choosemyplate.gov/food-groups/downloads/TenTips/DGTipsheet11KidFriendlyVeggiesAndFruits.pdf.)

BOX 18-3   RESEARCH FOR EVIDENCE-BASED PRACTICE

Atopic Eczema, Diet, and Toddlers—A Cure?

The toddler diet is a force with which to be reckoned since the toddler has tastes for non-nutritious and highly sweetened food. Imagine that same toddler with atopic eczema and the possibility of adding or excluding a food or food supplement might eliminate this inflammatory skin disease. Two meta-analyses were conducted: one meta-analysis investigated dietary exclusions and the effect on atopic eczema, whereas the other meta-analysis investigated the inclusion of dietary probiotics and the effect on atopic eczema.

The meta-analysis investigating dietary exclusions included 6 randomized, controlled trials (RCTs) for a total sample size of 288 participants who were not allowed to consume eggs and milk. There was no benefit of an egg- and milk-free diet on the atopic eczema; however, there may have been an improvement in the body surface area of infants with suspected egg allergies.

The meta-analysis investigating inclusion of dietary probiotics included 12 RCTs for a total sample size of 781 participants, who were all children. There was no change in the symptoms or severity of the eczema as rated by the parents or the investigator. However, adverse effects including infection and bowel ischemia did occur from the probiotics.

The hierarchical strength of the evidence from both studies is as powerful as possible for a study with randomization of the sample participants and the treatment modality, and the use of a control group. However, limits always occur with meta-analyses because of the various methodologies used within the studies. So even with RCTs, one must be cautious when interpreting the evidence.

Boyle, R. J., Bath-Hextall, F. J., Leonardi-Bee, J., Murrell, D. F., & Tang, M. L.-K. (2009). Probiotics for the treatment of eczema: A systematic review. *Clinical & Experimental Allergy,* 39:1117–1127. doi: 10.1111/j.1365-2222.2009.03305.x.

BOX 18-4   NURSING INTERVENTIONS TO PROMOTE HEALTHY EATING IN TODDLERS

- Offer simple, single foods, because mixtures of foods are often rejected.
- Serve your toddler's favorite foods along with new ones. Several introductions may be necessary before the toddler accepts a new food. Make sure you eat it, too.
- Encourage the use of utensils, but accept that toddlers still often need to use their fingers.
- Routines are important to toddlers. Serve scheduled meals and snacks. Parents are responsible for what, when, and where the toddler eats. The toddler decides whether to eat and how much.
- Turn off the TV. Mealtime should be a relaxed and pleasant time, free of distractions.
- Do not use food to bribe, reward, or punish your toddler.
- Schedule meals and sleep periods such that the child is awake and alert during mealtime.
- Serve small portions and let your toddler ask for more.
- Avoid foods that may cause choking, such as hard candy, mini-marshmallows, popcorn, pretzels, chips, spoonfuls of peanut butter, nuts, seeds, large chunks of meat, hot dogs, raw carrots, dried fruits, and whole grapes.
- Drinking more than 24 ounces of milk per day can reduce your child's appetite for other healthy foods. For those younger than age 2 years, do not use reduced-fat, low-fat, or fat-free (skim) milk because children younger than 2 need the extra fat for their developing nervous systems.

BOX 18-5   QUALITY AND SAFETY SCENARIO

Initiating a Toileting Program for Toddlers

- Interest in and awareness of bowel and urinary elimination usually begin by 18 months of age.
- Before beginning toilet training, parents should check their toddlers for the prerequisite skills, which include being able to walk well, stoop and recover, stay dry for at least 2 hours during the day, and communicate sensation before elimination, as well as the discomfort of wet or messy pants and the need for assistance.
- When these prerequisites are present, introduce the child to a potty seat or chair. The potty chair should provide secure seating with the child's feet touching the floor. The potty seat should be used with a small step stool to create the same effect.
- Because of the gastrocolic reflex, bowel elimination is more likely after a meal, so this is a good time to place the toddler on the potty. When a pattern of bowel or urinary elimination is noticed, use this pattern as a guide for placing the child on the potty.
- Encourage the toddler to stay on the chair for 2 to 3 minutes and always explain what to do ("Go potty") rather than what not to do ("Don't wet your pants"). Do not refer to elimination as dirty or yucky. Remember this is your child's first creation.
- Praise the child for desired behavior. Introduce underwear as a badge of success. Ignore undesired behavior and never punish the child by scolding, spanking, or other punitive measures.
- Anticipate that your toddler may want to touch his or her genitals.
- Remember that daytime dryness usually is achieved by 3 years of age and ahead of nighttime dryness, where the need to wear a diaper remains.

who can approach toilet training with a relaxed attitude, accepting some delays and frustrations, will have a better chance of success and a more positive outcome for the toddler.

Activity-Exercise Pattern

Toddlers are always busy—emptying wastebaskets and drawers, building and destroying towers, throwing, kicking, chasing after balls, or dressing and undressing. Many of their activities are repeated over and over, providing practice opportunities for their newly realized skills.

During the toddler period, children will advance from taking their first step to running, climbing stairs, and even pedaling a tricycle. They enjoy pushing and pulling, whether it is an unsuspecting laundry basket or a push-pull toy made for the job. They scribble spontaneously, usually with vigor, and will emerge from toddlerhood capable of copying a circle and creating tadpole-like figures. They learn to use a spoon and a fork with fairly good success and to wash their hands. They also advance from being dressed by others to dressing themselves with assistance, although at times they resist it.

Toddlers spend most of their waking hours at play—exploring their expanding environment, imitating others' actions, and creating a safety net of rituals around the routines of eating, sleeping, and everything in between. In their enthusiasm to try many activities, toddlers invariably take on tasks that are beyond their abilities, which can result in frustration and an occasional well-known temper tantrum. Their exploratory nature and limited, but advancing, skills also make them vulnerable to injury.

Most toddlers are interested in other children. However, this interest is limited because toddlers, although ready to be with other children, are not ready to share. Successful social encounters with toddlers are best described as **parallel play,** where children play side by side, doing similar things with similar toys, but each working independently (Berger, 2011). Sharing and cooperative play will not develop until well into the preschool age.

Nursing Interventions

When parents inquire about what toys and activities to provide for their toddler, the following are suggested:

- Provide toys that challenge the child to develop new skills: toys that require skills slightly above the child's present level, but not so advanced that the child cannot achieve some success.
- Provide opportunities for new learning. This may be as basic as a book with pictures of new animals or a walk through the produce section of the grocery store to point out fruits and vegetables.
- Provide opportunities for social encounters with other children, but do not force playing together. Creating separate, yet parallel space, with the use of small mats or hula-hoops as boundaries, is recommended.
- Follow the child's lead. Let the toddler choose and explore new toys or objects, within safe limits.
- Make sure the toy is safe for the toddler and does not have any parts that can be removed and swallowed, have lead paint, or can cause harm to the curious toddler.

The desire of some parents to raise the smartest, most coordinated, or most musically talented super kids often begins in the toddler period. The American Academy of Pediatrics (AAP) (2011b) recommends no screen time, including television, videos, and computers, for children under the age of 2. For older toddlers, the AAP recommends no more than 1 to 2 hours daily of high-quality screen time with the parent watching too. For interactive computer games that may include touch-screens, the parent needs to be there with the toddler so that two-way conversation occurs. Ideally, children should be allowed to explore their interests, with parents responding to their cues. It is interaction with parents and others in their environment that provides the advantage with cognitive development. Past research associated television watching by toddlers with interference at a critical time when language development occurs and suggested that this can cause a delay in that process. Current research indicates that audible television loud enough to decrease the child's exposure to discernible adult speech and decreased child vocalizations also led to delayed speech development (Christakis et al., 2009). Additionally, the more television shows with advertising watched, the more likely the child will become obese (Zimmerman & Bell, 2010). For more information on helping parents support their toddler's activity and exploration in a safe and educational way, go to the *Zero to Three* website at www.zerotothree.org.

Sleep-Rest Pattern

Toddlers' need for sleep decreases to 12 hours a day, including 1 or 2 naps of shorter duration. One of the naps usually is replaced by quiet time, a brief period to unwind from a busy or noisy activity. Occasionally the parents or caregivers need these rest breaks as much or more than the toddler. Sitting together in a rocking chair for a soothing song or quiet music or reading side by side or together can be suggested by the nurse.

The toddler may be involved in an activity and not be aware of fatigue, especially when visitors are in the home or some interesting new toys have been discovered. All parents are familiar with the child who is overtired but unable to relax enough to sleep. Parents can potentially avoid this dilemma by scheduling nap and quiet time even when there are house-guests or holidays that pre-empt the toddler's routine.

Rituals are characteristic of this age, and most toddlers have a nap and bedtime ritual. The following might be a typical pattern: eating a nutritious snack, followed by bathing, brushing teeth, listening to a story, getting a kiss, and having overhead lights turned off and the night light turned on. Following this ritual is important, because the toddler gets a sense of security when ending the day. Changing this ritual can be upsetting. The nurse encourages parents to establish and follow the sleep time ritual as closely as possible, even when visitors, family illness, or travel makes the routine more difficult. Also, incorporate rituals as much as possible when the toddler stays outside of the home, for instance staying overnight at their grandparent's house or during a hospitalization.

Many toddlers will try to delay sleep by calling for water, another story, or another kiss, or by making other requests. Parents should be certain that the toddler has ample opportunity for interaction with them during the day, follow the usual bedtime ritual, and be firm and consistent in resisting any requests for attention after the final good nights have been said. Encouraging toddlers to use transition or security objects, such as stuffed animals or blankets, helps them to self-quiet and console themselves both at bedtime and in new situations (Figure 18-4).

FIGURE 18-4 Toddlers need adequate sleep for healthy growth and their stuffed toys can help them feel more secure.

Night terrors may begin in toddlerhood. Night terrors are different from nightmares, which generally begin at a later age and result in the child awakening and being able to recall the frightening dream. The child who experiences night terrors does not waken completely, but cries out, looks terrified, and cannot be aroused for several minutes. Eventually, usually after 5 to 10 minutes, the child falls back into quiet sleep. Parents need to be reassured that these episodes will become less frequent as the child develops. The parents should talk in a soothing voice but should not try to awaken the child. If the child does waken, the parents should then provide comfort and tuck the child back in bed.

Cognitive-Perceptual Pattern

Toddlers who experienced the security of a nurturing and reliable source of protection and attachment during infancy have a strong base from which to begin to explore and learn about their expanding world. They begin toddlerhood in Piaget's sensorimotor stage of cognitive development and start moving to the preoperational stage. Their advancing thought-processing skills and abilities to use the language are heralded by the development of egocentrism, an inability to put oneself in another's shoes. Toddlers who come running into a room asking their parents "Where is it?" are confused when parents respond "Where is what?" They assume their parents and all others share their same thoughts and cannot understand why they do not.

Toddlers interpret and learn about objects and events, not in terms of general properties, but in terms of their relationship with them or their use to them. Their thoughts are dominated by what they see, hear, or otherwise experience, and they want to experience everything. Their two- to three-word phrases are most often related to present events, describing an action, a desire, or a possession (example: "Mommy, me up!").

Both receptive and expressive language skills are developing rapidly in toddlers; however, their receptive language skills far outweigh their expressive language ability, and toddlers often use gestures until words are found to represent the meanings already acquired. Toddlers also learn the use of inflection. "Mommy" may mean "Pick me up" on one occasion and "I'm scared" or "Where are you?" on another. Often frustrated by their limited repertoire of expressive language, which usually includes about 400 words, young toddlers default to using "NO" as a method of gaining control over a situation or expressing themselves (see the Think About It box at the beginning of this chapter).

By age 3, children have mastered the basics of language function, form, and content, and these fundamentals will continue to be refined throughout childhood and adolescence. Table 18-1 outlines the landmarks of speech, language, and hearing ability for this age group.

Toddlers have a solid understanding of object permanence and are no longer easily distracted when a desired toy, blanket, or parent is not to be found. Many toddlers will sit patiently in front of the washing machine while a favorite blanket is laundered or stare out a front window awaiting a parent's return. They can inadvertently put themselves in harm's way as they pursue an object or person they sense is just out of view.

The toddler period is dominated by play, but often referred to as "child's work," which is repetitive and ritualistic. When toddlers bounce a ball over and over and over again they are not trying to drive their parents crazy. They are trying to learn about balls, and repetition is the best teacher. Toddlers' ritualistic behaviors help them master skills and decrease anxiety, and the addition of a seemingly endless string of questions to these behaviors can test the limits of the most patient parents. These queries, however, must be acknowledged and answered in a manner that not only provides solutions but also validates and reinforces the toddler's burgeoning curiosity. The nurse explains the "terrible twos" by teaching parents and caregivers that toddlers might better be viewed as "young scientists" in need of a safe "laboratory" in which to conduct their trial and error research. Better now and in parents' close proximity than in adolescence, a developmental period that mirrors and repeats many of the parent-child challenges of toddlerhood. The American Academy of Pediatrics has recommended administering autistic screening at the 18-month preventive care visit (Hagan et al., 2008). At present, autism spectrum disorders are defined as pervasive developmental disorders with onset in infancy or childhood and characterized by impaired social interactions, impaired communications, and significantly restricted activities and interests. There is no known cause. The current prevalence is 1 in every 150 American children and almost 1 in 94 boys (Robins, 2008; Wetherby et al., 2008). See www.autismsociety.org and www.myautism.org for more information.

Hearing

The ability to hear and listen to others is critical for speech and language development. Listening includes attending to what is heard, discriminating among the various qualities of sound, cognitively associating what is heard with previously learned experiences, and remembering what is heard. The quantity and quality of language to which the toddler is exposed is thought to be more important for the development of listening ability and therefore receptive language skills than it is for the development of expressive language skills (Genesee, 2008). Toddlers often seek repetition of auditory input, as observed in their seemingly endless repetition of sounds, words, and combinations of words. This repetition is their way of practicing and organizing new language (Neuman & Dickinson, 2011) (see Table 18-1).

Hearing loss is one of the most common conditions present at birth. If undetected during early infancy, even mild hearing loss can impede speech, language, cognitive, and emotional development (Hagan et al., 2008). Health care providers need to continue to monitor, screen, and refer children for formal audiological evaluation if they develop signs of identified risk factors for hearing loss. The timing and number of hearing reevaluations for children with risk factors should be individualized. Infants who pass the neonatal screening but have a risk factor should have at least one diagnostic audiology assessment by 24 to 30 months of age (AAP, 2011a). Early and more frequent assessment may be indicated for children with cytomegalovirus (CMV) infection, syndromes associated with progressive hearing loss, neurodegenerative disorders, head trauma, or culture-positive postnatal infections associated with sensorineural

TABLE 18-1 GROWTH AND DEVELOPMENT

Landmarks of Speech, Language, and Hearing Ability During the Toddler Period

AGE (MONTHS)	RECEPTIVE LANGUAGE	EXPRESSIVE LANGUAGE	RELATED HEARING ABILITY
18	Up to 50 words; recognizes between 6 and 12 objects by name, such as *dog, cat, bottle, ball;* identifies three body parts, such as *eyes, nose, mouth;* understands simple, one-step commands such as *give me the doll, open your mouth, stick out your tongue*	Up to 20 words; jargon and echolalia are present; uses names of familiar objects and one-word sentences, such as *go* or *eat;* uses gestures; uses words such as *no, mine, eat, good, bad, hot, cold,* and expressions such as *oh-oh, what's that, all gone;* use of words can be quite inconsistent; 25% of speech intelligible	Has begun to develop gross discrimination by learning to distinguish between highly dissimilar noises, such as doorbell and train, barking dog and auto horn, or mother's and father's voices
24	Up to 1200 words; knows *in, on, under;* identifies *dog, ball, engine, bed, doll, scissors, hair, mouth, feet, nose, cup, spoon, car, key;* distinguishes between one and many and formulates a negative judgment (a knife is not a fork); understands simple stories; follows simple, two-step directions; is beginning to make distinctions between *you* and *me*	Up to 270 words; jargon and echolalia almost gone; average 75 words per hour during free play; talks in words, phrases, and two-word to three-word sentences; averages two words per response; first pronouns appear, such as *I, me, mine, it, who, that;* adjectives and adverbs are only beginning to appear; names objects and common pictures; refers to self by name, such as *Katrina go bye-bye;* uses phrases such as *I want, go bye-bye, want cookie, ball all gone;* 60% of speech intelligible	Refinement of gross discriminative skills
30	Up to 2400 words; identifies action in pictures and objects by use; carries out one-part and two-part commands, such as *pick up your shoe and give it to mommy;* knows what is used to drink liquids, what goes on the feet, what is used to buy candy; understands plurals, questions, difference between boy and girl, the concepts *one, up, down, run, walk, throw, fast, more, my*	Uses up to 425 words; jargon and echolalia no longer exist; averages 140 words per hour; names words such as *chair, can, box, key, door;* repeats 2 digits from memory; average sentence length is approximately 2½ words; uses more adjectives and adverbs; demands repetition from others, such as *do it again;* nearly always announces intentions before actions; begins to ask questions of adults; 75% of speech intelligible	—
36	Up to 3600 words; understands *both, two, not today,* what to do when thirsty (hungry, sleepy), why people have stoves; understands *wait, later, big, new, different, strong, today, another,* and taking turns at play; carries out two-item and some three-item commands, such as *give me the ball, pick up the doll,* and *sit down;* identifies several colors; is aware of past and future	Up to 900 words in simple sentences, averaging three to four words per sentence; averages 170 words per hour; uses words such as *when, time, today, not today, new, different, big, strong, surprise, secret;* can repeat three digits, name one color, say name, give simple account of experiences, and tell stories that can be understood; begins to use more pronouns, adjectives, and adverbs; describes at least one element of a picture; is aware of past and future; uses commands such as *you make it* and expressions such as *I can't, I don't want to;* verbalizes toilet needs; expresses desire to take turns; communication includes criticisms, commands, requests, threats, questions, answers; 85% of speech intelligible	Starts to distinguish dissimilar speech sounds, such as the difference between *ee* and *er,* although there may be some difficulty with the concepts of *same* and *different*

Modified from Hockenberry, M. J., & Wilson, D. (Eds.). (2011). *Wong's nursing care of infants and children* (9th ed.). St. Louis: Mosby/Elsevier; Ports, N. L., & Mandleco, B. L. (2011). *Pediatric nursing: Caring for children and their families* (3rd ed.). Clifton Park, NY: Thomson Delmar Learning; Pan, B. A., Rowe, M. L., Singer, J. D., & Snow, C. E. (2005). Maternal correlates of growth in toddler vocabulary production in low-income families. *Child Development, 76*(4), 763-782.

hearing loss (e.g., herpes viruses); for toddlers who spent more than 5 days in a neonatal intensive care unit (NICU) at birth or who received extracorporeal membrane oxygenation (ECMO), exchange transfusions, or chemotherapy; and for caregivers of toddlers who are concerned because there is a family history of hearing loss (AAP, 2007, 2011a).

Younger toddlers are screened using visual-reinforcement audiometry, in which stimulus tones and visually animated reinforcers (e.g., a lighted toy) are paired and presented together. After the toddler has been conditioned to expect this relationship, the visual reinforcer is withheld and the sound is presented alone. The toddler looks for the visual reinforcer in response to the sound, and the visual reinforcer is then presented as a reward. Conditioned-play audiometry is used for older toddlers and preschool children. The child is first taught to play listening games, using blocks or rings. The child learns to wait and listen for a sound and then perform a motor task (e.g., places a block, a bucket, or a ring on a stacking stick) in response. The motor task is followed by social reinforcement. Noncalibrated toys or noisemakers and signals that lack frequency specificity are inappropriate screening methods and should be used only as gross indicators for monitoring.

Otitis media, or middle ear infection, is one of the leading causes of visits to health care providers during the toddler years and the primary reason for which antibiotics are prescribed for these children. Discussing the current literature and evidence-based reports and recommendations often helps parents understand the proper use of antibiotics, which is also imperative in preventing antibiotic resistance. When it is deemed necessary to use an antibiotic, nurses teach how to administer the medication safely and stress the importance of taking the medication at the prescribed time and for the full duration of the course, which is indicated by an empty container of medication, not by the absence of initial symptoms.

Vision

Toddlers' visual acuity is usually around 20/40, although gaining their cooperation for screening is often difficult and not recommended unless parents, caregivers, or health care providers identify a concern. Depth perception is still immature, although more developed than in infancy.

Amblyopia is one of the major health care concerns of this age group and occurs in 2% to 5% of children. It is defined as diminished, or loss of, vision in an eye that has not received adequate use. The eye looks normal, but it is not being used normally. Because the brain favors the other eye, the term "lazy eye" is often used. The most common cause of amblyopia is strabismus, but it may also occur when one eye is more nearsighted, farsighted, or astigmatic than the other. Occasionally amblyopia is caused by other eye conditions such as a cataract.

Amblyopia is preventable and treatable especially if detected early. The earlier detection of amblyopia will contribute to the greater chance for a complete recovery. The American Academy of Pediatrics (AAP) and the American Academy of Ophthalmology strongly recommend that children have their eyes examined at the following times: newborn, 6 months, 3 years, and before starting school (American Association for Pediatric Ophthalmology and Strabismus, 2012; American Optometric Association, 2012). Management of amblyopia depends on the cause and may include surgery or paralytic, autonomic, and centrally acting pharmacological agents. However, no matter what the cause, management will involve making the child use the lazy eye, the eye with reduced vision. There are two ways to accomplish this: using atropine eye drops or patching the stronger eye (American Association for Pediatric Ophthalmology and Strabismus, 2012). If glasses are worn with the patch, the nurse will help the parents secure them with the active toddler. Researchers have found that not all children benefit from eye drop treatment for amblyopia. When the stronger eye is nearsighted, the atropine eye drops may not be as effective (American Association for Pediatric Ophthalmology and Strabismus, 2012) (Box 18-6: Innovative Practice).

Strabismus is a deviation of the line of vision from the midline resulting from extraocular muscle weakness or imbalance and is commonly referred to as crossed eye. One or both eyes may turn in, out, up, or down and can be constant or intermittent. Marked or continuous strabismus usually is noticed early by the parents and health care providers and is therefore treated early; the more subtle deviations are often unnoticed until older

---

✳ BOX 18-6   INNOVATIVE PRACTICE

The Eye Patch Club

It is estimated that 2% to 5% of all children suffer from amblyopia. Prevent Blindness America is creating a support group called the Eye Patch Club for families coping with a child's amblyopia treatment. *The Eye Patch Club News* is a newsletter featuring tips and techniques for promoting compliance, stories from and about children whose eyes are patched, and professional advice from optometrists, ophthalmologists, and orthoptists. Each issue also includes a Kid's Page, and there is a classroom guide for teachers with explanations for the classroom, as well as activities for everyone to learn more about their eyes. An Eye Patch Club calendar and stickers that allow children to track their patch-wearing activity, a refrigerator magnet with helpful hints, and pen pal opportunities are also available. To learn more about Prevent Blindness America and The Eye Patch Club, visit their website at www.preventblindness. org/children/EyePatchClub.html.

---

toddlerhood or the preschool years. Every toddler should be screened for strabismus as part of the routine eye examination that is performed by the physician or nurse practitioner during well-child visits.

Other signs of vision problems that the nurse observes or parents report in their toddlers include the following red flags:

- Rubs eyes excessively
- Shuts or covers one eye, tilts head, or looks sideways to view an object
- Has difficulty or is irritable when doing close work
- Blinks, squints, or frowns when viewing objects
- Holds books close to eyes
- Has red, encrusted, or swollen eyelids
- Has red, inflamed, or watery eyes
- Develops recurring **styes** (swelling at the edge of the eyelid)

Taste and Smell

Toddlers are beginning to take control of their world and have the capacity to taste and smell, new skills that are rapidly used. Toddlers often refuse to even taste something that looks or smells displeasing to them or eat something that they recall as tasting terrible. They are able to react accurately to a sensation that a taste or smell arouses in them, and they begin to learn conditioned association between certain smells and culturally acceptable values. Foods and smells found in one family or culture become palatable and accepted, and those that are unacceptable become displeasing. Many of our adult eating habits, food likes and dislikes, and visceral responses to odors have their roots in this period.

Self-Perception–Self-Concept Pattern

According to Erikson (1995, 1998), the developmental task of toddlers is to acquire a sense of **autonomy** while overcoming a sense of **doubt** and **shame.** To exert autonomy, toddlers must relinquish the dependence on others that was enjoyed during infancy. Continued dependency has the potential to create a sense of doubt in toddlers about their ability to take control of, and ultimately take responsibility for, their own actions. Toddlers seem to thrive when parents can accommodate their increasing autonomy yet maintain a strong parenting presence that includes a full measure of patience, enough parental self-confidence to set appropriate limits, and the ability to realize that their toddler's negative behavior is not directed at them and their egocentrism is not a reflection on them.

The toddler must explore the world, not only the physical aspects but also the interpersonal aspects of relationships, to develop a true sense of autonomy. Exploring the physical world involves poking into, climbing onto, crawling under, tasting, smelling, and taking apart the objects encountered. The child explores relationships with others by searching for the limits of the child's power: If a "no" or a temper tantrum means control of another person's behavior, the child learns that one's own self is more powerful than the other person's self. The toddler continually practices separateness to develop a sense of autonomy.

This process can be frustrating and confusing for parents. The toddler may say a vehement "no" when offered a drink and then scream and cry when the drink is taken away; the parents may wonder whether or not the toddler wants the drink. Likely the answer is "yes," but the toddler may also need to express autonomy by refusing it. Occasionally the same toddler who displays a strong need for autonomy spontaneously cuddles or even clings to a parent. These conflicting desires can be confusing to both the parent and the toddler. The toddler's need for more autonomy may conflict with parental expectations, safety limits, or the rights of other children or adults. Any of these conflicts results in feelings of frustration. A typical toddler response to frustration is the well-known temper tantrum.

Nursing Interventions

The nurse assesses the toddler-parent relationship to determine the following:

- How is the toddler expressing the need for autonomy?
- How do the parents perceive these actions?
- How does the toddler respond to frustration in exploring the environment or controlling personal and others' actions?
- How do the parents respond to the toddler's display of frustration?
- What provisions are the parents making to allow safe choices for the toddler?

The nurse's teaching focuses on the aspects that are troublesome for the toddler-parent relationship. The following examples are some general concepts to include:

- Match the environment to the child's needs and abilities. Childproof the home such that the child can explore safely. Provide toys that the child can master. Give opportunities to play with more challenging toys, but do not make these toys the rule.
- Give advance notice of a change in activity, such as lunch or nap time. Utilize transition rituals and objects.
- Do not offer a choice if there is not one. For example, rather than ask if the toddler wants to take a bath, say "It is time to take a bath, do you want to take it upstairs or downstairs, or do you want to start at the face and move down to the toes or start with the toes and wash the face last?" This allows for the toddler to be in charge and the task of bathing achieved.

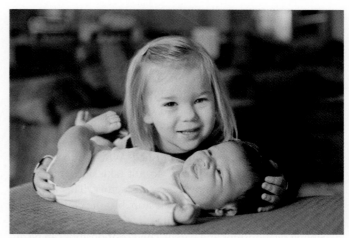

FIGURE 18-5 It's a big change for a toddler when a new baby is introduced.

- Set and enforce consistent limits such that the toddler will come to develop control within these limits.
- To prevent temper tantrums, keep routines simple and consistent, set reasonable limits and give rationales, avoid "head-on clashes," and provide choices.
- If temper tantrums occur, provide a safe environment for the toddler, identify the tantrum's cause, and help the toddler regain control. Do not reason, threaten, promise, hit, or concede. Respond consistently and follow through on discipline free of anger. Overcriticizing and restricting the toddler may dampen enthusiasm and increase feelings of shame and doubt.
- Praise the toddler's skills and abilities. Never miss an opportunity to catch your toddler being good. Be positive. Remember to say "yes" once in a while.

Roles-Relationship Pattern

By toddlerhood, children typically know their mother, father, and older siblings and have established some form of reciprocal relationship with them (Treyvaud et al., 2009). Toddlers' capability for relationships is limited and usually reflects their egocentric approach to everything else. Parents' and siblings' roles are understood, just like everything else in their lives, in terms of how those roles relate to the toddler. One family member may be the fixer of toys or the comforter of bruises, another the troublemaker who takes away toys.

Toddlers are interested in everything, and their parents' and siblings' activities and possessions are often imitated and preferred. Frequently the desire to be like or have something that belongs to a sibling creates sibling rivalry. This happens between toddlers and their older siblings, but even more when a new younger sibling is introduced (Figure 18-5). A new baby who is often loud, unable to play, unable to be touched or explored too vigorously, and demands and gets too much parental attention quickly becomes a nuisance to toddlers, who have been known to inform their parents that they can "Take the new baby back where it came from now." Realizing the new sibling is here to stay, toddlers often regress, reverting to earlier, previously abandoned infantile behavior such as losing toileting skills, wanting to be fed or dressed, or even communicating by "baby talk." They are usually trying to retain or regain a sense of mastery and, once reassured, will progress. This process is not the end of sibling rivalry, but only the beginning of what will assume many forms and require ongoing negotiation from all family members. Parents cannot stop sibling fighting by forbidding it, but reasonable limits can be established. One way to deescalate fighting is to remove the reward of the fight. Generally the desired outcome in the toddler's mind is to see the self rewarded and the sibling punished. When parents do not reward or punish, or when they do not take sides, the gain is missing and fighting becomes less satisfactory. This approach does not mean that all fighting will stop, but the child will look for other ways of getting approval.

Sibling relationships and parent-child relationships can be difficult subjects for parents to discuss. Parents may think that any hint of discord indicates an unhealthy family (Bergman & Harpaz-Rotem, 2004). The nurse includes normal family development and role relationships as part of the anticipatory guidance given during the toddler years (Warren et al., 2008). Toddler behaviors are frustrating for all parents, and discipline can often be influenced as much by parental emotions as by parenting knowledge and skill (Caughy et al., 2009). When parental anger, depression (Del Vecchio & O'Leary, 2008; Gartstein & Bateman, 2008; Treyvaud et al., 2009; Weinfield et al., 2009), criticism, and restrictions go unchecked, physical and emotional abuse can occur.

Child Abuse

Child abuse and maltreatment is not limited to a particular age or particular families (Siebel et al., 2008). However, it is more likely to occur with a major change or turmoil (Centers for Disease Control and Prevention, 2010c, 2012a; Norris, 2008) in the family and when parental role models were abusive. Toddlerhood is a trying time for the most patient of parents, and nurses are alert to family changes and stresses as well as to warning signs of abuse (Box 18-7). Many injuries are difficult to differentiate from accidental injury and, at times, may even be confused with culturally appropriate healing practices (Box 18-8: Diversity Awareness). However, the toddler years have the greatest

incidence of child maltreatment with 37% of nonfatal cases reported for children ages 1 to 3 years and 80% of deaths from child maltreatment occurring in children younger than 4 years (CDC, 2010a). Nonfatal cases appearing in emergency departments, pediatrician offices, and day care centers may be the only opportunity for health care providers to prevent later death from continued child maltreatment.

Typically parental responses to childhood injuries include a spontaneous reporting of the details of the illness or injury accompanied by concern, questions about progress and discharge, difficulty in leaving the child, and an attempt to identify with the child's feelings. These parents may also experience guilt for not protecting the child from the accident and may offer gifts to compensate for these feelings of guilt. In contrast, neglectful or abusive parents are often hesitant to provide information about the illness or injury; they may be evasive or even contradict themselves, irritated by the inconvenience of being asked questions. Abusive parents may not exhibit guilt feelings and often contend that the toddler was solely responsible for the injury.

Although these signs of potential abuse are certainly not present in all abusive parents, their presence alerts the nurse to assess and observe further. The nurse also remembers that some of these signs may be found in nonabusive parents, and that the presence of these signs serves only as a cue for further assessment. All nurses are required by law to report any and all suspected child abuse to the local child protective services agency.

BOX 18-7 WARNING SIGNS OF CHILD ABUSE

- Parental delay in seeking help
- Inconsistencies in the history of how the injury occurred
- Injury inconsistent with the history or child's developmental capability
- Old, unexplained fractures evident on radiographs
- Bruises confined to back surface of the body—neck to knees
- Bare spots and broken hair
- Pattern of injury or bruising descriptive of object used to inflict injury (belt or belt buckle, hand, cigarette, hot water)
- Burns with sharply demarcated edges or circumferential patterns
- Perineal injuries of any kind

From Centers for Disease Control and Prevention (2012).
Child maltreatment: Risk and protective factors and *Learning the signs, act early: Developmental milestones.* Retrieved July 1, 2012, from www.cdc.gov.

⊕ BOX 18-8 DIVERSITY AWARENESS

Evaluating for Child Abuse with Cultural Sensitivity

Nurses are required by law to report cases of suspected child abuse to Child Protective Services. The nurse who takes a careful health history may discover that what might appear to be characteristic burns or bruises associated with child abuse may instead be the product of a traditional culturally appropriate healing practice. The following are two examples of healing practices found in the Pacific Islander and Asian populations that might create such confusion.

Coining (CAO GIO)
Coining is a common healing practice used among Pacific Island and Asian families within the United States. Traditionally, coining is used for conditions associated with "wind" illnesses, as well as a wide variety of febrile illnesses. The lesions seen from coining are produced by rubbing a warm oil or balm on the skin and firmly abrading the skin with a coin or special instrument. The practice produces linear petechiae and ecchymosis on the chest and back that often resemble strap or belt marks. The appearance of the deep red-purple skin color is confirmation that the person had bad wind in the body.

Cupping (Ventouse)
Cupping involves creating a vacuum inside a special cup or glass by burning the oxygen out of it and then promptly placing it on a person's skin surface. Cupping draws blood and lymph to the body surface that is under the cup or glass, increasing local circulation. The purpose for doing this is to remove cold and damp "evils" from the body or to assist blood circulation, or both. The procedure frequently is used to treat lung congestion. The resulting circular ecchymotic marks are approximately 2 inches in diameter and resemble nonaccidental trauma.

Sexuality-Reproductive Pattern

The toileting process, during which attention is focused on the genital area, may precipitate the toddler's curiosity about genital organs. The nurse includes this aspect when teaching about toilet training, giving parents time to consider their feelings and decide on their approach to genital exploratory behavior and masturbation. Some parents accept the child's curiosity, whereas others see this as an opportunity to introduce their own sexual values and taboos.

The nurse encourages parents to approach this curiosity and exploration, as well as masturbation, as a normal developmental process. These behaviors provide toddlers with an opportunity to become better acquainted with their bodies. Many parents are uncertain about the vocabulary they should use and often create cute, unrelated words rather than provide the correct anatomical terms. The use of cute alternative words often is a reflection of parental discomfort or embarrassment. Using correct terms will help toddlers develop accurate knowledge about sexuality and communicate more effectively if inappropriate touching by others occurs. For example, a young boy was initially ignored by day care providers because he said an older boy ate his "pickle." After repeated episodes, the parents were contacted because the child seemed so upset (even though day care workers gave him a new pickle to eat). The parents shared that "pickle" was their name for penis.

Coping-Stress Tolerance Pattern

Perceptions of events and reactions to them are filtered through children's developing cognitive, emotional, and social capacities. The relevance of life events and the child's vulnerability to their impact depend on the given developmental period (see the Case Study and Care Plan at the end of this chapter). A child's temperament, which is defined as an individual's style of emotional and behavioral response across situations, especially those involving change or stress, serves as a foundation for coping (Burns et al., 2009). Although temperament generally has been accepted as inborn, it is influenced by environmental characteristics and exerts an influence on psychosocial adjustment by way of its effect on parent-child interactions. Nurses assist parents in recognizing their toddler's innate behavioral qualities as expressions of temperament and in developing management strategies (Box 18-9: Hot Topics).

Toddlers are developing new ways to cope with the myriad of new stresses that come with being a toddler. As is typical of their stage of development, coping is egocentric and reflective of their need for autonomy. Typical stressors include new siblings, babysitters, day care, toilet training, parental limit setting, and an endless string of tasks involving skills they have yet to develop.

Toddlers often imitate their parents' behavior and this includes their methods of dealing with stress. They also regress, at times, to earlier infantile behavior when overwhelmed, until they regain some sense of mastery. Parents can help to anticipate and prepare toddlers for stressful experiences before they happen. However, they need to remember that toddlers' sense of time and ability to recall are limited. Preparations should be honest, simple, and focused on what the toddler will experience.

Enough time should be allowed for the toddler to rehearse the coping behavior with the parent, but not so early before the event that the toddler forgets.

The nurse helps the parents anticipate developmental stressors and suggests age- and temperament-appropriate coping behaviors for toddlers. Early efforts at dealing with stress are an essential step to more mature coping responses as the child grows (Kolak & Vernon-Feagans, 2008).

Values-Beliefs Pattern

Healthy behaviors are expressions of positive values and beliefs. These values and beliefs are learned, and their recognition and acceptance are fundamental to the integrity of every child. Toddlers believe rules are absolute and behave, according to Kohlberg, out of a fear of punishment. However, toddlers' environments should not only help them become aware of right and wrong but also contribute to their sense of security, belonging, and autonomy. Development of moral integrity is enhanced if toddlers believe they are valued.

Because most of toddlers' developing values and beliefs depend on their interactions with parents, the nurse's assessment

BOX 18-9 HOT TOPICS

Coping with a Child's Temperament

Temperament is defined as the style of behaviors that a child habitually uses to cope with demands and expectations of the environment. Chess and Thomas (1986) originally described three common temperament patterns that they believe are innate: the easy child; the difficult child; and the slow-to-warm-up child. The easy child is cuddly, affectionate, and easy to manage. The way in which a child with an easy temperament elicits positive reactions from adults is obvious.

Children with a difficult temperament, however, are less adaptable, are more intense and active, and have more negative moods. These behaviors can be distressing to parents and caregivers and may cause them to feel ineffective in their roles.

Temperament affects development throughout the life span but is especially significant for toddlers when placed in the context of development. Toddlers are increasingly mobile and are striving for independence at a time when parents become more demanding. Various approaches to parenting, teaching, and providing health care, including the adults' own temperament styles, culture, and gender-related biases, can influence the way in which the child's behavior is viewed.

According to the goodness-of-fit interactive model of temperament, adults can accommodate their demands and expectations in ways that match the child's behaviors, including learning strategies to help toddlers adapt positively to social expectations.

Questions
- What are some of the consequences of labeling a toddler as difficult, easy, or slow to warm up?
- What are common reactions to girls who are extremely active and highly distractible? Boys who are clingy, cry often, and prefer to play with dolls? What influences these reactions in adults? What influence do these reactions have on children?

Data from Burns, C. E., Dunn, A. M., Brady, M. A., Starr, N. B., & Blosser, C. (2008). *Pediatric primary care* (4th ed.). St. Louis: W.B. Saunders; Chess, S., & Thomas, A. (1986). *Temperament in clinical practice.* New York: Guilford Press.

questions are often directed to or focused on the parent or caregiver. The following are some examples of questions asked by the nurse:

- What are the family's values and beliefs about what is right and wrong?
- How does the parental approach to limit-setting reflect these values and beliefs?
- What religious, spiritual, or cultural traditions and activities does the family have?
- How is the toddler included in these traditions and activities?

Children are exposed to and begin to participate in and imitate their family's religious rituals and practices during toddlerhood. They are often taught prayers and songs with a religious theme that are tied into what the family believes are right and wrong. Toddlers may be able to learn the words to these simple prayers and songs, but parents should be cautioned that knowing the words does not mean that toddlers understand the full meaning of what is said. This early introduction into the family's religious beliefs is important as a socialization factor but should not be assumed to produce a good child.

The creation of values and beliefs in young children is related to their developmental stage and reflected in their behaviors. An important aspect of teaching young children what is right and wrong involves stating what acceptable behavior is and then reinforcing the behavior when it occurs. Parents often attend to toddlers only when they are misbehaving, leaving them alone when they are being good. In this scenario, toddlers receive no attention for acceptable behavior but gain their parents' attention when they misbehave. The nurse can remind parents to catch their toddlers being good and give them the same or more attention.

ENVIRONMENTAL PROCESSES

Physical Agents

Accidents

"If a disease were killing our young children in the proportions that injuries are, people would be outraged and demand that this killer be stopped."

C. Everett Koop, MD, Former Surgeon General

Toddlers are at high risk for accidental injury, because they lack judgment and experience and have only rudimentary problem-solving skills, limited physical coordination, and a heightened level of curiosity about their environment (Garzon et al., 2007). Most parents think that it is natural for children to get hurt and that childhood injuries are just a part of growing up. However, most injuries are predictable and preventable and can cause disabilities requiring long-term care. Furthermore, they cause more deaths than all childhood diseases combined.

Of every 10 toddlers who come to the emergency department, 1 is treated for accidental injury. Male toddlers tend to have more injuries than their female counterparts, but the overall numbers of accidental injuries peak during toddlerhood for both males and females. A second peak occurs for males during adolescence. Major causes of accidental injury in toddlers involve structural hazards, sports, drowning, burns, motor vehicles, and poisoning.

Recent research indicates that although overall injury rates for young children have decreased over the past 20 years, mortality rates from injury remain higher in African American and American Indian/Alaskan Native children. The young children in these groups had higher injury and mortality risk for residential fires, suffocation, and poisoning. These findings suggest new strategies and approaches are needed to narrow the disparities that continue to exist.

Structural Hazards

Houses and other buildings can be hazardous for toddlers. Their desire to explore lures them to locations to which older children or adults would not consider. The toddler will climb onto furniture or fixtures, out of windows, or into small spaces. Injuries that result from these explorations can range from minor scrapes and bruises to fatal head injuries. Ideally, homes are "baby-proofed" before the infant begins scooting and crawling and toddler-proofed before the toddler becomes increasingly mobile. Parents should reassess the safety of their home as their child acquires new skills. Injuries to toddlers occur most often when they fall from furniture, high chairs, changing tables, stairs, windows, and playground equipment. When the child or family visits the home of a friend or relative, it must be inspected for hazards, or the toddler must be confined to one safe room. Many injuries occur in unfamiliar environments.

Preventive measures for structural hazards include the following:

- Do not leave a toddler unattended.
- Use gates at the top and bottom of stairways, and at doors.
- Keep chairs away from countertops and tables to prevent toddlers from climbing.
- Securely anchor large television monitors and other electronics that can fall onto toddlers.
- Lock doors to dangerous areas and use gates and window guards.

Toys

Toys commonly found in homes are another source of injury. Parents should inspect not only the toys that are in their own homes, but also the toys given to the toddler outside the home by relatives, friends, babysitters, or day care personnel (see the Case Study and Care Plan at the end of this chapter). Many toys that are likely to be safe for older children are extremely hazardous for the toddler. Of concern are small, removable parts, magnets and batteries, toxic paint or stuffing, sharp edges, and flammable material.

Sports

Although sporting and recreational equipment is recognized as a major source of accidents in older children and adolescents, parents and health care personnel occasionally forget that these items can also be dangerous to toddlers. Improper storage of this equipment is a primary danger. Firearms that are left loaded and unlocked are deadly hazards, and bodybuilding weights and other heavy equipment easily overwhelm toddlers who may pull these objects down on themselves. Toddlers should always be supervised closely, especially in new environments or on playground equipment.

As toddlers become more mobile, they are introduced to riding toys, tricycles, and bicycles. Nurses remind parents about the need for, and in most states the requirement of, bicycle helmets that are fitted properly and worn every time the toddler rides or is a passenger on a bicycle.

Drowning

Children between the ages of 1 and 3 years are at the highest risk of drowning, because most do not know how to swim and do not have the skills to keep their heads above water or to get out of the water. Toddlers can drown in water just deep enough to cover their noses and mouths. Although swimming pools and other natural bodies of water are a big part of the problem, even pails of water, toilets, bathtubs, and wading pools are dangerous. When toddlers fall into a pail of water or toilet it is hard for them to straighten up because all of their weight is forward. Toddlers should never be left unattended—even for a few seconds—near a bathtub, hot tub, wading or swimming pool, toilet, pail of water, or a small creek. All swimming pools should be fenced and have self-closing gates and latches. Toddlers must be supervised constantly and competently whenever they are near any body of water regardless of size and fitted properly with personal flotation devices whenever they are on a boat.

Burns

Each year more than 1 million U.S. children from birth to 6 years of age require emergency department treatment (D'Souza et al., 2009). Hot tap water, boiling water, coffee, tea, and food are the most common sources of injury resulting in scalds from hot liquids. These very painful and often debilitating injuries often occur as toddlers begin to gain mobility and explore their environments, inadvertently touching hot surfaces or spilling hot liquids on themselves. They may also put their mouths on live electrical cords or their fingers into electrical sockets and become seriously burned, as well as tip their walkers or themselves into fireplaces or woodstoves.

Nurses give parents the following reminders:

- Never eat, drink, or carry anything hot while holding a child.
- Lower the water heater temperature to 120° to 125° F.
- Never leave hot beverages or foods within a child's reach.
- Put children in a playpen while cooking.
- Never leave a toddler unattended in the bathtub. It takes only a moment to turn on the hot water.
- Put screens around fireplaces or woodstoves.
- Do not let children handle food directly from the microwave oven.
- Use burners at the back of the stove and turn pot handles in toward the stove.
- Install and maintain smoke detectors, replacing batteries annually.

Motor Vehicles

Motor vehicle–related injuries, which include both passenger and pedestrian injuries, are the primary injury in children from 1 to 4 years of age. For the toddler, passenger injury is more frequent and often involves the lack of use or misuse of child safety seats. Child safety seats, when properly installed and used, have reduced the risk of death and serious injury to children. Unfortunately, improper installation and use of child safety seats are widespread problems, with some experts reporting that more than 80% of them are misused in some way. Certified Child Passenger Safety Technicians are trained in installing car safety seats properly and can help parents make sure their children are as safe as possible on the road. To find the closest inspection station, the nurse can visit or direct parents to visit www.seatcheck.org or call toll-free 866-SEAT-CHECK (866-732-8243).

The rear-facing child safety seat supports a young child's head, neck, and spine; helps reduce stress to the neck and spinal cord in a crash; and is the car seat for a newborn. When children reach 2 years and their child safety seat's upper weight limit of 35 pounds, the nurse confirms with parents that they can switch to forward-facing child safety seats. Rear seat position is preferred and safer than the front seat for all child safety seats, and a special warning has been issued that no child should be seated in the front passenger seat if the car has airbags (AAP, 2011c) (www.exchange.aaa.com/safety/child-safety/safety-seat-guide).

During the toddler years, it is safest to keep your child in a forward-facing seat with a harness until he or she reaches the seat's maximum height or weight (40 to 65 pounds). Children can use a booster seat when they have outgrown the weight or height limit of their forward-facing harnesses. Children at this stage are not yet ready for adult safety belts and should use belt-positioning booster seats until they are at least 4 feet 9 inches tall and between 8 and 12 years old. Safety belts are designed for 165-pound male adults, so it is no wonder that research shows poorly fitting adult belts can injure children. When a child can sit with his or her back straight against the vehicle seat back cushion and knees bent over the seat edge without slouching, it is time to switch to an adult safety belt (AAP, 2011c) (www.exchange.aaa.com/safety/child-safety/safety-seat-guide). The nurse can provide a list of approved car seats and local retail outlets or agencies that sell, lend, or rent car seats.

Toddlers are also injured or killed when they are hit by drivers backing up in their own driveways and often by members of their family or nearby neighbors. They are too small to be seen by a driver backing up and quick to run out after a departing parent or relative who thinks they are still safely inside.

Biological Agents

Bioterrorism

Recent events have heightened concern about bioterrorism, and concerns about agents such as anthrax are becoming more common questions for health care providers. Nurses provide information that can assist parents in dealing with their toddler's and their own fears. Nurses encourage parents to:

- Talk about their fears and worries.
- Stick to family routines that help toddlers feel comfortable and secure.
- Supervise toddlers' television viewing.
- Educate themselves, the best protection against unnecessary fear. Toddlers will be less fearful if they see that parents are not afraid.

Many parents feel that toddlers, because of their exploratory nature and limited cognitive competence and understanding, are especially vulnerable to certain agents such as anthrax. This is accentuated by knowing that no anthrax vaccine exists for this age group. Fearful parents might request antibiotics that they can keep on hand, just in case. The nurse teaches parents that giving children antibiotics when they are not needed can do more harm than good. Many antibiotics, especially those identified for anthrax management, have serious side effects and using them when they are not needed can lead to the development of drug-resistant forms of bacteria. If this happens, the antibiotics will not be able to kill the resistant bacteria the next time the child needs the same antibiotic to treat common ear, sinus, or other infections.

The AAP website addresses numerous issues related to bioterrorism and children (www.aap.org), including the development of a teaching toolkit for parents to use with their children.

Chemical Agents

Poisoning

Studies have shown that poisoning happens 10 times more often among young children between the ages of 1 and 4 years than in their older counterparts. Toddlers between the ages of 1 and 2 years are at the greatest risk. They are becoming more mobile, enabling them to explore and discover poisonous substances in the home. These include prescription and over-the-counter medications, alcohol, household products, plants, cosmetics, lead-based paint, and cigarettes (Box 18-10). They are also at risk because they still use their mouths as a way of exploring. Although many parents take precautions against poisoning in their own homes, some forget that toddlers can be poisoned away from home, while visiting grandparents or other relatives (for example, see the Case Study and Care Plan at the end of this chapter).

The toddler, because of limited experience and cognitive level, is unaware that these items are harmful. Many emergency department calls and visits are precipitated by a toddler's ingestion of a potentially or actually harmful substance. These incidents are likely to occur in the kitchen, bathroom, bedroom, or work area and usually are discovered by the parent or caretaker who finds an open or empty container or a half-eaten leaf or other substance.

When parents or caregivers suspect that a toddler has ingested a poisonous substance, they should call the poison control center, even if the child appears perfectly healthy. Each

---

BOX 18-10   INTERVENTIONS TO PREVENT POISONING IN TODDLERS

- All household, garden, and car products should be kept out of reach.
- Keep medications out of reach in locked cabinets.
- Use childproof caps on medication.
- Keep all products and medication in their original containers for easy identification.
- No poisonous plants should be kept in the house. A list, which includes poinsettia, amaryllis, aloe vera, English ivy, mistletoe, mums, and spider plants, is available from local poison control centers.
- Avoid outdoor plants and shrubs that are poisonous, including azaleas and mums.
- Supervise toddler's activity at all times.
- Post the poison control center number (800-222-1222) next to every telephone, including your cell phone.

For more information on poison prevention and locating the closest poison control center, visit the American Association of Poison Control Centers at www.aapcc.org.

center is part of a nationwide effort to provide immediate information about poisonings. Parents should not attempt to induce vomiting without specific instructions from the center. Vomiting can cause further harm if the child is drowsy, unconscious, or convulsing; or if the substance ingested is corrosive, such as lye or a strong acid. When vomiting is recommended by the poison control center, instructions often are given to use ipecac syrup to stimulate the vomiting rapidly. This medication should be stored as carefully as any other medication or hazardous household product and replaced often because of its short shelf life.

Chronic poisonings, such as lead poisoning, are often undetected until irreversible damage has occurred. Primary prevention involves teaching parents about risk factors and dangers of lead poisoning and the importance of a diet that encourages decreasing fat intake, because lead is retained in fat. Vitamin C, calcium, and iron intake reduce lead levels in the body. Secondary prevention involves performing periodic screening of blood lead levels on all young children identified at risk. Consumer protection laws in the United States require that all toys and furniture manufactured for small children be free of lead-based paint products. However, imported toys and furniture or antique and older family furniture or paint in older houses may have been painted with a lead-based product.

DETERMINANTS OF HEALTH

Social Factors and Environment

Day Care

During the toddler years many parents return to work or decide that an experience in a group setting would be beneficial for their child. The nurse can provide counseling about the decision to place a child in day care and the resulting emotions, as well as guidelines for selecting a safe child care or day care provider (Siebel et al., 2008).

The U.S. Department of Health and Human Services Administration for Children and Families recommends a four-step approach as a guideline for selecting a child care provider or day care center (see www.acf.hhs.gov/programs/occ/parents/index.htm) (see Chapter 17):

- Interview potential child care providers and observe the program or setting.
  - Ask about cost; enrollment; ages served; daily activities; accreditation and licensing regulations; caretaker credentials and experience; and policies about visiting, illness, and nutrition.
  - Look at provider-child interactions, safety, and the quality of the learning material and toys.
- Check references.
  - Talk to parents with children in the center or being cared for by the provider about discipline and responsiveness to parents, and talk to local child care resource or referral agencies and licensing offices.
- Make a decision based on specific criteria.
  - Think about safety, values, fit for you and your toddler, and affordability.
- Get and stay involved.
  - Talk to the provider regularly about how your child is doing, to your child about what the children are doing each day, and to other parents.
  - Visit often, announced and unannounced, and at various times of the day.

Many organizations have developed guidelines and checklists on choosing child care. Child Care Aware (www.childcareaware.org or 1-800-424-2246) is a national initiative designed to improve the quality of care and increase the availability of high-quality child care in local communities. Services include helping to find child care and connecting parents with local child care resource and referral agencies. Their brochure, *Give Your Child Something That Will Last A Lifetime—Quality Child Care,* outlines the steps to finding child care and includes an observation checklist.

Regardless of the reasons for the parents wanting or needing day care for their child, the traditional expectation of caring for the young child at home continues to influence the parents' concept of what they should do for their child. Parents must be reassured that a day care environment congruent with the family environment is not detrimental to the child. If a child has been placed in a setting that is detrimental to physical or emotional development, the parent may need assistance in selecting an alternative setting. Changes in caregivers are difficult for toddlers, and regressive behaviors may surface during transition periods.

Culture and Ethnicity

Culture influences everything we do, know, and believe. Each culture possesses its own values, attitudes, and practices with regard to family and childrearing. Toddlers continue to be shaped by the cultural values and beliefs of their parents and families, the first of many socializing forces they will encounter. As their world expands, other forces and subcultures, including peers, the media, and their schools, will also be encountered.

Unlike older children, toddlers do not question the cultural practices of the family. The toddler who refuses to do certain expected things usually does so out of a need for autonomy and control rather than a questioning of beliefs. However, nurses remind parents of this, because parents may be feeling the pressure of cultural norms and expectations. This is especially true for families who have emigrated recently.

Nurses are prepared to provide culturally sensitive and competent care. Knowledge and respect for various cultural world views, customs, values, and traditions are needed to negotiate different approaches in developing a health-promotion plan with families. Health care practices are culturally influenced. For example, if a culture views immunizations as dangerous or unnecessary, the toddler may be unprotected from certain communicable diseases. Incorporation of knowledge, respect, and negotiation facilitates the development of a therapeutic relationship grounded in trust, as well as effective, high-quality health care outcomes (Burns et al., 2008).

Levels of Policy Making and Health

Toddlers are completely incapable of contributing to the economic resources of the family; however, a lack or paucity of economic resources is capable of affecting the toddler's health and well-being. Toddlers who live in poverty have higher mortality rates, poorer health, poorer growth, and more physical morbidity from respiratory tract infections, gastrointestinal tract infections, anemia, asthma, dental caries, otitis media, and visual loss, as well as higher rates of accidental injury and psychological and developmental disorders (Burns et al., 2008).

About 25% of all children in the United States are enrolled in Medicaid programs and another 10 million are uninsured. In 1997, the federal State Children's Health Insurance Program (SCHIP) was developed to address this need. Other services that are available to low-income families with toddlers include Temporary Assistance for Needy Families and the Special Supplemental Nutrition Program for Women, Infants, and Children (WIC). The nurse can play a critical role in mobilizing these resources for families.

Legislation

Local and state legislation specific to the toddler is directed primarily toward safety and injury prevention. Many states have passed laws requiring use of child safety seats, bicycle helmets, and temperature limits for household hot water heaters.

Each state has passed laws that provide protection for a child or developmentally disabled adult, define abuse and neglect, require that a report be made to a designated agency in the case of actual or suspected abuse or neglect, and define the responsibility of the protecting agency. These laws also provide for a central registry of reported cases of abuse. Nurses are aware that they are required by law to report suspected child abuse and should familiarize themselves with the child abuse and neglect laws in their states.

Based on current neuroscience and developmental research, as well as "data from a recent 50 state study of current health, child care, and family support policies," Knitzer 2008 (p. 18) proposes five care policy challenges: enacting a national family leave; expanding access to child and family programs such as Early Head Start; providing policy incentives and resources for high-quality infant and toddler child care; strengthening the early identification and treatment for infants and toddlers at risk for poor development; and building a policy framework to support, in every state, an infant and early childhood mental health infrastructure (Knitzer, 2008).

Another legislative issue for the toddler is the Education of the Handicapped Act amendment of 1986 (Public Law 99-457). This law creates programs that assist states in planning, developing, and implementing systems within states for handicapped children from birth to 3 years of age. Nurses who work with young children with disabilities need to investigate and familiarize themselves with the programs in their states.

Health Services/Delivery System

The health of toddlers is significantly affected by the health care delivery system in the place where they live (Burns et al., 2008). Private physicians, nurse practitioners, and public well-child clinics are the most frequently used resources for ongoing health maintenance or illness care for toddlers. Health professionals specializing in pediatrics often coordinate their efforts to provide optimal health care for young children. For young children who do not receive routine health care, some public clinics sponsor special immunization days. Retired health care professionals donate their time at free dental clinics for children.

Each health care visit includes an interval history, assessment of growth and development, physical assessment, discussion of age-appropriate developmental concerns, and anticipatory guidance. Immunizations are given according to the current CDC (2011) *Immunization Schedule for Children from Birth through 6 Years*. Both provider and parent schedules are easily found on the CDC website: www.cdc.gov/vaccines/schedules. The nurse informs parents that they can anticipate and keep track of their toddler's immunizations with the CDC Childhood Immunization Schedule.

Toddlers need to explore their environment to master it, and this is also valid for their health care encounters. They may need to observe and listen as their parents interact with the health care providers, be introduced to and allowed to manipulate examination equipment, and be given simple explanations and choices so that they can maintain some degree of control. Taking the time to enlist the cooperation of a toddler will make the health care visit more productive and conducive to information exchange and health care teaching.

NURSING APPLICATION

Educating parents about health promotion and disease prevention in the toddler age group is similar to that of the infant. The nurse involved with the family provides education that is focused on the physical and developmental changes that are expected to occur in the toddler stage. This is the period of life from approximately 18 months to 3 years of age.

In addition to providing education to the parents, the nurse is able to begin to teach some health-promotion activities to the toddler. Examples of this type of toddler education are nutrition and oral hygiene. At this stage of development, it is crucial that caregivers model healthy behaviors and eating patterns. Parents may need education from the nurse on providing age-appropriate food choices while discouraging the intake of empty calories.

The nurse dealing with the toddler and family can engage in screening activities. Assessments can be performed to evaluate for hearing loss and vision disturbances. Some conditions associated with vision or hearing can be treated if detected early.

As toddlers begin to explore their autonomy, they become at-risk for accidental injury. Parents should be educated about objects on which the child may climb, possibly creating a crush or entrapment injury. They should also be aware of hazardous toys, sports equipment, drowning, burns, poisoning, and motor vehicle safety. In addition to this, medical personnel must remain alert to the potential for child abuse and report any suspicious injuries.

Another important element of health promotion with the toddler age group is educating to the parents about routine health examinations and the childhood immunization schedule. Nurses need to remain informed about changes in immunization recommendations and educate families as the changes occur. Nurses working with families need to remain knowledgeable about resources available in the community that may provide free or low-cost injections.

CASE STUDY

Grandparents Provide Care: Jeremy

Mary and John are the parents of 18-month-old Jeremy. They plan to take a week-long vacation while leaving Jeremy with his grandparents at their house. Because Jeremy is the first grandchild, the older couple is eager to spend time with him, but they have expressed concern about caring for a toddler.

Reflective Questions
1. What do the parents need to discuss with the grandparents concerning safety issues?
2. What psychosocial issues of a toddler are important for both the parents and the grandparents to consider?
3. What resources are available for today's grandparents?

⊚ CARE PLAN

Grandparents Provide Care: Jeremy

*NURSING DIAGNOSIS: At Risk of Injury related to change in environment and change in primary caregiver(s)

Definition
At risk of injury as a result of environmental conditions interacting with the individual's adaptive and defensive resources

Related Factors
- Heightened level of curiosity about environment
- Lack of more mature judgment and experience
- Limited height and physical coordination

Risk Factors
- Heightened level of curiosity about environment
- Lack of more mature judgment and experience
- Limited height and physical coordination

Risk Factors
- Change in living environment to grandparents' home
- Grandparents home not "child-proofed"

- Change in primary caregiver(s) from parents to grandparents
- Grandparents not up-to-date with caregiver/safety knowledge for toddlers

Expected Outcomes
- Grandparents will receive instruction regarding toddler care/safety.
- Grandparents will take necessary precautions to childproof their home.
- Grandparents will identify available resources to assist in toddler care/safety.
- Toddler will remain free of injury while in grandparents' care.

Interventions
- Surveillance: Safety
  - Conduct a safety check in grandparents' home/community.
  - Provide a safety checklist for grandparents.
  - Assist grandparents in identifying resources/support.
- Risk Identification
  - Identify potential risk factors in grandparents' home/community.
- Teaching: Toddler Care/Safety
  - Teach grandparents about toddler care/safety issues.

Based on Johnson, M., Moorhead, S., Bulechek, G., & Butcher, H. (2011). *NANDA, NOC, and NIC linkages* (3rd ed.). St Louis: Mosby.
**NANDA Nursing Diagnoses—Definitions and Classification 2012-2014,* Herdman T.H. (ED). Copyright © 2012, 1994-2012 NANDA International. Used by arrangement with John Wiley & Sons Limited. In order to make safe and effective judgments using the NANDA-I nursing diagnoses it is essential that nurses refer to the definitions and defining characteristics of the diagnoses listed in this work.

SUMMARY

This period can be an exciting and challenging time for both toddlers and their parents. Parents who have encouraged their toddlers' desire to explore can now delight in their developing sense of adventure as they enter their preschool years. The world is a wonderful place for the toddler who has known and experienced support, affection, and protection.

REFERENCES

American Academy of Pediatrics (AAP). (2007). 2007 Position statement: Principles and guidelines for early hearing detection and intervention programs. Joint Committee on Infant Hearing. *Pediatrics, 120,* 898–921.

American Academy of Pediatrics (AAP). (2011a). *Ages & stages: Listen up about why newborn hearing screening is important.* Retrieved July 15, 2012, from www.healthychildren.org/English/ages-stages/baby/Pages/Listen-Up-About-Why-Newborn-Hearing-Screening-is-Important.

American Academy of Pediatrics (AAP). (2011b). Policy statement: Media use by children younger than 2 years. Council on Communication and Media. *Pediatrics, 128*(5), 1040–1045.

American Academy of Pediatrics (AAP). (2011c). Policy statement—child passenger safety. *Pediatrics, 127*(4), 788–793.

American Academy of Pediatrics (AAP). (2012). Policy statement: Breastfeeding and the use of human milk. *Pediatrics, 129*(3), e827–e841. doi: 10.1542/peds.2011-3552.

American Academy of Pediatrics, Healthy Children. (2012a). *Feeding and nutrition: Your two-year-old.* Retrieved July 14, 2012, from www.healthychildren.org/English/ages/Feeding-and-Nutrition-Your-Two-Year-Old.

American Academy of Pediatrics, Healthy Children. (2012b). *Juice boxes.* Retrieved July 14, 2012, from www.healthychildren.org/English/healthy-living/nutrition/Pages/Juice-Boxes.

American Academy of Pediatrics, Healthy Children. (2011c). *Where we stand: Fruit juice.* Retrieved July 14, 2012, from www.healthychildren.org/English/healthy-living/nutrition/Pages/Where-We-Stand-Fruit-Juice.

American Association for Pediatric Ophthalmology and Strabismus (AAPOS). (2012). *Amblyopia.* Retrieved July 23, 2012, from www.aapos.org/terms/conditions/21.

American Optometric Association (AOA). (2012). *Children's vision conditions.* Retrieved July 23, 2012, from www.aoa.org/x7854.xml.

Bath-Hextall, F. J., Delamere, F. M., & Williams, H. C. (2008). Dietary exclusions for established atopic eczema. *Cochrane Database of Systematic Reviews 2008, 1,* (CD005203).

Berger, K. S. (2011). *The developing person through the life span* (6th ed.). New York: Worth.

Bergman, A., & Harpaz-Rotem, I. (2004). Revisiting rapprochement in the light of contemporary developmental theories. *Journal of the American Psychoanalytic Association, 52*(2), 555–570. doi: 10.1002/14651858.CD005203.pub2.

Boyle, R. J., Bath-Hextall, F. J., Leonardi-Bee, J., Murrell, D. F., & Tang, M. L.K. (2008). Probiotics for treating eczema. *Cochrane Database of Systematic Reviews 2008, 4,* (CD006135). doi: 10.1002/14651858.CD006135.pub2.

Burns, C. E., Dunn, A. M., Brady, M. A., Stan, N. B., & Blosser, C. (2009). *Pediatric primary care* (4th ed.). St. Louis: W.B. Saunders.

Caughy, M., Huang, K., & Lima, J. (2009). Patterns of conflict interaction in mother-toddler dyads: Differences between depressed and nondepressed mothers. *Journal of Child and Family Studies, 18*(1), 10–20.

Centers for Disease Control and Prevention. (2010a). *Child maltreatment—Facts at a glance.* Retrieved July 1, 2012, from www.cdc.gov/ViolencePrevention/pub/CM_datasheet.html.

Centers for Disease Control and Prevention. (2010b). *Growth charts: CDC and WHO*. Retrieved July 1, 2012, from www.cdc.gov/growthcharts.

Centers for Disease Control and Prevention. (2010c). *Understand child maltreatment: Fact sheet*. Retrieved July 1, 2012, from www.cdc.gov/violenceprevention/pdf/CM-FactSheet-a.pdf.

Centers for Disease Control and Prevention. (2011). *Immunization schedules*. Retrieved July 1, 2012, from www.cdc.gov/vaccines/recs/schedules/default.htm#child.

Centers for Disease Control and Prevention. (2012a). *Child maltreatment: Risk and protective factors*. Retrieved July 1, 2012, from www.cdc.gov/ViolencePrevention/childmaltreatment/riskprotectivefactors.html.

Centers for Disease Control and Prevention. (2012b). *Learning the signs, act early: Developmental milestones*. Retrieved July 1, 2012, from www.cdc.gov/ncbddd/actearly/milestones/index.html.

Christakis, D. A., Gilkerson, J., Richards, J. A., Zimmerman, F. J., Garrison, M. M., Xu, D., et al. (2009). Audible television and decreased adult words, infant vocalizations, and conversational turns. *Archives of Pediatric and Adolescent Medicine, 163*(6), 554–558.

Del Vecchio, T., & O'Leary, S. G. (2008). Predicting maternal discipline responses to early childhood aggression: The role of cognitions and affect. *Parenting: Science & Practice, 8*(3), 240–256.

D'Souza, A. L., Nelson, N. G., & McKenzie, L. B. (2009). Pediatric burn injuries treated in U.S. emergency departments between 1990 and 2006. *Pediatrics, 124*(5), 1424–1430.

Erikson, E. H. (1995). *Childhood & society* (35th anniversary ed.). New York: Norton.

Erikson, E. H. (1998). *The life cycle completed*. New York: Norton.

Gartstein, M. A., & Bateman, A. E. (2008). Early manifestations of childhood depression: Influences of infant temperament and parental depressive symptoms. *Infants and Child Development, 17*(3), 223–248.

Garzon, D. L., Lee, R. K., & Homan, S. M. (2007). There's no place like home: A preliminary study of toddler unintentional injury. *Journal of Pediatrics Nursing, 22*(5), 368–375.

Genesee, F. (2008). Early dual language learning. *Zero to Three, 29*(1), 17–23.

Grummer-Strawn, L. M., Reinhold, C., & Krebs, N. F. (2010). Use of World Health Organization and CDC growth charts for children aged 0—59 months in the United States. *Morbidity and Mortality Weekly Report (MMWR), 59*(rr09).

Hagan, J. F., Shaw, J. S., & Duncan, P. M. (Eds.), (2008). *Bright futures: Guidelines for health supervision of infants, children, and adolescents* (3rd ed.). Elk Grove Village, IL: American Academy of Pediatrics.

Hockenberry, M. J., & Wilson, D. (Eds.), (2011). *Wong's nursing care of infants and children* (9th ed.). St. Louis: Mosby/Elsevier.

Holt, K., Wookdridge, N. H., Story, M., & Sofka, D. (2011). *Bright futures: Nutrition* (3rd ed.). Elk Grove Village, IL: American Academy of Pediatrics.

Knitzer, J. (2008). Giving infants and toddlers a head start: Getting policies in sync with knowledge. *Infants and Young Children, 21*(1), 18–29.

Kolak, A. M., & Vernon-Feagans, L. (2008). Family-level coparenting processes and child gender as moderators of family stress and toddler adjustment. *Infant and Child Development, 17*(6), 617–638.

More, J. (2008). Don't forget the undernourished children in our midst. *Journal of Family Health Care, 18*(5), 159–160.

Neuman, S. B., & Dickinson, D. K. (2011). *Handbook of early literacy research*. (Vol. 3). New York: Guilford Press.

Norris, F. W. (2008). Decision-making criteria in child custody disputes that involve requests for overnight visits with infants and toddlers: Derived from a review of the literature. *Journal of Child Custody, 4*(3–4), 33–43.

Pan, B. A., Rowe, M. L., Singer, J. D., & Snow, C. E. (2005). Maternal correlates of growth in toddler vocabulary production in low-income families. *Child Development, 76*(4), 763–782.

Robins, D. L. (2008). Screening for autism spectrum disorders in primary care settings. *Autism: The International Journal of Research and Practice, 12*(5), 537–556.

Rosales, F. J., & Zeisel, S. H. (2008). Perspectives from the symposium: The role of nutrition in infant and toddler brain and behavioral development. *Nutritional Neuroscience, 11*(3), 135–143.

Seidel, H. M., Ball, J. W., Dains, J. E., Flynn, J. A., Solomon, H. S., & Stewart, R. W. (2011). *Mosby's guide to physical examination* (7th ed.). St. Louis: Mosby.

Siebel, N. L., Gillespie, L. C., & Temple, T. (2008). The role of child care providers in child abuse prevention. *Zero to Three, 28*(6), 33–40.

Treyvaud, K., Anderson, V. A., Howard, K., Bear, M., Hunt, R. W., Doyle, L. W., et al. (2009). Parenting behavior is associated with the early neurobehavioral development of very pre term children. *Pediatrics, 123*(2), 555–561.

U.S. Department of Health and Human Services, & Office of Disease Prevention and Health Promotion. (2010). *Healthy People 2020*. Washington, DC: USDHHS. Retrieved July 1, 2012, from www.healthypeople.gov.

Warren, H. K., Denham, S. A., & Bassert, H. H. (2008). The emotional foundations of social understanding. *Zero to Three, 28*(5), 32–39.

Weinfield, N., Ingerski, L., & Moreau, S. (2009). Maternal and paternal depressive symptoms as predictors of toddler adjustment. *Journal of Child and Family Studies, 18*(1), 39–47.

Wetherby, A. M., Brosnan-Maddox, S., Peace, V., & Newton, L. (2008). Validation of the Infant-Toddler Checklist as broadband screener of autism spectrum disorders from 9 to 24 months of age. *Autism, 12*(5), 487–511.

Zimmerman, F. J., & Bell, J. F. (2010). Associations of television content type and obesity in children. *American Journal of Public Health, 100*(2), 334–340.

Preschool Child

Anne Rath Rentfro

ⓔvolve WEBSITE

http://evolve.elsevier.com/Edelman/

- Study Questions
- Glossary

- Website Resources
  19A: Recommended Literature for Preschool Children
  19B: Healthy Eating for Preschoolers
  19C: Childproof Your Home from Poisons

OBJECTIVES

After completing this chapter, the reader will be able to:

- Explain physical and psychosocial changes occurring during the preschool years that influence child and family health needs.
- Discuss the concepts of cognitive development of preschoolers using Piaget's theory.
- Review *Healthy People 2020* concepts that pertain to preschool children and their families.
- Describe family teaching and nursing support for the typical sleep disturbances of the preschooler years.

- Differentiate the nursing roles regarding vision and hearing screening for preschoolers.
- Compare coping skills of preschoolers with those of younger children.
- Outline primary prevention immunization requirements for preschoolers.
- Identify warning signs of cancer in preschoolers.
- List risk factors for asthma in preschoolers.
- Identify major causes of injuries during the preschool years.

KEY TERMS

Acquired lactase deficiency	Heterophoria	Otitis media
Acute lymphocytic leukemia	Heterotropia	Parental divorce
Amblyopia	Homeostasis	Peabody Picture Vocabulary Test
Asthma	Induction	Preoperational stage
Centering	Induction explanation	Preschool Readiness Experimental
Chloroma	Initiative	Screening Scale (PRESS)
Deduction	Irreversibility	Quiet
Doll or puppet play	Ishihara's test	Receptive language
Draw-a-Person and Draw-a-Family tests	Lactose intolerance	Refractive errors
	Mnemonic techniques	Retinoblastoma
Early and Periodic Screening, Diagnosis, and Treatment (EPSDT)	Mutual storytelling	Snellen E chart
	Myopic vision	Strabismus
Eccrine sweat gland function	Neuroblastoma	Transductive reasoning
Egocentrism	Nightmares	Vineland Social Maturity Scale
Expressive language	Night terrors	Wilms tumor

objectives related to this developmental stage (U.S. Department of Health and Human Services, 2011).

THINK ABOUT IT

Aggressive Behavior

Phillip, age 4, started preschool 2 weeks ago after spending his early years at home with his mother and his 18-month-old sister. His mother recently returned to her job as an accountant, works 9 hours a day, and is fatigued when she picks up Phillip at 5:00 PM. Phillip's father travels for his job but is home on weekends to spend time with his family. Although Phillip's mother always believed that Phillip was shy because he was quiet, during the last week at child care he started hitting his peers and becoming loudly vocal at story time. His mother, believing that Phillip's behavior is related to her return to work, feels embarrassed and frustrated by his behavior, especially because she enjoys her new job and the extra income.

- *What factors might be contributing to Phillip's changed behavior?*
- *How might you define Phillip's temperament? Why?*
- *What discussions might you have with Phillip's parents to help them understand, respond to, and change their son's behavior for the better?*

The preschool child (ages 3 to 6 years) has a more developed body structure, an ability to control and use the body, and a facility with language that more closely resembles that of the adult than that of the toddler. The major psychological thrust of this period of development is mastery of self as an independent human being, with a willingness to extend experiences beyond those of the family. Although historically the end of early childhood in the Western world was marked by entrance into the formalized educational system, increasing numbers of children in the United States begin formalized schooling during their preschool years. Box 19-1: *Healthy People 2020* presents

BIOLOGY AND GENETICS

The protuberant abdomen of the toddler disappears during the preschool years as the pelvis begins to straighten and the abdominal muscles develop. Hips gradually rotate inward, replacing out-toeing with straight or slight in-toeing. Mild in-toeing (metatarsus adductus) may remain during the preschool years, but anything beyond a mild level should be investigated and treated.

Growth rates remain steady from ages 3 to 6 years. Average preschoolers gain approximately 2 kg (4 pounds) of body weight and 7 cm (2 inches) of height each year, whereas head circumference increases less than 2 cm during the entire preschool period. During early childhood, skin matures in its ability to protect the child from outer invasion and loss of fluids. The skin's capacity to localize infection increases but remains less than that of a mature person. Negligible secretion of sebum makes the skin fairly dry. Changes occur both in color and in texture of the hair. Hair usually turns darker and becomes straighter. Eccrine sweat gland function, part of the body's heat-regulation mechanism, gradually matures, but the quantity of eccrine sweat produced in response to heat or emotion remains minimal. Apocrine sweat glands, located primarily in the axillae, areolas of the breast, and the anal area, remain nonsecretory during this period.

Kidneys reach full functional maturity by the end of infancy and early toddlerhood with only their size changing during the

BOX 19-1 HEALTHY PEOPLE 2020

Selected National Health-Promotion and Disease-Prevention Objectives for Preschool Children

- Increase the proportion of children and youth with disabilities who spend at least 80% of their time in regular education programs.
- (Developmental) Increase the proportion of preschool Early Head Start and Head Start programs that provide health education to prevent health problems in the following areas: unintentional injury; violence; tobacco use and addiction; alcohol and drug use; unhealthy dietary patterns; and inadequate physical activity, dental health, and safety.
- Reduce blood lead levels in children.
- Reduce exposure to selected environmental chemicals in the population, as measured by blood and urine concentrations of the substances or their metabolites.
- (Developmental) Increase the proportion of children who are ready for school in all five domains of healthy development: physical development, social-emotional development, approaches to learning, language, and cognitive development.
- Increase the proportion of parents who use positive parenting and communicate with their doctors or other health care professionals about positive parenting.
- (Developmental) Decrease the proportion of children who have poor quality of sleep.
- Reduce infections caused by key pathogens transmitted commonly through food. (FS–1.5: postdiarrheal hemolytic-uremic syndrome [HUS] in children under 5 years of age)

- Achieve and maintain effective vaccination coverage levels for universally recommended vaccines among young children.
- Reduce fatal and nonfatal injuries.
- Reduce child maltreatment deaths.
- Increase the proportion of children with special health care needs who receive their care in family-centered, comprehensive, coordinated systems.
- Increase the number of states with nutrition standards for foods and beverages provided to preschool-aged children in child care.
- (Developmental) Prevent inappropriate weight gain in youths and adults (11.1 children ages 2 to 5 years).
- Reduce iron deficiency among young children and females of childbearing age (21.1 children ages 1 to 2 years).
- Reduce the proportion of young children ages 3 to 5 years with dental caries experience in their primary teeth.
- Increase the proportion of children and adolescents ages 2 years through 12th grade who view television, watch videos, or play video games for no more than 2 hours a day. (PA–8.2.1: children ages 2 to 5 years)
- Reduce asthma deaths (1.1 children and adults under age 35 years).
- Reduce the proportion of nonsmokers exposed to secondhand smoke (11.1 children ages 3 to 11 years).
- Increase the proportion of preschool children ages 5 years and under who receive vision screening.

U.S. Department of Health and Human Services. (2011). *Healthy People 2020 topics and objectives.* Retrieved July 7, 2011, from www.healthypeople.gov/2020/topicsobjectives2020/default.aspx.

preschool years. By the end of the preschool years, urine excretion totals from 650 to 1000 mL (19 to 30 ounces). Under normal homeostatic conditions, the preschooler's renal system conserves water and concentrates urine on a level that approximates adult abilities. Under conditions of stress, however, their kidneys lack the ability to respond fully and to maintain homeostasis when compared with the more rapid response of the adult renal system.

Growth of gastrointestinal organs continues through the preschool years without functional changes. Children achieve full voluntary control of elimination. Lactose intolerance, intolerance to milk products manifested by diarrhea, often appears during the preschool years. This condition, more common in Black, Asian American, and Native American children, can be managed successfully by eliminating lactose from the diet.

Lung capacity continues to increase, with a gradual decrease in respiratory rate. Preschoolers make better decisions than toddlers about objects they place in their mouths, resulting in fewer instances of choking and obstruction. A gradual increase in the size and shape of the ears coincides with decreases in the incidence of otitis media (middle ear infection). Tonsils and adenoids are large compared to their throat, which may contribute to noisy breathing and upper respiratory tract infection in preschoolers.

The cardiovascular system enlarges in proportion to general body growth. Heart rate for preschoolers ranges from 40 to 70 beats per minute with a mean blood pressure of 100/60 mm Hg. Early hypertension develops in some children during the preschool years; therefore, measuring blood pressure routinely is indicated, particularly in children with a strong family history of hypertension (see Chapter 20). Preschool children maintain adequate hemoglobin levels when dietary intake is sufficient. Bone marrow of the ribs, the sternum, and the vertebrae become fully established as primary sites for red blood cell formation. The liver and spleen continue to form erythrocytes and granulocytes.

The immune system continues to develop. Preschoolers boost their immune response to common pathogens as exposure occurs. Group activities, such as joining preschool or play groups, increase exposure and subsequently escalate the incidence of common contagious illnesses during the time of exposure, regardless of the child's age. Initial encounters with such group activities usually result in increases in illness. Later these children may be less prone to common contagious diseases because of their early exposure to infectious illnesses and their consequent immunity.

Primary teeth finish erupting by late toddler or early preschool years. Initial permanent teeth generally erupt toward the end of the preschool period. Permanent teeth tend to erupt approximately 6 months earlier in girls than in boys. Older preschoolers usually take responsibility for dental hygiene, although all children need gentle guidance about proper brushing and appropriate nutritional intake for healthy teeth. Parents should continue to assist with brushing and supervise flossing and fluoride intake. Fluoride intake plays an in important role in the preschool period when development of tooth enamel presents a more sensitive environment for fluoride, resulting in opacity of the permanent teeth when the child ingests more than the recommended intake (Oganessian, Ivancakova, Lencova, & Broukal, 2011). Balancing between this risk of opacity and the prevention of caries involves assessing the amounts of fluoride the child receives from various sources. Fluoride sources include public water supply in some regions, foods, drinks, fluoride supplements, and accidently swallowed toothpaste (Oganessian et al., 2011). Because the preschool period is an age of caries formation, regular dental check-ups are essential. Nurses assess whether the child is receiving preventive dental care. Parents should be encouraged to begin or maintain this care. Suggestions for promoting good oral hygiene as part of general health-promotion teaching can be found in Chapter 20.

Musculoskeletal and neurological development reaches a level that allows for seemingly effortless walking, running, and climbing. Older preschoolers' ability to copy figures and draw recognizable pictures indicates their advancing fine motor abilities, and they are eager to demonstrate these skills to others. Practice, increases in muscle size, continuing associations among existing neural pathways, and the establishment of new pathways for already accomplished tasks are a few of the many complex factors that contribute to the advances in neurological function observed during early childhood. These advances in fine motor and gross motor skills are outlined in Table 19-1.

TABLE 19-1   GROWTH AND DEVELOPMENT

Developmental and Behavioral Milestones for Preschool Children

AGE	EXPECTATIONS
3 years	At this age, the typical child: • Opens doors • Kicks a ball; jumps in place; rides on a tricycle • Builds a tower of nine cubes; imitates bridge made from three cubes • Demonstrates speech that is mostly intelligible (The child who fails to speak in sentences or whose speech is unintelligible to strangers should be referred for speech, language, and hearing evaluation.) • Knows own name, age, and gender • May comprehend cold, tired, hungry; may understand the prepositions over and under; differentiates bigger and smaller; can convey the use of scissors, key, and pencil • Copies a circle, may imitate a cross, and begins to visually discriminate colors • Describes action in picture books and shows some early imaginative behavior • Puts on some clothing and shoes • Eats without assistance

Continued

TABLE 19-1   GROWTH AND DEVELOPMENT

Developmental and Behavioral Milestones for Preschool Children—cont'd

AGE	EXPECTATIONS
4 years	At this age, the typical child:

- Alternates feet when descending stairs; jumps forward; hops on one foot, and can stand on 1 foot for up to 5 seconds
- Climbs a ladder
- Rides a tricycle or a bicycle with training wheels
- Can walk on tiptoes
- Throws a ball overhand
- Holds and uses a pencil with good control
- Builds a tower of 10 or more cubes
- Is able to cut and paste
- Gives first and last name
- Engages in conversational give-and-take
- Asks, why, when, how, and inquires about meanings of words
- Talks about daily experiences and things that are used at home (food, appliances)
- Can name three or four primary colors
- Can count from 1 to 5
- Enjoys jokes
- Can sing a song
- Knows about things used at home (e.g., food, appliances)
- Washes and dries hands and brushes teeth
- Dresses and undresses with supervision, except for handling laces and buttons, when allowed sufficient time to dress; begins to be selective about clothes
- Initiates dramatic make-believe and dress-up play during which the child assumes a specific role
- Is imaginative and intensely curious
- Distinguishes between fantasy and reality
- Has formed gender identification
- Copies a cross and a circle
- Draws a person with two to three parts
- Enjoys the companionship of other children, plays cooperatively, and shows interest in other children's bodies
- Meets the challenges of kindergarten class
- Rides with training wheels
- Is aware of gender of others

5 years	At this age, the typical child:

- May be able to skip; can walk on tiptoes; broad jumps
- Can cut and paste
- Names four or five colors and can identify coins
- Tells a simple story and knows several nursery rhymes
- Defines at least one word (ball, shoe, chair, table, dog)
- Dresses and undresses without supervision
- Knows address and telephone number
- Can count on fingers
- Copies a triangle from an illustration
- Recognizes many letters of the alphabet
- Prints some letters
- Draws a person with a head, body, arms, and legs
- Begins to understand right and wrong, fair and unfair
- Engages in dramatic make-believe and dress-up play during which the child assumes a specific role; engages in domestic role playing and dressing up
- Enjoys the companionship of other children; plays cooperatively
- Has formed gender identification ("Are you a boy or girl?")

6 years	At this age, the typical child:

- Bounces a ball 4 to 6 times; throws and catches
- Skates
- Rides a bicycle
- Ties shoelaces
- Counts up to 10; prints own first name; prints numbers up to 10
- Understands right from left
- Draws a person with six body parts, with the figure depicted wearing clothing

Modified from American Academy of Pediatrics. Retrieved from http://brightfutures.aap.org/.

Gender

Boys tend to experience more childhood illnesses than do girls during ages 3 to 6 (see Chapter 18). Preschoolers are more aware of their sexual identity than are toddlers and may imitate societal stereotypes more closely. Traditionally boys have been encouraged to take more risks than girls have been and they have more accidents than do preschool girls, who may have been encouraged to choose more sedentary activities. For example, in their study of 476 preschool children (50% male), Brown and colleagues (2009) found that 3-year-old males were more active than 3-year-old females. In today's society, boys and girls have more opportunities to choose the same activities, but preschool activities can also be geared to be gender neutral to encourage more female participation. Gender-neutral activities such as tag, hide and seek, kick ball, duck duck goose, red rover, and obstacle courses may encourage physical activity for both boys and girls. Whether societal changes or preschool policy changes will reflect accident or obesity statistics in the future will be interesting to observe.

Race

Race, with its related economic and cultural issues, can influence health care practices at this age, as is the case during all ages. Cultural preferences and economic issues, therefore, influence the environments and other health-promoting behaviors, such as nutrition and recreation (Brown et al., 2009; Division of Adolescent and School Health, National Center for Chronic Disease Prevention and Health Promotion, 2011; Dogra et al., 2010; Lee & Im, 2010).

Genetics

Signs and symptoms of most genetic problems appear during infancy or the toddler years, whereas other genetic problems will be noted during adolescence. Those most likely to appear during the preschool years are cystic fibrosis, Duchenne's muscular dystrophy, fragile X syndrome, Williams syndrome, and autism, which is generally considered a genetic disorder with a high degree (90%) of heritability (Freitag et al., 2010). These disorders, characterized by aberrant social interaction, communication, and stereotyped patterns of behavior, affect 0.5% to 1.0% of the population and often are diagnosed or suspected in the preschool years when social interaction plays a larger role in development (Boyd et al., 2010; Freitag et al., 2010).

Genetic conditions diagnosed early in life affect the child's health, and nursing strategies focus on continuing parent education, assessing the child's development (including complications), and providing interventions to support family coping (Boyd et al., 2010).

GORDON'S FUNCTIONAL HEALTH PATTERNS

Health Perception–Health Management Pattern

Preschoolers have a fairly accurate perception of the external parts of their own bodies based on what they can see and do; they may be extremely curious about the body of a member of the opposite sex. Their concepts of what is inside the body

and how its internal functions operate are vague and inaccurate. Preschoolers view the internal part of the body as hollow. Most preschoolers can name one or two items inside the body (blood, bones). Many of their questions involve body functions. Anxiety surrounding the body and fear of mutilation and death pervade the children's concerns. Their size as compared with that of adults produces a sense of vulnerability and fear of loss of control (Price & Gwinn, 2008).

By age 4 or 5, children have amassed their beliefs about health from the family. They begin to understand that they play a role in their own health. The preschooler often becomes upset over minor injuries. Pain or illness may be viewed as a punishment. The preschooler's declaration, "If you don't put your seat belt on you will get in an accident" is a statement that reflects the idea of expected immediate and absolute cause and effect. The preschooler cannot conceive that the purpose of the seat belt is to prevent injury in the event of an accident, not prevention of the accident itself.

Although preschoolers are not completely responsible for their own health management, they certainly contribute by brushing their teeth, taking medication, wearing appropriate clothing for inclement weather, and performing other actions. Preschoolers' memory for these activities can be sporadic, but they are at least beginning to be their own health care agents (Yoo et al., 2010).

Reinforcement of health-promotion activities, which occurs in the home and child care environments, helps to instill behaviors that affect self-esteem, safety, and an individual's overall balance with life. For example, family support for active lifestyles provides one way for parents to assume a positive role to model for children (Division of Adolescent and School Health, National Center for Chronic Disease Prevention and Health Promotion, 2011). The National Association of Pediatric Nurse Practitioners has designed *Healthy Eating and Activity Together (HEAT)* resources to engage families in health-promoting behaviors (Gance-Cleveland et al., 2009).

In addition, the preschool environment influences health-promotion activities for many children in this age group. For example, when Brown and colleagues (2009) directly observed children in 20 preschool settings, they demonstrated that aspects of the preschool environment affected children's activity levels. Preschool settings with more resources also offered a greater variety of activities. Even these preschools with more resources were well below the physical activity time recommended (120 minutes per day) by the National Association for Sport and Physical Education (National Association for Sport and Physical Education, 2009). Their findings provide further support for those of Bower and colleagues (2008), who demonstrated that in preschool settings children participated in physical activity about 80 more minutes in settings with more resources than those children in settings with fewer resources. These findings indicate a need for health-promotion advocacy and policy development focused on environment. Many community bookstores carry health-promotion–focused books appropriate to the preschool population; these references provide information for discussion among parents, caregivers, and children on the importance of healthy behaviors for success in life. See **Website Resource 19A** for a detailed list of recommended books.

Nutritional-Metabolic Pattern

Establishing healthful nutritional and physical activity behaviors begins during childhood. Children should eat a variety of foods with at least five servings of fruits and vegetables per day. Children ages 3 to 5 years old should receive 1200 to 1600 calories per day depending on their activity level and gender (U.S. Department of Agriculture & U.S. Department of Health and Human Services, 2010). Preschool children should consume approximately half of their diet in carbohydrates, with the other half consisting of protein (≈5% to 20%) and fat (≈20% to 35%) (U.S. Department of Agriculture & U.S. Department of Health and Human Services, 2010). With more than half of the preschool diet consisting of carbohydrates, whole grains and other complex carbohydrates should be plentiful in order to attain a total fiber intake of 20 to 25 grams per day (U.S. Department of Agriculture & U.S. Department of Health and Human Services, 2010). Fat requirements in preschool children are higher than those for older children, but fat consumption should consist primarily of unsaturated fat, with saturated fat, trans fatty acids, and cholesterol intake as low as possible. Guidance for these recommendations along with types and amounts of foods is depicted in the systems called MyPyramid and Choose My Plate (www.choosemyplate.gov/). A child-friendly version of MyPyramid addresses the special needs of children 6 to 11 years old (Nappo-Dattoma, 2010). Preschoolers need approximately 90 kcal/kg of body weight per day for health maintenance, activity, and growth. **Website Resource 19B** lists suggestions for healthy eating including a daily food plan. Preschooler dietary patterns are unique to their age group, making estimates for consumption of nutrients difficult. Generally, estimates for preschoolers are adapted from food intake patterns of other age groups (Hockenberry & Wilson, 2010).

Specific issues that impact the preschool age include bone growth, iron-deficiency anemia, milk intake, salt intake, sugar intake, and dentition. Bone growth needs in 1- to 8-year-old children require a calcium intake of approximately 700 to 1000 mg. Although iron-deficiency anemia is decreasing generally, it is more prevalent in vulnerable populations (McCann & Ames, 2007). Studies that have been conducted, although small in number, demonstrate support for the idea that iron deficiency results in behavioral and cognitive deficits (McCann & Ames, 2007). Salt and sugar intake should be moderate. The contribution of sugar intake to caries development is well established. For example, Warren's study group (Warren et al., 2009) examined factors associated with cariogenicity in 128 children. Their study suggests that sweetened beverages, in particular, are associated with development of caries.

Nutrition and dentition impact health at all ages. Pain from dental caries, infection, and poorly maintained teeth affects appetite and chewing ability with a subsequent impact on future nutritional status. Dental caries in children have declined dramatically in recent years because of preventive measures such as use of fluoride toothpaste, fluoridation of community water supplies, implementation of sound dietary practices, and use of

dental sealants. Children from low-income families carry the bulk of the burden of these dental caries (Nappo-Dattoma, 2011). Oral health promotion involves self-care and population-based initiatives, along with professional care. Adequacy of professional dental care varies significantly by age, race, educational level, family income, and dental status (Nappo-Dattoma, 2011). Nurses interface with families in a variety of these settings and are therefore in an ideal position to impact dental health promotion.

As early childhood progresses, intense food preferences emerge. This behavior is a natural outgrowth of the increased physical capacity to react to the taste and textures of foods and the realization that expressing an opinion about food is a way to control the environment. Older preschoolers frequently refuse to try new foods. Favorite foods for this age are meat, cereal grains, baked products, fruits, and sweets. Selecting finger foods that facilitate independence helps the preschooler learn to eat without assistance. Examples of appropriate nutritional foods include cheese, crackers, small pieces of meat, and celery stuffed with cheese or peanut butter. Parents' support for food choices has been demonstrated to be an effective strategy to promote healthy food choices in this age group (Marshall et al., 2011). Parents should provide nutritious foods, avoiding salty and sweet foods. Parents should encourage good nutritional habits to help establish healthy eating behaviors. Increased consumption of fats and processed foods along with diminished physical activity have contributed to a significant increase in obesity and type 2 diabetes in children and adolescents (Liou et al., 2010; U.S. Department of Agriculture & U.S. Department of Health and Human Services, 2010; U.S. Department of Health and Human Services, 2011). Family tolerance for individual food preferences varies, and children vary in their tendency to develop strong likes and dislikes. When families reach extreme differences over food preferences, major conflicts may arise requiring insightful counseling to achieve a mutually satisfying solution. For example, some families may institute a "take a little taste before your refuse" standard for foods at the preschool age. Nurses collaborate with families to discover comfortable approaches to maintain nutritional adequacy of foods that children prefer. Community nurses use a variety of approaches and recognize the wide range of possibilities that exist for families of varying cultures.

Preschoolers begin to eat meals away from home more often than toddlers. Minimal standards require licensed child care centers and preschools to serve foods using recommended dietary allowances of basic nutrients. Parents should communicate regularly with agency personnel about foods eaten at home and away to provide healthy food variety. Preschoolers in group settings learn both positive and negative eating habits and food preferences from care providers and other children. School settings are ideal for community health nurses to impact nutritional patterns of the preschool child (Water, 2011). Communication about nutritional intake habits reinforces positive behaviors and discourages negative habits at home (Box 19-2: Innovative Practice).

Preschoolers struggle with the intricacies of using utensils. In the later years of the preschool period, children attain skill with spoons, demonstrate fair proficiency with forks, and manage knives for spreading soft foods on bread or crackers. Most preschool children, however, need help cutting meat and pouring from large, heavy containers. Preschoolers enjoy helping to prepare family meals and may be capable of simple tasks, such as washing fruits and vegetables. Involving young children in meal preparation teaches them about healthy nutrition. Sharing important family functions nurtures self-esteem and a sense of value.

The prevalence of food allergy in children in the United States continues to increase, affecting up to 8% of children. About 1 million preschool children are affected and one third of these children have the potential for a severe reaction (Fleischer et al., 2012; Gupta et al., 2011). Most allergies develop before the age of 2. Foods most likely to cause allergic reactions in the preschool age group include milk, eggs, and peanuts (Fleischer et al., 2012; Gupta et al., 2011). Reactions to peanuts tend to decrease over time; however, children who experience peanut allergy should avoid allergens and parents should receive written emergency plans along with instructions for epinephrine injection (Fleischer et al., 2012). Clear food labeling and education are essential for preventing allergic reactions. Many preschools have banned foods such as peanut products as a precautionary measure. Parents may

BOX 19-2 INNOVATIVE PRACTICE

Healthy Start

Risk factors for cardiovascular diseases are prevalent by 3 years of age, the most common of which are hypercholesterolemia and obesity. Healthy Start, a project located in Valhalla, New York, sponsored by the Child Health Foundation and the American Health Foundation, is a 3-year demonstration and research program to evaluate the effectiveness of interventions for reducing cardiovascular risk factors in preschool centers. Two interventions are recommended. The first is that the preschool food service be designed to reduce the total fat in the preschooler's meals and snacks to less than 30% of calories and to reduce saturated fat to less than 10% of calories. The second intervention is a comprehensive preschool health education curriculum, which focuses on nutrition and exercise.

The effectiveness of this program is evaluated using many components. Changes in the nutritional behaviors (including dietary intake of school snacks and meals of the preschoolers) are being recorded, as are those in snacks and meals consumed at home. Special attention is being given to the intake of total and saturated fat. Additionally, changes in the health knowledge of preschoolers are being assessed to evaluate the education component. Physical examination data include semiannual assessments of growth and body weight and blood lipid levels.

The specific details of the rationale and methods of the randomized, controlled trial studies within the Healthy Start project are described at its website: www.healthy-start.com.

Contact Information
Healthy-Start, LLC
Healthy-Start Preschool Education
PO Box 115
Huntington, NY 11743
Telephone: (631) 549-0010
Fax: (631) 549-0010
E-mail: info@healthy-start.com

need help identifying potential hazardous situations and communicating their child's needs to agency personnel. A food allergy action plan that includes a written emergency plan should be developed for parents to use to facilitate communication regarding the child's allergies. Educational resources are available at www.cofargroup.org/.

Elimination Pattern

Toilet training is an important milestone in child development (Kaerts et al., 2012). Older preschool children are capable of and responsible for independent toileting. Their verbal skills have developed to better communicate their needs, they begin to insist on performing independently, and they are proud of accomplishments (Kaerts et al., 2012). These developmental achievements provide additional signs for independence with elimination patterns. They may forget to flush the toilet or wash their hands when they are rushed, but they have the physical ability to perform the skills. Preschoolers should not be teased or punished when they are unable to perform independently. If their clothing becomes soiled, they should be responsible for changing their clothes and reminded gently and encouragingly of ways to avoid problems in the future. (Enuresis and encopresis are discussed in Chapter 20.)

Activity-Exercise Pattern

Play continues to be the primary activity for preschoolers as well as for toddlers; however, preschoolers explore intently and demonstrate increased coordination and confidence with motor activities. They venture farther from home than toddlers. Many activities involve other children (Figure 19-1) and involve modeling behavior. Particularly in group care settings, children should be monitored for safe activities that enhance gross and fine motor skills while creating fun in movement.

Most 4-year-old children separate easily from their parents, play simple interactive games, dress themselves, copy a number of basic geometric figures well, and draw recognizable people. Preschoolers enjoy using language skills to tell stories and ask questions. Their physical abilities include balancing on one foot, jumping, and running (Driscoll & Nagel, 2008). Generally,

FIGURE 19-1 Preschool children enjoy a new pet with their friends and teacher.

preschoolers appreciate an audience, enjoy practicing new skills, and demonstrate mastered skills to others. Play constitutes an important role in preschoolers' social and psychological development. Play offers a vehicle that allows them to explore while experimenting with who they are, who they might become, and how they relate to others socially. The drama of play allows preschoolers to view themselves from another perspective. Play often reveals the child's reality and complex perception of the world.

Children mimic the behavior of people familiar to them, expanding their representation beyond self and rehearsing what has been demonstrated to them as appropriate behavior (Driscoll & Nagel, 2008). Young children seldom assume the role of a younger child or infant while playing. They usually assume adult roles and use a doll for the younger child. Through play preschoolers learn to exert control over their own behavior. Assuming an adult role in play allows children to consciously adopt more mature behaviors. Patterns of behavior used in play can be transferred to actual situations. For example, children who express their anger in a play situation aggressively by vocalizing their distress, scolding the offending party, or using withdrawal of attention are likely to respond with aggression or tantrum behavior when facing frustration or anger in real life situations. Observing children at play, as seen by the study group Brown and colleagues (2009) employed in their research, reveals natural physical capacities of children better than observation in an examination or testing environment and provides further evidence of the child's social and inner development for use by practitioners in the field.

Observing symbolic play and imitation play in peer groups helps nurses assess social competency as their perceptions unfold (Driscoll & Nagel, 2008). At first the new child in a peer group may be expected to stand back and observe other children before manipulating a toy. Preschool children engage in more interactive play, particularly dramatic play, than at any other age. Two or more children may become involved in an imaginary plot, especially when toys and equipment support a particular scenario, such as toy kitchen equipment. Patterns emerge in the interactive processes of play: initiating, deciding with whom to play, play themes/roles/rules, and finally enactment or collaborative pretending. These patterns provide opportunities for support to facilitate play initiation and collaborative play (Driscoll & Nagel, 2008). Much of the preschooler's play involves fantasy. The young child frequently invents an imaginary companion who plays, eats, and sleeps with the child. The section about cognition and perception addresses more fully the aspects of fantasy during the preschool stage; however, the goal of symbolic or pretend play is to derive meaning from their play experience using their knowledge and skills acquired. The play is a way to integrate previously learned ideas and skills (Driscoll & Nagel, 2008).

Most preschoolers spend some time in a group setting each week. Ground rules at these facilities govern sharing, quiet times, and group activities. Although time orientation remains incompletely developed in preschoolers, they have an idea about past and future. They enjoy planning activities with their parents for the future. Visiting the library to review books about wild animals, packing lunches, and choosing what clothes to wear may preface a trip to the zoo.

The preschooler regulates body activities with more purpose and copes with limit setting better than the toddler, but has much energy and requires outlets for this energy during their day. During this period, physical play begins to be more organized and simple games can be learned such as "Ring around the Rosy." Although this age group needs physical activity, many preschoolers spend long periods each day watching television, videos, and playing electronic games. Occasionally parents use the electronic diversions inappropriately to entertain the child. Although some excellent television, video, and electronic game programming is available for preschoolers, many electronic entertainment options focus on adult themes and violence. Many experts agree that television, videos, and electronic games disengage the child's mind and support less learning (Frost et al., 2008) (see Chapter 20). Parents should remember that preschoolers who rely on television, videos, and electronic games do not have enough life experiences to interpret many of the issues presented in adult shows (violence, interpersonal relationships, moral decisions); might be missing opportunities for interacting with other children or adults and other opportunities for active learning; and cannot judge which shows are appropriate for them. In addition, these electronic activities usually offer sedentary recreation, hindering the development of an active healthy lifestyle. Parents should choose which electronic devices and activities are appropriate for their child, limiting time and promoting physical activity in lieu of sedentary play. Furthermore, taking time to share activities provides the child with an opportunity for discussion and for the child to ask questions (Frost et al., 2008). Nurses should explain to parents and preschoolers the relationship between watching television/screen time and lack of physical activity that leads to health problems such as obesity (Frost et al., 2008). Family support for engaging in physical activity has been shown to affect children's health-promoting behaviors. In a study of 93 children and their parents, Marshall and colleagues (2011) demonstrated that parental influence shaped children's physical activity and nutritional health-promoting behaviors. The literature review by Kornides and colleagues (2011) also describes factors that influence overweight in Latino children. Their review of 24 studies revealed that parental body mass index (BMI) provided the strongest predictor of BMI in Latino children.

Gordon's Health Promotion–Health Maintenance, Nutritional-Metabolic, and Activity-Exercise patterns clearly overlap and should be considered together during the assessment phase in order to plan and intervene successfully (Marshall et al., 2011). Resources for these patterns may be used together to provide optimal health promotion. One resource for physical activity is The Fitness Pyramid, which depicts typical situations intended to encourage physical activity among children. The pyramid website uses interactive strategies to produce more personalized recommendations. A figure climbing up the left side of the pyramid links to recommendations for physical activity (www.fitness.gov/10tips.htm).

Sleep-Rest Pattern

Most preschoolers sleep from 8 to 12 hours during the night, with wide variation among children (Hoban, 2010). Many children do not receive the recommended number of sleep hours and sleep problems in preschool children commonly occur (Vriend & Corkum, 2011). For many older preschoolers, a nap is not necessary. By age 5, most preschoolers no longer regularly nap during the day (National Sleep Foundation, 2011). Quiet time provides a welcome respite for the parent, along with a chance for the active preschooler to relax before afternoon activities. Many child care/preschool environments routinely provide rest periods, enhancing rest and relaxation with soft music and a story. An afternoon rest also gives the young child energy for the evening routine when family members have other duties beyond work and school.

Sleep time habits, falling asleep, and waking up during the night present challenges for families with preschool children (National Sleep Foundation, 2011). The preschooler's expanded imaginative play and increased physical activity during the day may provoke nighttime fears, nightmares, sleep walking, and sleep terrors that are at a peak during this stage of development (National Sleep Foundation, 2011).

Bedtime Ritual

Preschoolers usually require a ritual of activities at bedtime to move from playing and being with others to being alone and falling asleep. These children prolong bedtime routines more often than the toddler. They insist on sleeping with the light on, take a treasured object to bed, request parental attention after being told good night, and experience delays falling asleep. The bedtime ritual generally lasts 30 minutes or longer. Parents honor reasonable rituals, but repeated requests for attention afterward are handled firmly and consistently. Consistency with the routine helps to ameliorate bedtime battles (Hoban, 2010). Vigorous resistance to bedtime challenges parents more during the preschool period than at any other developmental stage. Behavioral insomnia in children occurs when this resistance is associated with a negative association to sleep (Vriend & Corkum, 2011). Preschoolers learn to use the behaviors that meet their needs and control the family regardless of the disruption created.

Nursing Interventions

When a demanding bedtime behavior extends beyond 1 year or an episode persists longer than 1 hour, the nurse explores the family situation. A comprehensive assessment in this case includes the following elements:

- Description of early episodes
- The manner in which these early episodes were managed and the progression of events since then
- Current bedtime behaviors of the child and siblings
- Identification of parental temperament and the resulting responses of parent and family members
- Feelings of the parents and child about each other and about the bedtime situation
- Stressful events and changes that have occurred over the past several years
- Behavior of the child at other times of the day
- Parents' thoughts about reasons why these episodes continue
- Parents' ideas about strategies to use now

The nurse observes interactions within the family. A home visit at mealtime provides an excellent method to observe active interaction. In the office or clinic setting the nurse can ask a parent to teach the child a task or give directions. The nurse remains as unobtrusive as possible while observing the interaction. The first-hand observation of parent-child interaction, along with the detailed history, usually provides the nurse with adequate baseline information to decide whether to manage the situation in the primary care setting or refer the family to a child behavior specialist. Sharing recent literature about management techniques for children with differing temperaments helps families understand more about the behaviors. For example, findings from a study of more than 1500 children by Prior's (Prior, Bavin, Cini, Eadie, & Reilly, 2011) research team provide support that temperament in children may be somewhat modifiable and that parents may consider strategies to influence their preschooler's behavior that focus on their temperament. Research-based strategies should be used to help parents reach their goals related to managing bedtime concerns.

Sleep Disturbances

Night terrors and nightmares characterize the nighttime wakening problems that generally occur during the preschool years. Night terrors manifest as frightening dreams that cause the child to sit up in bed, scream, stare at an imaginary object, breathe heavily, perspire, and appear in obvious distress (see Chapter 18). The child, not fully awake, may be inconsolable for 10 minutes or more, before he or she relaxes and returns to a deep sleep. In most cases the child does not recall the dream and in the morning does not remember the incident (Hoban, 2010). These night terrors can start at approximately age 2 years but are more common during the preschool years. Night terrors rarely occur in older children and adults, and only approximately 6% of preschool children have them. Night terrors and *nightmares* trigger apprehension for the parents (Hoban, 2010).

Nightmares (anxiety dreams) are a more common cause of night wakening. Although infants and toddlers likely have nightmares, their limited verbal skills hinder relating details of the incidents. After age 3, nightmares occur frequently. Approximately 20% of the night is spent dreaming. Dreams frighten preschoolers as they connect to the larger world with their active imaginations and fantastic ideas. These children can waken fully and feel fearful and helpless. Usually they provide vivid descriptions at the time, and they frequently remember the event the following morning. Consolation can be given by a parent who sits with the child, listens to descriptions and fears about the dream, and reminds the child that dreaming is natural and sleep will soon return (Hoban, 2010).

Helping children appreciate the meaning of the words *pretend* and *real* facilitates growth during this phase of childhood. When the parent reads a story to the child or the child tells a make-believe tale, the parents can specify that these are "pretend" and did not really happen. The parent relating a true event can say, "This is real." Children differentiate between the two concepts as they develop cognitively.

Recommendations

Parents of a preschooler can benefit from knowing the following facts:

- Bedtime rituals of 30 to 45 minutes are common for preschoolers. These rituals, because of their importance to children, are respected within reasonable limits. Maintaining a regular consistent and relaxing routine facilitates sleep (National Sleep Foundation, 2011).
- Night-wakening events are common during the preschool years. A consistent sleep environment with the same bed in a room that is cool, quiet, and dark without television promotes sleep (National Sleep Foundation, 2011). Children who waken at night are reassured and encouraged to return to sleep.
- Parents have clear rules about children sleeping with them if the children will not stay in their own beds.
- Restricting frightening television shows and stories and discussing "real" versus "pretend" ideas and stories can help lessen the incidence of nightmares.

Cognitive-Perceptual Pattern

During the preschool years, children cultivate their conceptual and cognitive capacities. The quality of the child's care environment enhances these gains. Family and cultural values influence preschoolers' perceptions and their reaction to events (Gonzalez-Mena, 2012). Internalization of family rules has been associated with social competency in this age group (Kochanska et al., 2010). Preschoolers gradually differentiate today from yesterday and define tomorrow and future more clearly as concepts of time emerge. The child becomes more oriented in space and develops an awareness of the location of the home within the neighborhood. The child also begins to structure daily activities and to value certain activities, objects, and people above others.

Piaget's Theory

The older toddler enters the first substage of the preoperational stage described by Jean Piaget (see Chapter 18). The hallmark of this preconceptual substage includes the ability to function symbolically using language. The preschool child demonstrates increased symbolic functioning during the intuitive substage, from age 4 to 7 years. The predominant feature of this and the following period is the concrete thought process, as compared with adult abstract thinking. As they experience symbolic mental representations, preschoolers process mental symbols as though they were actually participating in the event. Adults analyze and synthesize symbolic information without concrete connections between the mental process and the actual event. At this stage, mental abstraction, such as skipping from one part of an operation to another, reversing the operation mentally, or thinking of the whole in relation to the parts, is not feasible.

The egocentrism that is characteristic of the preschool years exemplifies this concept of concrete thinking. At this stage, children concentrate solely on their own perspective. They consider only their own personal meanings for symbols. The preschooler

wonders why another person fails to follow these idiosyncratic communications.

Furthermore, attention focuses solely on one part of an object without shifting. This behavior, termed centering by Piaget, illustrates the child's inability to consider more than one factor at a time when solving simple problems. For example, a child can be given two identical cups containing equal amounts of water and asked which cup contains the greater amount of water. During the preoperational stage, the child responds that they contain the same amount of water. The child is then asked to pour the water from each cup into two different containers (one flat and wide, the other tall and narrow). When asked which container has more water, the child always identifies one. The child usually selects the taller, narrower container with water at the higher height. When the water is again transferred to the identical cups and the experiment repeated, the child returns to the original conclusion that the amounts are equal.

This experiment also illustrates the trait of irreversibility. The child is unable to connect the reversible operation, the transfer of the water back into the original cup, to reach the logical conclusion that the differently shaped containers may hold the same amount of water. The child cannot mentally associate that the transformation from one state to another relates to the shape of the container, not the amount of the water.

Finally, Piaget describes the preoperative stage of thinking as transductive reasoning. The child cannot proceed from general to particular (deduction) or from particular to general (induction); rather, the child moves only from particular to particular in making associations and solving problems. For example, Piaget relates an association made by one of his children between being hunchbacked and being ill. When a hunchbacked neighbor was unable to visit one day because he had a communicable illness, the child understood that the neighbor was ill. However, when the child was told later that the neighbor was better and that she could go see him, her conclusion was that now his hunched back was straight and well. She thought in terms of the man being well or ill, but she placed the man in one or the other category and assumed that he possessed all the attributes and meanings that she linked symbolically with either trait.

The cognitive development of preschoolers is reflected in their symbolic games, which become significantly more orderly and representative of reality (Box 19-3). They begin to incorporate the reality of the world, as it exists outside the self. They increasingly seek play objects that represent models of authentic objects in their environment (Langevin et al., 2009). Preschoolers progressively imitate more social rules in their play. Social interactive play predominates as the young child develops a more secure sense of self.

Preschoolers may have one or more imaginary companions who exist for varying periods. These fantasy companions assume the form of another child, an animal, or some other friendly or fearsome creature. Preschoolers may save special chairs, insist that an extra place be set at the table, and talk at length to this companion. Imaginary companions serve an important function; they are controlled totally by the child and are not a threat. In this way, the preschooler

BOX 19-3 PLAY AS A METHOD OF LEARNING: PRESCHOOL-AGE CHILD

Throughout life, play develops cognitive, affective, and psychomotor skills that are important to the effective performance of life skills. For the preschool-age child, the following play activities provide the foundation for later competency and socialization-skill refinement:

- Arts and crafts (jewelry making, painting, drawing, ceramics, printmaking)
- Group sports (softball, volleyball, soccer, swimming)
- Skating, skateboarding
- Bicycling
- Puzzles
- Gymnastics
- Games (board, card, knock-knock jokes, computer)
- Secret clubs
- Imaginary play (being in playhouse productions)
- Horseback riding

practices social interactions, controls a fearsome beast, or blames someone for naughty behavior without fear of scolding, shame, or attack. Imaginary companions do and say only what the child wills.

Vision

Vision capabilities, which are well developed by 2 years of age, continue to undergo refinement during the early childhood period. By approximately age 6, the child should approach a 20/20 visual acuity level. The possibility of developing amblyopia decreases; it appears most frequently during infancy through approximately the fourth year (see Chapter 18). Depth perception and color vision become fully established, and the child recognizes subtle differences in color shading by the sixth year. Maximal visual capability usually is achieved by the end of the preschool years.

Visual capacity throughout the rest of life deteriorates rather than improves. This phenomenon relates partly to changes in the refractive power of the lens and developmental changes that occur in the shape of the eyeball. In the normal sequence of growth, the eyeball becomes increasingly spherical, losing the short shape typical of infancy and progressing to the point at which light converges accurately on the surface of the retina. This change occurs at approximately 6 years of age. When this change occurs before the sixth year, growth continues past the point of ideal light conversion, the eyeball lengthens, and the child may develop early myopic vision, which will progress with age. Glasses are always indicated for the child who develops myopia before approximately age 8.

Early detection requires regular screening with standardized tests such as the Denver Eye Screening Test or the Snellen Screening Test. The Snellen Screening Test, when administered under standardized procedures, has the advantage of rendering a reliable estimate of actual visual acuity (Hockenberry & Wilson, 2010). The child must be able to understand the test requirements of either pointing in the direction of the E or naming the letters. The Denver Eye Screening Test was designed

for preschool children and includes detection of the commonly occurring visual problems, such as refractive errors, strabismus (crossing of the eyes), and amblyopia.

The Snellen E chart is designed for preschool children; a version for home testing is available from the National Society for Prevention of Blindness. Home testing has been demonstrated to be reliable and offers the advantage of obtaining an estimate for younger children who might not cooperate with this type of testing in a strange environment.

The pupillary light reflex provides a screening approach for heterotropia, a condition in which the child's eyes do not focus together to transmit effective, coordinated binocular vision. When the child has heterotropia, the light from a penlight held approximately 20 inches from the eyes reflects off the pupil slightly off center. Consistent and observable strabismus may be noted. The cover test provides further evidence of a tendency for the child's eyes to cross, known as heterophoria. The child focuses on a spot 14 inches away, then 20 feet away. As the child gazes at the designated spot, one eye is covered completely for several seconds (the eye and eyelashes must not be touched), and then the cover is removed abruptly. If the covered eye moves from the line of vision of the uncovered eye, that eye has a tendency toward muscle imbalance and must be evaluated further. The American Optometric Association website offers resources that can be used to promote healthy vision (www.aoa.org/x9450).

Color blindness presents a particular problem for younger children, because many cues encountered at school depend on the child's ability to distinguish colors. With early detection, the child is able to receive assistance to interpret visual cues, thus minimizing the disadvantage of being color blind. The nurse screens for certain types of color discrimination difficulties by asking the child to respond to various colors in the environment; however, accurate testing for all types of color blindness requires a specialized tool, such as Ishihara's test, which uses a series of cards with color-tinted letters and figures.

Preschoolers may be aware of some discomfort or limitations with vision. The nurse gathers history from the parents, including the questions listed in the Vision section in Chapter 18, about signs of eye problems.

The preschooler is asked questions to elicit information about the following symptoms:

- Itching, burning, or "scratchy" eyes
- Poor vision
- Dizziness, headaches, or nausea after close eye work
- Blurred or double vision

Hearing

During the preschool years, hearing develops to the level of an adult's, when the ability to attend to and interpret what is heard becomes more refined. The 4-year-old preschooler begins to discriminate among remarkably similar speech sounds, such as the difference between sounds made with "f" and "th" or "f" and "s." It is generally accepted that hearing ability of preschoolers can be hindered by repeated middle ear infections (otitis media). Otitis media with effusion occasionally can result in temporary hearing loss. Parents who notice language delays because of ear infections should be referred to their health care provider for appropriate follow-up care for their children (Hockenberry & Wilson, 2010). Parental reports of difficulty should be taken seriously. Clear evidence supports that effective newborn hearing screening programs correct problems early and often correct developmental delay (Houston et al., 2011). The most effective programs have rigorous evaluation of their policies, procedures, processes, and outcomes (Houston et al., 2011; Yoshinaga-Itano, 2011).

Audiometric methods most accurately measure the child's ability to hear. Preschool children possess the developmental capability to perform the standard audiometric test. The child can follow directions by this age, and most preschoolers enjoy demonstrating their abilities and cooperate easily during vision and hearing screening examinations (Hockenberry & Wilson, 2010). Refractive error can be significant in the preschool child. The prevalence of refractive errors (5% to 7%) and amblyopia (2% to 4%) in preschool children places vision loss as an important public health concern; however, some screening tests reveal only refractive errors (O'Donoghue et al., 2012). Children younger than 7 years of age demonstrate significant improvement in amblyopia when treated, providing a rationale for screening and early recognition programs. The American Academy of Pediatrics on-line resources supply information for nurses and families and can be accessed at www.healthychildren. org/English/Pages/default.aspx.

To ensure success, the nurse encourages a positive experience by adhering to the following points:
- Use equipment skillfully.
- Use age-appropriate language. Avoid the word test to limit anxiety or fear of failure.
- Encourage the child to ask questions and scrutinize the equipment.
- Perform screening before other intrusive or painful procedures.
- Perform screening in a quiet, private area without distractions.
- Praise the child for cooperating.
- Allow rest periods when the child becomes distracted or tired.
- Discuss results with the child in age-appropriate language.

Sensory Perception

Sensory abilities contribute to preschoolers' skill to perceive and interact with the world. Both sensory acuity and sensory perceptual abilities mature during the preschool years. The nature of the visual stimulus determines the response. Preschoolers respond powerfully to visual illusions and have difficulty discriminating right and left mirror images. Confusion commonly occurs with the letters "b," "d," "p," and "q."

Language

Cognitive and sensory abilities contribute to preschool language development. Toward the end of the preschool period, expressive language rivals that of an adult except for minor deficiencies in refinement, vocabulary, and structure. Language ability depends on aptitude, opportunities to use language, quality and quantity of language used at home, and range of experiences. Regardless of expressive capacity, the child develops receptive language during the preschool years that provides a vital foundation for later communication. Throughout early childhood, receptive capacity exceeds expressive capacity. Children comprehend meanings of words and phrases not contained in their expressive vocabulary. Associations between concepts materialize, although the child lacks the ability to explain these concepts. Table 19-2 outlines the receptive and expressive language skills of preschoolers.

During the early childhood years, rhythm develops as an important dimension in speech capacity. Between ages 3 and 5 years, children practice speaking by mimicking adult language patterns. Practice expands neuromotor capacities, and verbal interaction develops vocabulary and sense of grammatical structure. Hesitations, repetitions, and frequent revisions in speech reflect attempts to expand language capacity. Adults may label such preparation as stuttering, but these inaccuracies actually represent normal speech maturation. Stuttering originates during this developmental period, associated with response and reaction from adults and other children to the normal preschool broken speech pattern (Langevin et al., 2009). Reactions of impatience while waiting for the child to express thoughts and negative social interactions decrease the child's opportunities to use language. Insisting children use correct speech before capacity for fluent speech develops may hinder normal speech development. As many as 60% of expressive language delays resolve during the preschool years (Conti-Ramsden & Durkin, 2012). As nurses help parents provide anticipatory guidance for language development, they should maintain vigilance to identify those children who are not outgrowing their language difficulties. These children encounter lifelong obstacles with learning and socialization. Suggestions for nurses to assist parents and to facilitate preschoolers' language development are listed in Box 19-4.

Memory

Memory plays an important role in language development and learning in general (Archibald et al., 2011). Archibald and colleagues (2011) examined 12 preschool students and demonstrated an association between memory and verbal ability. At the preschool level children label pictures, group objects, and mimic others as ways to aid memory, performing these tasks with less precision than the older child. Younger children benefit from suggestions about how to group items using characteristics to remember. Preschoolers remember pictures better by saying names of pictures rather than simply hearing the name of a picture when it is first shown. Preschoolers do not spontaneously use rehearsal or other mnemonic techniques for remembering, but they do use and benefit from rehearsal when it is suggested. The nurse tests memory by asking the child to repeat an arbitrary sequence of numbers. By approximately age 5, children are able to repeat four consecutively named numbers easily.

TABLE 19-2   GROWTH AND DEVELOPMENT

Landmarks of Speech, Language, and Hearing Ability During the Preschool Period

AGE (MONTHS)	RECEPTIVE LANGUAGE	EXPRESSIVE LANGUAGE	RELATED HEARING ABILITY
42	Up to 4200 words; knows words such as *what, where, how, funny, we, surprise, secret;* knows number concepts to 2; knows how to answer some questions accurately, such as, Do you have a dog? Which is the girl? What toys do you have?	Up to 1200 words in mostly complete sentences averaging 4 to 5 words per sentence; uses all 50 phonemes; 7% of sentences are compound or complex; averages 203 words per hour; rate of speech is accelerating; relates experiences and tells about activities in sequential order; such as *what, where, how, see, little, funny, they, we, he, she, several;* can recite a nursery rhyme; asks permission; 95% of speech is intelligible	
48	Up to 5600 words; carries out 3-item commands consistently; knows why people have houses, books, umbrella, key; knows nearly all colors; knows words such as *somebody, anybody, even, almost, now, something, like, bigger, too,* full name, one or two songs, number concepts to 4; understands most preschool stories; can complete opposite analogies such as brother is a boy, sister is a girl, and in daytime it is light and at night it is dark	Up to 1500 words in sentences averaging 5 to 6 words per sentence; averages 400 words per hour; counts up to 3, repeats 4 digits, names 3 objects, repeats 9-word sentences from memory; names the primary colors, some coins; relates fanciful tales; enjoys rhyming nonsense words and using exaggerations; demands reasons why and how; questioning is at a peak, up to 500 a day; passes judgment on own activity; can recite a poem from memory or sing a song; uses words such as *even, almost, something, like, but;* typical expressions might include "I'm so tired," "You almost hit me," "Now I'll make something else"	Begins to make fine discriminations among similar speech sounds, such as the difference between *f* and *th* or *f* and *s* Child has matured enough to be tested with an audiometer. At this age, formal hearing testing usually can be carried out. Not only has hearing developed to its optimal level, but listening has also become considerably refined
54	Up to 6500 words; knows what materials a house, window, chair, and dress are made of and what people do with eyes and ears; understands differences in texture and composition, such as hard, soft, rough, smooth; begins to name or point to penny, nickel, dime; understands *if, because, why, when*	Up to 1800 words in sentences averaging 5 to 6 words; now averages only 230 words per hour—is satisfied with less verbalization; does little commanding or demanding; likes surprises; about 1 in 10 sentences is compound or complex, and only 8% of sentences are incomplete; can define 10 common words and counts up to 20; common expressions are "I don't know," "I said," "tiny," "funny," "because"; asks questions for information and learns to manipulate and control people and situations with language	
60	Up to 9600 words; knows number concepts to 5; knows and names colors; defines words in terms of use, such as a bike is to ride; defines wind, ball, hat, stove; understands qualifiers such as *if, because, when;* knows purpose of horse, fork, and legs; begins to understand *left* and *right*	Up to 2200 words in sentences averaging 6 words; can define ball, hat, stove, policeman, wind, horse, fork; can count five objects and repeat four or five digits; definitions are in terms of use; can single out a word and ask its meaning; makes serious inquiries—"What is this for?" "How does this work?" "Who made those?" "What does it mean?"; language is now essentially complete in structure and form; uses all types of sentences, clauses, and parts of speech; reads by way of pictures, and prints simple words	

Modified from Hockenberry, M. J., & Wilson, D. (2010). *Wong's nursing care of infants and children* (9th ed.). St. Louis: Mosby.

Testing of Developmental Level

Parents of preschool children determine their child's readiness for school programs. The child's skill level, the child and family's psychosocial status, and the characteristics of the school program under consideration contribute to readiness determination. Questions about readiness should be answered considering all three of these components. Developmental testing modalities used during the toddler years appear less accurate as the child approaches school age. Tools designed for this purpose can help identify the child's skill level.

Historically, tools to evaluate readiness skills have been used. The Preschool Readiness Experimental Screening Scale

(PRESS) has been used in the past. This tool screens easily for developmental lags or abnormalities that might interfere with academic and social success in school. Constructed for use with 5-year-old children, it may also estimate readiness of slightly older or younger children. The test measures school readiness and addresses specific skills, not intellectual level.

Other components of readiness, family dynamics and school environment, have concerned experts. Testing in environments that account for these contextual issues should yield a more accurate estimate of the preschool child's readiness for school (Bagnato et al., 2011). Authentic testing or observation-based testing places the child in a natural setting for testing. Early

BOX 19-4 **NURSING SUGGESTIONS TO ENCOURAGE LANGUAGE DEVELOPMENT IN PRESCHOOLERS**

- Read to the child. Encourage the child to be an active listener. Pause during the story to ask questions, such as "What do you think will happen next?" and "Why do you think the boy said that?" and "What would you do now?" See **Website Resource 19A** for a list of suggested books to read aloud to a child.
- Praise the child's storytelling and creativity with stories.
- Always respond to the child's questions. Occasionally a response must be delayed; for example, when the parent is driving in heavy traffic and the child asks a question that requires a complex answer, the parent might say, "That's a very good question; let's talk about that as soon as we get home." The parent should remind the child of the question later and respond if the child still expresses interest.
- Never tease or criticize a child about speaking style. If the child speaks so fast as to be fumbling over words, then the parent might say, "I can't listen that fast. Slow down a little for me." This is much more encouraging than is the statement, "You talk too fast. No one can understand you."
- Play language-focused games, such as naming the colors of houses or kinds of flowers as parent and child walk to the store.

Child Intervention (ECI) experts recognize this type of testing as more informative than either standardized tests or tests with questionable reliability and validity (Bagnato et al., 2011). One such test, the *Assessment, Evaluation and Programming System for Infants and Children,* provides an instrument for this type of assessment and is recognized by ECI programs to be informative and to facilitate accurate assessment (Bagnato et al., 2011). In addition to the actual assessment, quality ECI programs require the ability to use portable technologies. Using recognized standards for assessment, qualified trained personnel aim to improve early referral and treatment, primary goals of ECI programs (Bagnato et al., 2011).

Children who are ready for school demonstrate competencies in areas other than measurable skill performance. Complex home environments with stable caring adults or safe, predictable physical environments with regular, stimulating activities, peers, and materials contribute to readiness. Social norms define expectations; therefore, home values that align with school values are more likely to result in children characterized as ready for school. Conversely, when school expectations differ from those at home, children are less likely to be considered ready for school (Conti-Ramsden & Durkin, 2012).

To obtain a more specific measure of developmental age, the nurse uses one of several screening tools designed for use with the preschool child. These validated instruments provide rough estimates of ability for school and help determine whether a child needs referral for further evaluation. The Peabody Picture Vocabulary Test examines verbal intelligence but also estimates verbal ability. When used with predominantly middle class children who have acquired standard English-speaking ability, accuracy is reliable (Conti-Ramsden & Durkin, 2012). Insufficient language stimulation or cultural differences may influence scores negatively. Children from bilingual backgrounds, nevertheless, acquire letter recognition

readily once they encounter an environment that emphasizes these abilities (Fabiano-Smith & Goldstein, 2010; Gutiérrez-Clellen et al., 2012; Hammer & Miccio, 2006; Hammer et al., 2007; Lugo-Neris et al., 2010). Also, children sometimes become disinterested with the process and randomly point to options to finish more quickly. Examiners must remain alert to eye movement to identify changes in children's response behaviors. Readiness tests continue to improve in their ability to predict performance.

Draw-a-Person and Draw-a-Family tests approximate intelligence and emotional development; however, scoring figure drawings requires standardized test conditions and analysis of findings by a psychometric specialist. Nurses, however, use these methods in conjunction with other information to help establish rapport and to provide a starting point to guide assessment (Goldner & Scharf, 2012; Selwyn et al., 2009).

Drawings may indicate general developmental level, fine motor control, and evidence of concept formation. Perceptions of family relationships can also be assessed. Preschool children will draw a person with at least six body parts in the appropriate locations. Normally children name the parts correctly. The representation may be an approximation, but it should resemble the actual body parts and be drawn with strong, evenly flowing lines. The family drawing may be less sophisticated than a drawing of a single person and may lack some family members. The normal child names the family members readily and describes unique characteristics of each member from a child's perspective. The nurse provides a pencil and plain sheet of paper and asks the child to draw (Goldner & Scharf, 2012; Selwyn et al., 2009) the best picture possible. The nurse explains that the picture will remain with the nurse for documentation, but that another sketch may be drawn to take home.

Autism Spectrum Disorders

The prevalence of developmental disabilities (1 in 6 children) has increased in the United States, with a higher prevalence in boys than in girls (Boyle et al., 2011). Disparity in prevalence is more likely when children live in low-income families and lack health insurance (Boyle et al., 2011). Autism spectrum disorders (autism, Asperger's syndrome, and pervasive developmental disorder) occur more frequently than any other developmental condition. Prevalence rates for this continuum of conditions have increased from 4% (1997) to 6% (2008) of the U.S. population (Boyle et al., 2011).

These conditions are considered genetically determined disorders and are only rarely associated with nongenetic risk factors, such as maternal valproic acid use during pregnancy, congenital rubella, and cerebral palsy (Freitag et al., 2010). Although the genetic foundation is well recognized, no single gene or gene family is linked to the disorders (LeBlanc & Fagiolini, 2011; Mefford, Batshaw, & Hoffman, 2012). Chromosome microarray analysis is a promising area for assessment of autism spectrum disorder and currently provides diagnosis 15% to 20% of the time (Mefford et al., 2012). Genetic counseling is recommended once the diagnosis is established; however, if the diagnosis is not established, other genetic diagnoses, such as fragile X syndrome, should be eliminated and the child should be reevaluated in 6 months (Mefford et al., 2012).

Currently, multiple studies have linked autism spectrum disorders with atypical birth weight (high or low), low Apgar scores, hemolytic disease, hyperbilirubinemia (jaundice), respiratory distress, advanced parental age, length of gestation, and environmental factors (viruses), all of which may be subtle and complicated by the genetic influence (May-Benson, Koomar, & Teasdale, 2009). In their study of 467 children with autism spectrum disorder, May-Benson and colleagues (2009) provided support for the idea that there is no unique combination of characteristics, but rather a composite of risk factors that provide suspicion for the disorders.

Careful observation is vital during this time of language and communication development to assess for autism spectrum disorders (autism, Asperger's syndrome, and pervasive developmental disorder), since most cases of autism spectrum disorder are diagnosed in children (LeBlanc & Fagiolini, 2011). The majority of children have symptoms in the first year of life (Shumway et al., 2011). This assessment includes family history, clinical history, and physical assessment with a focused neurological exam.

Manifestations vary considerably (Freitag et al., 2010; May-Benson et al., 2009). Assessment of cognitive and behavioral symptoms is the cornerstone of diagnosis and early detection may help families address advancing behavioral aberrations sooner (LeBlanc & Fagiolini, 2011). Families of these children manage multiple behavioral and physical challenges early in the child's life; therefore, health providers need to remain apprised of current trends in pediatric development connected to the disorders (May-Benson et al., 2009). Providers should consider the prenatal events mentioned earlier in this section along with childhood stressors (e.g., chronic ear infections, sleeping/eating problems, absent/brief crawling phase, language delays, atypical responses to sensory stimulation, lack of separation anxiety, and failure to attain motor skill developmental milestones) as warning signs that warrant further assessment (LeBlanc & Fagiolini, 2011; May-Benson et al., 2009). Resources for families and professionals are available at www.cdc.gov/ncbddd/autism/index.html.

Self-Perception–Self-Concept Pattern

During the preschool years, basic self-concept emerges from the child's personal struggle for autonomy. As children develop beyond the toddler years, they refine their sense of self through both task-oriented and socially-oriented experiences. By reinforcing skills and successfully accomplishing tasks, preschoolers build self-esteem, enhancing overall health. Social acceptance helps children feel successful in their role as child, sibling, and friend. Preschoolers investigate roles through rich imagination. Pretending to be the parent or baby allows preschoolers to imagine experiences and feelings of others (i.e., empathy) and safely experiment with new ideas (Hockenberry & Wilson, 2010; Price & Gwinn, 2008).

Preschool children learn about their roles in their child care environments and learn that being dependable within

BOX 19-5   QUALITY AND SAFETY

Health Promotion with Preschoolers: Environmental Accountability

Rationale for Teaching Preschoolers about Environmental Protection

- Environmental education at an early age will produce environmental practitioners of the future.
- Preschoolers can learn basic concepts of environmental accountability and gain a sense of empowerment when they perceive that they make a difference to the future world.
- Health care providers, in consultation with child care providers, can promote environmental education that is based on their knowledge of child growth and development and concerns about overall health.

Basic Ways for Preschoolers to Help the Environment and Promote Overall Societal Health

- Use water wisely.
- Use electricity only when necessary.
- Recycle.
- Avoid using balloons.
- Plant trees, protect plants, and grow a garden.
- Create a compost pile.
- Care for birds.
- Clean up the neighborhood.
- Decrease the amount of trash; say "no" to Styrofoam and plastic garbage bags, and use paper cups and reusable cloth bags for groceries.
- Recycle old toys by giving them to others.
- Buy and use only earth-friendly school supplies.
- Walk rather than ride in the car.
- Use live Christmas trees and replant.

their world is important. When children perceive their value in improving the world in which they live, they experience good feelings about themselves and, ultimately, demonstrate improved mental and physical health. Many simple ways to improve the environment are available, and when children learn ways to contribute to environmental health, they often reinforce these behaviors in their parents (Box 19-5: Quality and Safety Scenario).

Erikson's Theory

Preschoolers develop a sense of initiative through their vigorous motor activity and active imagination. Erikson views this growth as the most central developmental task in the emerging self-concept of the preschool years. By praising preschoolers' efforts and providing opportunities for new experiences, parents promote development of initiative. Rather than requiring a particular behavior, parents should provide avenues for experimentation. Preschoolers then feel mastery, thus encouraging repetition. With mastery, preschoolers become more confident about trying new actions.

Roles-Relationships Pattern

Family members continue to play a vital role in the preschooler's life, but peers become increasingly significant as development progresses. Preschoolers receive ideas and information from peers. They may subsequently question rules or expectations at home, comparing them to their friends' situations. Discussion about family values and behaviors that are acceptable one place but not another help them understand differences.

Preschoolers understand gender expectations regarding jobs, activities, and competencies of people in their lives. Ideas about gender differences in work roles or activities are based on models in the home, at child care or preschool centers, and on television. Parents and caregivers should be aware of the powerful influence that environment has on role perceptions (Bower et al., 2008; Brown et al., 2009; Kochanska et al., 2010). When inaccurate portrayals of male and female roles are depicted, parents and caregivers should discuss more accurate ones with children. Preschoolers experiment through play, including adopting family roles. These roles vary depending on family structure and function. For example, the role-play for a child of gay or lesbian parents may differ from that of heterosexual parents. As the mother or father in a play situation, the preschooler sets limits, punishes, praises, and makes outlandish demands on the invented child. Play represents an important strategy for preschoolers to use for stress reduction and experimentation with new roles. By playing different roles, children safely experience effects of their behavior and understand others' roles more clearly. Parents also better understand effects of their own actions when they observe the behaviors of their child. Nurses help parents use their observations to improve interactions with their child.

Compared with toddlers, preschoolers relate to older children in the family on a more equal basis. Although their cognitive, motor, and language skills are less refined, preschoolers participate in some activities with their older siblings. Younger children may admire and imitate an older sibling. This behavior flatters the older child initially, but with continued persistence may develop into a source of frustration for the sibling. The older sibling, in a more powerful position, may resort to violence (Phillips, Phillips, Grupp, & Trigg, 2009).

Social interaction during the preschool period prepares the child for school. Through experience within the family, with peers, and with other adults, the child acquires readiness to interact in group situations, follow directions, take turns, recognize others' rights, channel energy toward an assigned activity, and demonstrate increasing independence. School readiness can be assessed by using several relevant tests, as discussed in this chapter. The nurse who sees the child repeatedly in an office, clinic, or group care or preschool setting assesses progress as the child develops social competencies. Comparing the child's current, more mature behavior with previous behavior provides insight into preschoolers' readiness for school. This method of evaluation, however, prevents comparison with other children of the same age. For example, school personnel may view a child who reflects a quiet temperament and is introverted or subdued as overly attached to the mother in comparison with other children the same age. However, if the child's earlier social behavior is known, the behavior may be interpreted as a progression toward independence.

Evidence of social competency can be obtained by discussion and evaluation of the child's family drawings. Children can be given the opportunity to draw pictures while they are waiting for outpatient visits, and the drawings can be used to begin the assessment process. The nurse observes the drawing and responds to any comments or questions volunteered by the child. When asked for advice or assistance, the nurse encourages the child to proceed with drawing. Positive encouragement for the child's efforts may be used, particularly with reluctant children. After the drawing is finished, the nurse discusses the sketch with the child to identify the people and describe individual characteristics. The nurse writes the names of each family member on the picture and documents the perceptions the child describes. Open-ended questions such as "What do you like best about your brother?" or "When do you get angry with your sister?" can be posed to encourage the child to describe the family interaction patterns. When an adult family member is present, the nurse explains the purpose of the drawing and interview and requests that the adult withhold comments or questions until the activity is completed. Any areas of concern or questions should be discussed, assuring the parent that confidentiality will be maintained. The child's perceptions can be verified with the adult at the conclusion of the interview, or further information can be sought to clarify them.

The **Vineland Social Maturity Scale** provides an objective, standardized estimate of social functioning and social maturity (Scattone, Raggio, Raggio, & May, 2011). This tool profiles the child's self-help skills, self-direction, locomotion, communication, and social relations. The scoring system seems to be culturally and socioeconomically neutral. The investigator collects data by observing the child's behavior and interviewing the mother or primary caregiver. Designed to measure progression toward independence, this instrument uses direct observation of the child's behavior whenever possible, using the interview data only if needed to complete the assessment (Scattone et al., 2011).

These kinds of tools elicit cues indicative of family stress and strain. **Parental divorce** commonly creates disruption in family relationships. Discussion of results of the assessment offers the opportunity to discuss family situations that otherwise might have remained unmentioned. Children's responses to changes in family circumstances depend on their developmental stages and their relationships before the change. Divorce represents a final decision, usually culminating from a period of conflict, stress, and changing relationships. Although preschoolers definitely sense stress in the home, they cannot articulate their feelings or determine their origin. Children react to changes in various ways, including regression, confusion, or irritability. Asking the same questions repeatedly, such as, "Is Daddy coming home for supper tonight?" or "Why doesn't Daddy stay here anymore?" can be a child's way of expressing difficulty in coping with or comprehending the situation.

Parents in the midst of marital problems or divorce frequently lack the psychological energy or patience to deal with questions and altered behavior. Nonetheless, these children desperately need closeness, patience, and consistent responses from their parents. Nurses advocate for children by helping parents explore ways to address regression and irritability. As parents develop skills to explain situations, they realize children are deeply affected during times of family disruption, regardless of their behavior (Kaakinen et al., 2010). Parents need to connect emotionally with their children to demonstrate that love will continue for the child despite dissolution of the marriage. Books appropriate to the preschooler's cognitive and emotional level can help parents address children's feelings and needs during divorce.

Child Abuse

Social processes within families and communities that create child abuse are multifaceted and complex. Research focuses on the complexity of the abuse cycle and the challenges involved in resolution. In some communities, hitting children as a form of discipline remains socially acceptable. Parents and caregivers who experience workplace stressors, financial worries, and other frustrations may project their anger and abuse toward their children physically, emotionally, or sexually. Effective primary and secondary prevention interventions involve promoting awareness of violence as a social problem, opposing violence to women, and offering community or school programs to teach nonviolent conflict resolution skills to people of all ages. Prevention of child neglect and abuse is the focus of many health-promotion programs; however, recognition of signs of child abuse is important and must be reported (Howard & Brooks-Gunn, 2009). Although it is important for families to begin to teach children about how to respond to strangers, child abuse in general and sexual abuse in particular occur more often within a family than with a stranger as the perpetrator. Most children suffer the abuse from someone who is familiar to them. The American Psychological Association provides helpful information about abuse for families at www.apa.org/pi/families/resources/child-sexual-abuse.aspx.

Sexuality-Reproductive Pattern

Preschoolers recognize there are two genders and identify with their own gender. Appropriate and positive representations of both genders on television and in role models, such as working mothers, allow preschoolers to interpret gender roles broadly and define their own roles more realistically (Hockenberry & Wilson, 2010). Body image, a part of gender identity, also includes perception of sex organs. Preschoolers develop curiosity at this age, including inquisitiveness about bodies and sexual functions of others. Questions should be answered simply and factually. Teasing preschoolers about this interest or implying that sexual information is unacceptable or naughty promotes negativity. Positive feelings about all aspects of the self (including gender role) create positive self-esteem. Many children's books address self-esteem in young children and provide interesting and informative approaches to nurturing overall health promotion in this age group. See **Website Resource 19A** for a list of recommended books for preschool children.

Coping-Stress Tolerance Pattern

Play Approaches

Assessing self-concept in preschool children who struggle to articulate their feelings presents a challenge for the nurse. Play can elicit behaviors that indicate sense of self and self-esteem, future success or failure, sense of acceptance, and competence. Doll or puppet play provides valuable insight into a child's sense of self. Dolls or puppets, including those representing a young child of the same gender, race, and cultural background as the preschooler, should be available (Hockenberry & Wilson, 2010). If the child spontaneously begins to engage the dolls or puppets in imaginary activity, no further guidance should be given. With a reluctant child, the nurse begins to pretend, using examples for the child, such as going to the store, moving the dolls through the related activities, and then involving the child. Frequently preschoolers continue the scenario to tell their personal stories.

A related technique is mutual storytelling. The nurse begins a story for the child to finish. The nurse might begin with a standard line, such as, "Once upon a time there lived a [girl, boy, cow, monkey, etc.] who…" The nurse then pauses for the child to continue. If the child hesitates, the nurse resumes the story for another sentence or two and asks what the figure in the story is doing. As the child supplies details, the nurse offers encouragement to continue, asking questions such as "And then what happened?" or "How did the child feel?"

The child's inner nature can be explored along several dimensions. The emotional theme of the story is noted and should be congruent with the child's tone and expression. For example, a child who centers on a theme of aggression and destruction but describes the character's anger in a monotone is demonstrating incongruence between content and expression. The child's emotionless response suggests difficulty with expressing feelings. At the conclusion of the story, possible meanings can be revealed by asking whether the child feels similar to any of the characters or would like to be any of the characters.

Although these dimensions may be explored for meaning, interpretation of a child's behavior in these play situations remains highly speculative. Determining possible themes or estimating the child's self-esteem requires several encounters. Additionally, the nurse's personality and approach influence the child's spontaneity and ability to tell a story. Observed behavior and responses without associated interpretation should be recorded for future reference. Interpretations are avoided until validated by a specialist.

Coping Mechanisms

Preschoolers use coping mechanisms similar to those of the toddler (separation anxiety, regression, denial, repression, and projection). Protest behavior in the form of temper tantrums normally disappears as a stress response in the older preschooler. Temper tantrums that persist through the fifth year indicate a lack of matured coping responses. The child uses tantrums and continues to gain the desired result.

Preschoolers lack the cognitive awareness, social abilities, and motives for communication of adults and older children. They display temperaments and tantrums that appear oppositional

The Challenge of Temperament and Preschoolers

Temperament describes the way in which an individual behaves or responds to new situations and to life occurrences and has consistently been associated with psychopathology and family function since the early work of Terry Brazelton with maternal attachment in 1978 (Healey, Flory, Miller, & Halperin, 2011; Joosen, Mesman, Bakermans-Kranenburg, & van Lizendoorn, 2012). Most children can be defined as *easy, difficult,* or *hard to warm up to* based on how they react to their surroundings and to people. Temperament and parental stress are linked; however, multiple other factors influence interactions between parent and child, including the child's own temperament (Healey et al., 2011; Prior et al., 2011). For many adults the challenge in parenting is to learn how to work with a child's temperament, which can vary from the parents' or other children's temperaments, in efforts to attain family happiness. Coping skills and stress management for families, particularly those with children defined as difficult, may improve family function (Healey et al., 2011).

to older individuals. Through positive interactions with parents and caregivers, preschoolers frequently learn how to organize their bodies, abilities, and environment to move successfully to the next stage of development (Brown et al., 2009; Luby et al., 2009). A positive relationship between the child's temperament and the demands of the environment (also known as goodness of fit) can be attained by social interaction, which, in turn, prevents the development of problem behaviors later (Box 19-6: Hot Topics).

Preschoolers possess a considerable range of experiences and memories; therefore, they respond more maturely to stress than do toddlers. Positive coping resources are determined by some of the following variables:

- Availability of emotional comfort and the child's inner resilience
- Ability to work on task
- Availability of play materials and toys
- Opportunity to engage in activities (Kalpidou, Power, Cherry, & Gottfried, 2004)

Preschoolers use many of the coping mechanisms developed during their toddler years, but they generally show greater ability to verbalize frustration, have fewer temper tantrums, and display more patience in experimentation to resolve difficulty than the typical toddler. Preschoolers refine their problem-solving skills. Through fantasy play, they investigate solutions or responses to stressful events and find inner control for challenging situations.

Occasionally projection and fantasy lead parents to consider their child dishonest. When faced with the question, "Did you break this dish?" the preschooler might respond, "No, Teddy did it." The child might even relate a detailed story of the toy bear's mishap. Preschoolers tend to project blame. Active fantasies help tell the story. Parents should not accuse the preschooler of lying, but rather the adult should help the child decide whether the story is pretend or real. The concepts of pretend and real help encourage children to discuss nightmares, television shows, stories, and their own active imaginations (Garrison et al., 2011).

Compared with toddlers, preschoolers better perceive their ability to control and manage situations. Strict adherence to rituals or game rules controls situations. As discussed, preschoolers have longer and more rigid bedtime rituals than those of toddlers. Preschoolers also dislike losing games and may structure the rules to ensure winning. Older children and adults may be able to accept these structures, but these controlling behaviors frustrate other preschoolers, because they also need to win. Gentle, consistent direction by parents and caregivers about how to play games fairly and how to move toward positive group outcomes helps preschoolers develop a sense of morality, which is important for later life success and happiness. See the Case Study and Care Plan at the end of this chapter for an example of ineffective coping in a preschool child.

Values-Beliefs Pattern

Preschoolers, like toddlers, lack fully developed consciences; however, at age 4 to 5 years these children do demonstrate some internal controls on their actions. Immaturity limits the consistency and effectiveness of these internal controls. With the child's concrete perspective, the internal controls may be rigid; therefore, a preschooler may feel overwhelming guilt when behavior and internal controls conflict. Cognitive developmental level determines, for the most part, preschoolers' maturity and their feelings about their behavioral fluctuations. Cognitive development continues with dramatic transformation during these years, explaining the differences not only among children but also for different times in the same child. Modeling and induction explanation, moving from specific to general, influence moral behaviors appreciably. Modeling stems from many sources, not all of which leave positive impressions. Parents affect the availability of models by screening television shows, carefully selecting child care situations, and monitoring play sessions. Responsible parents verify suitability of the models. More detailed inductive explanations, based on the child's cognitive level, generally are comprehended by the preschool population.

Preschoolers control their behavior to retain parental love and approval. From their perspective, parental disapproval represents a decrease in the child's importance from the parent's viewpoint. The child therefore suffers a decline in self-esteem, which motivates a change in behavior. Guilt results from perceived reduction of self-esteem, a critical step in the development of conscience. Moral actions are demonstrated in simple activities, such as taking turns and sharing. These actions stem from the assumption that other people have rights and desires that are as important as the rights and desires of preschoolers.

Preschoolers frequently express their values by stating who or what they like or what they want to be when they become adults. These values change frequently, even within a few minutes. Preschoolers occasionally use statements of value as punishment for playmates or family members and display insensitivity to the effect of their remarks on others. Preschoolers ask endless questions. When they ask these questions about moral actions or feelings, they may simply be asking, "How does this work?" and not questioning the underlying parental value. The same intent exists when the child asks about the spiritual values that the parent may be teaching. Parents may enroll their child in Sunday school or other faith-oriented classes or activities. The preschool child generally enjoys the social aspects of these activities and receives some important modeling of values from the involved adults and from working with peers as they struggle to develop morality (Kochanska et al., 2010).

Life beginnings and death concepts fascinate preschoolers. Because of their limited emotional experiences with death, some ask about dead insects and the process of death with great interest, occasionally with insensitivity. Others become upset with the idea of dying, assuming that when someone becomes angry and wishes them dead, they will cease to exist. Many children worry about who will care for them if their caregivers die, whether pain comes with death, what causes death, and what happens after someone dies. Children who actually lose a loved one to death can experience sleep disturbances and other behavioral changes as part of the grieving process. Parents, based on their own religious and cultural values, should respond to children in a supportive and open manner to provide an accurate interpretation of death. In some cases, counseling may be needed if the parents are unable to cope with their duties or if the child has significant behavioral problems as a result of the family disruption. Assessment using the preschoolers' drawings in such situations provides an accepted method to explore their perceptions about family relationships, death, and the afterlife (Selwyn et al., 2009).

ENVIRONMENTAL PROCESSES

Physical Agents

For many children physiological, psychosocial, and environmental factors create health problems that interfere with physical, social, and educational activities of normal development (Hockenberry & Wilson, 2010). Major disruptions limit fulfillment of the child's potential in adulthood. Environmental processes that affect toddlers also affect preschoolers. Occurrence rates and outcomes of health problems differ in this age group, likely because of developmental differences (U.S. Department of Health and Human Services, 2011). Preschoolers have more refined problem-solving skills, are more coordinated, and have more experience with a variety of situations than do toddlers. Although preschoolers recognize and avoid some environmental hazards, they remain impulsive and immature. Population-based programs ensure that screening takes place at the most developmentally appropriate time (Box 19-7: Research for Evidence-Based Practice).

Because many preschoolers attend child care programs, many have been trained to use 911 and can access help in emergencies when this phone code exists. At this age, a child needs to know his or her name, address, and how to say "no" to strangers.

Injuries

Accidents and injuries are often predictable and preventable (Ingram et al., 2011; Centers for Disease Control and Prevention [CDC], 2007). As preschoolers become more independent,

BOX 19-7 RESEARCH FOR EVIDENCE-BASED PRACTICE

Effectiveness of Parents' Language Interventions for Preschool Children

Roberts and Kaiser (2011) conducted a systematic meta-analysis of 18 studies with subjects ages 18 to 60 months who met the following criteria: used a comparison group, employed a parental intervention, and included a child communication component with at least one language outcome measure. Almost half of the studies evaluated used the Hanen Parent Program and focused stimulation. Effect sizes were determined for each study, as well as seven language outcome variables. Intellectual disabilities and parent report vs. direct observation measures were also compared. This meta-analysis indicated that parent-implemented language interventions have significant positive influence on both receptive and expressive language skills in preschool children regardless of whether they have intellectual impairment. The findings from this analysis provide evidence to support the use of parent-implemented interventions for preschool children with language impairments.

Data from Roberts, M. Y., & Kaiser, A. P. (2011). The effectiveness of parent-implemented language interventions: A meta-analysis. *American Journal of Speech-Language Pathology, 20*(3), 180-199.

causes of injury change; they may chase a ball into a busy street or suffer from sports-related injuries. Preschoolers continue to need supervision to prevent injury related to their developmental age. Nurses guide families to provide a safe environment for preschoolers with opportunities to explore without negative consequences (Box 19-8).

Of all injuries, two thirds occur in children and adolescents. The rate of death from injuries is decreasing in the United States. On the other hand, death rates continue to be higher than in countries with long-term comprehensive preventive approaches that focus on widespread community change (e.g., Great Britain and Scandinavian countries) (Orton et al., 2012). Although preschoolers have fewer accidents than toddlers, accidental injury continues to be a predominant cause of morbidity in this age group (Orton et al., 2012). Preschoolers are most likely to sustain injuries related to falls, poisonings, and thermal injuries than any other accidental injuries; however, as the child's age increases toward school age, these injuries begin to decline in number (CDC, 2012a; Ingram et al., 2011; Orton et al., 2012). Motor vehicle accidents consistently remain the top ranked reason for death attributable to injury in the preschool age group (CDC, 2012a). Consequently, the *Healthy People* initiative has promoted using car seat restraint systems (*Healthy People 2020*: IVP-16.3).

Although many state laws mandate federally approved car seats for children who are less than 4 feet tall or weigh less than 40 pounds and booster seats for children up to the age of 6 years, many parents fail to place their children in appropriate restraint systems, or they use them incorrectly. Although parents may know that infants should be placed in the back seat, they do not always know that children in the front seat of a motor vehicle face danger, even if they are using restraint systems. Federal investigations concluded that children younger than age 13 should ride in the back seat of a motor vehicle, particularly because of potential injury or death from a passenger seat airbag

BOX 19-8   INJURY PREVENTION FOR PRESCHOOLERS

A safe and developmental-stimulating environment allows children of all ages to explore without negative consequences. When teaching parents how to modify their homes for preschoolers, the following requirements for child safety should be considered.

Safe Sleep Environment

Provide beds with guardrails (as needed), soft corners, and appropriate bedding to prevent suffocation.

Well-Ventilated but Optimal Temperature Environment for Play

Provide safe play areas by using electrical outlet covers, handrails in stairwells, toy boxes with lids that lock securely, nonslip floor materials, well-anchored furniture, and appropriate soft ground coverings and padding for outdoor play equipment.

Burn Prevention

Use only cool mist humidifier for management of upper respiratory tract infections; dress child only in flame-retardant clothing, particularly at bedtime.

Appropriate Installation and Use of Emergency Home Equipment

Discuss the importance of properly operating smoke detectors and fire extinguishers, and practicing an escape plan from the home in case of emergency.

Connection to Emergency Services

Post 911 on all phones; teach the child how to use 911 and how to report the child's name and address over the phone; parents should be trained in cardiopulmonary resuscitation and the use of abdominal thrusts.

Prevention of Aspiration

Monitor use of balloons and eating habits of preschoolers.

Safe Daily Home Environment

Close doors of dishwasher, oven, washer, and dryer; mark all glass doors with decals to delineate doors; use gates at the top and bottom of stairs for the younger child; set water heater temperature at a maximum of 120° F to avoid burns; store all poisonous substances out of the reach of children; discourage running in the house; avoid throw rugs on bare floors.

Prevention, Recognition, and Management of Poison Ingestion or Exposure

Know how to use syrup of ipecac and have the nearest poison control center phone number within easy access; learn how to evaluate burns or blisters around the mouth, odor of poisons, empty containers around the child, stomach distress, or changes in normal activity level that might indicate poison ingestion.

Water Safety

Monitor bathtub and pool activity; teach preschooler swimming skills (usually by age 4); ensure that all pools are fenced.

Bicycle Safety

Ensure that the child is riding a developmentally appropriate bicycle with a federally approved safety helmet and is schooled in the rules of riding in the street and interacting with strangers.

Lead Concerns

Avoid items with a high lead content in the home (paint, wrapping paper, earthenware, colored newspaper); ensure that children are monitored when lead exposure is a concern.

Environmental Contaminants Hazardous to the Child's Health

Avoid exposure to tobacco smoke, nitrous oxide from wood-burning stoves, asbestos, pesticides, radiation, and factory-produced irritants.

From Hockenberry, M. J., & Wilson, D. (2010). *Wong's nursing care of infants and children* (9th ed.). St. Louis: Mosby.

that could inflate in a severe car accident. Attention to this important issue has increased the correct use of child restraint systems to 43%, with the goal to increase further to 47% by 2020 (U.S. Department of Health and Human Services, 2011). Nurses actively participate in health-promotion programs in communities and emergency departments that help families use car restraints correctly. Internet resources are available to assist professionals and parents (www.safekids.org/safety-basics/little-kids/on-the-way/car-seats-and-booster-seats.html, www.kidsandcars.org/; www.healthychildren.org/English/safety-prevention/on-the-go/Pages/default.aspx, www.iowadot.gov/curbitclickit/parents.html). When families have to consider financial constraints in order to comply with the requirements to restrain their children, nurses often are the first line of information. Nurses provide information about resources available locally through agencies such as hospitals, physicians' offices, insurance companies, United Way, Salvation Army, the fire department, and other community organizations.

Household furniture and fixtures also remain a hazard for preschoolers, as do structural features such as stairs and windows. Nursery and toy injuries decrease during the preschool years. Sports and recreational injuries increase markedly. This elevated incidence likely reflects a change in many preschoolers being involved in group sports, riding bicycles, and using

playground equipment (CDC, 2012a). Preschoolers need a broad range of play areas and experiences. Conscientious parents supply age-appropriate limits and supervision (Ingram et al., 2011; Price & Gwinn, 2008). Preschoolers lack the skill or judgment to ride bicycles in the street. They need instruction about safe use of playground equipment. Adult supervision of most preschooler activities, group sports in particular, is required to prevent injury.

Preschoolers begin to safely handle basic tools, kitchen equipment, and cleaning supplies. Children at this age take pride in participating in household projects with a supervising parent. They spend much of their time in the home and in the preschool or child care center. The facilities pose the same potentially harmful environmental conditions as the home, as well as some additional threats to safety (CDC, 2007).

In response to concern about firearm safety in homes with small children, most states have passed Child Access Protection (CAP) legislation to encourage safe storage of firearms. For young children, CAP means a decline in the rate of deaths attributable to firearms. Nevertheless, the number of preschoolers killed by firearms in 2008 (88) was twice that of law enforcement officers (41) (Children's Defense Fund, 2012). Most deaths from firearms are preventable. The risk of death increases in the mere presence of the firearm. Preschool children are physically capable of pulling a trigger before they are able to cognitively depict cause and effect of their actions. Even if gun safety training occurs, most curious children will handle firearms given the opportunity, which may give families a false sense of security (Children's Defense Fund, 2012).

Burns

Scalds and direct flame burns are major hazards for preschoolers. For many young children thermal injury results in an emergency department visit or hospital admission (Ingram et al., 2011). Thermal injury ranks as the third highest cause of death from injuries in U.S. children, most of which stem from residential fires (CDC, 2012a). In preschool children the number of deaths in house fires is nearly double that of other ages. Children of this age experiment with matches and fire, and they may be unable to escape from a fire once it starts. Measures discussed in Chapter 18 to reduce scald burns in the home apply to this age group as well. Preschoolers should be taught about the dangers of matches, open flames, and hot objects. Parents and caregivers should model appropriate use of active and potentially dangerous burning devices.

Drowning

Children more than 3 years old are at lower risk for drowning in the bathtub, but at greater risk for drowning in a swimming pool, than the toddler. Drowning ranks as the second highest cause of death from injuries in U.S. children (CDC, 2012a). Preschool children ages 1 to 4 years are at highest risk for drowning with two near-drowning episodes for every fatality. Most children are close to safety when drowning occurs. With this in mind, it is important to supervise young children when they are near a body of water, install fencing to isolate a residential pool from the house, use personal floatation devices while bathing or playing near a natural body of water, and teach children how to swim and that swimming alone is unsafe. Preschoolers should receive instruction in water safety and swimming and should always be supervised by a trained adult or older person. Because a good outcome depends on early resuscitation, it is reasonable to encourage parents and pool owners to learn cardiopulmonary resuscitation.

Preschoolers have the cognitive ability to learn water survival. They should always wear a personal flotation device (i.e., life jacket) when they are on boats, even when they know how to swim, and they must be supervised when near water, even shallow water. Safety campaigns provide one effective measure to prevent unnecessary injury and death (Children's Defense Fund, 2012; Ingram et al., 2011; Orton et al., 2012; *Healthy People 2020, Improving the Health of Americans*).

Mechanical Forces

Bicycle accidents become a greater source of injury during the preschool years. Many bicycle accidents involve automobiles, and most of these accidents result from the child's errors. Parents should set reasonable and age-appropriate limits on bicycle use. The transition from tricycle to bicycle provides an excellent time to begin using a helmet. Federally approved bicycle helmets are effective in reducing head trauma, a major cause of death among young children (Figure 19-2).

FIGURE 19-2 The use of bicycles warrants the beginning use of safety helmets.

Preschoolers, as passengers or pedestrians, present with great risk for an auto-related accident. At this age, pedestrian injury is more likely to occur than is passenger injury. Preschoolers should be taught proper street-crossing techniques and, generally, should be supervised when crossing streets. Although there is current controversy about the benefit of a car seat over that of the seat belt, restraint of any kind results in decreased fatalities (Rice & Anderson, 2009). Approved car seat restraint systems continue to be recommended for use by preschool aged children at all times during car travel (Rice & Anderson, 2009). The back seat is safer than the front seat, and all car doors should be locked. If the preschooler refuses to use the seat belt or appropriate restraint, parents must insist that the outing be postponed. Parents who provide a good example by using their seat belts directly influence the child's acceptance, and it meets the child's desire at this age to imitate the parent. The child who uses a car seat since infancy will generally accept the seat belt quite well.

Biological Agents

Preschoolers seem healthier than toddlers, with fewer illnesses of the respiratory and gastrointestinal tracts. They have developed antibodies to many common organisms through exposure. Children usually become ill more often when they enter their first group situation, where they may be exposed to new organisms. This concerns parents and should be discussed by the nurse before the child begins attending a group setting. Increasingly, child care settings provide instruction to children about appropriate handwashing techniques to decrease disease transmission and provide relevant health-promotion teaching (Rosen et al., 2011).

Immunization recommendations are reviewed annually and updated with professional educational tools and parent-friendly resources. These resources for professionals and families can be found in a variety of formats, in both Spanish and English at www.cdc.gov/vaccines/schedules/index.html. The American Academy of Pediatrics (AAP) also publishes the most current recommendations annually with a particular focus on the immunization needs of children. The 2012 recommendations can be found at www.healthychildren.org/english/tips-tools/pages/default.aspx#immunization-schedules. The child with a full course of immunizations as an infant receives repeat doses of diphtheria, tetanus, acellular pertussis (DTaP); measles, mumps, rubella (MMR); and varicella (VAR) vaccines between the fourth and sixth year (Centers for Disease Control and Prevention, 2012b). Many states require that all children in a school setting be fully immunized. Parents who choose not to immunize their children usually make this choice for religious reasons, but some parents worry about the risk of the immunization itself (Gilmour et al., 2011). Although vaccines provide an extremely safe way to combat communicable disease, issues about safety do arise. Individual health providers should develop their own strategies to impart evidence-based information, and participate in professional and public educational campaigns to disseminate the information widely (Gilmour et al., 2011). Because autism is often diagnosed around the same time a child is vaccinated, some parents have connected the onset of their child's autism with the vaccine. The American Academy of Pediatrics position statement refutes this association as coincidental (see www.healthychildren.org/English/news/Pages/Thimerosal-in-Vaccines-Not-Linked-to-Autism.aspx for more information) (Johnson et al., 2007). The risk of consequences of the disease itself far outweighs any vaccine risk, but without first-hand experience with vaccine-preventable diseases such as measles, *Haemophilus influenzae* type b, or polio, families today may minimize their severity (Diekema, 2012). Nurses must remain informed about recommended vaccines, their schedule, and their risks and benefits to provide accurate evidence-based information to families.

Nurses who remain informed about reasons for avoiding immunization will be better able to increase parents' understanding of the possible consequences of omitting a dose. Incomplete immunization may also occur as a result of parental forgetfulness or procrastination. Mandatory immunization for school entry provides an effective incentive for these parents. Although immunization rates are improving, disparities exist in certain regions of the United States (Diekema, 2012). Advances on the horizon are more combination vaccines to decrease cost of administration. Noninjectable vaccines that could be inhaled or eaten would greatly enhance pediatric immunization programs with ease of administration and simplified storage.

Continued efforts to vaccinate all children are needed, especially children living in poverty, particularly in large cities, where they are traditionally undervaccinated (Diekema, 2012; Gilmour et al., 2011). Nurses use immunization registry programs to consolidate records, to remind parents, to evaluate the person's scheduled program, and to analyze issues for a particular population. Registry programs avoid duplication and are of particular value to the preschool age group that may not be involved in day care or preschool with mandated immunization. The Centers for Disease Control and Prevention (CDC) publishes recommendations for individuals who have omitted doses for some reason. These alternate schedules are updated regularly along with the routine schedules and are available at the CDC website mentioned previously (www.cdc.gov/vaccines/recs/schedules/child-schedule.htm). When immunizations

have been omitted or delayed, the immunization schedule continues from the dose of the last vaccine. Parents should be fully informed about the potential side effects of immunizations. In most office and clinic settings, parents sign state-developed informed consent documents that describe potential side effects.

Chemical Agents

Preschoolers face exposure to environmental pollutants. The young child's skin area relative to body mass is twice that of an adult's, which increases the risk of toxicity. Environmental exposure has been implicated in the increased prevalence of learning disabilities, because of the unique vulnerability of a child's brain to chemicals (Landrigan & Goldman, 2011; Trasande & Liu, 2011; Tucker, 2012). Disparities exist among populations with regard to their risk. Ethnicity, socioeconomic status, and geographical location all have an impact on the risk of exposure (Landrigan & Goldman, 2011).

In particular, lead is found in products used in folk remedies for many reasons. In the preschool group, lead may be found in products used to treat upset stomach *(empacho)*, constipation, diarrhea, and vomiting. In Hispanic traditional medicine, these products, known as *greta, azarcon, alarcón, coral, luiga, maría luisa,* or *rueda,* may contain extremely high lead contents. Lead has also been found in traditional remedies from cultures other than the Hispanic group. For example, *ghasard,* an Indian traditional tonic, and *ba-baw-san,* a Chinese herbal remedy for colic, have also been found to contain lead.

Sources of lead other than those found in traditional medicine include pottery, cosmetics, and food additives. Common sources of environmental lead are listed at the CDC website (www.cdc.gov/mmwr/preview/mmwrhtml/rr5809a1.htm) in the article titled *Managing Elevated Blood Lead Levels among Young Children: Recommendations from the Advisory Committee on Childhood Lead Poisoning Prevention.* Chemical agents of concern for toddlers, such as pesticides, lead, and passive smoke, continue to merit consideration in the preschool population. Preschoolers, however, become more independent and understand the concepts of safe and poisonous.

More than 90% of U.S. poisonings occur in the home (McGregor et al., 2009). Even though companies enclose many children's medications in childproof packaging, the product may be administered incorrectly by the caregiver, or the child may experiment with another family member's colorful pills. For example, the medication used to treat attention-deficit/hyperactivity disorder, methylphenidate, poisons many children. **Website Resource 19C** presents recommendations on how to childproof a home from poisons.

Many household products, drugs, carbon monoxide, pesticides, lead, mercury, polychlorinated biphenyls, ethers, and poisonous plants pose hazards to preschoolers. Secondary smoke and lead exposure represent negative chemical influences on the growing child.

Preschoolers should receive verbal explanations about poisonous or dangerous substances, but parents cannot rely on preschoolers to remember instructions. A poison control program from the University of Pittsburgh introduced a character called Mr. Yuk in 1971, and this symbol has continued to be used to increase awareness and access to poison control centers (www.chp.edu/CHP/mryuk). The ability to identify warning symbols such as Mr. Yuk helps preschoolers remain safe. Preschools and child care facilities often incorporate topics about environmental pollutants and dangerous substances into their curricula to promote the health of preschoolers. Information about poison control is widely available on-line (www.aapcc.org/dnn/default.aspx). The national, toll-free poison control center number is 800-222-1212. From that number the caller is directed to the nearest poison control center.

Parents should teach children about the four forms of poison, which are *solids:* air fresheners, pills, vitamins, aspirin, lipstick; *liquids:* cleaning products, fuel, alcohol; *sprays:* furniture polish, oven cleaner, room deodorizer; and *invisibles:* carbon monoxide, space heater fumes. Communication with parents about environmental dangers remains a major role of the child care provider.

Cancer

Cancer mortality in preschool children has declined over the past 20 years; however, disparities attributed to race, ethnicity, poverty, and lack of health insurance exist (Bhatia, 2011). About one fifth of childhood cancers occur in preschool aged children (Centers for Disease Control and Prevention, 2009). Most cancer deaths annually in children from newborns to 4 years of age are a result primarily of leukemia, brain/central nervous system (CNS), endocrine (primarily neuroblastomas), and soft tissue malignancies (National Cancer Institute, n.d.). Even though mortality has decreased, the incidence of brain and other CNS tumors has increased (Landrigan & Goldman, 2011). Acute lymphocytic leukemia, the most common childhood cancer, accounts for about one third of the cases of cancer in preschool children (CDC, 2009). Although less common than other solid tumors, retinoblastoma merits attention because of the possible loss of vision. Remarkable advances in long-term survival of children with cancer have occurred. Early detection remains the key to successful treatment; therefore, early, aggressive efforts have been invested in detection programs. Some of the increases in rates of diagnosis may be attributed to improved imaging techniques and early detection.

Leukemia

Acute lymphocytic leukemia (ALL) accounts for one third of the mortality from childhood cancer (CDC, 2009). The incidence of ALL rises from age 2, peaks at age 5, and diminishes through later childhood and adolescence. The dominant signs and symptoms of ALL appear suddenly, but often the child demonstrates a prodromal period of weakness, malaise, anorexia, fever, and tachycardia. Bone pain, petechiae, and hemorrhages after minor procedures such as dental extractions are encountered frequently. When an unexplained infection does not respond to management, suspicion should arise. Early detection and treatment of ALL has resulted in a marked increase in 5-year survival rates. Survival depends on age at diagnosis, with the best survival rates occurring when diagnosis occurs during the preschool years (Hockenberry & Wilson, 2010).

With suspected leukemia, the nurse institutes secondary prevention strategies with an assessment that includes the following parameters:
- Examination of the cervical and peripheral lymph nodes
- Palpation and percussion of the liver and spleen
- Inspection of the skin for systemic signs of leukemia, such as pallor, purpura, petechiae, and chloroma, which is a localized tumor mass that has a greenish appearance and may be found in the skin, orbits, or other tissues in granulocytic forms of leukemia
- Inspection of the mouth for enlarged tonsils; hyperplasia of the gums; and red, friable gingivae
- Palpation of the sternum, bones, and joints for tenderness and pain

The rate of leukemia is higher in children with Down syndrome; therefore, school nurses and public health nurses should monitor these children for early signs of the disease.

Wilms Tumor

Most cases of Wilms tumor occur in children younger than 5 years of age. A strong correlation exists between Wilms tumor and several congenital malformations. Genetic links may contribute to its occurrence in children with bilateral tumors and those who have family members with the disorder. When Wilms tumor, aniridia (a congenital malformation of the iris of the eye), genitourinary malformations, and mental retardation occur together, the genetic association strengthens. However, survivors of Wilms tumor that is unilateral at diagnosis possess a low risk for producing a child who will develop the disease. Information about the risk factors for Wilms tumor is not definitive. The 5-year survival rates for children with this disease are excellent (Hockenberry & Wilson, 2010).

Retinoblastoma

Even as the most common intraocular tumor in younger children, retinoblastoma affects only 300 children younger than 20 years of age each year in the United States. Most of these children are less than 5 years old. Genetic mutations contribute to the incidence of retinoblastoma, usually causing the bilateral form of the disease. Even though the tumor is uncommon, the scientific work surrounding its diagnosis and management has resulted in many of the methods used for treatment of other cancers. Survival rates are excellent (Hockenberry & Wilson, 2010).

The history usually reveals a slow symptom progression. To determine risk factors, the following questions should be asked:
- Do tumors of the eye run in your family?
- If tumors of the eye run in your family, which relatives were affected and how were they treated?
- Have you noticed that your child has eye problems (crossed or lazy eyes or difficulty seeing)?
- Have you noticed any changes in your child's eyes?

Screening eye examinations for high-risk children include the following:
- Visual acuity
- Red reflex, which appears whitish with retinoblastoma (cat's eye reflex)

- Ophthalmoscopic findings
- Lid lag, which is found with exophthalmos
- Strabismus, by doing the cover-uncover test

The cat's eye reflex and strabismus are the most common signs of retinoblastoma. Any suspicious findings indicate referral for further evaluation.

Neuroblastoma

Neuroblastoma, a cancer of the sympathetic nervous system, begins in the abdomen, primarily in the adrenal gland, approximately 70% of the time. The remaining 30% of cases originate in cervical, thoracic, or pelvic areas. Approximately one half of these cancers occurs in individuals younger than 2 years, suggesting the contribution of prenatal or perinatal factors (Urayama, Von Behren, & Reynolds, 2007). More than 90% of diagnoses occur by age 5. Unfortunately, many of the children have metastases when the cancer is identified. Frequently, symptoms of secondary distribution bring the child to the health professional. The survival rate for children diagnosed during the preschool years is improving, but in other age groups it has remained static. There is little convincing evidence of specific risk factors. Prenatal exposure to pesticides and hormones and use of certain medications suggest an increased risk (Landrigan & Goldman, 2011).

Cancer in a child can be frightening to parents, particularly if there is a strong family history of cancers of any kind. Early detection continues to be associated with increased survival rates. Secondary prevention programs should include the warning signs of cancer in children. Routine procedures, such as a bath, provide opportunities for parents to examine the child for physical symptoms of disease that are outlined in Box 19-9.

Asthma

The incidence of asthma, a chronic inflammatory disorder of the airways, is rising more rapidly in preschool-age children than in any other group (U.S. Department of Health and Human Services, 2011).The inflammation in this disorder contributes to a hyperresponsive airway, limited airflow, and respiratory symptoms that include breathlessness, wheezing, cough, and chest tightness. Causes include genetic predisposition, allergens such as animal dander or dust mites, and nonspecific precipitants such as infections, exercise, weather, or stress. Rates for boys exceed those for girls, and rates in the Black and Hispanic populations exceed those in the non-Hispanic White population. Poverty contributes significantly to asthmatic illness, disability, and death (Azad et al., 2012; Tucker, 2012). Multiple factors contribute to exacerbation of asthma symptoms. High levels of exposure to tobacco smoke, pollutants, and allergens contribute. In addition to the generally known allergens of house mite dust and pet and rodent dander, cockroach particles have been implicated. Access to quality medical care, financial resources, and social support to manage the disease on a long-term basis exist in significantly different proportions from one population to another in the United States (U.S. Department of Health and Human Services, 2011).

DETERMINANTS OF HEALTH

Social Factors and Environment

Some preschoolers become involved with groups outside their families, such as group child care settings, church groups, or family involvement in other activities, by age 3. Other children of the same age experience little outside contact. A preschool setting introduces the child to a wider social arena. Parents learn to release their child to encourage independent activity in a safe, supervised setting. Preschoolers test their independence, interactive skills, and self-discipline as they learn to function in a group. Preschool provides a transition to kindergarten and first grade, where group interaction skills are expected. Parents often select

BOX 19-9 WARNING SIGNS THAT MAY INDICATE CHILDHOOD CANCER

Cancer remains a leading cause of death in children under 15 years of age, second only to injuries.

General
- Continued unexplained weight loss
- Persistent poor appetite
- Tires easily or lack of energy
- Tires constantly
- Noticeably pale

Leukemia or Lymphomas: "Liquid Tumors" (Cancer of the Blood, Blood-Making System, Lymph Nodes)
- Persistent fever (more than 2 weeks)
- Bruising without injury and purple or red patches appearing on the skin
- Swollen glands (lymph nodes) unrelated to infection
- Persistent bone pain or limping
- Paleness of the lips, skin, nails, or lining of the eyes

Brain Tumor
- Headaches, frequently with early morning vomiting

- Reflection in the pupil of the eye (eye tumor)
- Unexplained, persistent changes in behavior

Kidney Tumors
- Lump in the abdomen or abdominal enlargement
- Blood in the urine
- Bulging of the eyes
- Unexplained, persistent cough or chest pain
- A firm mass in the muscles

Make Bath Time Examination Time
- These complaints or physical findings should be interpreted only as warnings of possible serious disease. When these warnings are present, you should consult your physician at once.
- Do not forget that your children must be examined by a physician every year. The earlier cancer is detected, the better the chances are for a cure. With current treatment methods of surgery, radiation therapy, and chemotherapy (administration of anticancer drugs), the survival rate of children with certain forms of cancer has improved dramatically.

Data from the Cancer Association of Greater New Orleans, Inc., New Orleans, LA, and Be Child Aware, Child Cancer Symptoms, www.bechildcanceraware.org/child-cancer-info/childcancersymptoms.

a preschool based on geographical closeness to their home or a friend's recommendation, using the most practical approach (Box 19-10). With many child care facilities and options now available, parents frequently visit and evaluate a number of settings to determine the most appropriate for their needs (Bower et al., 2008).

Culture and Ethnicity

Family cultural heritage continues to shape preschoolers. Health-promotion assessment should adapt to cultural differences (Box 19-11: Diversity Awareness). For example, a child who has never seen snow may not be able to know that it is cold. Unlike toddlers, preschoolers frequently ask why the family follows certain practices. These young children notice differences from one family to another. Their playmates may celebrate different holidays or practice family rituals different from their own. As preschoolers experience more activities outside their home, differences become more apparent. Discussion about the strength of cultural differences provides an excellent learning opportunity (Andrews & Boyle, 2008).

Preschoolers also notice ethnic differences in appearance and pronounce skin colors, eyes, and hairstyles as "pretty" or "ugly." The socialization process forms presumptions similar to those of their family or playmates. Parents and caregivers who teach and role model positive behaviors allow children to

see differences in others as being positive rather than negative. Mass media influences on physical attractiveness also contribute and become more significant to the adolescent.

Certain cultures apply more pressure for children to assume responsibility for younger siblings or household tasks. Confusion develops in preschoolers when the family's culture varies from that of most playmates. Disciplinary approaches vary from culture to culture. Uncertainty also results when parents integrate their cultural background into the community standards, but the grandparents adhere to traditional cultural practices, rituals, and childrearing ideas.

Levels of Policy Making and Health

Many safety-focused legislative bills have affected preschoolers (see Chapter 18). School issues, as discussed in Chapter 20, also affect this age group. With current concern about health care costs, financial programs that focus on children may lose when competing with the whole of health care. If overall funding for vulnerable populations such as the homeless and the poor decreases, child health care in general in this country suffers. In the United States, one in every four children under the age of 6 lives in poverty. Poverty is associated with homelessness, which places the child at greater risk for mortality and less participation in health-promotion and disease-prevention programs (Kerker et al., 2011). In addition, homeless children in this population-based study in New York City were less likely to have blood lead levels tested than the comparison populations in outlying metropolitan areas. These children were also more likely than those living outside the city to have high lead levels (>10 mcg/dL). Homeless children had lower blood lead testing rates and a higher proportion of lead levels >10 mcg/dL than did both comparison populations.

Economics

Poverty influences preschoolers as it does any child. Unlike toddlers, preschoolers become more aware of family economic status. A preschooler may know that the family lacks money for

BOX 19-10   EVALUATING A CHILD CARE SETTING

Child care that meets the needs and expectations of parents will most likely ensure a happy preschooler as well. Questions that parents should consider in evaluating and choosing a child care setting include the following:

- Will my needs and those of my child be best met with a caregiver in a family home, commercial center, or preschool, or by having a person come to my home to care for my child?
- What kinds of backup plans will I need or will be available if the provider becomes ill?
- What are my standards for nutrition, safety, sanitation, and health, and can these standards be met at the chosen child care facility?
- How important is it to my child to be with other children? How many children would be ideal for my child's socialization needs?
- What personality attributes and educational preparation do I desire in my child's caregivers? What attributes do I dislike and how will I deal with these attributes to maximize the care given to my child? How important is caregiver stability to me? Can I comfortably communicate with the staff to collaborate with my child's learning?
- What educational philosophy do I want in the setting? What involvement do I wish to have in the educational mission of the facility?
- Do the hours of the facility meet my personal and professional needs? Is close access to my job or home important to me?
- How are the children grouped, and what is the caregiver-to-child ratio?
- Does the cost of the service meet my financial needs? Can I pay part-time fees during vacation or when my child is ill for a lengthy period?
- Is accreditation of the facility mandatory for me to use it?
- What is my internal response or my general feelings about the setting when I visit it before my child's enrollment? Are the caregivers interacting with and responsive to the children? Are the children happy and interactive? Are the children's individual needs addressed appropriately? Is the environment supportive of my child's care? Is discipline appropriate?

BOX 19-11   DIVERSITY AWARENESS
Preschool

Three groups of 36 Chinese children (each with a mean age of 61 months) were studied to identify cognitive abilities that might distinguish children at risk for dyslexia: (1) teacher- or parent-reported (and health care professional–confirmed) language delay; (2) family history of dyslexia; and (3) not at risk.

The cognitive skills studied included syllable awareness, tone detection, rapid automated naming, visual skill, and morphological awareness. Compared to the control, the language-delayed group of children scored significantly lower on all measures. Children in the familial risk group performed significantly worse only on tone detection, morphological awareness, and word recognition.

Testing these skills may be important assessment tools for diagnosing risks for reading problems and may be associated with broader cognitive impairment as found previously in various Indo-European languages.

Data from McBride-Chang, C., Lam, E., Doo, S., Wong, S. W., & Chow, Y. Y. (2008). Word recognition and cognitive profiles of Chinese pre-school children at risk for dyslexia through language delay or familial history of dyslexia. *Journal of Child Psychology and Psychiatry, 49*(2), 211-218.

toys but recognizes less the comprehensive limits to resources that influence the family lifestyle. In some cases the family's financial history prevents attendance at preschool or influences exposure to expanded learning activities. Preschoolers realize money acquires food, toys, and clothes, but they do not yet have a concept of economic values. The child might trade an expensive item for a trinket that looks more interesting. A child who uses the earnings to buy something realizes that more must be earned to buy more things. The child thus begins to learn the concepts of earning and spending.

Health Services/Delivery System

Access to health care resources for preschoolers remains the same as that for toddlers. When preschoolers enter a school setting, admission may require that a health care worker screen them physically and developmentally. For indigent children Early and Periodic Screening, Diagnosis, and Treatment (EPSDT), a Medicaid program, may fund the visit. Screening for children under age 21 who meet the economic criteria for Medicaid occurs in private offices, local health departments, and community clinics. Medicaid provides one screening examination per year, which includes the following elements:

- Medical history
- Assessment of physical growth, nutritional status, and mental development
- Inspection of ears, eyes, nose, mouth, teeth, and throat
- Vision screening
- Auditory screening
- Screening for cardiac abnormalities
- Screening for anemia
- Screening for the sickle cell trait
- Urine sampling
- Blood pressure reading
- Assessment and updating of immunizations
- Tuberculosis screening, when indicated
- Referral to a dentist for diagnosis and treatment for children 3 years of age and older

Referral for a complete physical examination addresses any health or developmental concerns identified during this screening. Eligible children receive EPSDT as a comprehensive service administered by Medicaid. Enactment of the Affordable Care Act in 2012 ensures health coverage for all children and free immunizations, affecting preschool-aged children's health and health promotion (www.healthcare.gov/law/index.html).

NURSING APPLICATION

Preschoolers show much interest in the tools and procedures of a health screening examination (Price & Gwinn, 2008) (Box 19-12). These inquisitive children may play with the stethoscope, otoscope, and other diagnostic instruments. The nurse explains the tests in age-appropriate terminology and expects the child to cooperate for most of the visit. Preschoolers may show self-control during injections but definitely need a parent close by to offer support and encouragement. The nurse includes the preschooler in the history by directing questions about dietary intake and health practices, such as tooth brushing, favorite activities, and friends. At this age children begin taking some interest in health, developing the cognitive maturity to learn many health-promotion skills that they will use for the rest of their lives.

BOX 19-12   HEALTH-PROMOTION SCREENING FOR PRESCHOOL CHILDREN

Annually
- Health history
- Height and weight
- Blood pressure
- Vision screening (age 3 to 4 years)
- Developmental and behavioral assessment
- Physical examination

Periodically
- Immunizations based on recommended schedule
  - Ensure currency
  - Diphtheria, tetanus, pertussis
  - Oral poliovirus
  - Pneumococcal
  - Measles, mumps, rubella
  - *Haemophilus influenzae* type b
  - Hepatitis B
  - Varicella
- Hematocrit or hemoglobin level at least once after age 9 months
- Urinalysis at 5 years old

Screenings for High-Risk Children
- Lead
- Tuberculosis
- Cholesterol

Anticipatory Guidance
- Injury prevention
  - Child safety car seat (age less than 5 years) or seat belt
  - Lap and shoulder belt (age 5 years and older)
  - Use helmet and avoid traffic when bicycling
  - Smoke detectors, flame-retardant sleepwear
  - Hot water temperature less than 125° F
  - Window and stair guards, pool fence
  - Safe storage of drugs, toxic substances, firearms, matches
  - Close availability of syrup of ipecac, poison control phone number
  - Parents and caretakers trained in cardiopulmonary resuscitation
- Violence prevention
- Nutrition and exercise
  - Limit saturated fats; maintain caloric balance; and emphasize grain, fruit, vegetable intake
  - Regular fun physical activity
- Tobacco
  - Effects of passive smoking
  - Antitobacco messages
- Dental health
  - Floss, brush with fluoridated toothpaste at least daily
  - Regular visits to dentist

CASE STUDY

Preschool Child: Ricky

Ricky, age 4, arrives in the clinic with his mother. Ricky lives with his mother and father, who both work full-time, and his infant sister. Their extended family lives in a different state more than 100 miles away. Both parents are of average height and in good health. Ricky's mother mentions that Ricky often expresses frustration, particularly in regard to food. Conflict over food occurs every day. Mealtime is a battle to get him to eat, unless his mother feeds him. Ricky's baby sister eats no table food and seems to be able to tolerate any food given. Ricky's mother is quite frustrated and concerned that he will become malnourished.

Reflective Questions

1. What additional assessment information would you collect?
2. What questions would you ask and how would you further explore this issue with the mother?
3. In what ways does the distance of the extended family influence this family's approach to health promotion?
4. What factors would you consider to determine whether malnourishment is a factor in this family?

CARE PLAN

Ineffective Coping in Preschool Child: Ricky

***NURSING DIAGNOSIS: Ineffective Coping related to parental feedback for regressive behaviors and lack of consistent limits and fulfillment of appropriate responsibilities**

Defining Characteristics
- Parent verbalization of need for help
- Changes in the usual behavior patterns of the child

Related Factors
- Inconsistent methods of parental discipline
- Inadequate impulse control
- Lack of social skills

Expected Outcomes
- The child will separate from his parents without incident (tantrum, crying).
- The child will join a community or church peer group activity.
- The child will perform one household task (picking up his toys) before bedtime every evening.
- The child will demonstrate independent self-care behaviors (feed himself).
- The parents will have clear, consistent, and age-appropriate expectations for behavior.
- The parents will explain the rationale for limiting a socially unacceptable or unsafe behavior as soon as it is displayed.

Interventions
- Discuss with parents the process of growth and development and the child's need to learn how to compromise, take turns, and channel energy appropriately.
- Use a prescreening developmental questionnaire to validate general assessment data.
- Encourage the parents to leave the child in someone else's care while they go shopping or to see a movie.
- Encourage the mother to formulate a bedtime ritual with the child that does not include her sitting in his room until he falls asleep.
- Discuss with the parents and the child what "jobs" he can do at home and the expectation that they be performed daily.
- Suggest laying out the child's clothes so that he can dress himself. Set a time to be dressed, such as before or after a certain television program.
- Explore with the parents the availability of playgroups or community activities for the child.
- Encourage the parents to take the child to the neighborhood playground so that he can meet and play with other children.
- Have the child help around the house alongside his parents. Specify "work" and "play" times.
- Encourage the parents to praise the child for age-appropriate behaviors, being careful not to bribe him to perform.
- Discuss the principles of discipline consistency, immediacy, realistic expectations, and clear explanations.
- Recognize the parents' frustration and encourage them to try different approaches, such as limited choices, diversion, and incentives ("when you finish your meat, we'll play a game").
- Suggest that the parents keep a diary of how long an approach was tried and how consistently the child responded.
- Discuss the decrease in appetite and reliance of food fads that typify the child's age. Review the principles of nutrition, timing of snacks, and ways of making food attractive to children.
- Refer the parents and the child to a nutritionist for nutrition counseling.

Evaluation
- Parents make appropriate verbal, nonverbal, and eye contact.
- Parents demonstrate correct caregiver techniques.
- Parents verbalize intent to maintain relationships.
- Parents attend to routine well child care appointments.
- Parents provide developmentally appropriate play activities.
- Parents describe healthy ways to express frustration.

*NANDA Nursing Diagnoses—Definitions and Classification 2012-2014, Herdman T.H. (ED). Copyright © 2012, 1994-2012 NANDA International. Used by arrangement with John Wiley & Sons Limited. In order to make safe and effective judgments using the NANDA-I nursing diagnoses it is essential that nurses refer to the definitions and defining characteristics of the diagnoses listed in this work.

SUMMARY

Schedules for preventive health care during the preschool years include visits at 4 and 5 years of age. Each visit includes an ongoing history; growth, physical, and developmental assessment; and discussion of age-appropriate developmental concerns.

In addition to the office or clinic contact, the nurse may consult with a preschool nurse or a nurse for a primary school and preschool. Early exposure to and reinforcement of health care information as part of preschool education lays a foundation for later healthy lifestyle habits, which influence overall societal health. Health as a curricular subject during the school-age years continues this focus. The school nurse's role in health promotion and prevention of illness is discussed in Chapter 20.

REFERENCES

Andrews, M. M., & Boyle, J. S. (2008). *Transcultural concepts in nursing care* (5th ed.). New York: Lippincott.

Archibald, L., Joanisse, M., & Edmunds, A. (2011). Specific language or working memory impairments: A small scale observational study. *Child Language Teaching & Therapy, 27*(3), 294–312.

Azad, M. B., Lissitsyn, Y., Miller, G. E., Becker, A. B., Hayglass, K. T., & Kozyrskyj, A. L. (2012). Influence of socioeconomic status trajectories on innate immune responsiveness in children. *PloS One, 7*(6), e38669.

Bagnato, S. J., McLean, M., Macy, M., & Neisworth, J. T. (2011). Identifying instructional targets for early childhood via authentic assessment: Alignment of professional standards and practice-based evidence. *Journal of Early Intervention, 33*(4), 243–253.

Bhatia, S. (2011). Disparities in cancer outcomes: Lessons learned from children with cancer. *Pediatric Blood and Cancer, 56*(6), 994–1002.

Bower, J. K., Hales, D. P., Tate, D. F., Rubin, D. A., Benjamin, S. E., & Ward, D. S. (2008). The childcare environment and children's physical activity [Abstract]. *American Journal of Preventive Medicine, 34*(1), 23–29.

Boyd, B. A., Odom, S. L., Humphreys, B. P., & Sam, A. M. (2010). Infants and toddlers with autism spectrum disorder: Early identification and early intervention. *Journal of Early Intervention, 32*(2), 75–98.

Boyle, C. A., Boulet, S., Schieve, L. A., Cohen, R. A., Blumberg, S. J., Yeargin-Allsopp, M., et al. (2011). Trends in the prevalence of developmental disabilities in US children, 1997-2008. *Pediatrics, 127*(6), 1034–1042. 10.1542/peds.2010-2989.

Brown, W. H., Pfeiffer, K. A., McIver, K. L., Dowda, M., Addy, C. L., & Pate, R. R. (2009). Social and environmental factors associated with preschoolers' non-sedentary physical activity. *Child Development, 80*(1), 45–58.

Centers for Disease Control and Prevention. (2007). Surveillance summaries: Fatal injuries among children by race and ethnicity—United States, 1999-2002. *Morbidity and Mortality Weekly Report, 56*(SS-5), 1–20.

Centers for Disease Control and Prevention (CDC). (2009). *United States cancer statistics: Childhood cancer.* Retrieved July 7, 2012, from http://apps.nccd.cdc.gov/uscs/ChildhoodCancerData. aspx.

Centers for Disease Control and Prevention (CDC). (2012a). *Injury prevention and control: Data and statistics (web-based injury statistics query and reporting system—WISQRS).* Retrieved July 6, 2012, from www.cdc.gov/injury/wisqrs/index.html.

Centers for Disease Control and Prevention (CDC). (2012b). Recommended immunization schedules for persons aged 0-18 years—United States, 2012. *Morbidity and Mortality Weekly Report, 61*(5), 1–4. Retrieved July 6, 2012, from www.cdc.gov/mmwr/preview/mmwrhtml/mm6105a5.htm.

Children's Defense Fund. (2012). *Protect children not guns 2012.* Washington, DC: Author.

Conti-Ramsden, G., & Durkin, K. (2012). Language development and assessment in the preschool period. *Neuropsychology Review, 22*(7), 1–18.

Diekema, D. S. (2012). Improving childhood vaccination rates. *New England Journal of Medicine, 366*(5), 391–393.

Division of Adolescent and School Health, National Center for Chronic Disease Prevention and Health Promotion. (2011). School health guidelines to promote healthy eating and physical activity. *MMWR Recommendations & Reports, 60*(5), 1–78.

Dogra, S., Meisner, B. A., & Ardern, C. I. (2010). Variation in mode of physical activity by ethnicity and time since immigration: A cross-sectional analysis. *International Journal of Behavioral Nutrition & Physical Activity, 7*(10), 1–11.

Driscoll, A., & Nagel, N. G. (2008). *Early childhood education: Birth - 8: the world of children, families, and educators* (4th ed.). New Jersey: Allyn and Bacon.

Fabiano-Smith, L., & Goldstein, B. A. (2010). Phonological acquisition in bilingual Spanish–English speaking children. *Journal of Speech, Language & Hearing Research, 53*(1), 160–178.

Fleischer, D. M., Perry, T. T., Atkins, D., Wood, R. A., Burks, A. W., Jones, S. M., et al. (2012). Allergic reactions to foods in preschool-aged children in a prospective observational food allergy study. *Pediatrics, 130*(1), e25–e32.

Freitag, C. M., Staal, W., Klauck, S. M., Duketis, E., & Waltes, R. (2010). Genetics of autistic disorders: Review and clinical implications. *European Child & Adolescent Psychiatry, 19*(3), 169–178.

Frost, J. L., Wortham, S. C., & Reifel, S. C. (2008). *Play and child development* (3rd ed.). New Jersey: Prentice-Hall.

Gance-Cleveland, B., Sidora-Arcoleo, K., Keesing, H., Gottesman, M. M., & Brady, M. (2009). Changes in nurse practitioners' knowledge and behaviors following brief training on the healthy eating and activity together (HEAT) guidelines. *Journal of Pediatric Health Care, 23*(4), 222–230.

Garrison, M. M., Liekweg, K., & Christakis, D. A. (2011). Media use and child sleep: The impact of content, timing, and environment. *Pediatrics, 128*(1), 29–35.

Gilmour, J., Harrison, C., Asadi, L., Cohen, M. H., & Vohra, S. (2011). Childhood immunization: When physicians and parents disagree. *Pediatrics, 128*(Suppl. 4), S167–S174.

Goldner, L., & Scharf, M. (2012). Children's family drawings and internalizing problems. *The Arts in Psychotherapy, 39*(4), 262–271.

Gonzalez-Mena, J. (2012). *Child, family and community, family centered early care and education* (6th ed.). New Jersey: Prentice-Hall.

Gupta, R. S., Springston, E. E., Warrier, M. R., Smith, B., Kumar, R., Pongracic, J., et al. (2011). The prevalence, severity, and distribution of childhood food allergy in the United States. *Pediatrics, 128*(1), e9–e17.

Gutiérrez-Clellen, V., Simon-Cereijido, G., & Sweet, M. (2012). Predictors of second language acquisition in Latino children with specific language impairment. *American Journal of Speech-Language Pathology, 21*(2), 64–77.

Hammer, C. S., Lawrence, F. R., & Miccio, A. W. (2007). Bilingual children's language abilities and early reading outcomes in head start and kindergarten. *Language, Speech, and Hearing Services in Schools, 38*(3), 237–248.

Hammer, C. S., & Miccio, A. W. (2006). Early language and reading development of bilingual preschoolers from low-income families. *Topics in Language Disorders, 26*(4), 322–337, 385–90.

Healthy People 2020—Improving the health of Americans. Retrieved January 23, 2012, from www.healthypeople.gov/2020/.

Healey, D. M., Flory, J. D., Miller, C. J., & Halperin, J. M. (2011). Maternal positive parenting style is associated with better functioning in hyperactive/inattentive preschool children. *Infant & Child Development, 20*(2), 148–161.

Hoban, T. F. (2010). Sleep disorders in children. *Annals of the New York Academy of Sciences, 1184*(1), 1–14. doi:10.1111/j.1749-6632.1009.05112x.

Hockenberry, M. J., & Wilson, D. (2010). *Wong's nursing care of infants and children* (9th ed.). St. Louis: Mosby.

Houston, K. T., Bradham, T. S., Munoz, K. F., & Guignard, G. H. (2011). Newborn hearing screening: An analysis of current practices. *Volta Review, 111*(2), 109–120.

Howard, K. S., & Brooks-Gunn, J. (2009). The role of home-visiting programs in preventing child abuse and neglect. *The Future of Children/Center for the Future of Children, the David and Lucile Packard Foundation, 19*(2), 119–146.

Ingram, J. C., Deave, T., Towner, E., Errington, G., Kay, B., & Kendrick, D. (2011). Identifying facilitators and barriers for home injury prevention interventions for pre-school children: A systematic review of the quantitative literature. *Health Education Research, 27*(2), 258–268.

Johnson, C. P., Myers, S. M., & The Council on Children with Disabilities. (November 2007). Identification and evaluation of children with autism spectrum disorders. *Pediatrics, 120*(5), 1183–1215.

Joosen, K. J., Mesman, J., Bakermans-Kranenburg, M. J., & van Lizen-doorn, M. H. (2012). Maternal sensitivity to infants in various settings predicts harsh discipline in toddlerhood. *Attachment & Human Development, 14*(2), 101–117.

Kaakinen, J., Gedaly-Duff, V., Coehlo, D. P., & Hanson, S. M.H. (2010). *Family nursing: Theory, practice and research* (4th ed.). Philadelphia: F.A. Davis.

Kaerts, N., Van Hal, G., Vermandel, A., & Wyndaele, J. (2012). Readiness signs used to define the proper moment to start toilet training: A review of the literature. *Neurourology and Urodynamics, 31*(4), 437–440.

Kalpidou, M. D., Power, T. G., Cherry, K. E., & Gottfried, N. W. (2004). Regulation of emotion and behavior among 3- and 5-year-olds. *Journal of General Psychology, 131*(2), 159–178.

Kerker, B. D., Bainbridge, J., Kennedy, J., Bennani, Y., Agerton, T., Marder, D., et al. (2011). A population-based assessment of the health of homeless families in New York City, 2001-2003. *American Journal of Public Health, 101*(3), 546–553.

Kochanska, G., Koenig, J. L., Barry, R. A., Kim, S., & Yoon, J. E. (2010). Children's conscience during toddler and preschool years, moral self, and a competent, adaptive developmental trajectory. *Developmental Psychology, 46*(5), 1320–1332.

Kornides, M. L., Kitsantas, P., Yang, Y. T., & Villarruel, A. M. (2011). Factors associated with obesity in Latino children: A review of the literature. *Hispanic Health Care International, 9*(3), 127–136.

Landrigan, P. J., & Goldman, L. R. (2011). Children's vulnerability to chemicals: A challenge and opportunity to strengthen health and environmental policy. *Health Affairs, 30*(5), 842–850.

Langevin, M., Packman, A., & Onslow, M. (2009). Peer responses to stuttering in the preschool setting. *American Journal of Speech-Language Pathology, 18*(3), 264–276.

LeBlanc, J. J., & Fagiolini, M. (2011). Autism: A "critical period" disorder? *Neural Plasticity.* 2011, 921680.

May-Benson, T. A., Koomar, J. A., & Teasdale, A. (2009). Incidence of pre-, peri-, and post-natal birth and developmental problems of children with sensory processing disorder and children with autism spectrum disorder. *Frontiers in Integrative Neuroscience, 3*, 31.

Lee, S. H., & Im, E. (2010). Ethnic differences in exercise and leisure time physical activity among midlife women. *Journal of Advanced Nursing, 66*(4), 814–827.

Liou, Y. M., Liou, T., & Chang, L. (2010). Obesity among adolescents: Sedentary leisure time and sleeping as determinants. *Journal of Advanced Nursing, 66*(6), 1246–1256.

Luby, J. B., Sullivan, A., Hayen, J., McCadney, R., & Spitznagel, A. (2009). Shame and guilt in preschool depression: Evidence for elevations in self-conscious emotions in depression as early as age 3. *Journal of Child Psychology & Psychiatry, 50*(9), 1156–1166.

Lugo-Neris, M., Jackson, C. W., & Goldstein, H. (2010). Facilitating vocabulary acquisition of young English language learners. *Language, Speech & Hearing Services in Schools, 41*(3), 314–327.

Marshall, S., Golley, R., & Hendrie, G. (2011). Expanding the understanding of how parenting influences the dietary intake and weight status of children: A cross-sectional study. *Nutrition & Dietetics, 68*(2), 127–133.

McCann, J. C., & Ames, B. N. (2007). An overview of evidence for a causal relation between iron deficiency during development and deficits in cognitive or behavioral function. *American Journal of Clinical Nutrition, 85*(4), 931–945.

McGregor, T., Parkar, M., & Rao, S. (2009). Evaluation and management of common childhood poisonings. *American Family Physician, 79*(5), 397–403.

Mefford, H. C., Batshaw, M. L., & Hoffman, E. P. (2012). Genomics, intellectual disability, and autism. *The New England Journal of Medicine, 366*(8), 733–743.

Nappo-Dattoma, L. (2010). Dietary recommendations and guidelines during growth and development of the pediatric patient and eating patterns affecting oral health. *Access, 24*(2), 6.

Nappo-Dattoma, L. (2011). Updated dietary standards: The 2010 dietary guidelines for Americans, MyPlate and other nutrition education resources for the oral health professional. *Access, 25*(8), 16–19.

National Association for Sport and Physical Education. (2009). *Active start: A statement of physical activity guidelines for children birth to five years* (2nd ed.). Reston, VA: National Association for Sport and Physical Education Publications.

National Cancer Institute. (n.d.). *Cancer statistics.* Retrieved July 7, 2012, from http://seer.cancer.gov/statistics/index.html.

National Sleep Foundation. (2011). *Children and sleep.* Retrieved July 6, 2012, from www.sleepfoundation.org/article/sleep-topics/children-and-sleep.

O'Donoghue, L., Rudnicka, A. R., McClelland, J. F., Logan, N. S., & Saunders, K. J. (2012). Visual acuity measures do not reliably detect childhood refractive error—An epidemiological study. *PLoS ONE, 7*(3), e34441.

Oganessian, E., Ivancakova, R., Lencova, E., & Broukal, Z. (2011). Alimentary fluoride intake in preschool children. *BMC Public Health, 11*, 768.

Orton, E., Kendrick, D., West, J., & Tata, L. J. (2012). Independent risk factors for injury in pre-school children: Three population-based nested case-control studies using routine primary care data. *PLoS ONE, 7*(4), e35193.

Phillips, D. A., Phillips, K. H., Grupp, K., & Trigg, L. J. (2009). Sibling violence silenced: Rivalry, competition, wrestling, playing, rough-housing, benign. *Advances in Nursing Science, 32*(2), E1–16.

Price, D. L., & Gwinn, J. F. (2008). *Pediatric nursing.* St. Louis: Saunders Elsevier.

Prior, M., Bavin, E., Cini, E., Eadie, P., & Reilly, S. (2011). Relationships between language impairment, temperament, behavioural adjustment and maternal factors in a community sample of preschool children. *International Journal of Language & Communication Disorders, 46*(4), 489–494.

Rice, T. M., & Anderson, C. L. (2009). The effectiveness of child restraint systems for children aged 3 years or younger during motor vehicle collisions: 1996 to 2005. *American Journal of Public Health, 99*(2), 252–257.

Roberts, M. Y., & Kaiser, A. P. (2011). The effectiveness of parent-implemented language interventions: A meta-analysis. *American Journal of Speech-Language Pathology, 20*(3), 180–199.

Rosen, L., Zucker, D., Brody, D., Engelhard, D., Meir, M., & Manor, O. (2011). Enabling hygienic behavior among preschoolers: Improving environmental conditions through a multifaceted intervention. *American Journal of Health Promotion, 25*(4), 248–256.

Scattone, D., Raggio, D. J., & May, W. (2011). Comparison of the Vineland adaptive behavior scales, second edition, and the Bayley scales of infant and toddler development. *Psychological Reports JID - 0376475, 109*(2), 626–634.

Selwyn, N., Boraschi, D., & Ozkula, S. M. (2009). Drawing digital pictures: An investigation of primary pupils' representations of ICT and schools. *British Educational Research Journal, 35*(6), 909–928.

Shumway, S., Thurm, A., Swedo, S. E., Deprey, L., Barnett, L. A., Amaral, D. G., et al. (2011). Brief report: Symptom onset patterns and functional outcomes in young children with autism spectrum disorders. *Journal of Autism and Developmental Disorders, 41*(12), 1727–1732.

Sparks, S. M., & Taylor, C. M. (2010). *Nursing diagnostic reference manual* (8th ed.). Philadelphia: Lippincott Williams & Wilkins.

Trasande, L., & Liu, Y. (2011). Reducing the staggering costs of environmental disease in children, estimated at $76.6 billion in 2008. *Health Affairs, 30*(5), 863–870.

Tucker, P. G. (2012). *Principals of pediatric environmental health—Course WB2089.* Washington, DC: U.S. Department of Health and Human Services, Agency for Toxic Substances and Disease Registry. Retrieved July 12, 2012, from www.atsdr.cdc.gov/csem/csem.html.

Urayama, K. Y., Von Behren, J., & Reynolds, P. (2007). Birth characteristics and risk of neuroblastoma in young children. *American Journal of Epidemiology, 165*(5), 486–495.

U.S. Department of Agriculture, & U.S. Department of Health and Human Services. (2010). *Dietary guidelines for Americans 2010* (7th ed.). Washington, DC: U.S. Government Printing Office.

U.S. Department of Health and Human Services. (2011). *2020 Topics and objectives.* Retrieved July 7, 2011, from www.healthypeople.gov/2020/topicsobjectives2020/default.aspx.

Vriend, J., & Corkum, P. (2011). Clinical management of behavioral insomnia of childhood. *Psychology Research and Behavior Management, 4*(1), 69–79.

Warren, J. J., Weber-Gasparoni, K., Marshall, T. A., Drake, D. R., Dehkordi-Vakil, F., Dawson, D. V., et al. (2009). A longitudinal study of dental caries risk among very young low SES children. *Community Dentistry and Oral Epidemiology, 37*(2), 116–122.

Water, T. (2011). Critical moments in preschool obesity: The call for nurses and communities to assess and intervene. *Contemporary Nurse: A Journal for the Australian Nursing Profession, 40*(1), 60–70.

Yoo, J., Slack, K. S., & Holl, J. L. (2010). The impact of health-promoting behaviors on low-income children's health: A risk and resilience perspective. *Health & Social Work, 35*(2), 133–143.

Yoshinaga-Itano, C. (2011). Achieving optimal outcomes from EHDI. *ASHA Leader, 16*(11), 14–17.

School-Age Child

Leslie Kennard Scott

evolve WEBSITE

http://evolve.elsevier.com/Edelman/

- Study Questions
- Glossary
- Website Resources
  20A: Blood Pressure Levels for Girls and Boys by Age and Height Percentiles

- 20B: Development of Deciduous and Permanent Teeth
- 20C: Dental Health Education
- 20D: Helpful Information for Parents about Nocturnal Enuresis
- 20E: Common Developmental and Cognitive Tests

OBJECTIVES

After completing this chapter, the reader will be able to:

- Identify expected physical and developmental changes occurring in the school-age child.
- Explore stages of cognitive development of the school-age child, particularly its relation to academic skills and performance.
- Appraise relevant health-promotion needs and common health risk factors found in the school-age child.

- Analyze cultural, societal, peer influence, and stress on development in the school-age child.
- Describe common developmental problems that occur in the school-age child including ways to assist parents in the management of these common problems.
- Determine strategies for the family (parents) to improve the child's self-concept, socialization abilities, and stress reduction in the school-age child.

KEY TERMS

Astigmatism
Attention-deficit/hyperactivity disorder (ADHD)
Auditory acuity
Auditory learners
Child abuse
Chronic serous otitis media
Classifying and ordering
Concrete operation
Conservation
Coping strategies
Dental caries
Depression
Discipline
Disorders of arousal
Dyslexia

Encopresis
Enuresis
Gastroenteritis
Human papillomavirus (HPV)
Hyperopic (farsighted)
Hypertension
Individualized educational plan (IEP)
Individuals with Disabilities Education Act (IDEA)
Industry versus inferiority
Intelligence
Intelligence quotient (IQ)
Kinesthetic learners
"Latchkey children"
Learning disability
Lice (pediculosis)

Limit setting
Malocclusion
Menarche
Meningococcal vaccination
Moral development
Myopia (nearsightedness)
No Child Left Behind Act of 2001
Obesity
Orthodontic care
Ossification
Overweight
Peer group
Phonics
Preconventional level
Puberty

KEY TERMS—cont'd

Public Law 94-142 (Education for All Handicapped Children Act)	Self-esteem	State Children's Health Insurance Program (SCHIP)
Punishment	Sexual abuse	Talismans
Scabies	Sleep talking	Tooth eruption
Section 504 of the Rehabilitation Act of 1973, Amendment Act of 2008	Sleepwalking	Tympanograms
Self-concept	Snellen E chart	Visual acuity
Self-discovery	Socialization	Visual learners
	Somatization	Vision screening programs
	Standardized growth charts	

? THINK ABOUT IT

School-Age Shyness

Rebecca Sims, 7 years of age, has demonstrated withdrawn behavior. Her mother reports she has "always been a quiet and reserved child." She performs well in school; however, her teacher has reported that Rebecca is very quiet and withdrawn and speaks in a hesitant fashion when called on. Rebecca's stepfather has voiced frustration with her withdrawn behavior and has enrolled her in a cheerleading group and an after-school soccer team to combat her shyness. Rebecca will frequently not speak during cheerleading ("she'll just go through the motions") and her soccer coach reports she does not engage with the other players. This pressure has created an intense home environment that has Rebecca's parents feeling frustrated about her behavior. Her stepfather will frequently mention what others are saying about her shyness to Rebecca. "I don't know how else to get her involved with her classmates and get over this shyness."

Rebecca says that she prefers to be alone and is afraid to speak up in school. She has poor eye contact, speaks hesitantly, and shrugs her shoulders in initial response to assessment questions. "I'm afraid they'll laugh at what I say." She reports she "has no friends."

Her parents are divorced and both are remarried. She visits her father every other weekend and on various holidays. Her mother and stepfather are both employed full-time outside the home. They often try to engage her in conversation and include her in activities, but "she seems like she would rather be alone."

- Is Rebecca's behavior typical for a 7-year-old child?
- Discuss the values inherent in Rebecca's and her parents' behavior and how these might be related to the scenario as described.
- How might you, as the health care professional, guide this family in finding ways to encourage Rebecca and thus decrease family stress?
- Are there any further underlying issues that may be contributing to Rebecca's behavior?

"The school-age years" is a span of time between a child's entrance into kindergarten and the beginning of adolescence, a range from 5 to 12 years of age. During this time period observable differences in growth, development, and cognitive ability are prominent. Consider how different the child entering kindergarten is from the preadolescent, particularly the differences in size as well as mental ability. Children grow (physically) much more slowly during this time period as compared with growth during infancy and adolescence. Fine and gross motor skills are being perfected and mental abilities grow tremendously as the child learns to read, write, and compute mathematics in addition to other topics of interest. Relationships outside the family including peer groups are also developing during this phase of growth and development.

Most children are relatively healthy during this time period. Health-promotion and health-maintenance strategies are important. During this period of development children learn to accept personal responsibility and participate in the management of self-care tasks in the areas of personal hygiene, nutrition, physical activity, sleep, and safety. Nurses fill a significant role in the facilitation of parental roles and child roles in meeting growth, developmental, and self-care aspects of the school-age child (Hockenberry & Wilson, 2011; Krause-Parello & Samms, 2010).

BIOLOGY AND GENETICS

A child's growth and development is influenced by genetic inheritance, nutrition, and the physical-sociocultural environments in which the child lives. The school-age child has an overall slimmer appearance as compared with the preschool-age child. Their legs are longer as compared to the rest of the body, allowing greater strength, balance, coordination, and fluidity of motion in running, jumping, climbing, throwing, and riding a bicycle (Hockenberry & Wilson, 2011).

Most body systems reach adult level of function during the school-age years. Before 6 years of age, children use the diaphragm as the primary breathing muscle. After 6 years of age, thoracic muscles develop and the respiratory rate slows to 14 to 24 breaths per minute (Moses, 2011). The school-age child's head circumference continues to grow. However, after age 5 years head growth slows until puberty, at which time the head and brain reach adult circumference measurements (53 to 54 cm; 21 inches) (Hockenberry & Wilson, 2011). The heart slowly grows in size and the heart rate slows to an average rate of 60 to 160 beats per minute, approaching that of an adult. Mean blood pressure is lower in this age group than in adults and ranges from 95 to 105 mm Hg systolic and from 57 to 71 mm Hg diastolic (Moses, 2011). The gastrointestinal system is maturing with increased stomach capacity, resulting in less need for snacks and decreased calorie needs as compared to the preschooler. Bladder capacity improves. The immune system is better able to produce an antibody-antigen response (Hockenberry & Wilson, 2008). By puberty, the endocrine system (with the exception of reproductive function) approaches adult capacity and function.

Elevated Blood Pressure

The long-term effects of elevated blood pressure, **hypertension,** in adults are well-known and documented. The realization that adult hypertension often begins in childhood has encouraged efforts to screen young children for elevated blood pressure. The American Academy of Pediatrics and the American Heart Association recommend that children have their blood pressure measured annually, beginning at 3 years of age (Urbina et al., 2008). This recommendation has transpired as a result of concerns of higher blood pressure values in children over the past 2 decades, demonstrating risk of cardiovascular disease (Rodriguez-Cruz, 2011). About 5 of every 100 children have higher than normal blood pressure levels (American Academy of Pediatrics [AAP], 2011a). Blood pressure values among school-age children may vary greatly depending on height and weight of the child. See **Website Resource 20A** for detailed tables of blood pressure levels for boys and girls according to height and weight.

Black children and Mexican American children are followed closely because of earlier onset and end-stage organ damage in those with hypertension as compared to Caucasian children (American Academy of Pediatrics, 2011a; American Heart Association [AHA], 2011a; Hansen, Gunn, & Kaelber, 2007; Lande et al., 2008; Urbina et al., 2008). A family history of hypertension or identification of an elevated blood pressure in a child mandates close monitoring and assessment of cardiovascular risk factors at well-child check-ups during the school-age years (American Academy of Pediatrics, 2011a; Urbina et al., 2008). Differentiation between primary and secondary hypertension is determined in any school-age child with elevated blood pressure (Urbina et al., 2008).

Physical Growth

Although many children have "spurts" of growth alternating with periods of minimal growth, height and weight growth velocities assume a slower and steadier pace as compared with earlier years of growth. The school-age child gains approximately 5 cm (2 inches) per year in height and 2 to 3 kg (4.4 to 6.6 lb) per year in weight (Hockenberry & Wilson, 2011). Black children tend to be slightly larger and Asian American children somewhat smaller than their Caucasian counterparts, as plotted on growth charts that are believed to be standardized for various ethnic groups (World Health Organization [WHO], 2011). Before the onset of **puberty,** there is little difference in size between boys and girls. However, towards the latter part of this developmental stage, girls tend to grow more rapidly in height and weight (Tidy, 2011). A preadolescent increase in height and weight tends to occur around 10 years of age in girls and 12 years of age in boys. However, maturation rates vary, resulting in a wide range of sizes in both boys and girls, particularly among 10 to 12 year olds (Hockenberry & Wilson, 2011; Tidy, 2011).

Black and Mexican American children mature earlier than do Caucasian children (Rosenfield et al., 2009). Black children are often taller and heavier than their Caucasian counterparts. They also tend to have longer and denser bones, slimmer hips, more muscle, and less fat on their limbs than on their central body as compared to Caucasian children (Hockenberry & Wilson, 2008). Girls tend to mature, enter puberty, and stop growing earlier than boys. From birth, girls tend to have more fat than boys, and after puberty girls have a greater percentage of body weight devoted to fat. In fact, adiposity has a direct correlation to puberty onset in girls, yet conversely relates to a delayed pubertal onset in boys (Rosenfield et al., 2009).

School-age children tend to be concerned about their rate of growth, weight, time of menarche, and final height. These children need to understand that the timing and extent of their physical changes usually reflect their genetic inheritance. When assessing a child's height and weight and before referring to **standardized growth charts,** the height of the child's family must be taken into consideration (Centers for Disease Control [CDC], National Center for Health Statistics, 2010). For more information, see www.cdc.gov/growthcharts/. For example, the child whose height is in the third percentile may have parents who are shorter than average. Shorter height can be expected because of the family's genetic composition. Likewise, although the average age of **menarche** is around 12.5 years in Caucasian girls and 12.0 years in Black girls, most girls experience their menarche at about the same age their mothers did (Rosenfield et al., 2009). With sufficient body fat to stimulate hormones needed for menses, girls can have their first menstrual period between ages 11 and 15 and still be considered normal. As a result of better nutrition and differences in lifestyle, girls appear to experience menarche earlier than did girls of 30 years ago (Tidy, 2011). Although the school-age child experiences numerous physical changes before adolescence, changes in three physical areas are of particular interest: oral development, lymphoid tissue, and motor skills development.

Oral Development

Teeth enable a person to speak, chew, and smile. They also help give the face shape and form. The school-age child appears to be constantly losing or gaining a tooth. Deciduous or baby teeth are usually lost in the same order in which they initially erupted. School-age children begin shedding their first teeth when they are around 6 to 7 years of age, and the process is complete with the loss of the second molars at 11 to 13 years of age. The first permanent teeth, the 6-year molars, erupt at 6 to 7 years of age and continue to erupt until the third molars (wisdom teeth) appear at about 17 to 22 years of age. **Website Resource 20B** shows deciduous teeth and the 32 adult teeth and their average time of appearance. The child between ages 6 and 13 loses and gains approximately four teeth per year. A 13-year-old child should have 28 teeth, having lost 20 deciduous teeth (American Dental Association [ADA], 2011a; Hockenberry & Wilson, 2011). When deciduous teeth erupt, only the crown is lost; the root has been reabsorbed in the developing permanent tooth. As the child's mouth becomes filled with the larger, permanent teeth, the shape of the jaw and the facial appearance normally change. Girls tend to experience earlier permanent **tooth eruption** than do boys (ADA, 2011a).

Dental problems, primarily **dental caries** (cavities), periodontal disease, and **malocclusion,** are among the most common health problems in school-age children today. In fact, it remains the most common chronic disease of children 5 to 17 years of age, four times more prevalent than asthma (Centers for Disease Control and Prevention [CDC], 2011a). Present in up to 42% of children 2 to 11 years of age, untreated caries occur more frequently in poor and ethnically diverse children and in those who lack insurance or access to preventive dental care. School dental programs are necessary to educate school-age children on proper care and maintenance of their teeth. School-based oral health education programs and sealant programs are in line with the *Healthy People 2020* initiatives and interventions for reducing dental caries among children (American Academy of Pediatric Dentistry, 2011; U.S. Department of Health and Human Services [USDHHS], 2012a). Over the past decade of *Healthy People* initiatives it has been determined that community-based and school-based sealant programs can reduce new cases of tooth decay by up to 60% for 2 to 5 years after a single application in high-risk children (CDC, 2011a,b). These programs demonstrate an area in which child oral health can be affected to improve the overall health of children in the United States.

The rapid change in the number and type of teeth and the uneven growth in the child's jaw may cause malocclusion, an unacceptable relationship of the teeth in one jaw to those in the other. Dentists evaluate children with overbites, gaps between teeth, and other alignment problems that may influence speech and eating (American Dental Association [ADA], 2011b). Some children will grow out of these problems, but others may need orthodontic care and appliances (braces) to correct problems or improve their appearance. Peer reaction to braces is addressed as part of the teaching about body changes; this teaching may decrease problems with the child's self-concept or body image as a result of looking different. School dental programs include education about conscientious tooth care for the child who wears braces, because these frequently make brushing and flossing more difficult, especially for the school-age child who lacks manual dexterity (see **Website Resource 20C**).

Lymph Tissue

Lymph tissue grows rapidly throughout childhood, reaching maximal size before puberty, after which it begins to decrease in size, most likely as a result of changes in the concentrations of sex hormones. The amount of lymphoid tissue of a child up to 10 years of age often exceeds that of an adult (Kanwar, 2010). This is most often reflected in the size of the tonsils. As a result, tonsils that appear pathologically enlarged to a parent can be normal for the child's age. Additional lymphoid tissue during the school-age period generally helps this group to have a stronger immune response than do younger and older children. This is a result of the immune system being activated by environmental antigens and exposure to common organisms (Kanwar, 2010).

Motor Skills Development

Neurological, skeletal, and muscular changes combine to increase the child's overall motor abilities. With maturation of the nervous system by age 7 or 8 years, the brain's two hemispheres articulate to allow the child more control over and coordination with motor tasks (Hockenberry & Wilson, 2011).

The child grows taller because of lengthening of the long bones that continues into adolescence. Ossification, replacement of cartilage with bone, occurs throughout childhood but

is not complete until adulthood (Ott, 2008). Therefore special attention must be paid to well-fitting shoes, appropriately sized chairs and desks, and backpack loads to avoid strain on an evolving musculoskeletal system (American Academy of Pediatrics [AAP], 2011b; Hockenberry & Wilson, 2011). Children at this age also need protective sports equipment and conditioning exercises before sports to prevent sports fractures (AAP, 2011b). However, the child builds new bony tissue during the entire period of childhood, which generally allows for rapid healing of fractures. Overweight children typically have greater bone density as compared to their normal weight peers. Although they have greater bone density, this does not translate into reduced risk of fractures and joint pain. In fact, overweight children are more likely to suffer bone fractures and have more joint and muscle pain than their normal weight counterparts (Uusi-Rasi et al., 2010). The etiology of this finding is not clearly understood at this time.

Muscle mass also increases with muscle strength. During the school-age years, physically active boys are slightly stronger than girls, but this difference is not significant until adolescence. With these changes, the child has the potential to perform more complex fine motor and gross motor functions but must practice to perfect these skills. Children willingly exercise their newfound skills and feel pride when others see their improved skill level when bike riding, tying shoes, and engaging in team sports, for example.

GORDON'S FUNCTIONAL HEALTH PATTERNS

Health Perception–Health Management Pattern

The school-age child understands an abstract definition of health and sometimes the factors causing illness, but this understanding differs from that of an adult. Most school-age children perceive symptoms and show an ability to participate in health-promoting behaviors. Health-promoting behaviors taught at school and home must meet the school-age child's cognitive level (concrete operation) and moral level (external rules and forces) to be effective. Teaching strategies using cognitive, psychomotor, and affective senses can help children learn responsibility for their own health (Hagan et al., 2010). This knowledge provides an excellent foundation for health-promotion behaviors during the school years.

School-age children's understanding of illness is directly correlated with their cognitive development and follows a direct sequence of developmental stages. It is important for nurses to integrate the child's developmental views on illness because this has direct implications for plans related to health education. When specifically asked about their ideas on causes of illness, school-age children usually state the germ theory, the punishment theory, or the external forces theory. Although many younger school-age children know that germs play a role in illness, they have limited understanding of how germs work (Durani, 2011; Reeve & Bell, 2009). They may believe that a misdeed or misbehavior caused their illnesses.

Various cultural influences may also contribute to a child's understanding of illness. Hinduism ascribes to the theory of karma (law of cause and effect). Persons create their own destiny by thoughts, words, or deeds (Chattopadhyay, 2007). Illness, accident, or injury results from the karma one creates and is often seen as a means of purification. Belief in the "evil eye," another cultural influence, occurs in many cultures and manifests itself in slightly different ways depending on where it arises. Most cultures believe that the victims are primarily babies or young children because they are so often praised and commented upon by strangers. The evil eye is thought to be based on jealousy and can have significant implications for the health of the victim (Chattopadhyay, 2007; Woodburne, 1945). This belief is strongest in Middle-Eastern countries, Asia, Latin America, and Europe. Attempts to ward off the curse have led to the use of a number of talismans within the various cultures. It is important to be aware of such cultural and developmental beliefs of the school-age child in defining strategies for teaching health promotion.

School-age children face challenges in meeting health-promotion goals as defined by *Healthy People 2020* (USDHHS, 2012b). The *Healthy People 2020* initiatives present selected objectives related to this age group (Box 20-1: *Healthy People*

2020). However, people in the school-age child's life can facilitate societal attainment of these goals (Inman et al., 2011). Parents, caregivers, and teachers teach health-promotion concepts when they spend time monitoring and reinforcing preventive health practices, such as personal hygiene, dental care, and good nutrition. Role playing, reading an age-appropriate book, and modeling of health-promotion behaviors (e.g., washing hands) also may help children make the link between behavior and improved health. Unfortunately, by imitating some caregivers, children can become passive health care consumers, asking few questions, doing as they are told, and perpetuating poor choices. These responses may also be caused by children's developmental and cultural obligation to obey authority figures. Parents, caregivers, and teachers need to make commitments to demonstrate and teach healthy behaviors at home and in school; this helps children develop health values as part of their educational process toward reaching a healthy adulthood (Hagan et al., 2010).

Counseling the child and family on a broad definition of health, one that includes personal and environmental health and safety, requires an awareness of the school-age child's

♥ BOX 20-1 HEALTHY PEOPLE 2020

Selected National Health-Promotion and Disease-Prevention Objectives for School-Age Children

Oral Health
- Reduce proportion of children who experience dental caries in their primary or permanent teeth to 49% for all children in 2020. (Baseline: 54% of children ages 6 to 9 years from 1999 to 2004)
- Reduce proportion of children 6 to 9 years of age with untreated dental decay in primary or permanent teeth to 25.9% by 2020. (Baseline: 28.8% of children ages 6 to 9 years from 1999 to 2004)
- Increase proportion of children 6 to 9 years of age who have received dental sealants on one or more permanent teeth to 28.1% by 2020. (Baseline: 25.5% of children ages 6 to 9 years from 1999 to 2004)
- Increase the percentage of school-based health clinics with an oral health component including dental sealants to 26.6% by 2020. (Baseline: 24.1% of schools offered sealants for 2007 to 2008)
- Increase the percentage of school-based health clinics with a topical fluoride treatment (including fluoride rinse/varnish) program to 32.1% by 2020. (Baseline: 29.2% of schools offered fluoride program for 2007 to 2008)

Respiratory Illness
- Reduce hospitalizations for asthma among children to 8.6 hospitalizations/10,000 children under 18 years of age by 2020. (Baseline: 14.9 hospitalizations/10,000 children for 2007 to 2008)
- Reduce emergency department visits for asthma among children to 49.1/10,000 children by 2020. (Baseline: 56.4/10,000 children for 2007 to 2008)
- Reduce percentage of 5- to 17-year-old children who missed school because of an asthma attack in the previous year to 48.7% by 2020. (Baseline: 58.7% of children 5 to 17 years of age who had an asthma attack in the previous 12 months missed school in 2008)

Injury Prevention
- Increase percent of children 8 to 12 years of age who use safety belts to 86% by 2020. (Baseline: 78% of children 8 to 12 years used safety belt in 2008)

- Increase percent of 6- to 17-year-old children using appropriate protective eyewear to 18.2% by 2020. (Baseline: 16.5% of children wore protective eyewear in 2008)
- Reduce percent of children exposed to any form of violence, crime, or abuse to 54.5% by 2020. (Baseline: 60.6% exposed to crime/abuse in 2008)

Physical Activity
- Increase proportion of our nation's public/private elementary schools that require daily physical education for all students to 4.2%. (Baseline: 3.8% schools required physical education in 2006)
- Increase number of states that require regularly scheduled recess for all students to 17 states by 2020. (Baseline: 7 states required regularly scheduled recess in 2006)
- Increase proportion of children from 2 years to twelfth grade who view TV, videos, or videogames for no more than 2 hours/day to 86.8% by 2020. (Baseline: 78.9% children 6 to 14 years of age viewed TV, video, or played video games for more than 2 hours/day in 2007)
- Increase proportion of children 5 to 15 years of age who walk to school (up to a mile) or bike to school (up to 2 miles). (New objective, no data)

Nutrition
- Reduce the proportion of children and adolescents ages 6 to 11 years who are overweight or obese (defined as at or above gender-specific and age-specific 95th percentile) to 15.7%. (Baseline: 17.4% from 2005 to 2008)
- Prevent inappropriate weight gain in children 6 to 11 years of age. (New indicator, no data)
- Eliminate very low food security among children (target 0.2%) by 2020. (Baseline: 1.3% of households with children had very low food security in 2008)

From U.S. Department of Health and Human Services. (2012b). *Healthy People 2020: Leading health indicators.* [Online]. Retrieved January 2, 2012, from http://healthypeople.gov/2020/LHI/default.aspx.

normal perceptions of health (Inman et al., 2011). The nurse, in consultation with teachers, is in a prime position to use such information in order to present content in a manner beneficial to the school-age child's level of understanding. Topics may include some of the following content areas: cultural difference of causes and management of illnesses, causes of personal and environmental health problems, and critical issues affecting the school-age child's general health (e.g., backpack safety) (AAP, 2011b). All of these issues may be integrated into general academic studies to establish a foundation for teaching prevention as well as help the school-age child develop advocacy skills to become an assertive health care consumer.

Nutritional-Metabolic Pattern

School-age children, like all people, need a well-balanced diet. An average of 1200 to 1600 calories per day is recommended to meet growth requirements (based on sedentary behavior) (American Heart Association, 2011b). Usually these calories are consumed in three daily meals and one or two snacks. School-age children often eat foods low in iron, calcium, and vitamin C, and foods that have a higher fat and sodium content than foods their parents ate when they were this age. There is a disjuncture between current dietary practices and recommended dietary intake of children. These behaviors place children at risk for poor nutritional habits, obesity, iron deficiency anemia, and chronic illnesses such as diabetes and hypertension (American Academy of Child & Adolescent Psychiatry, 2011a).

Factors Influencing Food Intake

Access to food, the influence of mass media, and contemporary busy lifestyles play a role in poor food choices. At the final review of the *Healthy People 2010* initiatives, up to 98% of American households were food secure throughout the year, surpassing the initiative target rate of 94% (USDHHS, 2012c). Federal food assistance programs are in existence to assist in the achievement of these initiative targets.

A multitude of television and billboard messages pressure children to eat certain foods, many of which contain large amounts of salt, sugar, and calories. These messages comprise the bulk of food commercials seen by children. Unfortunately, children are now being exposed to more fast-food commercials than they were in 2003 (Powell et al., 2011). A majority of non–program content time is devoted to food-related advertisements. Frequent and lengthy watching of television and exposure to food-related advertisements has been linked to childhood obesity (Zimmerman & Bell, 2010). In 2005, American children watched an average of 3 hours, 19 minutes of television daily (Powell et al., 2011). In 2010, 50% of meals were eaten away from home and 1 in 5 breakfasts were consumed from McDonald's (Hayman, 2012). These behaviors contribute to more "fast food" consumption and food of poor nutritional quality. On a typical day, 33% of children consume fast food (Demory-Luce & Jensen, 2011). Healthy food often costs more and may be less accessible than unhealthy food (Yukhananov, 2011). Some cultures value food that has high salt and fat content.

Cultural factors as well as food access influence poor nutrition among the homeless and children in child care centers and contribute to the high level of obesity, especially among Hispanic, Black, and Native American children. These groups often lack access to safe and nutritious food. Thus, successful interventions for school-age overweight and nutrition must focus on economic, social, and cultural factors that influence access to and use of food.

Although some school-age children willingly try new foods, many continue to dislike vegetables, fruits, casseroles, spicy foods, and iron-rich foods and prefer a small range of foods. Some children may eat only raw vegetables and fruits and go through a phase of eating only one food at lunch, such as a peanut butter sandwich. These practices seldom hurt the child nutritionally. Unfortunately, at the final review of the *Healthy People 2010,* no progress has been made in initiatives focused on reducing dietary fat intake and increasing consumption of fruits and vegetables in children (USDHHS, 2012c).

Children frequently make their own after-school snacks and need supervision regarding the content. Foods high in vitamins A and C, fruits, and vegetables should be encouraged daily. With parental, caregiver, or teacher help and positive reinforcement, school-age children can learn to calculate nutrition needs, plan family meals, and eat better for their overall health. These activities also assist school-age children in developing wise decision-making practices, feelings of empowerment about health, and healthy food habits for the rest of their lives.

American families have such busy lives that they eat few meals together. A positive environment for nutrition and socialization during a shared meal time is important. Parents encourage positive food habits for each family member, and pressure to eat certain foods is avoided to prevent power struggles between parent or caregiver and child. A child's nutritional pattern usually reflects family patterns. For example, parents who skip breakfast tend to have trouble convincing their children to eat breakfast. Educating children as a group to eat healthy foods can be successful because of the powerful influence of a peer group (people of the same age, experience, and usually gender) (Stock et al., 2007). The child whose friend is eating a candy bar usually prefers the same rather than an apple for a snack.

Nutrition Education

Nutrition education incorporated into the general curriculum of school-age children throughout their educational experience is important. Despite evidence that the school can serve as an environment for nutritional health–promotion education, not all schools require nutrition education from kindergarten through twelfth grade (Hockenberry & Wilson, 2011). School nurses and teachers, as part of core concepts usually taught in school, teach students about choices related to weight control and health and help them understand the role of media and culture in nutritional choices (National Association of School Nurses [NASN], 2012). Teachers and school personnel also serve as role models for optimal eating and exercise habits for children in their charge. Lunch and breakfast programs exist in most schools and meet guidelines established by the U.S. Department of Agriculture [USDA] (2011). Many of these programs continue in after-school programs and during the summer when school is out of session to support needs

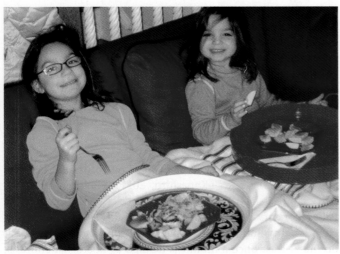

FIGURE 20-1 Children 9 to 13 years old should eat two or more portions of vegetables and fruit totaling 3 to 4 cups daily.

for quality food intake in 31 million U.S. children (Martin & Oakley, 2008; NASN, 2012; USDA, 2011).

The American Academy of Pediatrics and the American Heart Association have established dietary guidelines for children and adolescents. Daily nutritional needs of a child who is 9 to 14 years old include the following (AHA, 2011b) (Figure 20-1):

- Milk group: 3 cups (24 oz total) of fat-free milk
- Meat group: 5 oz of lean meat or beans; or equivalent combinations of these foods
- Vegetable group: 2 to 2½ cups of vegetables daily
- Fruit group: 1½ cups of fruit
- Grains group: 4 to 6 oz daily, of which half should be whole-grain items (AHA, 2011b)

Overweight and Obesity

Overweight and obesity are major nutritional problems that have reached alarming proportions among adults and children in the United States. The Expert Committee on the Assessment, Prevention, and Treatment of Child & Adolescent Overweight and Obesity lists the following definitions for use in children and adolescents (CDC, 2011c):

- Individuals 2 to 18 years of age with a body mass index (BMI) >95th percentile for age and gender or BMI exceeds 30 (whichever is smaller) should be considered obese.
- Individuals with a BMI >85th percentile, but <95th percentile, should be considered overweight.

The problem of overweight and obesity in children and adolescents has increased significantly over the last 50 years. Childhood obesity is now the number one concern for parents, surpassing drug abuse and smoking. One in three children is now considered overweight or obese (AHA, 2011c). Unfortunately, this demonstrates movement away from the *Healthy People 2010* initiative target of 15% (Hobson, 2010). Evidence suggests that adult obesity begins in infancy or childhood and results from both genetic and environmental factors. For example, a child whose overweight parents constantly use food as a reward faces a greater risk for obesity than does a child of thin parents who do not reward with food. Excessive food intake and lack of physical activity also lead to obesity, and once overweight these children tend to exercise even less. Overweight occurs more in Black and Hispanic children than in Caucasian children (35%, 37.9%, and 30%, respectively) (AHA, 2011c). These higher overweight and obesity rates may reflect less physical activity of Black and Hispanic children attributable to unhealthy living conditions and an inability to purchase higher-cost healthy food choices (Taveras et al., 2010).

Overweight increases the risk of hypertension, diabetes, sleep apnea, orthopedic problems, and heart disease. In fact, experts believe that overweight and sedentary behaviors are the primary risk factors for the development of insulin resistance, hyperlipidemia, hypertension, type 2 diabetes, and heart disease (AHA, 2011c). There is also evidence that postprandial hyperinsulinemia may result in excessive weight gain (Felszeghy, Juhasz, Kaposzta & Ilyes, 2008). Also, hormones released during the pubertal years make the situation worse in that these hormones cause the body to use insulin less effectively, leading to insulin resistance and thus increasing the risk for development of type 2 diabetes.

Current evidence suggests that overweight is associated with obstructive sleep apnea. Whether each disease state increases the expression of the other is unclear at this time (CDC, 2011c; Myers, 2009). The potential association between short sleep duration and childhood overweight has been described in the literature (Box 20-2: Research for Evidence-Based Practice). Longer sleep durations are associated with higher degrees of activity, which may assist with weight loss. Recent findings support the proactive approach of ensuring adequate sleep in the prevention of overweight in children (Bayer, Rosario, Wabitsch, & von Kries, 2009).

The overweight and obese child faces ridicule by peers and discrimination later in life. These responses reinforce an already low self-esteem and poor body image and cause a cycle of personal isolation that influences a child's success, current and future (American Academy of Child & Adolescent Psychiatry [AACAP], 2011a). Helping the overweight and obese child change lifestyle patterns requires intensive intervention, including the support of parents. Even with these interventions, few overweight children achieve or maintain significant weight loss because of the complexity of factors (environmental, cultural, economic, and psychological) involved (Hockenberry & Wilson, 2011). In addition, there are reports that failure of maintained weight loss may be associated with impulsivity behaviors (van den Berg, Pieterse, Malik, Luman, Williams van Dijk, Oosterlaan et al., 2011). Some success has been achieved by programs that include implementing reasonable caloric restriction; eating a variety of low-fat and low-cholesterol foods; and utilizing diet support groups, physical exercise, peer counseling groups, and habit changes (AACAP, 2011a). However, intervention sometimes fails because some school-age children do not show concern about being overweight. Nursing suggestions for parents who are interested in preventing obesity in their school-age children appear in Box 20-3.

BOX 20-2   RESEARCH FOR EVIDENCE-BASED PRACTICE

Sleep Duration Relation to Overweight in Children

The purpose of this study was to better describe the association between short sleep duration or sleep problems with childhood overweight. Emerging research has introduced the association between sleep and the regulation of many physiological functions including energy balance, appetite, and weight maintenance. The researchers sought to determine if the association of short sleep duration and overweight in children existed while controlling for measures such as quality of the home environment, parenting, and child behavior problems.

A longitudinal study of 785 children and their parents who were enrolled in the National Institute of Child Health and Human Development Study of Early Childcare and Youth Development was conducted. Data were collected regarding body mass index (BMI), gender, socioeconomic status, and race in third and sixth grade students. Questionnaires regarding sleep and home environment were completed by the participant's mother at the same time intervals.

Findings reported an association between short sleep duration in the sixth grade and overweight in the sixth grade. Shorter sleep duration in the third grade was independently associated with overweight in the sixth grade regardless of the child's weight in the third grade. For every additional hour of sleep received in the sixth grade, the child was 20% less likely to be overweight in sixth grade. For every additional hour of sleep in the third grade, the child was 40% less likely to be overweight in the sixth grade. Interestingly, sleep problems were not associated with overweight in children.

Adequate sleep duration in childhood may offer a protective effect on weight maintenance and overweight risk in children. One preventive approach to overweight in children may simply be to ensure adequate sleep in childhood.

Data from Lumeng, J., Somashekar, D., Appugliese, D., Kaciroti, N., Corwyn, R., & Bradley, R. (2007). Shorter sleep duration is associated with increased risk for being overweight at ages 9 to 12 years. *Pediatrics, 120*(5), 1020-1029.

BOX 20-3   NURSING INTERVENTIONS TO PREVENT OVERWEIGHT/OBESITY DURING THE SCHOOL-AGE YEARS

- Incorporate discussion of healthy food intake and daily activity into daily school life.
- Encourage parents to be a role model for their child—be active; plan physically active family outings.
- Make activity FUN!
- Limit the amount of TV, video games, time on computer/Internet use.
- Discourage eating while watching TV.
- Encourage parent(s) to consider cultural influences on dietary intake. Evaluate snacking habits and food choices. Balance healthy foods with ethnic food choices.
- Encourage family to assess "fast food" consumption and explore/develop eating habits that support a healthier diet as defined by MyPlate.
- Encourage child to participate in food/meal selection and preparation.
- Support lunch choices that meet overall healthy nutrition intake.

Sources: Hagan, J., Shaw, J., & Duncan, R. (2007). *Bright futures: Guidelines for health supervision of infants, children, and adolescents* (3rd ed.). Elk Grove, IL: American Academy of Pediatrics; Bruss, M., Applegate, B., Quitugua, J., Placios, R., & Morris, J. (2007). Ethnicity and diet of children: Development of culturally sensitive measures. *Health Education Behavior, 34*(5):735-747, 2007.

Elimination Pattern

Most children have full bowel and bladder control by 5 years of age. Control involves the ability to undress and dress and to wipe, flush, and clean hands. The child's elimination patterns are similar to the adult's, with urination occurring six to eight times a day and bowel movements averaging one or two times a day (Hockenberry & Wilson, 2011). For some school-age children, however, elimination continues to be a problem.

Enuresis

Involuntary urination at an age when control should be present is called enuresis (Kaneshiro, 2011). Children with primary enuresis have never achieved bladder control, and those with secondary enuresis have periods of dryness and recurrent enuresis. Involuntary nocturnal urination (bedwetting) that occurs at least once a month is defined as nocturnal enuresis, and wetting during the day has been termed diurnal enuresis (Ball & Bindler, 2008). Enuresis should not be considered a disease but a variation of normal development. Enuresis affects 7% of boys and 3% of girls at 5 years of age (Chakraburtty, 2012).

Nocturnal enuresis causes disruption for both child and family. The child may frequently experience teasing from classmates and siblings. It can have profound effects on life socially, emotionally, and behaviorally. Although many forms of enuresis do not pose any significant health risk, there are social stressors. A night away from home appears impossible because of fear of wetting. Parents may be angry about the frequent bed changes and laundering and may try punishments, thinking that the child should be able to control the problem. Parental stress places additional pressure on the child, who may already have low self-esteem and lack self-confidence as a result of a perceived inability to control the problem (Pillinger, 2011).

Often because they lack information, frustrated families seek help. Many therapies exist yet require a high degree of motivation from the child and parents. Their views must be taken into consideration when considering various treatment options. In addition to providing information, the nurse provides active support to facilitate coping. **Website Resource 20D** presents helpful information for parents about nocturnal enuresis. If a child does not have a urinary tract infection, various forms of management may be considered. These include wet alarm systems, bladder training and retention control, waking schedules, drug therapy, and hormone therapy. Each method has advantages, disadvantages, and cost considerations, but all require consistency and time from the child and parents, as well as positive reinforcement by the parents, to reach a successful outcome (Pillinger, 2011).

Diurnal enuresis is often called daytime dribbling. This term describes a urinary pattern most often seen in school-age girls. These children demonstrate "holding on" behaviors, including not voiding first thing in the morning, voiding only two or three times a day, and voiding exceptionally quickly (National Institute of Diabetes and Digestive and Kidney Diseases [NIDDK], 2010). It is not clear why children delay urination or empty their bladders only partially, thus promoting overflow incontinence. Evaluation of these children begins with a urine culture to rule out urinary tract infection. If no infection exists or symptoms persist after treatment, then the intervention is focused on increasing fluid intake to prevent "holding" and establishing a voiding routine of every 2 hours, with a conscious effort to empty the bladder completely. The nurse can be instrumental in helping the child and parents understand the problem and its management.

Encopresis

Another elimination problem that may occur in children is encopresis, defined as the persistent voluntary or involuntary passing of stool into the child's underpants after age 4 (Hockenberry & Wilson, 2011). In most cases, the problem has no discernible physiological cause and is not related to laxative use. There may be a history of inconsistent toilet training or early life stress in affected children. Encopresis is a common complication of chronic constipation. In fact, more than 90% of children with encopresis have a history of recent constipation and/or painful bowel movements (Gavin, 2012). Once children become constipated or have hard and painful stools, they begin to hold their bowel movements to prevent further pain. This creates a cycle that leads to fecal impaction and rectal distention. Stool then begins to leak around the impaction and leaks through the child's rectum, often times without the child's knowledge. In most cases, soiling occurs during the day when the child is awake and active. Soiling at night is uncommon.

Encopresis is often associated with complaints of recurrent abdominal pain and, for many, enuresis as well. Often these children have emotional difficulties that began before or resulted from encopresis. They experience poor peer relationships and self-esteem, perhaps attributable to their offensive odor. Awareness of this childhood problem is necessary to appropriately identify the affected child, refer the child for treatment, and support the child and family during a bowel management program and counseling.

Activity-Exercise Pattern

Physical activity in children is an important aspect of health and an integral component of health promotion. Childhood is considered to be a critical time in which regular physical activity behaviors are acquired and fostered (Figure 20-2). Generally, the school-age child is naturally active although many do not meet current activity recommendations (Mattocks et al., 2008). Boys are typically more active than girls (Figure 20-3). Also, those who perceive their neighborhood as unsafe or do not have at least one parent who exercises are less likely to exercise themselves. Physical activity and participation in sport activities tends to decrease with age, particularly among girls.

As previously discussed, impressive changes in motor skills occur between the ages of 6 and 12 years, allowing the child to engage in many activities that develop strength, balance, and coordination (Table 20-1). Exercise typically occurs through group activities and organized sports such as Little League baseball and soccer, through individual activities such as gymnastics and ballet, and through unorganized play such as bike riding, sledding, rollerblading, and imaginary play. Typically play provides important learning and health promotion and for this

FIGURE 20-2 Peer play is important during the school-age years.

FIGURE 20-3 Boys are typically more active than girls.

reason should be encouraged consistently during the school-age years. For many children, involvement in physical activities is fun and connects them to their peers, family members, and other important people in their lives (Milteer et al., 2012).

Play activities also promote social, personal, and cognitive development. School-age children frequently prefer interacting with peers rather than with family. This desire for peer interaction, usually with one of the same gender, extends beyond school and carries over to play and outside activities (Hockenberry & Wilson, 2011). A child's skill in motor tasks wins the respect of other children and provides a feeling of self-accomplishment (Williams, 2008). Organized sports such as baseball teach team cooperation, competition, and other social skills. Concerns exist that young children have experienced too much physical and psychological pressure to perform in sports. This has generated a renewed commitment by many parents to focus more on the fun of sports than on the winning of games (Craggs et al., 2011). In addition, organized activities such as Scouts and 4-H clubs teach children about group functioning, processes involved in carrying out a task, and the power of social relationships to create change. These lessons can prepare them for discipline needed for a job later in life. Overall, children who

TABLE 20-1 GROWTH AND DEVELOPMENT

Motor Development of the School-Age Child

AGE (YEARS)	GROSS MOTOR	FINE MOTOR
5	Dresses independently Runs well and jumps	Prints letters Ties shoes, buttons Draws triangle, square
6 to 8	Balances on one foot for 10 seconds Can perform tandem gait Pedals a bicycle Is skilled in physical activities, running, skipping	Spreads with knife Holds pencil with fingertip Draws a person with 3 to 6 parts Cuts and pastes Aligns letters horizontally Knows right from left
8 to 10	Has good body balance Enjoys vigorous activities Has increased coordination	Spaces words and letters with writing Draws a diamond Has good eye-hand coordination Bathes self Sews and builds models
10 to 12	Balances on one foot for 15 seconds Catches a fly ball May experience clumsiness from prepubertal growth spurt Possesses all basic motor skills similar to adult	Writes well Has skills similar to those of an adult

From Ball, J., & Bindler, R. (2008). *Child health nursing: Partnering with children & families.* Upper Saddle River, NJ: Pearson-Prentice Hall.

perform well in these activities, evidenced by prizes or trophies, feel good about themselves, their competence, and their sense of industry (Hockenberry & Wilson, 2011). Parents and teachers who compliment children when they perform well enhance self-esteem, as well.

As part of play, school-age children incorporate new cognitive skills, including the ability to count and sort objects. Children of this age express pleasure in their collections of stamps, rocks, or other objects. Understanding the concepts of fair and consistent rules found in games requires cognitive skills of memory, logical reasoning, and the desire to work with others (Hockenberry & Wilson, 2011). Many children like to read, which provides ideas about life and cultures that differ from their own, thereby enhancing their acceptance of human diversity. The nurse helps parents promote healthy play activities for children by encouraging the following (AAP, 2011c):

- Family activities that focus on physical activity and togetherness between parents or caregivers and children, such as daily reading (out loud or silently)
- Use of a library card to encourage reading on a variety of topics and to teach responsibilities involved with borrowing
- Purchase of personal magazines for children's learning and ownership

- Monitoring of daily television and computer use that detract from physical activity and more active mental activities
- Encouragement of both group and solitary activities to support the child's overall development

Sleep-Rest Pattern

Sleep Patterns

Most school-age children have no difficulties with sleep. Generally their sleep requirements and patterns are more similar to those of an adult than those of a younger child. Individual needs vary based on activity, age, and state of health, but most school-age children sleep between 10 and 12 hours a night without naps during the day (Gavin, 2011). Unlike younger children, school-age children experience few difficulties with going to bed. Most children and parents can agree on a bedtime with some flexibility on non–school nights and adhere to that agreement. When problems arise regarding bedtime, children may be testing parents who have not been clear and firm about their expectations for going to bed or have not been willing to discuss the arrangement with their children (Boyse, 2010). Although most Americans accept the idea that school-age children should sleep in their own beds, some Black, Hispanic, Chinese, and Japanese families may encourage the family or siblings to sleep together (Li et al., 2009). Studies have shown that in the school-age child, bed-sharing does not have any impact on sleep patterns, nor does it show any long-term effects towards health, positive or negative (Boyse, 2010).

Sleep Disturbances

The most common sleep problems that occur during the preschool and school-age years are night terrors (see Chapter 19), **sleepwalking, sleep talking,** and enuresis. As a group, these disturbances have been called **disorders of arousal** (Boyse, 2010) and share the following characteristics:

- They occur immediately before a REM, or rapid eye movement, state of sleep.
- Most occur 1 to 2 hours after going to sleep.
- There is a family history of sleep problems, and more boys experience sleep problems than girls.
- Problems reflect normal central nervous system (CNS) immaturity of the child.
- Problems may be influenced by fatigue and stress within the child.
- Problems do not involve the respiratory system.

Approximately one out of six children (15%) between ages 5 and 12 has sleepwalked at least once, but far fewer children walk in their sleep persistently. Sleepwalking is most likely due to the brain's inability to regulate sleep/wake cycles because of immaturity of the nervous system. It occurs more often in boys and often occurs with enuresis (Hopkins & Glaze, 2008). Shortly after going to sleep, the child may suddenly sit up in bed, make repetitive finger and hand movements, or walk, usually for a short time. In most cases, however, the child stays in bed. The child may mumble when talking to a parent or other person (sleep talking). The words tend to be simple but unclear to the listener. Often the child falls back to sleep quickly after talking or walking (Boyse, 2010; Hockenberry & Wilson, 2011).

Parents who are concerned about sleepwalking or sleep talking need to know that most children outgrow these episodes with CNS maturation. However, parents protect their child from injury by placing gates at the top of stairs and removing sharp objects from the child's path. Most parents find that the easiest solution is to direct the sleepwalker back to bed, where the child returns to a normal sleep (Hockenberry & Wilson, 2011). Occasionally parents can intervene effectively by implementing relaxation techniques for their child before bedtime, avoiding stressful and fatiguing situations, and providing consistency with sleep preparation patterns (American Academy of Sleep Medicine, 2006; Boyse, 2010). If a child has many episodes of sleepwalking or sleep talking or if parents express particular concern, he or she may need further evaluation and treatment by health care professionals.

Cognitive-Perceptual Pattern

The school-age child spends extensive time in settings that require mastery of new ideas and concepts. The child's basic intelligence, heredity, and environment encourage or discourage learning. Mastery of ideas and learning requires intact senses, such as vision, hearing, language, and memory capabilities that allow for cognitive development and acquisition of skills needed for later life success (Brannagan, 2010). Unfortunately, many children in society lack these capabilities and will have learning problems if not identified early through parental awareness, school observations, or routine health care assessments. For further information about school-age tests or procedural preparations, see www.nlm.nih.gov/medlineplus/ency/article/002058.htm (Manheim, 2010).

Piaget's Theory

Piaget (2001) refers to the age span of 7 to 11 years as the period of concrete operation, a stage when children learn by manipulating concrete objects and lack the ability to perform thinking operations that require abstraction. During this time, the child moves from egocentric interactions to more cooperative interactions and increased understanding of many concepts gained through environmental connections (Atherton, 2011). Children increasingly change their reasoning from intuitive to logical or rational operations (rule-governed actions) and engage in serial ordering, addition, subtraction, and other basic mathematical skills. The operations of this period are termed concrete because the child's mental operations or actions still depend on the ability to perceive specific examples of what has happened. Older school-age children use both concrete and recently acquired abstract operations, which add flexibility and control to their thinking and meet developmental needs of adolescence. Unlike the egocentric preschooler, a school-age child begins to take the other person's point of view into account. This trait does not emerge suddenly and completely (Hockenberry & Wilson, 2011). The new skill appears occasionally and then more frequently as the child's mental capacity and experience grow.

During the school-age period, the child understands a number of expanding concepts regarding objects, including the concept of conservation of substance (Atherton, 2011). When asked if a difference exists in the amount of liquid poured into two glasses of different shapes, the preschool, preoperational child focuses on the different shapes and says "yes." The concrete operational school-age child realizes that no change has occurred in the substance despite the change in shape (Hockenberry & Wilson, 2011). Conservation of numbers, weight, volume, and quantity, required to understand basic mathematics, sequentially develops as the school-age child gains chronological age and experience.

The concept of time also develops during this period. Children begin to learn to tell time and understand the passage of time. By age 8, most children understand the difference between past and present, and history becomes meaningful (Hockenberry & Wilson, 2011). The concept of human aging becomes increasingly understandable, and the child can comprehend the difference between an 18-year-old and an 80-year-old person.

Two major operations of the school-age period are classifying and ordering. The child classifies or groups objects by their common elements and understands the relationship between groups or classes (Hockenberry & Wilson, 2011). For example, when given 12 wooden beads, some brown and some white, the child understands that the beads may be grouped by their color and by their material. Conversely, the preschool child focuses only on one property of the beads, such as color. The newfound ability to classify shows in the school-age child's interest in collections, such as stamps or coins (Atherton, 2011). Children in school frequently "order" their world; they line up in school according to height, they repeat numbers and letters in their classic order, and they receive numbers in school to reflect an alphabetized surname. These two operations (classifying and ordering) must exist to learn to read, understand the concepts of numbers, and learn subjects based on relations, such as history (the relation of events in time) and geography (the relation of places in space) (Hockenberry & Wilson, 2011).

Vision

The child's sensory abilities continue to develop during the school-age years. Visual capacity should reach optimal function by the sixth or seventh year (Stephenson, 2010). Peripheral vision and the ability to discriminate fine color distinctions should be fully developed as well. Although many 4 year olds have 20/20 vision, a school-age child should have a visual acuity of at least 20/30 in each eye, as measured by the Snellen E chart, an assessment tool for children who can read some letters (Segre, 2011).

Physiological changes occur in the eye during the school-age years. Eyes in the preschool years are normally hyperopic (farsighted), a condition in which the visual image of an object falls behind the retina (Hockenberry & Wilson, 2011). However, unlike older individuals, preschool children do not need glasses because their eyes normally accommodate by adjusting their lenses. For most children, vision becomes normal as the shape of the eye changes and lengthens with maturation. However, many school-age children need visual correction to prevent academic difficulties and headaches and dizziness when reading or doing close work.

Twenty-five percent of school-age children have visual problems. Unfortunately, only about one third of all states in the United States require children have an eye examination or vision screening before entering school (American Optometric Association, 2012). **Vision screening programs** for school children are intended to help identify those children who have or may potentially have a vision problem that may affect physiological or perceptual processes of vision or that could interfere with school performance. Vision screenings are not diagnostic nor do they lead to treatment, but rather only indicate a potential need for further care. The school nurse is in an optimal position to ensure eye screenings are performed and the nurse encourages parents of children with deficits to seek further optometric care to correct these defects so that these children can learn more effectively.

Two visual problems are common in the age group of the school-age child. Many school-age children inherit **myopia (nearsightedness)**, a condition in which the visual image of an object falls in front of the retina, causing the child to have difficulty seeing distant objects (Hockenberry & Wilson, 2011). The other condition, **astigmatism**, causes blurred vision because the image is focused poorly on the retina because of changes in the surface of the cornea or lens (Hockenberry & Wilson, 2008). Eyeglasses correct the defects, but the problem must be identified before it can be solved (American Optometric Association, 2012). For example, a child with myopia may not realize that his visual images are impaired. Children with corrective lenses often express delight and surprise when they first see the fully focused and rich detail of the world after experiencing less refined visual acuity for some time.

Hearing

The child's hearing ability **(auditory acuity)** is nearly complete by 7 years of age, although some maturation continues into adolescence. Hearing deficits occur less frequently than visual deficits, but hearing loss affects more than 1 million children from birth to age 21 years in the United States (American Academy of Otolaryngology, 2011a). This deficit compromises learning in school and important socialization with peers. **Chronic serous otitis media,** or long-term fluid in the middle ear, remains a common cause of hearing deficit in both the preschool and the early school-age years (American Academy of Otolaryngology, 2011b; Hockenberry & Wilson, 2008). Fortunately, reduction in rates of otitis media in children has met the *Healthy People 2010* initiative targets (National Institute on Deafness and Other Communication Disorders, 2010). The success of meeting this initiative has been attributed to the introduction of heptavalent pneumococcal conjugate vaccine in 2000 (National Institute on Deafness and Other Communication Disorders, 2011). Additionally, concerns about the potential for long-term hearing loss in children who listen to loud music have been raised (Hockenberry & Wilson, 2011).

All school-age children, especially those with a history of recurrent ear infections or fluid behind the eardrum, should have periodic hearing evaluations performed as part of a health-promotion program in school and as required by many states. Various treatments exist for acute otitis media, including antibiotics and the recent discovery that Xylitol gum may be of some preventive benefit (Fuller, 2007). Additionally, work continues on a vaccination for prevention of otitis media infections. **Tympanograms,** used to measure the sensitivity of the tympanic membrane to vibrations induced by pressure and sound waves, help detect and monitor this problem as part of well-child and ill-child care. The nurse considers education on hearing protection for school-age children in order to maintain this important sense for the future.

Sensory Perception

Children learn simultaneously through many senses, and most teaching approaches incorporate this concept. For example, young school-age children see a letter, hear its sound, and feel its shape. With this approach, children learn in a number of ways to interpret an event. For example, some children learn best by listening **(auditory learners)**, others by doing **(kinesthetic learners)**, and others by engaging all sensory modalities (auditory, kinesthetic, and **visual learners**). Because no two children have exactly the same sensory acuity, sensitivity, or discrimination, all children build slightly different perceptions and conceptions of the world around them and do not follow the same timetable to grasp concepts. Therefore, teaching approaches must be individualized to meet the learning needs of most children.

Of all the senses, visual perception has been studied the most, primarily because of its role in helping children learn to read. Studies have examined children's abilities to discriminate parts of a picture (to see a figure within a picture). Children usually progress from the preschool stage, during which they perceive visual stimuli more as a whole, to the school-age stage, during which they perceive more details, and finally to the point at which they perceive and integrate both. This process helps children recognize letters, the first step needed for reading. Children may first be able to differentiate between obviously different letters, such as "h" and "o," but may have difficulty with letters similar in appearance, such as "b" and "d," until they can distinguish details more effectively (Hockenberry & Wilson, 2011).

Language

Language develops rapidly during the school years. Most school-age children enter this period with an ability to understand and speak a language, but with only a basic knowledge of reading and writing. By the end of the school-age period, most children have acquired at least a functional ability in both areas. Language development mandates that a child have visual perception for reading, auditory acuity and perception for understanding spoken language, and fine motor skills for both articulation and handwriting.

The full capacity to imitate sounds develops during the childhood years. Between 6 and 7 years of age, the child shows the ability to produce proper articulation for most vowel and consonant sounds. However, some have difficulty expressing sounds for "s," "l," "z," "sh," "ch," and "r" (Hockenberry & Wilson, 2011). By 7 years of age the child should be able to articulate all sounds for speaking and by age 12 years has a vocabulary of around 4000 words. Understanding of the syntax (grammar) and semantics (meaning) of language continues to develop. The child uses more complex sentences and understands multiple meanings for the same word and metaphors (Levene, 2010). The child should be able to recognize and correct spelling and grammatical errors by 8 or 9 years of age. The capacity to learn foreign languages is at an optimal level at this stage and provides rationale for foreign language instruction during the school-age years. Foreign language instruction also provides children with information about other cultures and an opportunity to understand people who are different from themselves.

Much of the child's time in school focuses on learning to read and write. Learning to read is a complex process, beginning with letter and sound recognition (Levene, 2010). Letters combine to form words that the child must learn to decode. Words combine to form sentences, and so on. Most children need help from teachers, peers, parents, or older children to learn to read effectively. Some researchers believe that children learn best by sounding out the individual letters of a word (phonics), whereas others think that learning the word as a whole unit is better. Both processes have value, and likely a combination of both is most effective (National Institute for Family Literacy, 2010). Considering the wide range of processes that support development of reading skills (conceptual, perceptual, verbal, and motor), it is not surprising that most children experience some difficulty in learning to read (National Institute for Family Literacy, 2010).

Handwriting requires eye-hand coordination, motor control, and perceptual abilities (Harron, 2011). Primarily a motor skill, handwriting does not reflect mental capacity. Many bright children and adults have poor handwriting, and vice versa. Boys tend to have more problems with legible handwriting than do girls. Writing style does not approach adult-level maturity until the end of late childhood, but the handwriting should reflect the child's handedness. No reversal of letter outlines should occur by age 7 or 8, and the relative size of letters should be uniform. By age 8 or 9, letter strokes should be firm, even, and flow with ease (Hockenberry & Wilson, 2008). The individual who has difficulty with handwriting may use a typewriter, computer, or graphics to produce a satisfactory written product. Tutoring by a handwriting specialist can help children with dyslexia, a term defining the tendency to reverse the normal appearance of letters and numbers in writing.

Memory

Memory abilities, both short term and long term, improve for school-age children. Strategies such as organizing, classifying, and labeling information help them retain information. Rehearsal, repeating an item to be learned, is also a helpful memorization strategy. At age 5 children use rehearsal when someone suggests or models it; at age 10 they rehearse spontaneously. Memory abilities improve with practice and through various strategies, such as placing the words that need to be remembered in a song or by rhyming words (Raghubar, Barnes, & Hecht, 2010).

Intelligence

Intelligence tests assess a person's mental abilities and compare them with the abilities of other people through the use of numerical scores. Although the term intelligence is used as if there is agreement on what it means, in reality there is much debate as to how this term should be and has been defined. For example, debate has surrounded whether intelligence should be considered an inherent cognitive capacity, an achieved level of performance, or a qualitative construct that cannot be measured. Psychologists have debated whether intelligence is learned or inherited, culturally specific or universal, or one or several abilities (Sacerdote, 2008). While these debates are ongoing, evidence is increasing that traditional intelligence tests measure specific forms of cognitive ability that are predictive of school functioning, but do not measure the many forms of intelligence that are beyond these more specific skills, such as music, art, and interpersonal and intrapersonal abilities. **Website Resource 20E** contains a list of common developmental and cognitive tests.

The concept of intelligence usually conveys an ability to think and process information learned earlier in life. Scores on an intelligence test should measure the child's basic abilities as compared with others of the same age and experience level and, ideally, should predict performance in school or society. However, this is not always the case. Intelligence test scores tend to differ because each test, or each form of the same test, measures slightly different samples of abilities and reflects the test author's philosophy on intelligence. It is important to note that some intelligence tests may be culturally insensitive (123Test, 2012). For example, the protectionism of the Asian culture may cause lower test scores on self-help skills and socialization among Asian children, who demonstrate in other ways that they are good students. Furthermore, words on the test may not be part of an ethnic group's usual vocabulary, causing children to miss these items on an intelligence test.

Children also take achievement tests that measure the amount of information learned in a specific area and offer insight into a child's overall intelligence. Although intelligence and achievement tests should measure different issues (basic ability versus learned achievement), their results correlate well. Some researchers believe this correlation exists because both tests actually measure the same thing (achievement, notability).

Reports from intelligence and achievement testing differ. Intelligence tests usually provide a number that represents intelligence quotient (IQ). An IQ of 90 to 110 is considered average (Logsdon, 2009). Achievement tests compare the child's performance with that of other children and report scores as percentiles. For example, a score in the 20th percentile of a test means the child scored better than only 20% of other children of the same age in that skill. Current beliefs accept that people inherit some of their intelligence but that environmental factors also influence opportunities for learning and overall intelligence. Most likely the greatest environmental influence is socioeconomic, reflected in the correlation in scores: children from low-income families tend to score lower on intelligence tests than do children from middle-income or high-income families. The reason for this probably relates to many subfactors, such as nutrition, language, parental reinforcement and encouragement, and sociocultural environmental stimuli. Social programs such as the federal nutrition program for Women, Infants, and Children (WIC) and preschool stimulation programs such as Head Start have attempted to address these subfactors to improve the potential of young children from diverse populations. Many people have suggested less focus on IQ tests, primarily because they label children early in life and influence, often negatively, their self-perception and their performance.

Learning Disabilities

Educators estimate that 10% of children 6 to 17 years of age have a learning disability (American Academy of Child & Adolescent Psychiatry, 2011b). Many terms and definitions have been used to describe the impairments of children who have normal or above-normal intelligence and usually do not have visual, hearing, or motor handicaps or emotional problems yet have difficulties in school learning. Some children have minor, almost unnoticeable difficulties, whereas other children are so impaired that they appear to be mentally retarded until diagnosed and helped. An individual child may have more than one developmental disorder. Some children will develop behavior and self-esteem problems as a response to their inability to function satisfactorily (Boyse, 2008).

One well-known condition that causes difficulty in the child's adjustment to the school setting is attention-deficit/hyperactivity disorder (ADHD), a behavior that reflects developmentally inappropriate degrees of inattention, impulsiveness, and hyperactivity (National Institute of Mental Health, 2007). ADHD is the most common neurobehavioral disorder of childhood and among the most prevalent chronic health conditions affecting school-age children. Frequently these children have high energy, intuitiveness, and creativity, personal characteristics that help them succeed in some facets of their lives. Despite diagnostic criteria for ADHD developed by the American Psychiatric Association (2000), the problem has been difficult to assess, primarily because the child manifests symptoms in varying degrees in different settings and with different people (Box 20-4). Treatment of children with ADHD has been controversial but includes behavior management, family counseling, classroom management, nutrition therapy, and medication (American Academy of Pediatrics, 2011d). These interventions may also be successful in management for ADHD-affected adults.

The nurse's role with the child who has a learning disability varies. The nurse may participate in detection of the problem, consultation during evaluations, collaboration with school administration on implementation of a treatment plan, referral to resources, assistance as a liaison between school and home environments, and source of instruction for both the child and the family to improve overall development and the family's adaptation to meet the needs of this unique child.

There are two laws protecting children with disabilities, including those with ADHD: the Individuals with Disabilities Education Act (IDEA) of 1997; and Section 504 of the Rehabilitation Act of 1973, Amendment Act of 2008 (Wright's Law, 2011). The IDEA is a special education law, whereas Section

---

BOX 20-4 DIAGNOSTIC CRITERIA FOR ATTENTION-DEFICIT/HYPERACTIVITY DISORDER

Note: Consider a criterion met only if the behavior occurs more frequently than that noted in most people of the same mental age as the child.
- A disturbance of at least 6 months exists during which at least six of the criteria for either inattentive behavior or hyperactivity-impulsivity behavior are met.*
- Some inattentive or hyperactive-impulsive symptoms that caused impairment existed before age 7 years.
- Some impairment for the symptoms exists in two or more settings (at school or at home).
- Clear evidence of clinically significant impairment exists in social or academic functioning.
- The symptoms do not occur only with a pervasive developmental disorder, schizophrenia, or other psychotic disorder and do not support another mental disorder (mood disorder, anxiety disorder, dissociative disorder, and personality disorder).

From American Academy of Pediatrics, Committee on Quality Improvement, Subcommittee on Attention-Deficit/Hyperactivity Disorder. (2000). Clinical practice guideline: Diagnosis and evaluation of the child with attention-deficit/hyperactivity disorders. *Pediatrics, 105,* 1158-1170; Leslie, L., Weckerley, J., Plemmons, D., Landsverk, T., & Eastmen, S. (2004). Implementing the American Academy of Pediatrics attention deficit/hyperactivity disorder guidelines in the primary care setting. *Pediatrics, 114,* 129-140.
*For specific criteria, refer to American Psychiatric Association. (1994). *Diagnostic and statistical manual of mental disorders (DSM-IV)* (4th ed.). Washington DC: Author.

---

504 is a civil rights statute. Both guarantee qualified students a free and appropriate public education and instruction in the least restrictive environment. This means that students are to be instructed among those who are not disabled and to the maximal extent appropriate for the student's needs.

The nurse plays a vital role in promoting the school-age child's overall cognitive and perceptual health, helping to prevent problems in these areas. The nurse must talk to parents and school administration personnel about any child who has language articulation problems beyond 6 or 7 years, because this child should be evaluated by a professional. The nurse helps parents understand their child's level of cognitive and sensory abilities so that learning expectations are realistic. Through educational materials sent home or provided during school meetings, the nurse may address the socialization needs and development of school-age children. The nurse also needs to help parents understand common tests used for child intelligence and achievement screening (National Institute of Mental Health, 2009). In addition, the nurse helps evaluate a child believed to have a learning disability when the child may actually suffer from a health problem, general immaturity, or an environmental deficit (poverty or divorce).

Self-Perception–Self-Concept Pattern

Through each of the developmental processes of physiological growth, cognitive development, and social development, children progressively engage in an important process of self-discovery. Through these processes, children actively build and create their own personalities, develop relationships with others, and expose themselves to a wide range of experiences that influence their behavior, attitudes, and values.

Erikson's Theory

The stage of personality development described by Erikson for the school-age child is industry versus inferiority (Learning Theories Knowledgebase, 2012). The major task to be accomplished is full mastery of whatever the child is doing (sense of industry). The child focuses on success in personal and social tasks and avoidance of a sense of inferiority. Inferiority occurs with repeated failures at attempted tasks and with little encouragement or trust from people important to the child (Hockenberry & Wilson, 2011). With mastery of the tools of the culture in relation to those of the peer group, a sense of worth and understanding of the self develops (Erikson, 1993, 1994).

Self-Concept

Self-concept develops over time and through a variety of experiences and relationships. For example, by being responsible for a pet's care and by showing love to this animal, the older school-age child nurtures a positive self-concept. The way in which others, especially peers, view the child influences the sense of self (Ferrer-Chancy & Fugate, 2007). Increasing cognitive abilities facilitate better understanding of the identifying factors of others (race, ethnicity, disability, or gender) and how those others compare with the child. Self-concept includes self-esteem, sense of control, and body concept.

Self-Esteem. Self-esteem has been defined as the extent to which an individual believes oneself to be capable, significant, successful, and worthy (Sheslow, 2008). The younger school-age child has a limited self-concept, but one that develops with successful completion of the tasks of this period (Erikson's sense of industry). Although engaged in more activities outside of the home, the child still depends on family, as defined by one's culture, to develop high self-esteem. In school, teachers or group leaders frequently reward those who have succeeded in a task with badges, stars, or privileges (tangible objects that validate success).

The peer group's influence on the school-age child's self-esteem is unquestionable. Acceptance by a peer group contributes to feelings of self-worth and a sense of belonging to a desired group. Competition or collaboration with peers in school, clubs, and activities also influences feelings of adequacy and feelings of success (Women's & Children's Health Network, 2010). Parents must be encouraged to expose their school-age children to interesting activities of their choice, involving peers, to nurture their self-esteem and sense of uniqueness.

Concern has been voiced about school-age girls suffering a decline in self-esteem that affects their school achievements. Some research indicates that boys receive more praise in school than do girls, and girls receive criticism on the content of their work whereas boys receive more criticism on the appearance of their work (Myers, 2009). Girls experience greater competition now than in earlier times, and they face pressures about personal appearance, particularly if they are White (Women & Children's Health Network, 2010). Various authors report that

girls need strong adults to support their ways of thinking and behaving in a world often built on "male values." Girls tend to have high self-esteem if they perceive parental harmony that supports perceptions of balance within themselves and promotes their emotional health (Myers, 2009).

In encouraging development of self-esteem in all school-age children, the nurse remembers that a child needs to experience success with tasks, and completely structured activities may not provide this opportunity for some children. A child who succeeds in some things and receives acceptance by peers gains a sense of competence and worth, is self-confident, and has high self-esteem, which are important qualities for life survival.

Sense of Control. As the school-age child matures and makes choices, a sense of control develops about the self and the environment. Children with an internal locus of control believe they are responsible for their behavior and accomplishments and tend to have higher levels of achievement than do children who believe in an external locus of control. The latter think that fewer reasons exist for them to try hard at a task, because others or fate determines life results. Hispanic and Black cultures may more often support an external locus of control based on a strong belief that God determines one's outcome (Tynan, 2011). Older children and girls tend to have a more internalized locus of control than do younger children and boys.

Body Concept. The school-age child's concept of the body and its functioning also changes from the preschool period and adds to overall self-concept. By ages 8 to 11, children know that parts of the body constitute a related whole (Hockenberry & Wilson, 2008). The 11-year-old child can name twice the number and functions of internal body structures that a 6-year-old child can and frequently understands the functions of the cardiovascular, musculoskeletal, and nervous systems. For example, the 7-year-old child knows that the heart is important and that it beats, whereas the 13-year-old child knows that the heart pumps blood. Changes or differences in the body may frighten the school-age child until one understands normal developmental processes such as losing deciduous teeth. Physical differences, such as freckles, can provoke ridicule and isolation. Children in this age group frequently feel threatened by others with deformities (Hockenberry & Wilson, 2011). Children with chronic illness worry that their peer relationships will be negatively influenced if others know about their illness. Children who learn about body differences, by meeting people with chronic health problems as well as by reading and discussion of anxiety about differences, increase their knowledge about the body and ways to maintain health. They also gain an understanding of the value of each person, despite their differences.

Roles-Relationships Pattern

The family environment provides a sense of security that allows the school-age child to cope with uncertainties in the external environment (Hockenberry & Wilson, 2008). Although many live in single, divorced, mixed-race, or same-gender parenting households, the family structure generally encourages a child's cognitive growth through exposure to a variety of experiences that bolster the desire to achieve and develop positive self-esteem.

Parents, caregivers, and children interact in a variety of ways to show love and companionship for each other. Caregivers, such as grandparents or extended family members, protect the dependent child and teach the learning child. The caregiver-child relationship is not equal, primarily because caregivers and parents serve as authority figures that establish the rules needed for the functioning of the family and safe growth of the child. During the school-age years, the child's increasing maturity, independence, and responsibility begin to reduce the amount of parental authority and structure needed. In some cultures parents set higher standards for child independence than parents of other diverse populations (Women & Children's Health Network, 2010). With increasing independence, the child prioritizes school and peer group relationships to develop socialization skills and understand group social mores (Sturaro et al., 2011). These connections will help prepare the child for future heterosexual relationships.

School-age children also begin to broaden their interests outside the home, often encouraged by parents. Unfortunately, some older children may become involved in gangs, behavior that causes much stress for both children and their parents. The child's changing world frequently alters family schedules and patterns, supporting studies that have found that parents express the least amount of parental satisfaction when their oldest child is between the ages of 6 and 13. The relationships between siblings vary, depending on birth order, culture, gender, and age differences and perceived power of siblings (Hockenberry & Wilson, 2011). Siblings interact with one another in a number of roles, such as playmates, teacher-learner, protector-dependent, and adversaries, based on feelings of jealousy and rivalry that often occur in families. School-age children cope with these feelings better than do preschool children because they have outlets outside the family, including school and friends. Parents can minimize conflicts by recognizing each child's needs and level of maturity and by providing guidance and support.

As children mature, they assume more responsibilities within the family and the community. School-age children learn responsibility for allowance, household chores, self-care, and pets and acquire a sense of empowerment as an integral part of the family (Hockenberry & Wilson, 2011). This is the period during which families often give allowances or children earn money through chores or small jobs, such as paper routes. The amount of an allowance may relate to cultural values. In one study, Asian children earned higher allowances than did other children from diverse population groups for completing fewer chores and for meeting higher standards of academic performance (Goldstein & Brooks, 2012). School-age children learn valuable life lessons by earning and spending their allowances.

Children learn socially accepted behaviors when their parents engage in limit setting (defining expected behavior and consequences when limits are not honored). Violent behavior must be discouraged, and nonviolent methods to reach resolutions for personal problems should be encouraged. Parents who express their feelings, explain why things happen, and listen to their children while setting limits encourage the development of self-control and positive self-esteem. Some families with school-age children find it helpful to have periodic family meetings during which everyone discusses family issues, rules, and responsibilities. Behavior contracts between parent and child provide direction and may also encourage improved behavior by delineating favorable consequences when the terms of the contract are followed.

Children frequently model their behavior after that of people they love or admire (parents, friends, and other adults). Positive reinforcement (rewards for good behavior) is an effective form of limit setting (i.e., discipline), used often by upper class parents. Punishment, a negative reinforcement as reflected in shaming a child in front of the child's community or family (seen with some Asian cultures), may stop an undesired behavior, but often only until the child repeats the action and is not caught. Lower-class parents tend to use more punishment directed toward misbehavior or failure to adhere to parental values and requirements (Hockenberry & Wilson, 2008).

Child Abuse

Child abuse (physical, sexual, or emotional exploitation of children) and neglect (lack of adequate food, shelter, or emotional support) continue to be significant societal problems. According to the U.S. Department of Health and Human Services (2011) and the American Academy of Pediatrics (2011e), more than 3 million cases of abuse or neglect in children are reported annually in the United States. Abused children have an increased likelihood of becoming violent adults and of abusing their own children. Factors that increase the risk of abuse include family poverty, culture, limited maternal education, needy child syndrome, presence of a stepfather, single-parent status, parental drug addiction, and teenage parenthood (American Academy of Pediatrics, 2011e). However, child abuse occurs in families that do not have these risk factors. Cultural factors must be considered in detecting abuse. For example, coin rubbing of the chest (used in the Asian ethnic group for treatment of respiratory tract infections) leaves abrasions that may be perceived as abuse by a nurse assessing an ill child (Hockenberry & Wilson, 2011). Both national governmental agencies and professional organizations recommend that health care providers report suspected abuse and participate in preventing, assessing, and treating victims. Many state nurse practice acts require nurses to report suspected cases of abuse. Ultimately, nurses help interrupt the vicious cycle of abuse by becoming involved in community coalitions and innovative evidence-based programs that prevent and intervene with child and family abuse.

Unfortunately, relationships between children and adults are not always positive. Sexual abuse, use of a child for sexual exploitative purposes, has become a more common but often hidden problem for a variety of reasons (American Academy of Pediatrics, 2011e; USDHHS, 2011): the child may be too frightened to talk about the situation, families and society do not want to admit its existence, Internet traffic has supported pornography and pedophilia, and fewer agencies exist to respond to these cases. Many victims know their abusers (many are parents), and people in positions of authority (e.g., physicians or clergy members) may be abusers. The child may comply for a variety of reasons, such as a need to be good or a

BOX 20-5 WARNING SIGNS OF CHILD ABUSE

- Physical evidence of abuse or neglect, including previous injuries
- Conflicting stories about the "accident" or injury from the parents or others
- Injury or complaint inconsistent with the child's history or developmental level (e.g., the child received a concussion and broken arm from falling off a bed)
- Signs and symptoms consistent with signs of abuse and inconsistent with history, vague recall of event (e.g., chief complaint is a cold when there is evidence of first-degree and second-degree burns)
- Inappropriate response of caregiver, such as an exaggerated or absent emotional response, refusal to give consent for additional tests or agree to necessary treatment, excessive delay in seeking treatment, or absence of the parents
- Inappropriate response of child, such as little or no response to pain, fear of being touched, excessive or lack of separation anxiety, or indiscriminate friendliness to strangers
- Child's report of physical or sexual abuse
- Previous reports of abuse in the family
- Repeated visits to emergency facilities with injuries

Source: Kellogg, N. D. (2007). Clinical report: Evaluation of suspected child physical abuse. *Pediatrics, 119*(6), 1232-1241.

need to keep the family together. Emotions are complex and change as the child grows, but they often lead to adult anxiety, depression, and physical symptoms and illnesses. Males less often report sexual abuse but are more likely than girls to suffer negative emotional effects from incest, a form of sexual abuse (Hockenberry & Wilson, 2008).

As in any type of suspected abuse, nurses assist these children by recognizing those at risk and those experiencing abuse and referring them to relevant resources. All people who work with young children must acknowledge the warning signs of abuse (Box 20-5). When sexual abuse is suspected, an in-depth interview and examination must be conducted by a multidisciplinary team that is sensitive to the needs of the child and can validate the abuse. Most authorities believe that children who describe sexual abuse are telling the truth, because the details are usually specific and trauma is evident. Therefore a child's story should be believed unless it is disproved.

Sexuality-Reproductive Pattern

The preschool child learns about gender and begins to model the general societal behaviors expected of a female or male child. The child enters the school-age years with a strong identification with the parent of the same gender. The child continues to learn the concepts and behavior of the gender role and incorporate these into the self-concept. This challenge is significant for all children, but more so for homosexual children. Societal stereotypes related to gender roles continue to influence the school-age child's ideas of male and female roles (Hockenberry & Wilson, 2011). Fortunately, most children receive early teaching about gender roles that emphasizes that gender does not determine one's choices, personality, or behavior. As a result of this teaching, children increasingly choose occupations based on their skills and interests, rather than on what appears appropriate because of their gender.

The school-age child's increasing awareness of the body, its functioning, and a need for sexual identity combine to foster a desire for knowledge about the biological aspects of sexual function. Late in the school-age period, when the physical changes of puberty have begun, concern and curiosity about sexual issues frequently develop. A child may become extremely attached to another of the same gender, and they may explore one another's sexual organs. This is common exploratory behavior and does not reflect true homosexuality, even though parents and children may express concerns about it. With the advent of physical changes of puberty, the school-age child desires more privacy in a bedroom shared with no one. As noted earlier, the physical changes of puberty appear gradually over several years.

Children frequently share questions about sexual matters with their peer group. Parents are often uncomfortable or unsure of what sexual information to give to their children and when to give it. Many health care agencies sponsor short programs to educate parents and older school-age children, in a supportive environment, about body and mental changes during preadolescence and puberty. An increasing number of age-appropriate books that focus on emotional and body changes can be used at home and in school to increase children's understanding. Particularly because menstrual cycles start earlier now than they did 50 years ago, education about body changes and puberty appears appropriate as part of later school-age education.

The nurse plays an important role in sex education in health care and education settings. This professional should be receptive to answering questions in this area and at each health care visit (Hockenberry & Wilson, 2011). The nurse employed in the school is in an ideal position to teach group sex education programs using literature and games. Children at this age appear to respond most favorably with gender-segregated classes, based on their general discomfort with sexual topics and unique needs and questions (Hockenberry & Wilson, 2011). Some schools appropriately incorporate these classes into school curricula as part of a health-promotion curriculum. Other schools have special programs focused only on sex education based on parental desires or school board policies. Most school-age children have the cognitive skills to respond to programs on responsible sexuality, including discussions on abstinence and condom use, pregnancy, sexually transmitted diseases, and the human immunodeficiency virus (Eisenburg et al., 2008). The nurse also wants to include program content specific to disabled children, who face unique body changes and concerns and need to understand ways others can express affection to them without causing accusations of abuse.

Coping-Stress Tolerance Pattern

The school-age child must learn to cope with stress as part of the developmental process. Through a health-promotion program, children can learn to identify symptoms of stress (pounding heart, stomach "butterflies," and sweaty hands) and ways to cope with these perceived stresses (e.g., deep breathing and walking) before they cause illness. The child actually faces many stressful experiences in life, including competition, homework deadlines, failure at home or school, and decisions whether to cheat, steal, or even join an unpopular peer group. The young school-age child may never have shared his or her life with other children the same age, and cultural values learned earlier in life may not be reflected in school or in peer relationships. Threats to the child's security (e.g., bullying) cause feelings of helplessness and anxiety that may affect the ability to function successfully (Reuschel, 2011). Grief over the death of a loved one, parental divorce, loss of a favorite activity because of misbehavior, or expulsion from a favorite peer group may cause negative behavior. Parents need to provide appropriate discipline in responding to this behavior but should also listen and analyze factors related to the problem in order to increase the child's feelings of control and decrease stress for the family (Box 20-6).

Children use a variety of coping strategies, healthy behaviors intended to buffer perceived stressful events. However, in a very stressful situation or many stressful situations, a child may be unable to move beyond the coping behaviors. In conversations with teachers and parents, the nurse may offer a variety of strategies for coping with a school-age child's problems, enabling the child to cope and learn from others. These strategies may involve role playing or referral to literature on the problem topic to interrupt the child's negative behavior cycle and improve family health (Table 20-2). The nurse may also refer a child to relevant religious and spiritual leaders, based on school-age children's belief that prayer will help them cope with an otherwise uncontrollable situation (Hockenberry & Wilson, 2008).

BOX 20-6 HOT TOPICS

The School-Age Child: Points for Effective Discipline

Effective discipline is essential to family harmony and individual child growth and reflects cultural beliefs. The goal of discipline is to encourage and reinforce positive child behaviors, eliminate inappropriate child behaviors, improve parent-child communication, and meet parental needs. Effective discipline requires these essential components: a positive, supportive, loving relationship between parent and child; use of positive reinforcement strategies to increase desired behavior; and removal of reinforcements or application of punishment to reduce/eliminate undesired behaviors.

Specifics of discipline strategies include the following:
- Ignoring the misbehavior and acknowledging the appropriate behavior
- Using distraction or substitution to avoid a problem situation
- Offering choices to prevent inappropriate behavior such as whining or emotional outbursts

- Using humor to decrease the intensity of a situation
- Modeling the appropriate behavior
- Setting age-relevant limits
- Giving specific and clear commands for behavior appropriate to the child's age
- Talking calmly, being a good listener, and encouraging negotiation, perhaps in a family meeting, to promote problem resolution
- Limiting a child's environment (distractions such as music and television)
- Setting clear and consistent consequences for misbehavior (withholding privileges, using contracts)
- Providing one-to-one time, focusing on positive attention
- Taking time for oneself to replenish one's energies as a parent and as an individual

Compiled from Hockenberry, M. J., & Wilson, D. (2008). *Wong's essentials of pediatric nursing* (8th ed.). St. Louis: Mosby; Hockenberry, M. J., & Wilson, D. (2011). *Wong's nursing care of infants and children* (9th ed.). St Louis: Elsevier; American Academy of Pediatrics. (2012). *Disciplining your child*. [Online]. Retrieved January 6, 2012, from www.healthychildren.org/English/family-life/family-dynamics/communication-discipline/pages/Disciplining-Your-Child.aspx.

TABLE 20-2 THE SCHOOL-AGE CHILD'S COPING STRATEGIES AND NURSING INTERVENTIONS TO PROMOTE COPING

COPING STRATEGIES	NURSING INTERVENTIONS
Use of defense mechanisms (regression, denial, repression, projection, displacement, sublimation)	Accept child's use of defense mechanisms as temporary, healthy coping responses; provide child options for moving to more age-appropriate ways of responding to stressors
Cognitive mastery (problem-solving, communication)	Ask children what they know of situation and how they might handle it; encourage questions; use diagrams and models to help explain; encourage child to verbalize feelings and use past successful strategies that might help deal with present stressors; try personalized approaches, such as books, puppets, and manipulation of equipment to increase feelings of control when faced with stressful situation; encourage praying and other communications to a chosen deity as appropriate
Controlling, holding behaviors	Encourage child to participate and to make decisions; accept child's need to direct as appropriate; set consistent age-appropriate limits; respond to signals for help; let child be responsible for self-care
Use of repetition	Use books, games, and other communication media to work through feelings; emphasize "ok" for child to continue to ask questions and to receive answers that assist in coping
Use of humor	Be a good listener and participate in riddles and jokes used by child; be a good sport with school-age children's desire to play jokes on each other; share stories and cartoons with child
Motor activity, aggression, protest behavior	Encourage physical activity to deal with stress; accept appropriate behavior; establish limits on behavior for group safety
Withdrawal (resurgence of separation anxiety)	When child is separated from family, may have separation anxiety; encourage close emotional contacts between child and significant others (friends, family, church members); allow favorite objects from home to be brought to hospital or new environment for child

Parental Divorce

More than half of all marriages end in divorce, leaving many school-age children to face stress related to their parents' separation. Often children experience a feeling of loss, although they may hope that their parents will reunite at some point. Box 20-7 discusses the effects of divorce on a school-age child. Children's responses vary with their level of development (Kim, 2011). Factors such as economic security; availability of both of their parents, other family, church, and school supports; and quality of interactions with their parents can influence the child's ability to cope with divorce. Unfortunately, many parents become so immersed in their own feelings that they fail to support their children (Pickhardt, 2011). Conflicts over custody, child support, and visitation rights add to the child's difficulty in coping. Sometimes the school system becomes the child's advocate to encourage the parents to provide a supportive environment during divorce proceedings. Despite this intervention, some children do not cope well with the divorce and have emotional consequences that result in juvenile behavior problems or require long-term counseling (see the Case Study and Care Plan at the end of this chapter).

Somatization and Depression

Children, like adults, use defense mechanisms to cope, with varying degrees of success. Two strategies used by the school-age child to respond to uncontrollable situations are somatization and depression.

Some children respond to a stressful situation by transferring their feelings to a physical problem (somatization). In this phenomenon, school-age children, unable to discuss their concerns, complain of stomachaches or headaches, symptoms reflective of functional or psychogenic pain. These children may also develop discrete, repetitive movement habits called tics. In many cases the child with these problems must be evaluated to determine whether an underlying physiological cause exists. The child and the family will then need assistance in understanding the child's concerns to define successful ways to cope with the behavior.

Depression occurs in up to 2% of school-age children (National Alliance on Mental Illness, 2010; National Institute of Mental Health, 2012), and more often in boys than in girls during the school-age period. Depression reflects a disturbance of mood, when a child displays sadness, guilt, or worthlessness, and other unusual behaviors that disengage the child from peers and family. In defining depression in children, most authors emphasize that they are referring to a more long-term syndrome in which the child's normal development and functioning become impaired, not a periodic sadness that all children occasionally experience. Factors that place a child at risk for depression include homelessness, death of a parent or significant other, divorce, long-term hospitalization, chronic illness, learning problems, or emotional turmoil at home. Parents and teachers look for symptoms of depression, including anorexia, sleeplessness, lethargy, changed affect, aggressive behavior, frequent crying, or withdrawal from previously enjoyed activities.

Although it has been concluded that there is insufficient evidence to routinely screen all school-age children for depression, the nurse can serve an important role in identifying any child who appears to be depressed and in notifying parents about the need for further assessment (National Institute of Mental Health, 2009). Depending on the child and the situation, varying amounts of counseling and individual child guidance may be required. Antidepressant medication may also be prescribed (National Institute of Mental Health, 2009). Nurses in schools and outpatient settings are often the ideal helpers, because they have the skills and time needed to help a child cope with a helpless feeling and its cause.

BOX 20-7 EFFECTS OF DIVORCE ON THE SCHOOL-AGE CHILD

School-age children tend to view life in black and white, and are likely to blame one parent for the break-up. Boys, especially, mourn the loss of their fathers and frequently express anger at their mothers. Both boys and girls have great difficulty accepting their parents' new dates. Crying, daydreaming, and problems with friends and school are common divorce-related behaviors in children this age.

Here are some suggestions that might help the school-age child cope with divorce of parents.

- **Discourage reconciliation fantasies.**
  Have parents avoid dinners, outings, or holiday celebrations with ex-spouse. This only fuels the child's fantasies. Instead, emphasize the finality of divorce.
- **Make sure the child has the phone number of the absent parent.**
  Both parents should encourage easy access and frequent conversations with the noncustodial parent.
- **Do not allow the child to manipulate parents into buying more possessions.**
  School-age children are likely to feel deprived. Although they may intensify requests for playthings or other possessions, do not try to retain child's affection through material objects. Even children of divorce need to be told "No!"
- **Talk to the child's teachers or school counselors about the divorce.**
  School personnel may better understand possible learning or behavioral problems and will likely offer extra support.

From University of Michigan Health System. (2006). Divorce: The effects on children. *Pediatric Advisor 2006.* [Online]. Retrieved from www.med.umich.edu/1libr/pa/pa_divorce_pep.htm.

Values-Beliefs Pattern

Children make decisions related to moral and ethical issues every day. Should they tell the teacher which classmate broke the rule? Should they share their candy with a younger sibling? For these situations, the child makes a decision based on the level of moral development. Moral development involves choosing the most appropriate behavior based on one's values and feelings related to the situation. Environmental factors and culture strongly influence a child's moral development, as do the type of family discipline, role models, people with whom the child identifies, and the child's rehearsal and practice of moral behavior (Hockenberry & Wilson, 2011).

Kohlberg's Theory

Most researchers agree that the younger school-age child is at the preconventional level, a level of moral development characterized by self-interest only. The child continues to do many things simply to avoid getting in trouble and does not understand the reason for rules, but also performs actions that will benefit the self (Kohlberg, 1981). During later childhood (10 to 13 years) most children progress to the conventional level, a stage of moral development defined by concern about group interests and values. The conventional level of moral judgment involves the child looking to others for approval and to societal authority for a definition of rules. Children 10 to 12 years old judge a behavior in terms of the intention of the offender, understand the "golden rule" concept, and engage in behavior that maintains a valued relationship. The conventional level coincides with Piaget's cognitive level of concrete operations and the child's increased social involvement with people outside the home (Hockenberry & Wilson, 2011; Kohlberg, 1981).

Moral Behavior Problems

Some moral behavior problems, such as lying, stealing, or cheating, are common during the school-age years. Cultural, religious, and parental values influence a child's moral development, concept of right and wrong, and consequences of not demonstrating moral behavior. Preschool and younger school-age children frequently lie as a result of fantasy, exaggerations, or inaccurate understanding. As children mature, they may use the defense mechanism of denial to block upsetting situations and maintain self-esteem. The lie then becomes an unconscious act. Older children often lie because they fear punishment or ridicule. Children may cheat because of a desire to win, do well in competitive society, or "look good" for their peers. Children usually steal when they think they will not be caught and they think that there is no other way to get what they want (Nucci, 2008). Although these actions can be quite upsetting for parents, they are common developmental behaviors. Parents frequently need reassurance that the child is normal and probably will outgrow the behavior with parental assistance. They may need help in developing fair rules for behavior and communicating their expectations for a child's behavior to meet parental and cultural values. Therefore the nurse encourages the parents to warn the child clearly not to steal, lie, or cheat; offer other, more socially acceptable, ways to cope with the stressor causing the behavior; and then apply appropriate punishment congruent with an understanding of the event (Hockenberry & Wilson, 2011).

ENVIRONMENTAL PROCESSES

Physical Agents

School-age children, similar to those of all other age groups, face daily exposure to environmental agents and factors that may cause injury, illness, or death. Many of these agents and factors are harmless if appropriately used or if there is minimal exposure. Examples include physical agents such as fires; mechanical agents such as bicycles, skateboards, and cars; biological agents such as bacteria; chemical agents such as asbestos; and radiological agents such as x-rays. Death rates from these agents vary among ethnic groups because of access to health care and environmental issues (Hockenberry & Wilson, 2011). For example, Native Americans and Alaska Natives experience higher death rates from motor vehicle accidents, residential fires, and drowning than do other groups. Blacks experience higher death rates for unintentional injury than do other ethnic group members (National Safety Council, 2011).

Accidents

Accidents are the leading cause of death in children more than 1 year of age in the United States (National Safety Council, 2011). Most accidents do not result in death, but many serious ones cause significant morbidity and disability. Because of this effect, the nurse has a significant role in educating parents and school personnel on ways to prevent dangers to school-age children and to become involved in public initiatives to create a safer society for them.

The agent, host, and environment must be considered in developing solutions to decrease the number of accidents. The type of agent varies with the child's age. Most fatal accidents during the school-age period occur from motor vehicle accidents when the child (host) is a passenger or pedestrian (walking or riding a bike). Other fatal accidents occur from fires and burns, bicycles, drowning, and firearm accidents. Most common nonfatal accidents tend to be caused by simple agents that produce simple injuries. Despite helmet laws in several states, many school-age children continue to experience head injuries related to recreational equipment, such as bicycles, swings, skateboards, and trampolines (Hockenberry & Wilson, 2011; Safe Kids, 2011). Slightly older children have an increased number of accidents from contact sports and cuts, falls, burns, and injuries from firearms.

Specific accident factors relate to the host—the school-age child (Box 20-8: Quality and Safety Scenario). Children in this age group tend to become hurt because of their carefree attitude, curiosity, love of mimicking older people, and intense oral tendencies. Typically, school-age boys have more accidents than girls, perhaps attributable to differences in personalities, societal expectations, childrearing practices, and increased propensity for risk-taking behaviors. The mechanism varies with the gender of the host. For school-age boys, drowning is the most common fatal accident; for girls, automobile accidents are the most common (CDC, 2008b; Safe Kids, 2011).

The physical environment of the child dictates the type or frequency of accidents, which occur in the home, neighborhood, and school. Most accidents happen outdoors, which means that school-age children face greater risk for automobile or bicycle accidents than for poisoning or falls, indoor accidents that occur predominantly in younger children. More accidents (drowning and pedestrian-vehicle accidents) occur in the summer than in the winter because of children's outside play. Socioeconomic level affects children's physical environments and access to dangers. For example, space heaters place children of low-income families at risk for burns, whereas skiing places wealthier children at risk for injury.

The social environment, which includes the family, school, and playmates, also plays a role in accidents. Although little research has focused on the physical trauma caused by heavy backpacks that many school-age children use, these bags exert significant pressure against functionally immature muscles of

BOX 20-8 QUALITY AND SAFETY SCENARIO

Safety Concerns Specific to School-Age Children

Because of increased independence, school-age children face significant exposure to situations threatening their health. Consequently, parents of these children must be involved in community and legislative activities that provide safe play environments. Additionally, at appropriate health visits, health care workers should provide anticipatory guidance to parents in the following areas:

Bicycle Safety

Each child should have a well-maintained bicycle, ride only in safe areas approved by parents, observe rules for vehicle traffic, ride on the side of road with traffic, "bike defensively," and use a federally approved riding helmet.

Street Safety

Children should look right, left, then right again to check safety of crossing a street; cross only at safe and well-monitored intersections, preferably with an adult present; ensure parental supervision when children play close to streets and heavy traffic areas.

Motor Vehicle Safety

Children should wear a seat belt or be in an age-appropriate booster seat as needed; older children should ride with restraint system and in back seat until age 12.

Pool Safety

All children should have swimming lessons and swim with a buddy or adult who swims well; all pools should have drain covers; children should avoid swimming after a heavy meal and avoid "roughhousing" behavior around the pool; children should be monitored by parents during swimming.

Firearm Safety

Adults need to lock away guns and ensure gun safety locks are intact; parents need to educate children NEVER to touch guns.

Playground Safety

All playground equipment should meet federally approved standards; children should be trained on how to use equipment safely; equipment should be evaluated for safety and repaired before children use it.

Fire Safety

Working smoke detectors should be in place in home and school; family needs to have a fire evacuation plan and practice it; children need to wear fire-retardant clothing at night; children should not play with matches, open fires, fireworks, or open wires that can cause injury and fire.

Toxin Safety

Children should avoid insecticides, radiation sources, inappropriate use of medications, and pollution sources; parents need to store all known toxins, chemicals, and household cleaning agents in an adequately ventilated location that is inaccessible to children.

Stranger Safety

Children should play with friends, have a plan for returning home, know home phone number and address, play in safe and known area, and report any suspicious activity threatening their safety to an appropriate adult; children should know how to say "no" and how to locate assistance when in an unsafe situation.

Sports Safety

Children need to engage in age-appropriate activities and wear protective equipment relevant to the sport; parents need to ensure safety and maintenance of all sports equipment; parents need to caution children against hazardous sports, such as trampolines.

Animal Safety

Parents should teach children to avoid strange animals, especially sick or injured ones, and ensure that personal pets receive vaccinations; they need to teach children not to mistreat pets and not to place their faces close to any animal.

Although nurses offer suggestions to parents to improve their children's play safety, studies have shown that few parents follow these suggestions. Reasons for this behavior include parental difficulty in assessing the safety of and age appropriateness of play equipment, the amount of effort involved, and a lack of money to create a safe play area. The nurse helps parents respond to these perceived barriers. With more children using skateboards and rollerblades, the nurse also encourages the use of child safety helmets and knee, elbow, and wrist guards to prevent muscle sprains and bone fractures. The school offers an on-site opportunity for teaching children, teachers, and parents about accident prevention. In addition to providing this guidance, nurses can participate in legislative and educational actions to increase community consciousness about child safety.

the back and torso. Daily carrying of bulging backpacks causes muscle strain, headaches, improper posture, shoulder slouch, and other physical problems. Also to be considered are teachers' expectations that all textbooks be available both in the classroom and at home. At least one study has shown that children will change their backpack carrying behaviors if involved in a school-based program focused on this topic (American Academy of Pediatrics, 2011b).

As part of the social environment, the family may influence the rate of accidents in the school-age child. Chronic familial stress (parental unemployment) or sudden acute stress (parental illness) may contribute to homicide as the third-leading cause of death among children ages 5 to 14 years (Child Trends, 2012). Homicide is a more common cause of death among Black and Hispanic children than White children. Children also face increased risk of accidents when parental supervision is limited, such as during holidays or a move to a new home.

Drowning

Fewer school-age children than infants and adolescents die from drowning. More Black children of this age drown than do White children (CDC, 2012a). Water safety measures can help reduce drowning, along with the many other injuries that occur around water, such as falls in slippery areas. Environment and safety teaching can influence the number of school-age children dying as a result of drowning.

Burns

Each year many children become victims of house fires, many of which occur during the winter months from Christmas trees, space heaters, and fireplace malfunctions. Many homes lack working smoke detectors because of incorrect installation or inadequate testing. If a fire occurs in a home with a smoke detector, the risk of death is decreased by 40% to 50% (CDC, 2011d). Most burned children survive, frequently with varying degrees of physical and psychological scars. Children need to learn about fire safety, including the importance of avoiding situations involving fire and practicing fire drills routinely at school and home (CDC, 2009). The nurse encourages parents to understand other practices to prevent fire-related problems, including parental purchase of flame-retardant sleepwear for children.

Firearms

People in the United States who use firearms frequently cause fatal injury through homicide, suicide, or accidents. Every 2 hours, 45 minutes someone's child dies from a gun accident (Child Trends, 2012). With many U.S. homes containing a handgun and because of recent shootings by adolescents, concern about children's safety remains well-founded. Possibly the best means of preventing accidents with firearms is to ban them from private ownership, as seen in England. However, because handgun ownership is an important individual right in this country, several states have passed legislation that allows handguns for individual protection. Families with firearms in the home should store guns in a locked area apart from ammunition and consider using nonlethal (wax) bullets. All family members should be knowledgeable about gun safety.

Sports and Recreation

Accidents from sports and other recreational activities increase during the school-age years and include lacerations, contusions, hematomas, concussions, sprains, and fractures. Some evidence exists that adolescents now have more musculoskeletal injuries because of involvement in repetitive team sports earlier in their lives. This suggests that society needs to examine the current emphasis on initiating young children with musculoskeletal immaturity into team sports such as football, hockey, soccer, and basketball. Intense social pressure for children to participate in these sports means that parents and school systems must ensure that each child has protective body devices to prevent injuries, as well as psychological support to allow a child to benefit from the team sport. There is a further need to increase safety by ensuring that each child fits the sport, has adequate hydration during the game, and engages in conditioning exercises before and after the game for prevention of injuries. Furthermore, literature supports societal need to focus more on the collaborative skills children learn by being part of a team, rather than the intense focus on winning philosophy found in many school-age team sports.

Recreation area injuries may be prevented by several measures. The National Bureau of Standards set guidelines in 1976 for home playground equipment, regulating objects such as sharp edges, moving parts, and equipment design. Nurses help prevent accidents by participating in decisions about school playground equipment and counseling families on a variety of issues. Playground safety has become an important issue because *200,000* children need emergency department assessment each year for related injuries (CDC, 2008b). Girls are slightly more likely to be injured on the playground than boys and many of these injuries occur in low-income neighborhoods where playgrounds fail to meet safety standards (CDC, 2008b).

Mechanical Forces

Motor vehicles and bicycles represent the two most common mechanical agents that cause injury to school-age children.

Motor Vehicles. The leading cause of death in the United States in all individuals from age 1 to 34 years is motor vehicle accidents (CDC, 2012b). Children die as passengers in cars, as pedestrians, and as bicycle riders. In this country, more children die from pedestrian-related accidents than passenger-related accidents (CDC, 2011e). Since 1999, 127 children have died each year in bicycle accidents, 80% of whom did not wear helmets to prevent head injury. Helmet use in children can reduce the risk of head injury by 45% (Safe Kids, 2011). Although not all accidents result in death, children may also sustain injury that causes permanent disability as a result of motor vehicle accidents.

Automobile passenger injuries can be prevented, or the severity reduced, by altering some aspects of the child's environment. Lower speed limits, stricter enforcement of alcohol-related laws, better automobile and highway designs, improved door lock mechanisms, and more effective restraint system requirements in all states have reduced the severity and number of accidents and injuries (USDHHS, 2007b). However, more injuries have been correlated to higher speed limits instituted in the United States several years ago. Furthermore, many children remain at risk for injury because various school districts and states do not require seat belts in buses used to transport students, despite a recommendation by the American Academy of Pediatrics to do so.

Studies indicate that proper and consistent use of federally approved belt-positioned booster seats for children ages 4 to 7 years decreases the likelihood of child death and serious injury significantly (American Academy of Pediatrics, 2011a). However, one study showed that only 19% of such children used these seats (National Highway Traffic Safety Administration, 2008). Less than 10% of children needing the protection of a booster seat ride in one, and younger, smaller school-age children (under 4 feet, 9 inches) often fail to use them correctly (National Highway Traffic Safety Administration, 2008). Reasons given by parents and children for not using seat belts or booster seats include forgetting to use the device, having difficulty reaching and fastening belts, feeling discomfort from wearing the belt or using the seat, and receiving misinformation about the need for the belt or seat for short trips. Clearly, consistent use of booster seats by young children and seat belts by older children and adults, who model seat belt behavior to their children, will occur only when legal enforcement occurs. Federal government and national professional groups recommend that all children under the age of 12 years ride in the automobile's back seat in an appropriate restraint because of the potential for death from an airbag activated in a motor vehicle accident (Hockenberry & Wilson, 2008; Daly, et al, 2010). Many families have difficulty meeting this recommendation because of long-term acceptance of older children riding in the front seat after they have outgrown booster seats.

Urban children younger than 15 years old experience more than half of all pedestrian-automobile accidents (Hockenberry & Wilson, 2011). These occur when using rollerblades, skateboards, and skate scooters and tend to be more severe (head injuries) than passenger injuries. Many factors cause pedestrian accidents: children often have difficulty interpreting traffic signs and judging the speed of cars, and they forget to look carefully before crossing the street. Although overcrowding, poverty, high volume of traffic, stress, and unsafe play areas influence children's street safety, various principles can direct interventions to decrease the number of street dangers.

Bicycles and Motorized Vehicles. Many accidents occur each year with young children on bicycles, motorized skateboards, and all-terrain vehicles (ATVs). Most of these are not serious, but deaths occur among young children who have suffered head trauma or significant body injury from inappropriate use of this equipment. The American Academy of Pediatrics (2012a) recommends that only people at least age 16 years ride ATVs and then only in rural areas with adult supervision. Bicycle accidents occur most frequently near the child's home and during the day and commonly involve injuries from the spokes when children ride behind the bike seat. More boys than girls experience these injuries from bicycles, motorized skateboards, and ATVs, perhaps based on their greater risk-taking behavior (Daly et al,. 2010).

In response to children's developmental behavior related to bicycles, motorized skateboards, and ATVs, the nurse addresses safety issues. Additionally, nurses encourage parents to teach and reinforce safe bicycling habits to their children and should sponsor helmet and bike programs within the school (Box 20-9).

Biological Agents

School-age children face constant exposure to bacterial, viral, and other biological agents that pose threats to or improve their overall health (e.g., immunizations). Compared with the preschool child, the school-age child has fewer illnesses. The most frequent illness continues to be upper respiratory infections (URIs), illnesses shared among school children who fail to practice good handwashing techniques and avoidance of ill peers. These illnesses cause children to lose school days and learning opportunities. Most URIs result from viruses, but bacteria can play either a primary or a secondary role. Two problems associated with URIs are streptococcal infection ("strep throat") and otitis media.

Strep throat occurs frequently among school-age children. A child with an infection from group A *Streptococcus* may have a severe sore throat, fever, and malaise or may have only a minor sore throat. A throat culture confirms the diagnosis, and antibiotic treatment typically cures the infection. Children are noninfectious after 24 hours of treatment and may return to school (Choby, 2009). If not treated, the affected child may develop rheumatic fever or acute glomerulonephritis as a secondary infection following the sore throat. Greater transmission

of streptococcal infection occurs in areas where there is close personal contact during colder weather. The school nurse's preventive efforts focus on teaching the children good handwashing techniques and identifying children who complain of sore throats. Children with throat infections caused by other strains of *Streptococcus,* such as group B, do not usually require treatment, because these infections generally do not cause the same serious complications.

The school-age child may experience other illnesses. The frequency of gastrointestinal tract infection (gastroenteritis) decreases during the school-age years but is still the second most common acute condition of childhood. Usually caused by a virus, gastrointestinal tract infections cause vomiting and diarrhea. Older and larger school-age children have little chance of rapid dehydration; they basically react to the illness the same as do adults and need to be treated similarly. Gastroenteritis is contagious and, therefore, the nurse should monitor school children for symptoms of illness and encourage proper handwashing to prevent transmission of the virus from one child to another.

Scabies and lice (pediculosis) are common skin disorders among school-age children. This problem causes extreme itchiness of either the body (scabies) or the head (lice) and is easily spread to other children. The nurse educates parents to visualize or use a lice comb to check their children for scabies and lice when they complain of itchiness or seem to be constantly scratching their heads (Durani, 2011a). Previously, children diagnosed with lice could not come to school until they were lice free. This isolated students from their peers and influenced state school funding based on student attendance. The American

Academy of Pediatrics now recommends that if children are undergoing treatment for the problem, they should be allowed in school (AAP, 2010).

A biological agent that many children know about is human immunodeficiency virus, or HIV, which causes acquired immunodeficiency syndrome (AIDS). Of all age groups, the young school-age child is at the lowest risk for contracting the disease, because AIDS acquired by the perinatal route emerges in infancy and toddlerhood, and most young school-age children do not use intravenous drugs or engage in high-risk sexual practices. However, the school-age child may know a person with AIDS or may have heard something about the disease from adults, older children, or the news media. The school-age child and school staff should know basic facts about the disease and its transmission and, most importantly, that it cannot be transmitted through casual contact, such as being in the same classroom with a child who has HIV or AIDS. As a result of widespread misinformation and fear, the U.S. Surgeon General has called for mandatory, explicit AIDS education beginning with children 8 years of age. The involvement of parents, students, and school personnel in AIDS education programs through age-appropriate materials will increase each group's knowledge and acceptance of people who have the disease. Accepting parents assist their own children in learning to accept others with special needs and in taking better control of their own health.

Children with AIDS may attend school as long as they will not be exposed to illness from other children. Most children with AIDS receive routine immunizations but may need further immunization if exposed to a typical childhood disease (CDC, 2008a). During outbreaks of contagious disease, the chronically ill child may have home tutoring; this approach will need to be evaluated annually to identify the risks versus benefits of school attendance. Certainly, long periods of isolation from peers will contribute to feelings of loneliness in the child with AIDS and may even appear to be a punishment for being ill. The school nurse undoubtedly has an important role in facilitating the multidisciplinary nature of AIDS care while maximizing the learning environment of affected children.

Most states require that the child's immunizations be current before entering kindergarten or the first grade and that additional tetanus immunization be given every 10 years or when an unclean wound is acquired. Other immunizations recommended by the American Academy of Pediatrics include a meningococcal vaccination at age 11 or 12 years and the series of three injections for hepatitis B and human papillomavirus (HPV) during the late school-age and early adolescent years (USDHHS, 2011). If the child has no history of chickenpox, a varicella immunization is also recommended (Hockenberry & Wilson, 2008). In many states, the school nurse has a responsibility to ensure that all students' immunizations are current, and if they are not current, the nurse informs the parents that the children may not attend school until their immunizations are up to date (CDC, 2008a; USDHHS, 2011). Any child lacking age-appropriate immunizations can "catch up" according to a schedule developed by

the American Academy of Pediatrics. Although 79% of American children receive immunizations by school entrance time (Child Trends, 2012), increasing numbers of immigrants and transient workers have deepened concern about exposure of Americans to previously conquered diseases (e.g., tuberculosis). Strides towards meeting the *Healthy People* initiative targets related to immunizations continue to be made according to the midcourse review and the 2020 objectives (USDHHS, 2012b).

Chemical Agents

A number of potentially toxic chemical agents exist in the environment, and the child is exposed to these through inhalation, ingestion, or direct contact. Children are particularly susceptible to chemical hazards. Food and drugs are two sources of chemicals ingested by children on a regular basis, and some older school-age children ingest tobacco as a result of cigarette smoking. Although normally safe, some foods and drugs can be harmful when used inappropriately. Other environmental hazards include pollution, heavy metals (lead and mercury), and pesticides.

The nutritional needs of the school-age child were discussed earlier in this chapter. As stated, children frequently eat foods with large quantities of sugar, salt, and fat and with chemical additives. The effects of some of these additives have been questioned, and concern has been expressed about the effect of biochemically altered food on children and future generations. On a short-term basis, some foods may cause allergic reactions; on a long-term basis, some may contribute to the development of coronary disease, hypertension, and cancer. Nurses are aware that the child's diet may contribute to future health problems, and therefore assess intake and counsel the child and parents accordingly about ways to improve it.

The incidence of poisoning decreases during the school-age years as children become more aware of the appropriate uses of drugs and other agents. Childproof containers have decreased exposure of children to dangerous poisons and chemicals in the home. However, children continue to face exposure to drugs (alcohol and glue inhalants) because of less monitoring by working parents, and older school-age children face exposure to recreational drugs, primarily through their peers and older children. In the school environment the nurse and school personnel need to encourage students to engage in wise decision-making about recreational drug use that will affect their future and overall health.

With pressure on older school-age children to smoke cigarettes, attention must be paid to effective strategies to prevent these behaviors. Every day, more than 6000 school students try to smoke a cigarette (Stop Smoking Update, 2009). Most students who smoke initiate their habit around 11 years of age (American Heart Association, 2008). White students start smoking at a younger age than Black students. Males tend to begin smoking earlier than females; however, girls catch up in smoking rates during middle school–age years (Stop Smoking Update, 2009). The Federal Tobacco Settlement Project (National Association of Attorneys General, 1998) provides funds to address the public health problem posed by tobacco smoke in the United States. Although funding for tobacco prevention and cessation programs has reached its highest level in 6 years, many states continue to fall short of the minimal recommendations by the CDC (Tobacco Free Kids, 2012). Attention to smoking as part of a health-promotion program seems merited because so many children begin smoking at a young age; in addition, because nicotine is highly addictive, many believe that this habit leads people to experiment with more risky drugs (cocaine and methamphetamines).

School policies have been instrumental in supporting a tobacco-free environment. By 2006, 63.6% of schools prohibited all tobacco use in all locations and those associated with school-sponsored events. To further assist in health-promotion efforts, many institutions require staff development and education programs related to the effects of tobacco use on health. By 2006, 67.6% of elementary schools had implemented required instruction on tobacco use prevention (CDC, 2009). Various governmental efforts to reduce exposure to environmental tobacco have occurred. For example, 22 states and numerous cities nationwide have enacted smoke-free laws.

Pollution has become a fact of life for many Americans and, particularly, for the 25% of urban-dwelling children who must breathe air that exceeds federal government levels for acceptable ozone (Breysse et al, 2010). Air pollution irritates the eyes and the respiratory tract, causing URIs, ear infections, and allergies. More children now experience asthma, and many inner city children face higher rates of this disease because of poor air quality, including secondary and tertiary smoke. Knowing the negative effects of air pollution and smoking to their health, many school-age children participate in school projects to improve their environmental health.

Children also face exposure to various toxic materials in their environment. Progress has been made over the past decades to reduce children's exposure to chemical hazards. Lead, for example, has been removed from gasoline and paint. This in turn has resulted in significant reductions in children's blood lead levels. Lead exposure continues to exist. Children are exposed to lead through parents' clothes, shoes contacting lead-infused soil, lead in older residential water pipes, traditional medications in some cultures, or in school building structures. Children living in poverty receive high exposure from lead-based paint used on older and less expensive homes. The long-term effects of these metals on children remain unclear, but some evidence indicates children suffer neurotoxic effects from this type of exposure. High lead levels in children contribute to dental caries and hearing loss.

Routine use of chemicals to control insects and undesirable weeds in landscaping has led to increasing concerns about children's exposure to these agents. With increased interest in more natural substances to control insects and gardening problems, perhaps less reliance will be placed on biological chemicals for these problems in the future. Knowing the primary source of exposure to the most hazardous materials and avoiding these materials are often sufficient to accomplish real risk reduction and offer substantial protection within the child's environment (Children's Health Environmental Coalition, 2008). Various behaviors can be implemented to create a safe environment

and minimize health risks associated with hazardous chemical exposure. Nurses are instrumental in the assistance and support of parents, schools, and community agencies in the implementation of these behaviors such as using nonhazardous cleaners and pesticide-free foods, and further monitoring of the environment for hazardous materials.

X-ray Exposure

The child receives exposure from both naturally occurring radiation and human-made ionizing radiation. Exposure occurs in varying degrees with radiographic examinations of teeth and bone, from nuclear power plants and explosions, and in the management of many childhood cancers. Children exposed to high levels of radiation risk developing breast or thyroid cancer or leukemia and compromised growth. With little advocacy in this area, nurses and other professionals improve children's health by becoming active in initiatives that focus on prevention of chemical and radiation hazards.

Cancer

Leukemia is the most common form of childhood cancer. Of those affected younger than 5 years of age, 90% will be cured with current medical treatment (Leukemia & Lymphoma Society, 2012). Among the 12 major types of childhood cancers, leukemia and cancers of the brain and central nervous system (second most common forms of childhood cancers) account for more than 50% of all new cases (National Cancer Institute, 2012). Lymphomas (Hodgkin's disease and non-Hodgkin's lymphoma) also affect school-age children and adolescents as the third most common group of malignancies. Non-Hodgkin's lymphoma is more common during the school-age years, and boys experience this malignancy 3 times more often than do girls. Mortality rates in the United States tend to be greater in densely populated areas, particularly where the more-educated and wealthy live (Hockenberry & Wilson, 2011). The most common symptom is abdominal pain caused by intestinal obstruction and symptoms resulting from organ compression. With effective treatment regimens, children with limited disease may be cured but may experience side effects of treatment later in life (e.g., development of cataracts, dental problems, learning difficulties). These children present a challenge to the nurse because they are in various stages of recovery, may be developmentally delayed, and may fear a recurrence of their disease. The nurse provides psychological and emotional support to affected children and their families, to help children develop peer relationships and meet developmental goals important to them during the school-age years.

The school-age child interacts daily with other children and adults to become more independent by age 12. Mutual problem-solving of child and parents or friends frequently occurs at this age related to a higher level of maturity in social relationships and concerns. Exposure to a variety of social roles and expectations of others strengthens the process of socialization so that the child develops social competence—the ability and skills to participate effectively in the social interactions of society. Social competence includes both the obvious social behaviors and an inner understanding of the appropriateness of behaviors.

Several elements play a role in the development of the child's social competence. The child's desire for a sense of industry encourages interactions, positive relationships, and accomplishments within society. Cognitive development supports understanding of relationships and effective problem-solving. Moral judgment helps the child understand consequences and fairness in relationships. Understanding and obeying authority help to maintain order in society. Social sensitivity is a result of social interactions and requires the child's ability to perceive the social cues of others, understand the roles of others, and communicate verbally with them. Social behaviors are also a part of social competence; these are learned most frequently through imitation, role modeling, and reinforcement of others' behaviors. The interaction of all these elements produces a level of social competence and simultaneously plays a role in the child's self-perception. Individuals frequently see themselves as others see them.

Social Factors and Environment

Peers

The strongest relationships that school-age children develop outside their families are with their peers (other children encountered in the neighborhood and school). The peer group acts as a new social system, becoming increasingly influential in the child's life. All children continue to be influenced significantly by the family, the culture of the family, and many other environmental factors, but the peer group begins to influence lifestyle, habits, and speech patterns and formulate standards of behavior and performance. The standards of the peer group become vitally important, and children attempt to conform to its rules. Being accepted by the peer group becomes more important than being accepted by anyone else. Conforming to the pressures of peers becomes an issue, especially when it interferes with the parents' expectations. When children realize that their own goals, desires, and aspirations might be quite different from those held by the peer group or the school, they must find ways to cope and perform according to the new standards if they are to succeed. The degree to which children fit in socially, learn to cope, and receive satisfaction from the group is a powerful determinant of healthy socialization.

A child may have one best friend or several important friends and a mutual understanding and willingness to help each other. Friendship groups that form during this age may change and become goal directed, such as groups composing a sports team. These groups frequently have set rules or rituals that connect the members. During the middle school–age years, friendships often revolve around same-gender relationships, videos, songs, books, and media shared by the group. Later in the school-age years, the development of sexual relationships with the opposite gender occurs during dating and mixed parties.

School-age children also become increasingly involved with adults outside the family, including teachers, coaches, and others who become role models, all of whom influence the child's view of the world and self. Although this influence may not be as significant as that of a child's peers, long-term ideas and beliefs frequently develop from these relationships. Children usually perceive some similarity between themselves and their models, those of the same gender with similar physical or behavior traits. During these years children may not maintain a strong identification with the parent of the same gender, but they tend to adopt other adult models with whom they can identify.

Working Parents

Both dual-career couples and single-parent families influence their children's safety when no adult is present to monitor the environment after school. Many "latchkey children" who are left alone until their parents return from work follow directions given by their parents. These directions may include beginning dinner in anticipation of their parents' return or completing homework while remaining inside the home with the doors locked.

Parents and school-age children often disagree about how old is "old enough" to be left at home alone or with an older sibling. Although the school-age child might consider being at home alone to be a real mark of maturity, children who look after themselves after school can become more isolated and miss peer relationships important to their development. Nurses give guidance to families who must cope with the issue of after-school care for school-age children to ensure that relevant and safe decisions are made.

Culture and Ethnicity

School-age children focus more on the influences of their culture on their lives than do younger children. Aspects of American culture that the child must confront include poverty and affluence, ethnic and racial differences, acceptance of these differences, and the power of media as a cultural phenomenon in American society.

Ethnic Groups

Preschool children may notice racial and ethnic differences, but school-age children increasingly show evidence of being aware of these differences. This is a time during which attitudes toward race develop based on family and community attitudes. Studies of children 5 to 7 years of age show that most identify with and prefer to play with members of their own race. As children get older, they may continue this behavior. Although prejudice exists among some school-age children, they may be encouraged to view people from different cultures and ethnic backgrounds in a positive light. Many schools appropriately focus on the importance of other cultures by having multicultural awareness weeks. During these times, children dress, eat, and live as other cultures do, allowing them to recognize the uniqueness of individual cultural beliefs and values (Box 20-10: Diversity Awareness).

Television and Video and Computer Games

Television and video and computer games exert a major influence on ideas and behavior in American culture. Unfortunately, many television programs and games pose harm to children

BOX 20-10   DIVERSITY AWARENESS
Expectations for Child Behavior Related to Culture

American Indian
Expect child to respect elders and take pride in heritage; develop natural talents as child matures; personal independence must balance with accountability to family, community, and tribe; help sought from family members, not outsiders

Mexican American
Family environment protects child; child expected to be obedient, respectful, and work hard to reach goals; "next" generation expected to do better than current generation

Filipino
Family raises child in protective environment; expect child to conform to values of culture and child shamed if fails to meet expected behaviors; child taught to avoid direct confrontation and hide emotions and to be respectful and shy; strong emphasis on education for personal and financial gain

Black
Child expected to complete family chores, complete schooling, and develop talents such as music or sports to improve self for future; discipline and respectful behavior encouraged

Chinese Americans
Child is highly valued, particularly male child; child expected to honor elders and family needs; high value of education to honor family and child

because of their messages and because such activities prevent children from engaging in physical activity. Recent advances in gaming offer an option for increased activity during gaming activities. New video games and gaming systems, such as Wii, have been developed that encourage movement during gaming. Energy expenditure more than doubled when sedentary screen times were converted to active screen time.

Computers connected to the Internet pose danger unless locking devices have been installed to prevent school-age children from accessing inappropriate websites. Additional concerns have focused on the violent themes of programming, persuasive television commercials, unrealistic depiction of the world, unhealthy food intake, and the passivity of television viewing.

Many times, certain ethnic or racial groups implement the violence in these media sources, leading children to stereotype these groups as the perpetrators of violence. Research has shown that television facilitates negative attitudes and values among children, increases their aggressive behavior, decreases their emotional sensitivity when aggressive acts occur, and leads them to accept aggressive acts (Adams, 2012). One positive note is that adults who discuss violence with children by pointing out that these acts are unacceptable and cause pain to others can help inhibit some childhood aggression. Discussion of recent acts of violence committed by young people in such a context also helps. Anger control programs, as part of school health-promotion programs, also help decrease societal violence and produce more collaborative workers needed for the future.

The average child views an overwhelming number of television commercials by age 18, and these commercials influence daily and future choices and behaviors. Many television commercials focus on sugary foods that cause damage to teeth, diminish overall healthy habits, and lead to increased rates of obesity. Young children cannot always separate the program from the commercials and believe that they must purchase products the television says to buy. Many childhood authorities question the ethics of exposing children to any type of advertising. Although concern about the effect of advertising has led to programming changes during children's watching time, more work is needed to send more socially responsible messages.

The world as presented on many television shows does not accurately reflect the real world. Despite an increasingly diverse and aging population, stereotypes of women and minority groups and a predominance of younger actors continue to make money for the media industry. Parents and health care providers should monitor television viewing to ensure the age appropriateness of the material, respond to television stations about inaccuracies in the content, and write letters to their newspaper or television networks to express concerns about the material presented. Parents may also participate with their children in responding to media presentations on learning and moral themes. Parents follow recommendations from the American Academy of Pediatrics—limit television and media viewing to 2 hours per day, have media-free bedrooms, disallow television viewing while eating, and participate in national "Turn Off the Television Week."

Some positive aspects of television viewing exist. A number of children's programs, such as "Sesame Street," "Wishbone," and "Kratt's Creatures" for younger children and "Bill Nye, the Science Guy," "Cyberchase," and "Zoom" for older children, have been deemed developmentally appropriate for children (Public Broadcast Station [PBS], 2008). Likewise, there are excellent websites for school-age children that stimulate their learning and promote their health.

Increasingly, parents engage their school-age children in learning and playing on a home computer. Although this technology serves as a good resource for locating information, writing papers, and organizing information, parents must limit the time students spend on computers. Likewise, limitations must be put on computer games that detract from socialization with peers and family and take time away from school work.

Levels of Policy Making and Health

Throughout this chapter, laws that support the health and well-being of the school-age child have been discussed. These laws include guidelines for the safe use of products, utilization of flame-retardant clothes, mandates against tobacco advertisements, and nutritional guidelines for federally supported school lunch programs. Another important law is mandatory public education for disabled children. The Individuals with Disabilities Education Act (IDEA), formally known as Public Law 94-142 (Education for All Handicapped Children Act), established in 1977, states that any child with special needs (disabled) aged 5 to 21 years has the right to free appropriate public education in the least restrictive environment and evaluation by school or health professionals to identify learning needs. Disability includes having a limitation in one or more functional areas (U.S. Department of Education, 2008) and affects as many as 10% of children ages 5 to 17 years.

Many states begin educational services for affected children at 3 years of age based on an individualized educational plan (IEP) for that child and as mandated by law (Hockenberry & Wilson, 2011). The school nurse is responsible for collaborating with other school personnel and parents in ensuring that the IEP, including the health care needs of the child and connection to resources addressing the unique learning needs, receives attention. However, some parents have expressed concern that their "normal" or "gifted" child receives less attention in school systems because of the cost and time expenditures associated with implementing IEPs for disabled children. To add further concern, with recent school budgetary shortfalls, lesser-trained people than the school nurse often have responsibility for implementing IEPs. Despite these concerns, the value of Public Law 94-142 has been that disabled people have had their problems addressed in the educational arena.

To ensure access to educational opportunities for every individual, the U.S. Department of Education was developed in 1980. Through the U.S. Department of Education, President George W. Bush enacted the No Child Left Behind Act of 2001, aimed at improving the academic achievement of the disadvantaged (U.S. Department of Education, 2008). The No Child Left Behind Act of 2001 intended to help ensure that all children have the opportunity to obtain a high-quality education and reach proficiency on challenging state academic standards and assessments. As a result of the No Child Left Behind Act of 2001, more reading progress was made by 9 year olds in 5 years than the previous 28 years combined. Reading and math scores of 9 year olds and fourth graders have reached all-time highs, and 46 states improved or held steady in all categories of students tested in reading and math (U.S. Department of Education, 2008).

Poverty

In the United States more than 22% of children less than 18 years of age live in families whose incomes are below the poverty level (National Center for Children in Poverty, 2009). Among diverse population groups, 50% of Black, 30% of Hispanic, and an unknown percentage of Native American children live in poor economic conditions that negatively influence their health. These conditions include unemployment, inadequate or crowded housing, poor sanitation, poor nutrition, low educational levels, and limited or sporadic access to health and social services perhaps attributable to lack of health insurance or contextual factors of these persons' lives. The number of uninsured children continues to be high, particularly among Hispanics (30%), and limits the number of children and families receiving primary health care (National Center for Children in Poverty, 2009). The lack of primary care among Black, Hispanic, and White children in rural areas prevents needed asthma management, dictating an expanded role for health care providers to connect families to resources for more effective disease control.

Many homeless children face poor living conditions and high rates of depression related to few friends and poor health status. Migrant children face more disease (e.g., tuberculosis,

scabies, ear infections), injury, and dental caries and pose treatment challenges because of their transient status (Hockenberry & Wilson, 2011). The effects of limited financial resources on children include higher mortality rates at all ages than in those who are not poor or migrant and more lost school days because of illnesses. Numerous problems exist for children in poverty, including greater developmental delay as a result of poor nutrition; increased peer rejection; poorer self-concept; increased risk of accidents, drug abuse, and abuse or neglect from parents; and greater overall poor coping abilities.

Nurses interacting with poor families and their children are familiar with federal health resources, such as the State Children's Health Insurance Program (SCHIP). This program, part of the Balanced Budget Act of 1997 and implemented at the state level, supports comprehensive care for newborns to young adults 18 years of age who do not meet Medicaid criteria but live in families too poor to afford private insurance. This program has advanced children's health by improving access for many groups (SCHIP Information Center, 2008). The nurse improves the overall health of poor children by encouraging relationships with appropriate role models and by reinforcing strong family relationships that help children develop resilient and positive self-images.

Family wealth may have a negative influence on the school-age child if there is frequent substitute caregiving of varying quality attributable to parental absence, extremely high or unreasonable parental expectations, availability of material possessions but little child awareness of relevant responsibilities, and easy access to drugs and alcohol and similar dangers. The nurse reinforces the need in wealthy families for consistent demonstration of parental love and support, firm limits on appropriate behavior, and the value of recognizing the child's unique abilities. The nurse also offers ideas that will help decrease risk-taking behavior (e.g., drugs) and increase parent-child connection until a parent is in the home.

When discussing children raised in poverty or affluence, the nurse remembers at least two points. First, many variables affect each child, often in different ways, to influence overall development. Second, although personality and support networks help a child in a socially poor environment to excel later in life, most authorities believe that problems of affluence are easier to overcome than are the all-pervasive problems of poverty.

Health Services/Delivery System
Well-Child Care

The American Academy of Pediatrics recommends that children 6 years and older have a well-child examination at least every 2 years by either a physician or a nurse practitioner (Hockenberry & Wilson, 2008). In the ideal situation, the child has a primary health care provider, one person or practice from which the child receives wellness and illness care coordinated by members of a health care team. Unfortunately, many American children still do not have this quality of care (see the earlier section on Poverty). With increasing numbers living in poverty because of family violence, single parenthood, and divorce, many lack a primary care provider for their physical and emotional needs often because of a lack of health insurance. In this situation, they often receive emergency care only when they are very ill or injured.

The nurse encourages the school-age child and parents to be active members of any health evaluation. Children may give some of their own history, answer questions, and discuss their health concerns. During the history, the child's privacy should be respected. Some children in this age group want a parent present during the examination; others do not. When possible, the nurse spends at least some time alone with the child to allow discussions that the child may not feel comfortable with when parents are present. The examinations can also be a time for education on how the body works and ways to keep it healthy. Preventive information on diet and exercise can be offered relevant to prevention of obesity, cardiovascular disease, and diabetes. Information also can be obtained on school adjustment and performance, particularly because this is a major portion of the child's life. School performance can reflect the child's cognitive and general development. If there are any concerns, the nurse obtains more information through separate testing or discussion with school officials. Health education is directed to both the child and the parents for the best results. Activities that the child performs alone and with the family can give a picture of relationships and adjustments that relate to the child's health (see the Care Plan at the end of this chapter).

A challenge for nurses who work with school-age children is to maintain their normal healthy status and prevent illness. This task is accomplished through a variety of health-promotion mechanisms, such as examination, guidance, education, and legislation. The success of this health-promotion approach has been illustrated in at least one study in which Black children improved lifestyle choices when engaged in an intervention focused on cardiovascular health. Many professionals have noted that school-age children guided by the nurse generally seek health and use various resources to attain, maintain, or regain optimal health for their future productivity. Aspects of the nursing process are implemented when structuring a program to maintain the child's health (such as seen with an assessment of immunization status), promote health habits (seen with teaching bicycle safety), and prevent illness (seen by obtaining throat cultures to detect streptococcal infection).

Nurses have many opportunities and settings to help carry out their interventions as consultants, board members, and active providers of care. For example, nurses and school-age children interact during well-child evaluations and at school. Nurses in other roles, such as in public health positions and in hospitals, also play a role in health promotion, although these nurses must often focus more on helping the child and family respond to an illness or a crisis. Local and national groups influence the health of children through their activities and regulations. These include organizations such as Boy Scouts and Girl Scouts, Big Brothers and Big Sisters, charities such as the Red Cross, and government agencies such as the Consumer Product Safety Commission.

As an integral part of the community, the school system has the responsibility to provide a healthy school environment and a comprehensive health-education program. In some areas,

nurses, physicians, and other health care personnel work as a team in the school health program, which includes health care and maintenance and education. The nurse advocates and searches for resources so that each child has a source of health care, or the nurse is a nurse practitioner who delivers care. School health programs range from an occasional mention of body care and the changes of puberty to a full program that integrates physical and mental health principles into all aspects of the educational experience.

Comprehensive school health services require an interdisciplinary, coordinated effort between health care providers and educators. Recommendations state that each school should have an on-site nurse to conduct and mentor students and faculty in health-promotion areas. Nevertheless, many schools share nurses because of budgetary concerns. However, when available, nurses offer educational and interpersonal skills to initiate health-promotion teaching that improves the overall health of consumers (students, parents, teachers, community). Nurses have a wide scope of practice, including that of referring parents to relevant resources aimed toward activities that improve the school environment and its inhabitants.

The nurse's role in planning health maintenance for children of a school varies, depending on the type of health maintenance program. In one system, the school nurse may refer children to resources available to provide a source of health care, whereas in another system, the school nurse functions as a nurse practitioner. Based on scope of practice and state legal requirements, the school nurse monitors and updates children's immunizations and identifies and intervenes with children who have acute or chronic health care problems, such as scoliosis, strep throat, common cold, or child abuse. Increasingly, school nurses provide sophisticated care according to evidence-based protocols for chronically ill school-age children who have been integrated into the regular academic environment. Based on state regulations, the nurse also engages in completing vision, hearing, and scoliosis screening at regular intervals. In most schools the nurse works with the school's physician, community physicians, and parents in meeting children's and community health needs.

For all school-age children, the school nurse plays a role in developing a healthy educational environment through promoting a comprehensive and age-appropriate health-education program focused on children becoming responsible for their own health. A program aimed at accident prevention in and around the school is part of the nurse's role. The program includes assessing the school for pedestrian and automobile traffic patterns, broken playground and classroom equipment, ice and snow dangers, poorly maintained toilet facilities, and inappropriately prepared food. Regular practice drills are held to acquaint teachers and students with emergency procedures (i.e., fire, bomb, or intruder threats or actual events). All people in the school are prepared to respond to chemical hazards. The nurse implements existing school-based programs on drug and alcohol abuse.

It is also important to consider the role of the nurse in fostering a healthy social environment in the school. The nurse examines the social interactions of the children and interacts with them to promote positive relationships. However, social

---

※ **BOX 20-11** **INNOVATIVE PRACTICE**

School Emergency Preparedness

Because children spend a significant portion of their day in school, pediatric emergencies such as exacerbation of a medical condition, behavioral crisis, and accidental/intentional injuries are likely to happen. As a result of the likelihood of such risks, the American Academy of Pediatrics and the American Heart Association recommend the implementation of a medical emergency response plan (MERP) (AAP Council on School Health, 2008). The purpose of a MERP is to establish procedures within the school for the administration of emergency first aid services, emergency treatments, and administration of emergency medications for students. A plan helps schools prepare to respond to life-threatening medical emergencies in the first minutes before the arrival of EMS personnel. All procedures established in the MERP are to be followed during school hours, at school-sponsored activities, and while on school buses and other school property.

Due to the fact that injuries are the most common life-threatening emergency encountered, teachers, trainers, school nurses, and other school personnel should be trained and know general principles of first aid. Schools now employ fewer nurses, and school nurses often rotate between schools, resulting in many schools without medical coverage for several hours/days each week. As a result, much of the emergency care is the responsibility of teachers and other school personnel.

The MERP should have the following core elements in place in order to save the greatest number of lives with the most efficient use of school equipment and personnel:

- Establish an efficient and effective campus-wide communication system for each school.

- Develop a coordinated and practiced medical emergency response plan with the school nurses, physicians, athletic trainers, and the EMS system, with appropriate evaluation and quality improvement.
- Reduce the risk of life-threatening emergencies by identifying students at risk and ensuring that each has an individual emergency care plan and by reducing the risk of injury and disease triggers at the school.
- Train and equip teachers, staff, and students to provide cardiopulmonary resuscitation (CPR) and first aid.
- Establish an automated external defibrillator (AED) program in schools.

A recent study assessing school disaster preparedness found only 12 states met the minimal standards of disaster preparedness in 2010 (Save the Children's U.S. Programs, 2012). School nurses play an important role and should participate in all phases of planning and implementing all emergency preparedness and management plans as they pertain to school health and student safety (National Association of School Nurses, 2011).

Although many schools are in compliance with many of the recommendations for emergency preparedness, specific areas for improvement exist such as practicing the MERP and ensuring the identification of authorized personnel in the case of an emergency. Preparedness of schools to manage life-threatening emergencies requires the commitment of the entire community. The nurse is in a prime position to facilitate these community efforts and orchestrate partnerships between school officials, local EMS, school personnel, and local pediatricians to ensure the planning and implementation of a disaster plan.

Modified from Olympia RP, Wan E, Evner JR. (2011). The preparedness of schools to respond to emergencies in children: A national survey of school nurses. *Pediatrics,* 116(6):e738-e745.

---

problems continue to constitute a major concern for many children during this time. Children may experience difficulty in making the initial transition away from family and gaining satisfaction from a group of peers. Children may make the initial adjustment but then have difficulties interacting with others (e.g., bullying). When problems such as these arise, the nurse, parents, and school system determine reasons for this behavior and intervene appropriately (Box 20-11).

NURSING APPLICATION

The nurse working with the school-age child has a unique and exciting opportunity to engage the child in health-promoting behaviors. Most school-age children are able to participate in the teaching strategies if the strategies are geared toward the child's appropriate cognitive ability. Since the age range of the school-age child is from 5 to 12 years, the nurse must consider the mental ability and comprehension of each developmental stage.

Nurses can teach health-promotion behaviors directly to the child through spending time demonstrating, monitoring, and reinforcing preventive health practices such as handwashing, dental hygiene, nutrition, and physical activity. These activities can be taught through age-appropriate reading materials, modeling, and role playing. Engaging the child in these practices may also help the child conceptualize the link between the behavior and disease prevention. The nurse must partner with parents to model healthy behaviors at home, at school, and in the community settings.

A variety of methods can be utilized to educate children on health and nutrition. Keeping culture, socioeconomics, and

media influences in mind, the nurse should teach children concepts about food choices, exercise habits, and ways overall health is impacted by those choices. Nutrition education can be individualized to the age of the child through utilization of games, activities, colorful food guides, and simple cooking activities.

Physical activity in childhood is crucial in promoting healthy behaviors that continue into adulthood. Exercise for this age group is generally provided in group activities and sports. Physical activity provides the school-age child with peer interaction and social relationships. This aspect of health promotion should be encouraged by the nurse as well as the family.

As with younger age groups, health promotion of the school-age child focuses on education about routine health examination and the childhood immunization schedule. The nurse provides the families with immunization recommendations and must remain updated on current guidelines. The nurse also focuses on prevention of childhood injuries by educating about seat belt and bicycle safety, as well as other topics with a potential for causing injury.

Screening for health problems is another aspect of caring for the school-age child. Screenings are generally conducted for problems with vision, hearing, height, weight, and oral health. The nurse may be the first person to identify a potential issue with regards to an acute or chronic condition. At that time, he or she gathers assessment data to determine if the child needs immediate treatment or a referral to another provider. For the nurse working with school-age children and their families, the role is often one of providing education, case management, consulting, counseling, and community outreach.

CASE STUDY

Change in Usual Communication Pattern in School: Joey

Joey is an 8-year-old boy in elementary school. His teacher has voiced a grow-ing concern regarding his classroom behavior. Over the past 2 months Joey has become more withdrawn from his classmates and rarely participates in class discussion. This is a new behavior in that he "used to talk all the time, and raise his hand to answer questions in class." His teacher reports that they were dis-cussing family and family roles in class this week. Joey became very aggressive and yelled, "My dad isn't at home anymore 'cause of my mom'." "I really miss dad. My mom's new boyfriend isn't nice and won't buy me stuff, like my dad does." His teacher determines Joey's parents are divorced. A parent-teacher conference has been scheduled to discuss Joey's behavior since it is now affect-ing his grades in school.

Reflective Questions

1. Is Joey's behavior appropriate for his age?
2. Joey's parents do not understand his change in behavior. His father yells, "If she would let me spend more time with MY son, Joey wouldn't be having trouble with school. She doesn't care about MY son now that *she* has *her* new boyfriend." How might the nurse respond to this situation?
3. What interventions might be effective for Joey's parents and teacher in improving his classroom behavior and school performance?

◎ CARE PLAN

Change in Usual Communication Pattern in School: Joey

*NURSING DIAGNOSIS: Ineffective Coping related to disruption of home environment

Defining Characteristics
- Frequent absences from school (1 day per week over the past 2 months)
- Change in quality of schoolwork: grades have deteriorated over the past month
- Verbal outbursts in class

Related Factors
- Parents separated 9 months ago
- Lives with mother; her boyfriend moved into home 2 months ago
- Mom reports, "He frequently complains of headaches and stomachaches, but his doctor can't find anything wrong." Results in frequent absence
- Visits father every other weekend
- No siblings

Expected Outcomes
- Child will decrease number of absences from school related to "headache/stomachache" complaints.

- Child's grades will improve over the 9-week period.
- Parents will become more involved with the school in order to establish a relationship with the school that addresses the needs of the child related to home and school.

Interventions (School Nurse)
- Assess level of family problems within the home regarding communication between parents and visitation with child.
- Assess somatic complaints by the child. Have child complete "headache diary"/"stomachache diary" to determine aggravating/alleviating factors. Document frequency of complaints and discuss/review with parents.
- Meet with child to assess academic and emotional needs as they relate to home and school. Discuss findings with child's parents.
- Meet with the parents to develop a plan to help child meet academic goals and address emotional needs of the child. Involve child's teacher in plan development.
- Offer community resources to address emotional needs for the child such as support groups for children of divorced parents, Boy's Club of America, and peer play groups. Include information for parent support resources as well.
- Offer after-school tutoring to facilitate meeting academic goals as desired.

*NANDA Nursing Diagnoses—Definitions and Classification 2012-2014, Herdman T.H. (ED). Copyright © 2012, 1994-2012 NANDA International. Used by arrangement with John Wiley & Sons Limited. In order to make safe and effective judgments using the NANDA-I nursing diagnoses it is essential that nurses refer to the definitions and defining characteristics of the diagnoses listed in this work.

SUMMARY

Many changes occur in children during the exciting period of the school-age years. The child's development progresses from the immaturity of the preschooler to the beginning of adoles-cence and eventual adulthood. Cognitive abilities increase dra-matically, adding to the desire to master tasks and the ability to develop moral judgment. The child's world expands beyond the family unit as school and peers begin to exert a major influence. Opportunities for nurses during this period occur primarily in ambulatory settings, with the school nurse frequently the most effective and influential health care provider for children of this age group and their families.

REFERENCES

Adams, N. (2012). *How TV violence affects kids*. [Online]. Retrieved December 28, 2012, from http://www.livestrong.com/article/221006-how-tv-violence-affects-kids/.

American Academy of Child & Adolescent Psychiatry. (2011a). *Facts for families: Obesity in children and teens*. [Online]. Retrieved Janu-ary 6, 2012, from www.aacap.org/galleries/FactsForFamilies/79_obesity_in_children_and_teens.pdf.

American Academy of Child & Adolescent Psychiatry. (2011b). *Chil-dren with learning disabilities*. [Online]. Retrieved January 6, 2012, from http://aacap.org/page.ww?name=Children+with+Learning+Disabilities&section=Facts+for+Families.

American Academy of Otolaryngology. (2011a). *Children's hearing health*. [Online]. Retrieved January 10, 2012, from www.entnet.org/HealthInformation/childshearing.cfm.

American Academy of Otolaryngology. (2011b). *What is otitis media and ear infection?* [Online]. Retrieved January 10, 2012, from www.entnet.org/HealthInformation/childrensEaraches.cfm.

American Academy of Pediatric Dentistry. (2011). *Policy on oral care programs for infants, children, and adolescents*. [Online]. Retrieved December 28, 2011, from www.aapd.org/media/Policies_Guidelines/P_OralHealthCareProg.pdf.

American Academy of Pediatrics. (2010). *AAP offers updated guidelines on treating head lice*. [Online]. Retrieved December 28, 2012, from http://www.aap.org/en-us/about-the-aap/aap-press-room/pages/AAP-Offers-Updated-Guidance-on-Treating-Head-Lice.aspx.

American Academy of Pediatrics. (2011a). *Health issues: High blood pressure in children*. [Online]. Retrieved December 27, 2011, from www.healthychildren.org/English/health-issues/conditions/heart/pages/High-Blood-Pressure-in-Children.aspx.

American Academy of Pediatrics. (2011b). *Back to school tips*. [Online]. Retrieved January 6, 2012, from www.aap.org/en-us/about-the-aap/aap-press-room/news-features-and-safety-tips/Pages/Back-to-School-Tips.aspx.

American Academy of Pediatrics. (2011c). *Helping your child learn to read*. [Online]. Retrieved January 10, 2012, from www.healthychildren.org/english/ages-stages/preschool/Pages/Helping-Your-Child-Learn-to-Read.aspx.

American Academy of Pediatrics. (2011d). Clinical Practice Guideline ADHD: Clinical practice guidelines for the diagnosis, evaluation, and treatment of attention-deficit, hyperactivity disorder in children and adolescents. *Pediatrics, 128*(5), 1007–1022.

American Academy of Pediatrics. (2011e). *Child abuse and neglect*. [Online]. Retrieved January 10, 2012, from www2.aap.org/sections/childabuseneglect/.

American Academy of Pediatrics. (2012). *Disciplining your child*. [Online]. Retrieved January 6, 2012, from www.healthychildren.org/English/family-life/family-dynamics/communication-discipline/pages/Disciplining-Your-Child.aspx.

American Academy of Pediatrics. (2012a). *Injuries, manufacturer warnings do not deter ATV use by children under age 16*. [Online]. Retrieved December 28, 2012, from http://www.aap.org/en-us/about-the-aap/aap-press-room/pages/Injuries-Manufacturer-Warnings-Do-Not-Deter-ATV-Use-by-Children-under-Age-16.aspx.

American Academy of Pediatrics, & Committee on Quality Improvement, Subcommittee on Attention-Deficit/Hyperactivity Disorder. (2000). Clinical practice guideline: Diagnosis and evaluation of the child with attention-deficit/hyperactivity disorder. *Pediatrics, 105*, 1158–1170.

American Academy of Sleep Medicine. (2006). *Sleep & children*. [Online]. Retrieved April 23, 2012, from http://yoursleep.aasmnet.org/topic.aspx?id=8.

American Dental Association. (2011a). *Eruption charts, primary/secondary*. [Online]. Retrieved December 28, 2011, from www.ada.org/2671.aspx.

American Dental Association. (2011b). *Oral health topics: Braces and orthodontics*. [Online]. Retrieved December 28, 2011, from www.ada.org/3061.aspx#overview.

American Heart Association. (2008). *Cigarette smoking in children*. [Online]. Retrieved January 30, 2009, from http://americanheart.org/presenter.jhtml?identifier=4549.

American Heart Association (AHA). (2011a). *High blood pressure in children: AHA recommendations*. [Online]. Retrieved December 27, 2011, from www.heart.org/HEARTORG/Conditions/HighBloodPressure/UnderstandYourRiskforHighBloodPressure/High-Blood-Pressure-in-Children_UCM_301868_Article.jsp#.

American Heart Association (AHA). (2011b). *Dietary recommendations for healthy children*. [Online]. Retrieved January 6, 2012, from www.heart.org/HEARTORG/GettingHealthy/Dietary-Recommendations-for-Healthy-Children_UCM_303886_Article.jsp.

American Heart Association (AHA). (2011c). *Overweight in children*. [Online]. Retrieved January 6, 2012, from www.heart.org/HEARTORG/GettingHealthy/Overweight-in-Children_UCM_304054_Article.jsp.

American Optometric Association. (2012). *Need for comprehensive visual examinations in preschool and school-age children*. [Online]. Retrieved January 10, 2012, from www.aoa.org/x5419.xml.

American Psychiatric Association. (2000). *Diagnostic and statistical manual of mental disorders* (4th ed.). Washington, DC: Author.

Atherton, J. S. (2011). *Learning and Teaching; Piaget's developmental theory*. [Online: UK]. Retrieved December 28, 2012, from http://www.learningandteaching.info/learning/piaget.htm.

Ball, J., & Bindler, R. (2008). *Pediatric nursing: Caring for children* (4th ed.). Upper Saddle River, NJ: Pearson-Prentice Hall.

Bayer, O., Rosario, A. S., Wabitsch, M., & von Kries, R. (2009). Sleep duration and obesity in children: Is the association dependent on age and choice of the outcome parameter? *Sleep, 32*, 1183–1189.

Boyse, K. (2008). *Learning disabilities*. [Online]. Retrieved January 10, 2012, from www.childdevelopmentinfo.com/learning/learning_disabilities.shtml.

Boyse, K. (2010). *Sleep problems*. [Online]. Retrieved January 10, 2012, from www.med.umich.edu/yourchild/topics/sleep.htm.

Brannagan, S. (2010). *Cognitive learning in children*. [Online]. Retrieved January 10, 2012, from www.livestrong.com/article/151537-cognitive-learning-in-children/.

Breysse, P. N., Diette, G. B., Matsui, E. C., Butz, A. M., Hansel, N. N., & McCormack, M. C. (2010). Indoor air pollution and asthma in children. *Proceedings of the American Thoracic Society, 7(2)*, 102–106.

Centers for Disease Control and Prevention (CDC). (2008a). *Recommended immunization schedule for persons 0-6 years, 7-18 years*. Retrieved from www.cdc.gov/vaccines/recs/schedules/child-schedule.htm#printable.

Centers for Disease Control and Prevention (CDC). (2008b). *CDC childhood injury report*. [Online]. Retrieved from www.cdc.gov/safechild/Child_Injury_Data.htm.

Centers for Disease Control and Prevention (CDC). (2009). High school students who tried to quit smoking cigarettes: US-2007. *MMWR, 58*(16), 428–431.

Centers for Disease Control and Prevention (CDC). (2010). *National Centers for Health Statistics: Clinical growth charts*. [Online]. Retrieved December 28, 2011, from www.cdc.gov/growthcharts/.

Centers for Disease Control and Prevention (CDC). (2011a). *Oral health: Preventing cavities, gum disease, tooth loss and oral cancer at a glance 2011*. [Online]. Retrieved December 28, 2011, from www.cdc.gov/chronicdisease/resources/publications/AAG/doh.htm.

Centers for Disease Control and Prevention (CDC). (2011b). *Data 2010…the Healthy People 2010 database*. [Online]. Retrieved January 6, 2012, from http://wonder.cdc.gov/data2010/focraceg.htm.

Centers for Disease Control and Prevention (CDC). (2011c). *Overweight and obesity: Basics about childhood obesity*. [Online]. Retrieved January 6, 2012, from www.cdc.gov/obesity/childhood/basics.html.

Centers for Disease Control and Prevention (CDC). (2011d). *Fire death and injuries: Fact sheet.* [Online]. Retrieved December 28, 2012, from http://www.cdc.gov/HomeandRecreationalSafety/Fire-Prevention/fires-factsheet.html.

Centers for Disease Control and Prevention (CDC). (2011e). *Pedestrian safety.* [Online]. Retrieved December 28, 2012, from http://www.cdc.gov/Motorvehiclesafety/Pedestrian_safety/index.html.

Centers for Disease Control and Prevention (CDC). (2012a). *Unintentional drowning: Get the facts.* [Online]. Retrieved December 28, 2012, from http://www.cdc.gov/homeandrecreationalsafety/water-safety/waterinjuries-factsheet.html.

Centers for Disease Control and Prevention (CDC). (2012b). *Child passenger safety: Fact sheet.* [Online]. Retrieved December 28, 2012, from http://www.cdc.gov/MotorVehicleSafety/Child_Passenger_Safety/CPS-Factsheet.html.

Chakraburtty, A. (2012). *Enuresis in children.* [Online]. Retrieved January 8, 2012, from www.webmd.com/mental-health/enuresis.

Chattopadhyay, S. (2007). Religion, spirituality, health, and medicine: Why should Indian physicians care? *Journal of Postgraduate Medicine, 53*(4), 262–266.

Child Trends. (2012). *Teen homicide, fire arms, and suicide.* [Online]. Retrieved December 28, 2012, from http://www.childtrendsdatabank.org/?q=node/174.

Choby, B. A. (2009). Diagnosis and treatment of streptococcal pharyngitis. *American Family Physicians, 79*(5), 383–390.

Council on School Health. (2008). Disaster planning for schools. *Pediatrics, 122*(4), 895–901.

Craiggs, C., Corder, K., van Sluijs, E., & Griffin, S. J. (2011). Determinants of change in physical activity in children and adolescents. *American Journal of Preventive Medicine, 40*(6), 645–658.

Daly, L., Kalian, M. J., Abogast, K. B., & Durbin, D. (2010). Risk of injury to child passengers in sport utility vehicles. *Pediatrics, 117*(1), 9–14.

Demory-Luce, D., & Jenson, C. (2011). *Fast food for children and adolescents.* [Online]. Retrieved January 6, 2012, from www.uptodate.com/contents/fast-food-for-children-and-adolescents.

Durani, Y. (2011a). *Head Lice.* [Online]. Retrieved December 28, 2012, from http://kidshealth.org/parent/infections/common/head_lice.html#.

Durani, Y. (2011). *What is a germ?* [Online]. Retrieved April 22, 2012, from http://kidshealth.org/kid/talk/qa/germs.html#.

Eisenburg, M. E., Bernat, D. H., Bearinger, L. H., & Resnick, M. S. (2008). Support for comprehensive sexuality education: Perceptions from parents of school-age youth. *Journal of Adolescent Health, 42*(4), 352–359.

Erikson, E. H. (1993). *Childhood and society* (2nd ed., reissued). New York: W.W. Norton.

Erikson, E. H. (1994). *Identity, youth and crisis* (35th ed., reissued). New York: W.W. Norton.

Felszeghy, E., Juhasz, E., Koposzta, R., & Ilyes, I. (2008). Alterations in glucoregulation in childhood obesity—Association with insulin resistance and hyperinsulinemia. *Journal of Pediatric Endocrinology and Metabolism, 21*(9), 847–853.

Ferrer-Chancy, M., & Fugate, A. (2007). *The importance of friendship for school-age children.* [Online]. Retrieved December 28, 2012, from http://edis.ifas.ufl.edu/fy545.

Fuller, C. (2007). Xylitol and ear infection treatment. *Ezine articles.* [Online]. Retrieved January 30, 2009, from http://ezinearticles.com/?Xylitol_and_Ear_Infection_Treatment&id=57l80l.

Gavin, M. L. (2011). *All about sleep.* [Online]. Retrieved January 12, 2012, from http://kidshealth.org/parent/general/sleep/sleep.html#.

Gavin, M. L. (2012). *Encopresis (soiling).* [Online]. Retrieved January 8, 2012, from http://kidshealth.org/parent/emotions/behavior/encopresis.html#.

Goldstein, S., & Brooks, R. (2012). *Raising resilient children.* [Online]. Retrieved December 28, 2012, from http://www.psychologytoday.com/blog/raising-resilient-children/201211/giving-children-allowance-nurturing-resilience.

Hagan, J., Shaw, J., & Duncan, P. (2010). *Bright futures: Guidelines for health supervision of infants, children, and adolescents* (4th ed.). Elk Grove, IL: American Academy of Pediatrics.

Hansen, M. L., Gunn, P. W., & Kaelber, D. C. (2007). Underdiagnosis of hypertension in children. *JAMA, 298*, 874–879.

Harron, W. (2011). *Your child's handwriting—Signs of handwriting problems.* [Online]. Retrieved January 10, 2012, from http://kidshealth.org/parent/positive/learning/handwriting.html#.

Hayman, M. (2012). *How eating at home could save your life.* [Online]. Retrieved January 6, 2012, from http://healthimpactnews.com/2011/how-eating-at-home-can-save-your-life/.

Hobson, K. (2010). *Early report card on Healthy People 2010: (Barely) a C.* [Online]. Retrieved December 28, 2012, from http://blogs.wsj.com/health/2010/05/05/early-report-card-on-healthy-people-2010-barely-a-c/.

Hockenberry, M. J., & Wilson, D. (2008). *Wong's essentials of pediatric nursing* (8th ed.). St. Louis: Mosby.

Hockenberry, M. J., & Wilson, D. (2011). *Wong's nursing care of infants and children* (9th ed.). St Louis: Elsevier.

Hopkins, B., & Glaze, D. (2008). Disorders of arousal in children. *Pediatric Annals, 37*(7), 481–487.

Inman, D. D., vanBakergem, K. M., Larosa, L. C., & Garr, D. R. (2011). Evidence-based health promotion programs for schools and communities. *American Journal of Preventive Medicine, 40*(2), 207–219.

Kaneshiro, N. K. (2011). *Bedwetting.* [Online]. Retrieved December 28, 2012, from http://www.nlm.nih.gov/medlineplus/ency/article/001556.htm.

Kanwar, V. S. (2010). *Lymphadenopathy.* [Online]. Retrieved December 28, 2011, from http://emedicine.medscape.com/article/956340-overview#showall.

Kim, H. S. (2011). Consequences of parental divorce for child development. *American Sociological Review, 76*(3), 487–511.

Kohlberg, L. (1981). *The philosophy of moral development.* San Francisco: Harper & Row.

Krause-Parello, C. A., & Samms, K. (2010). School nurses in New Jersey: A quantitative inquiry on roles & responsibilities. *Journal for Specialists in Pediatric Nursing, 15*(3), 217–222.

Lande, M. B., Pearson, T. A., Vermillion, R. P., Auinger, P., & Fernandez, I. D. (2008). Elevated blood pressure, race/ethnicity, and C-reactive protein levels in children and adolescents. *Pediatrics, 122*(6), 1252–1257.

Learning Theories Knowledgebase. (2012, December). Retrieved December 28, 2012, from http://www.learning-theories.com/.

Leukemia & Lymphoma Society. (2012). *Leukemia facts & statistics.* [Online]. Retrieved April 25, 2012, from www.lls.org/#/diseaseinformation/getinformationsupport/factsstatistics/leukemia/.

Levene, S. (2010). *Helping children learn to read.* [Online]. Retrieved January 10, 2012, from www.onlineworksheets.org/learntoread.html#ReadingStages.

Li, S., Jin, X., Yan, S., Wu, S., Jiang, F., & Shen, X. (2009). Factors associated with bed and room sharing in Chinese school-age children. *Child Care Health Development, 35*(2), 171–177.

Logsdon, A. (2009). *Average tests scores—Average test scores in special education.* Retrieved from http://learningdisabilities.about.com/od/ac/g/average.htm.

Lumeng, J., Somashekar, D., Appugliese, D., Kaciroti, N., Corwyn, R., & Bradley, R. (2007). Shorter sleep duration is associated with increased risk for being overweight at ages 9 to 12 years. *Pediatrics, 120*(5), 1020–1029.

Manheim, J. (2010). *School-age test or procedure preparation.* [Online]. Retrieved January 10, 2012, from www.nlm.nih.gov/medlineplus/ency/article/002058.htm.

Martin, J., & Oakley, C. B. (Eds.), (2008). *Managing child nutrition programs: Leadership for excellence* (2nd ed). Sudbury, MA: Jones & Bartlett.

Mattocks, C., Ness, A., Deere, K., Tilling, K., Leary, S., Blair, S. N., & Riddoch, C. (2008). Early life determinants of physical activity in 11-12 year olds: Cohort study. *BMJ, 336*(7634), 26–29.

Milteer, R. M., Ginsburg, K. R., & Mulligan, D. A. (2012). The importance of play in promoting healthy child development and maintaining strong parent-child bond: Focus on children in poverty. *Pediatrics, 129*(1), e204–e213.

Moses, S. (2011). *Pediatric vital signs.* [Online]. Retrieved December 28, 2011, from www.fpnotebook.com/cv/exam/pdtrcvtlsgns.htm.

Myers, B. (2009). *Helping your child develop self-esteem.* Retrieved from www.healthy/place.com/adhd/add-focus/helping-your-child-develop-Self-esteem.

National Alliance on Mental Illness. (2010). *Depression in children and adolescents fact sheet.* [Online]. Retrieved December 28, 2012 from http://www.nami.org/Template.cfm?Section=By_Illness&template=/ContentManagement/ContentDisplay.cfm&ContentID=88551.

National Association of Attorneys General. (1998). *Master settlement agreement.* [Online]. Retrieved December 28, 2012, from http://web.archive.org/web/20080625084126/http://www.naag.org/backpages/naag/tobacco/msa/msa-pdf/1109185724_1032468605_cigmsa.pdf.

National Association of School Nurses. (2011). *Emergency preparedness—The role of the school nurse (position statement).* Silver Spring, MD: Author.

National Association of School Nurses. (2012). *SCOPE—School nurse childhood obesity prevention education.* [Online]. Retrieved January 6, 2012, from www.nasn.org/continuingeducation/livecontinuingeducationprograms/scope.

National Cancer Institute. (2012). *Cancer trends progress report 2011/2012 update.* Retrieved December 28, 2012, from http://progressreport.cancer.gov.

National Center for Children in Poverty. (2009). *Ten important questions about child poverty and family economic hardship.* Retrieved from www.nccp.org/faq.htm/#question8.

National Centers for Health Statistics. (2000). *2000 CDC growth charts: United States.* Retrieved from www.cdc.gov/nchs/nhanes/growthcharts/clinical_charts.htm.

National Highway Traffic Safety Administration. (2008). *Child passenger safety.* Retrieved from www.nhtsa.gov/portal/site/nhtsa/template.

National Institute on Deafness and Other Communication Disorders. (2010). *Office visits to U.S. physicians resulting in primary diagnosis of otitis media.* [Online]. Retrieved April 17, 2012, from www.nidcd.nih.gov/health/statistics/Pages/officevisits.aspx.

National Institute on Deafness and Other Communication Disorders. (2011). *Healthy hearing objectives.* [Online]. Retrieved January 10, 2012, from www.nidcd.nih.gov/health/healthyhearing/what_hh/pages/objectives.aspx.

National Institute of Diabetes and Digestive and Kidney Diseases (NIDDK). (2010). *Urinary incontinence in children.* [Online]. Retrieved January 8, 2012, from http://kidney.niddk.nih.gov/kudiseases/pubs/uichildren/.

National Institute for Family Literacy. (2010). *The effect of family literacy interventions on children's acquisition of reading.* Portsmouth, NH: RMC Research Corp.

National Institute of Mental Health. (2007). *ADHD.* [Online]. Retrieved January 30, 2009, from www.nimh.nih.govlhealthjpubli-cationsladhdlcomplete-publication.shtml.

National Institute of Mental Health. (2012). *Depression in children and adolescents.* [Online]. Retrieved December 28, 2012, from http://www.nimh.nih.gov/health/topics/depression/depression-in-children-and-adolescents.shtml.

National Safety Council. (2011). *Safety & Health Facts Sheet.* [Online]. Retrieved December 28, 2012, from http://www.nsc.org/news_resources/Resources/Pages/SafetyHealthFactSheets.aspx.

Nucci, L. P. (2008). *Handbook of moral and character education.* New York, NY: Routledge, Taylor and Francis Group.

Ott, S. (2008). *Bone growth and remodeling.* [Online]. Retrieved December 28, 2011, from http://depts.washington.edu/bonebio/ASBMRed/growth.html.

Piaget, J. (2001). *Psychology of intelligence.* Florence, KY: Routledge, Taylor and Francis Group.

Pickhardt, C. (2011). *Impact of divorce on young children and adolescents.* [Online]. Retrieved December 28, 2012, from http://www.psychologytoday.com/blog/surviving-your-childs-adolescence/201112/the-impact-divorce-young-children-and-adolescents.

Pillinger, J. (2011). *Bedwetting (enuresis).* [Online]. Retrieved January 8, 2012, from www.netdoctor.co.uk/diseases/facts/bedwetting.htm.

Powell, L., Szczypka, O., & Chaloupka, E. (2011). Exposure to food advertising on television among U.S. children. *Archives of Pediatric Adolescent Medicine, 161*(6), 553–560.

Public Broadcast Station. (2011). *Strategies for talking and listening.* [Online]. Retrieved January 30, 2009, from www.pbs.org.

Raghubar, K. P., Barnes, M. A., & Hecht, S. A. (2010). Working memory and mathematics: A review of developmental individual differences and cognitive approach. *Learning and individual differences, 20*(2), 110–122.

Reeve, S., & Bell, P. (2009). Children's self-documentation and understanding of the concepts 'healthy' and 'unhealthy.' *International Journal of Science Education, 31*(14), 1953–1974.

Reuschel, L. M. (2011). *Generalized anxiety disorder in children and adolescents: Implications for practice.* [Online]. Retrieved December 28, 2012, from http://psychology.illinoisstate.edu/cc/Comps/Reuschel%20-%20GAD.pdf.

Rodriguez-Cruz, E. (2011). *Pediatric hypertension.* Retrieved December 27, 2011, from http://emedicine.medscape.com/article/889877-overview.

Rosenfield, R. L., Lipton, R. B., & Drumm, M. L. (2009). Thelarche, pubarche, and menarche attainment in children with normal and elevated body mass index. *Pediatrics, 123*(1), 84–88.

Sacerdote, B. (2008). *Nature and nurture effects on children's outcomes: What have we learned from studies of twins and adoptees?* [Online]. Retrieved January 10, 2012, from www.econ.nyu.edu/user/bisina/Chapter5_Sacerdote.pdf.

Safe Kids. (2011). *Injury trends fact sheet.* [Online]. Retrieved December 28, 2012, from http://www.safekids.org/our-work/research/fact-sheets/injury-trends-fact-sheet.html.

Save the Children U.S. Programs. (2012). *Disaster preparedness for children in the USA*. [Online]. Retrieved December 28, 2012, from http://www.savethechildren.org/site/c.8rKLIXMGIpI4E/b.7705371/k.10C/Disaster_Preparedness_for_Kids_in_the_USA.htm.

SCHIP Information Center. (2008). *SCHIP information center*. [Online]. Retrieved December 28, 2012, from http://www.schip-info.org/.

Segre, L. (2011). *The eye chart and 20/20 vision*. [Online]. Retrieved January 10, 2012, from www.allaboutvision.com/eye-test/.

Sheslow, D. (2008). *Developing your child's self-esteem*. Retrieved from www.kidshealth.org/parent/emotions/feelings/self_esteem.html.

Stephenson, M. (2010). *Eye exams of children*. [Online]. Retrieved January 10, 2012, from www.allaboutvision.com/eye-exam/children.htm.

Stock, S., Miranda, C., Evans, S., Plessis, S., Ridley, J., Yeh, S., et al. (2007). Health buddies: A novel, peer-led health promotion program for the prevention of obesity and eating disorders in children in elementary school. *Pediatrics, 120*, e1059–e1068.

Stop Smoking Update. (2009). *Helping your child to stop smoking*. Retrieved from www.stop-smoking-updates.com/quitsmoking/family/care/helping-your-child-Stop-Smoking.htm.

Sturaro, C., van Lier, P. A., Cuijpers, P., & Koot, H. M. (2011). The role of peer relationships in the development of early school-age externalizing problems. *Child Development, 82*(3), 758–765.

Taveras, E. M., Gillman, M. W., Kleinman, K., Rich-Edwards, J. W., & Rifas-Shiman, S. L. (2010). Racial/ethnic differences in early-life risk factors for childhood obesity. *Pediatrics*. [Online]. Retrieved January 6, 2012, from http://pediatrics.aappublications.org/content/early/2010/03/01/peds.2009-2100.

Tidy, C. (2011). *Normal and abnormal puberty*. [Online]. Retrieved December 28, 2011, from www.patient.co.uk/doctor/Puberty-Normal-and-Abnormal.htm.

Tobacco Free Kids. (2012). *Tobacco use among youth*. [Online]. Retrieved April 23, 2012, from www.tobaccofreekids.org/research/factsheets/pdf/0002.pdf.

Tynan, W. D. (2011). *Teaching your child self-control*. Retrieved January 4, 2012, from http://kidshealth.org/parent/emotions/behavior/self_control.html#.

Urbina, E., Alpert, B., Flynn, J., Hayman, L., Harshfield, G. A., Jacobson, M., et al. (2008). Ambulatory blood pressure monitoring in children and adolescents: Recommendations for standard assessment: A scientific statement from the American Heart Association Atherosclerosis, Hypertension, and Obesity in Youth Committee of the Council on Cardiovascular Disease in the Young and the Council for High Blood Pressure Research. *Hypertension, 52*, 433–451.

U.S. Department of Agriculture. (2011). *National school lunch program*. [Online]. Retrieved January 6, 2012, from www.fns.usda.gov/cnd/lunch/AboutLunch/NSLPFactSheet.pdf.

U.S. Department of Agriculture, Center for Nutrition Policy and Promotion. (2011). *Choose My Plate*. Retrieved April 17, 2012, from www.choosemyplate.gov/food-groups/downloads/TenTips/DGTipsheet11KidFriendlyVeggiesAndFruits.pdf.

U.S. Department of Education. (2008). *No Child Left Behind update*. [Online]. Retrieved January 30, 2009, from www.ed.gov/print/about/overview/mission/mission.html.

U.S. Department of Health and Human Services (USDHHS). (2007b). Healthy eating and physical activity across your lifespan. *Helping your child: Tips for parents*. [Online]. Retrieved January 30, 2009, from http://win.niddk.nih.gov/publicaaons/child.htm.

U.S. Department of Health and Human Services (USDHHS). (2011). *Child maltreatment 2010*. [Online]. Retrieved January 10, 2012, from www.acf.hhs.gov/programs/cb/pubs/cm10/cm10.pdf#page=31.

U.S. Department of Health and Human Services (USDHHS). (2012a). *Healthy People 2020: Oral health*. [Online]. Retrieved January 6, 2012, from http://healthypeople.gov/2020/topicsobjectives2020/objectiveslist.aspx?topicId=32#186.

U.S. Department of Health and Human Services (USDHHS). (2012b). *Healthy People 2020 leading health indicators*. [Online]. Retrieved January 6, 2012, from http://healthypeople.gov/2020/LHI/default.aspx.

U.S. Department of Health and Human Services (USDHHS). (2012c). *Healthy People 2020: Nutrition and weight status: Food access*. [Online]. Retrieved January 6, 2012, from http://healthypeople.gov/2020/topicsobjectives2020/objectiveslist.aspx?topicid=29.

Uusi, K., Kannus, R., Pasanen, M., & Sievanen, H. (2010). Is childhood obesity associated with bone density and strength in adulthood? *Journal of Osteoporosis*, article ID 904806. doi:10.4061/2010/904806.

Van den Berg, L., Pieterse, K., Malik, J. A., Luman, M., Williams van Dijk, K., Oosterlan, J., & Delemarre-van de Waal, H. A. (2011). Association between impulsivity, reward responsiveness and BMI in children. *International Journal of Obesity, 35*(10), 1301–1307.

Williams, H. K. (2008). *How to boost self-esteem through play*. [Online]. Retrieved January 10, 2012, from http://ezinearticles.com/?How-to-Boost-Self-Esteem-Through-Play&id=1028608.

Women & Children's Health Network. (2010). *Self-esteem*. Retrieved January 10, 2012, from www.cyh.com/HealthTopics/HealthTopicDetails.aspx?p=114&np=141&id=1702.

Woodburne, A. S. (1945). The evil eye in south Indian folk-lore. *International Review of Mission, 34*, 237–247. doi:10.1111/j.17586631.1945.tb04321.x.

World Health Organization. (2011). *Growth reference data for 5-19 years*. [Online]. Retrieved December 28, 2011, from www.who.int/growthref/en/.

Wright's, Law (2011). *Discrimination: Sections 504 and ADA*. [Online]. Retrieved January 5, 2012, from www.wrightslaw.com/info/sec504.index.htm.

Yukhananov, A. (2011). *Eating healthy food costs more money in the U.S.* [Online]. Retrieved January 6, 2012, from www.reuters.com/article/2011/08/04/us-food-costs-idUSTRE7734L620110804.

Zimmerman, F. J., & Bell, J. F. (2010). Associations of television content type and obesity in children. *American Journal of Public Health, 100*(2), 334–340.

123Test. (2012). *Culture fair intelligence tests*. [Online]. Retrieved January 10, 2012, from www.123test.com/culture-fair-intelligence-tests/.

Adolescent

Yi-Hui Lee, Ali Salman, and Tawna Cooksey-James

⊖volve WEBSITE

http://evolve.elsevier.com/Edelman/
- Study Questions
- Glossary

OBJECTIVES

After completing this chapter, the reader will be able to:

- Distinguish between the terms *puberty* and *adolescence*.
- Summarize the physical growth, developmental, and maturational changes that occur during adolescence.
- Outline the recommended schedule of health-promotion and preventive health visits and the appropriate topics for discussion with the adolescent during each visit.

- Analyze factors that contribute to risk-taking behaviors and situations during adolescence.
- Develop a health teaching plan addressing some of the physical, emotional, social, and spiritual challenges facing adolescents.

KEY TERMS

Acne	Gynecomastia	Peer group
Adolescence	Idealism	Primary sexual characteristics
Anorexia nervosa	Identity	Puberty
Binge eating disorder	Identity versus role confusion	Purge
Body image	Introspection	Risk-taking behaviors
Bulimia nervosa	Klinefelter syndrome	Scoliosis
Depression	Menarche	Secondary sexual characteristics
Egocentrism	Menstruation	Sexually transmitted diseases (STDs)
Ejaculation	Nocturnal emissions	Tanner staging
Emancipated minors	Obesity	Turner syndrome
Formal operations	Overweight	

❓ THINK ABOUT IT

Risk Behaviors in Adolescents

The mortality rate for adolescents is three times higher than it is for school-age children. Suicide rates in adolescents are increasing across all ethnic groups. Increasing numbers of young adolescents not only are becoming sexually active but also are choosing not to use any protection or contraception.

- *What growth and developmental factors make adolescents susceptible to these risky situations?*
- *What anticipatory guidance and strategies might be offered to adolescents and their families to prevent this risky behavior?*

The term adolescence is commonly used to describe the transitional stage between childhood and adulthood. The period of **adolescence** is defined as beginning with the onset of puberty, around age 11 to 13 years. Many researchers and developmental specialists in the United States use the age span 10 to 24 years as a working definition of adolescence. The term adolescence refers to the psychosocial, emotional, cognitive, and moral transition from childhood to young adulthood, while **puberty** refers to the development and maturation of the reproductive, endocrine, and structural processes that lead to fertility.

Rapid change in physical, psychosocial, spiritual, moral, and cognitive growth—the most characteristic trait of adolescence—creates an extremely tenuous sense of balance. A pivotal developmental period, adolescence offers health care providers unique opportunities for health-promotion and preventive services. Providing knowledge about the changes, challenges, and choices adolescents will encounter, as well as the tools with which to approach them, encourages and reinforces developing competencies and sense of responsibility (American Academy of Pediatrics [AAP], 2008; Berger, 2011; Seidel et al., 2010). Box 21-1: *Healthy People 2020* presents objectives related to adolescent health.

BIOLOGY AND GENETICS

In contrast to the slow, steady growth of childhood, adolescents experience accelerated growth that dramatically alters their body size and proportions. The most noticeable changes in adolescence involve physical and sexual growth, including the appearance of **secondary sexual characteristics.** These changes occur in a predictable sequence, but the onset and duration of the sequencing vary among individuals. Females usually begin puberty 2 years earlier than males and experience their growth spurt earlier. The appearance and sequence of secondary sexual

♥ BOX 21-1 HEALTHY PEOPLE 2020

Selected Health-Promotion and Disease-Prevention Objectives for Adolescents

- Increase the proportion of adolescents who have had a wellness check-up in the past 12 months.
- Increase the proportion of adolescents who participate in extracurricular and out-of-school activities.
- Increase the proportion of adolescents who are connected to a parent or other positive adult caregiver.
- (Developmental) Increase the proportion of adolescents and young adults who transition to self-sufficiency from foster care.
- Increase the proportion of schools with a school breakfast program.
- Reduce the proportion of adolescents who have been offered, sold, or given an illegal drug on school property.
- Increase the proportion of adolescents whose parents consider them to be safe at school.
- (Developmental) Increase the proportion of middle and high schools that prohibit harassment based on a student's sexual orientation or gender identity.
- Decrease the proportion of public schools with a serious violent incident.
- Reduce adolescent and young adult perpetration of, as well as victimization by, crimes.
- Reduce the proportion of children and adolescents who have dental caries in their primary or permanent teeth.
- Reduce the proportion of children and adolescents with untreated dental decay.
- Increase the proportion of adolescents who meet current federal physical activity guidelines for aerobic physical activity and for muscle-strengthening activity.
- Increase the proportion of adolescents who participate in daily school physical education.
- Increase the proportion of children and adolescents who do not exceed recommended limits for screen time.

- Reduce the proportion of adolescents and young adults with *Chlamydia trachomatis* infections.
- Increase the proportion of sexually active females ages 24 years and under enrolled in Medicaid plans who are screened for genital *Chlamydia* infections during the measurement year.
- Increase the proportion of sexually active females ages 24 years and under enrolled in commercial health insurance plans who are screened for genital *Chlamydia* infections during the measurement year.
- Reduce the proportion of females ages 15 to 44 years who have ever required treatment for pelvic inflammatory disease (PID).
- Increase the proportion of students in grades 9 through 12 who get sufficient sleep.
- Reduce the proportion of adolescents who report that they rode, during the previous 30 days, with a driver who had been drinking alcohol.
- Increase the proportion of adolescents never using substances.
- Increase the proportion of adolescents who disapprove of substance abuse.
- Increase the proportion of adolescents who perceive great risk associated with substance abuse.
- Reduce physical fighting among adolescents.
- Reduce bullying among adolescents.
- Reduce weapon carrying by adolescents on school property.
- Reduce suicide attempts by adolescents.
- Reduce the proportion of adolescents who engage in disordered eating behaviors in an attempt to control their weight.
- Reduce the proportion of children and adolescents who are considered obese.
- Reduce tobacco use by adolescents.
- Reduce the initiation of tobacco use among children, adolescents, and young adults.
- Increase smoking cessation attempts by adolescent smokers.

From U.S. Department of Health and Human Services. (2011). *Healthy People 2020.* Washington, DC: Author. For information on the upcoming *Healthy People 2020*, go to http://healthypeople.gov/2020/.

TABLE 21-1 GROWTH AND DEVELOPMENT

Sexual Maturity Rating, Tanner Stages: Developmental Stages of Secondary Sexual Characteristics

STAGE	MALE GENITAL DEVELOPMENT	PUBIC HAIR DEVELOPMENT	FEMALE BREAST DEVELOPMENT	OTHER CHANGES
1	Prepubertal	No distinction between hair over pubic area and hair over abdomen		
2	Initial enlargement of scrotum and testes; reddening and texture changes of scrotum	Sparse growth of long, straight, downy hair at base of penis or along labia	Enlargement of areolar diameter; small area of elevation around papillae (breast bud)	Usual time of peak height velocity for girls
3	Initial enlargement of penis, mainly in length; further growth of testes and scrotum	Hair becomes dark, coarse, and curly; spreads sparsely over entire pubic area	Further elevation and enlargement of breasts and areolas, with no separation of their contours	Usual time of menarche; facial hair begins to grow on upper lip and voice deepens in boys
4	Further enlargement of penile diameter, testes, scrotum, and glans	Further spread of hair distribution, not extending to thighs	Areolas and papillae project from breast to form secondary mound	Usual time of peak height velocity for boys; axillary hair begins to grow
5	Adult in size and contour	Adult in amount and type; spreads to inner surface of thighs	Adult, with projection of papillae only; recession of areolas into general breast contour	

Modified from Hockenberry, M. J., & Wilson, D. (2010). *Wong's nursing care of infants and children* (9th ed.). St. Louis: Mosby.

characteristics and pubertal events are summarized in Table 21-1 and later illustrated in Figure 21-3 on p. 518.

The physical changes experienced during adolescence are mediated primarily by the hormonal regulatory systems in the hypothalamus, pituitary gland, gonads, and adrenal glands (Pinyerd & Zipf, 2005) (Figure 21-1). The hypothalamus releases gonadotropin-releasing hormone (GnRF), which stimulates the anterior pituitary to release the gonadotropin hormones luteinizing hormone (LH) and follicle-stimulating hormone (FSH) (Ball & Bindler, 2008). In females, this stimulates ovarian development and estrogen production. Estrogen produces all secondary sexual characteristics except axillary and pubic hair, which are controlled by adrenal androgens. In males, luteinizing hormone results in testicular enlargement and the development of Leydig cells in the testes, which produce testosterone. Follicle-stimulating hormone stimulates the development of the seminiferous tubules of the testes, leading to spermatogenesis and fertility. Once sexual maturation is completed, the ongoing release of hormones controls menses, pregnancy, and lactation. Menarche, the onset of menses in females, usually occurs late in puberty as the growth spurt is subsiding (Ball & Bindler, 2008). Adolescents who do not follow the normal sequence or who have not begun pubertal development by age 14 years, for males, and age 13 years, for females, should have an endocrine evaluation (Herman-Giddens & Kaplowitz, 2010). However, racial and ethnic differences in ages of achieving pubertal milestones vary (American Academy of Pediatrics, 2008).

Before the growth spurt, many adolescents experience a transient increase in body fat or adipose tissue. As puberty progresses, the proportion of total body weight composed of fat usually declines, particularly in boys. Body fat begins to accumulate again in both genders after their growth spurt, but at a slightly higher rate in females.

The heart grows in size and strength. Blood volume and blood pressure increase, and the heart rate decreases to adult levels. These cardiovascular changes occur earlier in females and parallel puberty. Compared to adolescent males, adolescent females also generally have higher pulse rates and slightly lower systolic blood pressure measurements. Adolescents are identified as hypertensive when their systolic or diastolic blood pressure is at or above the 95th percentile (based on age, gender, and height) on three separate occasions.

Respiratory rate decreases throughout childhood, reaching an average rate of 15 to 20 breaths per minute during adolescence. Respiratory volume and vital capacity increase, particularly in males. The larynx and vocal cords grow, producing the characteristic voice changes of puberty. Both male and female voices become deeper and laryngeal cartilage enlarges, with both effects more pronounced in males.

The gastrointestinal system reached functional maturity during school-age years. However, it continues to grow along with the growth spurt (Ball & Bindler, 2008; Guyton & Hall, 2011).

Permanent teeth begin erupting around 6 years of age, and all 32, except the third molars, or wisdom teeth, are in place by 13 to 14 years of age. Third molars are often pulled during adolescence to make space for the other permanent teeth. However, it is increasingly common for them never to develop (Burns et al., 2009).

Both the sweat and sebaceous glands become more active during adolescence. The sweat glands are located primarily in the axillary, genital, and periumbilical areas and are the primary source of body odor. The sebaceous glands are located primarily on the face, neck, shoulders, upper back, chest, and genitals. They can become clogged and inflamed, leading to the common teenage condition called acne. Acne occurs in up to 80% to 85% of all adolescents and young adults (Burns et al., 2009).

Acne

Adolescents typically are concerned about their skin changes. The sebaceous glands increase production of sebum, a primary factor in the pathogenesis of acne. The sebaceous follicles

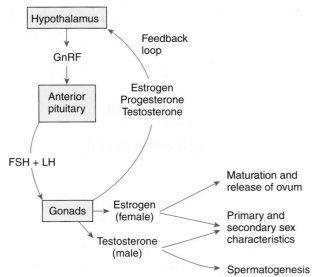

FIGURE 21-1 Hormonal interaction among hypothalamus, pituitary, and gonads. (From Hockenberry, M. J., & Wilson, D. [2010]. *Wong's nursing care of infants and children* [9th ed.]. St. Louis: Mosby.) *FSH,* Follicle-stimulating hormone; *GnRF,* gonadotropin-releasing hormone; *LH,* luteinizing hormone.

FIGURE 21-2 Scoliosis screening. So that the entire back can be seen, the adolescent should remove all clothing from the upper body when being assessed for scoliosis. **A,** While the adolescent stands up straight, check for any asymmetry; observe and palpate for differences in shoulder or scapular height, prominence of either scapula or hip, waist asymmetry, and misalignment of the spinous processes. Lateral curvature and thoracic convexity of the spine indicate scoliosis. **B,** With feet together, legs straight, and arms hanging freely, the adolescent bends forward until the back is parallel with the floor. Check for prominence of the ribs, or rib hump, on one side only and hip and leg asymmetry. With scoliosis, the chest wall on the side of convexity is prominent, and the scapula on the side of convexity is elevated.

become clogged with sebum and debris, forming open (blackheads) or closed (whiteheads) comedones. The incidence of acne within families suggests that hereditary factors are involved.

Thorough examination of the adolescent's skin and a discussion of its impact on the overall body image are necessary to determine appropriate management strategies. Intervention should include teaching the individual about the pathophysiological nature of acne. Knowledge allows the adolescent to become instrumental in its management and helps dispel common myths about acne and its care.

Washing with soap and water two or three times a day is the best way to remove dirt and oil. Vigorous scrubbing should be discouraged, because the skin can become irritated, leading to follicular rupture. The adolescent should not attempt to remove the pustules and papules that form. Squeezing the lesion can result in further irritation of the gland and permanent injury to the tissue. Many nonprescription topical medications contain benzoyl peroxide, which is bacteriostatic and comedolytic. Unfortunately, these agents cause drying and peeling; therefore, therapy is begun with application of 5% strength once a day. If tolerated, after 2 weeks the application is increased to twice a day.

Adolescent females need to be careful when selecting makeup. Most preparations, when applied extensively over the face, prevent adequate exposure to air and light, especially those that have a fat base. Sunlight can have a beneficial effect on acne; however, prolonged exposure should be avoided. Stress can exacerbate acne in some adolescents. In these cases, stress-management techniques should be considered. The effect of diet on acne is a highly controversial issue. Evidence indicates that dietary restrictions specific to acne are unnecessary.

Adolescents with acne need support and understanding. The nurse can help adolescents and their families understand that

management does not result in immediate improvement. In fact, topical agents may make acne appear worse initially, with any improvement occurring slowly over several months.

Scoliosis

A common skeletal deformity found in adolescents is scoliosis, a lateral S-shaped curvature of the spine (Figure 21-2). The curve is typically convex to the right. Classifications of scoliosis include secondary or functional, congenital, neuromuscular, constitutional, and idiopathic, which has an infantile, juvenile, or adolescent onset. Approximately 10% of all adolescents have a mild truncal asymmetry; however, curves greater than 15 degrees are abnormal and can progress to significant curvature during the growth spurt (Burns et al., 2009). Idiopathic scoliosis is the most common type and is significantly more prevalent in females. Early intervention is important, because untreated scoliosis can result in disfigurement, impaired mobility, and cardiopulmonary complications.

The nurse includes scoliosis screening in the assessment of both prepubertal and pubertal adolescents, paying close attention to the timing of the growth spurt. Most adolescents with scoliosis will require only observation; however, bracing and surgical correction may be necessary and early referral to an orthopedic surgeon is important. Early identification

FIGURE 21-3 Diagram of sequences of events at adolescence in girls **(A)** and boys **(B)**. Single numbers *(2, 3, 4, 5)* indicate stages of development. The average is represented. A range of ages when each event may begin and end is indicated by inclusive numbers listed below each event. (Modified from Marshall, W. A., & Tanner, J. M. [1969]. Variations in pattern of pubertal changes in girls. *Archives of Disease in Childhood, 44,* 291-303; Hockenberry, M. J., & Wilson, D. [2010]. *Wong's nursing care of infants and children* [9th ed.]. St. Louis: Mosby.)

can help avoid more invasive care and prevent the long-term consequences.

Gender

During puberty, **primary sexual characteristics** begin to develop and secondary sexual characteristics emerge. Primary sexual characteristics involve the organs necessary for reproduction, such as the penis and testes in boys and the vagina and uterus in girls. Secondary sexual characteristics are external features that are not essential for reproduction. Breast development, facial and pubic hair growth, and lowering of the voice are examples of secondary sex characteristics (see Table 21-1). Sexual maturity rating, also referred to as **Tanner staging**, is used widely to assess and monitor the degree of maturation of an adolescent's primary and secondary sexual characteristics. Each of the characteristics, breast, pubic hair, and genitals, is staged separately (from 1 to 5) and compared with the expected sequencing (Figure 21-3).

Breast development usually is confined to females; however, some degree of unilateral or bilateral breast enlargement, termed **gynecomastia,** may appear early in male puberty, just before the growth spurt. Gynecomastia is usually temporary and typically disappears. However, occasionally it persists and leads to body image problems and can be surgically reduced if psychological assessment warrants it.

The first sign of puberty in males is a thinning of the scrotal sac and enlargement of the testicles. **Ejaculation** is considered a milestone of male puberty and precedes fertility by several months. **Nocturnal emissions,** or "wet dreams," can concern adolescent males, because the event happens beyond their control.

For females the first sign of puberty is the appearance of breast buds, followed by the growth spurt. The onset of **menstruation,**

or menarche, occurs approximately 2 years after the appearance of the breast buds and near the end of the growth spurt.

Familiarity with the stages of development of sexual characteristics and their expected sequence helps the nurse monitor the adolescent's progression through puberty and detect any variations that might herald an alteration in normal growth and development.

Genetics

Most genetic problems are discovered during infancy and early childhood. Some syndromes, however, may not be diagnosed until adolescence. These genetic disorders frequently are discovered during the assessment of an adolescent with delayed or irregular pubertal development. Family history not only can help physicians make a diagnosis if the adolescent shows signs of a disorder but also can help to reveal whether there is an increased risk for a disease for the adolescent (Box 21-2: Innovative Practice).

Turner syndrome (XO) is a female disorder in which only one X chromosome is present instead of two. Assessment findings include short stature, a webbed neck, a low posterior hairline, low-set ears, a shield-shaped chest with widely spaced nipples, and gonadal-ovarian dysgenesis, resulting in a lack of sexual development and menses during puberty. Cardiac and renal anomalies are often present. Learning disabilities are common. Management consists primarily of administration of growth hormone, to increase height, and estrogen therapy to help develop secondary sexual characteristics and menses. However, the female with Turner syndrome remains sterile. Ongoing emotional support for the adolescent and her family is important.

Klinefelter syndrome (XXY) is seldom diagnosed before puberty. Males have an extra X chromosome and typically are

✴ BOX 21-2 INNOVATIVE PRACTICE

My Family Health Portrait

Teens can create a simple pedigree with the Surgeon General's *My Family Health Portrait* at www.hhs.gov/familyhistory/. *My Family Health Portrait* is a downloadable, web-based tool for use on a personal computer. It helps individuals create their own family health history and is a part of the National Human Genome Research Institute (NHGRI) and the U.S. Surgeon General's Family History Initiative. Because it is web-based, teens may be the family member best prepared (or most technologically comfortable) to coordinate the input of data. With their family's help, teens gather their family health history, and then, using any type of computer, build a drawing of their family tree and a chart of their family health history. Both the chart and the drawing can be printed and shared with other family members and health care providers.

Each year since 2004, the Surgeon General has declared Thanksgiving to be National Family History Day. In 2006, the Centers for Disease Control and Prevention (CDC) arranged a workgroup to explore the use of family history information in pediatric primary care and public health. For more information about tools and resources regarding use of family history please visit www.cdc.gov/ncbddd/pediatricgenetics/family_history.html.

In 2009, the National Institutes of Health hosted the Family History State-of-the-Science Conference to provide health care providers, patients, and the general public with a responsible assessment of current available data on family history and improving health. It had been pointed out that family history has been and will continue to be a core component of clinical and public health practice. For access to more information about this conference, please visit http://consensus.nih.gov/2009/familyhistory.htm. In addition, the National Coalition for Health Professional Education in Genetics (NCHPEG) has published a summary of other family history tools at www.nchpeg.org/index.php?option=com_content&view=article&id=61&Itemid=74.

tall, initially thin, and do not develop secondary sexual characteristics. They often have gynecomastia. Klinefelter syndrome is associated with learning or behavior problems during childhood. As with Turner syndrome, management typically involves androgen therapy and counseling; however, the adolescent remains sterile.

When the nurse recognizes signs of either of these syndromes during routine screening, the adolescent is referred to specialists who are qualified to diagnose and manage the physical, social, spiritual, and emotional aspects of these problems.

Most adolescents with delayed development do not have a genetic disorder; their pattern of growth merely falls at the far end of the normal curve and is referred to as a constitutional delay. Whatever the cause, delays can have a tremendous effect on psychosocial development, and these adolescents need ongoing assessment and support to promote development of positive self-esteem.

GORDON'S FUNCTIONAL HEALTH PATTERNS

Health Perception–Health Management Pattern

Teens have fewer acute illnesses than do younger children and fewer chronic illnesses than adults. They are seen in health care facilities less frequently than younger children and adults, and they rarely are hospitalized. Yet they need to be monitored, because adolescence is a pivotal developmental period

with numerous physical, psychosocial, and spiritual changes. Box 21-3 lists interventions recommended for periodic health examinations for adolescents.

A crucial component for understanding adolescent health is an adolescent's own perceptions of health, illness, and health care services. Too often, their sense of invincibility and "Peter Pan" ideology couples with typical adolescent experimentation and risk-taking behaviors to produce deleterious health care choices and outcomes. Caught somewhere between childhood and adulthood, teens may no longer feel as if they are being attended to by pediatricians, pediatric nurse practitioners, and pediatric nurses, yet, at the same time, are often misunderstood by adult health care providers. Health care services for adolescents need to be developed that are available, visible, confidential, and flexible. For information regarding health care services for adolescents, visit the National Adolescent and Young Adult Health Information Center (NAHIC) at http://nahic.ucsf.edu.

Adolescents are in the process of developing health habits and patterns of problem-solving that are likely to last a lifetime. The cognitive and psychological changes that they experience can affect their adherence to health-promotion and disease-prevention strategies. Teens do not always consider the health risks of their behavior and have an overall sense of invulnerability to illness or injury. Peer influence is primary, and parental input often is rejected. Nurses need to be sensitive to the changes that occur as adolescents become increasingly capable of more independent decisions about their health behavior.

Parents, teachers, and health care providers will be more successful in assisting teens to manage their health needs wisely if they treat them as joint partners in planning the care for which the adolescents, themselves, will assume responsibility. Key components of successful health supervision include respect for individual differences, support for the adolescent's emerging autonomy, a developmental approach, and a focus on the individual's strengths (American Academy of Pediatrics, 2008).

Nutritional-Metabolic Pattern

Many teens have concerns about their body, proper nutrition, and exercise. The media not only portrays the ideal body as thin, lean, or muscular, but at the same time promotes fast food, soda pop, sweets, and alcohol consumption (Dixon & Stein, 2005). Asserting their newfound autonomy, teens may choose dietary intake as a mechanism to gain control over their changing bodies, exert independence, or experiment with a new identity or cause, such as becoming a vegetarian. All of this occurs as their body's nutrient and energy demands increase in preparation and response to the adolescent growth spurt. Teen activities, including sports and other vigorous extracurricular physical activity, can further increase these demands. Gymnasts, runners, body builders, rowers, wrestlers, dancers, and swimmers are particularly vulnerable to eating disorders because their sports necessitate weight restriction. Complicating matters are teens' overwhelming desire to "fit in" with their peers, which often prevails and can lead to unhealthy dietary practices.

In the United States, up to 10% of adolescent females suffer from an eating disorder (American Academy of Child & Adolescent Psychiatry [AACAP], 2008) and 62% of female and

BOX 21-3 INTERVENTIONS RECOMMENDED FOR THE PERIODIC HEALTH EXAMINATION: 11 TO 21 YEARS OF AGE

Screening
- Height, weight, and BMI
- Blood pressure
- Scoliosis
- Vision and hearing
- Tanner stage
- Anemia
- Hyperlipidemia
- Urinalysis
- TB
- Eating disorders
- Sports injuries
- Tattoos and piercings
- If sexually active, Pap test and STD screening
- Counseling

Injury and Violence Prevention
- Lap and shoulder belts in car
- Bicycle, motorcycle, all-terrain vehicle helmets
- Protective gear for sports, work, and other physical activities
- Learn first aid and CPR
- Skin cancer, sun exposure, sunscreen SPF 15 or higher
- Safe storage and use of firearms

Substance Use
- Avoid tobacco, alcohol, and drug use
- Avoid alcohol or drug use while driving, swimming, boating, riding a bike or motorcycle, or operating farm equipment or other machinery

Sexual Behavior
- Abstinence, resisting sexual pressures, saying no
- STD prevention and protection
- Unintended pregnancy, contraception
- Date rape

Diet and Exercise
- Choose a variety of healthy foods
- Balance caloric intake and energy expenditure
- Limit fat and cholesterol; emphasize grains, fruits, vegetables
- Adequate calcium, iron, and folic acid

Dental Health
- Regular (every 6 months) visits to dental care provider
- Brush at least twice a day and floss daily
- Avoid tobacco products

Immunization
- DT vaccine: booster if at least 5 years since last dose of DTP, DTaP, or DT
- Hepatitis B virus vaccine (if not given previously)
- Hepatitis A virus vaccine (if indicated)
- MMR vaccine
- VAR vaccine (if not given previously or no reliable history of chickenpox; if 13 or older, two doses 4 to 8 weeks apart)
- Meningitis vaccine
- HPV vaccine

BMI, Body mass index; *CPR*, cardiopulmonary resuscitation; *DT*, diphtheria tetanus; *DTaP*, diphtheria, tetanus, acellular pertussis; *DTP*, diphtheria, tetanus, pertussis; *HPV*, Human papillomavirus *MMR*, measles, mumps, rubella; *Pap*, Papanicolaou; *SPF*, sun protection factor; *STD*, sexually transmitted disease; *TB*, tuberculosis; *VAR*, varicella.

20% of male adolescents participate in "fad" dieting (Dixon & Stein, 2005). Adolescents who meet the criteria for eating disorders should be referred to an interdisciplinary team that is experienced and skilled in working with these disorders (Dixon & Stein, 2005). Research shows that early identification and treatment at either end of the spectrum leads to more favorable outcomes (AACAP, 2008).

Eating Disorders

At one end of the eating disorder spectrum is anorexia nervosa and bulimia nervosa. At the other end is binge eating disorder and obesity. Adolescents with anorexia nervosa are typically female, perfectionists, and high achievers with families that tend to be achievement oriented and experiencing marital discord. Symptoms or warning signs include a relentless pursuit of thinness, self-starving with significant weight loss, lack of menstruation (in females) and decreased sexual interests (in males), compulsive physical activity, preoccupation with food, portioning food carefully, eating only small amounts of only certain foods, and a distorted body image.

The adolescent may also have brittle hair and nails; dry, yellowish skin; growth of fine hair over the body; constipation; mild anemia and muscle weakness; and often complains of feeling cold. The onset of anorexia is typically in response to low self-esteem and real or imagined obesity. Needing mastery, the teen with anorexia nervosa experiences a sense of control when able to say no to the body's normal food demands (AACAP, 2008). Eventually, the teen becomes dangerously malnourished and in some cases dies.

Another eating disorder, bulimia nervosa, also affects females more than males. The symptoms or warning signs are different from those of anorexia nervosa. Teens with bulimia nervosa typically binge on huge quantities of high-caloric foods and then purge by self-induced vomiting and/or laxatives. Binge episodes may alternate with diets, resulting in dramatic weight fluctuations. These teens often try to hide the signs of vomiting by running water as a sound cover. Purging poses serious threats to the teen's health, including dehydration, sometimes fatal electrolyte imbalances, and erosion of teeth enamel.

At the other end of the eating disorder spectrum is *binge eating disorder* and obesity. Binge eating disorder is a relatively newly recognized disorder that is often referred to as compulsive overeating (AACAP, 2008). Similar to bulimia nervosa, the teen with binge eating disorder frequently consumes large amounts of food while feeling a lack of control over eating. However, this disorder is different from bulimia nervosa because these teens usually do not purge their bodies of the excess food they consume during their binge episodes, often leading to obesity.

The obese adolescent consumes too many calories for the amount of energy expended. Studies have shown a strong correlation between inactivity, such as viewing television, playing computer games, and Internet surfing, and the tendency to be **overweight**. Other research has identified depression as one of the strongest predictors of adolescent obesity. Obesity can be detrimental to adolescents' self-esteem and social development, because they often become trapped in a vicious cycle of social rejection, isolation, inactivity, and continued obesity. Adolescent obesity has a poor prognosis, with most obese adolescents becoming obese adults. In addition, obesity increases the risk of and occurrence of type 2 diabetes mellitus.

Obesity, Type 2 Diabetes, and Teens

Soaring obesity rates are making type 2 diabetes, a disease that used to be seen mostly in adults over age 45, more common among teens and young people. Diabetes is a group of diseases marked by high levels of glucose in the blood, which left unattended lead to blindness, kidney failure, amputations, heart disease, and stroke. Type 2 diabetes, formerly called adult-onset diabetes, is the most common form. People can develop it at any age. However, being overweight and inactive increases your risk. Teens can access information about weight control with *Take Charge of Your Health! A Teenager's Guide to Better Health* available at www.win.niddk.nih.gov/publications/take_charge.htm. Further, the National Diabetes Education Program (NDEP) has now developed a new *Tips for Teens with Diabetes* series that includes a tip sheet on how to *Lower Your Risk for Type 2 Diabetes* that is "teen-friendly." Nurses can direct high-risk teens or teens with type 2 diabetes to visit their website at http://ndep.nih.gov/teens/LowerYourRisk.aspx.

More than anything, adolescents need reassurance about their bodies. Parents, teachers, and health care providers will be more successful in helping teens assume responsibility and manage their ongoing health needs if they approach and treat them as partners in planning their care. Nurses need to engage adolescents and help them create an individualized wellness plan that addresses body image, diet, weight concerns, and physical activity.

Elimination Pattern

The renal and gastrointestinal systems are functionally mature by adolescence, and elimination patterns are consistent with those found in adults. Abnormal variation can occur in teens with eating disorders. It is important to remember that an adolescent's need for privacy or self-protection may inhibit normal elimination in public places, such as schools.

Activity-Exercise Pattern

During adolescence, the alterations in body composition and growth of lean muscle mass allow the teen to experience increased physical strength and endurance. All adolescents should be taught that regular exercise can improve their endurance, appearance, and general state of health and that these positive effects can extend into adulthood.

Many teens participate in organized sports, and the preparticipation sports examination is one of the most common reasons to seek primary care (Figure 21-4). This examination

FIGURE 21-4 Adolescents frequently participate in organized activities, especially sports.

BOX 21-4 ADOLESCENT PREPARTICIPATION SPORTS EXAMINATION

Areas for Special Concern
- Previous trauma, including concussion
- Cardiovascular disease
- Hypertension
- Asthma
- Seizure disorder
- Splenomegaly, or enlarged spleen, often seen with infectious mononucleosis
- HIV infection
- Absence of paired organs: eye, kidney, testicle, or ovary

HIV, Human immunodeficiency virus.

offers an opportunity for nurses to identify adolescents at risk, evaluate their general state of health, and promote healthy lifestyle behaviors (Box 21-4). Frequent injuries, stress fractures, secondary amenorrhea, extreme dietary measures to gain or lose weight, exclusion of other activities, deteriorating school work, and chronic pain are a few of the signs of overuse, overexertion, or overinvestment (Dixon & Stein, 2005).

Sleep-Rest Pattern

During adolescence, the amount of time needed each night for sleep declines in comparison to earlier childhood needs. Although their sleep patterns vary greatly, adolescents need at least 8 hours of sleep per night. Adolescents who are employed, those involved in extracurricular sports, and those who have "too much on their plate" are at increased risk for sleep deprivation. They stay up late and are then forced to wake up before their sleep cycles have finished because the high school day has such an early start. Many adolescents send and receive text messages at night after room lights are turned off and they are going to bed, which can interfere with a good night's sleep. Even a moderate level of nighttime texting can greatly increase the likelihood of having long-term fatigue. Adolescents without sufficient sleep can find it difficult to concentrate and learn, or even stay awake in classes. Too little sleep also might contribute to mood swings and behavioral problems. Adolescents who drive when they are sleep-deprived can cause accidents, which could lead to death. Nurses can suggest that adolescents keep their cell phones out of their bedrooms at night. Nurses also can suggest strategies for daily living that help adolescents cope with the challenge of balancing their varied responsibilities while preventing exhaustion or burnout.

Cognitive-Perceptual Pattern

Piaget's Theory of Cognitive Development

Adolescence is characterized by a shift in cognitive abilities to Piaget's stage of formal operations. Piaget's theory used the term *formal* to represent the emergence of ability to focus on the "form" of thoughts, objects, and experiences rather than on the exact content, which in turn lays the groundwork for abstract thinking. These new cognitive abilities are reflected in adolescent behaviors in several ways.

The first change is that, because of their new ability to "think about their thinking," adolescents become highly introspective. As introspection increases, they develop an internalized audience that provides them with a means to evaluate questions such as "Who am I?" "How do others see me?" and "Where am I going?" Introspection also combines with a reemergence of egocentrism, leading to their sense of being the primary focus—special, unique, and exceptional. Being exceptional to the adolescent means being the exception, giving rise to the risk-taking behaviors for which they are well-known:

- I can get drunk on weekends and not develop a drinking problem.
- I won't get pregnant; I've had sex for 6 months and haven't gotten pregnant yet.
- I can take those turns at 60 miles per hour and not lose control.

Another behavioral manifestation of adolescents' formal operations is an intolerance of things as they are. They are able to conceptualize things as they might or could be, rather than how they are, and can think of elaborate means for achieving these changes—now. With this newfound capability, they constantly challenge the ways things are and challenge themselves to consider the way things can or should be. Teens can

be vehement in trying to convince others of their viewpoints and untiring in their support of causes that align with them. This idealism can lead to a rejection of family beliefs, religion, or social causes, which do not appear to the adolescent to be working fast enough to solve the problems of society. Although this idealism appears to most adults to be a flight from reality, it is a necessary stage in formal thinking. Reality is recognized, but only as a subset of many other possibilities that needs to be aligned with their own thinking. Eventually, their thinking becomes less egocentric and omnipotent, giving way to an appreciation of differences in judgment between themselves and others. This becomes the basis of an adolescent's ability to think about politics, law, and society in terms of abstract principles and benefits rather than focusing only on the punitive aspects (Burns et al., 2009).

Erikson's Theory of Psychosocial Development

According to Erikson's theory of psychosocial development, the central task of adolescence is the establishment of identity, with the primary risk being role confusion. Although it may appear that adolescents are involved in a final, rather than a transient or initial, identity formation, adolescence provides a means of moving into and through what might be termed an identity crisis.

This crisis involves a restaging of each of the previous stages of psychosocial development. Development of trust in self and others, as emphasized in infancy, is encountered again as the adolescent searches for people and ideologies in which to have faith. Toddlerhood, and its search for autonomy, is also revisited as adolescents search for autonomy from their primary family units. However, searching for autonomy while avoiding shame and doubt leads to an interesting paradox for adolescents. They would rather behave shamelessly in the eyes of their parents than be forced into behavior that would bring ridicule from their peers. The preschooler's challenge, a sense of initiative rather than guilt, resurfaces as the adolescent searches for direction and purpose. The school-age child's developing sense of industry is carried into the adolescent period also, as teens make choices in social, recreational, volunteer, academic, familial, and occupational activities. The confusion and hesitation in making these choices arise from fears of participating in activities that will not afford them the opportunity to excel or win the approval of their peers.

The extent to which these earlier tasks were accomplished successfully influences an adolescent's resourcefulness and success in experimenting with the new identity. When the threat of identity confusion is exceedingly great, delinquent behavior and alterations in mental health can occur. This threat is enhanced by conditions of poverty, racism, and other social inequities (see Box 21-12 on p. 531).

The pursuit for something to which to be devoted and the search for a meaningful ideology frequently create a puzzling combination of shifting devotion and sudden extremes in action (Box 21-5). Erikson views this behavior as an attempt to try on various roles and to search for some stable principle that might last through the testing of extremes and be carried into adulthood.

BOX 21-5 HOT TOPICS
Body Piercing and Tattooing

Adolescence is a developmental period full of identity experimentation and risk-taking behavior. Body piercing and tattooing have become popular forms of expression of identity, particularly among adolescents. Each carries health risks and potentially fatal complications.

There are very few sites on adolescent bodies that have not been pierced. Ears, nipples, navels, noses, and eyebrows have all succumbed to metallic rings, rods, studs, and barbells. However, approximately one in three piercings suffers a complication. Most commonly these include localized infection, bleeding, and dermatitis. Intraoral soft tissue piercing of the lips, cheek, uvula, and tongue harbor additional and potentially fatal complications, including a constant risk of aspiration, hemorrhage, and swelling leading to airway compromise, nerve damage, keloid scar formation, abscess, and tetanus. There is also an increased risk of hepatitis and HIV, as well as tooth injury, gingival recession, and difficulty with speech, taste, and swallowing.

Tattooing carries similar risks of infection, with a heightened concern for the transmission of blood-borne diseases including hepatitis and HIV, especially with colorful tattoos. Color ink is expensive and is often reused to cut costs, increasing exposure risks. Tattoos are also permanent markings and do not age well.

Nurses need to provide health education that allows adolescents to make informed decisions about body piercing, tattooing, and other forms of self-expression.

TABLE 21-2 DECIPHERING AND CONVERSING IN THE LATEST TEXT MESSAGING LINGO

MESSAGE	MEANING
GR8	Great
LOL	Laughing out loud
BRB	Be right back
AFC/AFK	Away from computer/keyboard
POS/MOS/DOS	Parent over shoulder/Mom over shoulder/Dad over shoulder
9	Parent watching
99	Parent no longer watching
CD9	Code 9: Parent watching or in room
RUOK	Are you ok?
XLNT	Excellent
F2F	Face to face
Zzz	Sleeping, bored, tired
Y	Why
B4N	Bye for now
YYSSW	Yeah yeah sure sure whatever
PCM	Please call me

Time Orientation

Adolescents look at time differently than they did as younger children. They realize that the response to a problem can, and sometimes should, be delayed to think through the possibilities for approaching the problem. Additionally, teens develop a future orientation and are able to delay immediate gratification to gain more satisfaction in the future.

Language

Advances in cognitive skills are reflected in an increased understanding of language. Formal operations and more abstract thought processes require expression in different words than did the more concrete thoughts of younger children. Adolescents give complex definitions, frequently including all possible meanings or uses. Interpretations of pictures or stories are complex and abstract. Older teens are capable of using and understanding complex sentence structure, although they, like adults, may not use these complex sentences routinely in their speech.

Both receptive and expressive vocabularies increase during adolescence. As with all ages, receptive far exceeds expressive vocabulary. The adolescent's vocabulary frequently includes slang. Slang may be centered on topics such as drug use, popular dress, music, and certain peer activities, or it may be more pervasive, in which case adults or "outsiders" may have difficulty following a conversation between two teens. The surge in cell phone use, instant and text messaging, and on-line chat rooms has given rise to an entirely new set of communications to decipher (Table 21-2).

Self-Perception–Self-Concept Pattern

The term *self-perception*, which often is used interchangeably with the terms *self-concept* and *self-esteem*, refers to both the description of the self and the evaluation of that description. Body image, on the other hand, specifically refers to the picture of and feelings about one's body. Tied together and brought to the forefront in adolescence, both self-perception and body image dominate, influence, and are influenced by individual, peer, and societal norms and expectations.

Assessment, anticipatory guidance, education, and counseling are strategies the nurse can use to guide the adolescent in developing a healthy self-perception that incorporates a healthy body image. It is important for parents, teachers, and health care providers to remember to praise adolescents for who they are rather than for what they do, value each of them as unique, demonstrate belief in their abilities to grow and develop, and delight in their discoveries of themselves and their unique means of expressing it.

Roles-Relationships Pattern

Until adolescence, the younger child is highly dependent on the parents and other adults. Striving for identity and increased independence, the adolescent begins to spend increased time away from the family. Parents sense a narrowing of their influence as their teen not only begins to prefer the company of peers and other adults but also begins to question familial beliefs and values. Parents may respond by setting unreasonably strict limits and asking intrusive questions about their teen's activities, friends, and ideas or decide to drop all rules and limits and assume that the adolescent can now manage alone. Neither of these approaches works well.

While adolescents strive for a sense of identity and independence, their parents try to learn how to let go. Each is temporarily unsure of the relationship with the other, and the family unit may experience more stress than at any previous time. Further, this period is often prolonged since more teens remain financially dependent on their families as they move into young adulthood.

Some families experience better outcomes than do other families. Families in which parents maintain a willingness to listen and demonstrate an ongoing affection for and acceptance of their adolescent, yet still maintain some consistent limits experience more constructive, positive outcomes during this period. This situation does not mean that parents necessarily agree with their teen's ideas or actions, but rather that they are willing to hear what the adolescent has to say and to negotiate some limits. Parents may need assistance in determining negotiable versus nonnegotiable rules and in developing ways to voice their concerns in an honest, open way. Even when teens do not want to "discuss" a topic, they need to know why their parents are concerned.

Peers

Faced with the need to become autonomous, achieve identity, and become productive, the adolescent often turns from family to peer group to find a safe psychosocial shelter in which to develop. Belonging to an informally organized clique, crowd, gang, or group is the primary means with which to make the transition from primary allegiance as a young child in the family to a member of a group. Identification with a group is proclaimed through conformity to standards of clothing, behavior, language, and values. This feature of the adolescent subculture persists despite the strong inclination in society as a whole toward greater levels of individuality.

The peer group is a vehicle for movement out of and away from the family unit and, as such, provides a means of achieving the goals of independence and individualization. It provides a sounding board against which young teens can test ideas, as well as a barometer for their own growth and development (Dixon & Stein, 2005).

Adolescents talk a great deal with their peers. Whether on the phone, on-line, or in person, they can discuss a 10-minute situation for hours on end. This sharing of thoughts and impressions is important. The telephone or computer can provide a "safe" mechanism for the teen to interact with members of the opposite sex as they share intimate ideas and concerns and begin to experience the closeness and caring that develops into the capacity to form a future intimate relationship.

Sexuality-Reproductive Pattern

The emergence of secondary sexual characteristics increases adolescents' awareness of themselves as sexual human beings. They fantasize about relationships and sex and gradually experiment with dating and a myriad of noncoital physical contacts, as well as coital contacts. Adolescents become sexually active for a variety of reasons. They have sex for affection, because of peer pressure, as a symbol of maturity, as spontaneous experimentation, to feel close, because it feels good or right, and at times without their consent (see the Case Study and Care Plan at the end of this chapter). In the process of establishing a sexual sense of themselves, it is not uncommon for them to question if they are homosexual. Same-sex arousal or experimentation with same-sex physical activity does not necessarily indicate homosexuality or future sexual orientation (Dixon & Stein, 2005).

The technological revolution has opened up a limitless world of unmediated information to adolescents and led to increased issues of on-line risky behaviors. The use of on-line social networks like Facebook and Twitter continues to increase rapidly among all age groups and segments of our society, presenting new opportunities for the exchange of sexual information as well as for potentially unsafe encounters between predators and the vulnerable or young. Sexting has been a recognized increasing occurrence for several years and is a global practice among teens and young adults. Sexting refers to sending a text message with sexually explicit content or a sexually explicit picture. This type of texting can cause emotional pain for the person in the picture, as well as the sender and receiver.

Knowing adolescents are heavily invested in these and other sexual issues, nurses are capable and willing to discuss them. Nurses need to be comfortable with their own sexuality; able to discuss the subject of sex and sexual orientation, contraception, protection against STDs; and aware of their own limitations, beliefs, and biases. Anticipatory guidance about the decision to become sexually active, to use contraception, and to obtain protection from sexually transmitted diseases (STDs) needs to be provided before adolescents encounter a situation in which they need this information (see Tables 22-2 and 22-3 on pp. 551 and 552). This is also a good time to introduce the adolescent to breast and testicular self-examinations (Box 21-6: Quality and Safety Scenario). Nurses help adolescents understand that text messages should not contain pictures of naked people or of people kissing or touching each other, and that sending such type of text message is considered a crime in some areas.

Adolescent Pregnancy

For health care providers adolescent pregnancy is viewed as a high-risk situation, because of the serious health risks and potential complications for both the mother and the infant. For politicians and governmental agencies it is a social problem that makes overwhelming demands on social and economic resources. For adolescents and their families it may be seen as positive and normal or the worst disaster imaginable. No matter what the perspective, adolescent pregnancy represents a myriad of concerns with far-reaching effects.

According to the *National Vital Statistics Reports,* the preliminary estimate of teens giving birth in 2009 was more than 400,000 teen girls ages 15 to 19 years (Martin et al., 2011). The overall birth rate for U.S. teenagers ages 15 to 19 dropped 6% to 39.1 per 1000 in 2009; this represents the lowest level reported in the United States in nearly 7 decades (Martin et al., 2011). The birth rate for ages 15 to 19 was highest in Hispanic teenagers (70.1%), followed by non-Hispanic Blacks (59.0%), American Indian/Alaska Native (55.5%), non-Hispanic Whites (25.6%), and Asian/Pacific Islanders (14.7%). These birth rates represent a significant decrease in all ethnic subgroups from 2008 to 2009 (Martin et al., 2011).

The National Campaign to Prevent Teen and Unplanned Pregnancy (2004) emphasizes the likely negative outcomes of adolescent pregnancy in outreach efforts. For the mother, these include a significant decline in her future prospects, especially

BOX 21-6 QUALITY AND SAFETY SCENARIO
Performing Breast and Testicular Self-Examination

BSE or TSE should be performed once a month, so that teens become familiar with the usual appearance and feel of their breasts or testicles. This routine makes noticing any changes from 1 month to another easier. Finding a change from "normal" is the main idea behind regular self-examination. The best time for females to perform a BSE is 2 or 3 days after their period ends, when breasts are least likely to be tender or swollen. For males, the best time for a TSE is during or right after a warm shower.

Breast Self-Examination
- Stand in front of a mirror. Inspect both breasts for anything unusual, such as any discharge from the nipples, puckering or dimpling of the skin, or marked asymmetry.
- While watching closely in the mirror, clasp your hands behind your head and press your hands forward, and inspect again.
- Next, press your hands firmly on your hips and bow slightly toward the mirror as you pull your shoulders and elbows forward, and inspect again.
- Next, raise one arm. Use three or four fingers to explore the breast firmly, carefully, and thoroughly. Beginning at the outer edge, press the flat part of your fingers in small circles, moving the circles slowly around the breast.

Gradually work toward the nipple. Be sure to examine the entire breast. Pay special attention to the area between the breast and the armpit, including the armpit itself. Feel for any unusual lump or mass under the skin.
- Gently squeeze the nipple and look for a discharge. Repeat the examination on the other breast.

The last two steps should be repeated lying down. This position flattens the breast and makes examination easier. Some women perform BSE in the shower. Fingers gliding over soapy skin make concentrating on the texture underneath easier.

Testicular Self-Examination
- Cup or support the testicles with one hand and feel with the other.
- Gently roll each testicle between the thumb and fingers. There should not be any pain. Feel for any swelling or hard lumps on the surface of the testicle. Testicles are normally oval, firm, smooth, and rubbery. One may be slightly larger than the other.
- A natural tubelike structure, the epididymis, is along the back of the testicle. Learn what it feels like.

Sources: Lowdermilk, D. L., Perry, S. E., & Cashion, M.C. (2011). *Maternity nursing* (8th ed.). St. Louis: Mosby; Neinstein, L. S., Gordau, C. M., Katzman, D. K., Rosen, D. S., & Woods, E. R. (2008). *Adolescent health care: A practical guide* (5th ed.). Philadelphia; Lippincott Williams & Wilkins. *BSE*, Breast self-examination; *TSE*, testicular self-examination.

BOX 21-7 COPING MECHANISMS OF ADOLESCENTS

Cognitive Mastery
The adolescent attempts to learn as much as possible about the situation or stressor. This strategy is common for the adolescent with a chronic illness. The nurse can assist by clarifying any misinformation, sharing research findings, and encouraging a discussion of feelings.

Conformity
The adolescent attempts to be a mirror image of peers, which includes dress, language, attitudes, and actions. The nurse must respect this need for sameness and can also encourage discussion of feelings about differences among teens.

Controlling Behavior
Adolescents must be in charge of some aspects of life and can no longer accept family and school rules without question as they did in the past. This need

to control extends to health care. The nurse cannot simply give directions or instructions, but rather should present the options and allow the adolescent to partner with the nurse to work out an acceptable plan.

Fantasy
The adolescent may use fantasy as a way to escape or experiment. The nurse can encourage the teen to use fantasy constructively to develop creative plans to deal with a stressful situation.

Motor Activity
Engaging in sports, dancing, running, or other physical activity can be an effective tension-releasing strategy, and can also provide an instant peer group. The nurse can encourage physical activity and offer information about protective gear and injury prevention.

educational and economic; serious health risks, including an increased risk of obesity and hypertension; single parenthood; and poverty. For the child born to adolescent mothers there is a higher risk of low birth weight. Low birth weight is associated with infant mortality and other health problems, including cerebral palsy, mental retardation, dyslexia, and hyperactivity. Further, these children often fall victim to abuse and neglect and suffer from poor school performance.

When pregnancy occurs, adolescents and their families deserve honest and sensitive counseling about all of the options available to them, as well as the support systems available for them throughout the pregnancy, birth, and subsequent parenting. Nurses not only need to reinforce reproductive health education efforts, but also need to encourage adolescents to build on the strengths in their lives and opportunities available to them.

Coping-Stress Tolerance Pattern

When all of the changes that occur in adolescents are aligned with their need to separate from their parents and gain a sense of their own independence, their ability to cope is put to the test over and over again. Common coping mechanisms, and the strategies the nurse can use to encourage teens to use them in adaptive ways, are listed in Box 21-7.

However, too often adolescents are unable to balance the stresses, lacking the appropriate skills and outlets, adequate support systems, or available mental health intervention. Depression, suicide, and substance abuse emerge as life becomes overwhelming and the future unimaginable.

Depression
As with many other diseases, the rate of **depression** increases with age and the incidence continues to increase during

adolescence. Based on the data from the National Comorbidity Survey-Adolescent Supplement (NCS-A), about 11% of adolescents have a depressive disorder by age 18. Moreover, girls are more likely than boys to experience depression (National Institute of Mental Health, 2011). The term depression includes both major depressive and dysthymic disorders. A depressive disorder is defined as a depressed or irritable mood or a diminished interest and pleasure in usual activities, whereas dysthymia is a depressed or irritable mood that extends over a year with symptom relief for no more than 2 months (Burns et al., 2009).

Depression is suspected when the adolescent uses words such as down, sad, low, blue, hopeless, worried, bored, or discouraged and exhibits several of the following symptoms:
- Change in weight or appetite
- Insomnia or hypersomnia
- Decreased energy or fatigue
- Loss of interest and pleasure in usual activities
- Out-of-proportion feelings of self-reproach or guilt
- Difficulty concentrating; declining school performance
- Preoccupation with death or suicidal ideation

The nurse needs to refer the adolescent with depression to a mental health specialist. Nurses should lead the way in screening for and assessing children and teens for mental health problems, including depression. Moreover, nurses may promote mental health promotion in both children and teens by teaching them effective coping skills and stress-reduction techniques.

Suicide

Adolescence is a period of considerable stress, and when coping mechanisms and social supports are inadequate, suicide may emerge as an outcome. Suicide is the third leading cause of death in persons between 10 and 24 years of age (CDC, 2009). A national survey revealed that 15% of youths in grades 9 to 12 in the United States reported that they were seriously considering suicide, 11% reported creating a plan, and 7% reported trying to take their own life in a 12-month period (CDC, 2009).

These figures may not even reflect the full scope of the problem, because many suicides are classified as accidental deaths. Suicide attempts are not included in these statistics, although estimates show that 50 to 200 attempts occur for every successfully completed suicide. Attempts are three to nine times more common in females, but males are four times as successful (Evans et al., 2005). Many researchers are convinced that suicide during adolescence is not an impulsive or spontaneous act: it is selected carefully only after other problem-solving methods have failed and suicide is viewed as the only option.

Adolescent suicide can be prevented. Distressed adolescents tend to give clues, both verbally and nonverbally. Any single clue may mean nothing, but when several clues are noted, they should be recognized as important warning signs. Box 21-8 outlines vigilant warning signs for parents, teachers, health care providers, and peers to prevent adolescent suicide.

When the nurse suspects that an adolescent is suicidal, immediate referral is made to a mental health specialist. A suicide threat should never be ignored, and the adolescent who is in immediate danger of committing suicide should never be

BOX 21-8   WARNING SIGNS OF SUICIDE RISK IN ADOLESCENTS

Behavioral Changes
- Increased risk taking
- Increased incidence of accidents
- Substance use and abuse
- Physical violence to self, others, or animals
- Decreased appetite
- Alienation from family or peer group
- Giving away personal items
- Writing letters or notes, essays, and poems with suicidal content

Cognitive and Mood Changes
- Expression of hopelessness
- Increasing rage or anger
- Dramatic swings in affect
- Sleep disorders
- Preoccupation with death
- Difficulty concentrating
- Hearing voices, seeing things or people
- Newfound interest in religion or cult

left alone (American Academy of Pediatrics, 2008; Shaw et al., 2005).

Values-Beliefs Pattern

Values and beliefs are learned phenomena that serve as guides for decision-making and actions. With the development of abstract thought, adolescents begin to expand their understanding of good and bad or right and wrong, to include autonomous moral principles that have validity apart from the authority of parent or society and instead are based on the individual's beliefs. Their newly discovered maturity in moral reasoning is situational and relational and often is superceded by psychosocial developmental needs and influences. Adolescents may think or feel something is wrong or bad yet may act contrary to that belief because of peer pressure or the need to declare their independence.

Adolescents often align their values and beliefs with a particular religion, philosophical school of thought, social movement or cause, or other formal system, using it to make decisions about what is right or wrong, best or worst, and important or trivial. During adolescence these alignments can change drastically and often, causing strife and concern for parents, yet providing the teen with different ranges of experience from which to base eventual and lasting choices.

According to Kohlberg's theory of moral development (Kohlberg, 1981), the adolescent begins to make the transition to the postconventional stage, equating what is right with the idea of justice and basing actions on the recognition of the universal principles underlying laws and social agreements. Gilligan, who developed a parallel theory of moral development for females, proposes that the female adolescent sees "good" as involving self-sacrifice and caring for the relationships in her life (Gilligan et al., 1990). As moral reasoning matures, the female adolescent learns to achieve a balance between what is good for her and what is good for others in her network of relationships.

As adolescents struggle with their journey to discover who they are, parents, teachers, and health care providers need to provide positive role modeling, reinforce positive behaviors, and remember the difficulty of their own journeys. It is often when we like them the least that they need us the most.

ENVIRONMENTAL PROCESSES

Because adolescents are in developmental transition, their lifestyle choices may have significant effect on their current and future health. These choices are particularly sensitive to the immediate physical and social environments. These environmental influences include their family members, friends, and community and their school, neighborhood, and work environments as well. Several critical types of adolescent health behaviors—including alcohol and drug use, injury and violence, tobacco use, nutrition, physical activity, and sexual behaviors—have been identified to contribute to the leading causes of death and disability among adults and youth.

Physical Agents

Accidents

Accidents, along with suicide and homicide, continue to be the leading cause of death and injury during adolescence. Approximately 30% of all deaths among adolescents ages 10 to 24 years are attributed to injuries caused by motor vehicle crashes (Centers for Disease Control and Prevention [CDC], 2010a). The risk of motor vehicle crashes is four times higher among 16- to 19-year-olds than among any other age group (CDC, 2010c). Whether drivers, passengers, pedestrians, or cyclists, few adolescents take measures to reduce their risk of injury, with 9.7% rarely or never using a safety belt and 84.7% rarely or never using a bicycle helmet (CDC, 2010b). Research also suggests that distractions, such as talking or texting on cell phones, eating, or playing with the radio, increase teen drivers' risk of being involved in a crash.

Nurses talk to teens about the consequences of texting while driving, encourage teens to wear their safety belts, and avoid driving, or riding with someone, under the influence of drugs or alcohol. The tendency to play loud music and change the tune or disc often, as well as the pressure to answer cell phones, can also be distracting, as can a car full of other teens. Recognizing this and that teens have a much higher nighttime crash fatality rate, many states have enacted new driver restrictions and nighttime curfews.

Sports Injuries

Organized sports in and out of school provide adolescents with experiences in competition, teamwork and effort, and conflict resolution. They also provide a valuable means for adolescents to develop self-esteem. However, adolescents are particularly vulnerable to sports injuries. Their coordination skills are developing, their judgment often immature and inadequate, their epiphyses not yet closed, and their extremities poorly protected by stabilizing musculature. They can also become obsessed or driven to perform beyond their capabilities or to

the exclusion of all other activities. The use of performance-enhancing substances, such as steroids, which have been unfortunately modeled by many professional athletes, can create another potential extreme scenario that places the adolescent at risk for injury.

The nurse advocates for the proper use of protective gear during all activities and a thorough preparticipation sports examination and also monitors for overuse, overexertion, or overinvestment on the part of the adolescent.

Violence

Adolescents today face an unprecedented risk of injury (American Academy of Pediatrics, 2008) and death from violence in their homes, schools, and communities. Becoming increasingly independent, they test the limits of authority, experiment with a variety of roles, question adult values and authority, and look to peers for affirmation. They may feel pressure to join gangs or feel threatened by them. Many teens report carrying weapons to protect themselves or intimidate others. Adolescents often report a fear of violence and try to avoid situations where they might be vulnerable to it, including home or even the bathroom at school.

Many studies suggest that witnessing or observing violence, whether in person or projected on the TV, video, or movie screen, results in a higher incidence of violent behaviors. Graphic violence in current music lyrics and videos has also been implicated.

In his documentary *Bowling for Columbine*, filmmaker Michael Moore made a compelling case that what endangers America most today is not the act of violence or the crime, but our fear of it. Fear is stoked by a media that trumpets every street murder and bank robbery as an imminent threat and elevates shark attacks and escalator mishaps to a national crisis. Children and adolescents with fears that remain unresolved have been shown to have an increase in violent behaviors, and fear about others often surfaces as racism. Figure 21-5 outlines the interrelationships of internal and external precipitating factors that increase an adolescent's vulnerability to and for violent behaviors.

Teenagers may be involved in cyberbullying. Cyberbullying refers to sending harassing texts, e-mails, or instant messages and posting intimidating or threatening websites or blogs (National Crime Prevention Council, 2012). Receiving bullying text messages can make a teen feel insecure and may lead to school absences.

Nurses engage adolescents, examining and discussing the messages in videos, songs, movies, and television shows. Discussing their developing sense of self, their sense of belonging and where that sense is found, and their fears may help to intercept an adolescent who might otherwise turn to violence. Teens who are valued and nurtured by caring adults have the best chance of emerging from adolescence unscathed. Nurses may also discuss cyberbullying with adolescents; encourage them to talk to a trusted adult if he or she receives harassing text messages and to consider options such as rejecting texts from unknown numbers; and tell them that it is inappropriate to send harassing text messages to others.

FIGURE 21-5 Factors contributing to adolescent violence.

Biological Agents

Infection

Infectious mononucleosis is a self-limiting viral infection transmitted by direct contact of oropharyngeal secretions. It is prevalent among adolescents and often referred to as the "kissing disease"; however, it can occur in younger children. It is caused by the Epstein-Barr virus. Typically adolescents complain of a sore throat, lymph node enlargement, and lethargy. Both splenomegaly and hepatomegaly can occur, creating a risk for injury.

Rates of meningococcal disease remain highest for infants, but in the past decade rates have increased among adolescents. Reports have identified an increased risk for meningococcal disease among college freshmen who live in dormitories or residence halls. As adolescents prepare for college, nurses need to review their risk and provide them with information on available vaccines.

Adolescents are at the period of life with high sexual energy that may lead to high levels of risk-taking behaviors attributable to an increased sense of invulnerability. As adolescents experiment with and explore their sexual development and emerging independence, they engage in risky sexual behavior and expose themselves to increased risk of acquiring sexually transmitted diseases (STDs). STDs most commonly include gonorrhea, syphilis, chlamydia, herpes simplex virus, human papilloma virus, *Trichomonas,* hepatitis B, and human immunodeficiency virus (HIV). An estimated 8300 young people ages 13 to 24 years in 40 states reported HIV infection in 2009, and near

half of the 19 million new STD cases each year are among young people ages 15 to 24 years (CDC, 2011a).

Considered an epidemic, STDs have the highest rates in adolescents, with minorities, especially African Americans, disproportionately affected (Burns et al., 2009). Many contributing factors have been identified and found to negatively impact this significant public and adolescent health problem. Factors such as inconsistent use of contraceptive and protective devices, increasingly earlier age and more frequent sexual activity, lower self-esteem, depression, social and peer pressure, and an adolescent's sense of invincibility were related to higher risks of STDs. On the other hand, factors such as self-efficacy, parent-child communications, and sexual knowledge could be significant protective factors to prevent STDs in adolescents. Higher self-efficacy has been found as a significant protecting factor associated with less sexual risky behaviors in adolescents. Not only in Western societies, similar findings were also reported in adolescents living in other cultures (Lee et al., 2009).

Several theories have been employed to guide the practices of preventing sexual risk-taking behaviors in adolescents. The Health Promotion Model (Pender et al., 2010) was used by nurses for developing sexual risk-reduction interventions for adolescents, and these interventions were found effective. Most of the cognitive-behavioral interventions that stem from these theories report effectiveness in reducing risk of HIV infection. Scientific studies show that well-designed and well-implemented HIV/STD prevention programs can decrease

BOX 21-9 RESEARCH FOR EVIDENCE-BASED PRACTICE

Effective Prevention Programs for Adolescents' Sexual Health

Regardless of advances in prevention and treatment, sexually transmitted infections (STIs) continue to be a significant cause of morbidity and mortality in the United States. Promoting the ability of children and adolescents to avoid risk-taking sexual behaviors is considered a significant approach to encourage sexual health in adolescents. Positive youth development (PYD) programs may provide youth with the motivation and confidence needed to use skills and knowledge they need to abstain from sex or to practice safer sexual behaviors.

A systematic review of the published data was conducted to identify and describe positive youth development (PYD) programs that improve adolescent sexual and reproductive health. Eight databases were searched for articles about PYD programs published between 1985 and 2007. A total of 30 programs were found that met the following inclusion criteria: fostered at least 1 of 12

PYD goals in multiple socialization domains or addressed 2 or more goals in at least 1 socialization domain; allocated at least half of the program activities to promoting general PYD outcomes; included participants younger than 20 years old; and used an experimental or quasi-experimental evaluation design. Among the 30 programs, 15 of them had evidence of improving at least 1 adolescent sexual and reproductive health outcome. Results revealed that effective programs were significantly more likely than those that did not have an impact to strengthen the school context and to deliver activities in a supportive atmosphere. Moreover, effective programs were also more likely to build skills, enhance bonding, strengthen the family, engage youth in real roles and activities, empower youth, communicate expectations, and be stable and relatively long-lasting.

Source: Catalano, R. F., David-Ferdon, C., Gloppen, K. M., & Markham, C. M. (2010). A review of positive youth development programs that promote adolescent sexual and reproductive health. *Journal of Adolescent Health, 46,* S75-S91; CDC. (2011). *Effective HIV and STD prevention programs for youth.* [Online] Retrieved from www.cdc.gov/healthyyouth/sexualbehaviors/effective_programs.htm.

sexual risk behaviors among adolescents (Box 21-9: Research for Evidence-Based Practice).

Nurses are aware of the cultural issues that may play a significant role in the prevention of STDs in adolescents, such as HIV/acquired immunodeficiency syndrome (AIDS) infections. While nurses develop interventions for reducing STD-related sexual risk behaviors, they take adolescents' cultural/ethnic backgrounds into considerations. For example, a recent study (Lee et al., 2010) identified barriers and suggested strategies for approaching Chinese American adolescents for studies/interventions related to HIV, STDs, and sexual activity.

Moreover, although adolescents can be evaluated and treated for STDs, diseases must be reported and the nurse must be aware of the government rules about reporting.

Chemical Agents

Substance Use and Abuse

Adolescents are influenced by a complicated interaction between biological and psychosocial development, environmental messages, and societal attitudes regarding the use of substances such as alcohol, tobacco, or marijuana. Society as a whole is increasingly oriented toward using chemicals such as drugs, alcohol, and tobacco to feel better, look better, act more sociable, stay awake, sleep, be sexy or erect, or lose weight. Some of the most famous music, movie, and sports stars openly model substance use and abuse. It is no surprise that adolescents are making the choice to experiment with and use substances at earlier and earlier ages.

Substance use is a precursor to abuse, which emphasizes the need for health care providers to be alert and screen for its presence. Identifying an adolescent with substance use or abuse requires a careful nursing assessment that is conducted in an accepting manner (Boxes 21-10 and 21-11).

Tobacco Use

Most teens begin smoking during adolescence, especially if a close friend, sibling, or parent also smokes (Burns et al.,

BOX 21-10 SIGNS OF SUBSTANCE ABUSE

- Accidents
- Agitation
- Appetite loss
- Blackouts
- Bleeding gums
- Chronic cough
- Delusions
- Depression
- Diarrhea
- Dyspnea
- Eye drops
- Headache
- Hoarseness
- Hyperactivity
- Inability to concentrate
- Insomnia
- Lethargy
- Memory loss
- Muscle weakness
- Paranoia
- Rhinorrhea
- Seizures
- Somnolence
- Sore tongue
- Stomach pain
- Taste loss
- Violent outbursts
- Vomiting
- Weight loss
- Withdrawal

From Payne, W. A., & Harm, D. B. (2010). *Understanding your health* (11th ed.). Boston: McGraw-Hill.

2009). The highest rate of smoking is among White females, while "smokeless" tobacco, such as snuff and chewing tobacco, is more popular among males. Adolescents begin using tobacco for a variety of reasons, including wanting to appear older or wanting to imitate their friends, adult role models, or media images. Advertising by the tobacco industry directed at adolescents has been shown to encourage adolescent smoking.

The nurse's primary prevention focus is on keeping nonsmokers from starting and helping smokers to stop. The National Institutes of Health has published guidelines for health care providers to follow, titled *The 5 A's for Brief Intervention in Adolescents Who Use Tobacco*, which are:

- *Ask* about tobacco use.
- *Advise* to quit.
- *Assess* willingness to attempt quitting.
- *Assist* in quit attempt.
- *Arrange* for follow-up.

See www.ahrq.gov/clinic/tobacco/clinhlpsmksqt.htm for more information (Agency for Healthcare Research and Quality, 2008).

Cancer

Adolescents are affected by many of the same cancers as are younger children, such as leukemia, osteogenic sarcoma, lymphomas, and central nervous system tumors. Older adolescents are entering the period of their lives during which cancer of the reproductive and related organs is more common. For females, the focus is on cervical and breast cancer; for males, testicular cancer is of concern.

Peak incidence of breast and cervical cancer is during middle age and is actually rare in the teenage years. Breast self-examination (BSE), which has been highly recommended for more than 30 years, has recently been questioned as a routine practice for most adolescents. The extremely small incidence of breast cancer in teens has caused some health care providers to deemphasize this practice for them. However, most still feel that regular examination of the breasts begins a lifelong habit that should begin as soon as the female adolescent develops (see Box 21-6).

Cervical cancer is detected with a Papanicolaou (Pap) smear, obtained from the cervix during a pelvic examination. According to the Center for Young Women's Health at Boston Children's Hospital (www.youngwomenshealth.org), factors that increase the risk for cervical cancer include sexual intercourse before age 20, multiple sexual partners or a sexual partner who has had many partners, any history of STDs or exposure to exogenous hormones, and smoking. Sexually active adolescents should have a Pap test performed annually and the American College of Obstetricians and Gynecologists recommends annual pelvic examinations by age 18, even when the young woman is not sexually active. The nurse can explain the purpose and the process involved in conducting a pelvic examination and Pap test.

Administration of a vaccine to prevent cervical cancer and other diseases caused by certain types of genital human papillomavirus (HPV) has been recommended by the Advisory Committee on Immunization Practices (www.cdc.gov/hpv/). HPV vaccination is recommended for preteen girls and boys at age 11 or 12 years. The vaccine is also recommended for all teen girls and women through age 26 who did not receive all three doses of the vaccine when they were younger and for all teen boys and men through age 21 who also did not complete the vaccine series in their younger ages (CDC, 2011b). Ideally, females should get the vaccine before they are sexually active. This is because the vaccine is most effective in girls/women who have not yet acquired any of the four HPV types covered by the vaccine. Girls/women who have not been infected with any of those four HPV types will obtain the full benefits of the vaccine.

Females who are sexually active may also benefit from the vaccine, but they may receive less benefit since they may have already acquired one or more HPV type(s) covered by the vaccine. Few young women are infected with all four of these HPV types; therefore they would still procure protection from those types they have not acquired. It is not yet known if the vaccine is effective in boys or men. It is possible that vaccinating males will have health benefits for them by preventing genital warts and rare cancers, such as penile and anal cancer. It is also possible that vaccinating boys/men will have indirect health benefits for girls/women. When more information is available, this vaccine may be licensed and recommended for boys/men as well.

Testicular cancer is the number one cancer in adolescent and young adult males. Adolescent males should learn to perform a testicular self-examination and continue this practice monthly (see Box 21-6). Nurses introduce and teach methods of self-examination to adolescents, who naturally are interested in their developing bodies.

DETERMINANTS OF HEALTH

Social Factors and Environment

School

Junior high and high school are a new social experience, introducing the adolescent to changing classes, multiple teachers and teaching styles, variable class schedules and homework load, and a variety of peer influences. Adolescents must learn to become accustomed to greater anonymity as they navigate the corridors of larger, more impersonal institutions (Dixon & Stein, 2005). Yet despite these challenges, junior high and high school settings also provide meaningful in-school and after-school learning, peer contact, intellectual stimulation, and activities.

Schools and peers, as opposed to home and parents, become the primary setting through which expectations are shared and standards communicated. Adolescent peer groups serve as sounding boards against which teens test their ideas and gauge their physical, intellectual, psychological, and moral growth (Dixon & Stein, 2005). Nurses ask adolescents about school and their friends, and how they are doing with both. The nurse can also monitor adolescents as they prepare for and make the

Barriers of Recruiting Chinese American Adolescents for Future Development of HIV Interventional Programs: A Lesson Learned

It has been suggested that there is an imperative need to deliver culturally sensitive programs for HIV/AIDS prevention. To oppose health disparities in the United States, recruiting participants with ethnic minority background in health care research is essential. Chinese Americans comprise the largest ethnic group of Asian Americans and have been rarely separated from a combination of various Asian American populations to address issues related to HIV/AIDS prevention. Given the fact that there are many distinct and separate cultures within the Asian American community, this misclassification makes Chinese Americans an underrepresented population in HIV/AIDS research and has resulted in limited public awareness and deprived HIV/AIDS preventive service for this population. It is important for nurses to know about the recruitment strategies or challenges specific to enrolling Chinese Americans in order to have capabilities to efficiently approach Chinese American adolescents and deliver culturally sensitive HIV/AIDS prevention programs.

The purpose of this newly published article was to report identified barriers and challenges experienced in the recruiting process of Chinese American adolescents to a cross-sectional designed HIV/AIDS-related study. The sexual topic, a taboo in Chinese culture, was the major barrier to recruiting Chinese American adolescents. Barriers of the recruitment were also found related to unawareness and denial of HIV/AIDS risks, authoritarian parenting style in Chinese culture, and the required informed consents. The most successful recruitment strategy was found to be associated with the assistance of Chinese American adolescent participants. Providing educational programs targeting Chinese American parents and community leaders to enhance their awareness of the risks and to improve parent-child communication regarding sex-related issues was suggested as the first step to successfully approach and recruit Chinese American adolescents to an HIV/AIDS-related preventional program or research.

Information from Lee, Y.H., Salman, A., & Wang, F. (2012). Recruiting Chinese-American adolescents to HIV/AIDS related research: A lesson learned from a cross-sectional study. *Applied Nursing Research* 24(1):40-46.

transition to their next social arena and role whether it is college, vocational training, the military, or another career choice.

Culture and Ethnicity

Cultural and ethnic influences operate throughout childhood and continue into adolescence. The primary difference in adolescence is that teens question, modify, or reject these influences, exchanging them for those of their peers or of the dominant cultural group. First-generation adolescents of immigrant parents have to negotiate two cultures, languages, and sets of expectations. These adolescents live a double life that results in increased stress. Adolescents from minority groups, such as African Americans, Hispanics, Asian Americans, Native Americans, Russian Americans, or Arab Americans, may experience discrimination and rejection as they try to fit in to the dominant adolescent culture. Additional stress may also be experienced when their attempts to fit in to the dominant culture are offensive to the values and beliefs of their own culture.

Young people from minority groups have a particular problem in relation to the culture of adolescence. These teens may desire strongly to fit in to the predominant adolescent culture, which in society is often middle class, White, and Protestant, and they may be able to meet one or two of these criteria but be unable to meet the others because of economics, different appearance, or different education and experiences. Advertising does not emphasize the economically depressed or ethnic-looking model, and the teens' peers are trying every means possible to look and act similarly to the dominant culture adolescent. Further pressure comes from their own minority culture when they emulate the majority culture in ways that the family views as offensive to their ideas and beliefs.

The growing ethnic diversity in the adolescent population influences how adolescent health will be approached. According to reports from the U.S. Census Bureau, the Asian population increased by 43% between 2000 and 2010, growing faster than any other major race group between 2000 and 2010

(Humes et al., 2011) (Box 21-12). With fast growth in the numbers of Hispanic and Asian American youth, cultural awareness of health care needs and the highlighted attention to health disparities and academic outcomes especially among adolescents from racial minorities and ethnic groups are required. Nurses need to recognize and assess for additional stresses experienced by adolescents as they wrestle not only with their own but also with their cultural identities.

Levels of Policy Making and Health

Many laws and regulations are aimed at adolescents and deal with the minimum age at which they can assume adult responsibilities and decision-making. The rationale for these restrictions is that adolescents, although capable, lack the experience, perspective, and judgment to recognize and avoid choices that might be detrimental to them, so they require protection. A question raised frequently when considering minimum age is whether strict age criteria are appropriate for any adolescent, particularly because development is variable and experiences are diverse.

The restrictions that have recently been questioned most strongly deal with issues related to sexual activity. The U.S. Supreme Court affirmed the right of all individuals to have equal access to contraceptive service, regardless of age or marital status. However, variations occur from state to state and the nurse must be aware of legal age determinants, as well as variations in definitions of emancipated minors.

The emancipated minor provision of certain laws recognizes that some adolescents become independent from their families at an early age and assume adult responsibilities. An emancipated minor is an adolescent who has not reached the standard legal age for certain activities, such as consenting to marriage or seeking certain kinds of health or illness care, but who is permitted to accept full responsibility for these decisions because the individual is economically and emotionally separate from the family.

Most often confidentiality is the more important issue for adolescents. The nurse can assure them that information shared will be kept confidential unless the teens pose a risk to themselves or others or state laws mandate that the information be shared (Burns et al., 2008). For example, abuse must be reported, STDs need to be reported, and some states require report of adolescent sexual activity if an age difference of 3 or more years exists between the sexual partners.

Nurses need to familiarize themselves with the legal rights of adolescents in their state and the resources available in their community.

Economics

Identification with peers, the essence of self-image during adolescence, includes dressing alike, having similar possessions, and doing similar things, all of which require economic resources. This can be a major conflict between parents and adolescents. Parents may think that they should have the power to decide how their adolescent spends money. Adolescents may believe, just as strongly, that they know the best ways to allocate resources and determine the amount of money they need.

Ideally, parents and adolescents should negotiate economic questions, with the parents becoming less controlling as the teen gains more experience and expertise in these matters. However, the family with limited economic resources has fewer choices, and adolescents from these families may feel trapped by their circumstance. Poverty is particularly hard on children, and as they become adolescents they often develop a fatalistic view of life.

Some adolescents seek employment to earn their own money and have control over it. Others work because their families need the income. It is important for the nurse to assess the economic resources of each adolescent's family and work within them when partnering with the adolescent in health care planning.

Health Services/Delivery System

Many health care resources are available to the adolescent. Teens can continue to see their child health care providers in a pediatric center as they did as younger children, but this setting usually is rejected because of the young-child atmosphere.

School-based clinics frequently are available in junior high and high school, and adolescent-focused clinics are available in many communities through both public and private agencies. Each of these clinics serves only adolescents, and the staff is oriented to the needs of this age group. Adolescents frequently have a stronger sense of comfort in these settings than in those in which young children or adults are also served.

Adolescents can also make use of services such as family planning clinics. These settings may designate certain days and hours for teens, whereas other facilities integrate them into the adult-oriented protocols. The pregnant adolescent typically finds prenatal care in an adult-focused setting, although more adolescent-specific programs are being developed. The physical needs of pregnant adolescents may be the same as those of the pregnant adult, but the psychosocial needs are different and should be approached by a professional who has a comprehensive knowledge of their development and responses to stress.

BOX 21-13   HEADSSS ASSESSMENT

The HEADSSS Assessment provides a mnemonic that guides health care providers through an adolescent's psychosocial assessment. Responses should be interpreted as those that are indicators of strengths or protection from risk and those that are indicators of risky behavior or situations.

Home and health
Education, employment, eating
Activities, affiliations, aspirations
Drugs
Sexuality
Suicide, depression, self-image
Safety

Data from Goldenring, J. M., & Rosen, D. (2004). Getting into adolescent heads: An essential update. *Contemporary Pediatrics,* 21(1):64-90

The adolescent is a rapidly changing individual. The nurse who works in an adolescent-focused practice is well prepared in adolescent health-promotion strategies. The nurse should have a thorough understanding of adolescent physical and psychosocial growth and development and recognize each teen as a person.

Adolescents not only tend to be fearful about procedures or possible diagnoses but also need to stay in control of the situation. These conflicting feelings can be difficult to manage simultaneously. By establishing the adolescent as a partner with the health care providers in promoting good health and screening for health risks, the nurse facilitates the adolescent's sense of control (Box 21-13).

The adolescent's questions should be answered thoroughly and honestly. In many instances the adolescent is hesitant to voice concerns, so information is offered even when questions are not asked. An effective indirect approach to learning about adolescent concerns, especially about potentially embarrassing or stressful topics, is to say, "Many teenagers ask me about [a topic]. Have you ever thought about this?" or "A lot of young people want to know about [a topic]."

Direct questions are also important, even about sensitive topics: "Have you ever thought about suicide?" "Are you depressed?" "Are you sexually active?" "Do you use birth control and/or protection?" However, asking first about friends and the adolescent's feelings about them may be a good lead-in approach: "Are any of your friends doing drugs?" "How do you feel about it?" Vague or circuitous questions may be interpreted as a sign of discomfort or lack of understanding and may cause the adolescent to be equally vague when responding.

Correct anatomical terms and descriptions of laboratory tests, disease processes, and possible outcomes are essential components in treating adolescents as individuals who are capable of being responsible for their own bodies.

NURSING APPLICATION

Adolescence is a period of rapid growth and development with changes occurring physically and psychosocially. Nurses play a pivotal role in influencing health promotion, preventive screening, and disease prevention activities. The primary responsibility for the nurse dealing with the important period of time known as the transition from childhood to adulthood is to provide education about some of the expected changes and how to deal with them.

Primary prevention methods are effective when the nurse is able to partner with the adolescent in recognizing his or her health needs. Treating the teen in a respectful manner enables the teen to assume more responsibility. Nurses must remain sensitive to the changes the adolescent is encountering and understand the need for guided independence.

Some important health-education topics for the adolescent population include proper nutrition, exercise, teen pregnancy, and protection from sexually transmitted diseases. Teens are taught about the significance of their lifestyle choices on future health. Drug and alcohol use, injury prevention, violence, and tobacco use are all behaviors that are known to contribute to illness and death among teens. Nurses use educational tools that appeal to the age group by conducting Internet searches for resources. Teens are able to relate to Internet resources, celebrities, and social media sites. Peers have the greatest influence on teenagers.

Nurses need to educate teens in partnership with parents about the fact that accidents are the leading cause of death and injury in the adolescent population. Nurses should reinforce research regarding distracted driving, seat belt use, and texting, adjusting the radio, and listening to loud music while driving.

Adolescent girls are educated about breast self-examinations, cervical cancer, and human papillomavirus. Adolescent males are educated about testicular self-examination. Both sexes are encouraged to obtain physical examinations and follow the recommended vaccination schedule.

Various screenings are utilized by the nurse as a secondary prevention measure for the adolescent. Scoliosis screening is conducted in prepubertal and pubertal adolescents because early identification and treatment is important to prevent long-term disability or disfigurement. Nurses also screen for eating disorders, type 2 diabetes, pregnancy, and sexually transmitted diseases.

Adolescents respond better when they feel that they are regarded as young adults and a partner in their health-promotion efforts. The nurse needs to become skilled at discussing difficult or embarrassing topics with teenagers. It is essential that adolescents feel that they are treated with respect and regarded as an individual.

CASE STUDY

Drug-Facilitated Sexual Assault: Jessica

Sexual assault includes any type of sexual activity to which an individual does not agree. Because of the effects of some drugs, commonly called date rape drugs, victims may be physically helpless, unable to refuse, or even unable to remember what happened.

Jessica, a 16-year-old high school sophomore, expresses concern to the school nurse that she knows someone who might have had sex "without knowing it." How can the nurse answer these common questions?

Reflective Questions
1. What are date rape drugs and how can a person be unaware that such a drug has been ingested?
2. What can you do to protect yourself?
3. What do you do if you think you have been sexually assaulted?
4. What can you do when someone you care about has been sexually assaulted?

◎ CARE PLAN

Drug-Facilitated Sexual Assault: Jessica

*NURSING DIAGNOSIS: Risk for Powerlessness related to suspected rape/rape trauma syndrome

Definition
At risk for perceived lack of control over a situation and/or one's ability to significantly affect an outcome

Risk Factors (R/T)
- Suspected date rape/rape trauma syndrome
- Acute injury (rape)
- Deficient knowledge
- Disturbed body image
- Situational low self-esteem

Expected Outcomes
- Acknowledges personal strength
- Perceived control

- Perceived resources
- Participation in health care decisions
- Increase healthy lifestyle choices

Goal: Increase individual's sense of power over potential/actual situation for self/others.

Interventions
- Active listening
- Risk identification
- Health care information exchange
- Support system enhancement
- Rape trauma treatment
- Decision-making support
- Health education

Based on Johnson, M., Bulechek, G. M., Dochterman, J. M., Maas, M. L., Moorhead, S., Swanson, E., et al. (2006). NANDA, NOC and NIC linkages: Nursing diagnoses, outcomes & interventions (2nd ed.). St. Louis: Mosby.
* NANDA Nursing Diagnoses—Definitions and Classification 2012-2014, Herdman T.H. (ED). Copyright © 2012, 1994-2012 NANDA International. Used by arrangement with John Wiley & Sons Limited. In order to make safe and effective judgments using the NANDA-I nursing diagnoses it is essential that nurses refer to the definitions and defining characteristics of the diagnoses listed in this work.

SUMMARY

Adolescence is a period of rapid change, when the integration of family, peer, educational, social, cultural, and community experiences begins to take form in the teen's sense of self. Many view adolescence as a construction site in its early stages. Onlookers assume that eventually a recognizable structure will emerge but have no idea what that structure will be. Although many parents, teachers, and health care providers feel that hard hats and steel-reinforced shoes are needed, each is better equipped with an understanding and respect for the adolescent's developmental struggles with physical and cognitive changes, autonomy, body image, peer relations, and identity. The goal, after all, is for the teen to emerge in young adulthood with a healthy body, mind, and spirit.

REFERENCES

Agency for Healthcare Research and Quality (AHRQ). (2008). *Helping smokers quit: A guide for clinicians.* Retrieved January 1, 2012, from www.ahrq.gov/clinic/tobacco/clinhlpsmksqt.htm.

American Academy of Child & Adolescent Psychiatry (AACAP). (2008). *Teenagers with eating disorders. Facts for families (no. 2).* Washington, DC: Author. Retrieved January 5, 2012, from www.aacap.org/cs/root/facts_for_families/teenagers_with_eating_disorders.

American Academy of Pediatrics (AAP). (2008). *Bright futures: Guidelines for health supervision of infants, children, and adolescents* (3rd ed.). Elk Grove, IL: Author.

Ball, J. W., & Bindler, R. C. (2008). *Pediatric nursing: Caring for children* (4th ed.). Upper Saddle River, NJ: Pearson/Prentice-Hall.

Berger, K. S. (2011). *The developing person through the life span* (8th ed.). New York: Worth.

Burns, C. E., Brady, M. A., Dunn, A. M., Starr, N. B., & Blosser, C. (2009). *Pediatric primary care* (4th ed.). New York: Saunders.

Centers for Disease Control and Prevention (CDC). (2009). *Suicide prevention: Youth suicide.* Retrieved April 1, 2012, from www.cdc.gov/violenceprevention/pub/youth_suicide.html.

Centers for Disease Control and Prevention (CDC). (2010a). *Healthy youth! Injury and violence.* Retrieved January 10, 2012, from www.cdc.gov/healthyyouth/injury/index.htm.

Centers for Disease Control and Prevention (CDC). (2010b). Youth risk behavior surveillance—United States, 2009. *MMWR, 59*(SS-5), 1–142.

Centers for Disease Control and Prevention (CDC). (2010c). *Teen drivers: Fact sheet.* Retrieved January 10, 2012, from www.cdc.gov/Motorvehiclesafety/teen_drivers/teendrivers_factsheet.html.

Centers for Disease Control and Prevention (CDC). (2011a). *Sexual risk behavior: HIV, STD, & teen pregnancy prevention.* Retrieved January 1, 2012, from www.cdc.gov/healthyyouth/sexual behaviors/index.htm.

Centers for Disease Control and Prevention (CDC). (2011b). *Human papillomavirus (HPV): HPV vaccines.* Retrieved January 10, 2012, from www.cdc.gov/hpv/vaccine.html.

Dixon, S. D., & Stein, M. T. (2005). *Encounters with children* (4th ed.). New York: W.B. Saunders.

Evans, E., Hawton, K., Rodham, K., & Deeks, J. (2005). The prevalence of suicidal phenomena in adolescents: A systematic review of population-based studies. *Suicide and Life Threatening Behaviors, 35,* 239–250.

Gilligan, C., Lyons, N., & Hanmer, T. (1990). *Making connections: The relational worlds of adolescent girls at Emma Willard School.* Cambridge, MA: Harvard University Press.

Guyton, A. C., & Hall, J. E. (2011). *Textbook of medical physiology* (12th ed.). Philadelphia: W.B. Saunders.

Herman-Giddens, M., & Kaplowitz, P. B. (2010). Sexual maturity stage. In *Performing preventive services: A bright futures handbook.* Elk Grove, IL: American Academy of Pediatrics. Retrieved January 1, 2012, from http://brightfutures.aap.org/pdfs/Preventive%20 Services%20PDFs/Physical%20Examination.PDF.

Humes, K. R., Jones, N. A., & Ramirez, R. R. (2011). *2010 Census briefs. Overview of race and Hispanic origin: 2010.* Retrieved January 1, 2012, from www.census.gov/prod/cen2010/briefs/c2010br-02.pdf.

Kohlberg, L. (1981). *The philosophy of moral development.* San Francisco, CA: Harper & Row.

Lee, Y.-H., Salman, A., & Fitzpatrick, J. J. (2009). HIV/AIDS preventive self-efficacy, depressive symptoms, and risky sexual behavior in adolescents: A cross-sectional questionnaire survey. *International Journal of Nursing Studies, 46*(5), 653–660.

Lee, Y.-H., Salman, A., & Wang, F. (2010). Recruiting Chinese-American adolescents to HIV/AIDS related research: A lesson learned from a cross-sectional study. *Applied Nursing Research* 10.1016/j.apnr.2010.02.001.

Martin, J. A., Hamilton, B. E., Ventura, S. J., Osterman, M., Kirmeyer, S., Mathews, T. J., et al. (2011). Births: Final data for 2009. *National Vital Statistics Reports 2011, 60*(1), 1–104.

National Campaign to Prevent Teen and Unplanned Pregnancy. (2004). *Why it matters—Teen pregnancy.* Retrieved January 10, 2012, from www.thenationalcampaign.org/why-it-matters/wim_teens.aspx.

National Crime Prevention Council. (2012). *Cyberbullying.* Retrieved April 12, 2012, from www.ncpc.org/cyberbullying.

National Institute of Mental Health. (2011). *Depression in children and adolescents (fact sheet).* Retrieved January 12, 2012, from www.nimh.nih.gov/health/publications/depression-in-children-and-adolescents/index.shtml.

Pender, N. J., Murdaugh, C., & Parsons, M. A. (2010). *Health promotion in nursing practice* (6th ed.). Upper Saddle River, NJ: Pearson/Prentice-Hall.

Pinyerd, B., & Zipf, W. B. (2005). Puberty—timing is everything. *Journal of Pediatric Nursing, 20*(2), 75–82.

Seidel, H. M., Ball, J. W., Dains, J. E., & Benedict, G. W. (2010). *Mosby's guide to physical assessment* (7th ed.). St. Louis: Mosby.

Shaw, D., Fernandes, J. R., & Rao, C. (2005). Suicide in children and adolescents: A 10-year retrospective review. *American Journal of Forensic Medicine and Pathology, 26,* 309–315.

http://evolve.elsevier.com/Edelman/
- Study Questions
- Glossary

OBJECTIVES

After completing this chapter, the reader will be able to:
- Analyze specific health requirements of the young adult.
- Identify attitudes, behaviors, and habits that frequently compose the lifestyles of young adults.
- Define tasks that are consistent with the adult development achieved during this period.
- Describe the nurse's role in reducing the rate of unintentional pregnancies in young adult women.
- Determine occupational hazards that infringe on the young adult's welfare.
- Evaluate strategies that the nurse can use to reduce the risks associated with young adult behaviors.
- Analyze occupational, cultural, and ethnic risk factors that may affect young adults.
- Differentiate the nursing roles in preventive intervention for healthy young adults in home and community environments.
- Discuss proposed suggestions for preconceptual care.

KEY TERMS

Achievement-oriented stress	Genetic impairments	Metabolic syndrome
Aerobic exercise	Genital herpes virus	Orchitis
Basal metabolic rate	Hepatitis B	Papanicolaou (Pap) smear
Binge drinking	Human immunodeficiency virus (HIV)	Postconventional level of moral
Breast self-examination (BSE)	Human papillomavirus (HPV)	reasoning
Congenital defects	Hypertension	Rubella
Congenital rubella syndrome (CRS)	Infertility	Stress
Coronary artery disease (CAD)	Intimacy versus isolation	Sunscreen protective factor (SPF)
Fetal neural tube defects (FND)	Maternal mortality rate	Testicular self-examination (TSE)

THINK ABOUT IT

Using Private Information in Shared Living Arrangements

Young adults in communal living arrangements (for example, college dormitories, the military) are often placed with other individuals who have different cultural, language, or other values. The use of cell phones and computers with video and audio taping capabilities has opened the possibility that private behavior may be videoed or taped without consent and then may be shared through a form of social networking (Facebook, Twitter, instant messaging, other shared computer sites).

These situations are expected to become more prevalent in the future.

- What are the implications of this for violation of privacy for individuals and even groups (e.g., military, fraternities, sororities)?
- What are the legal implications? Some states have laws against unauthorized taping.

The young adult period encompasses the ages from 18 to 35 years, a time that spans from the end of adolescence to the beginning of middle adulthood. Formal education beyond high school to college and graduate school, as well as military experience, and the major milestones of marriage and beginning a family may be included in this phase of development. The major task accomplished in this period is preparing for, and assuming adult responsibilities, rights, and privileges.

BIOLOGY AND GENETICS

The young adult period is a time of many physical and emotional changes and is an opportunity for learning by experience and experimentation (Box 22-1: Quality and Safety Scenario).

Young adulthood is characterized by greater complexity of thinking, further organization of emotional and cognitive development, and decision-making based on impact on others and future consequences. All phases of young adult development garner considerable interest. Judging by the increase in books about self-development, more adults are exploring topics in holistic healing and spiritual health and development. Health behaviors, safety practices, diet, exercise, weight control, sexuality, and addictions are widely discussed topics. Preventive health concerns for young adults can be separated into two categories: developing behaviors that promote a healthy lifestyle and decreasing the incidence of accidents, injuries, and acts of violence. *Healthy People 2020* reports that 72% of all deaths among children and young adults are due to injuries from four causes: motor vehicle crashes (30%), all other nonintentional injuries (15%), homicide (15%), and suicide (12%) (U.S. Department of Health and Human Services [USDHHS], 2010).

In 2010, approximately 20.5% of the American population was composed of adults ages 20 to 34 (U.S. Census Bureau, 2011). The young adult population is projected to be approximately 20.6% of the general population by the year 2015 and 19.4% by the year 2025. The percentage of young adults ages 20 to 24 years shows a decline from 9.4% in 1980 to a projected 6.5% in 2025 (U.S. Census Bureau, 2011). A decline in this age group is influenced by birth rates, and the U.S. Census Bureau (2011) reported that the birth rate per 1000 people for women of all ages in 2008 was 14.0; this rate has been dropping since 1990, when it was more than 16.7 live births per 1000. Health-promotion efforts are particularly important for young adults, because health teaching for this age group has the significant potential to directly influence subsequent generations (Box 22-2: *Healthy People 2020*).

BOX 22-1 QUALITY AND SAFETY SCENARIO

Topic: Examining Problematic College Drinking Behaviors in Young Adults

A recent study of 211 college students indicates that 63% of female and 83% of male college-aged students (mean age 20.7 years) engaged in binge drinking. Associated with these intermittent excessive drinking "binges" were various disordered and unhealthy weight-reducing behaviors (skipping meals, fasting, using diet pills, and self-induced vomiting) (Kelly-Weeder, 2011).

You are the clinic director and nurse at a small liberal arts college. Mary, a 19-year-old freshman, has generally been a good student, easily making the adjustment to living away from home during her first 2 months in the dormitory. She comes to you to talk about an episode that occurred the previous weekend and that frightened her. On Saturday night she was at a party at a private residence in a rural, wooded setting away from the campus. She remembers consuming five or six alcoholic drinks; however, any memory after midnight is missing. She woke up in a fellow female student's dormitory room without any memory of leaving the party or returning to the dormitory. She was able to piece together information from her friends, who told her that she consumed at least nine alcoholic drinks that night and that she left the party with others who were returning to the dormitory, but they were not the friends with whom she had been seen with all evening. She is concerned that she may have been drugged

or that she may be having memory lapses. Assessment of her alcohol use in the past reveals that she can recount at least four occasions during which she drank more than seven drinks at a party or family gathering. She describes her family as "social drinkers." On days that she anticipates drinking, she restricts her caloric intake. Last June, she was involved in a minor car accident that might have been related to her consumption of at least three drinks that afternoon. The road to this rural college has two road side shrines dedicated to students who have died in automobile crashes near the college. To further analyze Mary's situation, you formulate the following questions:

- Do you think that Mary has a problem with drinking? Would you classify her as a binge drinker? How do you clarify what she values?
- Is Mary engaging in risky behavior especially if she drives while drinking?
- What kind of physical assessment might assist you in making a determination that Mary has a drinking problem?
- What kinds of preventive educational programs could you advise?
- What kinds of monitoring and follow-up mechanisms might assist Mary in keeping her safe and in a treatment plan?

Kelly-Weeder, S. (2011). Binge drinking and disordered eating in college students. *Journal of the American Academy of Nurse Practitioners, 23(1)*, 33-41; Quality and Safety Education for Nurses (QSEN). (2012). Retrieved April 28, 2012, from www.qsen.org; Institute of Medicine (IOM). (2003). *Health professions education: A bridge to quality.* Retrieved December 29, 2011, at www.iom.edu/Reports/2003/Health-Professions-Education-A-Bridge-to-Quality.aspx.

Young adulthood is generally the healthiest time of life. Physical growth is mostly complete by the age of 20; most concerns related to physiological development are focused on ensuring the optimal functioning of body systems. The young adult's physical abilities are in peak condition, and compensatory mechanisms operate optimally during illness to provide minimal disruption in health patterns. Nursing goals for individuals of this age group are oriented toward prolonging this period of optimal physical energy; developing the mental, emotional, spiritual, and social potential; encouraging proper health habits; anticipating and screening for and, therefore, being able to treat the onset of chronic disease at an early stage; and treating disease when appropriate.

Full adult stature in men is reached at approximately age 21; in women, full growth occurs earlier, typically by age 17. Optimal muscle strength occurs during ages 25 to 30, and then gradually declines by approximately 10% from ages 30 to 60.

Manual dexterity peaks in young adulthood and begins to decline in the middle thirties.

Women have greater longevity than do men. Women are considered biologically stronger than men, outlive men, and naturally outnumber men. On the average, in the United States women live 5 years longer than do men; an increase of about 3 years within the past decades (U.S. Census Bureau, 2011). These statistics may be a result in part of female genetic composition or men's greater exposure to environmental and occupational hazards. Men also seek health care services less frequently than do women. Females generally seek preventive care more often than men. Although some of this reflects the inclusion of multiple prenatal visits, it also supports better health practices.

A classic public health indicator of a nation's health resources and services is the maternal mortality rate. Since 1980, maternal mortality has been fairly stable in the United States. In 1980 the rate was 9.2 per 100,000 live births; then mortality dropped

---

♥ BOX 22-2 HEALTHY PEOPLE 2020

Selected National Health-Promotion and Disease-Prevention Objectives for the Young Adult

- Increase the proportion of adults who engage in regular aerobic activity of moderate intensity. (In 2008, 43.5% of adults performed the recommended amount of physical activity and the target is 47.9%.)
- Increase the proportion of adults who perform muscle-strengthening activities on two or more days of the week. (In 2008, 21.9% of adults performed those activities and the target is 24.1%.)
- Increase the proportion of adults who are at a healthy weight. (From 2005 through 2008, 30.8% of adults ages 20 and older were at a healthy weight and the target is 33.9%.)
- Reduce the proportion of adults who are obese. (From 2005 through 2008, 34% of adults age 20 and older were considered obese and the target is 30.6%.)
- Reduce cigarette smoking by adults. (In 2008, 20.6% of adults 18 and older were current cigarette smokers and the target is 12%.)
- Reduce the proportion of adults using any illicit drug during the preceding 30 days. (Illicit drug use in adults age 18 or older in 2008 was 7.9% and the target is 7.1%.)
- Increase the proportion of males and females who have received formal instruction on HIV/AIDS prevention before the age of 18. (From 2006 through 2008, 88.3% of females and 89.0% of males had received instruction and the target is 97%.)
- Reduce the proportion of college students engaging in binge drinking of alcoholic beverages during the past 2 weeks. (In 2008, 40.9% of college students reported binge drinking in the past 2 weeks and the target is 36.0%.)
- Increase the proportion of females or their partners at risk of unintended pregnancy who used contraception at the most recent sexual intercourse. (From the years 2006 through 2008, 83% of sexually active females or partners used contraception and the target is 91.3%.)
- Increase the proportion of adults with recognized depression who receive treatment. (In 2008, 58% of adults who were diagnosed with depression received treatment and the target is 64.6%.)
- Reduce deaths caused by motor vehicle crashes. (In 2007, 13.8 deaths/100,000 population occurred and the target is 12.4.)
- Increase the number of states that have adopted a graduated driver licensing model law. (In 2009, 35 states had adopted graduate driver licensing and the target is 51 states including the District of Columbia.)

- Increase the proportion of motorcycle operators and passengers using helmets. (In 2008, the baseline was 67% and the target is 73.7%.)
- Reduce sports and recreation injuries. (In 2008, there were 45.6 medically consulted injuries per 1000 population and the target is 41.0 injuries per 1000 population.)
- Reduce firearm-related deaths. (In 2008, there were 10.2 firearm-related deaths per 100,000 population and the target is 9.2.)
- Reduce the number of homicides. (In 2007, 6.1 homicides/100,000 population occurred and the target is 5.5/100,000 population.)
- Increase the proportion of persons with a usual primary care provider. (In 2007, 76.3% of all individuals had a usual source of health care and the target is 83.9%, a 10% improvement.)
- Increase the proportion of pregnancies that are intended. (In 2002, 51% of pregnancies were intended and the target is 56%; this target represents a 10% improvement.)
- Increase the proportion of women who receive early and adequate prenatal care. (In 2007, 70.8% received early and adequate prenatal care and the target is 77.9%.)
- Reduce the proportion of pregnancies conceived within 18 months of a previous birth. (From 2006 through 2008, 35.3% of pregnancies were conceived within 18 months and the target is 31.7%.)
- Increase the proportion of adults 20 years and older who are aware of signs of heart attack and the importance of accessing rapid emergency care. (In 2008, 39.2% of adults were aware of signs of need for, and access to, emergency care; the target is 43.1%.)
- Increase the proportion of adults ages 18 and older who have had their cholesterol level measured in the last 5 years. (In 2008 74.6% of adults 18 or older had their blood cholesterol level checked and the target is 82%.)
- Reduce the proportion of adults ages 18 and older reporting using artificial sources of ultraviolet light for tanning. (In 2008 15.2% of adults ages 18 or older reported using artificial tanning and the target is 13.7%.)
- Increase the proportion of adults ages 18 and older who follow protective measures that may reduce the risk of skin cancer. (In 2008 was 72.8% of this population used protective measures and the target is 80.1%.)

From U.S. Department of Health and Human Services. (2010). *Healthy People 2020.* Washington, DC: U.S. Government Printing Office.

to 6.6 in 1987 and rose to 8.9 in 2002. In 2007 the maternal mortality rate was much higher, 12.7 per 100,000 live births (USDHHS, 2010), reflecting inclusion of pregnancy status as a separate item on death certificates in some states. *Healthy People 2020* (USDHHS, 2010) set a target goal of 11.4 maternal deaths per 100,000 live births, but to reach this goal there is a need for much more national and statewide action to identify gaps in disparities, early prevention, treatment, and research.

GORDON'S FUNCTIONAL HEALTH PATTERNS

Health Perception–Health Management Pattern

Because excellent physical health frequently is taken for granted, concern about health and well-being is relatively low in individuals in their twenties but begins to increase in individuals in their thirties. Monitoring of specific health parameters is both necessary and appropriate to determine health needs and incipient problems. After the middle thirties, an increased sense of the finiteness of life develops with limitations imposed by work choices, well-being, monetary resources, and the deterioration of physical abilities. For more specific health care management, the young adult age span is split into two age groups (18 to 24 and 25 to 35), according to the preventive services that are required.

The assumption that all adults should have an annual physical examination has been supplanted by increased scientifically based information about health screening measures. Screening services provided in a health-monitoring program need to meet cost-effective criteria. Evidence-based practice uses best practices' information for clinical decisions instead of intuition and unmethodical clinical experience and, as such, forms the current recommended standard of care. Evidence-based approaches ultimately will determine which screening measures are best supported by scientific data (randomized controlled treatment studies), reduce regional variations in use of diagnostic and therapeutic modalities, and close the gap between practice and research (Melnyk & Fineout-Overholt, 2011).

Behavioral Health History

A behavioral health history is particularly important for young adults. This type of history focuses on risk factors for unintentional injuries, such as accidents, seat belt use, and alcohol consumption, which are major causes of death and disability in this age group. The safety focus of nursing health promotion for the younger adult takes different forms, from the simple—monitoring helmet and seat belt use—to more complex concerns—threats such as bioterrorism and globally spreading infections (USDHHS, 2010). Figure 22-1 lists questions and content that may be appropriately included in a health history for young adults focusing on likely age-specific behaviors.

Preventive Care

Basic goals of preventive care are to maximize the period of optimal health status and detect incipient health problems at an early stage. At age 18 (approximately the time of graduation from high school), a full health appraisal is recommended.

Table 22-1 illustrates preventive care that is important during the young adult period, along with recommended frequency of screening. As a rule, the recommendation for most procedures is a repeat health history and visit at approximately 2-year intervals. Appropriate intervention in the younger age group is directed toward correcting health issues through history assessment and counseling about avoidance of adverse health behaviors. Subsequent counseling sessions focus on rechecking and updating information gathered in earlier meetings.

A physical examination includes measurements of height, weight, body mass index (BMI), blood pressure, and blood tests, with an emphasis on the need to avoid inactivity and obesity, which are risk factors for many health problems. Clinicians who advise women to perform breast self-examination (BSE) to screen for breast cancer should understand that currently the U.S. Preventive Services Task Force (USPSTF) recommends against teaching BSE and concludes that the current evidence is insufficient to assess the additional benefits and harm of clinical breast examination (CBE) beyond screening mammography for women 40 and older. Screening is strongly recommended for cervical cancer in women who have been sexually active (Papanicolaou [Pap] smear). Testicular self-examination (TSE) may be taught to men in this age group, although there is little evidence to assess accuracy, benefits, or effectiveness (U.S. Preventive Services Task Force, 2010) since early testicular cancers often present as benign inflammations such as epididymitis or testicular trauma. A rectal examination is not recommended unless symptoms are present.

The typical young adult health examination also looks for signs of chronic disease. The most common chronic diseases reported by young adults are asthma, arthritis (including rheumatic diseases such as lupus and fibromyalgia), and hypertension (Figure 22-2). Although the percentage of young adults reporting chronic disease is small, more women than men (17.4% versus 12.9%) reported having at least one of the six most highly selected young adult chronic disease conditions (arthritis, asthma, cancer, diabetes, heart disease, and hypertension) (Centers for Disease Control and Prevention [CDC], 2009).

After age 25, the preventive emphasis is on modifying coronary disease risk factors. Recommendations for screening for young adults are undergoing revision as more information becomes available about the interactive risks of sedentary lifestyle, high cholesterol levels, familial high lipid levels, diabetes mellitus, and smoking. USPSTF recommends screening for young adults ages 20 to 35 for lipid disorders if they are at increased risk for coronary disease (U.S Preventive Services Task Force, 2010). Aging is responsible for some degenerative changes in respiratory and cardiac function, but during the young adult years this decline amounts to less than 1% per year and is largely determined by an individual's fitness level (Huether & McCance, 2012). Cardiovascular assessment of the young adult includes determining the presence of hyperlipidemia, hypertension, diabetes, chest pain, or heart disease. A *Healthy People 2020* target is to reduce the mean total blood cholesterol levels among adults to 177.9 mg/dL; the baseline between 1988 and 1994 for adults 20 and older was 197.7 mg/dL

Well Young Adult Behavioral Health History Content

Sociodemographic content and questions:

What organizations (community, church, lodge, social, professional, etc.) are you involved in?_____
_____

How would you describe your community?_____
_____

Hobbies, skills, interests, and recreational activities? _____

Military service? No_____   Yes_____   From _____ to_____

Overseas assignment? No_____   Yes_____

Close friends or immediate family members who have died within the past two years? _____
_____

Names and addresses of relatives or close friends in the area. _____
_____
_____

Marital status: S M D W   Length of time _____

Environmental content and questions:

Do you live alone? No_____   Yes_____

When did you last move? _____

Describe your living situation. _____

Number of years of education completed: _____

Elementary?_____   High school?_____   College?_____

Occupation?_____   Employer?_____

How long have you worked for this employer? _____

Are you satisfied with your work situation? No_____   Yes_____

Do you consider your work risky or dangerous? No_____   Yes_____

Is your work stressful? No_____   Yes_____

Over the past two weeks, have you felt depressed or hopeless? No_____   Yes_____

Biophysical content questions:

Have you smoked cigarettes? No_____   Yes_____

How much? Less than ½ pack per day? About one pack per day? More than 1½ packs per day?

Are you smoking now? No_____   Yes_____   Length of time smoking?_____

Have you ever smoked cigars or a pipe? No_____   Yes_____

If yes, how long?_____   Do you smoke cigars or a pipe now? No_____   Yes_____

Do you drink alcohol (wine, beer, or whiskey)? No_____   Yes_____

If you do, how much each day on the average?_____   Each week?_____

Do you consume large amounts occasionally (binge drinking)? No_____   Yes_____

Have you been drunk on work days? No_____   Yes_____

Have you had alcoholic drinks in the morning sometime in the past year? No_____   Yes_____

How much coffee, tea, or cola do you drink? _____

Do you use seat or lap belts? No_____   Yes_____

What type of exercise do you do each week? Describe type and amount. _____
_____

Are you satisfied with your weight? No_____   Yes_____   Body image? No_____   Yes_____

Do you use a bicycle or motorcycle helmet? No_____   Yes_____   Helmet and pads while rollerblading? No_____   Yes_____

How much sleep do you usually get each night?_____

Meals: Do you generally eat: three regular meals per day? two meals per day? irregular meals?

Are you sexually active? No_____   Yes_____

If so, are you aware of the risks of sexually transmitted diseases? No_____   Yes_____

For women: Do you perform breast self-examination (BSE) each month? No_____   Yes_____

For men: Do you perform testicular self-examination (TSE) regularly? No_____   Yes_____

FIGURE 22-1 Common well young adult behavioral health history content. (From U.S. Preventive Services Task Force. [2010]. *Guide to clinical preventive services*. Rockville, MD: Agency for Healthcare Research and Quality. Retrieved April 28, 2012, from www.ahrq.gov/clinic/uspstfix. htm; Somers, A. R., & Breslow, L. [1979]. Lifetime health monitoring program. *Nurse Practitioner, 4*[40], 50, 54.)

TABLE 22-1 WELL YOUNG ADULT HEALTH MONITORING

HEALTH ISSUE	AGES 18 TO 24		AGES 25 TO 35	
	INTERVENTION	FREQUENCY (YEARS)	INTERVENTION	FREQUENCY (YEARS)
Tobacco use	History and counseling	Each visit	History and counseling	Each visit
Obesity/nutrition/body mass index (BMI)	History, weight, and counseling	Each visit	History, weight, and counseling	Each visit
Avoid alcohol while driving, swimming, engaging in activities that involve mental and physical alertness	History and counseling	At least once	History and counseling	Every 2
Accidental injury, lap and shoulder belts, bicycle or motorcycle helmets, smoke detectors, safe firearm use	History and counseling	At least once	History and counseling	Every 2
Unintended pregnancy	Counseling	At least once	History and counseling	Every 2
Contraception	Counseling	Individually determined	Counseling	Individually determined
Illegal drug use	History and counseling	At least once	History and counseling	Every 2 to 4
Regular physical activity	History and counseling	At least once	History and counseling	Every 2 to 4
Blood pressure, hypertension	Blood pressure measurement	Every 2	Blood pressure measurement	Every 2 to 4
Breast or testicular cancer	BSE or TSE counseling	Every 1 to 2	BSE or TSE counseling	Every 1 to 2
Vision defects	Examination	Once and refer	Examination	Every 4
Tetanus/diphtheria/pertussis (Tdap)	Booster	Once if 10 yr since last one	Immunization	Every 10
Hepatitis B	Immunization	If not immunized	Immunization	If not immunized
Diabetes, proteinuria, bacteriuria	Urinalysis	Once	Urinalysis	Every 4
Coronary artery disease	Serum cholesterol level determination, triglyceride level	Once	Serum cholesterol level determination	Every 5
Dental care	Dental examination and cleaning	Every year	Dental examination and cleaning	Every year
Cervical dysplasia	Gynecological exam; Pap smear	Every 2, start age 21	Gynecological exam; Pap smear	Every 2
STD prevention	Counseling Offer HPV vaccine	Individually determined	Counseling	Individually determined
Chlamydia (women)	*Chlamydia* screen	At gynecological examination, if sexually active	*Chlamydia* screen	At gynecological examination, if sexually active
Gonorrhea (women)	Vaginal culture	At gynecological examination, if sexually active	Vaginal culture	At gynecological examination
Influenza	Seasonal flu vaccine	Each year	Seasonal flu vaccine	Each year

Modified from U.S. Preventive Services Task Force. (2010). *Guide to clinical preventive services.* Rockville, MD: Agency for Healthcare Research and Quality. Retrieved April 28, 2012, from www.ahrq.gov/clinic/uspstfix.htm; U.S. National Library of Medicine. (2011). *Health screening for women/men ages 18-39.* Retrieved April 28, 2012, from www.nlm.nih.gov/medlineplus/ency/article/007462.htm.
BSE, Breast self-examination; *TSE,* testicular self-examination; *Pap,* Papanicolaou; *STD,* sexually transmitted disease.

(USDHHS, 2010). This 2020 target set a goal of 10% improvement. From 1999 to 2002, 17% of persons age 20 years and older had high total blood cholesterol levels (greater than 240 mg/dL), down from 21% for the 1988 to 1994 period. A comprehensive health history should also elicit pertinent information about hypertension and **coronary artery disease (CAD)** in parents and relatives. A pregnancy history of pregnancy-induced hypertension (PIH) or preeclampsia makes a female at increased risk for cardiovascular disease (Box 22-3: Research for Evidence-Based Practice).

Hypertension results from increases in cardiac output or increases in peripheral resistance, or a combination of both, and is the third leading cause of death worldwide. According to the *Seventh Joint National Committee Report (JNC VII),* the focus of blood pressure assessment is on systolic hypertension and the risks from systolic hypertension, which rise beginning with systolic pressures of 115 mm Hg. The risk from diastolic hypertension starts to rise at 75 mm Hg. The focus of attention is on lowering blood pressure toward the new lower normal goal of 120/80 mm Hg or less (Chobanian et al., 2003; USDHHS, 2010). USPSTF highly recommends (Grade A) screening of young adults for hypertension. Each increase in blood pressure over this level exerts a consistent rise in risk for heart attack, stroke, and heart failure. *JNC VII* also established a new category of "prehypertension" to better identify individuals at risk for developing treatable hypertension to encourage lifestyle changes before vascular disease is present (USDHHS, 2010).

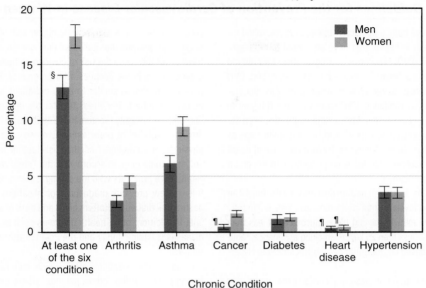

**Percentage of Young Adults Aged 18–29 Years*
with Selected Chronic Conditions,† by Sex**

* Overall respondents: 6898 men and 8532 women

† Estimates are based on household interviews with a sample of the civilian, noninstitutionalized, adult U.S. population. The prevalence of diagnosed chronic conditions was
determined by asking respondents if a doctor or other health professional ever told
them that they had a specified condition. Asthma estimates are for current asthma and
are based on the additional question "Do you still have asthma?" Arthritis includes arthritis, rheumatoid arthritis, gout, lupus, and fibromyalgia. Cancer excludes nonmela-
noma skin cancer or skin cancer of unknown type. Diabetes includes all types with the
exception of diabetic conditions related to pregnancy. Heart disease includes coronary
heart disease, angina or angina pectoris, or heart attack or myocardial infarction. Hypertension is based on respondents indicating that on two or more separate visits they
were told by a doctor or health professional that they had hypertension. Young adults
who reported more than one condition are counted in each category.

§ 95% confidence interval.

¶ Estimate is statistically unreliable; data have a relative standard error of 20%–30%.

FIGURE 22-2 Percentage of young adults ages 18 to 29 years with selected chronic conditions,
by gender. (From *National Health Interview Survey, United States, 2005-2007.* Retrieved April 28,
2012, from www.cdc.gov/mmwr/preview/mmwrhtml/mm5825a3.htm.)

The Mexican American population has the lowest percentage of high blood pressure individuals (25.5%); the
White-only/non-Hispanic population is intermediate at
28.8%; and the non-Hispanic/Black African American population has the highest (42%) level of hypertension (USDHHS,
2010). The prevalence of treatment and control of hypertension was also lowest in young adults (31%) and Mexican Americans (37%). This may be related to lack of a usual
source of care, but most surveyed had health insurance, so
health insurance alone is not sufficient to correlate with better hypertension control (Gillespie et al., 2011). Gillespie and
colleagues (2011) also report that adoption of healthy behaviors, particularly of reducing dietary salt intake from an average of 3400 mg to 2300 mg daily, could dramatically reduce
the incidence of hypertension.

Although for the entire population deaths attributable to
coronary heart disease have declined since the 1960s (CDC,
2011b), the mortality rate remains higher for American Indi-
ans/Alaska Natives and Blacks. A prevention target of *Healthy
People 2020* (USDHHS, 2010) is to increase the proportion of

young adults 18 years and older with hypertension whose blood
pressure is under control from 18% (in 1988 to 1994) to 61.2%
(USDHHS, 2010). From 2005 to 2008, 43.7% of adults 18 and
older had control of their blood pressure. A related target goal
of *Healthy People 2020* is to increase the proportion of adults
ages 20 and older who are aware of the importance of accessing rapid emergency care for either heart attack or stroke. In
2008, 92.9% of young adults were aware of this and the target
for improvement was 94.9%, a 2% improvement (USDHHS,
2010).

The metabolic syndrome includes a group of cardiovascular risk factors associated with overweight and obesity, particularly abdominal obesity. This syndrome includes the lethal
risks of high lipid levels, insulin resistance, and hypertension.
A prominent sign of metabolic syndrome is central or waist-
centered obesity. Currently, at least one fifth of U.S. adults are
estimated to have this cluster of risk factors and the prevalence
increases with age. First-step therapy involves lifestyle alterations, including weight management and increase in physical
activity (USDHHS, 2010).

BOX 22-3   RESEARCH FOR EVIDENCE-BASED PRACTICE

Effectiveness-Based Guidelines for the Prevention of Cardiovascular Disease in Women—2011 Update*

During the last decade, there have been a number of randomized controlled trials, such as the Women's Health Initiative, that have attempted to differentiate how cardiovascular disease (CVD) preventive strategies should be altered for women. The myth that CVD is a "man's" disease has been abolished. CVD caused more deaths in women than cancer, chronic lower respiratory disease, Alzheimer's disease, and accidents combined. CVD deaths are much higher in Black females than in White females. These guidelines thoroughly dispelled the conventional wisdom that as far as CVD, women should be treated the same as men. This is also a global problem. Heart disease is the leading cause of death in women worldwide. These guidelines also focus on preventive efforts and a long-term risk analysis in younger women.

The "ideal cardiovascular health" long-term pattern described by the American Heart Association (AHA) includes levels of total cholesterol less than 200 mg/dL, blood pressure less than 120/80 mm Hg, fasting blood glucose level less than 100 mg/dL, lean body mass index less than 25 kg/m^2, smoking abstinence, regular physical activity, and a diet based on the Dietary Approaches to Stop Hypertension (DASH) concept.

An important newer recommendation of these guidelines is that pregnancy history provides the health care professional with a criterion to predict future CVD risk. Women with a history of pregnancy-induced hypertension (PIH) or preeclampsia have a significantly higher risk of CVD. The panel reviewed a large meta-analysis that indicated that women with a history of preeclampsia have about the twice the risk of developing heart disease, stroke, and thrombolytic events in the decades after pregnancy. Pregnancy may induce a temporary state that is similar to early metabolic syndrome, and as such, could be considered a failed stress test for the development of CVD in the future. Therefore it is highly recommended that the delivering health care personnel provide a referral of preeclamptic women after delivery to the primary care physician or cardiologist so that risk factors for CVD can be observed and adjusted to be more in accord with the "ideal cardiovascular health" pattern. Health care providers who are seeing females during a first visit should carefully review previous pregnancy complications including preeclampsia and gestational diabetes, preterm birth, and birth of an infant small for gestational age. In addition, other health disorders such as depression and autoimmune diseases (systemic lupus and rheumatoid arthritis) may also elevate the risk for CVD.

These recommendations also include cultural differences. An interesting finding points out the "ethnic paradox" where the female Hispanic population, despite the stresses of immigration and less access to medical care, has a longer life expectancy than non-Hispanic Whites and non-Hispanic Blacks.

*Guidelines from the American Heart Association (AHA). (2011). Effectiveness-based guidelines for the prevention of cardiovascular disease in women—2011 update. Data from *Circulation, 123*(11), 1243-1262. doi:org/10.1161/CIR0b013e31820faaf8. These guidelines have also been published in other journals and at National Institutes of Health (NIH) Public Access; the guidelines represent the work of many participating organizations and sponsors including the Nurse Practitioners in Women's Health. Also from Melnyk, B., & Fineout-Overholt, E. (2011). *Evidence-based practice in nursing & healthcare.* Philadelphia: Lippincott Williams & Wilkins.

Diabetes is seventh on the list of leading causes of death in the United States; it is also one of the six major chronic diseases affecting young adults (CDC, 2009). Currently, 23.6 million Americans have the disease and about 25% of Americans with diabetes are undiagnosed (USDHHS, 2010). Minority populations (Blacks, Native American/Alaska Natives, and Hispanics) are disproportionately affected with Native American populations experiencing twice the rate for new cases recorded in White non-Hispanic populations (USDHHS, 2010). The incidence of diabetes, especially type 2 diabetes (adult onset), and related complications (cardiovascular disease, blindness, lower limb amputations, and kidney disease) is increasing in the United States (USDHHS, 2010). Of those diagnosed with diabetes, only a few have their blood pressure, glucose levels, and cholesterol levels sufficiently controlled to avoid or delay vascular disease. Diabetes lowers life expectancy by up to 15 years. Because careful control can delay the beginning and progression of long-term complications, early detection and monitoring of diabetes in young adults is important.

Decision-Making and Risk-Taking

The decision-making of a young adult directly affects health and well-being. Peak physical skills stimulate young adults to be venturesome, daring, enterprising, and aggressive. Young adults have less experience with the death of significant people in their lives, and they may take inordinate risks. The leading causes of death in individuals 15 to 24 years of age are unintentional injuries, homicide, and suicide (USDHHS, 2010). The prevalence of adverse behaviors associated with sudden death illustrates a developmental lack of fear in young adults. Underuse of seat belts and helmets by motorcyclists and bicyclists is a cause of many accidental injuries and deaths. Some states still do not have laws that require helmets.

Communicable Diseases and Adult Immunization

Communicable (infectious) diseases affect young adults with varying degrees of severity. Although the increased availability of better drug treatments and/or vaccines, improved hygiene and food handling, and provision of cleaner water supplies have promoted prevention and control of infectious disease, new disease threats are continually emerging at a rate of approximately one per year. Much of this increase is due to improvements in travel and changes in social, sexual, and other behaviors that expose broader populations of individuals to emerging pathogens. Newer threats include seasonal influenza, drug-resistant tuberculosis, H5N1 bird flu, diarrhea caused by *Escherichia coli* 0157:H7, and Hantavirus pulmonary disease or syndrome (HPS). A more recent goal of *Healthy People 2020* is to increase the percentage of adults who are vaccinated for seasonal influenza from 29% to 80% (USDHHS, 2010). Increasingly, new cases of tuberculosis are occurring in foreign-born individuals (USDHHS, 2010), even as the incidence of this disease declined overall from 6.8 cases per 100,000 to 4.9 in 2005; the target is 1.0 new case per 1000,000 population. An increase in tuberculosis rates, particularly in some minority groups (Asian American/Pacific Islanders, Blacks, and Hispanics), illustrates that preventive activities must be reinforced and constant vigilance maintained over monitoring and effectiveness for all communicable diseases. The focus of tuberculosis surveillance is moving toward tracking of full completion of drug protocols. New infectious agents and diseases continue to be detected and must be understood in a global context because of increasing travel and migration, importation of foods, agriculture practices, and bioterrorism (USDHHS, 2010).

Cases of acute hepatitis B (HB) infection declined in young adults because of vaccination programs aimed at children, adolescents, and adults in high-risk groups (USDHHS, 2010). A primary way of achieving high levels of vaccination coverage is to identify settings in which unvaccinated young adults can be vaccinated, such as correctional facilities, drug treatment centers, and clinics treating sexually transmitted diseases (STDs) (USDHHS, 2010). An objective of *Healthy People 2020* is to continue to reduce hepatitis B infections in adults 19 and older from 2.0 cases per 100,000 persons in 2007 to a target goal of 1.5 cases per 100,000 persons (USDHHS, 2010).

Rubella in young adults is generally a minor disease; however, when the disease is contracted during the first trimester of pregnancy, miscarriage, stillbirth, or congenital rubella syndrome (CRS) can result. CRS is associated with loss of hearing, ocular defects, developmental delay and growth retardation, and cardiac malformations. In 2008, there were no cases of confirmed rubella reported in the United States and the future target for 2020 is total disease eradication (USDHHS, 2010). All women of childbearing age should be screened (titer monitored) for rubella antibodies and those who are not immune should be immunized. Nurses inform women of childbearing age that antibody testing is recommended before pregnancy and that vaccination is available.

Another target of *Healthy People 2020* is to keep the incidence of hepatitis C stable at 0.2 new symptomatic cases in 100,000 people (USDHHS, 2010). Chronic hepatitis became a nationally reportable disease in 2003. Individuals most at risk are those who have injected illicit drugs, are undergoing hemodialysis, are seropositive for human immunodeficiency virus (HIV), or have elevated liver function studies.

Although most outbreaks of meningococcal disease are sporadic, young adults living in college/university dormitories or crowded conditions may be more susceptible than young adults not living in close settings. Although meningococci are sensitive to the penicillins and many antibiotics, the case fatality rate is high in otherwise healthy adults, and many survivors may have substantial neurological disabilities or loss of hearing. Most susceptible are college freshmen living in dormitories, who have a higher case ratio (Bilukha & Rosenstein, 2005; Wu, 2010). Approximately 44% of persons ages 13 to 15 years were vaccinated against meningococcal infection and the *Healthy People 2020* goal is more comprehensive coverage of 80% (USDHHS, 2010).

Other viral agents, such as genital herpes virus and human papilloma virus (HPV), commonly affect young adults. Genital herpes virus infections occur frequently in young adults because of the escalation of sexual activity during this period. HPV is spread through sexual contact, and some forms of the virus in combination with smoking are strongly related to the later development of cervical dysplasia and cancer. The prevalence of HPV infection is 45% among 20 to 24 year olds (Fontenot et al., 2007). The first vaccine to prevent cervical cancer, Gardasil® HPV vaccine, is effective against four types of the virus (HPV types 6, 11, 16, 18); it is available and is recommended for individuals from 9 to 26 years old. *Healthy People 2020* recommends three doses of HPV vaccine for females 13 to 15 years of age. Seventeen percent were vaccinated in 2008 and the target is 80% (USDHHS, 2010).

Pertussis (whooping cough) is part of the original vaccine series offered to infants. Since it is now known that the antibody titer protection for pertussis diminishes with age, pertussis vaccination is recommended with the 10-year tetanus booster injection. This newly formulated vaccine recommended for adults is known as Tdap (tetanus, diphtheria, acellular pertussis). Adults younger than 65 who have never received Tdap should substitute it for their next 10-year interval booster dose (www.cdc.gov/vaccines/pubs/vis/downloads/vis-td-tdap.pdf).

Nutritional-Metabolic Pattern

In the earlier *Healthy People 2010 Midcourse Review* (USDHHS, 2006), the sheer magnitude of the obesity problem is described and reinforced by the findings that none of the objectives in the Nutrition and Overweight section met or exceeded their targets. Obesity in the United States is attaining epidemic proportions and is a pressing public health problem. From 2005 to 2008, 30.8% of young adults 20 years and older were at a healthy weight and the target set for 2020 is 33.9% (USDHHS, 2010). It is unlikely that future overweight/obesity targets will be met, because lifestyle factors and nutritional habits within the American culture are difficult to change.

Most young adults value slimness, defined muscle tone, and athletic ability. Emphasis on body "thinness" seen in entertainment news can lead to improper eating. Regular physical activity increases muscle and bone strength, decreases body fat, aids in weight control, enhances well-being, and reduces depression (USDHHS, 2010). Physical activity levels are positively influenced by structural environments, such as sidewalks, bike lanes, and parks, and by legislative policies that improve access to physical activity facilities (USDHHS, 2010). An optimally functioning basal metabolic rate in the young adult allows for adequate oxygen intake during normal activity and rest periods. A young adult male requires approximately 1600 to 1800 calories a day to meet his body's basal metabolic needs, and a young adult female only 1200 to 1450 calories a day. After growth in height stops in the late teens, the basal metabolic rate declines.

During the young adult years, caloric intake increases substantially, particularly in men. Increased caloric intake without a corresponding increase in energy expenditure can lead to obesity, which is a precursor to hypertension, coronary disease, and diabetes.

According to information from 2005 to 2008, 17.4% of children and adolescents ages 6 to 19 years were overweight or obese and 30.8% of adults age 20 and older were obese (USDHHS, 2010).

Although trends toward increasing weight occurred in all major racial and ethnic groups, the increase was more pronounced in the White non-Hispanic population (32.1%) and the Mexican American population (23.7%) (USDHHS, 2010). In the same survey period, the prevalence of obesity among males age 20 years and older was 26.2% and in 20-year-old females and older was 35.1% (USDHHS, 2010). To stop or decrease these trends, new lifestyle behaviors must be practiced, learned, and adopted for nutrition and physical activity.

For many Americans, food sources are abundant, portion sizes have increased, and lifestyles are becoming increasingly sedentary. More specifically, young adult diets should contain a variety of nutrient-dense foods, especially whole grains, fruits, vegetables, low-fat or fat-free milk, lean meats, and protein sources. Caloric intake and the intake of saturated and trans fats, cholesterol, added sugars, sodium, and alcohol should be limited. Food-label information (now includes trans fats) should be read on all processed and packaged foods. Another challenge is the increasing consumption of food prepared and eaten away from home, which is generally higher in fats, cholesterol, and sodium, and lower in fiber and calcium than that prepared in the home (USDHHS, 2010). This suggests that the composition of food prepared outside the home promotes weight gain (Frank, 2007). Many states have legislation pending that would require restaurants and fast food outlets to list food composition on menus (Frank, 2007). Collective national action and community involvement are needed to promote healthful diets among all Americans and to reverse the increasing trend to be overweight and obese. With increased obesity and its associated health problems, there will be more access to better pharmaceuticals and increased use of bariatric surgery, although these treatments also must be evaluated for risks and benefits (Burke & Wang, 2011). Young adults, in particular, are influenced by the body shapes of celebrities, and "celebrity worship" may be an important motivator to seeking change in body shape and plastic surgery alternatives (Maltby & Day, 2011).

Health professionals are counseled to investigate weight problems by monitoring waist circumference measurement, blood pressure level, cholesterol levels, and activity levels rather than solely monitoring weight, to the frustration of many people. Assessments are made of weight and height to calculate body mass index (BMI). Those with a BMI of 25 or less (male waist size of 40 inches or less, women 35 inches or less) should have weight maintenance teaching. Individuals with a BMI of 30 or greater who have tried diets and exercise may be considered for weight-reducing drugs (CDC, 2010; LeBlanc et al., 2011). A BMI of 40 or more meets the criteria for bariatric surgery in psychologically stable individuals. In persons with comorbidity, bariatric surgery may be suggested with a BMI of 35 or greater (CDC, 2010; LeBlanc et al., 2011). The focus of professional advice is conservative at first, recommending careful diet appraisal and increase in exercise patterns. Repetitions will probably be necessary, because long-term weight management is a frustrating process. In 2005 to 2006, 30.8% of adults older than age 20 were within healthy weight guidelines and the target for 2020 is 33.9% (USDHHS, 2010). Changing the upward obesity trend is one of the most difficult goals to achieve (Jiang et al., 2011).

Proper nutrition is particularly necessary for the young adult female during the childbearing years. Contributing factors to iron deficiency in this age group are regular loss of blood (during menses) and pregnancy. The prevalence of anemia in women of childbearing potential was 24.5% in 2003 to 2006 and the 2020 target is 22.1% (USDHHS, 2010) (see Case Study and Care Plan at the end of this chapter). A blood loss of 2 to 4 mL per day (1 to 2 mg of iron) can cause iron deficiency anemia; young women who do not eat a healthy diet and have heavy periods or use nonsteroidal antiinflammatory drugs are specifically at risk for iron deficiency anemia. Iron supplementation is recommended during pregnancy for optimal growth of the fetus and supporting structures (Perry et al., 2010). The CDC and USDHHS (2010) recommend that all women of childbearing age consume 0.4 mg of folic acid daily to reduce the risk of **fetal neural tube defects (FND)**, including spina bifida. Supplementation should include at least the month before pregnancy and the first trimester during pregnancy. The CDC and Food and Drug Administration recommend folic acid fortification of food to prevent neural tube defects (USDHHS, 2010). In the years 2003 to 2006, only 23.8% of nonpregnant females ages 15 to 44 reported a daily intake of folic acid of 400 mcg from fortified foods or dietary supplements and the target for 2020 is 26% (USDHHS, 2010). Efforts are also being made to reduce health disparities in neural tube defects including the use of better communication modalities with the Hispanic population and other groups that have higher rates of neural tube defects (USDHHS, 2010).

Most adolescents and adult women fail to meet their calcium requirements, placing them at risk for osteoporosis and bone fractures in later life. Low calcium intake is a direct result of low milk consumption related to soft drink ingestion. An increase in calcium-containing foods is therefore recommended, particularly for teens and young women (see Chapter 11).

Elimination Pattern

Patterns of elimination are generally well established by young adulthood. Although eating disorders (anorexia and bulimia) typically begin at an earlier stage of development, they can persist during young adulthood. The fashion industry is widely criticized for using underweight women as young female models, thereby emphasizing excessive thinness as the ideal female standard. Assessment of young adults is directed toward teaching about the common complaints of constipation, hemorrhoids, and occasional diarrhea. Although the risk of colon cancer is low in this age group, young adults should be aware that changes in elimination patterns or blood in the stool should be reported to their primary care provider. Young adults should be counseled about drinking adequate amounts of fluid and eating fruits and vegetables, which are sources of fiber, to promote bowel health.

Activity-Exercise Pattern

Inactivity is a predisposing factor to cardiovascular disease and obesity; increasing access to and promoting locations for physical activity are increasingly emphasized. A *Healthy People 2020* goal is to reduce the proportion of adults who engage in no leisure-time physical activity to 32.6% from approximately 36.2% in 2008, and to increase the proportion of adults who engage in moderate physical activity for 150 minutes a week to 47.9% from 43.5% in 2008 (USDHHS, 2010).

Aerobic exercise, in which oxygen is metabolized to produce energy, develops an optimally functioning cardiorespiratory system. Aerobic conditioning achieves cardiovascular fitness through five periods of moderately intense exercise weekly for about 30 minutes or more (Physical Activity and Public Health, 2007; USDHHS, 2010) at a heart rate of approximately 220 minus the age of the person multiplied by 65% to 85%. Although this formula is controversial and there may be individual variations, it seems a reasonable first approach. Young adults are encouraged to engage in fitness activities that increase the heart rate to approximately 150 or more beats per minute. After 5 minutes of activity at this rate, the body is required to make adjustments in cardiovascular capacity by enlarging the lungs and the capillaries in the muscles and the heart. Repeated aerobic exercise, such as swimming, cycling, running, skipping rope, and walking, produces physical fitness and decreases the likelihood of problems caused by inactivity. Muscle-strengthening activities should also be stressed. The major barriers to increasing physical activity seem to be lack of time, lack of access to exercise facilities, and inability to find safe environments in which to exercise (USDHHS, 2010).

Radiation and Excessive Sun Exposure

Nurses need to educate young adults about the risks of sun exposure and tanning, the preventive use of sun-blocking agents, and the awareness of skin symptoms that might indicate cancer. Sun-blocking agents reduce sunburn or other skin damage with the goal of lowering the risk of skin cancer. A number of the agents are rated based on skin type and sensitivity to burning. Many lotions and creams are available with differing radiation protection levels. Sunscreen protective factor (SPF) index is a calculation of the effectiveness of various preparations. The agents are rated on a scale by the U.S. Food and Drug Administration (FDA). For example, a rating of 30 means the sunscreen provides 30 times the protection of unprotected skin. Newer guidelines for sunscreen protection were adopted for June 2012 by the FDA. New sunscreens should provide broad-spectrum protection, sun protection factor (SPF) of 30 or greater, and water resistance (American Academy of Dermatology, 2011). Women's makeup preparations and moisturizers now include sun-blocking agents. Young adults should avoid sunbathing during the 2-hour period before and after noon, because two thirds of the day's ultraviolet light comes through the earth's atmosphere during this time. Ultraviolet light is stronger at different times of the day depending on geographical location. Sunscreens that block both ultraviolet A (UVA) and ultraviolet B (UVB) light are more effective in preventing cancer than those that block only ultraviolet B light (American Academy of Dermatology, 2011). Best protection is achieved by applying agents 15 to 30 minutes before exposure, and then reapplying every 15 to 30 minutes during exposure to the sun. Further application may be necessary if activities involve swimming, sweating, or rubbing of skin. Sun-protective measures such as use of sunscreen, utilization of sun-protective clothing, and avoidance of ultraviolet light are an essential part of young adult education.

Sports

Bicycling and motorcycling are encouraged by environmentalists to decrease automobile pollution; this trend is also promoted to relieve traffic congestion, avoid the high costs of fuel and car maintenance, and increase interest in healthy exercise. Cyclists are at risk of being involved in accidents with automobiles. Head injury is responsible for many bicycle-related fatalities. In 2009, only 19 states had mandatory helmet requirements for riders under 15 years of age (USDHHS, 2010). Bicycle helmets are believed to be the single most effective preventive measure available to decrease the incidence of brain and head injury (USDHHS, 2010).

Motorcycles have less occupant protection than do automobiles but are appealing to young adults, primarily because they have high-performance and speed capabilities. Using a motorcycle helmet reduces the chance of dying in an accident by 29% (USDHHS, 2006). A target of *Healthy People 2020* is to increase the proportion of motorcyclists using helmets from 67% in 2009 to 74% in 2020 (USDHHS, 2010).

Accidental deaths from drowning are also common in young adults. USDHHS (2010) estimates 1.2 drownings/100,000 population occurred in 2007. Swimming, boating, and scuba diving are associated with the high number of water-related fatalities. Hang gliding, parachuting, and flying small aircraft are responsible for a large number of outdoor fatalities. Mountain climbing, hiking in poor weather conditions, downhill ski racing, and bobsledding are other hazardous activities. Most so-called accidents are not random, uncontrollable events, but predictable and preventable if precautions and risks are analyzed (USDHHS, 2010).

Amateur and professional sports activities generally pose few hazards when rules and safety precautions are observed. Relatively few fatalities are associated with the professionally organized contact sports, such as football, hockey, or boxing, but chronic injuries can cause degenerative brain diseases. In 2008, 45.6 medically consulted injuries occurred per 1000 population and the target for 2020 is 41/1000 population (USDHHS, 2010). Also in 2009, Boston University researchers (Daniloff, 2010) and other investigators linked sports-related head injuries to an increased risk of dementia, memory-related diseases, and chronic traumatic encephalopathy (CTE). This has resulted in significant changes in professional National Football League policies and sports concussion protocols. Many of these policy changes have been adopted for college, high school, and amateur sports programs (Daniloff, 2010).

A comprehensive history of recreational activities alerts the nurse to specific needs about safety education. Young adults are encouraged to learn and abide by the rules of the sport in which they are engaged. Rules in many sports have evolved from health and safety concerns, enabling the individual to learn the sport well with appropriate instruction.

Sleep-Rest Pattern

Young adults are subject to fatigue induced by work, stress, or inactivity. Changes in activity or stressors can help reduce fatigue. Attempting new and challenging tasks can help reduce mental stress. New physical activities, such as learning a new sport or form of exercise, can also provide stimulation.

Cognitive-Perceptual Pattern

Physical and Mental Patterns

Visual acuity is highest at approximately age 20 and begins to decline at approximately age 40, when farsightedness frequently develops. Hearing is also best at age 20; the ability to distinguish high-pitched tones decreases with age. The other senses—taste, smell, touch, and awareness of temperature and pain—remain stable until age 45 to 50.

Further maturation requires young adults to learn skills and behaviors that improve the performance abilities gained as adolescents. Factors that an individual young adult may perceive as essential to learn will depend on specific goals, values, attitudes, and practices as influenced by intrinsic (constitutional) and extrinsic (environmental or community) factors. Executive decision-making becomes more developed: calculation of risks versus rewards, prioritizing, self-evaluation, self-correction, and long-term planning become more sophisticated. The development of intellectual maturity influences the selection of behaviors and attitudes that affect health and well-being practices.

Piaget's Theory

Jean Piaget's stage of formal operational thought evolves from concrete operational thought in adolescence and extends through the reasoning process of young adults (Piaget, 1972). Achievement of formal operational thinking allows a person to analyze all combinations of possibilities and construct hypotheses that can be tested. Young adult thought becomes more perceptive and insightful; issues can therefore be evaluated realistically and objectively. Young adults are energetic and can therefore contribute substantially to social and occupational decision-making. Although they tend to take greater risks, young adults typically demonstrate the use of appropriate reasoning, anticipation, and analytical approaches.

Intellectual Growth

Organization of information influences memory. Evidence shows that recall performance diminishes with age: at its peak in the twenties, memory starts to diminish during the thirties. Improved strategies for organization of information, however, can enhance recall, and limitation of memory with increasing age is likely a result of retrieval rather than storage mechanisms.

Erikson's Theory

A major goal for young adults is the development of an increased sense of competency and self-esteem (Erikson, 1993). In developing self-esteem, the individual learns to be truly open and capable of trust through the formation of intimate relationships that are characteristic of this period. In Erikson's classic theory (1993) this stage is described as a phase of psychosocial development termed intimacy versus isolation and loneliness.

Erikson's concept of genuine intimacy extends beyond sexual relations to a broader view of mutual psychosocial intimacy with a spouse or lover, parents, children, and friends. Characterized by the reciprocal expression of affection, intimacy requires mutual trust. These interchanges are spontaneous for the young adult; relationships should be free and allow for self-disclosure. Young adults who are unsure of their identity may avoid intimate contact or engage in promiscuous behavior lacking in true intimacy, which can result in isolation and consequent self-absorption. Healthy adults search for continuity, regularity, or unity of meaningful relationships, while avoiding situations of little commitment.

Moral Development

Young adults who have successfully mastered the previous cognitive, social, and moral stages are usually able to recognize or use principled reasoning. Lawrence Kohlberg identifies this ability as the postconventional level of moral reasoning (Kohlberg & Lickons, 1986). During this phase, the individual is able to differentiate the self from the rules and expectations of others and to define principles regarding rights in terms of self-chosen principles. The interests of individuals can be weighed against the needs of society and the state, and violations of law can be justified when individual interests are in accord with principles. Gilligan (1982, 2002, 2011), who studied the development of moral reasoning in women and girls, asserts that their moral judgments reflect less of a "rights" perspective and more of an emphasis on responsibilities in relationships. Newer framing of this theory of women's emotions and relationships is now essential to understanding intelligence and self-awareness (Gilligan, 2011).

Although development of principled moral reasoning is possible during young adulthood, it may never occur if the cognitive and social factors that stimulate higher reasoning are not present. Acts of personal violence representative of lower moral reasoning should not be present; however, such acts do occur during this period, illustrating the need for addressing moral developmental concerns at earlier stages of education and socialization.

Self-Perception–Self-Concept Pattern

In non-Western cultures the entrance to adulthood generally is defined and marked by social events such as marriage. In Western societies, maturation is defined through the individual's achievement of financial and residential independence, and is a more drawn-out, gradual process. Two emotional themes regarding the value of work become evident during young adulthood. During their twenties, young adults yearn to explore and experiment, keeping structures temporary and reversible. These individuals may move from job to job and relationship to relationship, remaining in a transient state. At the opposite extreme is the urge to prepare for the future by making firm commitments. During this period, both men and women question their value to society, the merit of their accomplishments, their success as sexual beings, and the probability of attaining their unfulfilled goals.

The U.S. Census Bureau (2011) reports that more than 74.7% of women ages 25 to 35 were employed in 2010; this percentage is expected to be about the same (74.2%) in 2018. As more mothers enter the labor force, the need for child care increases. The gap in earnings, or pay differential, between men and women is also significant. Recent legislation signed by President Barack Obama ensures women equal pay in the workforce. Access to insurance and retirement benefits is not always available, especially to high-risk groups such as minorities or people receiving the minimum wage. Even when there is sufficient access to health care, some types of employment expose individuals to occupational risks and hazards.

Many young adults are high achievers and seek opportunities to be challenged. Employment problems can be stressful and traumatic to an individual's self-esteem and self-worth, particularly in the current economic environment. The failure to receive a promotion or a pay raise can accelerate the degree of stress. Employment is more than a source of income; it provides self-esteem and social interaction. Because the adjustment to the job market influences many other aspects of daily living, young adults frequently require assistance in developing coping mechanisms to manage stress. Properly managing the initial stress prevents further complications that can arise if the young adult uses unhealthy stress relievers such as alcohol or drugs.

Young women have many of the same concerns about employment and success as do young men. Many young women postpone childbearing until they have established their careers; many are absent from the job for only a standard maternity leave. Women who return to work when their children are very young frequently risk the emotional strain caused by guilt feelings and role strain. In addition to helping parents cope with the stress of being absent from their children, nurses can help them identify ways to provide high-quality supervision in their absence, either through private baby-sitters, through day care programs, or through neighbors, friends, and relatives.

The U.S. workforce is changing dramatically as companies restructure, downsize, "right size," and shift employees around to meet changing market conditions, company mergers, and buyouts. The nature of work is changing with a continued trend toward longer hours, increased use of contracted and temporary workers, and increased telecommuting (USDHHS, 2010). There is increasing concern about "globalization," outsourcing, and jobs, especially in the computer industry, moving overseas. Since the recession began in the fall of 2008, overall unemployment rates have been higher than 9%; young adults, particularly recent college graduates, have been particularly affected (Rampell, 2011). This lower paying employment trajectory may last for years. New hires may start at lower salaries and begin their employed years with firms who pay less or have less potential for advancement. Nursing interventions in employment and industrial settings are directed toward improving both working conditions and employer-employee relationships. Healthy work sites increase the chance that young adults will have access to comprehensive health-promotion programs.

Roles-Relationships Pattern

Young adult friendships are more enduring than are earlier relationships. The focus of the relationship is the sharing of feelings or confidences as well as common interests. True friendship is characteristic of a person who wants to give rather than receive. Friendships are necessary in a constantly changing society; they provide a source of emotional support and a basis of stability for developing the self-concept. Social networking services such as Facebook, MySpace, and Twitter allow young adults to interact quickly with one another to organize events and share photos,

experiences, thoughts, and perceptions. Some young adults use Internet dating services to widen their pool of possible significant other prospects.

Establishing interpersonal relationships involves agreeable and purposeful interactions with others. Interpersonal relationships can be created with people of the same or the opposite sex; there tend to be more friendships with individuals of the opposite sex. Age is typically a less important factor than it was during adolescence. The formation of intimate relationships develops within or outside a family context and occasionally in the work environment. High-speed (4G) cell phone and wireless Internet access facilitate maintenance of relationships through text messaging, e-mail, and instant messaging.

For some the significant other is a person of the same sex. Coming to realization that a significant other is of the same sex often causes emotional upheaval and distress. Same-sex marriage (also known as gay marriage) legislative proposals are active in many states; these would legitimize the legal rights of same-sex couples through same-sex marriage or civil union statutes. Currently six states (mostly in the northeast) and the District of Columbia allow same-sex marriage. Proposals favoring same-sex marriage argue that civil recognition reduces the legal discrimination involved in such unions. Major resistance to legalization of same-sex marriage comes from individuals who note that historically the term "marriage" has been reserved for a union between a man and a woman. This issue has been fiercely debated politically and is currently the subject of court and jurisdictional challenges.

One example of the types of services available to gay and lesbian persons is the multidisciplinary educational program at the Tanger Center sponsored by the Lesbian and Gay Advisory Committee at Beth Israel Deaconess Medical Center in Boston. In 2004, Massachusetts became the first state to implement legislation allowing marriage between individuals of the same sex. The following are some educational topics offered at the Tanger Center: understanding the dynamics of the workplace and openness about being "out at work"; sensitivity training about the wording of forms and materials used in the workplace; building a trusting and comfortable health care communication dialogue between health care providers and gay and lesbian persons; and supporting and communicating with a gay or lesbian child.

In addition to achieving intimacy, the young adult must accomplish other developmental tasks to achieve true psychosocial maturation (Figure 22-3). Decision-making about life and career directions is the developmental milestone that heralds the transition from adolescence to adulthood. Decisions usually entail establishing independence from the family of origin. This transition may involve an actual physical move from the parents' home (going away to college, joining the military, or getting an apartment); however, movement away is not the sole indicator of independence. Young adults frequently remain in their parents' home for economic reasons, particularly when life choices involve continued schooling, unemployment, or remaining unmarried. In some cultures, unmarried adults live with their parents until they are married, and newly married

FIGURE 22-3 Young adults enjoy gathering in a local café to socialize together.

young adults share the home of their parents until they begin having their own children.

Young adults, including college graduates, are facing the highest unemployment rates since the Great Depression. A greater proportion of young adults are enrolled in higher education than ever before (Pew Research Center, 2012). Many low-income young adults are enrolled at for-profit institutions, which has become the fastest growing sector of U.S. higher education (Institute for Higher Education Policy, 2011). Since college loan repayment typically begins 6 months after graduation, new graduates have to face the harsh realities of trying to find employment and ways to begin repayment. Some reports indicate that up to 85% of new graduates are moving home (Byrne, 2011). Others will start or attend graduate school to wait out the recession.

Individuals in the later years of this age group typically choose life partners and begin families; they make decisions about childbearing and the number and education of children. Additional consideration must be given to decisions related to childbearing, such as finances, safety, family support, housing, the relationship with extended family members, and the roles and responsibilities within the nuclear family unit. Young adults who are establishing a family must have open communication about self-development, which includes issues of dual careers, childrearing practices, and domestic duties.

Family harmony and development are major goals for many young adults. Although family size and structure have undergone dramatic changes in recent decades, concern about each member's health and safety continues to be a primary focus. Family life is influenced by the qualities of individual family members. Typically, economic security, status, place in the community, and healthy patterns of living, such as good nutrition, personal hygiene, and physical fitness, are associated with healthy family adjustment.

Separation and Divorce

About one half of marriages terminate in divorce (U.S. Census Bureau, 2011). About one quarter of all children in the United States are living in single-parent, mother-led families, and one

---

✳ BOX 22-4 INNOVATIVE PRACTICE

Use of Internet and Mobile Phone Delivery Systems to Deliver Behavioral Components for STD/HIV Prevention

The use of technology is changing practice patterns and the way that health communications may be transmitted. The transference of technology has often been slowed by the reluctance of policymakers, administrators, providers, advocates, or consumers. Some biomedical innovations for sexually transmitted diseases (STDs) and HIV prevention have been adopted (such as use of electronic health records and cell phones/Internet to trace contacts), but full compliance by the person seeking care is often hindered by behavioral factors. Technological interventions allow behavioral supports and educational programs to be delivered with less cost and more convenience. These include STD/HIV testing and partner interventions, behavioral interventions, self-management strategies, and provider care information. These technological interventions have been demonstrated to be as effective as face-to-face interventions. Text messaging is also possible. Over the next years, smartphones will be more widely used, connecting many individuals domestically and globally. This will allow the dissemination of more active engaging STD/HIV treatment.

Data from Swendeman, D., & Rotheram-Borus, M. J. (2010). Innovation in sexually transmitted disease and HIV prevention: Internet and mobile phone delivery vehicles for global diffusion. *Current Opinion in Psychiatry, 23*(2), 139-144; Clutter, P. C. (2009). AHRQ healthcare exchange: Promoting adoption of innovations. *Critical Care Nursing Quarterly, 32*(1), 62-68.

half of the children affected by divorce frequently never see their fathers again. Many stressors contribute to divorce. It is a difficult process, and lingering anger and hostility may remain for years. Socioeconomic factors often place unreasonable stress on marriages. Age at the time of marriage is correlated with duration of marriage, and young adults whose parents have divorced have an increased rate of divorce. Employment has enabled women to leave unhappy marriages that they formerly would have been forced to tolerate.

Although dissatisfaction and unhappiness are frequent precursors to separation and divorce, the decision to dissolve a marriage is not easy. Considerable emotional strain exists for both partners, their children, their families, and close friends. Divorce requires that young adults reevaluate their basic values, individual personality, spiritual beliefs, and ego strength, job potential, and socioeconomic factors to ensure future security for themselves and their children. Divorced young adults frequently suffer severe emotional strain and depression. Some young adults are unable to adjust to role and status changes and to threats of self-concept. For these reasons, support systems in the form of groups, individual counseling, or special social activities are critical (Box 22-4: Innovative Practice). As a result of divorce, many women and their young children are forced to seek emergency shelter in publicly operated homes, including welfare hotels and group shelters.

Many people need support from the nurse to help them work through this difficult period. Nurses help to identify the feelings of guilt, grief, and loss that young adults experience during a separation or divorce. Suggesting that young adults read articles or books on issues related to divorce is helpful, because they provide a reference point for their experiences. The nurse recommends marital counseling by a qualified professional; this may be the most beneficial source of support.

Male and Female Risk of Violence

Violence is a global and national health problem. Violent deaths are intentional deaths that occur from physical force or power exerted against self, others, or a community (CDC, 2011a). Although the World Trade Center bombing in 2001 and violent events in other countries such as Iraq and Afghanistan are examples of organized terrorism, worldwide only about one fifth of violent acts are related to organized events. The overthrow of governments in the Middle East in Egypt and Libya was largely accomplished by young adults. Young adults can be involved as both the perpetrators and the victims of violence.

In the United States, there are about 51,000 violent deaths a year, and these deaths affect all Americans not only in emotional terms (from the preanticipated death) but also through additional medical costs and lost employment productivity (CDC, 2011a). Domestically, in the United States, the recipients of violence may be older adults, children, and women with whom they are familiar (USDHHS, 2010). Identification, education, and strategies to prevent bullying, dating violence, and sexual violence among young adults require more dissemination (USDHHS, 2010). Homicide (assault) is the second leading cause of death in the 15-year-old to 24-year-old age group and the leading cause of death for Black men in the same age category (U.S. Census Bureau, 2011). Between 1999 and 2007, the homicide rate has remained fairly static at 6.1 deaths/100,000 population; this is a significant decline from the rate seen in the early 1990s and there are ongoing efforts to understand what has contributed to the improvement (USDHHS, 2010). Firearms are involved in approximately two thirds of these deaths, and men have twice the risk of dying as do women (U.S. Census Bureau, 2011). When compared with the general population, mortality statistics are higher for men in poorer populations, in urban areas, and with less formal education. Homicide is closely associated with alcohol and drug abuse and frequently is related to other violent acts, such as robbery. Other risk factors include history of loss of employment, detention or prison experience, access to firearms, abuse in the home, mental illness, social isolation, and homelessness. The presence of firearms in the home is associated with the increased risk of unintentional and intentional injury to children. A target in *Healthy People 2020* is to reduce firearm-related deaths from 10.2 per 100,000 population in 2007 to 9.2 per 100,000 population and to reduce the number of nonfatal firearm-related injuries from 20.7 per 100,000 (USDHHS, 2010). The firearm-related death rate for young Black men and boys was nearly five times the rate for young White men and boys.

Intimate partner violence has serious health consequences for women and men; however, because of social and legal factors, it is probably the most underreported form of abuse (Box 22-5: Hot Topics). Abuse crosses all socioeconomic, racial, ethnic, religious, gender, and age boundaries. About 3 in 10 women and 1 in 10 men during their lifetime reported intimate partner violence or abuse. Women reported higher lifetime and recent-year

intimate partner violence than men (Black et al., 2011; Breiding et al., 2008). Nurses and other primary health care providers often fail to assess, detect, or treat violence or abuse in an optimal manner, and more efforts must be made to recognize the scope of the problem and to provide appropriate counseling (Box 22-5: Hot Topics). Physical assaults by intimate partners decreased in the last decade; this improvement is attributed to increased economic opportunities for women, increasing age at first marriage, and better access to domestic violence services. A target in *Healthy People 2020* is to reduce the rate of physical assault to 14.7 assaults per 1000 from 16.3 assaults recorded in 2008 (USDHHS, 2010).

Sexuality-Reproductive Pattern

By young adulthood the menstrual cycle generally is well established in the woman. Cyclical hormonal function is responsible for regularity of the cycle and normal functioning of the ovaries and uterus. The normal duration of menses is 4 to 5 days (range of 2 to 7 days, with a blood loss of 40 mL). Blood loss of greater than 80 mL per cycle is abnormal and may lead to anemia. Irregularities such as painful menstruation, premenstrual syndrome, and prolonged or heavy bleeding need further assessment. Although these problems are not always abnormal, the symptoms and the individual's reaction to them can signal functional disorders and the need for further investigation and treatment.

Reproductive Problems

Infertility is defined as the lack of conception in the presence of unprotected sexual intercourse for at least 12 months. Approximately 10% to 15% of couples of reproductive age in the United States are believed to be infertile (Perry et al., 2010). Infertility has become more of a public issue since the advance of assistive reproductive technologies, such as in vitro fertilization and gamete intrafallopian transfer, which can enable couples with known reproductive problems to conceive children. These technologies frequently create great stress for the couple and often result in marital conflicts and distress. Generally, infertility is not an issue for those 18 to 25 years old (peak fertility ages are 20 to 35); however, after the age of 30 infertility is a more frequent finding and in vitro fertilization or some type of assisted reproductive strategy may be indicated.

Common problems of the male reproductive system include orchitis, epididymitis, and varicoceles and hydroceles. Mumps in the postpubertal male can cause swelling of the tests, orchitis, and subfertility. External conditions such as fungal infections, contact dermatitis, and eczema; parasites such as scabies and lice; and nonvenereal diseases such as erysipelas, abscesses, and fistulas can occur in the scrotum.

Unintended Pregnancy

According to the U.S. Census Bureau (2011), the teen birth rate in the United States has been dropping since 1990. Improved child health and development is associated with healthy planned pregnancies (USDHHS, 2010). Unwanted or unplanned pregnancies can be a considerable source of stress to young adults. Unintended pregnancy is an important public

Intimate Partner and Family Violence

Assessing the Problem

Epidemiological researchers have attempted to determine the risks for intimate partner and family violence. Intimate partner violence includes four behaviors: physical violence, sexual violence, threats of physical or sexual violence, and/or emotional abuse. Understanding the roots of partner violence has been more difficult than ascertaining determinants of physical disease. Victims of family violence usually are children, female spouse, intimate partners, and the elderly (Black et al., 2011). Factors associated with intimate partner violence include young age, low income, pregnancy, mental health problems, separation or divorce, and history of abuse (U.S. Preventive Services Task Force, 2010). The unequal position of women in a relationship and the manner in which conflict is managed, as well as differences in education and prestige associated with the partners' occupations, are related to risk of violence. Domestic violence is a problem in all age, ethnic, and religious groups; in some cultures attitudes toward women even legitimize the practice. Women who have gained positions of respect and power outside the home through activities in their neighborhood or community are less likely to be abused. In men and women, viewing abuse as a child increases the likelihood that abusive behaviors are used by these same individuals as adults (Landenburger & Campbell, 2012).

Are Nurses Willing to Take Action?

Some studies indicate that nurses have been reluctant to take action regarding violence against women or men. Some of the traditional reasons for not taking action are based on paternalistic attitudes, in which the victim is blamed for her part in the social situation that becomes violent. Nursing's strong advocacy stance and emphasis on the communication of nonjudgmental, genuine concern should provide a strong foundation to avoid blaming the victim and to focus on pathological factors that have been identified by much of the health profession's research in this area.

How Can Nurses Recognize Abuse?

Research demonstrates that nurses should be more aware of indicators of partner violence (U.S. Preventive Services Task Force, 2010). These include the presence, as revealed by a health history, of separation or divorce, alcoholism, frequent verbal disagreements, and high levels of conflict. Other warning signs include repeated visits to the emergency departments, complaints of headaches or backaches, psychiatric illness, and incidents of bruises, sprains, and lacerations. Abusers are more likely to have hostile personality styles with aggressive tendencies. As children, they may have had unattainable goals, and their achievements may have been met with harsh criticism and toxic and depersonalizing behavior (Landenburger & Campbell, 2012). Abusers also may use passive aggressive tactics, turning passive withdrawal and blaming behaviors against the helping individual in an effort to portray the abuser as a victim. Currently, the U.S. Preventive Services Task Force does not recommend additional routine screening for intimate partner violence.

What Do You Think?

- Are nurses less than helpful in their detection and management of domestic violence? Why do you think this occurs?
- Are nurses, because of their education and sensitization to people with mental problems, more or less likely than others to experience violence in their own domestic settings? Explain.

Sources: U.S. Preventive Services Task Force. (2010). *Guide to clinical preventive services*. Rockville, MD: Agency for Healthcare Research and Quality. Retrieved April 28, 2012, from www.ahrq.gov/clinic/pocketgd1011/gcp10s2c.htm#Family; Black, M. C., Basile, K. C., Breiding, M. J., Smith, S. G., Walters, M. L., Merrick, M. T., et al. (2011). *National Intimate Partner and Sexual Violence Survey (NISVS): 2010 Summary Report*. Atlanta, GA: National Center for Injury Prevention and Control, Centers for Disease Control and Prevention; Landenburger, K. M., & Campbell, J. C. (2012). Violence and human abuse. In M. Stanhope & J. Lancaster (Eds.), *Public health nursing: Population-centered health care in the community* (pp. 828-853). Maryland Heights, MO: Elsevier.

health issue and can be related to increased risks of delayed prenatal care, depression, and other personal and relationship problems (USDHHS, 2010). Family planning is one of the biggest public health achievements of the twentieth century. Despite the advent of modern contraceptives, unintended pregnancy remains a persistent problem. Approximately half of all pregnancies are intended (USDHHS, 2010); in 2002, 51% of all pregnancies among females ages 15 to 44 years were intended and the target for the United States in 2020 is 56%. Although most young adults consider family planning services as an essential basic health service, health insurance plans historically have tried to manage and limit such services (USDHHS, 2010); currently, about 86% of employment-based health plans cover contraceptive supplies and equipment (USDHHS, 2010). The current lower pregnancy rates among teens seem to result from more involvement in school activities, contracts between young unmarried couples, effective birth control and pregnancy prevention programs, and expanding job opportunities.

Approximately half of unintended pregnancies are the result of contraceptive failure (Kaplan, 2007). Both married and unmarried young adults need information about contraceptives (Table 22-2) to decrease the number of unwanted pregnancies and the need for abortions. The nurse's role in contraceptive counseling involves helping individuals to choose the method most appropriate to their needs (PDR staff, 2008). New and improved contraceptive agents are continually becoming available, so the nurse continues to learn about current information; for example, two types of intrauterine devices are now available, the ParaGard T 380A (copper) and the Mirena hormonal device (levonorgesterol-releasing), and once inserted they are 99% effective (Kaplan, 2007). Laws and policies in some settings restrict nurses and other health care providers from engaging in certain types of counseling, including providing abortion information. Increasing the proportion of publically funded planning clinics is also important. In 2003, 38.3% of publically funded planning clinics offered the full range of FDA-approved methods and the target for 2020 is 47.9%, a 25% improvement (USDHHS, 2010).

Emergency contraception (EC) can reduce the number of unintended pregnancies. In 2003, 79.7% of family planning clinics offered emergency contraception and the target is 87.7% for 2020, a 10% improvement (USDHHS, 2010). There is a generic two-dose form, Next Choice, and a one-dose form, Plan B One-Step (Teva®). Both require a prescription for girls under 17. The FDA approved over the counter use for women of all ages reporting that Plan B One-Step is safe and effective.

TABLE 22-2 SUMMARY OF EFFECTIVENESS, RISKS, AND NONCONTRACEPTIVE BENEFITS OF SELECTED CONTRACEPTIVE METHODS

CONTRACEPTIVE METHOD	RISKS OF USE	NONCONTRACEPTIVE HEALTH BENEFITS
OCs (combined and progestin only)	Thromboembolic disorders, CVA, coronary artery disease especially with smoking, hypertension, diabetes, breast cancer	Reduced risk of functional pelvic inflammation, endometriosis, uterine fibroids, endometrial cancer, ovarian cancer, iron deficiency anemia, ectopic pregnancy, irregular cycles
Transdermal (contraceptive patch)	Similar to OCs	Easy verification of presence, weekly application
Implants (Implanon, single rod)	Similar to OCs, data more limited	Similar to OCs, data more limited
Injectable progestin (Depo-Provera)	Prolonged amenorrhea, venous thrombosis, thromboembolism	Bone loss especially in adolescents, unsure of lifetime risk of osteoporosis
Vaginal ring (NuvaRing)	Probably similar to OCs, but data more limited	Low-dose hormonal option
Intrauterine contraceptive device (IUD)	Bleeding, anemia, difficult removal, PID, ectopic pregnancy, cramping	Reduced risk of anemia, low cost for long term
Emergency contraception (Next Choice, Plan B One-Step)	Nausea, abdominal pain, delay of menses	Not for routine use
Diaphragm	Toxic shock syndrome, allergy to latex or spermicide, urinary tract infection	Reduced risk of vaginitis, cervicitis
Condom	Allergy to rubber, latex, or spermicide	Reduced risk of STD and HIV transmission
Spermicides*	Sensitivity to agent	Antiviral activity against HPV, decreased activity of other STDs, decreased risk of PID
Sponge	Toxic shock syndrome	Decreased activity of STD organisms
Female sterilization (tubal ligation)	Anesthesia, infection, hemorrhage	One-time procedure
Male sterilization (vasectomy)	Complication rates low, reversal may be difficult	One-time procedure

From Hatcher, R. A., Trussell, J., Nelson, A. L., Cates, W., Kowal, D., & Policar, M. (2011). *Contraceptive technology* (20th ed.). West Sussex, England: Bridge the Gap Foundation.
CVA, Cerebrovascular accident; HIV, human immunodeficiency virus; HPV, human papillomavirus; OCs, oral contraceptives; PID, pelvic inflammatory disease; STD, sexually transmitted disease.
*Often used in combination with other methods.

However, the Health and Human Services Commissioner overruled the FDA findings (December, 2011); for the present, girls 16 and younger must talk to a health provider before obtaining a prescription. Emergency contraception must be started within three days of unprotected sex; it works by either altering tubal transport of either sperm or ova, or inhibiting implantation. It will not terminate an existing pregnancy and it does not provide protection against STDs. The choice to use emergency contraception is frequently made with the partner and may involve complex decision-making centering around responsibility, relationship power, and a woman's right to choose and autonomy over her body (Beaulieu et al., 2011).

Prenatal Care

Access to prenatal care and financing of sufficient care are critical concerns. High-risk and minority women do not receive sufficient prenatal care. Lack of insurance coverage and less-than-adequate referral mechanisms exist. The well-being of mothers and their infants affects the next generation. Racial and ethnic disparities exist, especially for African American infants (USDHHS, 2010). In 2007, the proportion of mothers receiving care during the first trimester of pregnancy was 70.8%; the target in *Healthy People 2020* is to increase this to 77.6% (USDHHS, 2010). The proportion of mothers receiving early prenatal care needs to increase most in Native American, Hispanic/Latino, and Black non-Hispanic mothers (USDHHS, 2010). Another target of *Healthy People 2020*, which reviewed both *early* and *adequate* prenatal care, indicated that as of 2007,

70.5% of pregnant females received adequate care and the 2020 target hopes to raise this to 77.6% (USDHHS, 2010). Reasons why women do not seek early prenatal care are varied, but may include insensitivity and cultural biases of providers.

Sexually Transmitted Diseases

Sexually transmitted diseases (STDs) are a leading cause of infection and almost half of the new infections each year affect persons ages 15 to 24 years (USDHHS, 2010). Young adults ages 20 to 24 are the highest risk group for STD infection (USDHHS, 2010). Women ages 15 to 19 and ages 20 to 24 have the highest reported rates of chlamydia and gonorrhea (USDHHS, 2010; USPSTF, 2010). The list of STDs includes HIV, *Chlamydia trachomatis* infections, genital herpes, HPV, genital mycoplasma infections, cytomegalovirus infections, HB, and bacterial vaginitis, in addition to the more widely known diseases of syphilis and gonorrhea (Table 22-3). In particular, chlamydia screening efforts should focus on all sexually active nonpregnant and pregnant women ages 24 or younger in whom the prevalence of chlamydial infection is highest (Meyers et al., 2007). The presence of multiple STDs increases the risk of HIV infection (USDHHS, 2010). STDs cost billions of dollars in screening, treatment, and reporting. In addition to creating a substantial problem for young adults, STDs impose tremendous demands on health care facilities (USDHHS, 2010). Many cases are unreported and untreated for lack of screening or failure to recognize symptoms. Many young adults do not understand that STDs can be transmitted from oral and anal sex, not just vaginal

TABLE 22-3   SUMMARY OF SELECTED SEXUALLY TRANSMITTED DISEASES

DISEASE	CAUSATIVE AGENT	DIAGNOSTIC METHODS	TREATMENT	RISKS OR COMPLICATIONS	NURSING TEACHING
Viral Diseases	Treatment does not eradicate underlying infection				
Acquired immunodeficiency syndrome (AIDS)	Human immunodeficiency virus (HIV)	Enzyme immune assay, Western blot, viral tests	Current recommendations	Opportunistic infections, perinatal transmission	Monitor CD4 T-lymphocyte analysis and HIV plasma viral load, monitor MSM, early pregnancy testing strongly recommended
Hepatitis B	Hepatitis B virus (HBV)	Hepatitis B antibody test	No specific therapy available	Perinatal transmission	Routine vaccination or vaccine before pregnancy
Genital herpes	Herpes simplex virus (HSV)	HSV antibody test, culture, viral test	Acyclovir at first diagnosis or episode	Urethral stricture, lymph node enlargement	Examine partners, abstain from sex while symptomatic
Genital warts	Human papilloma-virus (HPV)	Clinical inspection, colposcopy, biopsy	Podophyllin, trichloroacetic acid (TCA), cryotherapy/laser, valacyclovir, tamiciclovir	Cervical dysplasia, cervical cancer	Offer Gardisil or Cervarix vaccine and counseling, return for treatment as necessary, treat partner
Bacterial/Other STDs					
Gonorrhea	*Neisseria gonorrhoeae*	Culture	Ceftriaxone, cefixime, some strains becoming resistant	PID, infertility, ectopic pregnancy	Monitor antibiotic treatment, examine partner, repeat culture, check for chylamydia infection
Syphilis	*Treponema pallidum*	Fluorescent antibody tests of lesion or exudates, VDRL, RPR	Benzathine penicillin G	Secondary/late syphilis	Monitor treatment, test and monitor partner
Chlamydia	*Chlamydia trachomatis*	Culture, chlamydia monoclonal antibody test	Azithromycin, doxycycline	Infertility, ectopic pregnancy, urethral scarring, PID, endocervicitis, neonatal infection	Refer partners for evaluation, condoms to prevent future infection
Bacterial vaginosis (BV)	*Gardnerella vaginalis*	Clinical criteria, wet mount (clue cells)	Metronidazole (Flagyl)	Asymptomatic infection	Sexual transmission not proven
Trichomoniasis	*Trichomonas vaginalis*	Trich Rapid Test, culture (protozoa)	Metronidazole (Flagyl)	Recurrence, excoriation of genital area	Use condoms to prevent new infection
Vulvovaginal candidiasis (VVC)	*Candida albicans*, non–*C. albicans*	Wet mount/KOH test (hyphae and spores)	Antifungal medication: butoconazole, miconazole, clotrimazole	Recurrence of disease	Reduce moisture/heat in genital area, recheck in 14 days

Based on information from Centers for Disease Control and Prevention. (2010). Sexually transmitted diseases treatment guidelines, 2010. *Morbidity and Mortally Weekly Report, 59*(RR-12), 1-116. Retrieved December 30, 2011, from http://www.cdc.gov/STD/treatment/2010/STD-Treatment-2010-RR5912.pdf (incorporates the 2006 guidelines); Hatcher, R. A., Trussell, J., Nelson, A. L., Cates, W., Kowal, D., & Policar, M. (2011). *Contraceptive technology*, 20th ed., Bridge the Gap Foundation; Perry, S., Hockenberry, M., Lowdermilk, D., & Wilson, D. (2010). *Maternal-child nursing care*. St. Louis: Elsevier.

KOH, Potassium hydroxide; MSM, males who have sex with men; *Pap,* Papanicolaou; *PID,* pelvic inflammatory disease; *RPR,* rapid plasma reagin test; *VDRL,* Venereal Disease Research Laboratory test.

intercourse. A study sponsored by the Centers for Disease Control and Prevention found that young adults rarely discussed STDs at home or with partners or close friends; however, young women may look to these intermediary sources if they are worried about having a STD (Friedman & Bloodgood, 2010). Neighborhood structural supports can also be associated with acquisition and incidence of STDs (Ford, 2011; Ford & Browning, 2011). Most of the information about STDs came from

health providers; this emphasizes the importance of health information provided by nurses about STDs to young adults (Friedman & Bloodgood, 2010).

Human Immunodeficiency Virus

More than 1 million persons were estimated to be living with HIV infection in the United States (USDHHS, 2010): improved longevity of infected persons and better treatment have made

HIV infection more like a chronic disease. Meeting the treatment or prevention needs of this large group of chronically infected persons, especially HIV-positive low-income Americans, has become a priority. An important challenge is to develop more effective strategies to prevent new infections and improved case finding (USDHHS, 2010). In 2010, the White House published a three-pronged HIV/AIDS strategy to reduce the number infected; increase access and care for affected individuals; and reduce HIV health-related disparities. HIV is transmitted by sexual intercourse (oral, vagina, anal), shared needles, and infected blood. Another less common source of transmission is from mother to baby across the placental barrier or through breast milk. The higher level of worry about contracting HIV and other STDs in young adults is correlated with the implementation of risk-reduction behaviors. The incidence of STDs is greatly reduced with proper use of condoms. In the *Healthy People 2020* report, use of condoms in various age groups surpassed targets (USDHHS, 2010), and condom use is considered to be increasing. Prevention education is aimed at all high-risk groups including heterosexuals and men who have sex with men. All sexually active individuals are counseled on the hazards of unprotected sexual activity and on the effective use and limitations of condoms, stressing that they must be used properly and can fail. Condom failures occur at an estimated rate of 10% to 15%; therefore, counseling should stress that condom use is not foolproof. Another success is the decline in perinatal transmission. Rates of HIV perinatal transmission are greatly reduced by drug therapy during pregnancy, changes in obstetric practice, and prohibition of breastfeeding in infected mothers. The U.S. Public Health Service highly recommends voluntary testing for HIV and counseling as a part of basic prenatal care (U.S. Preventive Services Task Force, 2010).

The nurse's role in intervening for STDs includes providing treatment and education, early diagnosis, and treatment. When an individual is suspected of having an STD, the nurse obtains a complete history, including sexual history, sexual contacts, previous treatment and test results, any signs or symptoms of a current infection, recent use of antibiotics, and allergic reactions to antibiotics. When treatment is required, the nurse ensures that the person understands the goals of treatment in an attempt to gain cooperation including follow-up care with partners and adherence to the plan of care.

The nurse is an educator not only of the individual but also of the general public (Ford & Browning, 2011). Appropriate health education for the individual with an STD includes mode of transmission, incubation periods, signs and symptoms, methods of treatment, complications resulting from lack of treatment, and signs of recurrent infections.

Coping-Stress Tolerance Pattern

Assessment of Stress Levels

Stress, the result of forces operating on the individual that disrupt physiological or psychological equilibrium, is an integral part of young adulthood; therefore, a comprehensive health assessment should include questions to determine stress levels. Anxiety, nervousness, depression, or somatic complaints

FIGURE 22-4 Young adults spend time learning in a center for higher education.

are indicators of stress, as are events such as divorce, loss of employment, failure to be promoted, or financial difficulties. The role of the nurse is to listen, offer support, and demonstrate concern. The nurse also suggests referrals to appropriate health providers and support groups.

Achievement-Oriented Stress

Achievement-oriented stress differs from the stress of situational crises in that the stress of an overachiever is derived from internal pressures to succeed as measured by self-defined goals. Among many other stressors, young adults are often engaged in higher education programs at the college or university level (Figure 22-4). Achievement-oriented stress frequently causes workaholic habits, including loss of sleep and omission of meals. When this behavior becomes extreme, serious physical and emotional consequences can occur, such as nutrition problems or burnout, which, in turn, leads to severe emotional and physical exhaustion. Workaholic behaviors may not be perceived by the individual and may not be apparent until changes in body functions or behavior occur. Young adults are generally health conscious and willing to alter personal lifestyles and behavior patterns to reduce stress and become healthier. Many people have responded to campaigns for physical fitness, exercise, and nutritional adjustment, which increase their well-being and life expectancy.

Suicide and Depression

Suicide is a leading cause of death in the young adult age group. Suicide occurs because many young adults are unable to cope with the pressures of adulthood. For some people, pressure arises when dealing with interpersonal conflicts such as marital problems, family discord, or the loss of a close relationship; for others, the precipitating event is a lack of personal resources, unemployment, or dissatisfaction with work or school. Many young adults try to solve their problems before the fatal incident but see no positive solutions; in many cases, a prior suicide attempt was a signal for help.

Suicide rates are higher for men than for women; approximately four to five times as many men as women (18.4 versus 4.7 deaths per 100,000 population in 2007) take their own lives (U.S. Census Bureau, 2011). However, more women are known to suffer from depressive disorders and to unsuccessfully attempt suicide. Young adults are more likely as a group to attempt suicide than are older individuals, and professionals are more likely to attempt suicide than are nonprofessionals. Suicide is more common among single, widowed, and divorced individuals. Chronically ill young adult males may also be more at risk for depression than young adult females because social support systems are more robust within female relationship networks (Kiviruusu et al., 2007).

A quick screening method for young adults who may be depressed requires the nurse to ask two questions. First, the nurse asks whether in the last month the young adult has been bothered by little interest or pleasure in doing things. Second, the nurse asks whether the young adult has felt down, depressed, or hopeless in the last month (U.S. Preventive Services Task Force, 2010). A "no" answer to both questions indicates a negative screening result. However, at this point the USPSTF does not recommend for or against routine screening for suicide because positive research support for routine screening is not clear.

In 2007, approximately 13 per 100,000 population-specific deaths between the ages of 25 and 34 were classified as suicides (U.S. Census Bureau, 2011). Nursing interventions are directed toward identifying behaviors in individuals who may be contemplating suicide. Physical clues include self-neglect, depression, slowed gait, slumped shoulders, and droopy faces. Presuicidal individuals also tend to exhibit impaired reality testing; feelings of hopelessness, helplessness, and rejection; impaired judgment and decision-making; anxiety; weight loss; insomnia; or a radically changed affect. In addition to identifying presuicidal behaviors, the nurse also investigates relationship patterns to determine behaviors that are complicated by feelings of worthlessness and defeat. When the nurse identifies a young adult at risk for a suicide attempt, referrals to other professionals are indicated.

If the health care provider becomes more concerned that the young adult may be at risk for suicide, the following two questions may be asked: "Have these symptoms or feelings that you have been talking about led you to think that you might be better off dead?" "What thoughts have you had about hurting yourself or even killing yourself?" To question further the nurse can ask, "Have you actually done anything to hurt yourself?" (Depression Management Tool Kit, 2001; U.S. Preventive Services Task Force, 2010). Even with education of the public and health care providers about the incidence of suicide in the young adult population, suicide continues to be a major health problem and annual rates, especially for men, remain high.

Values-Beliefs Pattern

Young adults enter their twenties with habits, values, and beliefs acquired during childhood and adolescence. Many acquired habits foster continuance of practices that are hazardous to health and well-being in later life. Prevention is directed toward altering value and belief patterns that encourage poor health practices, and reorienting them toward those that support optimal health behaviors. Nursing interventions are more effective when the nurse can describe, discriminate, identify, and align value and belief patterns consistent with practices known to maximize health.

Values Involved in Parenting

Parenthood is envisioned as an important developmental stage by most young adults; therefore, health-promotion and health-protection activities to ensure healthy offspring are crucial (see Case Study and Care Plan at the end of this chapter). Genetic impairments, or congenital defects caused by abnormal chromosomes, are responsible for 4% to 6% of perinatal deaths (Perry et al., 2010). Tests are available for about 200 genetic diseases (Perry et al., 2010). Most of the offered genetic testing is for single-gene impairment to mothers and fathers who have a family history of genetic disease. Young adults with a genetic disease must make many important decisions; predicting the transmission of the disease to potential offspring is essential to future planning.

Values Regarding Prenatal Diagnosis and Genetic Impairment

Extensive prenatal diagnostic procedures commonly used have been available since the middle 1960s. This capability has enabled the identification of high-risk pregnancies and requires the cooperation and education of childbearing women and their partners, both of whom must provide accurate family health and obstetrical histories and comply with suggested screening and follow-up measures. Decisions about the advisability of reproduction are based on current information on genetics and known deleterious genetic factors.

The finding of a malformed or genetically impaired fetus may result in a parental decision to terminate the pregnancy. Theological and political debates in addition to legislative mandates have greatly influenced family control over many of these decisions. Genetic counseling is an important nursing intervention for young adults. A genetic specialist gives technical explanations of genetic disorders; however, nurses have a supportive role in helping young adults decide whether to have children or to carry through a pregnancy that is at risk.

ENVIRONMENTAL PROCESSES

Physical Agents

Ethnicity, Race, and Culture

The young adult whose ethnic background is different from that of the dominant culture may encounter prejudice and discrimination, which can occur because of differences in race, creed, language, attitudes, values, preferences, or behaviors. The young adult is susceptible to these prejudices at work, at school, in health care delivery systems, and in the community. Young adults must meet not only personal needs but also the needs of children or older adults; therefore, nurses continue to consider the values that are common to specific cultures and ethnic backgrounds.

Race and ethnicity are closely connected to educational and work-related decisions, which subsequently affect choice of residence. Many minority families live in substandard housing or crowded living spaces. A lifestyle of this type, when combined with insufficient economic resources, frequently affects health. Poverty is more common among Black families, which often leads to unmet basic needs of food, clothing, and housing and, in turn, leads to decreased regard for health needs.

Accidents

Injuries are the highest cause of death in young adults and individuals under age 44 (USDHHS, 2010). Motor vehicle accidents cause more fatalities than all other causes of death combined. Reducing speed limits contributes to lower fatality rates. Most states have seat belt laws, and all states have seat belt requirements for children. All individuals in the car need to use seat belts, because an unrestrained occupant can cause harm to another passenger in a crash. In 2009, 84% of motor vehicle drivers and front seat occupants used seat belts and the target for 2020 is 92.4% (USDHHS, 2010). Driving distracted, texting while driving, and using cell phones while driving cause motor vehicle crashes (USDHHS, 2010). Some states require "hand-free" or "Bluetooth" remote audio for car cell phone use. The continued high incidence of vehicle accidents in the young adult age group is related to accessibility of cars to young adults and peer pressure on driving behavior; reckless driving and driving under the influence of alcohol and drugs are now viewed as closely connected to violent and abusive behavior (USDHHS, 2010).

Accident-prevention education, long considered appropriate for young children, is an important part of young adult instruction. Most young licensed drivers have participated in driver education courses, and a number of states have adopted progressive licensing programs. "Graduated driver licensing" (GDL) programs have the potential to reduce younger driver crash rates by 20% to 40% (Shope, 2007). In 2011, 35 states had banned texting while driving. The young adult must understand the potentially fatal consequences of aggressive tendencies or thoughtless risk-taking. When young adults are encouraged to reflect on the consequences of their actions, they tend to be more willing to control and change unsafe driving behaviors.

Biological Agents

Noise Pollution

Young adults are exposed to high levels of noise in occupational and recreational settings. Long-term exposure to loud noise is directly related to impaired hearing and can increase irritability and stress. Young adults can be exposed to noises in the work setting from industrial machinery and equipment. Although industrial exposure can be difficult to mitigate, many young adults worsen the situation through recreational exposure, by listening to music or videos at excessively high decibel levels. Ear protection is necessary in some situations to prevent hearing disability. Recognition of hazards and corresponding appropriate preventive education are early nursing strategies for decreasing excessive noise exposure.

Air Pollution

Motor vehicles are the largest source of air pollution; vehicles release more than 90 million tons of particles and noxious gases each year, most of which is either carbon monoxide or hydrocarbons. Carbon monoxide in high concentrations is deadly; in lower concentrations it causes headaches, dizziness, and heart palpitations. In sunlight and low-lying areas, automobile exhaust becomes photochemical smog that contains ozone, which irritates the eyes and the respiratory tract. Although air pollution is not a problem only for young adults, but also they frequently work in dirty, entry-level jobs in industrial settings and may be among the age group that is most affected.

Occupational Hazards and Stressors

Occupational hazards pose a threat of illness, injury, or death in all age groups, and occupational safety standards have contributed greatly to the reduction of work-related accidents. The Occupational Safety and Health Act (OSHA) (1970), has resulted in the improvement of work conditions, along with the provision of health care facilities, in many companies.

Young adults should not be allowed to work in certain industrial settings without vocational training to reduce hazards. Young adults frequently want a challenge and high wages; therefore, they work at hazardous jobs—for example, on offshore drilling rigs, on high bridges, or in nuclear plants. Because of their age, physical stamina, and agility, young adults are suitable candidates for positions that require extreme physical abilities. Occupational training should include education about personal exposure risks, identification of work-related hazards, and identification of situations in which the severity of accidents is connected to personal behaviors or habits. For example, drivers of heavy construction machinery should be particularly observant, avoid reckless behaviors, and avoid fast driving. Working women who are pregnant can expose their fetuses to industrial substances. Proper evaluation and temporary reassignment may be necessary.

Occupational preventive intervention requires that known work hazards and risks be identified early. Health histories should include questions about the place of work, type of work, and young adults' understanding of the risks associated with their occupations. Occupational risk and health are closely related; stress associated with work, the use of alcohol or drugs, and a negative attitude toward work are predictive of occupational injuries. Job counseling aimed at changing the nature of employment can be an appropriate referral for some people with health conditions. Employees in industrial settings should visit a health care provider on a periodic basis for health assessment, update of the health history, and counseling.

Chemical Agents

Drug Use

Misuse of drugs, a major risk for young adults, is associated with injury, disability, violence, homicide, and suicide and is related to social problems (criminal behaviors and maladjustment to accepted norms). Drug abuse may be closely related to an inability to cope appropriately with adult responsibilities. Physical health problems associated with drug misuse account for more than 50% of the major acute and chronic problems of young adults. Heroin users have increased mortality rates because of overdosage or chronic disability associated with hepatitis infections. Drug use is an independent risk factor involved in HIV infections (USDHHS, 2010).

Use of drugs, such as anabolic steroids, to improve athletic performance is increasing. The risks of using steroids are enormous, and preventive education should focus on healthier sports and exercise values. Nursing activities include preventive strategies to curb the problem of drug misuse. Distribution of information on drugs, early treatment of complications, and information regarding drug treatment centers are only part of the answer. Nursing efforts aimed at increasing individual awareness and altering drug-taking attitudes and behaviors are of critical importance (Box 22-6: Diversity Awareness).

Alcohol Use

Alcohol-related accidents among individuals ages 15 to 24 continue to be a leading cause of preventable morbidity, disability, and death. Heavy alcohol use, that is, consuming five or more drinks on at least one occasion within a month, is more common in 18 to 25 year olds than it is for younger or older adults (USDHHS, 2010). Raising the legal drinking age to 21 reduces not only deaths and injuries connected to motor vehicle accidents

but also homicides and other violent deaths. A nationwide legal standard of 0.08% blood alcohol concentration maximal levels for driving while intoxicated (DWI) enforcement and prosecution was achieved (USDHHS, 2010). Alcohol abuse is directly related to chronic conditions such as cirrhosis of the liver. Modifying alcohol consumption in young adults can decrease the frequency of chronic and disabling conditions in later life.

Alcohol consumption is increasing in the young adult population. In 2008, 27% of young adults ages 18 and older reported that they have engaged in binge drinking in the last 30 days (USDHHS, 2010). Also, approximately 7% of young military veterans had a substance abuse problem in the last year (USDHHS, 2010). Although young adults may drink less frequently than older adults, there is a tendency to consume larger amounts of alcohol at one time; the tendency is toward binge drinking, which causes increased loss of control and is related to an additional risk of automobile crashes. Teens with work schedules of more than 10 hours per week are more often involved in heavy or binge drinking, or both. Working longer hours increases the money available to purchase alcohol and exposes the teen to older adults who drink.

Tobacco Use

Smoking is a leading cause of preventable death in the United States; therefore, smoking cessation is the single most important counseling topic for all people because of its potential to lower the risk of contracting many preventable diseases. More than one third of current smokers ages 18 to 24 years started

BOX 22-6   DIVERSITY AWARENESS

Pharmacogenetics: Predicting Variation in Drug Response

Various studies, although limited, indicate genetic differences may be important factors to consider when prescribing certain drugs. Different genetic types tend to metabolize drugs differently, have different binding receptors, or have different environmental influences that change the utilization and uptake. This field of study is called pharmacogenetics. Early clues to variation in drug response were seen when comparing populations from different racial and ethnic backgrounds, so there are important cultural awareness implications of these avenues of study. DNA (nucleotide) gene variations are known as SNPs (single nucleotide polymorphisms) and are cause by the substitution of one nucleotide base for another. When these SNPs direct liver metabolic enzymes, the polymorphism or form of the gene inherited causes differences in drug metabolism.

In many ways, gene variation and selection had positive effects on evolution and favored the chances of a population to survive. For example, sickle cell trait developed through selection factors that favored resistance to malaria. Similarly, gene selection factors also favored the prevalence of glucose-6-phosphate dehydrogenase deficiency, which also provides resistance to malaria but causes drug-related red blood cell hemolysis. In related studies of warfarin response, ethnic differences were shown to affect bioavailability and distribution, which could be controlled through more precise clinical management and dosage regulation. Warfarin dosing is significantly altered by polymorphisms in the liver and enzymes affecting vitamin K synthesis.

In studies of people with hypertension, Black individuals responded with a greater decrease in systolic pressure in response to thiazide diuretics (hydrochlorothiazide) and calcium channel blockers. Black individuals have a blunted response to alpha-blockers, which can be improved by adding a diuretic. Many Black individuals have renin sensitivity, which would have favored survival in warmer climates.

The situation in Asian persons appears to be the exact opposite. In a study of the effectiveness of propranolol in Chinese and White men, the Chinese men had at least twice as much sensitivity as did the White men to propranolol administered at several dosage levels. Studies indicate that Asians are more sensitive to alcohol and its drug effects than are Whites. The most outstanding difference is in the amount of facial flushing, which was experienced by a substantial percentage of Asians compared with the White sample. The alcohol dehydrogenase enzyme is reported to be absent in about one half of Asians.

These examples suggest that nurses should be very attuned to diversity awareness and potential genetic variations that may affect drug metabolism and effectiveness. In individuals who do not respond to certain drugs as expected, the nurse may consider whether this might be related to constitutional factors within the person's genetic makeup. Pharmacogenetic research also invites rethinking of managed care practices that restrict diversity of drug use with prescribed drug formulary listings.

Sources: Kudzma, E. & Carey, E. (2009). Pharmacogenomics: Personalizing drug response. *American Journal of Nursing, 109*(10), 50-58; Barnes-Jewish Hospital at Washington University Medical Center & NIH. (2011). *Warfarin dosing.* Retrieved December 30, 2011, from www.warfarin-dosing.org/Source/Home.aspx; Flockhart, D. A. (2009). *Drug interactions: Cytochrome P450 drug interaction table.* Indiana University School of Medicine. Retrieved from http://medicine.iupui.edu/clinpharm/ddis/table.aspx; Shah, S. H., & Buehler, B. (2011). *Warfarin dosing and VKORC1/CYP2C9.* Retrieved December 30, 2011, from http://emedicine.medscape.com/article/1733331-overview.

smoking before the age of 16. Cigarette smoking rates among persons 18 and older continued to decline from the 1998 baseline of 24% to a 2008 level of 8.3% (USDHHS, 2010). An ancillary goal of *Healthy People 2020* to keep the smoking rate low is to increase tobacco cessation counseling in office-based ambulatory settings and hospital ambulatory settings.

Individuals employed in high-risk occupations are informed of the synergistic relationship between smoking and other environmental exposures including asbestos, coal dust, and radiation. Fear tactics, nagging, preaching, and threats are generally ineffective in convincing people to stop smoking. Major barriers to smoking cessation are the presence of other smokers, particularly in situations where alcohol is also being used.

State enforcement of no smoking policies is important. Lung cancer death rates declined in states with strong tobacco control enforcement and increased in states where tobacco control measures were weak. Measures of tobacco control are strongly correlated with smoking cessation rates of young adults ages 30 to 39. Nurses are familiar with the antismoking resources in their communities, enabling them to make the appropriate referrals.

Carcinogens

Young adults can be exposed to environmental carcinogens in their work settings or through unhealthy practices such as having multiple sexual partners. In the work setting, environmental regulations have limited exposure to some hazardous chemicals, but long-term effects on health of exposure to many industrial chemicals remains unknown. In health care, latex, long considered inert and safe, has now been shown to cause long-term immune system disease in some nurses exposed to the agent (or the chemicals that bind it) in surgical gloves.

DETERMINANTS OF HEALTH

Social Factors and Environment

Neighborhood Resources

The environment of the community strongly influences the well-being of the young adult and sets the standard for the health of people and families living within a neighborhood. Neighbors can be an excellent source of support, which can be especially important to a young mother who does not have immediate family nearby. Nurses working in the community facilitate the contact of individuals with common interests through community and religious activities and support groups. Community resources for exercise and recreation can make important contributions to the young adult's physical and emotional health. When these resources are available, the young adult can have the opportunity to exercise and release stress in a positive fashion.

Levels of Policy Making and Health

Young adults are one of the major political constituencies in the United States, as seen in the 2008 presidential election; they support many causes and have the time and energy to publicize issues related to the common good. Some of these issues involve unemployment, college debt, sustainability, pollution, the environment, nuclear energy, and war. Relative to health, predominant issues have involved housing and health care in neighborhoods and rural areas and health, agricultural, and sanitation concerns in foreign countries. Through these efforts, young adults can influence and improve living conditions for future generations.

One of the young adult's age-related tasks is to choose and develop a lifelong career. This choice is directly related to economic factors; young adults want satisfying occupations that also yield adequate economic returns. To manage financially and maintain a lifestyle in which personal needs can be met, young adults may elect to have fewer children. Caring for aging parents can also cause physical, psychosocial, spiritual, and economic stress.

Although goals vary greatly among young adult couples, they generally are concerned with acquiring material comforts; the desire for housing, transportation, clothing, or recreation generally necessitates that both partners are employed to meet financial obligations. This desire necessitates the changing of roles and the sharing of responsibilities, and open communication becomes a crucial component. For single parents these challenges can appear insurmountable.

New career opportunities and the economic expansion in the United States during the 1990s allowed young adults obtaining first jobs more career choices. The growing technology industry provided employment in a wide variety of occupations and start-up companies. Work styles within these companies tend to be different from those in the traditional workplace, including an expectation of longer and more fluid workdays. Internet-based companies provide young adults with jobs that have the potential to give them rapid financial rewards at the cost of long-term job stability. Since the economic downturn in 2008, young adults have learned to adapt to an economic realization that employment will be less available. Since 2012, the employment rate of young adults ages 18 to 24 (54%) has been at its lowest since data were collected in 1948. Employed young adults have also experienced more of a decline in weekly paychecks (decline of 6%) than any other employed age group over the last 4 years (Pew Research Center, 2012). Because of the high cost of housing, many young adults have multiple roommates, creating additional demands and health risks. Some young adults are interested in giving back to society by taking employment at lower salaries in nonprofit agencies involved in education and social issues, such as Habitat for Humanity, and going abroad in the Peace Corps to promote human rights in countries where such rights are nonexistent.

For many young adult couples, the increase in unemployment for one or both, different careers, friends, and varying maturity levels place additional strains on their relationship. These circumstances can provide a basis for domestic difficulty. Domestic arguments can precede family disruption, leading to marital separation or divorce. In addition to the emotional strain placed on family members, domestic arguments can result in aggressive acts of abuse and personal injury. Young adults can also be faced with decisions about day care facilities; the couple or mother may need support to resolve guilt feelings related to the separation from the child. Some young adults may also bear responsibilities for caring for aging parents or relatives.

Lifestyles may also include living arrangements with individuals of the same gender or the opposite gender. Although these lifestyles are becoming more acceptable in today's society, attitudes toward varied lifestyles contribute pressures that lead to further stress and uncertainty.

Health Services/Delivery System

The availability of health services is important. Economic realities, however, influence the effectiveness of resources, particularly for the young adult who lives in an economically depressed area. In some communities, health services are lacking or, when available, are not culturally sensitive or adapted to the customs and beliefs of the people who are served. In other communities, access to public transportation can be a critical problem, affecting the ability of the young adult to keep appointments. Young adults ages 18 to 24 years are the least likely of any age group to have a usual source of care; thus, a target of *Healthy People 2020* is to increase the proportion of young adults with a usual primary care provider (USDHHS, 2010). Gaps in health care insurance coverage that occur between the end of schooling and the achievement of full employment with health insurance coverage can reduce the access of young adults to primary care. The Affordable Health Care for All Americans Act passed in 2010 (March 23, 2010, Obama Care, www.healthcare.gov) mandates coverage for young adults up to the age of 26 within family health insurance coverage. This act has maintained 2.5 million young adults insured on their parent's health plans.

Health delivery methods in the United States are based primarily on Western belief systems, which tend to be rigid in their applications. For example, women seeking birth control information and prescriptions are expected to use health clinics and adhere to their schedule of return visits. Because health care provider systems have removed many traditional barriers once assumed to be responsible for poor utilization of services by low-income or minority groups (location and scheduling), nonattendance at scheduled clinic visits frequently is interpreted as noncompliance. Nurses need to be able to identify health practices and health system gaps that are barriers to care and harmful to people.

Nursing comprises the largest group of professionals within the U.S. health care system. However, nurses cannot deliver care optimally within changing health care settings because of barriers to practice and ineffective workforce planning, data, and information infrastructure. A recent Institute of Medicine report (IOM, 2010) noted that the nursing profession cannot contribute optimally unless there is full participation in team planning and health care redesign with physicians and other health care professionals. In addition, business, government, health delivery agencies, and the insurance industry must all participate in a newly designed health care system that provides accessible, affordable quality care, leading to increases in measureable health outcomes (IOM, 2010) (see Case Study and Care Plan at end of chapter).

NURSING APPLICATION

Young adulthood is generally considered to be the most healthful period of life. In terms of physical changes, growth is complete by this stage. The physical abilities of the young adult are in peak condition so the goals of the nurse are aimed at maintaining optimal physical condition, encouraging healthy habits, screening for disease, and treating illnesses.

Preventive care is recommended to young adults in the form of screenings. Health examinations at recommended intervals are a crucial component of screening for potential health concerns and providing education about measures to avoid disease and disability. Women are taught about breast self-examinations whereas testicular self-examinations are taught to men utilizing photos, models, and return demonstration.

It is necessary to screen for cardiovascular conditions after the age of 25 as well as provide education about risk factor modification. Intervention efforts should reflect diversion of age, gender, ethnicity, and socioeconomic status. As the nurse obtains an assessment of the individual and family history, the necessity of further screening, education, or monitoring is determined. Elements of education include smoking cessation and dietary modifications.

Immunizations are important for the young adult age group. Young adults are educated about recommended vaccinations for seasonal influenza, hepatitis B, and rubella. Nurses also provide screening for tuberculosis, food-borne illnesses, diseases related to travel, and sexually transmitted diseases.

Young adults are encouraged to engage in physical activity and muscle-strengthening exercise. Some barriers may be a lack of time or lack of access. The nurse working with the young adult population should consider implementing work site wellness programs. Group fitness or weight loss programs can be an effective means of promoting wellness at work while increasing employee satisfaction and productivity. Some workforce programs utilize an incentive system where points are awarded for the achievement of particular milestones. Once a set level of points is reached, the employee is given a reward in the form of gift cards or movie tickets. These types of programs are often effective for smoking cessation, weight loss, and exercise. In addition, some companies encourage the formation of facility-sponsored sports teams such as bowling leagues, softball teams, or a running club. This encourages camaraderie among colleagues and increases participation for people who respond well to group motivation. Nonworking young adults looking for a group fitness or sports program should be directed to resources within the community via Internet research.

The nurse working with young adults provides education about skin cancer risk, the need for adequate sunscreen, and signs and symptoms of skin cancer. Safety education is provided about recreational and sports-related injuries and how to prevent them. Additional education is required for young adult females. The nurse may be in a position of providing counseling or referrals for contraception, prenatal care, sexually transmitted diseases, and HIV. It is imperative that women receive early prenatal care in order to maintain optimal health for herself and the unborn child.

The nurse working with the young adult population often becomes a counselor. Stressors are important to assess as prolonged stress, anxiety, or depression can negatively affect the health of the individual. Stressors may be related to relationships, divorce, employment, layoffs, or financial concerns. The nurse listens, offers support and concern, and provides the individual or family with resources or support groups specific to the stressor. The nurse also utilizes depression screening to evaluate for suicide risk. The nurse assesses for:

- Physical clues of self-neglect
- Depression or anxiety
- Slow gait
- Slumped shoulders

- Saddened or droopy face
- Feeling of helplessness or hopelessness
- Impaired judgment or decision-making
- Weight loss
- Insomnia

Once the nurse identifies a person at risk for suicide, an immediate referral is made to the appropriate professional.

CASE STUDY

Preparing for Childbearing: Kirsten

Kirsten is a healthy 22-year-old whose favorite sport is running. Since this spring, Kirsten believes that her breathing capacity is diminishing and her levels of energy are decreasing. During her period these symptoms appear to worsen. Last week, while running up a rather steep course, Kirsten became much weaker, dizzier, and more fatigued than usual, and her best friend and running partner recommended that she make a physician's appointment for a physical examination. Kirsten's running partner also noted that she has appeared pale lately.

In the physician's office, Kirsten is noted to have a normal temperature, elevated heart and respiratory rates, and a blood pressure of 90/60 mm Hg. Kirsten's description of her period is that it tends to be heavy and has been this way for 5 years. For muscle aches and pains caused by running, she usually takes

two aspirin tablets every 3 to 4 hours for as long as 7 days. When her running increases during the summer, she takes aspirin continually for 2 to 3 months. Diagnostic testing indicates that her hemoglobin level is 7 g/dL, and her red blood cells are pale and small. Kirsten has been in a long-term relationship for several years, her wedding is in several months, and there has been discussion of preconceptual health planning and future children.

Reflective Questions
1. What common health alteration in young adult women is most likely for Kirsten?
2. What contributing factors place Kirsten at risk?
3. What lifestyle modifications can Kirsten implement to decrease her risk?

CARE PLAN

Preparation for Childbearing: Kirsten

*NURSING DIAGNOSIS: Health-Seeking Behaviors related to preconceptual assessment and preparation for childbearing

Defining Characteristics
- Expressed desire to improve overall health to prepare for childbearing
- Expressed thoughts about planning for pregnancy in the near future
- Desire to improve nutritional status before childbearing
- Desire to improve nutritional intake of essential vitamins and minerals (iron and calcium)
- Plan to take multivitamin each day
- Plan to limit foods high in sodium and fat
- Plan to limit alcohol consumption
- Plan for exercise program to increase stamina and flexibility
- Seeks physical examination to rule out problems that might negatively affect pregnancy
- Seeks information on pregnancy risk factors (biophysical, psychosocial, sociodemographic, and environmental)

Related Factors
- Expressed desire to improve the quality of relationship with husband or partner
- Desire to attend education classes to improve knowledge of childbearing and positive health practices
- Plan for room or housing to accommodate children
- Plan for employment arrangements that accommodate child care

Expected Outcomes
- Increase in indices of well-being in person
- Healthy pregnancy and future child

- Increase in self-confidence and awareness preparation for childbearing
- Management of pregnancy risk factors before becoming pregnant
- Making the person aware of resources available for pregnancy and child care

Interventions
- Assess current level of wellness regarding preparation for childbearing.
- Identify community resources that provide information regarding preconceptual planning and preparation.
- Identify primary health provider, midwife, or obstetrician, and hospitals with delivery services.
- Assess biophysical risk factors (genetic disorders, nutrition problems, and current medical problems).
- Assess for history of pregnancy loss.
- Test for blood type and Rh factor.
- Screen for sexually transmitted disease, tuberculosis, rubella titer, sickle cell trait.
- Review immunization history, including hepatitis B.
- Assess need to augment diet, particularly to increase intake of calcium and iron.
- Take a multivitamin daily.
- Assess for psychosocial risk factors (mental problems, use of drugs, alcohol, caffeine, and smoking).
- Counsel to avoid alcohol consumption.
- Assess for possible sociodemographic risk factors (poverty, first pregnancy risks of dystocia or PIH, residence [rural or urban], and ethnicity).
- Assess for environmental risks (exposures to chemicals, drugs, pesticides, pollution, smoke, stress, and radiation).
- Assess current employment situation.
- Identify child care arrangements.

PIH, Pregnancy-induced hypertension.
* *NANDA Nursing Diagnoses—Definitions and Classification 2012-2014,* Herdman T.H. (ED). Copyright © 2012, 1994-2012 NANDA International. Used by arrangement with John Wiley & Sons Limited. In order to make safe and effective judgments using the NANDA-I nursing diagnoses it is essential that nurses refer to the definitions and defining characteristics of the diagnoses listed in this work. *Retired NANDA Nursing Diagnosis.*

SUMMARY

Nurses promote health care measures and behaviors at all places where young adults come into contact with the health care delivery system. In community colleges and university settings, efforts can be directed toward health-education curricula with an emphasis on implementation of positive health behaviors, use of appropriate social networking skills, establishment of peer counseling groups, and better utilization of sports and exercise facilities. Workshops on alcoholism, substance abuse, sports or exercise, mental health and self-expression, relationships, and various aspects of sexual care are effective in college and graduate school populations. At the work site, programs of employee counseling, blood pressure monitoring and treatment, exercise recommendations, smoking reduction, cafeteria nutrition management, and stress reduction techniques have also been effective. Insurance programs are in continued flux to provide appropriate levels of integrated care and coverage. Preventive care, mental health, dental health, and maternity and infertility benefits are being analyzed and increased when necessary. Young adults are generally healthy, which challenges the nurse to be even more creative, sensitive, and insightful in implementing care for individuals within this age group.

REFERENCES

Affordable Healthcare for All American's Act. (2010). Retrieved April 28, 2012, from www.healthcare.gov.

American Academy of Dermatology. (2011). *Sunscreens.* Retrieved April 28, 2012, from www.aad.org/media-resources/stats-and-facts/prevention-and-care/sunscreens.

Beaulieu, R., Kools, S. M., Kennedy, H. P., & Humphreys, J. (2011). Young adult couples' decision making regarding emergency contraceptive pills. *Journal of Nursing Scholarship, 43*(1), 41–48.

Bilukha, O., & Rosenstein, N. (2005). Prevention and control of meningococcal disease. Recommendations of the Advisory Committee on Immunization Practices (ACIP). *Morbidity and Mortality Weekly Report, 54*(RR-7), 1–21.

Black, M. C., Basile, K. C., Breiding, M. J., Smith, S. G., Walters, M. L., Merrick, M. T., et al. (2011). *National Intimate Partner and Sexual Violence Survey (NISVS): 2010 summary report.* Atlanta, GA: National Center for Injury Prevention and Control, Centers for Disease Control and Prevention.

Breiding, M., Black, M., & Ryan, G. (2008). Prevalence and risk factors of intimate partner violence in eighteen U.S. states/territories, 2005. *American Journal of Preventive Medicine, 34*(2), 112–118.

Burke, L., & Wang, J. (2011). Treatment strategies for overweight and obesity. *Journal of Nursing Scholarship, 43*(4), 368–375.

Byrne, J. A. (2011). Eighty-five percent of college grads return to nest. *New York Post.* May 9, 2011.

Carpenito-Moyet, L. J. (2009). *Handbook of nursing diagnosis* (13th ed.). Philadelphia: Lippincott Williams & Wilkins.

Centers for Disease Control and Prevention (CDC). (2009). Quick-Stats: Percentage of young adults aged 18-29 years with selected chronic conditions, by sex—National Health Interview Survey, United States, 2005-2007. *Morbidity and Mortality Weekly Report, 58*(25), 699. Retrieved April 28, 2012, from www.cdc.gov/mmwr/preview/mmwrhtml/mm5825a3.htm.

Centers for Disease Control and Prevention (CDC). (2010). *Defining overweight and obesity.* Retrieved April 28, 2012, from www.cdc.gov/obesity/defining.html.

Centers for Disease Control and Prevention (CDC). (2011a). *Cost of violent deaths in the United States, 2005.* Retrieved April 28, 2012, from www.cdc.gov/ViolencePrevention/violentdeaths/index.html.

Centers for Disease Control and Prevention (CDC). (2011b). Prevalence of coronary heart disease—U.S., 2006-2010. *Morbidity and Mortality Weekly Report, 60*(40), 1377–1381. Retrieved April 28, 2012, from www.cdc.gov/mmwr/preview/mmwrhtml/mm6040a1.htm.

Chobanian, A. V., Bakris, G. L., Black, H. R., Cushmen, W. C., Green, L. A., et al. (2003). The Seventh Report of the Joint National Committee on Prevention, Detection, Evaluation, and Treatment of High Blood Pressure: The JNC 7 Report. *Journal of the American Medical Association, 289*(19), 2560–2572.

Daniloff, C. (2010). Game changers: How dramatic brain discoveries are influencing American's most popular sport. *Bostonia, 2010*(3), 24–31.

Depression Management Tool Kit. (2001). *MacArthur initiative on depression and primary care.* Retrieved April 28, 2012, from www.depression-primarycare.org.

Erikson, E. H. (1993). *Childhood and society.* New York: W.W. Norton.

Ford, J. L. (2011). Racial and ethnic disparities in human papillomavirus awareness and vaccination among young adult women. *Public Health Nursing, 28*(6), 485–493.

Ford, J. L., & Browning, C. R. (2011). Neighborhood social disorganization and the acquisition of trichomoniasis among young adults in the United States. *American Journal of Public Health, 101,* 1696–1703. doi:10.2105/AJPH.2011.300213.

Fontenot, H., Fantasia, H., & Allen, J. (2007). HPV in adolescents: Making the wake-up call. *ADVANCE for Nurse Practitioners, 15*(10), 73–76.

Frank, G. (2007). Good nutrition on the go. *ADVANCE for Nurse Practitioners, 15*(11), 55–57.

Friedman, A. L., & Bloodgood, B. (2010). "Something we'd rather not talk about": Findings from CDC exploratory research on sexually transmitted disease communication with girls and women. *Journal of Women's Health, 19*(10), 1823–1831. doi:10.1089/jwh.2010.1961.

Gillespie, C., Kuklina, E. V., Briss, P. A., Blair, N. A., & Hong, Y. (2011). Vital signs: Prevalence, treatment, and control of hypertension—United States, 1999-2002 and 2005-2008. *Morbidity and Mortality Weekly Report, 60*(4), 103–108.

Gilligan, C. (1982). *In a different voice.* Cambridge, MA: Harvard University Press.

Gilligan, C. (2002). *The birth of pleasure.* New York: Alfred A. Knopf.

Gilligan, C. (2011). *Joining the resistance.* Malden, MA: Polity Press.

Hatcher, R. A., Trussell, J., Nelson, A. L., Cates, W., Kowal, D., & Policar, M. (2011). *Bridge the Gap Foundation contraceptive technology.* (20th ed.). Sussex, United Kingdom: West.

Huether, S. E., & McCance, K. L. (2012). *Understanding pathophysiology* (5th ed.). St. Louis: Elsevier.

Institute for Higher Education Policy (IHEP). (2011). *New research shows more low-income young adults begin their higher education experience at for-profit colleges.* Retrieved April 29, 2012, from www.ihep.org/press-room/news_release-detail.cfm?id=203.

Institute of Medicine (IOM). (2003). *Health professions education: A bridge to quality.* Retrieved April 28, 2012, from www.iom.edu/Reports/2003/Health-Professions-Education-A-Bridge-to-Quality.aspx.

Institute of Medicine (IOM). (2010). *The future of nursing: Leading change, advancing health.* Retrieved April 28, 2012, from http://iom.edu/Reports/2010/The-Future-of-Nursing-Leading-Change-Advancing-Health.aspx.

Jiang, N., Kolbe, L. J., Seo, D., Kay, N. S., & Brindis, C. D. (2011). Health of adolescents and young adults: Trends in achieving the 21 critical national health objectives by 2010. *Journal of Adolescent Health, 49*(2), 124–132.

Kaplan, C. (2007). Intrauterine contraception. *ADVANCE for Nurse Practitioners, 15*(11), 47–52.

Kelly-Weeder, S. (2011). Binge drinking and disordered eating in college students. *Journal of the American Academy of Nurse Practitioners, 2*(1), 33–41.

Kiviruusu, O., Huurre, T., & Aro, H. (2007). Psychosocial resources and depression among chronically ill young adults: Are males more vulnerable? *Social Science Medicine, 65*(2), 173–186.

Kohlberg, L., & Lickons, T. (1986). *The stages of ethical development: From childhood through old age.* San Francisco, CA: Harper.

Kudzma, E., & Carey, E. (2009). Pharmacogenomics: Personalizing drug response. *American Journal of Nursing, 109*(10), 50–58.

Landenburger, K. M., & Campbell, J. C. (2012). Violence and human abuse. In M. Stanhope & J. Lancaster (Eds.), *Public health nursing: Population-centered health care in the community* (pp. 828–853). St. Louis: Elsevier.

LeBlanc, E. S., O'Connor, E., Whitlock, E. P., Patnode, C. D., & Kapka, T. (2011). Effectiveness of primary care-relevant treatments for obesity in adults: A systematic evidence review for the U.S. Preventive Services Task Force. *Annals of Internal Medicine, 155,* 435–447.

Maltby, J., & Day, L. (2011). Celebrity worship and incidence of elective cosmetic surgery: Evidence of a link among young adults. *Journal of Adolescent Health, 49*(5), 483–489.

Melnyk, B., & Fineout-Overholt, E. (2011). *Evidence-based practice in nursing and healthcare.* Philadelphia: Lippincott Williams & Wilkins.

Meyers, D., Halvorson, H., & Luckhaupt, S. (2007). Screening for chlamydial infection: An evidence update for the U.S. Preventive Services Task Force. *Annals of Internal Medicine, 147*(2), 134–141.

Perry, S., Hockenberry, M., Lowdermilk, D., & Wilson, D. (2010). *Maternal-child nursing care.* St. Louis: Elsevier.

Pew Research Center. (2012). *Young, underemployed and optimistic: Coming of age, slowly, in a tough economy.* Retrieved April 29, 2012, from www.pewsocialtrends.org/2012/02/09/young-underemployed-and-optimistic/.

Physical Activity and Public Health. (2007). Updated recommendations for adults from the American College of Sports Medicine and the American Heart Association. *Circulation, 116,* 1081–1093. Retrieved April 28, 2012, from http://circ.ahajournals.org/cgi/reprint/CIRCULATIONAHA.107.185649.

Piaget, J. (1972). Intellectual evolution from adolescence to adulthood. *Human Development, 15,* 1–12.

Quality and Safety Education for Nurses (QSEN). Retrieved April 28, 2012, from www.qsen.org.

Rampell, C. (2011). Many with new college degrees find the job market humbling. *New York Times.* May 18, 2011, A1.

Shope, J. T. (2007). Graduated driver licensing: Review of evaluation results since 2002. *Journal of Safety Research, 38*(2), 165–175.

U.S. Census Bureau. (2011). *Statistical abstracts of the United States: 2012* (131th ed.). Washington, DC: U.S. Government Printing Office. Retrieved April 28, 2012, from www.census.gov/compendia/statab/.

U.S. Department of Health and Human Services (USDHHS). (2006). *Healthy People 2010: Midcourse review.* Retrieved December 29, 2011, at www.healthypeople.gov/2010/data/midcourse/default.htm.

U.S. Department of Health and Human Services (USDHHS). (2010). *Healthy People 2020.* Retrieved April 28, 2012, from www.healthypeople.gov.

U.S. Preventive Services Task Force. (2010). *Guide to clinical preventive services.* Rockville, MD: Agency for Healthcare Research and Quality. Retrieved April 28, 2012, from www.ahrq.gov/clinic/uspstfix.htm.

Wu, H. (2010). *CDC commentary: Meningococcal disease—Prevention, diagnosis and management.* Retrieved December 28, 2011, from www.medscape.com/viewarticle/718595.

Middle-Age Adult

Dee Coover

evolve WEBSITE

http://evolve.elsevier.com/Edelman/
- Study Questions
- Glossary
- Website Resources
  23A: Community Resources for Health Promotion During Middle Adulthood

OBJECTIVES

After completing this chapter, the reader will be able to:
- Name three psychosocial and spiritual changes that frequently occur during middle age.
- Explain the normal biological changes that occur as a result of the aging process.
- Identify the major causes of mortality in the middle-age adult.

- Describe frequently occurring health patterns of middle-age adults.
- Discuss the unique health problems related to the occupations of the adult between ages 35 and 65 years.
- Analyze the influence of psychosocial stressors on the middle-age adult and the ways the individual's culture and occupation can affect these stressors.

KEY TERMS

Advance directive	Gingivitis	Osteoarthritis
Body mass index (BMI)	Glaucoma	Osteopenia
Calcium	Health care agent	Osteoporosis
Cardiac output	High blood pressure	Overweight
Cataracts	Kyphosis	Perimenopause
Constipation	Living will	Periodontitis
Degenerative joint disease	Macular degeneration	Presbycusis
Durable power of attorney	Menopause	Presbyopia
Functional aerobic capacity	"Midlife crisis"	Sleep disorders
Generativity versus stagnation	Obesity	Vitamin D

Terminal Illness

Charlie Shelton is dying of lung cancer. His wife, Sarah, finds that she must manage a household and provide for their two children (ages 15 and 18) on her own. The elder child plans to enter college next fall, but the Sheltons wonder whether they will be able to afford this. Although Charlie and Sarah worked hard and saved money all their lives, Charlie's long illness continues to deplete their savings. Their parents are helping as best they can, but they live on limited incomes themselves. The hospital bills continue to come, and the Sheltons are overwhelmed.

- What types of health care providers would be helpful to the Sheltons?
- What can health care providers do to guide and support the Sheltons during this stressful time?
- What health-promotion strategies might be suggested and implemented to help them?
- What community organizations might the health care provider recommend to meet the needs of this family?
- What responsibilities do health care providers and policymakers have to provide health promotion to middle-age adults?

Many adults living during their midlife years experience expanded responsibilities and increased productivity. In most cases, there is a concomitant increased sense of accomplishment. Middle adulthood spans a 30-year interval between 35 and 64 years of age. Within this age interval, significant biological, physiological, social, psychological, and spiritual changes occur. Vital Statistics Reports published by the Center for Communicable Diseases (2012) divide the middle adult into three categories for ease of describing mortality and morbidity data. These are 35 to 44 years, 45 to 54 years, and 55 to 64 years. This age group (30-year span) comprises nearly 40% of the population of the United States (Boston Women's Health Book Collective & Norsigian, 2005; Centers for Disease Control and Prevention [CDC], 2010a; U.S. Department of Health and Human Services [USDHHS], CDC, National Center for Health Statistics, 2007).

There are many changes related to aging and health that occur during this time frame that will be discussed in this chapter. Health promotion addresses choices in behavior and practices that optimize health and well-being for the adult in midlife. This concept is the central focus of the presentation of materials and related figures and study aids.

An examination of gains achieved for *Healthy People 2010* will be compared to the goals and objectives that lay ahead for this health-promotion initiative by 2020. Along with analysis of these findings, the role of nurses will be interwoven throughout the text. Nurses are integral to the health of the American people, hence, to fostering health promotion and health maintenance.

BIOLOGY AND GENETICS

Although their onset varies, biological changes come to the forefront during the middle years, affecting most body systems. The hair of the adult begins to thin and turn gray. The skin's moisture and turgor decreases, and with the loss of subcutaneous fat, wrinkling occurs. Excessive sun exposure through the years makes some changes more pronounced, especially increased coarseness of facial features.

Fat deposition increases during these years often with concomitant increases in weight. Body height decreases as a result of decreased bone density and mass. This combination of changes results in increased body mass index (BMI) values. The body contour changes as "love handles" and "saddlebags" appear. Sedentary lifestyles and unchanged dietary habits contribute considerably to these changes.

The inactive lifestyle is further compromised by a decrease in energy; "I'm not as young as I used to be" is a common remark. This proclamation is legitimate, because the capacity for physical work actually decreases. As **functional aerobic capacity** decreases, there is a resulting decrease in **cardiac output.** For individuals who maintain regular exercise programs that provide stretching and strengthening of skeletal muscle, cardiac output remains essentially undiminished for many years.

In the musculoskeletal system, bone density and mass progressively decrease. When 55-year-old adults say that they were 1 inch taller when they were 18, the observation is likely to be true. A 1 to 4 inch (2.5 to 10 cm) loss in height occurs as a person ages; thinning of the intervertebral disks accounts for approximately 1 inch. However, dramatic losses in height (more than 4 inches) can occur with thoracic **kyphosis,** an angulation of the posterior spine (commonly known as *"hunchback"*). The wear and tear on joints predisposes the adult to **degenerative joint disease,** deterioration of the joint(s), with more frequent painful backaches. The general decrease in muscle tone, categorized by many as *"flab,"* reduces physical agility.

Degenerative joint disease, specifically **osteoarthritis,** has its peak onset in middle age and can greatly influence activity and endurance, which impacts employment. Most frequently the knees and hands, followed by hips, spine, shoulders, and ankles, are involved. In *Healthy People 2010,* four objectives about arthritis moved toward their targets: activity limitations attributable to arthritis, counseling of adults for weight reduction and exercise, effects of arthritis on paid work, and activity limitations attributable to chronic back pain (USDHHS, 2000, 2005).

Osteopenia is a condition of subnormally mineralized bone, usually as a result of a rate of bone lysis that exceeds the rate of bone matrix synthesis. **Osteoporosis** is a disorder characterized by abnormal loss of bone density and deterioration of bone tissue, with an increased fracture risk. It occurs most frequently in postmenopausal women who have fair complexions and are small, in sedentary individuals, and in people using corticosteroids on a long-term basis. It increases with age.

The functional capacity of all organ systems generally decreases. For example, in the gastrointestinal tract, the following chain of events occurs: decreased metabolism leads to less enzyme production, resulting in lower hydrochloric acid levels, which decreases tone in the large intestine. As a result, the middle-age adult may complain of acid indigestion with increased belching.

When the adult leads a sedentary lifestyle as well, the effects of the diminished motility through the gastrointestinal tract can be more pronounced. It is well-known that Americans eat more refined foods (foods that are low in bulk) than residents of third-world nations. A low-bulk diet can contribute to the problem of constipation, a change in bowel habits characterized by decreased frequency or passage of hard, drier stools and difficult defecation, and is believed to be a primary contributor to the increased incidence of colon cancer in the United States. Between ages 25 and 85, a 35% loss of nephron units occurs. The remaining nephrons increase in size and undergo degenerative changes. The entire weight of the kidneys decreases. Because blood supply is also diminished, the glomerular filtration rate is decreased by nearly half.

Significant changes occur in the cardiovascular system as the blood vessels lose elasticity and become thicker. This process predisposes middle-age adults to coronary artery disease, hypertension, myocardial infarctions, and strokes. Heart disease is the second leading cause of death in middle-age adults (Heron, 2007).

When a previously menstruating woman does not have a period for 1 year, she has reached menopause. The median age for menopause is 51 to 52 years. Women now expect to live one third of their lives after menopause. A great deal more must be learned about what causes many of the symptoms that occur in menopause (Mendelsohn & Karas, 2007). Sheehy (1993) conducted interviews of 100 women from their middle forties to their sixties and also interviewed 75 physicians and other experts. Her analysis showed that many of these people felt there was a renewed sexual vitality and surge of mental energy for menopausal women. She characterized menopause as a gateway to a second adulthood. Northrup (2008) and Sheehy (1993) reiterate the importance of taking time to rethink and reprioritize one's life once menopause is in process (Boston Women's Health Book Collective et al., 2006).

During this time, production of ovarian estrogen and progesterone ceases; the remaining estrogen is produced by the adrenal glands. As a result of the diminished estrogen level, a woman's secondary sex characteristics regress, such as loss of pubic hair and decrease in breast size. The female reproductive organs shrink, and vaginal secretions decrease, requiring additional lubrication.

As they approach the end of the middle years, men experience changes in their sexual response cycle as testosterone levels plateau and then decrease. The testes undergo degenerative changes, the number of viable spermatozoa diminishes, and the volume and viscosity of semen decrease. In men, sexual energy gradually declines; achieving an erection takes longer, but it is sustained longer. Stress, however, can significantly diminish function (Rice, 2000).

Life Expectancy and Mortality Rates

In the last decade (2001 to 2010), life expectancy has increased for all groups of Americans in the middle adult years. Across the 30-year age span, there is a decrease in mortality for all racial and ethnic groups with the most significant decreases seen in the 35- to-44-year-age category (Arias, 2011). Life expectancies for American men and women are now at record highs—80.4 years for women and 75.2 years for men (USDHHS, 2007c).

BOX 23-1 LEADING CAUSES OF DEATH IN MIDDLE-AGE ADULTS*

Ages 35 to 44 Years
- Unintentional injuries (40.2)
- Malignant neoplasms (31.9)
- Heart disease (28.3)

Ages 45 to 54 Years
- Malignant neoplasms (116.3)
- Heart disease (88.0)
- Accidents (45.5)

Ages 55 to 64 Years
- Malignant neoplasms (321.2)
- Heart disease (207.3)
- Bronchitis/emphysema (39.2)

Data from Office of Disease Prevention and Health Promotion. (2012). *A closer look at health disparities.* Washington, DC: Office of the Secretary of the Department of Health and Human Services. Retrieved from http://odphp.ososph.dhhs.gov/.
*Deaths per 100,000 population.

The leading causes of death during middle adulthood are heart disease, cancer, and accidents (National Center for Health Statistics, 2011). Box 23-1 shows a breakdown for each decile or 10-year interval for the middle-age adult. Reducing disabilities and deaths from these chronic conditions are national health-promotion and disease-prevention objectives (Lubkin & Larsen, 2006; USDHHS, 2011). In Box 23-2: *Healthy People 2020,* selected objectives and target goals for 2020 are outlined to give the reader some perspective of the scope of the task and opportunities that lie ahead for Americans. In addition, knowledge of the direction of the program offers professional nurses an incentive to focus their practice and teaching to help Americans achieve the goals specified in the *Healthy People Initiative.*

Most of the leading indicators identified in *Healthy People 2020* (2011) are preventable, or at least, modifiable. Gains in combating heart disease and stroke and many types of cancer during the 10 years up to 2010 are evident because of the efforts of nursing professionals. Health education, often conducted by professional nurses, is effective with adults who want or must change their lifestyle behaviors. This section addresses the changes that have occurred in the past 10 years; in some cases there have been progression toward the target goals and in other cases regression. The *Healthy People Initiative* was established in 1980 to provide structure for health-promotion and disease-prevention programs. For 30 years, objectives and goals have been established every 10 years. In an on-line article by Harston (2010), *Healthy People 2010: How have Americans fared?"* the author identified gains that were made as a result of the influence of the overall health promotion program since its inception.

While the data analysis showed some progress toward reaching the *Healthy People 2010* goals, there were a number of areas of "backsliding." Most notably, greater proportions of Americans are obese and have symptoms of high blood pressure compared to findings reported for *Healthy People 2000.* Hypertension and obesity are conditions that significantly affect the

❤ BOX 23-2   HEALTHY PEOPLE 2020

Selected National Health-Promotion and Disease-Prevention Objectives for the Middle-Age Adult

Overall Goals
- Improve health and well-being for all age groups.
- Reduce disparities across all racial and ethnic groups of Americans.

Objectives
- Improve access to high-quality health services.
- Increase the numbers of persons with health insurance to 100%. (Baseline* was 83.2% in 2008.)
- Increase the proportion of adults who have a specific source of ongoing care. (Target goal is 89.4%, a 10% improvement over 2010 expected by 2020. Baseline in 2008 was 81.3% of adults.)
- Reduce the overall cancer death rate. (Target goal in 2020 is 160.6 per 100,000 population. Baseline was 176.8 per 100,000 population cited in 2007.)
- Reduce the annual number of new cases of diagnosed diabetes to 7.2 per 100,000 population ages 18 to 84 years. (Baseline data reported in 2009 [National Health Interview Survey] were 8.0 new cases per 100,000 population.)
- Increase the proportion of adults with disabilities who report sufficient social and emotional support. (Target goal is 76.5% with a baseline at 69.5% reported in 2008.)
- *New developmental goal:* Increase the proportion of local health departments that have established culturally appropriate and linguistically competent community health-promotion and disease-prevention programs.
- Increase the proportion of persons served by community water systems who receive a supply of drinking water that meets the regulations of the Safe Drinking Water Act. (Target goal is 91% with a baseline of 89% reported in 2005.)
- Increase the proportion of pregnancies that are intended to 56%. (Baseline of 51% reported in 2002; National Survey of Family Growth, CDC & NCHS.)
- *New developmental goal for health-related quality of life and well-being:* Increase the quality, availability, and effectiveness of educational and community-based programs designed to prevent disease and improve health and quality of life.
- Reduce the proportion of adults with hypertension. (Target goal for 2020 is 26.9%. Baseline of 29.9% of adults ages 18 years and older had high blood pressure or hypertension in 2005-2008 reported in data collected from the National Health and Nutrition Examination Survey, CDC.)
- Reduce coronary heart disease deaths. (Target goal is 100.8 deaths per 100,000 population. Baseline data gathered in 2007 showed 126.0 deaths per 100,000 population.)
- Reduce the number of new cases of AIDS among adolescents and adults to 13.0 per 100,000 population. (The baseline of 14.4 new cases per 100,000 population ages 13 years and older with newly-diagnosed cases was reported in 2007.)
- Increase the percentage of adults (noninstitutionalized high-risk adults ages 18 to 64 years) who are vaccinated against pneumococcal disease. (Target goal: 60%.)
- Reduce unintentional injury deaths to 36.0 per 100,000 population compared to 40.0 deaths per 100,000 reported in 2007 in National Vital Statistics System-Mortality.
- Improve the health and well-being of women, infants, children, and families.
- Increase the proportion of adults with mental health disorders who receive treatment. (Target goal is 64.6% in 2020. Baseline data indicate that 58.7% of adults ages 18 years and older with serious mental illness received treatment in 2008.)
- Reduce the proportion of adults who are obese. (Target goal is 30.6%. Baseline data show that 34.0% of persons ages 20 and older were obese in 2005-2008.)
- Reduce the number of new cases of work-related, noise-induced hearing loss. (Target goal is 2.0 cases per 10,000 workers compared to 2.2 new cases per 10,000 persons in 2008.)
- Increase the proportion of adults who engage in aerobic physical activity of moderate intensity on a regular, preferably daily, basis for at least 30 minutes per day to 47.9%. (A baseline of 43.5% was reached in 2008.)
- Increase the proportion of adults who get sufficient sleep. (Target goal is 70.9%. A baseline of 69.6% was reported in 2008 among persons ages 22 years and older.)
- Increase recent smoking cessation success by adult smokers. (Target goal is 8.0% with a baseline of 6.0% of adult smokers ages 18 years or older who last smoked 6 months to 1 year ago reported in 2008.)
- Reduce substance abuse to protect the health, safety, and quality of life for all persons.
- Increase the proportion of people who have a comprehensive eye examination, including dilation, every 2 years. (Target goal is 60.5% of adults ages 18 years and older. Baseline data reported in 2008 showed that 55.0% of adults had eye examinations that included dilation.)

From U.S. Department of Health and Human Services. (2012). *Healthy People 2020*. Washington, DC: U.S. Government Printing Office.
*Baseline year is variable as noted for 2020 Objectives.
AIDS, Acquired immunodeficiency syndrome.

---

middle-aged adult. They often lead to heart disease, stroke, and development of diabetes. Harton (2010) suggests that the 2010 goals perhaps were too ambitious, but findings of other research positively confirm that more Americans are obese in 2010 than earlier in the decade (CDC, National Center for Health Statistics, 2002).

Areas of improvement in reaching the target goals for *Healthy People 2010* were encouraging because there were decreases seen in cancer deaths and in numbers of injuries at work (Sondik, 2009). Furthermore, laws that discourage or forbid smoking are having a wider impact in populations.

In sum, there was evidence of some progress shown in about 670 of 955 goals. Projecting ahead for 2020, efforts must be directed towards the following: increasing awareness of the *Healthy People 2020 Initiative* as a tool to improve the overall health of Americans; expanding knowledge of the *Initiative* in schools, tribal communities, and local health agencies through the use of public service announcements carried on radio, television, and Internet-based programs; and linking the objectives and goals to preventive health provisions associated with work sites (occupational health programs) and features included in health insurance policies. The good news is that the *Healthy People 2020* target goals are more achievable (less ambitious than projected for 2010), and that the objectives focus on individuals more than on "big" programs. There are goals that involve health counseling and behavior modification strategies provided by nurses, advanced practice nurses, and mental health nursing specialists in addition to physicians. In the larger picture, Americans will benefit when nurses, in all roles, incorporate the *Healthy People 2020* objectives into their practice.

Gender and Marital Status

In the midlife years, the death rate for men is higher. They are more likely than women to die from heart disease for all age categories (35 to 44, 45 to 54, and 55 to 64 years) and all racial and ethnic groups (*Healthy People 2020,* 2012). Although death rates for cardiovascular disease are declining for both genders, heart disease remains one of the primary causes of death. Risk factors for heart disease include obesity, lack of physical activity, smoking, high total cholesterol level, hypertension, and genetics. Among American adults, 68.3% are overweight or obese (CDC, 2010b). See Chapter 11 for a discussion of overweight, obesity, and *Healthy People 2020* target goals.

Nearly 60% of adults in the United States are married. Married adults report better health than divorced, widowed, or never-married adults. Marriage rates for White adults (61%) are higher than for Hispanic adults (58%) or Black adults (38%). Married adults report they are less likely to smoke, drink heavily, or be physically inactive (U.S. Census Bureau, 2006). Findings from the most recent census (2010) show that the number of interracial and interethnic married couples has increased by 28% in the last decade. Among unmarried, opposite-sex partners, 18% described their union as interracial or interethnic whereas 21% of same-sex couples reported they are interracial (U.S. Census Bureau, 2010).

Race, Gender, and Ethnicity

Black Americans represent the second largest racial group in the United States. They comprise 12.6% of the U.S. population (U.S. Census Bureau, 2010). In actual numbers, there are slightly less than 40 million Black Americans.

Cancer is the leading cause of death for Black men and Black women (combined incidence rates) in middle age. Findings in recent years show an encouraging decrease in both the incidence and the mortality rates for cancer among Black adults since 1993. Black adults are less likely to survive 5 years after diagnosis than White adults. Researchers believe that this disparity is largely related to factors associated with a significantly lower income level than other racial or ethnic groups. Although Black Americans comprise 13% of the U.S. population, they represent 24% of the nation's poor (ACS, 2008). Black households have the lowest median income ($31,969), compared to non-Hispanic Whites ($52,423), Hispanics ($37,781), and Asians ($64,238) (DeNavas-Walt et al., 2007).

Hispanics are the largest ethnic group in the United States, comprising about 16.3% of the total population. The U.S. Census Bureau 2010 survey findings show that this group is the fastest growing with currently more than 50 million people. Mortality numbers from the National Center for Health Statistics indicate accidents (unintentional injuries) are the leading cause of death for 35- to 44-year-old Hispanics; malignant neoplasms rank first among combined numbers of males and female Latinos whose ages range between 45 and 55 years. Most interestingly,

mortality statistics show the set of leading causes of death for White, middle-age Americans is the same as that for Hispanics.

Individuals who describe their ancestry as Asian/Pacific Islander comprise about 5% of Americans. Across all age groups representing "the middle-aged adult," malignant neoplasms and heart disease ranked as the leading causes of death. The types of cancer found most often among Asians are liver (including intrahepatic bile duct) and stomach.

American Indian and Native Alaskan people represent about 1% of the American population. Mortality statistics for both genders 35 to 44 years of age show accidents to be the leading cause of death; heart disease kills more 45 to 54 year olds, and in the oldest group (55 to 64 year olds), malignant neoplasms, notably cancer of the kidney and renal pelvis, cause the greatest number of deaths.

Access to Health Care

Individuals who are poor, defined as having an annual income less than $20,000 for family of four, generally have less accessibility to medical care compared to people earning a greater income. In a recent on-line publication, people who were unemployed self-reported a "poor psychological and physical health status" more often than individuals who were employed (Driscoll & Bernstein, 2012). Further, this finding was true among people with and without health insurance. There has been a trend in the last 5 years that shows a growing proportion of people without health insurance. This observation may be related to an increase in the percentage of Americans who are unemployed or underemployed. Government reports also show that the cost of health insurance premiums has increased. The gravity of the situation increases because of the lost benefits, including health insurance, when individuals become unemployed (USDHHS, 2007a).

Blacks are more likely to be uninsured than non-Hispanic Whites. In an analysis conducted by the American Cancer Society, those without health insurance were less likely to have had a recent mammogram to detect breast cancer or to have been screened for colorectal cancer, two of the most common cancers in the United States. In addition, those without insurance who were diagnosed with cancer were more likely to have been diagnosed at an advanced stage, when cancer is more difficult to treat (American Cancer Society [ACS]). Although poverty and lack of health insurance are important reasons for ethnic and racial disparities in cancer outcomes, there are other reasons as well, including differences in tumor biology and a higher prevalence of coexisting conditions (ACS, 2005). More research is needed on ways to address the racial and ethnic disparities in cancer outcomes.

The second leading cause of death for Black Americans is heart disease. Of concern is that Black Americans are less likely to be diagnosed with heart disease, but they are 30% more likely to die from it compared to the population in general. Hypertension and overweight/obesity are risk factors for heart disease and stroke. Black adults are 50% more likely to have hypertension. A high proportion (77%) of Black women is overweight, compared to 57% of White women. Black adults are 50% more likely to suffer a stroke, compared to White adults.

Black Americans share a disproportionate burden of human immunodeficiency virus/acquired immunodeficiency syndrome (HIV/AIDS). Black men are eight times more likely than non-Hispanic White men to have HIV/AIDS. Black women are 23 times more likely to have HIV/AIDS than non-Hispanic White women. Blacks account for 47% of all persons living with HIV/AIDS in the United States (USDHHS, 2007c) according to findings reported by the CDC for 2009.

Latino/Hispanic Americans are the largest ethnic minority group in the United States. They comprise 16.3% of the population. There are more than 50 million Hispanic Americans. Most Hispanics (60%) are born in the United States. A disproportionate number of Hispanics are poor and lack health insurance.

Hispanic Americans have the highest uninsured rate of any racial or ethnic group in the United States. Findings reported by the American Cancer Society in 2006 indicate that twice as many Hispanic men under the age of 64 (32.7%) report no regular source of health care compared to non-Hispanic White men (14.9%). Results of a major population survey showed that approximately one third of Hispanics were uninsured at the time they were interviewed or had been uninsured for at least part of the past year. More than one fourth of Hispanics surveyed had been without health insurance for more than 1 year (Cohen & Martinez, 2007).

Cancer is the second leading cause of death for young (35 to 44 years) middle-aged Hispanics, surpassing unintentional accidents. As the Hispanic population ages (into the 45 to 64 age range), neoplasms become the leading cause of death. Breast cancer is the most common type of cancer in Hispanic women. Hispanic women with breast cancer are less likely to be diagnosed when the disease is at a local stage, and are approximately 20% more likely to die than non-Hispanic White women even when they are diagnosed at a similar age and stage of disease.

Heart disease ranks second as a cause of death among Latino/Hispanics who are 45 to 64 years. Hispanic adults are less likely to smoke than non-Hispanic White adults, but almost 80% of Mexican Americans are overweight; 42.3% of all Mexican American women are obese. Mexican Americans comprise approximately 60% of the Hispanic population in the United States. Obesity increases the risk of diabetes, hypertension, heart disease (American Heart Association, 2012; American Obesity Association, 2004), and premature death. Obesity is also associated with increased risk of breast, prostate, colon, and uterine cancer (ACS, 2006).

Genetics

The middle-age adult is at greater risk than the young adult for diseases known to be associated with genetics (i.e., familial characteristics). These conditions include diabetes, hypertension, Huntington's chorea, arteriosclerosis, gout, obesity, heart disease, and alcoholism. There are some malignancies that are related to genetics; for example, women with a personal or family history of breast cancer are at a higher risk for developing this type of malignancy. In addition, individuals with a family history of colorectal cancer, rectal or colon polyps, or ulcerative colitis have an increased risk for developing this type of cancer.

GORDON'S FUNCTIONAL HEALTH PATTERNS

Health Perception–Health Management Pattern

To promote health in the middle-age adult, the nurse performs a health assessment that includes the person's values and beliefs, lifestyle patterns, general perceptions of health, and health practices (see the health-promotion model by Pender et al, 2011).

Habits

The self-destructive habits of the middle-age adult that have been practiced for years (cigarette smoking, excessive alcohol use, and overeating) begin to have visible consequences. As pressures increase, adults are tempted to turn to substances such as these as a crutch for coping with stress. Prevention is extremely important, primarily because withdrawal from any of these substances is a difficult process.

Risk Factors

The major risk factors for adults in the middle years are environmental and behavioral; they can be changed through teaching, counseling, and utilization of other nursing interventions (USDHHS, 2000, 2007d). Helping adults to take care of themselves and to change, when indicated, can be accomplished on an individual or group basis.

Some of the health-promotion needs of the middle-age adult include acceptance of aging, the need to exercise, and weight control. Decreasing or stopping cigarette smoking and alcohol consumption can also be identified needs. Preventive health screening is vital. The adult needs input into and control of as many of these behaviors as possible.

Health risks of middle-age adults overall are categorized as group risks (age, gender, race) and personal risks. Precritical secondary prevention includes periodic selective screening for the detection of disease before it becomes clinically apparent, such as performing a breast self-examination. A suggested screening examination appears in Box 23-3.

Chronic conditions are defined as those that last for more than 3 months. Approximately 20% of the population age 45 to 64 reports limitations caused by chronic conditions (Lubkin & Larsen, 2006). A significant increase is seen between the ages of 45 and 64. Chronic conditions found in the middle-age adult include heart conditions, arthritis, impairments of the back and spine, chronic obstructive lung disease, diabetes, mental and nervous system conditions, and dental disease (Lubkin & Larsen, 2006).

Nutritional-Metabolic Pattern

Dietary factors are correlated with 5 of the 10 leading causes of death in the United States: coronary heart disease, some cancers, stroke, non–insulin-dependent diabetes mellitus, and atherosclerosis (Centers for Disease Control and Prevention, National Center for Health Statistics, 2010b).

Physical activities and nutritional patterns frequently are correlated. The middle-age adult typically leads a more sedentary lifestyle than does the young adult, primarily because of increased responsibilities at work and home and the many convenience devices that are found in homes and workplaces.

BOX 23-3   SCREENING EXAMINATION: AGES 35 TO 65

Database
- Health history: initial update with nurse or PE
- Health hazard appraisal: initial screening
- Psychological inventories as needed

Physical Examination (Every 3 to 5 Years Until Age 40, then Annually) Emphasizing
- Weight and height
- Blood pressure, pulse rate
- Breasts
- Pelvis
- Prostate
- Testicles
- Eyes
- Mouth
- Skin

Laboratory Procedures
- Pap smear
- Hemoccult: three stools for hemoccult with PE after age 50
- Colonoscopy or sigmoidoscopy every 3 to 5 years after age 50 as indicated
- Mammography screening at age 35 every 2 years, then yearly after age 50
- Urinalysis: examined at the time of PE
- Lipid profile (men ages 35 to 65; women ages 45 to 65)

- Chest radiograph with PE if heavy smoker
- Tetanus and diphtheria booster every 10 years
- Influenza vaccine: follow current recommendations
- Counseling and testing for HIV as indicated
- Rubella serology (women of childbearing age)

Self-Care Education and Counseling
- With physical examination; individualized according to individual's risk factors
- Injury prevention: seat belts, helmets, firearms, smoke detectors
- Stress reduction
- Exercise
- Diet: cholesterol, fat, sodium, fiber, multivitamins with folic acid (women of childbearing age)
- Calcium
- Breast self-examination
- Testicular self-examination
- Dental care
- Mouth care
- Sexually transmitted diseases
- Contraception
- Skin protection from ultraviolet light
- Alcohol and other substance abuse
- Smoking cessation
- Possible hormone prophylaxis (perimenopausal and postmenopausal women)

Data from American Cancer Society (Massachusetts Division), U.S. Department of Health and Human Services. (2000). *Healthy People 2010.* Washington, DC: U.S. Government Printing Office.
HIV, Human immunodeficiency virus; *Pap,* Papanicolaou; *PE,* physician examination.

Research findings published on the Centers for Disease Control and Prevention website show that the incidence of obesity is increasing among men and boys compared to women and girls. Linked with less activity is the lack of attention to modification of food intake and calorie consumption, resulting in obesity, one of the major health problems of the middle years.

Obesity

Obesity is defined as a body mass index (BMI) of 30 kg/m^2 or more, and being overweight is a BMI greater than 27.8 kg/m^2 for adult males and greater than 27.3 kg/m^2 for adult females. In 2009, an estimated 35.7% of the American population was considered obese (Ogden et al., 2012). Of note is the finding that the target goal of *Healthy People 2010* of 15% was *not* attained. In fact, the progress report on *Healthy People 2010* goals published by the U.S. Department of Health and Human Services (2005) indicates that there was an increase in the incidence of obesity to 34% of the adult population compared to 25% in the year 2000.

Overweight and obesity substantially raise the risk of illness from high blood pressure, high cholesterol, type 2 (non-insulin-dependent) diabetes, heart disease and stroke, gall-bladder disease, arthritis, sleep disturbances associated with breathing problems, and endometrial, breast, prostate and colon cancers. Individuals who are obese often suffer from social stigmatization, discrimination, and lowered self-esteem (USDHHS, 2005, p. 29).

Women with less education and low incomes and Black and Hispanic women are at an increased risk for being overweight. In addition to gender, race, and socioeconomic status, genetics may be a contributing factor. The most significant variables, however, are health behaviors, particularly food intake and exercise and activity patterns. Although an abundance of health information is available, these challenges persist.

As much as 40% of a typical American family's food budget is spent on food in restaurants or for take-out foods, both of which are usually higher in fat (including saturated and trans fats) and salt content than foods prepared at home (AHRQ, 2012). Losing and maintaining weight loss may require an individual to change eating and activity behaviors, but the social, food preparation, and consumption behaviors of the family must change as well.

Prevention of obesity is the goal of weight management during the middle years. When the adult is obese, a clear-cut history of the onset is imperative. A lifelong history of obesity is significantly more arduous to alter than that of adult-onset obesity. A decrease in calories should be accompanied by at least 30 minutes of exercise 5 times a week. When calories are reduced and exercise is increased, weight loss is achieved and maintained.

Weight-management resources available to the adult are plentiful. Weight-management programs using behavior modification can be found in varied settings, such as universities and work sites, Weight Watchers, Overeaters Anonymous, and Take Off Pounds Sensibly. If the nurse identifies a need for weight management and no program is available, a self-help group can be initiated. A suggested list of topics generated by the group is assembled. A discussion of basic nutrition with appropriate handouts is a good place to start. Having adults record their individual goals and keep a 1-week diet log is nonthreatening and helpful for future planning; it also gives them some responsibility in the program. Intake food journals assist the individuals in maintaining weight loss outcomes.

High Saturated Fat Diet

Lipid levels and ratios have a significant influence on cardiovascular and cerebrovascular morbidity and mortality rates. The National Heart, Lung and Blood Institute considers a total blood cholesterol level less than 200 mg/dL as desirable. For the first time in more than 40 years, the average total cholesterol level for adults in the United States is now 199 mg/dL (Japsen, 2007). Much of this success is attributed to the use of statin drugs that lower the level of low-density lipoproteins (LDLs) in the blood. The reference *Coronary Primary Prevention Trial* demonstrates that men at high risk are able to reduce coronary heart disease by approximately 2% for every 1% lower blood cholesterol level. Before using medication to reduce cholesterol level, persons with high cholesterol levels are advised to reduce their intakes of saturated fat, total fat, and dietary cholesterol; normalize their weight; and increase their level of physical activity. If lifestyle changes are not successful, medication is often advised. Some studies demonstrate the benefits of estrogen administration on heart health (Parker-Pope, 2007). One pharmaceutical company is currently seeking FDA approval to sell its cholesterol-lowering drug over-the-counter (Japsen, 2007; USDHHS, 2000).

Calcium

Adequate calcium intake is essential for developing and maintaining bone mass. Additionally, calcium is needed for other physiological processes, including muscle contraction and blood pressure regulation. Men and women need a minimal daily intake of 1000 mg of calcium. Pregnant and nursing women need 1200 mg, and postmenopausal women need either 1000 mg (when taking estrogen) or 1500 mg (when not taking estrogen). Vitamin D enhances the absorption of calcium (Karch, 2003). When daily intake of calcium is less than adequate, the serum calcium level will be maintained by leaching calcium from bone, resulting in osteoporosis. Exercise also contributes to bone mass by increasing mechanical stress on the bones.

Caffeine

Caffeine is a popular stimulant found in coffee, tea, and some soft drinks, such as colas. Caffeine prolongs the amount of time that physical work can be performed and appears to decrease boredom and increase attention span. On the negative side, coffee has recently been the subject of significant scrutiny from the media, with reports of a link between cancer of the pancreas and coffee consumption. There is controversy regarding whether daily moderate intake of caffeine has any detrimental effects.

Like alcohol and nicotine, caffeine is readily available and has become an accepted part of daily living. Because caffeine is a strong stimulant with effects that typically are taken for granted, its importance as an addictive substance must be emphasized. Ingestion of 0.5 gram of caffeine (3 to 4 cups of coffee) can increase the basal metabolic rate an average of 10%, and possibly as much as 25% for some people.

Long-term stimulation of the central nervous system results in restlessness, sleep disturbances, cardiac stimulation, and withdrawal effects. Nurses' assessment should screen for stimulating and addicting substances that may be producing these symptoms.

High-Sodium Diet

High-sodium diets play a significant role in hypertension, especially when consumed over many years. The result may be an increase in the amount of total body fluids, which increases peripheral vascular resistance. Salt contains approximately 40% sodium and is a contributing factor for hypertension in the 10% to 20% of Americans who are at risk. On average, Americans consume 4 to 5 g of sodium per day. A major contributor of dietary sodium is the salt found in processed foods.

Over the past 3 decades, many clinical studies have demonstrated the effectiveness of lowering blood pressure measurements by lowering dietary sodium intake. Other studies have described the relationships between urinary and sodium excretion and the change of blood pressure with age (Joint National Committee, 2003).

Alcohol Abuse

Substance abuse can be a devastating habit. Many adults abuse prescription and illicit drugs and, especially, alcohol. Twenty-three million Americans struggle with a drug or alcohol problem but 85% do not feel they need treatment (USDHHS, 2005).

Initially alcohol appears to be a stimulant, but actually it is a central nervous system depressant and anesthetic. Chronic alcohol use produces tolerance, thereby necessitating a gradual increase in dose to achieve the same effect. Alcohol contributes to problems with safety because of decreased reaction time and depression of the central nervous system.

Alcohol is frequently treated as a nondrug, but alcohol addiction is second only to nicotine addiction. Alcohol is readily available, reasonably inexpensive, and considered a part of social exchange; its long-range physiological and psychological effects are well documented. In the United States, two thirds of adults consume alcohol, and 18 million are problem drinkers. Presently, men outnumber women as alcohol abusers by approximately 5:1, but this ratio is decreasing as more women are exceeding low-risk drinking guidelines (USDHHS, NIH, 2005).

The *Dietary Guidelines for Americans*, issued jointly by the U.S. Department of Agriculture and the U.S. Department of Health and Human Services (www.nutrition.gov), defines moderate drinking as no more than one drink a day for women and no more than two drinks a day for men. Women are more vulnerable than men to the effects of alcohol because, pound for pound, women have less water in their bodies and they tend to weigh less than men. This means that a woman's brain and other organs are exposed to more alcohol and to the toxic by-products of alcohol as it is metabolized. The death rate for female alcoholics is 50% to 100% higher than for male alcoholics. A woman is more likely to drink excessively if her parents, siblings, or other blood relatives have problems with alcohol; if her partner drinks heavily; if she was abused physically or sexually as a child; if she has a history of depression; or if she is able to "hold her liquor" more than others (USDHHS, NIH, 2005).

Alcohol abuse is associated with motor vehicle accidents, homicides, suicides, drownings, heart disease, cancer, liver disease, pancreatitis, and fetal alcohol syndrome. It is a major cause of mental retardation in children (USDHHS, 2000). The alcoholic person is at greater risk for cancer of the larynx, oral cavity, and liver.

The alcoholic may complain of symptoms such as heartburn and gas, stomach distention, poor eating habits, nausea and vomiting, gastric pain, right upper quadrant pain, and irritation of the mouth, throat, and esophagus. Two additional subtle findings are spider angiomata and palmar erythema.

Primary prevention for substance and alcohol abuse is complex, especially because adults consume these agents for many reasons, including peer pressure, loneliness, alienation, frustration, anxiety, and low self-esteem. Heavy drinkers may also be following the example established by influential people in their lives. Merely telling people about the potential physical, emotional, and legal hazards appears to have little effect as a preventive measure. Promoting more realistic portrayals of substance abuse through the media is difficult to implement. Although techniques such as assertiveness training and teaching adults to resist persuasion are helpful, more useful approaches might include helping them learn to manage anxiety and increase their self-esteem. Less anxious and more confident people have greater skills in resisting peer influences to participate in substance abuse; they also are more likely to have fewer episodes of isolation and loneliness.

Early detection and intervention can decrease ongoing and future physical and psychosocial problems resulting from alcohol abuse. Nurses use a variety of screening strategies to identify individuals' perceptions and consequences of drinking. The CAGE questionnaire is the most popular screening tool used in primary care (Dunphy, 2004). The Michigan Alcohol Screening Test (http://counselingresource.Com/quizzes/alcohol/-mast/index.html) and Alcohol Use Disorders Identification Test (http://pubs.niaaa.nih.gov/publications/Assessing%20Alcohol/InstrumentPDFs/14_AUDIT.pdf) are examples of other screening instruments.

Abnormal laboratory test results, including elevations in aspartate aminotransferase level, erythrocyte mean corpuscular volume, and serum glutamyltransferase level, are not adequately sensitive and specific and may be a result of other causes including trauma, disease, and medications.

A variety of treatments are known to be effective, but no single "best" intervention has been identified. Effective treatments may be to address other problems using interventions such as pharmacological agents, stress management, acupuncture, individual and family therapy, and supportive environments.

Oral Health

Gingivitis. Gingivitis is found commonly among adults who fail to brush their teeth and use dental floss regularly. Redness and swelling develop around the teeth. Bleeding of the gums, while brushing the teeth, is an early sign of gingivitis. The gums may or may not be tender. When inflammation is not adequately treated and controlled, **periodontitis,** involving bone destruction, can develop in addition to tooth loss.

Dental Hygiene and Decay. Dental health is essential to overall health. Brushing the teeth and flossing after eating, receiving routine dental check-ups, and consuming fewer carbohydrates (especially simple sugars) are important interventions to prevent dental caries. Adults in the middle-age years have responsibility not only for their own regular dental care but also for the care of their children and parents. Fluoridation of water (versus bottled or tap water) and use of applied sealants are additional health choices that support prevention of dental caries and, possibly, tooth loss.

Dental health is one of the leading indicators identified in *Healthy People 2020* (2011). There is increasing evidence to show that periodontal, or gum disease is closely linked to diabetes, heart disease, and stroke. For the middle age woman, poor oral health can cause premature births and low-birth-weight infants (Bensley, Van Eehwyk, and Ossiander, 2011).

There are many conditions that begin with changes in the oropharyngeal mucosa such as cancer of the mouth and esophageal cancer. Consequently, annual dental check-ups are important because dental professionals (dentists or dental hygienists) may be the first to detect a symptom or irregularity that points to a potentially dangerous condition.

Findings described in the *Healthy People 2020* oral health web page indicate that approximately 44.5% of Americans representing all racial and ethnic groups receive annual health care by a dentist. Target goals for oral health services usage (OH-7 outlined in Objectives for *Healthy People 2020*) indicate an expectation of 10% improvement in the proportion of adults and children ages 2 and older who receive dental care annually. The target goal is 49.0% of the population seeking dental care on an annual basis compared to the baseline of 44.5% reported in 2007.

People who are in vulnerable populations—individuals whose annual income is below the poverty line, others who are chronically ill or disabled, or still others whose medical or psychiatric treatment plans are very complicated—may not receive adequate or proper oral health care. In a recent article, the Surgeon General addresses a proposed *Oral Health Care Initiative.* She says that while there is evidence of progress being made to increase access to oral health services for a greater proportion of the population, those who are vulnerable because of their illness, such as people with HIV and AIDS, still find difficulty in obtaining proper and adequate oral health care (Benjamin, 2012). The *Oral Health Care Initiative* will help address the multilayered complexities that people with HIV and AIDS face—for instance, the combination of lack of dental insurance, lack of transportation, limitations of disability, increasing costs of treatment, inability to afford the cost of oral health care, and discrimination on the part of dental health care providers. In sum, "the lack of dental care for individuals with HIV and AIDS undermines their treatment and diminishes their quality of life which in turn, can affect the overall outcomes of their overall treatment regimen" (USDHHS, Surgeon General, 2010).

However, other data indicate that about 15% of adults refrain from dental care because of cost of dental examinations and treatment. In 2009, working age adults, ages 18 to 64 years, were more likely to report unmet dental needs (within the previous 12-month interval) compared to children. Women more than men in the same age category neglected dental needs because of cost considerations (CDC, National Center for Health Statistics, 2002). Other findings discovered from this extensive health survey showed the percentage of reporting unmet dental concerns attributable to costs of examination and/or treatment increased 7% compared to 10 years earlier. These survey findings represent all races and ethnic groups.

Findings from the National Health and Nutrition Examination Survey (2002) show that dental health often is poor among smokers (currently smoking) compared to former smokers and to those who have never smoked. Smokers who were interviewed said that they had three or more dental problems. Also, current smokers reported infrequent visits to their dentist (in some cases, more than 5 years) or never seeing a dentist. The USDHHS (2010) website shows research findings that indicate the prevalence of gum disease is three times greater in individuals who smoke cigarettes compared to individuals who have never smoked.

In summary, oral disease is preventable. Regularly scheduled dental care with a dentist and dental hygienist is highly recommended for good dental hygiene and early treatment of dental decay and periodontal diseases, such as gingivitis. In addition, dentists can provide screening for oropharyngeal cancer. Oral health is essential in the overall digestive and elimination processes.

Elimination Pattern

Aging brings a gradual decrease of tone in the large intestine. This change, accompanied by a sedentary lifestyle, lack of fiber in the diet, and inadequate fluid intake, can predispose the adult to constipation. Advertising on television and forms of media present strong arguments that encourage individuals to rely on external controls rather than on exercise and dietary means to solve this problem. Consequently, many adults are dependent on taking fiber products as well as laxatives for regular bowel movements.

In the kidneys, degenerative changes in the nephron units gradually increase during the middle-aged years. In most cases, adults do not have any appreciable alteration in kidney function unless the person has experienced repeated infections, trauma, or the long-term effects of diabetes mellitus or hypertension.

Alteration in bladder control (incontinence) can occur in both women and men because of weakening of the muscles of the pelvic floor or damage to pelvic nerves. Urinary incontinence is problematic in women who have experienced multiple births. In men, urinary incontinence frequently occurs as a complication of surgery for prostate cancer. Incontinence can be socially embarrassing but the condition can be improved with Kegel exercises (Landefeld et al., 2008); Newman & Giovannini, 2002).

Activity-Exercise Pattern

Regular physical activity increases life expectancy and the quality of life. Exercise helps to prevent coronary heart disease, hypertension (American Heart Association, 2012), diabetes, osteoporosis (National Osteoporosis Foundation, 1998), and depression. Research findings show there is a strong correlation between physical exercise and lower rates of osteoporosis (National Osteoporosis Foundation, 1998), back injury, stroke (American Heart Association, 2012), and colon cancer. Weight loss programs that incorporate physical activities also make significant contributions to health promotion as evidenced by increased life expectancy and quality of life (Kriketos et al., 2000; USDHHS, 2000, 2007e).

One of the objectives for *Healthy People 2020* is to continue to decrease deaths related to heart disease. There is still evidence that a significant percentage of Americans in the middle-adult age bracket do not engage in regular moderate physical activity for at least 30 minutes, 5 or more days a week. Only a fraction of adults perform the recommended level, and slightly more report no leisure-time physical activities. Sedentary behavior increases with aging (USDHHS, 2007a). This finding may be due to the onset of conditions that affect mobility and strength.

Continuous, rhythmic exercise maintained for a sufficient period to stress the cardiac system (increase heart rate and blood pressure) is desirable. Some suggested activities include brisk walking, jogging, swimming, bicycling, and skipping rope as well as walking or biking to work. Activities that focus on skill and coordination should be attempted by the adult older than age 40 rather than activities necessitating speed and strength. Moderation is key for all groups of individuals. Caution is recommended for adults nearing age 65 to prevent muscle strains and/or falls. Overexertion—as evidenced by dizziness, chest pressure or chest pain, and unresolved shortness of breath—should be avoided. Also, in hot weather, strenuous exercise should be balanced with rest periods and increased intake of fluids to prevent heat stroke.

Nurses play significant roles in assessing, teaching, and evaluating individuals relative to activity-exercise programs. Advanced practice nurses often are instrumental in creating and guiding weight loss programs; nurses working in the community may see local citizens at health fairs or health-promotion events; and other nurses or therapists visit persons at home for care following hospitalization for surgery or acute illness as home health professionals. Activity programs are initiated to restore health (following heart attack) or to improve cardiac function (such as cardiac and pulmonary rehabilitation), and in some cases to control blood glucose levels. A thorough assessment, including a cardiac stress test, is necessary when an individual has not exercised regularly in the past. Parameters for heart rate, blood pressure, and length and frequency of exercise sessions are set in advance by a cardiologist. Nurses support and guide individuals by helping them determine program goals, by monitoring their progress, and by teaching individuals how to modify lifestyle behaviors to obtain particular objectives.

To achieve maximal effectiveness, physical exercise should involve as many muscles as is possible, and be performed on a regular basis. Adults should spend 30 minutes or more of brisk physical activity every day for a total of 3 to 4 hours per week. Optimal performance level varies for each individual, and should be based on parameters set by one's physician in advance of starting a fitness program. The following formula to calculate target heart rate is shown on the American Heart Association website (2012). Begin by subtracting one's age from the value 220 and then multiplying this number by 0.75 to determine a heart rate value that is within safe limits. For example, for an individual who is 50 years old: $(220 - 50) = 170$; $170 \times 0.75 = 127.5$ (or 128 beats/min) for the optimal heart rate. Comparatively, the cardiac muscle capacity of a person younger than 50 would be greater than 128 beats/min; and as one increases their functional aerobic capacity, the target heart rate required to tone the cardiac muscle would be increased.

To summarize, routine exercise is essential to the health of the heart and overall muscle strength. The type of activity and style is an individual choice. Program goals are achieved more readily when exercise is incorporated into leisure activities or is a part of a group activity.

Sleep-Rest Pattern

Middle-age Americans may not get as much sleep as young adults because of increased demands in their lives. Caring for immediate family, children, and sometimes parents as well as employment responsibilities consume most of a 24-hour interval.

Insomnia is a common finding in this age category. This condition may be the result of overstimulation resulting from drinking too many caffeinated beverages, strenuous exercise within 2 hours of bedtime, or failure to have a regular sleep/wake schedule in a 24-hour period (National Sleep Foundation, 2012). Frequently occurring insomnia can lead to distractibility and irritability and fatigue during the daytime hours.

Rest is essential to allow restorative functions of the body to occur. The effects of insomnia can be counteracted by regularly scheduled, high-quality sleep and occasional napping when fatigued. If insomnia becomes a chronic problem, cognitive-behavioral therapy has also been demonstrated as an effective treatment option (Jacobs, 1998; Jacobs et al., 2004). The National Sleep Foundation (www.nationalsleepfoundation.org) offers detailed information about treating insomnia and other sleep disorders with medications if those modalities are indicated.

Cognitive-Perceptual Pattern

Learning is a phenomenon that occurs across the life span. Needs for increasing knowledge or information and acquiring new skills are constants as adults develop through a variety of experiences. Employment demands or new roles in life, such as becoming a parent or suddenly needing to care for an elderly family member, thrust the middle-age adult into numerous different learning situations. The ability to learn a range of skills or to acquire knowledge through observing, performing, or participating in play activities begins in childhood as described by

> **BOX 23-4   DEVELOPMENTAL TASKS OF MIDDLE AGE**
>
> - Helping children become responsible, happy adults
> - Rediscovering or developing new satisfaction in the relationship with one's spouse (for the single adult, this can occur in a relationship with a sibling or significant other)
> - Developing an affectionate, but independent, relationship with aging parents
> - Reaching the peak in one's career
> - Achieving mature social and civic responsibility
> - Accepting and adapting to biological changes
> - Maintaining or developing friendships
> - Developing leisure-time activities

Gardner (1983, 1993) and extends into the middle years. The capacity to perform intellectually (i.e., reason through critical thinking, use/increase vocabulary, and apply spatial perception skills) stays constant through the 35- to 64-year-old age range. However, some decreases in reaction time and cognitive flexibility become more apparent as age increases.

Intellectual Ability

The ability to acquire new knowledge or skills, or "learning intelligence," accumulates through formal education and life experiences and continues to increase throughout life. The evidence of this phenomenon is demonstrated by the many scholars and artists who become more productive in their middle years than when they were young adults. Some individuals discover "new talents" later in life since there is more leisure time or motivation to explore new areas or interests.

The theories of Piaget (1970), Bloom (1984), and Havighurst and Orr (1956) are relevant to the middle-age adult. These theorists conclude that the prime time to be in the learner role is when the developmental task for that role is to be accomplished. The adult in the middle years as the learner-performer is a case in point. For example, to balance the responsibilities of caring for children and parents and being employed outside the home, the adult may explore new career options or creative endeavors.

Havighurst defines developmental tasks as the basic tasks of living that must be achieved for the adult to live successfully. These tasks are dictated by the expectations of society, the physiological changes of the body throughout life, and the individual's own value system and goals. Although initially described in 1956, Havighurst and Orr's developmental tasks of middle age remain timely (Havighurst & Orr, 1956) (Box 23-4).

If career goals have been previously identified, then attaining them can be highly rewarding, both psychologically and financially. In addition to career activities, the mature adult has an increased social awareness and often assumes more civic responsibility.

In Piaget's theory of cognitive development, formal operations are the highest or most complex level. This stage begins at approximately age 12 and continues throughout life. Piaget describes the thoughts of adults as being both flexible and effective. The adult can deal efficiently with complex problems of reasoning, including hypothesis testing (Piaget, 1970).

Bloom (1984) developed a hierarchy of cognitive levels in the adult learner. Knowledge is the simplest or most basic cognitive level. Knowledge is the acquisition of information. The adult learner defines "high blood pressure" in lay terms.

Comprehension is the second level, as indicated by the learner grasping the meaning of the communicated message and relating the term(s) to other material. For example, the individual can state one way that obesity influences high blood pressure.

The third level is application of knowledge. At this level the learner demonstrates understanding of ideas and concepts by extending them to describe or relate to real-life situations. For example, the individual with hypertension becomes involved in an exercise program.

The fourth level is analysis. At this level, all aspects of learning are united in thought and the individual is cognizant of the relationships and interactions of all the parts. For example, the individual considers his or her values and life goals when making decisions about taking action in regard to understanding health care needs.

The highest order of learning involves synthesis and evaluation. The person is able to combine various elements to form a plan, and then is able to judge the extent to which the actions and results satisfy the original objectives. For example, people may develop plans to improve their health status and increase their disease self-management responsibilities. The next step is to validate the results of ongoing health care programs in relation to their projected expectations. Genetic and personality factors, in combination with environmental conditions and lifestyle practices, account for the large difference in the ways in which individuals maintain mental abilities. Schaie and Willis (2005) have identified seven of these factors that maintain cognitive function in later life:

- Absence of chronic diseases
- Living with favorable socioeconomic factors, including maximal occupational complexity, a low degree of routine, and an intact family
- Involvement in complex social activities
- Flexible personality style
- Marriage to a spouse with high cognitive function
- Maintaining high levels of performance speed
- Personal satisfaction with accomplishments in midlife and early old age (Box 23-5: Research for Evidence-Based Practice)

Perceptual Changes

Presbyopia (farsightedness) is common in middle-age adults, even in individuals who have had no previous problems with their vision. This condition occurs because of the loss of elasticity in the lens of the eye so that the adult cannot focus on objects that are in close range, such as reading without using their prescription lenses (Glanze et al., 2008).

Presbyopia is corrected with prescription lenses, which may be needed only for reading or for close work. *Lasik surgery*, a surgical intervention to correct refraction, is currently employed widely, and is favored by individuals who do not want to use standard eyeglasses.

Other visual conditions that may not be as easily corrected include decreased peripheral vision and decreased visual

sensitivity in the dark. Both conditions are a result of the cornea becoming less transparent, and both are slow and insidious in their development. Because all of these conditions are not readily detected by the individual, middle-age adults should undergo a routine professional eye examination every year.

Glaucoma occurs as a result of increased intraocular pressure, which can damage the optic nerve. Damage to the optic nerve is irreversible, but visual loss can be prevented if damage is identified early and treatment is initiated. Peripheral vision is affected with glaucoma. Information available at EyeCareAmerica.org shows that glaucoma is the leading cause of blindness among African Americans in the United States. A current estimate is three times the number of African Americans have glaucoma compared to White Americans; also, the rate of blindness attributable to glaucoma is four times greater in African Americans relative to White Americans. The importance of regular eye exams by an ophthalmologist cannot be underestimated.

A cataract, opacity of the lens, can develop and cloud the vision in later years of middle age. Often cataracts develop in people who have diabetes. Another disorder, diabetic retinopathy, gradually causes rupture of vessels in the retina, which leak into the eye, causing lack of color differentiation and central vision changes.

Macular degeneration is a progressive deterioration of the maculae of the retina and choroid structures of the eye (Glanze et al., 2008). This condition is very serious because it represents the effects of several disorders. Once a diagnosis of macular degeneration has been made, retinal ophthalmologists should be involved in the care of the individual.

Another common perceptual change in middle age is presbycusis (impaired auditory acuity). The first sounds to be lost are higher frequencies, such as a woman's voice. This is important in the work environment and situations that require social interaction. Because this process is subtle, middle age is a time for auditory evaluations as a part of routine examinations.

Beginning in the middle years, the sense of taste also diminishes. A progressive loss of taste buds occurs, first affecting those located more anteriorly on the tongue, which detect sweet and salt. When the effectiveness of the posterior taste buds declines, detection of bitter and sour flavors is lost. Consequently, this change can alter a person's food preferences and present problems for people who insist on adding salt to compensate for the deficit. Nurses involved in the care of the middle-aged adult, perhaps in the community or in home health, can show the individual how using various herbs and spices can enhance flavor.

Self-Perception–Self-Concept Pattern

Levinson's Theory

In Levinson's research on men (1986a,b) and women (1996), a theory on "individual life structures" is posed. Levinson describes age-associated seasons or eras. The midlife transition, beginning at ages 38 to 40 years, appears to include reappraising one's life, integrating the polarities, and modifying one's life structure toward being who one wants to be. Middle-age adults struggle with meaning, value, and direction of their lives.

Erikson's Theory

In Erikson's eight stages of the life cycle (Erikson & Erikson, 1998), the last three stages are related to adulthood. Stage 7, generativity versus stagnation or self-absorption, most frequently is associated with the middle-age years.

Erikson identifies generativity as the primary task during this stage. Generativity includes a sense of productivity and creativity, as evidenced by reaching previously established goals (Hornstein, 1986; Reifman et al., 1991; Thomas, 1995). Generativity also encompasses a desire to care for others and is the opposite of stagnation, which is the result of a lack of accomplishment during middle-age's developmental tasks, and self-absorption, the tendency to direct most of one's interest and attention to oneself, thereby excluding others.

Middle age is a time of critical self-review, and some people are sad and disappointed in themselves and their accomplishments. Both women and men question their value to society, the merit of their accomplishments, their success as sexual beings, and the probability of attaining unfilled life goals. Women generally make this life assessment between ages 35 and 50, whereas men do not usually begin until approximately age 40. Because

BOX 23-6 HOT TOPICS
Skin Health Care for Middle-Age Adults

Wrinkling, xerosis (dry skin), and lentigines (sun spots, liver spots, age spots) begin to be more evident during the forties and fifties, sometimes being manifested even earlier depending on individual amounts of sun exposure, skin irritation, and genetics. Sloughing of the stratum corneum with aging has been projected to happen about twice as quickly as one reaches middle age. There also are changes occurring in the fat and dermis layers that begin around age 40. This causes sagging as the layers separate from each other.

Some middle-age individuals have one or more benign lesions called *seborrheic keratoses,* which are brown or black wartlike papules. Precancerous lesions such as actinic keratoses begin to manifest during the forties, and skin malignancies are more common with aging. There are about 400,000 new cases of basal cell carcinoma each year. These lesions typically occur on sun-exposed areas and have a 99% cure rate with treatment. There are 100,000 new cases of squamous cell carcinomas diagnosed every year. These lesions also have a high cure rate if treated.

Many people use over-the-counter anti-aging creams, lotions, sprays, and pills to moisturize and revitalize their skin. For these products to be effective, they must contain at least 5% to 10% α-hydroxy acids (Kučera, 2004). Eye cream should not contain oil but must have antioxidants such as coenzyme Q10 and an antiinflammatory agent such as vitamin C (Kučera, 2004). Creams containing collagen are not effective, because collagen cannot penetrate the skin. People need to be educated about these over-the-counter products.

Botox (botulism toxin A), a neurotoxin, is effective in managing wrinkles for 4 to 6 months. Another prescriptive treatment is tretinoin (Retin-A), which will decrease pigmented areas such as age spots and hyperkeratosis.

From Kučera, K. (2004). Managing common skin problems in the elderly. *Clinical Advisor, 7*(6), 23-30.

the male life assessment tends to begin later, there is a potential problem for couples of approximately the same age. Women begin looking at changes they may want to make in their lives (Apter, 1995), whereas men remain content with the status quo. This type of self-evaluation and lack of effective communication of personal needs to the spouse is a threat to marriage stability (Erikson & Erikson, 1998; Vaillant & Vaillant, 1990).

Physiological Changes

The effect of physiological changes on mental health is nearly as critical during the middle years as it is during adolescence. Some of the most obvious changes that influence self-esteem are graying hair, an increase in numbers of wrinkles, decreased visual and auditory acuity, and changes in body shape (Box 23-6: Hot Topics). The extent to which these changes are tolerated depends largely on the person's level of self-satisfaction and acceptance. Some people try to "hold on" to youth by dressing as more youthful counterparts dress, whereas others adapt their attire to their age and position in life.

Before 2002, hormone therapy (estrogen alone or estrogen and progesterone) was given to millions of postmenopausal women. Estrogen is still the only therapy approved by the FDA for the treatment of hot flashes associated with menopause. Millions of women took hormone therapy not only to relieve hot flashes, but also with the hope that it might prevent heart disease, the number one cause of death in postmenopausal women. All of that changed in 2002, however, when data from the Women's Health Initiative (WHI) showed that postmenopausal women who took estrogen and progesterone actually had higher rates of heart attacks and other health problems including stroke, blood clots, and breast cancer. The mean age of women in the WHI study was 63 years. Almost overnight, millions of women stopped using hormone therapy (AACE, 2006; Rossouw et al., 2007).

Follow-up analysis of the WHI data showed that the effects of hormone therapy vary based on a woman's age and the length of time since menopause. In younger postmenopausal women, between the ages of 50 and 59 years, hormone use did not increase the risk of cardiac events, as it did for older women. There is new evidence that hormone therapy may actually turn out to be beneficial for younger postmenopausal women, but for now, hormone therapy is not recommended for the prevention of heart disease (Mendelsohn & Karas, 2007).

Health benefits of hormone therapy include decreased risk for osteoporosis and decreased rates of colorectal cancer (Seaman, 2003). Research is ongoing regarding the risks and benefits of hormone therapy. Currently, the only approved indication for postmenopausal hormone therapy is for the relief of moderate to severe vasomotor symptoms (hot flashes). Only short-term use is advised (1 to 3 years) (Lowdermilk & Perry, 2012).

Increasing numbers of women are now looking for non-hormonal ways to treat hot flashes and other symptoms associated with menopause. Between 1998 and 2000, menopausal women in the United States had more than 100 new natural health products from which to choose (Légaré et al., 2007). The law passed in 1994 to regulate dietary supplements does provide some oversight for natural health products but does not require manufacturers to prove that dietary supplements are either safe or effective (AACE, 2006).

Because there are little scientific data, many midlife women find it difficult to make decisions about using alternative products. Black cohosh, soy, and vitamin E are just a few of the products marketed to women. Even if these products are effective, women must be cautious about drug interactions that may occur. The use of prescription medication increases with age. The benefits of using alternative therapy may outweigh the risks but more research is needed on the safety profile of natural remedies (AACE, 2006).

It is difficult to separate menopause from the physical and psychological changes that women experience as they age. Stressors common to women in their forties and fifties include raising a family, helping parents as they age, coping with divorce or death of a spouse, retirement, and financial insecurity. Menopause happens in the midst of this. All the events in a woman's life influence her experience of menopause and the **perimenopause,** a period of time that precedes menopause and lasts approximately 4 years. Symptoms such as mood swings, nervousness, agitation, fatigue, and depression are often ascribed to the decline in estrogen levels that occurs during this time. The physiological changes are important, but a woman's experience in menopause is profoundly affected by all the events in her life (Lowdermilk & Perry, 2012).

Men also experience physical and psychological reactions to middle age. The hormonal changes in men are gradual, typically beginning between ages 40 and 55. The symptoms are similar to those experienced by women, with the emotional effects related to other life events, past coping patterns, and general feelings of self-esteem.

Roles-Relationships Pattern

Middle age is frequently a time of reassessment, turmoil, and change. This time has been called "midlife crisis." The turning point occurs for several reasons. Middle-age adults recognize that their physical agility is decreasing; the inevitability of one's own death is recognized, perhaps for the first time. Lifestyle choices have been made and are less flexible than are those made at age 25. The adult identifies mistakes made in the past.

Family

Duvall and Miller (1985) delineate 8 stages of the family life cycle, with stages 5, 6, and 7 in the middle years (see Chapter 7):
- Stage 5: families with children, with the oldest child age 13 to 20; lasts approximately 7 years
- Stage 6: families launching young adults, from the first leaving until the last; lasts approximately 8 years
- Stage 7: families from empty nest to retirement; lasts approximately 15 years

The developmental tasks identified for the families in stages 6 and 7 are similar to those described by Havighurst; they focus on changes from a nuclear family to a marital couple with other responsibilities. For example, in stage 6, the parents who are helping their children become independent may also be caring for their aging parents. Additionally, middle-age adults fulfill multiple complex responsibilities within a variety of career, social, and civic positions.

These transitions can be even more challenging for the family headed by a single parent (most typically the mother), which is true of more than 10 million American households (out of a total of 35 million). The single most significant health risk in families headed by a single mother is poverty (USDHHS, 2007c). Nearly half of all of these families live in poverty, and the median family income for families with two parents is three times that of a family headed by a single mother. These inadequate resources make it extremely difficult for middle-age mothers, who are frequently raising grandchildren as well, to fulfill their responsibilities.

Families with young adolescent or young adult children have been described in research studies as both *postparental* and *launching families.* In contrast, criticism of this emphasis on the separation of children (regardless of age) from their families is increasing. Gilligan (1982) criticizes the work of many human development theorists who identify human development in terms of separation from the family. Apter (1990) also challenges the conventional view that adolescent girls must reject their mothers as part of a healthy development. Middle-age parents are encouraged to continue to care for and nurture their adolescent and adult children while recognizing the increasing interdependence of their relationships.

Although many adolescent and young adult children move out of their homes of origin to complete educational or career training, create their own living arrangement, or pursue a career, almost 16 million families had at least one child older than 18 years living at home in 2003, an increase of 7% since 1995 and of 14% since 1985 (*USA Today*, 2005). Many children of families in these age groups remain dependent on parental help for many more years.

By supporting their children's efforts, parents can increase the self-esteem of their children while being effective role models. The parent assumes less of a parent-child relationship, interacting more on an adult-to-adult level. As the children are "launched," the parents may have uninterrupted time alone and time to share activities. Parents who remove too much care too quickly place their children at risk for depression, substance abuse, violence, and suicide (Silverstein & Rashbaum, 1995).

Family life may also be threatened by older children living at home, opposition to a child's partner, or the inability to establish satisfactory relationships with potential or actual partners or sons-in-law and daughters-in-law. For many parents, the idea of their children leaving home is anticipated with relief that the heavy care responsibilities of parenting are over or with dread over having to fill the void of time and inactivity. The empty nest syndrome may be exacerbated if the husband and wife have never learned to communicate effectively and to enjoy each other's company without the children.

At the other end of the family spectrum, aging parents can place demands on the adult child, primarily because older adults frequently are beset with health problems. A caring relationship is in order, in which the aging parent's need for independence is recognized.

Because of society's emphasis on youth, the adult must associate feelings of self-worth with personal integrity rather than with body appearance or physical prowess. Friends of both genders can provide invaluable support systems. With the newly found free time after children have left home, the middle-age adult can share favorite activities and learn new ones. Middle-age adults should remind themselves how much and how well they are doing, especially considering the complexity of the demands placed on them. Never before in history have families pursued such varied and individual-oriented goals as they do today.

Although for many Americans the concept of family remains of major importance, the perceptions are different from those held by previous generations. Parents and children in most families are involved in numerous activities, as evidenced by a "let's-hurry-or-we'll-be-late" orientation. Even younger children frequently have schedules that must be met if they are to get to their dance, drama, play, or enrichment classes. None of these activities necessarily has a negative effect, but the cumulative influence places heavy demands on all family members. Additionally, many activities in which both children and adults are involved have a certain degree of competitiveness. For example, parents frequently become emotionally involved in the athletic activities of their children to the extent that the failure of a 6 year old to play a winning softball game causes a great deal of parental anguish. One only has to listen to the cheering of parents at a Little League baseball game to note whose self-esteem is at stake. Shouts of "Kill her," "Grab the third baseman," and so on do not tend to engender feelings of team spirit

or a notion of playing for the sake of having a good time (Erikson & Erikson, 1998).

Work

Perhaps the most common role that middle-age adults share is that of a worker. Much of their pride and sense of satisfaction is derived from their work. Work is equated with being "grown up"; one can easily recall the "What do you want to be when you grow up?" questioning of youth. Success and achievement are evaluated in terms of careers and family life. The work ethic still persists, especially with individuals born during the Great Depression and many of their offspring. Much of their conversation evolves from what they do, such as, "My name is Leslie Smith. I am a real estate agent." To be mature is to be a responsible, hard-working individual (Erikson & Erikson, 1998). Research has shown that middle-age adults are more satisfied with their jobs than are younger adults.

Middle-age adults comprise most of the workforce of 110 million people. Vocations play a major role in their levels of wellness. Approximately 10 million work-related injuries occur every year; 3 million of these are severe, including 3400 to 11,000 deaths and 1.8 million totally disabling injuries (Hunt, 2011). More than 22% of fatal occupational injuries involve motor vehicles; other injuries include falls, nonvehicular injuries, blows, and electrocutions. In decreasing order, workers in mining, agriculture, forestry, fishing, construction, and transportation are at an increased risk of dying from a work-related injury. Although the number of fatal injuries appears to be decreasing, work-related illness and injuries appear to be increasing. The highest nonfatal injuries occur in construction and manufacturing, with high rates also in health services. Thirty percent of nonfatal injuries and illnesses with days away from work continue to be due to overexertion and repetitive motion (Nicholson, 2011; USDL, 2010). Poor housekeeping and poor design predispose workers to falls and other accidents, expose them to noises and toxic chemicals, and make them susceptible to other illnesses. Many injuries that contribute significantly to the morbidity and mortality of adults can be prevented. Fixing faulty steps, repairing faulty electrical wires, and securing carpets are only a few of the many preventive measures.

Accidents are twice as high among smokers than among non-smokers. Possible explanations include the loss of attention, the use of one hand for smoking, and irritation of the eyes. Other work-related problems include exposure to harmful substances resulting in lung diseases, cancers, and workplace violence (Box 23-7: Quality and Safety Scenario).

The effect of life events on mental health depends on the personal strength of the individual, the availability of supports, and the nature and number of events and their significance for the person. Three common examples of life events with potential disruptive effects are getting a divorce, having two or more jobs, and caring for aging parents. Their negative effects may be alleviated if assistance is provided early in the process of a change. In some organizations, resources for managing problems of addiction, life transitions, emotional issues, financial problems, stress reduction, and grief counseling are available off-site to all employees. These resources are offered without cost to the

BOX 23-7 QUALITY AND SAFETY SCENARIO

Lifetime Prevention of Cardiovascular Disease in Women

- Stop smoking and avoid environmental exposure to tobacco smoke.
- Incorporate at least 30 minutes of moderate-intensity exercise on most, preferably all, days of the week. For women trying to lose weight or sustain weight loss, 60 to 90 minutes of exercise each day is best.
- Eat a variety of fruits and vegetables and whole-grain, high-fiber foods. In addition, consume oily fish twice a week, limit alcohol to one drink per day, and consume less than 2.3 grams of sodium each day.
- Manage body weight.
- Administration of daily aspirin, 75 to 325 mg, for women at high risk for cardiovascular disease is recommended unless contraindicated. For low-risk women whose blood pressure is controlled, consider daily aspirin, 81 mg, or aspirin every other day, 100 mg, if the benefits are likely to outweigh the risks of gastrointestinal bleeding and hemorrhagic stroke.
- Folic acid should not be used for primary or secondary prevention of cardiovascular disease, although folic acid should be used during childbearing years to prevent neural tube defects in children.
- Neither postmenopausal hormonal therapy nor selective estrogen receptor modulators should be used to prevent cardiovascular disease.

Data from Sherman, C. (2008). Reducing the risk of heart disease in women. *Clinical Advisor, 11,* 49-53.

individual and, in some cases, to their family members or support persons.

Two-or-More-Job Family: Family and Work Responsibilities

More and more women are in the workforce for their own financial well-being or that of their family, especially with the increased cost of living, health care insurance, and college expenses and the decreased availability of employer-sponsored pension. Other women, who are postmenopausal and have launched their last child, have a newfound freedom and begin to rediscover themselves, sometimes through a new career. The husband may be a support person in this venture or he may feel threatened by his wife's new pursuits. These role changes and life transitions can be stressors to the family.

The balance between marital status, with or without children at home, caring for older parents, and employment obligations can significantly affect the psychological well-being of the woman in her middle years. In recent years, changes in family patterns with adult children moving back into their parents' home, sometimes with their offspring, bring new challenges to relationships, resources, and responsibilities within the home.

Historically, women worked with their husbands within the family farm or business. Only in the few decades immediately after World War II did many middle-class White women stay at home while their husbands went to work. Currently, women make up a significant portion of the workforce. Additionally, many women are able to become highly educated and motivated to pursue careers. Both men and women are increasingly taking jobs that do not end at 5:00 PM. The problems and challenges of the workplace are experienced at home as adults bring projects and problems home with them.

Job-related travel has also increased during the last few years for both men and women. Travel by either partner means additional responsibilities for the one who remains at home. Additionally, if one spouse travels far more than the other travels, feelings of resentment may develop, or the common ground for discussion of work events may be altered. The one who stays at home may feel "put upon" when the spouse is perceived as having fun. In contrast, travel is tiring and is not usually as exciting as it appears to observers. The traveling spouse can come home tired and irritable and desire peace and quiet, which may conflict with the expectations of other family members.

Men may feel threatened by highly successful and visible women. For some families, the post–World War II prototype was for the husband to support the family financially and gain status through achievements of work outside the home. As women gain recognition and acclaim for their career accomplishments, even the most "enlightened" man may experience twinges of envy and discomfort. Men have few role models in learning the ways to be a participant in a successful two-career family. Men may need as much, if not more, support than do women in adapting to contemporary family styles. Opportunities to discuss what it means to be a man in today's society can be helpful, such as in support groups with volunteers or professionals who provide services to various agencies and community resources.

In addition to the changes in women and the effect on families of each adult working at one or more jobs, the nature of the parental work environment is critical to family coping ability. Work that is emotionally draining, particularly when it is filled with conflict, poses special threats to family stability. When parents come home tired, angry, or frustrated from their experiences at work, they likely have limited emotional support to share with other family members.

When people gain self-esteem from their jobs and generally enjoy going to work, they tend to experience less frustration and dissatisfaction with themselves and their positions, enabling them to give more of themselves to other members of the family (Reifman et al., 1991).

Middle age is important when looking at the career clock. Issues that need to be considered include midcareer changes and preretirement planning. Retirement is a major turning point; to many people, it is the transition from middle age to old age and the period of work to the period of leisure or different work.

Adults are working up to and beyond the age of retirement, and many are entering new careers later in life because they are living longer and are in need of more financial resources to successfully enter the older adult years. As adults progress through the middle years, they become increasingly aware of the time remaining until retirement: "Can I readjust my goals?" "Is there disparity between where I am in my career and where I would like to be?" An example might be the 60-year-old veteran nightclub singer whose goal to cut a solo album remains to be achieved. The heightened awareness of age and the decreased likelihood of finding another suitable job can precipitate increased anxiety or depression in this singer.

FIGURE 23-1 Middle-age children and their older parents can develop meaningful relationships with one another.

Comprehensive health-promotion programs at the work site contain these elements: " health education that focuses on skill development and lifestyle behavior change in addition to information dissemination and awareness building, preferably tailored to employees' interests and needs; supportive social and physical work environments, including established norms for healthy behavior and policies that promote health and reduce the risk of disease, such as work site smoking policies, healthy nutrition alternatives in the cafeteria and vending services, and opportunities for obtaining regular physical activity; integration of the work site program into the organization's administrative structure; related programs, such as employee assistance programs; and screening programs, preferably linked to health care service delivery to ensure follow-up and appropriate treatment as necessary and to encourage adherence. Optimally, these efforts should be part of a comprehensive occupational health and safety program" (USDL, 2010).

Caring for Aging Parents

The needs of aging parents and of the adult's own children can create additional demands during the middle years (Figure 23-1). The middle-age adult can feel caught between one's children and one's parents. Both children and older parents can present unrealistic, excessive demands and be difficult to please.

Middle-age adults may be faced with having frail and ill parents live within their own family unit or placing them in a nursing home. These dilemmas are complicated by the reality that their parents are growing older and may not have long to live. The recognition of the parents' impending death heightens middle-age adults' awareness of their own aging and mortality.

Difficulties in caring for older parents can be somewhat lessened when potential situations are discussed before a crisis arises. This is particularly true when all members of the middle-adult family are working, space in their home is limited, and the community has few resources for the well or ill older adults. Although institutionalization is undesirable to many families, the care of ill, older parents may eventually require it. By anticipating these needs and preparing for them, middle-age children

and their older parents can develop further meaningful relationships with one another.

Divorce

Divorce is a major disruption to the marriage and family and to each individual's short-term and long-term health. As the divorce rate has risen in recent years, individuals and families have been faced with new and multiple problems. When a divorce occurs, each family member must confront the necessity to examine and, in many cases, modify an accustomed style of living and adapting.

In the early 1970s, Wallerstein and her colleagues began a longitudinal study of 131 children of divorce through extensive interviews with the children and their parents. The children are now adults with families of their own and Wallerstein is still following their development through life. The most significant findings of this ongoing study are the long-lasting cumulative and demonstrative effects of divorce, which continue for decades. Although Wallerstein found healing in adults is more or less complete 3 years after divorce, this is not so for the children, who experience the divorce differently from their parents. Even as adults, the children have undercurrents of fears about their abilities to commit to relationships (Wallerstein et al., 2000).

Some of the limitations of Wallerstein's research are anecdotal methodologies versus double-blind interviews; the children are primarily White, educated, upper middle class; and the findings are not differentiated from those of high-conflict families, nor are distinctions made between the influences of conflict that caused the divorce and the actual divorce itself. There are many other studies that continue to illuminate these initial findings on the long-term effects of divorce (Fabricius & Luecken, 2007). Continuing research is being done on ways to prevent long-term health problems in the children of divorced parents (Fabricius & Luecken, 2007).

Death

Similar to divorce, death of a spouse can result in grieving for the loss of companionship and the lost anticipated future, free from the responsibilities of work and children. The surviving spouse may be unprepared to be single again, to be the only parent, or to live alone. The loneliness may be exacerbated by ill or dying peers or parents. Middle-age adults become increasingly aware of the finite nature of life, thinking not only of the number of years since birth but also of the number of years left to live. The midlife review is a common outcome of this recognition.

Sexuality-Reproductive Pattern

Men and women can continue to have a satisfactory pattern of sexual functioning throughout the middle and older adult years. As they would in any other developmental phase, middle-age adults may need counseling to make health-promoting decisions about their sexual and reproductive behaviors and health (Lowdermilk & Perry, 2007).

Unintended pregnancies are high in all ages of American women, but are the highest (77% of all pregnancies) in middle-age women. In contrast, women planning to have children during the fourth and fifth decades of life should know that fertility rates decrease and infant mortality rates increase, especially when mothers are age 44 years and older (USDHHS, 2000). Mothers ages 35 years and older, and those who are Black, had the highest rates of labor and delivery complications (USDHHS, 2005). Additionally, the maternal death rate in women 35 years and older is higher (16.1 per 100,000 live births) than for younger women (USDHHS, 2000). Achieving the *Healthy People 2020* target goal of reducing maternal deaths will require that national, state, and local policies address women's needs before and during pregnancy, and that gaps in research and prevention programs be identified through improved monitoring (USDHHS, 2011).

Median red blood cell folate level for nonpregnant females ages 15 to 44 years exceeded its target of 220 ng/mL. In addition to food fortification, the "Folic Acid Education Campaign" has contributed to this progress (USDHHS, 2011).

Changes in the reproductive systems of men and women result in changes in sexual function throughout adulthood. During middle adulthood, sexual arousal is slower, orgasms are less intense, and a return to prearousal levels is more rapid, with men having longer refractory periods between erection and ejaculation. When a person continues to be sexually active, these functional changes occur over decades and are minimally noticeable until later in adulthood, unless external factors are present, such as the negative effects of some antihypertensive and antidepressant agents.

After menopause, many women enjoy sex more, especially because no risk of pregnancy exists. Conversely, menopause can bring many challenges to a woman. American culture values women largely for their youth, beauty, and childbearing ability. Middle-age women may confront their own aging for the first time and may be perplexed as to the symptomatic factors and possibly changing roles. Women can experience vaginal dryness, difficulty finding a partner, less interest in initiating sex, and longer times to reach orgasm. No data exist that report decreases in postmenopausal women's interest in and physical capacity for sex (Nelson et al., 2006; Northrup, 2008).

Although men and women frequently enjoy satisfactory sexual relationships throughout the middle adult years, men in their middle age are more vulnerable to sexual dysfunction than are women. Frequently, men first experience problems with premature ejaculation, impotence, and retrograde ejaculation between ages 40 and 50 (Dunphy, 2004).

Abnormal genital bleeding and secondary amenorrhea are common gynecological complaints that indicate serious physical problems. Abnormal genital bleeding is the most common reason for gynecological office visits by adult women. Although pregnancy and menopause are the most common causes of secondary amenorrhea, other conditions related to abnormal pregnancy, functional disorders, physiological changes, and pathological factors must be considered (Eliopoulos, 2010).

As for adolescents and young adults, in the middle-age adult sexually transmitted diseases continue to be a major public health problem. Women and children bear an inordinate share of the burden: sterility, ectopic pregnancy, fetal and infant deaths, birth defects, and mental retardation. Human papillomavirus (HPV), a sexually transmitted disease, causes 90% of all cervical cancers (Lowdermilk & Perry, 2007). As with many other health behaviors and diseases, the full effect on the life of an individual and family may not be realized until middle age.

Adults in middle age represent 71% of all new cases of HIV/AIDS. Nearly three fourths of all people currently living with HIV/AIDS in the United States are men (CDC, 2007). Since the early 1980s, the demographics of HIV/AIDS have changed. An increased proportion of those infected are women, persons under the age of 20, heterosexuals, persons of racial or ethnic minorities, and people who live outside major metropolitan areas (Leone, 2007).

Considered by some to be a "hidden" HIV risk group, adults older than age 50 now comprise 19% of all people living with HIV/AIDS in the United States. They represent 13% of all new cases (Lindau et al., 2007). The actual numbers may be higher because HIV/AIDS is misdiagnosed, underreported, and undertested in this population. Studies show that older Americans know less about HIV/AIDS than younger people. They are also less likely to discuss sexual behavior with their health care providers. Many health care providers believe it is offensive to ask an older person about her or his sexual activity (amfAR, 2002). Homosexual/bisexual contact (36%) is the most common mode of HIV/AIDS transmission in adults older than 50, followed by injection drug use (19%) and heterosexual contact (15%). The CDC now recommends that all persons ages 13 to 64 years, in all health care settings, receive routine testing for HIV (Leone, 2007).

Coping-Stress Tolerance Pattern

Kobasa (1979) studied the concept of stress hardiness, which she identified as including control, commitment, and challenge. Her studies have strong clinical relevance because they strive to answer the following question (Harig, 2007): "Why do some people's illness progress while others improve despite both groups having similar level of stress?"

In a 45-year longitudinal study of 173 men, Vaillant and his colleagues (1990, 2003) found that the extent of tranquilizer use before age 50 was the most powerful negative predictor of both mental and physical health outcomes at age 65. Another important predictor for health outcomes was the maturity of defenses against stress (e.g., sublimation, anticipation, altruism, and humor).

Stress and Heart Disease

As reiterated throughout this chapter, heart disease is the second leading cause of death in the middle-age adult. In landmark studies, Haynes and colleagues (1978) describe the relationship of psychosocial factors to coronary heart disease using the Framingham study (Haynes et al., 1978, 1980). In the study, 24 measures of psychosocial stress were used. In men, aging worries correlated significantly with systolic and diastolic blood pressure values. Marital disagreement and personal worries correlated significantly with diastolic blood pressure values. Both diastolic and systolic pressure values correlated significantly with work changes and anxiety in employed women between

45 and 64 years of age. Anger suppressed, anger discussed, tension, and anger symptoms correlated significantly with diastolic blood pressure measurements in this age group.

Among white collar men in this age group, the Framingham type A and ambitiousness scales also correlated significantly with elevated diastolic blood pressure values. The correlation of anger symptoms and anger discussed with diastolic pressures was significant for white collar women between ages 45 and 64. The initial findings by Haynes and her colleagues have been supported by many other studies, including those of Spielberger and colleagues (1983), Kawachi and colleagues (1996), and Williams and colleagues (2000).

The death of a parent enhances awareness of one's vulnerability to illness and death. The more opportunities and time people have to prepare for these stressful events, the more likely they will be to feel in control and less likely to feel anxious and helpless. When individuals assume more responsibility for their life, decisions lead to concrete behaviors, such as drafting a will, developing an advance directive (which includes living will, health care agent, and appointing a durable power of attorney), and making funeral prearrangements. An advance directive is a legal document prepared when an individual is alive, competent, and able to make decisions to provide guidelines for health care providers in the future, when the individual is not able to make decisions because of physical disability (being unconscious) or mental incompetence. By appointing a durable power of attorney, the individual designates another person (spouse, son, daughter, or friend) to make health care decisions (especially about how aggressive treatment should be in forestalling death) when an individual becomes unable to make such decisions. The nurse helps middle-age adults anticipate stressors so that they are better prepared to cope and to prevent additional physical, psychosocial, and spiritual stressors, thereby optimizing their health.

Values-Beliefs Pattern

When adults make decisions affecting their lives, it is usually the result of a personal, complex pattern of values and beliefs (McFadden & Gerl, 1990). Much of what people value or believe to be true is formed early in life and can be the most difficult to alter (Rippe, 1996). Normally people do not spend a great deal of conscious thought on abstract explanations of the meaning of life and why certain things are valued. During times of illness or crisis, however, they frequently take time to review their value systems and seek meaning about what is important (Spector, 2003; Stuart et al., 1989) (Box 23-8: Innovative Practice).

A crisis at any age can be a turning point during which both increased vulnerability and increased potential are present. When the crisis is managed successfully, a virtue or strength will evolve. Erikson names *caring* as a middle-age adult virtue that can be developed.

※ BOX 23-8 INNOVATIVE PRACTICE
Benson/Henry Mind Body Institute of Massachusetts General Hospital, Harvard Medical School

Mind/Body Medical Symptom Reduction Programs
Research demonstrates that 60% to 90% of health care visits are for symptoms such as headaches, insomnia, weakness or fatigue, and gastrointestinal symptoms, all of which are frequently stress related. The Mind/Body Medical Symptom Reduction Programs are designed to help individuals who have chronic illnesses (including life-threatening illnesses) or stress-related symptoms to better manage their health problems and optimize their quality of life. The interventions combine conventional medical care with knowledge about the effects of behaviors and attitudes on health.

The following are included in the biopsychosocial-spiritual approach of the assessment and treatment plans:
- Eliciting the relaxation response, a state of deep rest that changes responses to stress (decreases vital signs and muscle tenseness, increased mindfulness)
- Enhancing coping skills through cognitive-behavioral strategies
- Encouraging exercise or physical activity
- Providing nutritional counseling
- Monitoring and adjusting medication, when necessary, in consultation with the physician

Insurance claims for these outpatient visits are submitted directly to each person's insurance carrier. Because health insurance policies differ, coverage and reimbursement vary. An advocate helps persons seeking care research their specific health insurance coverage and billing requirements.

Research demonstrates the following results may occur after these interventions:
- Persons with pain reduced their number of physician visits by 36%.
- Visits to an HMO were reduced by approximately 50% after a relaxation response–based intervention, resulting in significant cost savings.

- Blood pressure was lowered and use of medications decreased in 80% of hypertensive persons; 16% were able to discontinue all of their medications.
- Sleep patterns were improved for 100% of persons with insomnia; 90% reduced or eliminated the use of sleep medication.
- Infertile women reported decreased levels of depression, anxiety, and anger, along with a 35% conception rate.
- Women with severe premenstrual syndrome experienced a 57% reduction in physical and psychological symptoms.
- Health-promoting behaviors, such as nutrition, social supports, self-esteem, health responsibility, and exercise, increased after the program and were maintained by the 6-month follow-up visit.
- Six months after the program, 80% of persons continued to experience improvement of their physical symptoms.
- Anxiety and depression normalized for most participants and were maintained 6 months following the program.
- Women with menopause reported fewer hot flashes, lower blood pressure, improved sleep, and decreased depression, anxiety, and anger.

Contact Information
Benson/Henry Mind Body Institute
Massachusetts General Hospital
Harvard Medical School
824 Boylston Street
Chestnut Hill, MA 02467
Telephone: 617-732-9130

Committed responsibilities for the care and welfare of others promote moral development. When middle age is lived with generativity, many opportunities are afforded to live life by one's higher principles. The middle adult can differentiate among personal wants and needs, duties demanded by society, and principles by which to live. Kohlberg's work on moral development delineated these phases as conventional and postconventional. His studies of men described stage 3 as an interpersonal definition of morality, whereas stage 4 is a societal definition based on law and order. Kohlberg concludes that most American adults are in these phases of moral development. In contrast, stage 5 is the concern and willingness to sacrifice for the well-being of others (Kohlberg & Lickona, 1986). Subsequent studies by Gilligan on moral development in women and men demonstrate gender differences in describing high morality. Women discussed issues of selfishness versus responsibility, of exercising care with decision-making and avoiding hurting others. Men described terms of *justice, fairness,* and *rights of individuals.* Gilligan (1982, 1990) concludes that women possess a process of moral development different from that of men.

Valuing others, having relationships, and being responsible to others enable middle-age adults to make the transitions of moral development. This process is accomplished through raising children, developing more junior employees, and serving the community. As people fulfill these commitments, they increasingly treat others as equals and gradually develop a sensitivity and desire to change barriers to human worth and equality, such as racial prejudice, homelessness, inadequate access to health care, and the availability of weapons' stockpiles.

ENVIRONMENTAL PROCESSES

Environmental factors are significant variables in health promotion. Cleanliness in home, work, and school environments helps control the spread of infectious diseases such as influenza. The effect of handwashing in controlling illness cannot be understated. In a larger context, continued efforts at improving sanitation and controlling pollution (air, water, noise) will result in a reduction of health problems such as lung disease, transmission of bacterial and viral infections, and hearing loss.

Because there are approximately 100 million workers in the United States, occupational hazards are a serious threat to national health. Exposures to toxic chemicals, asbestos, coal dust, cotton fiber, ionizing radiation, physical hazards, excessive noise, and stress can precipitate numerous health problems. For the middle-age worker, these problems include cancers, lung and heart diseases, decreased hearing, physical injuries, and mental health problems (USDL, 2010).

Physical Agents

Ionizing radiation is a physical agent that can cause cancer. One example of this is cancer caused by medical procedures that include the use of diagnostic radiography and therapeutic radiation.

Water pollution has become another major concern. Many industrial and agricultural wastes, such as benzene and chlordane, have been recovered in rivers and lakes from which drinking water is obtained. These substances can lead to potential carcinomas and other health problems.

Air pollution from auto emissions, burning fuels, and industrial incineration has warranted smog alerts and air pollution indices. This issue is especially important to the individual with chronic respiratory or cardiovascular disease (USDL, 2010).

Noise pollution in industry is a potential problem for the middle-age adult worker. Hearing loss is the most common occupational disease, but it can be prevented if federal guidelines are followed with regard to noise exposure levels and hearing conservation programs, especially prevention activities aimed at miners and construction workers for whom hearing loss is a major problem.

Exposure to excessive noise, radiation, sunlight, and vibration can produce problems such as chronic obstructive lung disease, cancer, and degenerative diseases (Goines & Hagler, 2007).

Biological Agents

As noted throughout this text, health and disease are influenced by the interactions among the agent, host, and environment. Agent factors can be biological, physical, chemical, or psychological. The biological causes of diseases include bacteria, viruses, rickettsiae, fungi, parasites, and food poisoning. Because these causes are often limited to identifiable occupations, they can be readily diagnosed, treated, and prevented. Many of these agents are transmitted through the air or by contact with certain media, such as water, food, blood, or feces.

Hepatitis A is caused by viral infection, with transmission occurring primarily through the fecal-oral route. This host-agent interaction typically occurs in the middle-age adult living in an environment with poor sanitation and having close contact with an infected person. The person may also be exposed through contaminated food and water. Hepatitis B is transmitted primarily in the blood or plasma of the infected individuals, which is particularly significant for the adult who is employed in a health care setting.

Among medical and dental personnel (with surgeons, oral surgeons, and pathologists at the highest risk), the risk of contracting hepatitis B is six times higher than that of the general population.

There are two other infections that are of particular concern for middle-age adults: pneumonia and varicella/herpes zoster ("shingles"). Both can be prevented through vaccinations, which adults ages 60 years and older are advised to receive (Harpaz et al., 2008; Targonski & Poland, 2007).

Chemical Agents

Chemicals include a wide variety of substances that increase the risk of morbidity and mortality in the middle-age adult. When a home is located near an industry, there is the risk of exposure to toxic chemicals that pollute the air. Contaminants can also be carried home on the clothing from the workplace.

Workers at increased risk include coal miners, wood handlers, and those who work with asbestos and coke. Pneumoconiosis is found in approximately 15% of coal miners, with "black lung disease" implicated in 2430 deaths in 2005 (the *Healthy*

People 2020 target is 10% improvement). Wood handlers have increased risk of certain cancers. The asbestos worker has an increased risk of mesothelioma and asbestosis. Approximately 2 million workers each year have been exposed to benzene and vinyl chloride, which may be carcinogens. Among American industrial workers, 9 out of 10 may be inadequately protected from exposure to at least 10 of the 163 most common hazardous chemicals. More than 2000 of the 50,000 chemicals found in the workplace are suspected human carcinogens (USDL, 2012).

Tobacco

Currently, 23% of men and 18% of women in the United States smoke (USDHHS, 2007a). Many 50-year-old adults have a 30-plus-year history of cigarette smoking. Cigarette smokers have nearly twice the heart disease death rates of nonsmokers, with the risk being proportional to the amount of smoke inhaled directly and passively and the number of cigarettes smoked (Brownson et al., 1992). Smoke recipients are at increased risks for heart disease, as well as colds; chronic bronchitis; emphysema; and cancers of the mouth, lungs, esophagus, pancreas, and bladder.

Few smokers realize that cigarettes contain 2000 known chemicals, including tar, nicotine, hydrogen cyanide, formaldehyde, and ammonia. Cigarette smoking is, for most smokers, an addiction to nicotine, which is absorbed into the bloodstream. Nicotine acts on the two divisions of the nervous system: central (brain and the spinal cord) and peripheral (autonomic nervous system and motor and sensory fibers to the arms and legs). Effects of nicotine stimulation can be observed both in electroencephalographic changes and in hand tremors. Nicotine also stimulates the heart, leading to an increased pulse rate and elevated blood pressure. Although smokers frequently believe that cigarettes have a calming effect, this notion is misleading. Nicotine stimulates the body, whereas carbon monoxide causes lethargy. Smokers may feel calm, although they are actually having their sensations dulled by carbon monoxide. Additive effects such as those from chlorine, cotton dust, and γ-radiation can lower mid-expiratory flow values. Profound effects can also be observed with asbestos interaction.

DETERMINANTS OF HEALTH

Social Factors and Environment

Spector (2008) describes culture as the "sum of beliefs, practices, habits, likes, dislikes, norms, customs, rituals...we have learned from our families during the years of socialization" (p. 1). Spector further relates the ways in which one's cultural background is a component of one's ethnic background. The major ethnic groups of the United States are Asians, Blacks, Native Americans, and Hispanics.

Nurses understand the potential influences their own ethnic cultures have on those of others. The middle-age adult may not interpret dizziness as a possible symptom of hypertension; for example, it may be described simply as a spell. The Black adult's definition of health may be completely different from that of the White health care provider or the Asian person (Perez & Luguis,

2008). The obese adult who has received positive reinforcement throughout life for being pleasingly plump is less motivated to lose weight than is the adult who defines health as being svelte.

The health problems of middle-age adults, even within major ethnic groups, are varied. Recent immigrants who live in crowded urban areas have higher mortality rates than do earlier immigrants of the same cultural group who live in healthier environments. Immigrants' working conditions continue to be poor, with long hours and minimal wages. Modern preventive health care is difficult, if not impossible, to obtain.

Poverty is reported in approximately one third of Native Americans. The middle-age adult Native American is faced with a high rate of tuberculosis, alcohol abuse, inadequate immunization, mental health problems such as depression, and dental problems (Spector, 2008; USDHHS, 2005).

For many women in society, the cessation of menses is associated with aging; the role of the middle-age woman may be shaped by her culture. Nurses who have attained cultural competency can ensure that appropriate health promotion is provided, especially for vulnerable populations and those individuals, families, and communities who have special health care needs.

Levels of Policy Making and Health

Adults in the middle years are frequently at the peak of their careers. Although their net income may be greater than it was during early adulthood, they frequently have significant additional financial obligations. For many individuals in their late fifties or early sixties, retirement is a life-stage they have dreamt about and anticipated for years (Figure 23-2). Leaving full-time employment for a less strenuous daily routine has become beyond their reach. A number of reasons are offered to account for this relatively new trend:

- The high quality of health care in the United States provides technological advances that extend the limits for life expectancy. Individuals are living longer than previous generations, and therefore they cannot "afford" to retire in their mid-fifties to early sixties because they have a financial need to "fund" another 25 to 30 years of life.

FIGURE 23-2 Middle-age adults enjoy travel after retirement.

- Quality health care is expensive. Costs of health care are mounting because research and development expenses associated with medical treatments including pharmaceuticals are escalating. When diagnosed with an illness, consumers expect "the best" type of care and interventions, which, in turn, influences the financial burden borne by most all Americans.
- Changes in the American economy in the past 10 years have necessitated significant changes in family patterns. Increasingly, more than one generation lives together in the same home in order to afford the rising costs of commodities that have been taken for granted. For example, the costs of a college education funded by middle-aged adults are not necessarily balanced by a full-time position at the end of the 4 or 5 years needed to obtain a college degree. Young adults are not leaving home at 22 or 23 years of age. Consequently, their parents, if still employed, must continue to work to support adult children and to pay the debt of the college educational experience also.
- Individuals may have accrued increasing debt to pay for health insurance that is becoming more costly. As people develop health conditions that are related to accumulated stress and the aging process, they require more use of their benefits from their health insurance companies. In addition, they may be supporting elderly parents, whose health conditions have consumed their savings and home investment to pay for their parents' medications, hospitalizations, and/or nursing home expenses. When the adult or family members have ongoing health problems, the economic status of the family can be compromised further (Box 23-9: Diversity Awareness).
- Unemployment statistics show an increasing rate of unemployment across the United States. When people lose their jobs, often they are without health insurance, and when they develop illness or conditions that are associated with the middle years, they rely on their savings or must resort to less expensive housing. Such changes can cause extreme mental

strain and possibly lead to mental health problems. The individual's economic status plays a role in the incidence of mental illness, with higher rates of anxiety, depression, and phobias evident in adults at the lower socioeconomic level.
- Technological changes have opened opportunities for individuals to work at home and/or remote sites. These extensions of the workplace often necessitate individuals to change their routines, and to take educational courses to keep current with job requirements, or to be competent to take on more responsibilities. Training to increase skills or knowledge can be expensive and often must be funded by the individual.

Health Services/Delivery System

There are numerous agencies that are geared to providing information and other resources for the middle-aged adult. These can be categorized as official, voluntary, and service agencies. Councils of community services frequently publish a directory. Official agencies include those that are state and federally funded, such as public health departments and drug treatment centers. Voluntary agencies include the American Heart Association, the American Cancer Society, the American Lung Association, and Alcoholics Anonymous. Many educational and self-help programs are sponsored by these organizations. The American Lung Association sponsors a "Stop Smoking" program, which can be conducted on a group basis in a work or community setting. Service agencies include professional organizations, such as state nurses' associations, the American Medical Association (sponsor of the Tel-Med program), bar associations, Young Men's Christian Association (YMCA), hospice programs, and the Women's Occupational Health Resource Center. **Website Resource 23A** presents a detailed list of these agencies. The Affordable Care Act of 2010 is a law with provisions (Affordable Care Act Tax Provisions, 2012) that meet one of the primary objectives of *Healthy People 2020*; that is, increasing access to health care for all Americans (*Twelve Reasons to Support Health Care*, 2012). The implications of this statute are most significant for middle-aged adults who are currently uninsured and/or have preexisting health conditions. Preventive screening will allow individuals to receive testing for the detection of cancer and other conditions that can influence initiation of treatment at an earlier stage of illness. Thus the financial expense of treatment will be less potentially, and the stresses on the individual and family considerably eased. In addition, costs for unemployment benefits where individuals work will be reduced.

From another perspective, the Affordable Care Act already has expanded coverage for individuals less than 26 years of age who are still carried on the health insurance policy held by their parents. This provision is particularly relevant for young adults who are still in college or who have not found employment after college graduation. In the previous section, the economic impact of unemployment among this age group on families with middle-aged parents cannot be understated (Jarrett, 2012). The website www.irs.gov/newsroom/article/0,,id=220809,00.html gives specific details of the Affordable Care Act of 2010. The full implementation of the Act begins in 2014 (*Healthcare.gov*, July 12, 2012), and it is predicated that

BOX 23-9 DIVERSITY AWARENESS
Health Care for Middle-Age Gypsies

Culturally competent and effective health care is imperative for all, especially people with several comorbid conditions who do not have a consistent primary care provider or clinic. Middle-age gypsies, or Roma, are in need of consistent health care. However, because they tend to travel from one place to another and do not put down roots, health providers need to understand their beliefs so the episodic interactions will be most productive. It is important to realize the Roma prefer to involve their family when it comes to their health. Hence a family member should be allowed to participate in each interaction with a health provider. This involvement with family will increase the person's compliance with the health regimen. In an excellent study by Vivian and Dundes (2004), the researchers conclude that health care providers be aware that the following variables may affect the Roma's health care: pollution, cleanliness, ideal weight, views on death, and medical procedures.

From Vivian, C., & Dundes, L. (2004). The crossroads of culture and health among the Roma (gypsies). *Image: The Journal of Nursing Scholarship, 36*(1), 86-91.

the overall influence of this statute will not be realized for at least 5 to 10 years. In the meantime, however, the objectives and goals for *Healthy People 2020* that relate to the middle-aged adult may be more fully realized by 2020 than for initiatives proposed in previous years.

NURSING APPLICATION

Interventions focused on health promotion span the gamut for nurses working in the community or on location at work sites. Consequently, there are many ways nurses interact with middle-aged adults.

Individuals in this middle-age range, very possibly, will need the services of a professional nurse *several times* before they reach their sixties. They may meet with a nurse when seeking care for themselves in a physician's office or primary care center. As a parent, they are likely to accompany their school-age child or their own elderly parent to the emergency department to obtain care for a sports-related injury or trauma following a fall. In the employment realm, some individuals will have their initial experience with a nurse through a preemployment evaluation visit. As a company employee, the same person may receive first aid for a minor injury, or have their blood pressure monitored periodically by a nurse working in the occupational health department.

If the individual needs surgery or hospitalization, they may meet a home health nurse after discharge. Nurses also are available in rehabilitation settings to instruct and coach people regarding lifestyle changes following a heart attack or other acute events. Community health nurses provide health-promotion activities such as senior health fairs that include "flu clinics" where adults are vaccinated against influenza. Life events such as death of a partner, sudden unemployment, or disability may cause anxiety, depression, or other stress-related symptoms. Nurses who specialize in mental health can provide counseling and other forms of treatment for grief support or mental disorders resulting from trauma or sudden losses.

In a variety of settings, nurses are health educators. For example, the nurse who works in the community or in occupational health initiates events that raise awareness to identify health risks among middle-aged adults. She teaches strategies for controlling symptoms, and accepting responsibility for changing potentially dangerous health habits. These interventions can be provided on a one-to-one or group basis; or as a lecture presented in a health seminar.

Target groups identified by occupational health nurses frequently have common needs for information, interventions, and periodic monitoring. Some of the following problems are identified in the workplace: exposures to a particular chemical or toxic substance; cigarette smokers who must stop their unhealthful behavior; substance abusers whose habits interfere with their productivity; ongoing problems with fatigue attributable to frequent changes in scheduled shifts.

The occupational health nurse has a wide range of responsibilities. For example, he or she may evaluate patterns of absenteeism to identify a source for infection that is affecting a group of employees. The nurse participates in policy development focused on preventing or reducing the incidence of work site injuries or incidents. In another instance, the nurse provides clarification to Occupational Safety and Health Administration (OSHA) regulations when new machinery is incorporated into operation. The nurse is wise to invite a broad spectrum of employee-participants to join a company safety committee. Their primary purpose is focused on keeping the work site safe for employees. Strategies to achieve that objective include determining health hazards that exist in each department of the company and developing or refining procedures that promote safety, such as creating policies that address infection control or procedures for fire drills. If the nurse has certification from the American Heart Association, he or she can offer classes in cardiopulmonary resuscitation (CPR) and use of the automated external defibrillator (AED).

The scope of practice for community health nurses (CHNs) varies from state to state. They may be employed by a city or town, or derive their authority through the State Health Department. The role of the CHN focuses on health promotion and disease prevention for a population living in a specific area. The CHN interfaces with nurses working in the municipality and surrounding areas such as medical offices, state health department offices, hospitals, urgent care clinics, schools, emergency services, YMCA/YWCA, and local businesses. Frequently, lectures or demonstrations are sponsored by the CHN at the request of service organizations in communities such as the LIONS or Kiwanis Club. The CHN may combine efforts with nurses who volunteer as parish nurses. Together they may present an annual health fair or senior health fair to serve a broad scope of health-information needs of the local community. Features of the fair would include 15 to 20 displays that offer some of the following: demonstrations in the use of car seats and seat belts; short presentations on fall prevention; screening measures to identify risk factors of heart disease, cancer, and diabetes; town planning guides for emergency preparedness; massage therapy for stress reduction; informational guides for the regional poison control center; and "flu shots" against influenza for anyone who desires one— all on a single occasion. Such events allow the CHN to generate interest and enthusiasm among people who are interested in improving the health and well-being of residents living in their local community.

Health-promotion strategies will become more widely recognized as the objectives and target goals for *Healthy People 2020* are incorporated into health plans supported by health insurance policies, employers, wellness programs, and health care providers. With the passage of the Affordable Care Act in 2010, accessibility and utilization of health care services, especially to minorities, are expected to increase. Nurses will be in leadership roles to organize and implement early detection and screening programs. They will survey communities and identify needs of the specific populations, and evaluate the effectiveness of current public health measures already in place. They will be called upon to develop educational programs and create online information sites that disseminate current medical research findings to the public showing how changes in lifestyle behaviors can positively influence health outcomes. Progress toward target goals for *Healthy People 2020* can be incorporated in these websites or blogs so that the American people can see, and learn first-hand, how important changes in their own lifestyle will affect the overall health of our nation.

In summary, better health and enhanced well-being of the American people are expected by-products of health promotion. *Healthy People 2020* objectives and target goals provide the framework and direction for improving health awareness and practices among U.S. residents.

In this chapter, health needs and potential diseases and conditions relevant to middle-aged adults are addressed along with strategies to mitigate symptoms, prevent complications, and foster well-being. Normal changes expected with the aging process also are presented. Selected objectives and target goals set for *Healthy People 2020* are compared to findings published for outcomes of *Healthy People 2010*. Also, the impact of social processes—such as relationships, family, work, values and belief systems, disability and death, and finances—completes the discussion.

Nurses provide important strategies for fostering health promotion. They are employed in most settings where middle-aged adults live, work, play, and raise their families. Because of this integral position in society, nurses are highly influential in identifying health concerns, organizing interventions, and evaluating the effectiveness of program outcomes. *Healthy People 2020* is presented as one approach for health professionals to use in their mission to improve the health and well-being of the American people.

This sequence of information gives the reader an overview of the disease conditions and health concerns that predominate during the 35- to 54-year-old age range.

The Occupational Safety and Health Administration (OSHA) mandates that the employee have a healthy and safe work environment. Therefore a complete health history is essential. Is there a history of hypertension, arthritis, cancer, or hernia? Is there significant family history? Is the person a smoker? How many packs per day are smoked? Does the person take medications? Medical limitations must be addressed; for example, decreased visual acuity means no driving, and dermatitis means no skin exposure to oils, chemicals, or solvents. Removing a worker from a particular job may be indicated if the worker might endanger coworkers, if the worker has a disease condition that might be aggravated by the job, or if the worker is taking prescribed medications with potentially harmful side effects.

The nurse in the community and in industry should reiterate some key safety issues to the adult, such as wearing seat belts and observing speed limits. With a decrease in visual acuity, driving at night can be hazardous. The middle-age adult's reaction time is also decreasing, which reinforces the need for periodic driving testing as recommended by the National Highway Traffic Safety Administration.

With an increase in leisure time, the middle-age adult is at greater risk for recreational accidents. As noted, moderation should be stressed. Alcohol is a depressant and should be avoided in activities that require attentiveness.

Protection from burns is essential; 56% of fatal residential fires are cigarette related, such as from smoking in bed. Falls can occur

at any age, and safety measures should be considered for the entire family, with preparatory planning for aging parents. A few suggestions to the adult might be to avoid highly waxed floors, poor lighting, high beds, and bathtubs without nonslip bottoms.

Handgun availability is controversial at best; however, approximately 20% of American households have them. When the person believes strongly that it is necessary to have a firearm, safety measures to avoid accidental injury should be discussed, such as security locks and proper storage.

The Occupational Safety and Health Act (1970) was designed to ensure that workers are employed under safe and healthy working conditions. The Act is applicable to every employer who is engaged in a business that affects commerce. The employer must ascertain that the workplace is free from recognized hazards and must comply with the Act. OSHA has offices in most major cities and can provide recommended standards for occupational agents.

Nurses can participate actively in the safety committee of the industry in which they are employed. When no such committee exists, many protection measures will fall on the nurse. The following are some suggestions:

- Tour the facilities on a regular basis. Be familiar with resource books, laws, and codes.
- Develop a toxicology chart with symptoms of overexposure and recommended treatment. Update this chart frequently.
- Be a role model in safety issues; wear safety glasses, protective footwear, and gloves; and do not smoke.
- Discuss the preemployment physical with the employee, with an emphasis on risk factors. Monitor health problems and exposure levels in the work setting.

The worker must be aware of the protective clothing that should be worn, sanitation measures for the work environment, general hygiene measures, and proper immunization. The food handler, for instance, should have an annual tuberculosis skin test, wear clean clothing and appropriate hair protection, and use good handwashing techniques. The nurse should not assume that workers know how to protect themselves and others.

Since 1996, the National Occupational Research Agenda (NORA) has become the research framework for the National Institute for Occupational Safety and Health (NIOSH) and the nation. Partners work together to identify, research, and address the most critical issues in workplace safety (http://cdc.gov/niosh/about.html).

A major challenge for the nurse is to encourage workers to assume responsibility for protecting their own health. Increasingly, organizations are interested in promoting the health of their employees for many reasons, including enhancing their recruiting efforts and minimizing lateness, absenteeism, turnover, physical and emotional inability to work, disability costs, and health and life insurance costs. Health-promotion programs are increasingly recognized for their vital contributions to the financial viability of organizations. It has been validated that providing health care to middle-age adults in homeless centers, showing health-promotion videos during meals, and giving incentives for participating in wellness programs improve health outcomes (Clark, 2002).

Health-promotion programs within an organizational setting can be categorized in one of three levels: awareness; lifestyle change; and supportive environment. The goal of a health program at the level of awareness is to increase the individual's knowledge or interest in a particular health issue, such as smoking cessation. Examples of awareness programs include special events, flyers, lunch seminars, meetings, and newsletters. Changing health behaviors or status are not the goals of awareness programs, but are goals of lifestyle change programs.

Lifestyle change programs last at least 8 to 12 weeks and include assessment, education, and evaluation components to help individuals implement long-term modifications in health behavior and experience the results of their instituted changes. To maintain these long-term changes and to develop a healthy lifestyle, a supportive organizational environment is needed. This type of environment includes health-promoting physical settings, corporate policies and culture, ongoing programs, and employee ownership of programs (USDHHS, 2011).

Five models of nurse-managed primary health care delivery at the work site have been proposed as part of the American Nurses Association's program for reform of this nation's health care system, known as Nursing's Agenda for Health Care Reform. Each model is developed to enable employers to fulfill the goal of providing accessible, high-quality, affordable care at locations that are familiar and convenient for employees. These designs help employers introduce or expand health care services at the work site, control health care costs, and meet the health care needs of their employees (*Nursing facts: Nursing's agenda for health care reform*, 2005).

CASE STUDY

Caregiver Role Strain: Graham A.

Graham A., a 47-year-old divorced woman, was diagnosed with stage 3 ovarian cancer 4 years ago, for which she had a total hysterectomy, bilateral salpingo-oophorectomy, omentectomy, lymphadenectomy, and tumor debulking followed by chemotherapy, consisting of cisplatin (Platinol), paclitaxel (Taxol), and doxorubicin (Adriamycin). She did well for 2 years and then moved back to her hometown near family and underwent three more rounds of second-line chemotherapy. She accepted a less-stressful job, bought a house, renewed old friendships, and became more involved with her two sisters and their families.

She developed several complications, including metastasis to the lungs. Then she could no longer work, drive, or care for herself. She had been told by her oncologist that there was nothing else that could be done and that she should consider entering a hospice. She met with her attorney and prepared an advance directive and completed her will. She decided to have hospice care at home and, with the help of her family, set up her first floor as a living and sleeping area. She was cared for by family members around the clock for about 3 days.

Graham A. observed that she was tiring everyone out so much that they could not really enjoy each other's company. At this time she contacted the Visiting Nurse Association (VNA) to seek assistance. Her plan was to try to enjoy her family and friend's visits. After assessment the VNA nurse prioritized her problems to include fatigue and caregiver role strain. Other potential problem areas that may need to be incorporated into the care plan include anticipatory grieving and impaired comfort.

Reflective Questions

1. What are some of the stresses on her middle-age sisters and their families?
2. What resources are available to manage these stresses and support the sisters in caring for their dying sister?
3. Describe Graham A.'s feelings about dependency and loss of autonomy because she is unable to do her own activities of daily living any longer.

CARE PLAN

Caregiver Role Strain: Graham A.

*NURSING DIAGNOSIS: Risk for Caregiver Role Strain related to sister's terminal cancer

Defining Characteristics
- Ms. A. and sisters are tired of doing all of the daily care for Ms. A.
- Ms. A. and family are at a point where they are accepting Ms. A.'s terminal status.
- Ms. A. and family want to prepare for a death at home.

Related Factors
- Sisters are missing work and neglecting their own families.
- Sisters need assistance with Ms. A.

Expected Outcomes
- Ms. A. and sisters will contact the VNA to assist in planning daily hospice care at home.

- VNA and family will plan realistic care.
- Ms. A. will have enjoyable time with sisters and friends.
- Sisters will have quality time to spend with Ms. A.
- Sisters will be able to voice their grief and anger about their sister's upcoming death.

Interventions
- Home health aides are scheduled for 24 hours a day.
- A psychiatric nurse practitioner will meet with Ms. A. and family to schedule therapy time for anticipatory grieving.
- The sisters will meet with a support group for families involved in hospice care at home.
- A schedule will be made to allow each sister time at home, time with Ms. A., and time for rest.

SUMMARY

Nurses help middle-age adults improve their quality of life, both for the present and for the future, through the identification of risk factors, health promotion, and other nursing interventions. Nurses work in a variety of health care settings available to middle-age adults: outpatient clinics, occupational health clinics, and private practice.

Health promotion and disease prevention are aimed at the personal habits and lifestyles of adults to improve their biological, spiritual, and psychosocial development. Strategies to help an adult achieve a higher level of health include individual and group counseling based on identified risk factors, providing self-help information that is most relevant to the middle-age adult, and describing available resources. Using these strategies, the nurse can motivate middle-age adults to prioritize their own health and quality of life for the individual middle-age adult, including it as a prerequisite for their own present and future health and particularly preceding the responsibilities in promoting the health and quality of life of younger and older generations. After years of poor health practices, adults can make changes that reduce their risk of disability from chronic disease and promote functioning and quality of life.

REFERENCES

AACE Menopause Guidelines Revision Task Force. (2006). American Association of Clinical Endocrinologists Medical Guidelines for Clinical Practice for the Diagnosis and Treatment of Menopause. *Endocrine Practice, 12*(3), 315–337.

Affordable Care Act Tax Provisions. (2012). Retrieved June 14, 2012, from www.irs.gov/newsroom/article/0,=220809,00.html.

Agency for Healthcare Research and Quality. (February 22, 2012). Closing the quality gap: A critical analysis of QI strategies: volume 3 – Hypertension care. AHRQ Publication No.12 EHC003. Retrieved from www.effectivehealthcare.ahrq.gov/.

American Cancer Society. (2005). *Cancer facts & figures for African Americans 2005-2006*. Atlanta, GA: Author.

American Cancer Society. (2006). *Cancer facts & figures for Hispanics/Latinos 2006-2008*. Atlanta, GA: Author.

American Cancer Society. (2007). *Report links health insurance status with cancer care*. Retrieved December 20, 2007, from www.cancer.org/docroot/NWS.

American Cancer Society. (2009). *Cancer facts and figures 2009*. Atlanta, GA: Author.

American Heart Association. (2012). *Calculating target heart rate*. Retrieved April 9, 2012, from www.americanheartassociation.org.

American Obesity Association. (2004). Retrieved April 14, 2012, from www.obesity.org.subs/fastfacts/health_effects.shtml.

amfAR AIDS Research. (2002). *Seniors hidden HIV risk group*. Atlanta, GA: American Cancer Society. Retrieved December 29, 2007, from www.amfar.org.

Apter, T. (1990). *Altered loves: Mothers and daughters during adolescence*. New York: Ballantine Books.

Apter, T. (1995). *Secret paths: Women in the new midlife*. New York: Norton.

Arias, E. (September 28, 2011). United States Life Tables, 2007. *National Vital Statistics Reports, 59*(9). Retrieved April 17, 2012, from www.cdc/nchs.gov.

Benjamin, R. M. (2012). *Healthy People 2010*: The Surgeon General's perspective: Oral health care for persons living with HIV/AIDS. *Public Health Reports, 127*(Suppl 2). Retrieved April 22, 2012, from www.publichealthreports.org/issueopen.cf.

Bensley, L., Van Eehwyk, J., & Ossiander, E. M. (2011). Association of self-reported periodontal disease with metabolic syndrome and a number of self-reported chronic conditions. *Prevention of Chronic Disease, 8*(30), A50.

Bloom, B. S. (1984). *Taxonomy of educational objectives: Handbook 1, cognitive domain*. New York: Longman.

Boston Women's Health Book Collective & Norsigian, J. (2005). *Our bodies, ourselves: A new edition for a new era*. New York: Simon & Schuster.

Boston Women's Health Book Collective, Norsigian, J., & Pinn, V. (2006). *Our bodies, ourselves: Menopause*. New York: Simon & Schuster.

Brownson, R. C., Alavanja, M. C., Hock, E. T., & Loy, T. S. (1992). Passive smoking and lung cancer in non-smoking women. *American Journal of Public Health, 82*(11), 1525–1530.

Centers for Disease Control and Prevention. (2010). *Gender, race, age tables*. CDC Wonder, DATA2010…the Healthy People 2010 Database. Retrieved April 12, 2011, Hyattsville, MD: Author.

Centers for Disease Control and Prevention. (October 2011). *Healthy People Final Review*. Atlanta, GA: Centers for Disease Control and Prevention. Author.

Centers for Disease Control and Prevention. (2011). *Disparities in HIV? AIDS*. Retrieved from www.cdc.gov/nchhstp/healthdis. Atlanta, GA: Author

Centers for Disease Control and Prevention. (2007). *HIV/AIDS surveillance report*, 2005. (Vol. 17 rev. ed.). Atlanta, GA: U.S. Department of Health and Human Services, Centers for Disease Control and Prevention.

Centers for Disease Control and Prevention. (2009). *HIV among African Americans*. Atlanta, GA: Author.

Centers for Disease Control and Prevention. (2010a). *Health, United States, 2010 with special features on death and dying*, Washington, DC: Author. Retrieved April 13, 2012, from www.cdc.gov/nchs/data/hus/hus10.pdf.

Centers for Disease Control and Prevention. National Center for Health Statistics. (2010). *Health, United States, 2011, Socioeconomic status related to access to care*. Atlanta, GA: Author.

Centers for Disease Control and Prevention. (2010b). *CDC vital signs: Adult obesity*. National Center for Health Informatics. Retrieved April 23, 2012, from www.cdc.gov/vitalsigns/AdultObesity/.

Centers for Disease Control and Prevention, National Center for Health Statistics. (2002). *National Health and Nutrition Examination Survey, Health, United States, 2002*. Retrieved July 31, 2005, from www.cdc.gov/nchs/nhanes.htm.

Clark, C. (2002). *Health promotion in communities: Holistic and wellness approaches*. New York: Springer.

Cohen, R., & Martinez, M. (2007). *Health insurance coverage: Early release of estimates from the National Health Interview Survey, January-June 2007*. Washington, DC: CDC.

DeNavas-Walt, C., Proctor, B., & Smith, J. (2007). *U.S. Census Bureau, Current population reports, P60–233, Income, poverty, and health insurance coverage in the United States: 2006*. Washington, DC: U.S. Government Printing Office.

Driscoll, A. K., & Bernstein, A. B. (January, 2012). Health access to care among employed and unemployed adults: United States 2009-2010. National Center for Health Statistics, *News Briefs, 83*. Washington, DC: U.S. Department of Health and Human Services, Centers for Disease Control and Prevention. Retrieved April 15, 2010, from www.cdc.gov/nchs/data.

Dunphy, L. (2004). *Management guidelines for nurse practitioners working with adults* (2nd ed.). Philadelphia: F.A. Davis.

Duvall, E. M., & Miller, B. (1985). *Marriage and family development* (6th ed.). New York: Harper Collins.

Eliopoulos, C. (2010). *Gerontological Nursing: Common Aging Changes*. Philadelphia, PA: Wolter Kluwer, Lippincott, Williams & Wilkins.

Erikson, E. H., & Erikson, G. M. (1998). *Life cycle completed*. New York: W.W. Norton.

Exploredia. (May 6, 2011). *Ethnic groups in America*. Retrieved from http://exploredia.com/ethnic-groups-in-America.

Fabricius, W., & Luecken, L. (2007). Post-divorce living arrangements, parent conflict, and long-term physical health correlates for children of divorce. *Journal of Family Psychology, 21*(2), 195–205.

Gardner, H. (1983). *Frames of mind: The theory of multiple intelligences*. New York: Basic Books.

Gardner, H. (1993). *Multiple intelligences: The theory in practice*. New York: Basic Books.

Gilligan, C. (1982). *In a different voice: Psychological theory and women's development*. Cambridge, MA: Harvard University Press.

Gilligan, C. (1990). *Mapping the moral domain*. Cambridge, MA: Harvard University Press.

Glanze, W. D., Anderson, K., & Myers, T. (2008). *Mosby's medical, nursing and allied health dictionary* (8th ed.). St. Louis: Mosby.

Goines, L., & Hagler, L. (2007). Noise pollution: A modern plague. *Southern Medical Journal, 100*(3).

Harpaz, R., Ortega-Sanchez, I. R., & Seward, J. E. (2008). Prevention of herpes zoster: Recommendations of the Advisory Committee on Immunization Practices (ACIP). *MMWR Recommendation, 57*(RR-5), 1–30.

Harig, P. T. (2007). Stress management: A guide for senior leaders. Stress hardiness: beyond jogging. In *Executive wellness: A guide for senior leaders*. Carlisle Barracks, PA: US Army Physical Fitness Research Institute.

Harston, B. (January 18, 2010). *A look at Healthy People 2010: How did Americans fare?* Retrieved April 14, 2012, from www.healthypeople2010.us.

Havighurst, R. I., & Orr, B. (1956). *Adult education and adult needs*. Chicago, IL: Center for Study of Liberal Education for Adults.

Haynes, S. G., Levine, S., Scotch, N., Feinleib, M., & Kannel, W. B. (1978). The relationship of psychosocial factors to coronary heart disease in the Framingham Study. I. Methods and risk factors. *American Journal of Epidemiology, 107*(5), 362–383.

Haynes, S. G., Feinleib, M., & Kannel, W. B. (1980). The relationship of psychosocial factors to coronary heart disease in the Framingham Study. III. Eight-year incidence of coronary heart disease. *American Journal of Epidemiology, 111*(1), 37–58.

Healthy People 2020. (2012). *A closer look: Health disparities*. Washington, DC: U.S. Department of Health and Human Services. Updated April 17, 2012. Retrieved April 22, 2012, from www.HealthyPeople.gov.

Heron, M. (2007). Deaths: Leading causes for 2004. *National Vital Statistics Reports, 56*(5), 1–95.

Hornstein, G. (1986). The structuring of identity among midlife women as a function of their degree of involvement in employment. *Journal of Personality, 54*, 551–575.

Hunt, S. (2011). *The most common injuries and causes of accidents at work*. Retrieved April 30, 2012, from Occupational and Safety Health Act website.

Jacobs, G. D. (1998). *Say goodnight to insomnia*. New York: Henry Holt.

Jacobs, G. D., Pace-Schott, E. E., Stickgold, R., & Otto, M. W. (2004). Cognitive behavioral therapy and pharmacotherapy for insomnia: A randomized controlled trial and direct comparison. *Archives of Internal Medicine, 164*(17), 1888–1896.

Japsen, B. (2007). Cholesterol levels attain milestone. Retrieved January 4, 2008, from www.chicagotribune.com/business/chi-thu.

Jarrett, V. (2012). Affordable Care Act: Making a difference. *St Louis American*. Retrieved April 27, 2012, from www.stlamerican.com/news/columnist.

Joint National Committee. (2003). The Seventh Report of the Joint National Committee on detection, evaluation and treatment of high blood pressure. *Journal of American Medical Association, 289*. Retrieved April 21, 2005, from http://jama.ama-assn.org/cgi/content/full/289,19.2560VI.

Karch, A. (2003). *Focus on nursing pharmacology* (2nd ed.). Philadelphia: Lippincott Williams & Wilkins.

Kawachi, I., Sparrow, D., Spiro, A., Vokonas, P., & Weiss, S. T. (1996). A prospective study of anger and coronary heart disease: The Normative Aging Study. *Circulation, 94*, 2090–2095.

Kobasa, S. (1979). Stressful life events, personality and health: An inquiry into hardiness. *Journal of Personality and Social Psychology, 37*, 1–11.

Kohlberg, L., & Lickona, T. (1986). *The stages of ethical development: From childhood through old age*. New York: Harper Collins.

Kriketos, A. D., Sharp, T. A., Seagle, H. M., Peters, J. C., & Hill, J. O. (2000). Effects of aerobic fitness on fat oxidation and body fatness. *Medicine and Science in Sports & Exercise, 32*(4), 805–811.

Kučera, K. (2004). Managing common skin problems in the elderly. *Clinical Advisor, 7*(6), 23–30.

Landefeld, C. S., Bowers, B. J., Feld, A. D., Hartmann, K. E., Hoffman, E., Ingber, M. J., et al. (2008). National Institutes of Health State-of-the-Science Conference Statement: Prevention of fecal and urinary incontinence in adults. *Annuals of Internal Medicine, 148*(6).

Légaré, E., Stacey, D., Dodin, S., O'Connor, A., Richer, M., Griffiths, E., et al. (2007). Women's decision making about the use of natural health products at menopause: A needs assessment and patient decision aid. *Journal of Alternative and Complementary Medicine, 13*(7), 741–749.

Leone, P. (2007). *Expanded HIV testing: Practical screening cases to meet new CDC recommendations*. Retrieved December 27, 2007, from www.medscape.com.

Levinson, D. (1986a). A conception of adult development. *American Psychologist, 41*, 3–13.

Levinson, D. (1986b). *The seasons of a man's life*. New York: Ballantine.

Levinson, D. (1996). *The seasons of a woman's life*. New York: Knopf.

Lindau, S., Laumann, E., & Levinson, W. (2007). Sexuality and health among older adults in the United States. *New England Journal of Medicine, 357*(26), 2732–2733.

Lowdermilk, D., & Perry, S. (2012). *Reproductive system concerns. Maternity and women's health care* (10th ed.) St. Louis: Mosby.

Lubkin, I. M., & Larsen, P. D. (2006). *Chronic illness: Impact and interventions* (6th ed.). Boston: Jones & Bartlett.

McFadden, S., & Gerl, R. (1990). Approaches to understanding spirituality in the second half of life. *Generations, 14*, 35–38.

Mendelsohn, M., & Karas, R. (2007). HRT and the young at heart. *New England Journal of Medicine, 356*(25), 2639–2641.

National Center for Health Statistics. (2011). *Healthy People 2010 Data, DATA2010*. Hyattsville, MD: Author.

National Center for Health Statistics. (2004). *Married adults are healthiest, New CDC report shows*. Retrieved September 4, 2007, from www.cdc.gov/nchs/pressroom/04facts/marriedadults.htm.

National Osteoporosis Foundation. (1998). *Boning up on osteoporosis: A guide to prevention and treatment*. Washington, DC: The Foundation.

National Sleep Foundation. (2012). *Insomnia and sleep disorders.* Retrieved April 9, 2012, from www.nationalsleepfoundation.org.

Nelson, H., Vesco, K., Haney, E., Fu, R., Nedrow, A., Miller, J., et al. (2006). Nonhormonal therapies for menopausal hot flashes. *Journal of the American Medical Association, 295*(17), 2057–2071.

Newman, D. K., & Giovannini, D. (2002). The overactive bladder: A nursing perspective. *American Journal of Nursing, 102*(6), 36–46.

Nicholson, J. (2011). *Five leading causes of workplace injury: Occupational Safety and Health Act.* Retrieved April 29, 2012 from ehow.com/info_7933497.

Northrup, C. (2008). *The secret pleasures of menopause.* New York: Hay House.

Nursing facts: Nursing's agenda for health care reform. (2005). Washington, DC: American Nurses Publishing. Retrieved July 31, 2005, from www.nursingworld.org/readroom/rnagenda.htm.

Office of Disease Prevention and Health Promotion. (2012). *A closer look at health disparities.* Washington, DC: Office of the Assistant Secretary and Office of the Secretary of the United States Department of Health and Human Services. Retrieved April 23, 2012, from http://odphp.osophs.dhhs.gov.

Ogden, C. L., Carroll, M. D., Kit, B. K., & Flegal, K. M. (January 2012). *Prevalence of obesity in the United States, 2009-2010.* National Center for Health Statistics Data Brief, 82. Retrieved April 16, 2012, from CDC website.

Parker-Pope, T. (2007). Estrogen shows benefit for heart health. *Wall Street Journal Online.* Retrieved August 12, 2007, from www.wsj.com.

Pender, N., et al. (2011). *Health promotion in nursing practice.* Stamford, CT: Appleton & Lange.

Perez, M. A., & Luguis, R. R. (2008). *Cultural competence in health education and health promotion.* San Francisco: Jossey-Bass.

Piaget, J. (1970). *Structuralism.* New York: Basic Books.

Reifman, A., Biernat, M., & Lang, E. (1991). Stress, social support, and health in married professional women with small children. *Psychology of Women Quarterly, 15,* 431–445.

Rice, V. (2000). *Handbook of stress, coping, and health: Implications for nursing research, theory, and practice.* London: Sage.

Rippe, J. M. (1996). *Fit over forty: A revolutionary plan to achieve lifelong physical and spiritual health and well-being.* New York: William Morrow.

Rossouw, J., Prentice, R., Manson, J., Wu, L., Barad, D., Barnabei, V., et al. (2007). Postmenopausal hormone therapy and risk of cardiovascular disease by age and years since menopause. *Journal of the American Medical Association, 297*(13), 1465–1477.

Schaie, K. W., & Willis, S. L. (2005). *Intellectual functioning in adulthood: Growth, maintenance, decline, and modifiability.* Philadelphia: American Society on Aging.

Seaman, B. (2003). *The greatest experiment ever performed on women: Exploding the estrogen myth.* New York: Hyperion.

Sheehy, G. (1993). *Menopause: The silent passage.* New York: Random House.

Silverstein, O., & Rashbaum, B. (1995). *The courage to raise good men.* New York: Penguin.

Sondik, E., et al. (2009). Progress toward the *Healthy People 2010* Goals and Objectives. *Annual Review of Public Health,* December 2009.

Spector, R. E. (2003). *Culture care: Guide to heritage assessment and health traditions.* East Norwalk, CT: Appleton & Lange.

Spector, R. E. (2008). *Cultural diversity in health and illness* (6th ed.). East Norwalk, CT: Appleton & Lange.

Spielberger, C. D., Jacobs, G., Russell, S., & Crane, R. S. (1983). Assessment of anger: The state-trait anger scale. In J. N. Butcher & C. D. Spielberger (Eds.), *Advances in personality assessment.* (Vol. 2). Hillsdale, NJ: Lawrence Erlbaum Associates.

Stuart, E., Deckro, J., & Mandle, C. L. (1989). Spirituality in health and healing: A clinical program. *Holistic Nursing Practice, 3,* 35–46.

Targonski, P. V., & Poland, E. A. (2007). Pneumococcal vaccination in adults: Recommendations, trends, and prospects. *Cleveland Clinics Journal of Medicine, 74*(6), 408–410, 413, 414.

Thomas, S. P. (1995). Psychosocial correlates of women's health in middle adulthood. *Issues in Mental Health Nursing, 16,* 285–314.

Twelve Reasons to Support Health Care. (2012). Blog retrieved June 14, 2012, from www.standupforhealthcare.org/learn-more/wuick-facts/12reason=to-support-health.

U.S. Census Bureau. (2006). *Statistical abstracts of the United States: 2007* (126th ed.). Washington, DC: U.S. Government Printing Office.

U.S. Census Bureau. Centers for Disease Control and Prevention (2010). *Minority Health: Hispanic health: Demographics.* Retrieved April 3, 2012, from http://cdc.gov/minorityhealth/populations/REMP/hispanic.html). Washington, D.C.: Author.

U.S. Department of Health and Human Services. (2000). *Healthy People 2010.* Washington, DC: U.S. Government Printing Office.

U.S. Department of Health and Human Services. (2005). *Healthy People 2010: Midcourse review.* Retrieved January 29, 2008, from www.healthypeople.gov/data/midcourse/html.

U.S. Department of Health and Human Services. (2006). *A closer look: Health disparities.* Retrieved April 5, 2012, from www. Healthy People 2000.gov/chart. Washington, D.C.

U.S. Department of Health and Human Services. (2010). *Reports of the Surgeon General, U.S. Public Health Service Oral Health Initiative.* Washington, D.C: Author.

U.S. Department of Health and Human Services. (2011). *Office of Disease Prevention and Health Promotion. National Prevention Strategy.* Washington, D.C: Author.

U.S. Department of Health and Human Services. (2007a). *Every American insured.* Retrieved December 26, 2007, from www.hhs.gov/everyamericaninsured/.

U.S. Department of Health and Human Services. (2007b). *The office of minority health.* Retrieved December 26, 2007, from www.omhrc.gov/templates/browse.

U.S. Department of Health and Human Services, Centers for Disease Control and Prevention, National Center for Health Statistics. (2007c). *Health, United States 2010.* Hyattsville, MD: Author.

U.S. Department of Health and Human Services, Health Resources and Services Administration. (2007). *Women's health USA 2007.* Rockville, MD: Author.

U.S. Department of Health and Human Services. National Institutes of Health (NIH), National Institute on Alcohol Abuse and Alcoholism. (2005). *Alcohol: A woman's health issue.*

U.S. Department of Health and Human Services. *Healthy People 2020: Improving the health of Americans.* (October 31, 2011). Leading Health Indicators. Washington, DC.

U.S. Department of Health and Human Services. *Healthy People 2020.* (2009). *Leading health indicators: Oral health.* Retrieved January 6, 2013, from http://www.healthypeople/2020/LHI.

U.S. Department of Labor. Occupational Safety and Health Administration. (2010). *You have a right to a safe workplace.* Occupational Safety and Health Administration. Washington, DC.

U.S. Department of Labor. Occupational Safety and Health Administration. (2012). *Toxic and hazardous substances.* Occupational Safety and Health Administration. Washington, DC.

USA Today. (January 11, 2005). *Why grown kids come home.* Retrieved from www.usatoday.com/educate/college/careers/news4.htm.

Vaillant, G. (2003). *Aging well: Surprising guideposts to a happier life from the Landmark Harvard Study of Adult Development.* New York: Little, Brown.

Vaillant, G., & Vaillant, C. (1990). Natural history of male psychological health, XII: A 45-year study of predictors of successful aging at age 65. *American Journal of Psychiatry, 147*(1), 31–37.

Vivian, C., & Dundes, L. (2004). The crossroads of culture and health among the Roma (gypsies). *Image: The Journal of Nursing Scholarship, 36*(1), 86–91.

Wallerstein, J. S., Lewis, J., & Blakeslee, S. (2000). *The unexpected legacy of divorce: A 25 year landmark study.* New York: Hyperion.

Williams, J., Paton, G., Siegler, I. C., Eigenbrodt, M. L., Nieto, E. J., & Tyroler, H. A. (2000). Anger proneness predicts coronary heart disease risk: Prospective analysis from the Atherosclerosis Risk in Communities (ARIC) Study. *Circulation, 101*(17), 2034–2039.

Older Adult

Kathleen Blais

OBJECTIVES

After completing this chapter, the reader will be able to:
- Discuss various theories of aging.
- Discuss *Healthy People 2020* objectives as they relate to older adults.
- Describe normal aging changes in the older adult.
- Evaluate morbidity data according to age, gender, and race.
- Discuss nutritional factors that affect the health of the older adult.
- Recognize risk factors that could lead to health problems in older adulthood.
- Enumerate the five most prevalent health conditions and the five leading causes of mortality among older people.
- Analyze environmental, physical, biological, and chemical agents that contribute to disability, morbidity, and mortality in later adulthood.
- Analyze social and political issues that influence the well-being of the older adult.
- Identify major resources that are available for older adults.

KEY TERMS

Activities of daily living	Ego differentiation versus work role preoccupation	Mini-Mental State Examination (MMSE)
Alzheimer's disease (AD)		Multi-infarct dementia
Atrophy	Ego integrity versus despair	Osteoporosis
Body transcendence versus body preoccupation	Ego transcendence versus ego preoccupation	Physician-assisted suicide
Cataracts	Elder mistreatment	Polypharmacy
Cerumen	Euthanasia	Presbycusis
Cognition	Glaucoma	Presbyopia
Constipation	Health literacy	Reminiscence
Decubitus ulcer	Impotence	Sclerosis
Delirium	Influenza	Stress incontinence
Dementia	Instrumental activities of daily living	Urge incontinence
Depression	Life review	Urinary incontinence
	Mild cognitive impairment (MCI)	

❓ **THINK ABOUT IT**

Older Adult Smokers

You are the director of a senior center in which 10 of your 40 members smoke. Several of the smoking individuals currently experience health problems. One older woman has chronic obstructive pulmonary disease and avoids using her oxygen because she is not supposed to smoke while the oxygen tank is in the room. One older gentleman has high blood pressure; another one of the smokers has been diagnosed with lung cancer. As director of the center, you would like to help these older adults to stop smoking. You have referred them to their physicians to obtain assistance with smoking cessation. All involved are on limited incomes and cannot afford to pay the charge of either a behavior-management class or nicotine-replacement therapy.

- *What additional information do you need to determine the potential efficacy of a smoking cessation program in your center?*
- *What types of resources are available to help you obtain the necessary assistance for these smokers?*
- *What provisions are available under Medicare and the Affordable Health Care Act of 2010 to assist a person with smoking cessation?*
- *What policy changes might be instituted within the senior center to prevent secondhand smoke from harming the residents in the center's care?*

Because older adults are living longer and healthier as a result of health-promotion and technological advances, health care professionals now enjoy the gift of caring for an older population. To be caring for a group of human beings that was virtually nonexistent 100 years ago is truly extraordinary. The current standard of living, options in nutritional choices, prevention and treatment of infectious diseases, and progress in medical care have dramatically increased the expected longevity for people living in the United States. Once these individuals reach adulthood, they are likely to live to old age. In 2010 the number of Americans age 65 and older was approximately 39 million, or 12.7% of the population (U.S. Census Bureau, 2011a). By the year 2050 the percentage is projected to increase to more than 20% of the population (U.S. Administration on Aging, 2011).

The fastest-growing group within the older adult population is 85 years and older. According to the U.S. Census Bureau, an individual who was 65 years of age in 2009 could expect to live 19.2 more years, for a total of 84.2 years. Individuals aged 85 years in 2009 could expect to live an average of 6.3 more years, for a total of 91.3 years (CDC, 2012a).

The percentage of White Americans in the population of adults 65 and older is expected to decrease over the next 30 years, while the percentages of African Americans, Hispanics, and Asian Americans will continue to rise. Considering this shift in population characteristics, it is imperative that health care providers develop an awareness of the cultural diversity of the population and identify the cultural beliefs that influence the health care decisions of older adults.

During the past few decades, older adults have used the most health care dollars in the last 7 years of their lives. Older adults waited until they became sick before seeking health care. Health care providers focused more on illness care than health promotion and wellness care. Introduction into the health care system along with insurance reimbursement has come late for many, resulting in a high prevalence of illness and limited health-promotion interventions. The misconceptions surrounding health promotion for older adults impede the ability of nurses and other health providers to provide the best possible care. It is time to overcome these misconceptions and begin to promote the health of older adults rather than wait until they are ill to provide them with health services. Health promotion is as important in later adulthood as it is in childhood. Older adults can derive the same benefits from health-promotion activities as do their younger counterparts; they are not "too old" to stop smoking, start exercising, change their diet, or relinquish other bad health habits. The potential for improvement is great, and nurses have a key role in changing common societal misconceptions and in creating new understandings regarding health promotion and older adults.

The diversity of cultural backgrounds in the United States influences the many biological, psychological, social, and economic changes as well as the spiritual and life transitions associated with aging that will be discussed in this chapter. Older adults who have immigrated to the United States have brought with them different languages, spiritual and cultural beliefs, eating preferences, and views about health and illness that may seem foreign to the American culture. Further, people of different cultures may value older adults differently based on their cultural perspective. Older adults may be viewed as a source of family and cultural history and wisdom. Throughout this chapter, cultural norms and behaviors will be discussed within each functional health pattern.

HEALTHY PEOPLE 2020

In 2005, halfway through the *Healthy People 2010* project period, a midcourse review of the status of the national objectives was conducted. Data were collected to measure the progress of the goals and to revise and reword the goals to make sure they were accurate and scientifically relevant. Through this process it was determined that many goals focusing on older adults were being met. Importantly, the life expectancy and quality of life continue to improve throughout the nation. Years in good or better health and years free of activity limitations and chronic illness have also increased slightly. At the same time it was determined that new goals, topic areas, and topic-specific objectives needed to be developed. In December 2010, the U.S. Department of Health and Human Services (USDHHS, 2010) released *Healthy People 2020*. The overall goals of *Healthy People 2020* expanded on previous goals and are to:

- Attain high-quality, longer lives free of preventable disease, disability, injury, and premature death.
- Achieve health equity, eliminate disparities, and improve the health of all groups.
- Create social and physical environments that promote good health for all.
- Promote quality of life, healthy development, and healthy behaviors across all life stages.

As part of the development of *Healthy People 2020,* several new topic areas were added, several of which focus on the health and wellness of older adults. These new topic areas are Dementias, including Alzheimer's Disease; Health-Related Quality of Life and Well-Being; Healthcare-Associated Infections; Sleep

Health; and a unique category—Older Adults—which recognizes the unique needs of this population. Selected national health-promotion and disease-prevention objectives for the older adult are listed in the accompanying box (see Box 24-1: *Healthy People 2020*). These objectives focus on increasing health-promotion programs and decreasing morbidity and mortality related to various disease states. It must be remembered that other specific topic areas also provide objectives that address the needs of older adults. Some of these will be addressed later in this chapter.

As the population of older adults continues to increase, the cultural diversity within this population will also increase. Cultural background and race have an effect on the prevalence of disease in the United States. The Centers for Disease Control and Prevention (CDC, 2012a) report that the five major racial groups—African Americans, Asian Americans, Hispanic Americans, Native Americans, and White Americans—share eight leading causes of death. Heart disease and cancer are the first and second leading causes, respectively, with stroke, respiratory diseases, flu, pneumonia, Alzheimer's disease, diabetes, and other causes following with varying disease rates depending on racial background.

BIOLOGY AND GENETICS

Although there is a great need to promote the health of the older population, there are numerous challenges in meeting this need. One of the great challenges to health promotion for older

---

♥ BOX 24-1   HEALTHY PEOPLE 2020

Selected National Health-Promotion and Disease-Prevention Topics and Objectives Relevant for Older Adults

Older Adult
- Increase the proportion of older adults who are up to date on a core set of clinical preventive services.
- Increase the proportion of older adults with one or more chronic health conditions who report confidence in managing their conditions.
- Increase the proportion of older adults who receive Diabetes Self-Management Benefits.
- Reduce the proportion of older adults who have moderate to severe functional limitations.
- Increase the proportion of older adults who engage in light, moderate, or vigorous leisure time activities.
- Increase the proportion of the health care workforce with geriatric certification.
- Reduce the proportion of noninstitutionalized older adults with disabilities who have an unmet need for long-term services and supports.
- Reduce the proportion of unpaid caregivers of older adults who report an unmet need for caregiver support services.
- Reduce the rate of pressure ulcer–related hospitalizations among older adults.
- Reduce the rate of emergency department visits attributable to falls among older adults.
- Increase the number of states, the District of Columbia, and tribes that collect and make publicly available information on the characteristics of victims, perpetrators, and cases of elder abuse, neglect, and exploitation.

Dementias, Including Alzheimer's Disease
- Increase the proportion of persons with diagnosed Alzheimer's disease and other dementias, or their caregiver, who are aware of the diagnosis.
- Reduce the proportion of preventable hospitalizations in persons with diagnosed Alzheimer's disease and other dementias.

Hearing and Other Sensory Communication Disorders
- Reduce the proportion of adults who have elevated hearing thresholds, or audiometric notches, in high frequencies (3, 4, or 6 kHz) in both ears, signifying noise-induced hearing loss.
- Increase the proportion of adults bothered by tinnitus who have seen a physician or other health care professionals.
- Increase the proportion of adults for whom tinnitus is a moderate to severe problem who have tried appropriate treatments.

- Increase the proportion of adults with balance or dizziness problems in the past 12 months who have ever seen a health care provider about their balance or dizziness problems.
- Increase the proportion of adults with moderate to severe balance or dizziness problems who have seen or been referred to a health care specialist for evaluation or treatment.
- Reduce the proportion of adults with chemosensory (smell or taste) disorders who as a result have experienced a negative impact on their general health status, work, or quality of life in the past 12 months.
- Increase the proportion of persons with communication disorders of voice, swallowing, speech, or language who have seen a speech-language pathologist (SLP) for evaluation or treatment.
- Increase the proportion of persons with communication disorders of voice, swallowing, speech, or language who have participated in rehabilitation services.

Sleep Health
- Increase the proportion of adults who get sufficient sleep.

Respiratory Diseases
- Reduce activity limitations among adults with chronic obstructive pulmonary disease (COPD).
- Reduce deaths from chronic obstructive pulmonary disease (COPD) among adults.
- Reduce hospitalizations for chronic obstructive pulmonary disease (COPD).
- Reduce hospital emergency department visits for chronic obstructive pulmonary disease (COPD).
- Increase the proportion of adults with abnormal lung function whose underlying obstructive disease has been diagnosed.

Vision
- Reduce visual impairment.
- Increase the use of personal protective eyewear in recreational activities and hazardous situations around the home.
- Increase vision rehabilitation.
- (Developmental) Increase the proportion of Federally Qualified Health Centers (FQHCs) that provide comprehensive vision health services.

Source: U.S. Department of Health and Human Services. (2012a). *Healthy People 2020: Topics and objectives.* Retrieved February 26, 2012, from www.healthypeople.gov/2020/topicsobjectives2020/default.aspx

adults lies in the misconceptions about the benefits of disease prevention and health promotion. Another challenge relates to the difficulty separating the normal changes of aging from pathological processes and illness. Normal age-related changes frequently are regarded as inevitable and irreversible. However, there is a large amount of variability in age-related changes within each individual. Environmental, economic, physiological, genetic, psychological, social, and cultural factors combine to influence the aging process. Most researchers agree that biological changes show that growth and development peak during early adulthood, with subsequent linear decline until death. These normal changes must be distinguished from pathological changes to focus health-promotion interventions on behaviors that can be changed. For example, it is normal for older adults to experience a decline in their respiratory vital capacity. Therefore when recommending exercise programs, older people must start gradually, allowing them to experience the exercise free from respiratory distress. Selected changes will be discussed specifically under Gordon's Functional Health Patterns.

Another challenge to promoting the health of older adults lays in the prevalence of chronic illness and multiple health problems. Although chronic illness is not a normal change of aging, years of environmental assault, poor health behaviors, and stress have placed older adults at a high risk for developing these illnesses. Generally health deteriorates with aging through an accumulation of chronic disorders and disabilities. Table 24-1 lists the percentage of older adults with chronic conditions.

Illness influences the individual's capacity and motivation to learn new health-promoting behaviors. According to the Centers for Disease Control and Prevention (CDC, 2012a), in 2010, 35.4% of adults age 65 years and older had some physical limitation, 12.1% had limitations with independent activities

of daily living (IADLs), and 29.8% had difficulty with one or more activities of daily living (ADLs). Most of these limitations are associated with physical changes of aging and chronic disease such as arthritis, heart disease, stroke, and respiratory disease. The prevalence of preventable illness and the concomitant physical limitations associated with chronic disease clearly indicate that there is a great need for health-promotion and disease/injury-prevention activities in this population. It is important to note that health-promotion practices among older adults may vary because of the individual's self-perception of health status and their economic and cultural background (Box 24-2: Diversity Awareness).

TABLE 24-1	AVERAGE PERCENTAGE OF PEOPLE AGE 65 AND OLDER WHO HAVE CHRONIC HEALTH CONDITIONS	
CHRONIC CONDITION	**AGE 65-74**	**AGE 75 AND OLDER**
Hypertension	54.2	57.3
Arthritis	49.0	54.1
Heart disease	16.5	25.8
Cancer	20.4	27.2
Diabetes	22.0	21.7
Asthma	8.7	7.4
Chronic bronchitis or emphysema	11.4	12.6
Stroke	6.1	10.7

From Centers for Disease Control and Prevention, National Center for Health Statistics. (2010). *Summary health statistics for U.S. adults: National Health Interview Survey 2010.* Retrieved May 20, 2012, from www.cdc.gov/nchs/data/series/sr_10/sr10_252.pdf.

⊕ BOX 24-2 DIVERSITY AWARENESS

Perceptions of Health Status, Need for Assistance with Routine Needs, and Need for Assistance with Activities of Daily Living Related to Race

Data from the *National Health Interview Survey* conducted by the Centers for Disease Control and Prevention in 2010 (CDC, National Center for Health Statistics, 2010) provide interesting information about the perceptions of older Hispanic, non-Hispanic Black, and non-Hispanic White adults regarding their health status, their need for assistance with routine activities, and their need for assistance with activities of daily living.

When asked about health status, 42.7% of White adults 65 years or older stated that their health was excellent or very good, 34% described their health as good, and 22.9% described their health as fair or poor; 44% of Asian American older adults reported their health as excellent or very good, 34.4% stated their health was good, and 21.6% stated their health was fair or poor. In contrast, 25.3% of Black older adults reported their health as excellent or very good, 36.4% stated good, and 38.2% stated that their health was fair or poor. Of Hispanic older adults, 28.1% reported that their health was excellent or very good, 33.8% reported their health as good, and 38.2% stated their health was fair or poor. In all groups, those who described their health as fair or poor were also more likely to be financially poor, with 40% of White older adults, 51.6% of Black older adults, 53.4% of Hispanic older adults, and

45.6% of Asian older adults who reported their health status as fair or poor also being financially poor.

Respondents were also asked about their need for assistance with activities of daily living, such as bathing, showering, dressing, eating, getting in and out of the bed or chair, using the toilet, or getting around inside the home; and their need for assistance with routine activities, such as performing everyday household chores, doing necessary business, shopping, and getting around for other purposes outside the home. Results indicated that 11.2% of White non-Hispanic older adults reported needing assistance with routine needs, 18.1% of Hispanic and 17.1% of Black non-Hispanic older adults reported needing assistance, and 6.2% of White non-Hispanic older adults reported needing assistance with activities of daily living, whereas 11.5% of both Hispanic and Black non-Hispanic older adults reported needing assistance.

Nurses must be aware of racial disparities in the incidence of chronic disease, perceived health status, and perceived need for assistance with activities of daily living and routine tasks in the persons for whom they provide care. Assessing older adults holistically and planning interventions that focus on health promotion, illness and injury prevention, and effective management of chronic illness will help to ensure improved quality of life for all older adults.

Data from Centers for Disease Control and Prevention, National Center for Health Statistics. (2010). *Summary health statistics for U.S. adults: National Health Interview Survey 2010.* Retrieved May 20, 2012, from www.cdc.gov/nchs/data/series/sr_10/sr10_252.pdf.

Theories of Aging

The study of how and why people age has continued over many years and has been the source of a great deal of debate. Until fairly recently the cause of death on many older adults' death certificates was listed simply as "old age." At the 55th Annual Meeting of the Gerontological Society of America, Butler and Olshansky (2002) explored these questions in a presentation entitled, *Has Anyone Ever Died of Old Age?* As the study of gerontology has progressed, researchers have begun to question the physiological, social, and psychological reasons why people die.

Despite this attention, the debate among those studying biological, psychological, and sociological theories of aging continues. There is no formula to predict how a person will age or how long that individual will live. Many theories continue to be examined today, including metabolism, free radicals, stress, the role of the immune system, genetics, epigenetics (the blending of nature/genetics and nurture/environment), and diet. It is postulated that genetic markers may predict the development of disease and play a large role in determining how a person will age and how long the person will live. In addition, researchers report that calorie-restricted diets have shown an increase in longevity in animals; however, there is debate regarding whether caloric restriction alone or caloric restriction in the presence of genetic markers increases longevity. The role of antioxidants in binding free radicals is also being researched as an important influence on increasing longevity. Although no consensus has yet been reached that describes the entire aging process, theories continue to be forthcoming and are very exciting (National Institute on Aging, 2011). Detailed explanation of each of these theories is extremely interesting but beyond the scope of this book. Some of the theories used to explain aging are briefly described in Box 24-3.

GORDON'S FUNCTIONAL HEALTH PATTERNS

Health Perception–Health Management Pattern

An important factor in maintaining health is the older adult's motivation. Nurses who care for older adults know that all the best nursing in the world cannot make an individual do something he or she believes to be unnecessary. A primary factor in the older adult's motivation to promote personal health is the perception of health and its subsequent management.

The *Harvard Women's Health Watch* (Harvard Medical School, 2003) reports five major activities older adults can engage in to promote health and prevent frailty. These include maintaining healthy weight and diet; staying active; practicing fall prevention; maintaining relationships; and keeping regular medical appointments. Additionally, the Centers for Disease Control and Prevention (2011a) recommend clinical preventive services for older adults that include immunizations (influenza and pneumococcal) and screenings for early detection of breast cancer, colorectal cancer, diabetes, lipid disorders, and osteoporosis; and smoking cessation counseling for those who

---

BOX 24-3   THEORIES OF AGING

Biological Theories of Aging
- Programmed Theories of Aging—Aging is the result of predictable cellular death.
  - Immunity theory—Aging is a programmed accumulation of damage and decline in the function of the immune system resulting from oxidative stress.
  - Neuroendocrine control/pacemaker theory—Aging is a programmed decline in the functioning of the nervous, endocrine, and immune systems. The cells lose their ability to reproduce.
  - Gene theory—Longevity may be associated with a genetic trait or a "longevity gene," "juvenescent" genes mediate youthful vigor and mature adult well-being, "senescent" genes promote functional decline and structural deterioration.
- Error Theories of Aging—Aging is the result of an accumulation of random errors in the synthesis of cellular DNA and RNA.
  - Oxidative stress theory (free radical theory)—Errors are a result of random damage from free radicals.
  - Cross-linkage theory—Aging is a product of accumulated damage from errors associated with cross-linked proteins where cross-linked proteins become stiff and thick.
  - Wear-and-tear theory—Cellular errors are the result of deterioration over time because of continued use.
- Caloric Restriction Theory—In animal models, calorie restriction increased the life span and the health of the subjects.

Sociological Theories of Aging
- Activity Theory—Continued activity is an indicator of successful aging.
- Disengagement Theory—In the course of aging, the individual slowly withdraws from former roles and activities.

- Role Theory—The ability of an individual to adapt to changing roles throughout life is predictive of adjustment to the changing roles associated with aging.
- Continuity Theory—In normal aging, personality remains consistent. Personality influences role activity and life satisfaction.
- Age Stratification Theory—Focuses on the relationship between age as an element of social structure and aging people as a cohort.
- Subculture Theory—Older people have their own norms, habits, and beliefs and interact better among age peers than with other age groups.

Developmental Theories of Aging
- Erikson's Developmental Theory—There is a predetermined order of development and specific tasks are associated with specific periods in a person's life. For older adults the developmental stage is integrity versus despair.
- Peck's Developmental Theory—This theory expanded on Erikson's theory with identification of discrete tasks of late life that when accomplished together result in ego integrity.
- Havighurst's Developmental Theory—There are specific tasks associated with aging, including adjusting to the losses of aging (e.g., health, income, death of spouse and age peers), adapting to change and new roles, and accepting life's experiences.
- Tornstam's Theory of Gerotranscendence—Aging is viewed as the movement from birth to death and maturation toward wisdom. Gerotranscendence involves achieving wisdom through personal transformation.

smoke. Under the Affordable Care Act of 2010, many of these services are provided at no cost to older adults who have Medicare. Helping an older adult to understand the importance of these factors for maintaining health is an essential nursing role needed to form positive health perceptions and effective health management patterns.

Health maintenance behaviors include exercise, good nutrition, sexual safety, and appropriate sleep-rest patterns. Health maintenance practices also include regular health care checkups, which will provide early detection and management of disease. Although these behaviors are important for all older adults, the perception of these activities and the ability to practice good health behaviors vary by cultural group. It is essential that nurses are culturally competent and understand the cultural values that guide behavior. In so doing, the nurse will be most effective in helping the older adult form a positive health perception and practice good health behaviors (Box 24-4: Innovative Practice).

Nutritional-Metabolic Pattern

Ogden and colleagues (2012) report that 39.7% of adults 60 years of age and older are obese, with older women having a greater incidence of obesity (42.3%) than older men (36.6%). Obesity is associated with several chronic health conditions including hypertension, diabetes, and heart disease. The National Resource Center on Nutrition, Physical Activity & Aging (2012) states that between 35% and 50% of older residents living in long-term care facilities are malnourished and approximately 65% of older adults in hospitals may be malnourished. These data underscore the problems of maintaining good nutrition. For independent seniors, barriers that may interfere with the ability to obtain adequate and nutritional food include limited transportation, income, and social support resources. Problems with access to food are compounded by the effect of normal changes of aging. Declines in gastrointestinal organ function can lead to changes in digestive metabolism and the absorption and elimination of nutrients. A deterioration of the smell, vision, and taste senses and the high frequency of dental and swallowing problems make maintaining adequate daily nutrition even more difficult. Additionally, side effects of required medications may affect appetite. Cultural food preferences and lifelong eating habits, such as diets high in fat and cholesterol, are other obstacles to maintaining optimal nutrition.

The living environment further affects nutritional status. Community-dwelling seniors are at high risk for nutritional disorders because access to food may be limited. Institutionalized older adults do not have a problem with availability of food, but the meals served in institutions frequently contain excessive fat, cholesterol, or salt, and lack sufficient fiber. Additionally, fresh fruit and vegetables are less available, and

---

☀ BOX 24-4   INNOVATIVE PRACTICE

Geriatric Assessment

The health care system, with its emphasis on acute care, busy office schedules, and fragmented delivery systems, often frustrates older people and their families. The very old or frail person's health problems often are overlooked, ignored, or only partially treated. Many communities have a health care service that uses a team approach to meet the special needs of older adults. This service is known as geriatric assessment.

Goals of Geriatric Assessment
- Maintain health and health maintenance practices.
  - Promote disease prevention through routine immunizations and health screenings.
  - Implement fall prevention strategies to decrease the incidence of falls and fall-related injuries.
- Minimize hospitalizations.
- Establish complete diagnoses that are often missed or overlooked, including hearing impairment, vision deficits, early dementia, depression, and poor nutrition.
- Decrease over-prescription and misuse of medications including prescription, over-the-counter, vitamins/minerals/supplements, and herbal remedies.

Geriatric assessment uses an interdisciplinary team consisting of a geriatric nurse practitioner, physical therapist, and a social worker. Each member of the team evaluates the person from a health care, functional, cognitive, or psychosocial perspective. Additional members of the team might include a geriatric psychiatrist, geriatrician, nutritionist, pharmacist, dentist, or podiatrist. The program team evaluates the home environment, risk for falls, incontinence, vision and hearing impairments, memory loss, depression and anxiety, functional decline, physical deconditioning, caregiver stress, economic resources, advance directives, and quality-of-life issues. The team is coordinated by the geriatric nurse practitioner.

Geriatric assessment is not meant for all older people. The people who benefit are those who are frail. An older person who might benefit from geriatric assessment is one who:
- Is older than age 80
- Has a history of frequent falls
- Is losing weight
- Is depressed
- Has mild memory loss
- Has been hospitalized 3 times in 2 months
- Takes more than five medications regularly and frequently gets them confused
- Has no close family or other support persons in the community
- Is in need of health teaching

Geriatric assessment usually identifies the strengths and weaknesses of the older adult and evaluates their situation including family and other social support. Following the assessment, the geriatric nurse practitioner begins developing a plan of care to incorporate usable strengths and assist with weaknesses.

The primary care physician, family physician, internist, geriatrician, or geriatric nurse practitioner is a key link between the geriatric assessment team and the individual, primarily because this provider carries out the team's recommendation and monitors the person's progress. In most cases the nurse practitioner coordinates between the team and the person's primary physician and family.

Geriatric assessment clinics are available in many larger cities. As the U.S. health care system changes from its costly system of treating acute health problems with frequent office and hospital visits to a more cost-controlled, coordinated, comprehensive health management system, geriatric assessment will play a key role in identifying individual strengths, correcting problems, and maintaining the health and quality of life of older citizens.

Courtesy Carole Lium Edelman.

the nutritional value of produce is reduced significantly when the food is canned or frozen. Finally, institutional food tends to be unappealing, and most institutions may not be able to adapt their meals to the cultural and religious preferences of their residents.

Anorexia, or lack of appetite, can accompany disease. Medications, poor dentition, difficulty swallowing, or a lack of dentures can also cause older people to eat less than is optimal. Those in acute care hospitals or long-term care facilities may experience a lack of appetite as a result of illness. The hospital stay is a time during which good nutrition is most important to heal wounds and to restore energy; however, a lack of interest in or energy for eating during hospitalization places the older adult at a high risk for developing nutritional disorders.

Proper nutrition helps prevent cancer, obesity, and gastrointestinal disorders and provides older adults with the energy required to function in all activities of daily living. Good nutrition can be measured by ascertaining whether the individual is meeting the recommended daily allowance (RDA) for caloric intake. The U.S. Department of Agriculture (USDA, 2010) established the RDA of 2000 to 2800 calories for men age 51 and older: 2000-2200 for sedentary men, 2200-2400 for moderately active men, and 2400-2800 for active men. The range for women age 51 and older is 1600 to 2200—1600 for sedentary women, 1800 for moderately active women, and 2000-2200 for active women.

The nurse assists the older adult in maintaining the highest possible nutritional level. Teaching about the food needed to maintain optimal nutritional status is of utmost importance. The American Association of Retired Persons (2008) reports that 18% of all households participating in the Supplemental Nutrition Assistance Program (SNAP) include at least one person older than age 60. Older women were more likely to be users of SNAP than older men. One half of older SNAP participants were non-Hispanic White. Many older persons are unaware that they are eligible to participate in SNAP. In addition to SNAP, there are several other federally supported nutrition assistance programs available to older adults, including a commodity supplemental food program, child and adult food program, older adult nutrition program (Meals-on-Wheels), and the emergency food assistance program. However, Wellman and Kamp (2004) report that only 6% to 7% of the people who really need these programs use them. The nurse may assist the older adult in acquiring information about and transportation to obtain food and applying for these programs. Nurses who work in institutional settings are charged with the difficult task of encouraging good nutrition on the resident and administrative level. The dietitian or nurse can assess the person's food preferences and any difficulties in eating and plan an appropriate menu to meet the person's nutritional needs. Encouraging family members to bring in food that the resident enjoys is helpful. A pleasant setting with social interaction can also enhance the desire to eat. The reader may refer to Chapter 11: Nutrition Counseling for Health Promotion for more information to help older adults achieve improved levels of nutrition.

Elimination Pattern

Bowel and bladder functions in the older adult are altered by normal changes of aging. The bladder retains its tonus, but its capacity decreases. Gastrointestinal motility decreases as people age. In addition to some of the normal changes of aging, diet plays a significant role in problems with intestinal motility and constipation. Increased incidence of nutritional disorders, particularly decreased intake of fluids and fiber, contributes in large part to elimination problems. Many medications taken by older adults can cause elimination concerns. Lack of physical activity and changes in the environment that decrease privacy for toileting also contribute. To maintain healthy bowel hygiene, the nurse encourages the older adult to ingest adequate fluids and fiber, and to exercise routinely.

Constipation is a major problem for older adults and has far-reaching effects on their quality of life. There are several bowel elimination problems that are described by persons as constipation: hard stools, infrequent stools, the need for excessive straining, and a feeling of incomplete bowel evacuation often associated with abdominal cramping or feeling bloated. Although diet and activity are common causes of constipation, the nurse must also consider whether constipation in the older adult person is related to metabolic disease such as hypothyroidism, neurological disease such as Parkinson's disease, psychological illness such as depression, or medications. Nurses can conduct a careful assessment of the cause of constipation and develop an appropriate plan of care. By encouraging older adults to exercise and increase their fluid and dietary intake, nurses can help reduce the incidence of constipation. Exercise has a rapid and favorable effect on constipation. Dietary modifications, such as increasing fiber and fluid intake, can stimulate the colon and resolve constipation.

Urinary incontinence (UI) affects 50% or more of older adults who live at home or in long-term care facilities (Agency for Healthcare Quality and Research [AHQR], 1996). Incontinence is classified as either acute (transient) or chronic (established) (Touhy & Jett, 2012). Acute incontinence has a sudden onset, has been present for less than 6 months, and is usually secondary to a treatable condition. Chronic incontinence has either a sudden or a gradual onset and is categorized into four major types: stress incontinence, which is the most common and occurs during exercise, laughing, coughing, or sneezing; urge incontinence, or the inability to delay voiding after the bladder is full; **urge, mixed, or stress UI with high post-void residual incontinence,** which occurs when the bladder does not empty completely and becomes overdistended, which may be caused by an obstruction in the urinary elimination tract, such as that caused by an enlarged prostate gland; and **functional incontinence,** which is associated with environmental barriers, physical limitations, or cognitive impairment where the person is unable to reach the toilet.

Incontinence results in threats to both psychological and physical health, including depression, urinary tract infections, skin breakdown, and falls. The nurse can help older adults to understand and accept incontinence as a manageable problem. Implementing appropriate management is important for the older adult's continued good health and self-esteem.

For the chronically incontinent person, AHRQ (1996) recommends scheduled toileting, prompted voiding, improved access to toileting facilities, management of diet and fluids, and the use of disposable absorbent undergarments. Voiding schedules are most effective when the person can select specific times during the day for urination. Prompted voiding is another method to decrease incontinent episodes. The individual is reminded or asked about voiding. Improving access to toileting facilities can include providing adaptive equipment for ambulation; installing raised toilet seats and safety handrails; and providing bedside commodes for those who have difficulty getting to the toilet. Eliminating dietary caffeine can help persons with urge incontinence and increasing fiber in the diet may help those whose incontinence is related to constipation. Providing disposable absorbent undergarments can help older adults with UI stay dry and decrease their feeling of embarrassment related to potential "accidents." Anti-incontinence devices, such as pessaries, also are often helpful. In addition, pelvic floor or Kegel exercises can be taught to improve the musculature of the urinary system.

Activity-Exercise Pattern

According to the Centers for Disease Control and Prevention (CDC, National Center for Health Statistics, 2012a,b), 41.2% of adults age 65 to 74 years and 27.7% of adults 75 years of age and older met federal physical activity guidelines for aerobic activity through leisure-time aerobic activity. Men were more likely to meet the guidelines than women, and White older adults more likely than Black or Hispanic older adults. Benefits of regular exercise in promoting health and preventing disease are widely accepted. The overwhelming evidence of the positive effects of exercise has led the U.S. Department of Health and Human Services to develop within its program *Healthy People 2020* national objectives for increasing the percentage of adults who exercise regularly. Regular physical activity can help or prevent many chronic health problems associated with aging, including hypertension, obesity, diabetes, and depression. Regular physical activity can increase both the years of life and the quality of those years. Strength training can improve balance and reduce the risk of falls, strengthen bones, and reduce blood glucose levels. Although exercise is not popular among this age group, no physiological or psychological explanation has been found to explain this decline in interest. Normal changes of aging, pathological conditions, and environmental deterrents do not prevent the older adult from exercising (Figure 24-1).

The Centers for Disease Control and Prevention (CDC, 2011b) recommends a combination of aerobic exercise and muscle-strengthening activities every week. Aerobic exercise may range from moderate intensity to vigorous intensity depending on the older person's level of fitness, and muscle-strengthening activities can include exercises that work all major muscle groups. Teaching the many benefits of exercise is the first lesson in motivating older adults to engage. With respect to the role that culture plays on the value of exercise, individual counseling is needed to identify exercises that can be enjoyed and continued (Figure 24-2). The nurse or physical therapist

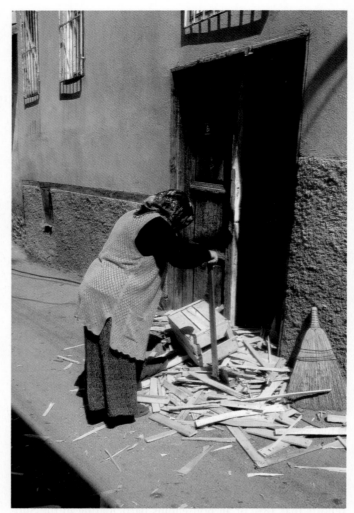

FIGURE 24-1 Normal changes of aging and environmental deterrents do not prevent older adults from exercising.

assists in designing an appropriate exercise program that will help to maintain strength, flexibility, and balance. Walking, which can be done in both community settings and health care facilities, is broadly reported as the most widely accepted form of exercise among older adults.

Other popular activities for older adults include swimming, weight-bearing exercises, and aquatic exercises. Weight-bearing and muscle-building exercises help to maintain functional mobility, promote independence, and prevent falls. Weight-bearing exercises are shown to be highly effective in reducing bone wasting associated with osteoporosis. Regular exercise promotes maintenance of bone mineral density in older adults. Exercising in the water is also an effective and enjoyable activity for those with arthritis. Older individuals who suffer from arthritis find aquatic or water exercise a pain-free way to increase their functional ability. The effects of exercise on the older adult are extensive. Box 24-5 lists many benefits that can be derived from participating in an exercise program.

Before beginning any exercise program, an older person who has not been exercising should consult a physician or nurse practitioner. After the program begins, activity levels

Bed   Sitting   Standing

Exercises

FIGURE 24-2 Bed-lying, sitting, and standing exercises. (Redrawn from Ebersole, P., & Hess, P. [1998]. *Toward healthy aging: Human need and nursing response* [3rd ed.]. St. Louis: Mosby.)

BOX 24-5	BENEFITS OF EXERCISE IN THE OLDER ADULT

- Better sleep
- Reduced constipation
- Lower cholesterol level
- Lower blood pressure
- Better digestion
- Weight loss
- Socializing opportunities
- Greater sense of well-being

can be increased gradually. Adherence to an exercise program is a major problem for all populations. The best strategies to encourage continued exercise among older adults are to communicate the importance of exercise in maintaining quality of life, and to help them choose an exercise that they can enjoy and is easily accessible.

Sleep-Rest Pattern

Inability to sleep is a frequent concern of older adults. Neikrug and Ancoli-Israel (2010) reported that "approximately 50% of older adults complain of difficulty sleeping." The Trans-NIH Sleep Research Coordinating Committee (AHRQ, 2005) found that 40 to 70 million Americans experience intermittent or chronic sleep disturbances. Older adults are more likely to experience insomnia in some form, including sleep apnea, the inability to fall asleep, the inability to stay asleep, the inability to fall back to sleep when awakening in the night, or the feeling of not being refreshed when awakening in the morning. Sleep-disordered breathing or sleep apnea may affect 20% to 40% of older adults and is associated with increased risk of stroke and mortality (Redline et al., 2010). In conjunction with insomnia, older adults are more likely to report excessive sleepiness, defined by Umlauf and colleagues (2008) as "somnolence, hypersomnia, excessive daytime sleepiness, and subjective sleepiness." The high prevalence of sleep disorders in older adults indicates that there is a great need to assist them in improving the quality of their sleep.

The benefits of a good night's sleep are numerous. Quality sleep results in overall increases in energy, motivation to continue a high quality of life, and improved immune function. Because of the problem with sleep, *Healthy People 2020* added a new topic related to sleep health with the goal to "increase public knowledge of how adequate sleep and treatment of sleep disorders improve health, productivity, wellness, quality of life, and safety...." Nurses assist older adults in achieving a good night's sleep through assessment that might reveal possible causes of sleep disturbances. The Pittsburgh Sleep Quality Index (PSQI) is a subjective tool that is helpful in assessing the quality and patterns of sleep in older adults. The tool measures seven areas: subjective sleep quality, sleep latency, sleep duration, habitual sleep efficiency, sleep disturbances, use of sleeping medication, and daytime dysfunction (Smyth, 2008). Teaching about normal changes can reassure older adults that their sleep patterns have changed but are not necessarily harmful. Having this information may decrease anxiety. Identifying normal bedtime rituals, such as drinking a glass of milk, taking a relaxing bath, reading, or meditating, and ensuring that the person is able to continue these practices may help to establish normal sleep routines. Increasing physical activity during the day can also help them fall asleep more readily at night. Taking pain medication or using alternative pain-relief methods before going to bed can help those who suffer from painful conditions obtain better rest at night.

Residents of nursing facilities or people in acute care facilities may have difficulty adjusting to the environment at night. Adjustments in noise and lighting can help these individuals sleep better. Emotional disorders frequently interfering with sleep can be identified, and therapy and medication can be administered during the day to help people experiencing these problems sleep peacefully at night. Finally, daytime napping has been viewed as inhibiting a good night's sleep in this population. Although a nap may be beneficial, one can insure the amount of daytime napping is not excessive so as to interfere with night-time sleep (Box 24-6: Hot Topics).

Sleep medications may be helpful for short-term use; however, the American Geriatrics Society Beers Criteria (2010) recommend avoidance of long-term use of benzodiazepines, barbiturates, and chloral hydrate for treatment of insomnia in older adults because of older adults' increased sensitivity to these drugs, increased risk of dependency, and the decreased metabolism of long-term agents resulting in an increased risk for cognitive impairment, falls, and overdose.

Cognitive-Perceptual Pattern

Cognition

Thinking processes (cognition) in old age have been the subject of intensive study over the past few decades. Brain weight decreases with aging, and a shift occurs in the proportion of gray matter to white matter. The ways in which these changes are manifested in individuals vary because of culture, heredity, lifestyle, environmental exposures, and many other factors. No consensus has been reached as to the ways in which these changes translate into human behavior.

There is a common belief that most older adults will eventually develop dementia; however, cognitive problems are not a normal change of aging and many live well into old age without ever experiencing dementia. It is important that the nurse be cautious in assessing the older person who presents with confusion, because confusion is not always indicative of dementia, but can be the result of many treatable health problems including electrolyte imbalances, diabetic ketoacidosis, and hypoxia. Mild cognitive impairment (MCI) is a pathological collection of symptoms that results in memory loss, language difficulties, and impairments in judgment and reasoning. A review of instrumental activities of daily living will help the nurse identify changes in higher executive functions, such as paying bills, taking medications as ordered, using the phone, and driving safely. It is estimated that 10% of adults older than age 65 will develop

---

🔥 **BOX 24-6   HOT TOPICS**

Measures to Promote Sleep

Sleep problems can be caused by many things, including stress; medications; medical conditions such as angina, asthma, anxiety, or depression; poor sleeping habits; and sleep disorders. The following are some suggestions to improve sleep in older adults.

Do
- Plan a regular bedtime and wake-up schedule.
- Participate in exercise, hobbies, and other activities during the day.
- Develop specific bedtime rituals, such as reading, meditating, drinking a glass of milk, or taking a warm bath. These tell the body it is almost time for sleep.
- Ensure a comfortable and quiet sleep environment, which is dark except for night safety lights.
- Sleep on a comfortably firm mattress with comfortable pillows and bedclothes.
- Use bed only for sleep and sexual activities.
- Check with physician about prescription and over-the-counter medications that may interfere with sleep.

Avoid
- Daytime naps; naps are considered part of the sleep total for the day
- Exercise or vigorous activity immediately before bedtime
- Caffeine after mid-morning
- Drinking alcohol before going to bed
- Sleep medications
- Tobacco products
- Driving when tired or sleepy

When Sleep Problems Persist
- Keep a sleep log, recording times and duration of sleep throughout the 24-hour period for at least 1 week.
- Ask sleep companion about sleep habits, such as snoring or restlessness.
- See health care provider.

Alzheimer's disease with this number increasing to 50% in the 90 and older age group (Beatty, 2006).

Dementia is an illness of the cognitive system and is not accepted as a normal change of aging. Dementia is defined by the Centers for Disease Control and Prevention (2011c) as a "group of cognitive disorders characterized by memory impairment, marked difficulty in the domains of language, motor activity, object recognition, and disturbance of executive function" (p. 1). Cognitive alterations are key symptoms that indicate changes in physiological function among older persons. Alzheimer's Disease International (2009) estimated that there were 35.6 million people globally living with dementia and that number was expected to double every 20 years. The greatest increases in dementia were found in low- and middle-income countries. The incidence of dementia and Alzheimer's disease in the elderly prompted the U.S. Department of Health and Human Services (2012b) to add *Dementia, including Alzheimer's Disease* as a new topic in *Healthy People 2020* with the goal to "reduce the morbidity and costs associated with, and maintain or enhance the quality of life for, persons with dementia, including Alzheimer's disease" (p. 1).

Two main types of dementia exist. The first type is **multi-infarct dementia**, which is caused by the death of brain tissue and diagnosed through brain imaging. Tissue death may be caused by a lack of blood flow to the brain from a cerebral vascular accident (CVA) or from another cause. The other main type of dementia is **Alzheimer's disease (AD)**, the most common type, which makes up about 50% of all dementia diagnoses. The Alzheimer's Association estimates that approximately 5 million U.S. adults have Alzheimer's disease. Other dementias include Parkinson-related dementia, Huntington's disease, Creutzfeldt-Jakob disease, Pick disease, and Lewy body dementia. Each one involves cognitive processes as defined earlier, although cognitive symptoms may vary depending on the area(s) of the brain affected by the disease (Alzheimer's Association, 2012).

The symptoms of dementia include forgetfulness, inattentiveness, disorganized thinking, altered levels of consciousness, perceptual disturbances, sleep-wake disorders, psychomotor disturbances, and disorientation. Assessment for dementia can be made part of the routine assessment of older adults especially if any of these symptoms arise. One tool that has been used successfully to screen for cognitive impairments among older adults is the **Mini-Mental State Examination (MMSE)** (Folstein et al., 1975) (Figure 24-3).

Mini Mental Status Examination Sample Items

Orientation to Time
"What is the date?"

Registration
"Listen carefully,
I am going to say three words.
You say them back after I stop.
Ready? Here they are...
HOUSE (pause), CAR (pause), LAKE (pause).
Now repeat those words back to me."
[Repeat up to 5 times, but score only the first trial.]

Naming
"What is this?"
[Point to a pencil or pen.]

Reading
"Please read this and do what it says."
[Show examinee the words on the stimulus form.]
CLOSE YOUR EYES

FIGURE 24-3 Mini-Mental State Examination sample items. (Reproduced by special permission of the Publisher, Psychological Assessment Resources, Inc., 16204 North Florida Ave., Lutz, FL 33549, from the Mini-Mental State Examination, by Marshal Folstein and Susan Folstein, Copyright 1975, 1998 by Mini Mental LLC, Inc. Published 2001 by Psychological Assessment Resources, Inc. Further reproduction is prohibited without permission of PAR, Inc. The MMSE can be purchased from PAR, Inc., by calling 800-331-8378 or 813-968-3003.)

BOX 24-7   RESEARCH FOR EVIDENCE-BASED PRACTICE
Evidence-Based Transitional Care for Chronically Ill Older Adults and Their Caregivers

Unplanned readmissions within 30 days of discharge are estimated to be at 90%. A multidisciplinary research team developed a Transitional Care Model (TCM) to focus on the needs of very-high-risk chronically ill older adults who are transitioning from hospital to home following an acute illness. The TCM is led by an advanced practice nurse (APN) using a holistic person-centered and family care–centered approach. The APN acts as the "point person" throughout the episode of care, facilitating timely exchange of information across all settings. Criteria identified to determine high-risk persons include those who are 80 years or older, those who have moderate to severe functional deficits, and those who are unable to complete self-care or manage daily tasks.

Tools used to assess potentially affected persons include the Hospital Admission Risk Profile (HARP), the Katz Index of Independence in Activities of Daily Living (ADL) or the Lawton Instrumental Activities of Daily Living (IADL) Scale, and the Mental Status Assessment of Older Adults (Mini-Cog). Potential persons are also screened using the Geriatric Depression Scale—Short Form (GDS) to assess symptoms of depression. The following risks associated with readmission have been identified: having four or more active coexisting health problems, being treated with six or more prescribed standing medications, having two or more hospitalizations within the previous 6 months, being hospitalized within the previous 30 days, having been hospitalized with baseline dementia, being treated for delirium, lacking formal or informal family caregiver support, and having low health literacy.

With APN services under the TCM, mutual goals are developed, there is improved communication and collaboration among health care providers, there is improved medication and dietary adherence, there are decreased numbers of rehospitalizations during the 52 weeks of follow-up, and there is high person, caregiver, and physician satisfaction. Barriers to widespread adoption of the TCM identified include the organization of current systems of care, barriers of regulation, lack of quality and financial incentives, and culture of care issues.

Source: Bixby, M. B. (2011). Evidence-based transitional care for chronically ill older adults and their caregivers. *Journal of Geriatric Care Management, 21*(2), 20-24.

This instrument was developed to assess the baseline mental status of older adults and to evaluate change or decline in mental functioning. The MMSE is based on a 30-point scale that measures level of awareness and orientation, appearance and behavior, speech and communication, mood and affect, disturbances in thinking, problems with perception, and abstract thinking and judgment. The higher the older adult scores on the examination, the more intact the mental status is presumed to be. When the result of the exam is 23 or lower, the individual is determined to have a problem with cognition. It is important to note that this instrument has been criticized for its cultural insensitivity, and it is difficult to use among individuals who speak languages other than English and among those with visual impairment and low literacy.

The MMSE is relatively easy to perform after a little practice and has been used for initial and subsequent evaluation of older adults in a variety of settings. The most effective way to perform the assessment is to make the person comfortable and establish a rapport. Eliminating extraneous noise and promoting attention and concentration will allow individuals to answer questions to the best of their ability. After the examination, the score can be computed and used as a basis for care planning and further evaluation.

At present, there is no cure for Alzheimer's disease. Treatment for AD includes the use of medications for memory loss including cholinesterase inhibitors and memantine, treatments for behavioral changes associated with AD, and treatment for sleep changes. Medications to treat Alzheimer's disease are known as cholinesterase inhibitors. These medications are most effective during the early stages of the disease and act by increasing the levels of acetylcholine in the brain to prevent further loss and improve cognitive status.

Nonpharmacological techniques for managing the problems associated with dementia include developing and keeping routines; working in a calm, gentle, and unhurried manner; encouraging self-care activity; and reducing sensory overload.

Interventions to keep the older adult safe include curtailing wandering behavior and preventing falls and other injury.

Stereotypes suggest that older people are less capable of learning and lose their intellectual capacity, but research has not supported this notion. Wood and Roberts (2006) found that expectations for intellect increased from adolescence to young adulthood; however, these expectations did not then decline from middle age to old age, instead appearing to increase nearly linearly across all age groups. Also, as expected, the expected mean-level differences across age groups appeared smaller in this study than previous studies following the separation of target age and role information. Nonetheless, the majority of the findings again showed strong agreement between the pattern of personality expectations for age and the actual pattern of personality changes exhibited over the life span.

Nurses encourage older individuals to take classes, read, engage in stimulating conversation and entertainment, keep their minds active, and continue learning throughout their lives. They are encouraged to continue with self-care activities rather than to relinquish them to caregivers. Because some memory impairment may be present in cognitively healthy older adults, memory aids and familiar environments are to be encouraged (Box 24-7: Research for Evidence-Based Practice).

Sensory Factors

Older adults experience several age-related changes in vision, hearing, taste, smell, and touch sensation. Because of the normal changes and potential pathological changes associated with the senses, older adults of all cultural backgrounds and in all settings can benefit from routine assessment and appropriate nursing interventions. A variety of structural changes cause visual acuity to decrease, color discrimination to become less acute, pupil size and constriction ability to decrease, and peripheral vision to diminish. Presbyopia is a loss of accommodation that occurs as people age and results in the inability to maintain focus on objects close to the eye. The lens of the eyes thickens and becomes yellow and predisposes the older adult to cataracts. The older adult is at increased risk for glaucoma, a group of eye disorders characterized by increased intraocular pressure. Because of the normal changes in the aging eye and the high risk for disease, a baseline eye assessment should be done early in this stage of life. Based on the normal changes and any disease processes identified, it is recommended that follow-up eye appointments be scheduled at least annually.

Hearing deficits are common in old age, resulting from inner ear atrophy or sclerosis of the tympanic membrane. The inner ear can also undergo a number of changes, including those that are cell degenerative and nerve related. Presbycusis is a progressive sensorineural hearing loss associated with aging and results in difficulty filtering background noise and understanding higher pitched voices. Sound threshold changes, with an associated difficulty in understanding what others are saying. Similar to the changes of the eye, changes in hearing and the increased risk for pathological conditions indicate that older adults begin regular ear and hearing screening tests early in this stage of life. On the recommendation of the audiologist, audiological testing is conducted at least annually. Hearing aids can assist those with hearing loss to communicate more effectively. Loss of hearing results in decreased quality of life and is associated with decreased function, miscommunication, loss of self-esteem, depression, falls, safety risks, and cognitive decline (Wallhagen & Pettengill, 2008). The nurse routinely assesses for the accumulation of cerumen (earwax) to ensure optimal hearing (see the Case Study and Care Plan at the end of this chapter). Safety, particularly while driving, is a concern for older adults and society. Normal vision and hearing changes affect the older person's ability to drive safely. Nurses can encourage older adults to take senior driving classes to learn how to become safer drivers as these changes occur.

Taste changes with aging because of a loss of taste buds. The flavors of sweet, sour, salty, and bitter become blurred with this loss. The sensations brought about by touch may also diminish with the decrease in sensory nerve endings, especially in the presence of debilitating diseases such as diabetes, stroke, or Parkinson's disease. The ability to smell and the acuity of the olfactory nerve also decrease with age. Because of the loss of smell and taste sensations, older adults have the tendency to increase the amounts of salt and sugar in their food, possibly negatively affecting chronic health conditions. Teaching about safe cooking and the use of alternate seasonings in food may be appropriate. Additionally, the sense of smell is impaired, which may result in the older adult not sensing common danger signals such as smoke or rotten food. Teaching older adults to check the dates on their food packages frequently and to be attentive when cooking and preparing meals ensures safety. The United States Department of Agriculture (USDA, 2010) recommends that infants and young children, pregnant women, older adults, and those who are immunocompromised should not eat or drink raw (unpasteurized) milk or any products made from unpasteurized milk, raw or partially cooked eggs or foods containing raw eggs, raw or undercooked meat and poultry, raw or undercooked fish or shellfish, unpasteurized juices, and raw sprouts.

The decline in taste and smell sensations, combined with problems of obtaining adequate nutrition, makes dental care of vital importance to this population. Lack of fluoridated water and preventive dentistry during the developmental years has caused tooth and periodontal problems to prevail in the older population. Periodontitis, or gum disease leading to tooth loss among adults, is a common contributor to decreased taste sensation and poor nutrition. In fact, *Healthy People 2020* established Oral Health objectives OH-4-2, to reduce the proportion of older adults ages 65 to 74 years who have lost all of their natural teeth; and OH-5, to reduce the proportion of adults ages 45 to 74 years with moderate or severe periodontitis (USDHHS, 2012c). The inability to chew and swallow food in a comfortable manner works synergistically with decreased smell and taste sensations and other problems that inhibit proper nutrition. The American Dental Association recommends that adults be seen for oral hygiene and counseling at least twice a year. During the initial evaluation, follow-up visits are scheduled to ensure that teeth and gums remain in good condition and that appropriate dental care devices are being used.

The skin of the older adult changes, becoming thinner, less elastic, wrinkled, and more fragile. Although sweating decreases and injuries take longer to heal, the skin remains capable of sensing and carrying out its protective role. Chronic disease, however, can place an individual at risk for decreased sensation throughout the body. Cerebrovascular accidents (CVAs) (strokes) or neuropathies resulting from diabetes are two examples of diseases that disrupt the ability to feel pain and pressure through the skin. This lack of sensation can threaten safety. When older adults are homebound, the nurse provides information about safety when cooking on a hot stove and the appropriate temperature for bathing and showering in order to prevent burns. The nurse performs frequent skin assessments to detect alterations in skin integrity at an early stage and implement appropriate interventions.

The potential for skin impairment is common for those who suffer sensory impairment from physical disease or dementia. A pressure sore (decubitus ulcer) is a localized area of tissue necrosis that develops when soft tissue is compressed between two bony prominences or between a bony prominence and an external surface for a prolonged period. In addition to prolonged pressure on the skin, friction, moisture, shearing, and inadequate nutrition place the older adult at risk of developing a decubitus ulcer, which is difficult to treat. Preventing the ulcer is the best method for maintaining intact skin. People at risk for decubitus ulcers should change their position at least every 2 hours to redistribute pressure appropriately throughout all areas of the skin. Elevating the lower extremities and maintaining proper body alignment are imperative to prevent decubitus ulcers. Specialty beds are readily available in most care settings to decrease pressure and assist in positioning individuals who are at risk. Positioning pillows and other orthopedic devices provide ways to help maintain the proper support of body parts and body alignment. Proper nutrition, including adequate amounts of zinc and vitamins C and E, will help prevent this skin problem.

Self-Perception–Self-Concept Pattern

The variability of self-concept in the older adult is similar to the variability that is seen in the general population. As in all aspects of health, culture, environment, family, lifestyle factors, and heredity combine to form self-concept. Self-concept includes an individual's attitudes, perception of abilities (cognitive, affective, or physical), body image, identity, general sense of worth, and general emotional pattern. Personality traits tend to remain constant throughout life.

Erikson's Theory

Many believe that adults no longer grow either emotionally or physically in their later years. In truth, although the rate of physical decline exceeds the rate of physical growth, no evidence was found that emotional growth declines in any way. One needs only view the classic film *Driving Miss Daisy* to understand that older adults go through many developmental changes in the 30 to 40 years that often make up older adulthood. Erikson's theory of development (1982) asserts that older adults must pass through developmental stages as do infants, children, and younger adults. As in all stages of psychosocial development, unsuccessful passage through a stage can result in psychological illness, and successful passage through the stage promotes health (Erikson, 1982).

   Ego integrity versus despair is the developmental stage of older adults (Erikson, 1982). The quality associated with successful passage of this stage is to achieve a balance between integrity and despair. "The process of bringing into balance feelings of integrity and despair involves a review of and a coming to terms with the life one has lived thus far" (Erikson et al., 1986, p. 70). Based on the increasing life span, this stage of development was expanded into three additional stages: **ego differentiation versus work role preoccupation,** which involves achieving identity apart from work; **body transcendence versus body preoccupation,** which focuses on adjusting to normal aging changes; and **ego transcendence versus ego preoccupation,** which involves accepting death (Erikson, 1997).

   Nurses working in all settings are charged with helping older adults accomplish the task of balancing ego integrity and despair. Two successful methods of assistance for older adults at all cognitive levels are *reminiscence* and *life review.* Touhy (2012a) states that reminiscing "is an umbrella term that includes any recall of the past." Haight (2005), a leader in nursing research on reminiscence, defines **reminiscence** as "a multifaceted, multipurpose, naturally occurring mental phenomenon manifested across the life span in a variety of forms and contexts" (Haight, 2005). **Life review** is a more formal therapy technique taking the person through their life in a structured and chronological order.

Roles-Relationships Pattern

Although the general framework of self-perception remains constant throughout the life span, the source of an individual's self-perception often changes with older adulthood. The formation of the self that has focused on a person's role in the family changes when the children become independent or a spouse dies. Roles such as daughter, son, sister, brother, wife,

FIGURE 24-4 The loss of roles can create new roles such as grandparenting.

or husband may be lost because of death or illness. The loss of these roles can result in grieving and sadness, and potentially depression in the older adult. In contrast, with the loss of these roles, new roles, such as grandparenting, evolve (Figure 24-4).

   In the United States in 2009, slightly more than 1.8 million, or 2.5%, children were being raised by their grandparents (U.S. Census Bureau, 2011b). The role of grandparent frequently brings great joy and happiness at a time when the older adult feels loss; however, grandparents who rear grandchildren encounter several issues. A study by Ross and Aday (2006) examined the degree of stress in 50 African American grandparents (median age = 63.12 years) who were raising their grandchildren and identified the importance of caregiver characteristics, the caregiving situation, and specific coping strategies that influence stress. Data were collected via interview at senior centers and churches in Harris County, Texas. The instruments used to measure stress and coping were the Parenting Stress Index and the Ways of Coping Questionnaire. Of the grandparent participants, 94% reported a clinically significant level of stress. Factors associated with less stress in the grandparents were using professional counseling, taking advantage of special school programs, and caring for the grandchild longer than 5 years. Coping strategies significantly correlated with less stress included accepting responsibility, confrontive coping, self-control, positive reappraisal, planned problem solving, and distancing. This study adds to the information about custodial grandparents and suggests use of counseling, support groups, and education to help them more effectively manage stress associated with their caregiving situation. Encouraging and supporting older adults in this role is important to help them fill the void left by the loss of their job or spousal roles, and to prevent the stress and strain of this caregiver role.

   With the average life span increasing, older adults can spend many more years in retirement than previous generations. There were approximately 54 million Social Security beneficiaries at the end of 2010 (Social Security Administration, 2012), of whom approximately 37 million were retired workers or the spouses of retired workers. In a large government study regarding retirement influences (USDHHS, 2007), respondents who said they were completely retired in 2002 were asked about four possible influences on their decisions to stop working: having poor health, wanting to do other things, not liking their work, and wanting to spend more time with family. More than one third of those who retired between 2000 and 2002 said that spending more time with their families was a very important reason for retirement, and approximately one fourth also cited "wanting to do other things." Poor health was a very important factor for 35% of retirees in the 55- to 59-year age category, but the importance of poor health as a motivating factor for retirement dropped consistently with increasing age. In keeping with findings noted earlier in this chapter about enjoyment of work, fewer than 10% of respondents were motivated to retire by a strong dislike of their work.

Hooyman and Kiyak (2011) found that several factors were predictors of satisfaction with retirement. Those factors included good health and functional ability, adequate income, a suitable living environment, a strong social support system, and a positive outlook. An important factor was the autonomy of the retiree in choosing retirement and the preparation for the retirement while still working. For married retirees, having a good marital relationship and sharing similar interests with one's spouse supported satisfaction with retirement. Having retirement activities that provide an opportunity to feel useful, to learn and grow, and to enjoy oneself are important. Many retirees enjoy sports and hobbies developed during their working years, whereas others become actively involved in volunteerism and other community and civic activities.

Volunteering can be an effective method for older adults to continue to feel engaged in the community as a productive, contributing member of society. Older adults who volunteer have an external incentive for getting dressed in the morning; they take a great amount of pride in their work. Filling a volunteer position can provide a feeling of self-worth and remedy any negative feelings about retirement and other role changes.

Federal and state funding has created a number of subsidized work programs for older adults. With the assistance of this funding through private agencies and local Area Agencies on Aging, older adults are given the opportunity to work for pay. Although the pay may not be comparable to that earned before retirement, the earnings can be a necessary supplement to Social Security benefits. These programs allow older adults to work with children in day care centers, with disabled and ill older adults at home, and in administrative positions. Nurses can provide interested individuals with information about these programs.

Downsizing from the family home to a smaller residence, widowhood, retirement, and relocation can elicit profound feelings of loss. Older adults who remain engaged in a variety of activities and relationships are happier and healthier. Personality, and its expression over time, is considered a major determinant of how engaged or active a person will be late in life. Other variables such as culture, health, bereavement, and habit affect activity as well.

Health-promotion activities center on an understanding of the individual's usual behavior and any unexpected or unexplained deviation from that behavior. Nurses can help older

adults identify the meaning of their lost roles and the results of those losses, and work through reactions to the losses. In more traumatic cases, support groups, such as bereavement groups, can be helpful. The nurse supports those going through role changes by eliciting reactions and facilitating communication about these reactions. Significant others, such as children, neighbors, and friends, can provide important support. The nurse is integral in helping older adults develop and explore their new roles in their older years.

Sexuality-Reproductive Pattern

The Centers for Disease Control and Prevention (CDC, 2012b) defines sexual health as "a state of physical, emotional, mental and social well-being in relation to sexuality; it is not merely the absence of disease, dysfunction or infirmity. Sexual health requires a positive and respectful approach to sexuality and sexual relationships, as well as the possibility of having pleasurable and safe sexual experiences" (p. 1). Much debate has taken place regarding the presence or absence of sexual desire among older adults. Many believe that older adults do not participate in sexual relationships. According to the AARP (2012) myths regarding sexual activity among older adults include the following: older men have erectile dysfunction (impotence) and are unable to have sexual intercourse; after menopause, older women no longer have sexual desire; there are physical and psychological reasons that older adults are unable to have sexual intercourse; an aging body is not sexy; and older people should not have sex.

The most accurate predictor of sexual interest in older adulthood is the enjoyment and frequency of sex at a younger age. No data were found to show that men or women lose interest in sexual activity as they age. Older adults also need to fulfill the human need for intimacy and love, and to touch and be touched. Touch is an overt expression of closeness and an integral part of sexuality. Although the need to express sexuality continues, older adults are susceptible to many chronic medical conditions, such as cardiac problems, arthritis, and normal aging changes that can make sexual intercourse difficult. In both genders, reduced availability of sex hormones results in less rapid and less extreme vascular responses to sexual arousal. The lack of circulating hormones in both men and women results in changes in four areas of the sexual system: arousal, orgasm, postorgasm, and extragenital changes. In women, the vagina becomes narrower, shorter, and thinner, and there is less natural lubrication. Men experience less intense and slower erections, increased difficulty regaining an erection, decreased force of ejaculation, and an extended refractory time. Medications and other management of a medical condition can hinder sexual response.

Nurses are in an ideal position to help older adults fulfill their sexual desires by helping them to compensate for normal aging changes and chronic medical conditions and medications. Knowledge is essential to the successful fulfillment of sexuality needs. After making a sexual assessment, nurses can intervene to prevent or correct problems, but they frequently choose not to consider sexuality when planning care. One of the reasons for this hesitation is that nurses may believe the societal myths about older adults' sexuality. Without proper education and experience, they are not sufficiently confident to venture into this delicate area.

One way in which nurses can gain knowledge about the sexual needs of older adults is through a staff development program using role play to discuss and process feelings associated with an older person's limitations in fulfilling intimate and sexual relationships. The expression of intimacy and sexuality among older adults results in a higher quality of life achieved through fulfilling a natural desire. In long-term care facilities, the need to address sexual needs of residents is great because of difficulties related to their chronic illnesses and because of a lack of resident privacy to engage in intimate and sexual relationships. Long-term care facilities can develop policies to assist residents in effectively fulfilling the need for intimacy and sexuality.

Many nurses believe that acquired immunodeficiency syndrome (AIDS) and other sexually transmitted diseases are not problems for older adults. However, the number of cases of HIV (human immunodeficiency virus) and AIDS in older adults continues to increase because greater numbers of older adults are becoming newly infected with the HIV virus and an increasing proportion of those who have been living with the virus are reaching their older years (www.HIVoverfifty.org). Older adults should use proper precautions, such as a condom or other barrier method, to prevent the spread of sexually transmitted disease. It is important that older adults follow the safer sex guidelines recommended by the CDC (2012b). Nurses use universal precautions to protect themselves from HIV and other blood-borne pathogens.

Coping-Stress Tolerance Pattern

An individual's ability to cope with the common stresses of older adulthood is a key factor in maintaining self-concept. As people age, they tend to encounter many losses, such as the loss of a home, spouses, friends, and siblings. They also experience declines in income, and in health and physical functioning. The nurse who cares for the older adult can be helpful in the coping process. In a sample of 99 older adults, it was found that continually thinking about a loss or bad event was not as effective as trying to find the positive and developmental benefits of losses. In a study exploring the relationships between cognitive-emotion regulation strategies and depressive symptoms, significant relationships between depressive symptoms and the cognitive-emotion regulation strategies of rumination, catastrophizing, and positive reappraisal were found. Whereas rumination and catastrophizing were positively related (the more the strategy was used, the more depression symptomatology expressed), positive reappraisal was negatively related. In addition, self-blame showed significant positive effects in all samples but the older adults. None of the samples showed significant relationships between depressive symptoms and other-blame (Garnefski & Kraaij, 2006). After assessing the most appropriate way in which the individual desires to cope with a situation, the nurse may help create a suitable environment for coping. The spirituality of older adults is also an important consideration for their care. Spirituality is very individual and may be exercised privately or through a religious framework. However, the impact of spirituality on quality of life

has been well documented among older adults and often has a strong relationship with older adults' ability to cope with the changes and losses of aging.

Depression

Among older adults, depression mainly affects those with chronic illnesses and cognitive impairment, and results in suffering, family disruption, and disability. Depression can worsen the outcomes of many illnesses and increase mortality (Alexopoulos, 2005). Aging-related and disease-related processes, including arteriosclerosis and endocrine and immune system changes, compromise the integrity of frontostriatal pathways, the amygdala, and the hippocampus, and increase vulnerability to depression. Heredity factors may also play a part. Psychosocial adversity—economic impoverishment, disability, isolation, relocation, caregiving, and bereavement—contributes to physiological changes, further increasing susceptibility to depression or triggering depression in already vulnerable older individuals (Alexopoulos, 2005).

From 2005 to 2006, according to the Centers for Disease Control and Prevention (CDC, 2011d), 4% of the population 60 years of age and older experienced depression. The National Institute of Mental Health (NIMH, 2007) states that the risk of depression increases in older adults as they experience chronic illnesses and when their ability to function becomes impaired. The numerous losses experienced by older people may be partly to blame. Depression is also caused by physiological changes in the aging body. Although depression appears to affect older adults in much the same way that it affects younger individuals, certain patterns of symptoms and older adults' overall susceptibility are different from those of younger counterparts.

Nurses are integral in helping to diagnose and manage depression in older adults. Depression can be found in all care environments. Some common behaviors include sullen affect, lack of appetite and weight loss, sleep disorders, fatigue, decreased ability to think or concentrate, psychomotor agitation, decreased participation in daily living and social activities, social withdrawal, and suicidal ideation. Many instruments are available to assist nurses in assessing for this commonly occurring disorder. The Geriatric Depression Scale (Yesavage et al., 1983) is available in several formats, with 30, 15, 5, or 1 question, and is easily administered (**see Website Resource 24A**). Positive results on the screening examinations require referral to social services for a diagnostic workup. After depression is diagnosed, successful management may include implementation of antidepressant medications and psychosocial therapy.

Suicide

According to the CDC (n.d.) "the rate of suicide for adults 75 years of age and older was 16 per 100,000, and there were approximately four suicide attempts for every completed suicide." The suicide rate for men is highest in those who are age 75 or older, at a rate of 36.1 per 100,000. non-Hispanic White men 85 years of age and older were the most likely to die by suicide with a rate of 49.8 per 100,000 (NIMH, 2007). Firearms (71%), overdose (liquids, pills, or gas) (11%), and suffocation (11%) were the three most common methods of suicide used by persons 65 years and older (National Strategy for Suicide Prevention, 2007).

The reason for the high number of suicides in the older adult population continues to be explored. The elevated rate of depression helps the medical community understand the motive of many older adults. Many older adults have serious medical illnesses that provide an explanation for wanting to die. Risk factors for suicide include social isolation, alcohol and substance abuse, psychosis, bereavement, and serious medical illness. Many who committed suicide were found to have alcohol and/or pain-killing drugs in their bodies on autopsy.

The importance of different aspects of life also varies by culture. Some older adults may visit a health care provider with a somatic complaint before the suicide attempt as, perhaps, a final call for help. Nurses working with older adults must be aware of the high rate of suicide in this age group and be alert for the risk factors. Older adults exhibiting signs of depression must be asked about possible suicidal thoughts. Suicide threats must be taken seriously and appropriate interventions implemented to keep the older adult safe.

The incidence of chronic illness that frequently accompanies old age raises a concern for ethical care. Many members of society believe that with the increased life span, individuals may be subjected to more suffering. A solution to ending the suffering of those with chronic illness has been euthanasia, or physician-assisted suicide. In many states, people are lobbying to legalize physician-assisted suicide. Nurses help society to understand the many benefits of older adulthood and celebrate the extended life span rather than deeming it wasteful. Nurses caring for chronically ill older adults have the added responsibility of determining who is at risk for wanting physician-assisted suicide and helping them to be as comfortable as possible and free of pain through the use of pharmacological and nonpharmacological interventions. Nurses are instrumental in ensuring that the older person experiences a pain-free death by advocating for an appropriate pain-management program and working with other health care professionals toward this goal.

Values-Beliefs Pattern

Every person that nurses care for will have a different sense of spirituality, which will have an influence on the way the person chooses to live and the decisions made by the person about health care. Hodge and colleagues (2010) found that the majority of older adults describe themselves as both spiritual and religious. The life of the spirit may help older adults to overcome the pain and suffering of chronic health and psychosocial problems encountered in their later years.

Nurses may find themselves in the providential but difficult position in attempting to promote the spiritual health of individuals. One reason for this perceived difficulty may be the nurse's discomfort with the person's belief system. Spirituality can play a significant role in meaning-making in relation to attitudes and beliefs about the world, self, and others. A spiritual process of meaning-making (or seeking significance in an event) can touch on all aspects of life, including work, interpersonal relationships, general philosophy of living, attitudes, and/or whatever that person's "God" may be (Gall et al., 2005).

There may be as many different spiritual values and beliefs as there are individuals. Varying spiritual values make helping older adults actualize their spirituality, and thus acquire a high quality of life, difficult for nurses. Because of the highly personal quality of spirituality, an unobtrusive and sensitive presence by the nurse is needed to allow the person in any setting to achieve spiritual health. Spiritual assessment tools are available to guide nurses with questions to better understand the person's spirituality. Open-ended questions, such as, "What is your perception of a higher being and spirituality?" can encourage discussions about the person's innermost spirituality. The nurse can provide an environment that is supportive to the practice of the person's spirituality. Assisting older persons to actualize their spirituality can provide great comfort to the person and lead nurses to a deeper understanding of their own spirituality.

ENVIRONMENTAL PROCESSES

Physical Agents

Accidents

Falls are a leading cause of morbidity and mortality among older adults (Box 24-8: Quality and Safety Scenario). According to the CDC (2011e), "falls are the leading cause of injury death and are the most common cause of nonfatal injuries and hospital admissions for trauma for older adults. In 2008, more than 19,700 older adults died from unintentional fall injuries." In 2009, there were 2.2 million emergency department visits related to nonfatal fall injuries among older adults. Injuries that occur with falls—including lacerations; fractures, especially of the hip, spine, arm, leg, pelvis, and hand; and traumatic brain injury—can result in decreased mobility, decreased ability to live independently, and increased risk of an early death. Falls account for 40% of admissions to nursing homes each year. Even if the person is not injured in a fall, they may develop a fear of falling, and therefore limit their activities and increase their risk for future falls. Governmental concern about falls among older adults has resulted in a *Healthy People 2020* objective to "prevent an increase in the rate of fall related deaths" (USDHHS, 2012d).

Some of the causes of falls in older adults are neuromuscular dysfunction, osteoporosis, stroke, and sensory impairment. Although a fall in a younger individual may not be problematic, a fall in an older adult can have devastating consequences. Because of the higher risk of osteoporosis in the older population, a fall can result in a fracture. Osteoporosis is a disease of bone loss common to women age 70 and older and men age 80 and older. The disease develops six times more frequently in women than it does in men. The rapid decline in estrogen secretion at the onset of menopause signals the calcium in the bones to move into the bloodstream, which allows the bones to become weak and brittle. Because of this weakness, falls in older adults with osteoporosis frequently result in fractures, which place these individuals in a spiral of iatrogenic risk, beginning with weeks of decreased mobility and possibly resulting in decubitus ulcers, psychological trauma, pneumonia, and even death.

Risk factors for osteoporosis include a small, thin frame; White or Asian ancestry; family history; excessive thyroid

BOX 24-8 **QUALITY AND SAFETY SCENARIO**

Current Approaches to Fall Risk Assessment in Nursing Homes

Falls are the most frequently reported adverse events in nursing homes; however, fall risk assessment is not standardized or regulated. There is a need for validated fall risk assessment tools to assist nursing home staff in assessing residents who are at risk for falls. The purpose of this study was to examine the types of fall risk assessment tools used in nursing homes to identify which are used and the domains included. Content analysis was done on 137 completed surveys and 54 fall risk assessment tools (FRATs), revealing little consistency among the nursing homes in type of FRAT used. Domains contained in the various FRATs examined intrinsic factors, treatment-related or extrinsic factors, mobility status, cognitive status, sensory abilities, history, behavior/attitude, age of resident, gender of resident, date of admission, and first week on unit.

Intrinsic factors included were continence, blood pressure measurement, secondary diagnosis, elimination alteration, neurological disease, orthopedic disease or problems, other disease problems, history of vertigo/dizziness/

hypotension, medical history/health, orthostasis, alteration in pathophysiology, seizures, generalized weakness, nutritional/hydration status, strength measurements, and joint difficulties/deformities/pain. Treatment-related or extrinsic factors included medications, intravenous therapy/heparin lock or saline lock, interventions, and attached equipment. Behavior/attitude factors included agitation, anxiety or emotional lability, ability to communicate, wandering, compliance, unwillingness or inability to call for help, attempts to get out of the bed or wheelchair, fatigue, sleep disturbance, and level of cooperation. History included fall history, history of fractures in the previous year, history of syncope, history of falls resulting in injury.

Not only can fall risk assessment be used to identify which residents are at high risk for falls but also fall risk assessment upon admission and throughout a resident's stay can enable staff to plan resident-specific interventions to prevent falls.

Source: Wagner, L. M., Scott, V., & Silver, M. (2011). Current approaches to fall risk assessment in nursing homes. *Geriatric Nursing, 32*(4), 238-244.

medication or high doses of cortisone-like drugs for asthma, arthritis, or cancer; a diet low in dairy products and other sources of calcium; physical inactivity; smoking cigarettes; and drinking alcohol. Osteoporosis typically is diagnosed after an older adult sustains a fracture. However, bone density testing is readily available to diagnose individuals at risk before a fracture occurs. Sufficient calcium intake remains vitally important and will continue to reduce the normal bone loss of aging. Most women need 1000 mg a day before menopause and 1500 mg daily after menopause. Consuming this amount of calcium from today's average diet is difficult; therefore, a calcium supplement is essential. Vitamin D is also essential for bone health. Although one can obtain adequate vitamin D by daily exposure to the sun, because of concerns about the amount of sun exposure necessary, 400 to 800 international units of vitamin D supplements are usually recommended in conjunction with calcium. For the prevention of osteoporosis and the optimal maintenance of both psychological and physical well-being in the older adult, regular physical activity is necessary.

A program to prevent falls is essential in the care of older adults. Because many factors contribute to falls, risk assessment is essential. Touhy (2012b) recommends that all older adults be screened for falls using valid and reliable fall assessment instruments. Moreover, if a prior fall was sustained, the older adult is at increased risk for falling again and fall prevention strategies must be implemented. Several fall risk assessment tools have been developed. These instruments are easy to use and can be employed in acute- or long-term care or in home settings. After completing the assessment, scores can assist in preventive care planning. Nurses in all settings will then be prepared to implement environmental, physiological, and psychological interventions. By identifying the risks for falls and assessing an older adult's vision, hearing, medication usage, blood pressure, mobility, and other factors, falls can be predicted and prevented (CDC, 2011e).

Table 24-2 lists frequent causes of accidents that occur in the home and nursing interventions to prevent them. Home

TABLE 24-2	SAFETY RISK AREAS AND RELATED INTERVENTIONS
AREA OF ATTENTION	**INTERVENTION**
Stairways	Secure handrails
	Illuminate stairways with light switches at both top and bottom
	Eliminate clutter on all steps and stair landings
	Use nonskid treads on steps
Bedroom	Use nightlights
	Tack-down carpet
	Discourage use of throw rugs
	Arrange furniture so that it will not obstruct clear pathways
	Secure extension cords and telephone wires and remove them from walking areas
	For smokers: never smoke in bed
Bathroom	Use handrails near tub and toilet
	Use nonskid mats in tub area and on floor
	Use a bath thermometer to measure hot water in tub
	Use nightlights
Kitchen	Wear nonflammable, lightweight clothing when cooking
	Place dishes and cooking utensils at reasonable heights
	Use stepstools with handrail according to specifications and only when not alone
	Keep off wet floor and refrain from using slippery wax
	Never climb on chairs
	Keep emergency numbers near the telephone
	Ensure locks can be easily opened in times of emergency
	Cook at front of the stove rather than at the back
	Do not use electrical appliances with frayed cords
Living room	Use furniture that is easy to get in and out of
	Eliminate clutter on all floor areas
	Install fire detectors at appropriate places
Outdoors	Make sure stairs are free of breaks and cracks, and clear of snow and ice
	Use safe handrails
	Provide good lighting for stairs and walkways

From AARP Driver Safety.

BOX 24-9   NURSING INTERVENTIONS FOR HYPOTHERMIA

Symptoms	Interventions
• Cold to touch	• Warm hands and feet
• Slow respirations	• Cover with blanket
• Bradycardia	• Set room temperature to 70° F
• Low blood pressure	• Wear cap to bed at night
• Slurred speech	• Wear socks to bed at night
• Drowsiness	• Wear several layers of clothing
• Temperature 95° F rectally	• Increase activity
	• Decrease alcohol intake
	• Use extreme caution with space heaters, heating pads, or electric blankets

BOX 24-10   WHEN TO STOP DRIVING

Poor driving skills that are warning signs of unsafe driving include:
- Not using turn signals correctly or not using them at all.
- Having trouble making turns.
- Having difficulty moving into or maintaining the correct lane of traffic.
- Having trouble judging the space between vehicles in traffic on highway entrance or exit ramps.
- Parking inappropriately.
- Hitting curbs when making right turns or backing up.
- Unpredictable stopping in traffic.
- Driving too slowly; other drivers often honk horns.
- Failing to stop at stop signs or stop lights.
- Failing to notice important activity on the side of the road.

care nurses are in an ideal position to prevent injuries. During the initial and subsequent assessments, the nurse can evaluate individuals' homes for common factors leading to fires, poisoning, and falls, such as frayed wires on electrical appliances that can produce sparks and start fires, improperly labeled cleaning products that can be accidentally ingested, loose rugs on the floor, absence of handrails on stairs or in bathrooms, and poor lighting that can cause falls. Appropriate health teaching incorporates the concept of accident prevention for all older adults living not only in the community but also in acute-care and long-term care facilities.

The older adult's ability to feel changes in heat and cold may be impaired as a result of normal and pathological changes of aging. This process can cause older adults to die from the effects of excessive heat or cold. During periods of high heat and humidity, older people should increase fluid and salt intake, stay in a cool and shaded environment, remain calm, have more rest periods, and refrain from going outdoors when the temperature is higher than 90° F. Sweating, which is reduced in older adults, can be accommodated by wearing light-colored, lightweight cotton clothing. If sweating ceases or is inadequate, the older person is at risk for heat stroke. Heat stroke can contribute to sepsis, myocardial infarction, and cerebrovascular accidents (CVAs), particularly in people with diabetes. Reduced body heat can also present problems in the older adult. Symptoms of and interventions for hypothermia are listed in Box 24-9.

Preventing Injury

According to the U.S. Consumer Product Safety Commission (CPSC, n.d.), "falls and fires are the two leading causes of unintentional injury and death in people 65 years of age and older." Other unintentional injuries and deaths in older adults are caused by motor vehicle accidents, suffocation, and poisoning. Because of normal age-related changes and the increased incidence of chronic illness, older adults can experience decreased muscle strength and delayed reaction time and subsequently become more vulnerable to environmental hazards. Decreased sensory acuity and impaired balance further diminish their ability to interpret the environment.

As the percentage of older adults living in the United States increases, the number of older drivers also increases. The CDC (2011f) reports that in 2009 there were 33 million licensed drivers 65 years of age and older, a 23% increase from 1999. The National Highway Traffic Safety Administration (2010, p. 2) states that it "is important to distinguish between healthy older drivers and older drivers who are medically at risk." Age-related changes in vision, joint mobility, and cognitive changes may affect the older person's ability to drive. Because of these changes older adults often avoid driving at night, in bad weather, in heavy traffic, on long trips, or on highways or high-speed roads. Older individuals are at increased risk for severe injury resulting in hospitalization, disability, or death from motor vehicle injuries because of the many changes in their neuromuscular and sensory abilities, which slow response time in emergency situations. In 2008 more than 5500 older adults were killed and more than 183,000 were injured in motor vehicle crashes; older males had a substantially higher death rate than older females. The National Center for Statistics and Analysis (2005) reports that most traffic fatalities involving older adults occur during the daytime and involve other vehicles. Interestingly, in two-vehicle fatal crashes involving both older and younger drivers, the older driver's vehicle was more than twice as likely to be struck than the younger person's, indicating a decline in defensive driving as opposed to an increase in aggressive driving among older adults. Older drivers involved in fatal automobile accidents had the lowest blood alcohol level.

Older adults are encouraged to take a Seniors Driving Safety Course to learn how aging changes can affect their driving and strategies for safer driving. Nurses working in the community may encourage older drivers to contact AARP or the American Automobile Association for driving classes designed to meet their needs. Attending these classes often provides savings on vehicle insurance. At some point, it may be better for the older adults to stop driving. Box 24-10 offers warning signs that suggest when an older adult should limit or stop driving.

Elder Mistreatment

Elder abuse (elder mistreatment) refers to intentional or neglectful acts by a caregiver or "trusted" person that results in, or may lead to, harm of a vulnerable elder. The National Center for Elder Abuse (2012) lists the following forms of elder abuse and mistreatment: physical abuse, neglect, emotional or psychological abuse, verbal abuse and threats, financial abuse and exploitation, sexual abuse, and abandonment. In many states, self-neglect is also considered mistreatment. *Women's Health USA 2010* (USDHHS, Health Resources and Services Administration, Maternal and Child Health Bureau, 2012) reported that in 2004 caregiver neglect accounted for 20.4% of elder abuse and self-neglect for 37.2%. Emotional or psychological abuse—described as threats or other verbal attacks, isolation, rejection, or denigrating acts that cause or could cause mental anguish, pain, or distress—accounted for 14.8%; financial abuse and exploitation including theft, fraud, misuse or neglect of authority, and use of undue influence to gain control over an older person's money or property accounted for 14.7%; physical abuse including the use of physical force that may result in injury, physical pain, or impairment accounted for 10.7%, and sexual abuse, which includes any type of nonconsensual sexual contact with an elderly person, including those who cannot give consent, accounted for 1.0%.

Victims of elder abuse are more likely to be single women older than age 75 who are dependent on the caregiver for food and shelter. They are more likely to be frail, to be incontinent, or to have mental disability. The abuser is usually the adult son or daughter of the victim who has poor impulse control and low self-esteem (Nies & McEwan, 2011). Nurses have a responsibility to identify abuse, provide appropriate care for injuries, and report suspected abuse to appropriate state agencies or law enforcement personnel. The nurse may consult social services to find a more suitable living arrangement for the victim. The most important consideration is to provide a safe environment for the older adult who is in immediate danger.

Biological Agents

Because of decreased immune system response, older adults are susceptible to bacterial and viral disease. In many cases, older adults have not received primary immunization against diphtheria and tetanus. A large emphasis is placed on immunizing young children against communicable disease; however, older adults can also be protected by commonly available vaccines that have been shown to lower both morbidity and mortality. Two disease processes that are associated with higher mortality and morbidity are influenza and pneumonia.

Influenza

Influenza has been a significant cause of morbidity and mortality in older adults. In 2009, there were 638 deaths caused by influenza and 42,831 deaths from pneumonia in people 65 years of age and older (CDC, 2011g). In 2010, the hospitalization rate for influenza among older adults 65 years of age or older was 62.1 per 100,000. The CDC (2012g) reports that influenza vaccination levels among older adults increased from 33% in 1989 to 67% in 2008, but less than the *Healthy People 2010* target of

90%. The vaccine, composed of inactivated whole virus or viral subunits grown in chick embryo cells, is given annually to older adults, especially those with chronic conditions such as pulmonary or cardiac problems and those in long-term care facilities. Vaccination is contraindicated in people who have experienced a reaction to it, and caution must be exercised in administering the vaccine to people who have allergies to eggs. A *Healthy People 2020* objective (IID-12-7 and 4-2) is "to increase the percentage of older adults who are vaccinated annually against influenza and to decrease the incidence of pneumococcal infections among older adults to 31 new cases per 100,000" (USDHHS, 2012).

Pneumococcal Infections

Estimates indicate that pneumococcal infections were responsible for approximately 52,306 deaths in 2007, a significant decline from previous years (U.S. Census Bureau, 2010). The decline in deaths from pneumonia indicates the value of the public health initiatives to make information widespread about the importance of immunization against pneumonia and influenza, and the implementation of immunization programs in public places such as supermarkets and drugstores in addition to physicians' offices and clinics. Nevertheless, many older adults remain unvaccinated. The CDC recommends that older adults receive the pneumococcal vaccination. Boosters are recommended for older adults who received the vaccine before the age of 65, if more than 5 years have passed; and for older adults who have received an organ transplant, have chronic kidney disease, or have a compromised immune status. It is important that nurses inform the public about the importance of immunizations and counteract the myth that receiving the vaccination will result in the disease, which often prevents older adults from receiving immunization.

Cancer

Cancer rates for older adults are disproportionately high in the United States. Although only 12% of the population is considered older adult, more than 50% of all diagnosed cancers are found in this population and the death rate for cancer is highest among adults 65 years of age and older. The reason for the large proportion of cancer in this country is unknown. Theories include longer exposure to carcinogens, increased susceptibility to cancer in the older body, decreased cellular healing ability, loss of tumor-suppressing genes, and decreased immune function. Although the exact cause cannot be determined, cancer is a significant problem for older adults in the United States.

The types of cancer common to older adults are listed by gender in Table 24-3. Prostate cancer is the leading cancer among men of all races and ages and is clearly the most common male cancer and the second leading cause of death from cancer in men in the United States. Estimates are that 8% of all men in the United States will be diagnosed with prostate cancer during their lifetime. Early detection of prostate cancer allows treatment while it is still localized in the prostate gland and highly curable. Evidence suggests that by using a combination of screening techniques, more cases of prostate cancer can be detected earlier. There are three key components of an

TABLE 24-3 2010 ESTIMATED U.S. CANCER DEATHS

MEN	N/%	WOMEN	N/%
All causes	299,490	All causes	270,290
Oral cavity and pharynx	5,430/0.018	Oral cavity and pharynx	2,450/0.009
Digestive system	79,010/0.263	Digestive system	60,570/0.224
Respiratory system	89,550/0.299	Respiratory system	72,120/0.266
Bones and joints	830/0.002	Bones and joints	630/0.002
Soft tissue including heart	2,020/0.006	Soft tissue including heart	1,900/0.007
Skin	7,910/0.026	Skin	3,880/0.014
Breast	390/0.001	Breast	39,840/0.147
Genital system	32,710/0.109	Genital system	27,710/0.103
Urinary system	19,110/0.063	Urinary system	9,440/0.035
Brain	7,120/0.023	Brain	5,720/0.021
Endocrine system	1,140/0.003	Endocrine system	1,430/0.005
Lymphoma	11,450/0.038	Lymphoma	10,080/0.037
Myeloma	5,760/0.019	Myeloma	4,890/0.002
Leukemia	12,660/0.042	Leukemia	9,180/0.034
Other	23,690/0.079	Other	20,340/0.075

Sources: American Cancer Society. (2010). *Cancer facts & figures 2010*. Atlanta: Author. Retrieved from www.cancer.org/acs/groups/content/@ epidemiologysurveilance/documents/document/acspc-026238.pdf; Centers for Disease Control and Prevention (CDC) (2012a) *National Vital Statistics Reports: Deaths: Preliminary Data for 2010*, 60(4). Retrieved February 22, 2012, from www.cdc.gov/nchs/data/nvsr60/nvsr60_04.pdf.

appropriate prostate screen: symptomatology, prostate-specific antigen level measurement, and a digital rectal examination. The four major treatment options for prostate cancer are surgery, radiation therapy, watchful waiting, and hormone therapy.

Breast cancer is the most common cancer in women of all ages and races in the United States. It is surpassed only by lung cancer as the cause of mortality in women. Reports suggest that one in nine women will develop breast cancer in her lifetime. Three quarters of all breast cancers occur in women older than 50 years of age. The risk is increased in women whose close female relatives (mothers or sisters) have had the disease. Women who have never had children or had their first child after age 30 appear to have an increased risk. The causes of breast cancer remain unclear. The best protection is early detection and prompt treatment. The American Cancer Society recommends that women have annual mammograms and breast examinations beginning at age 40 and practice monthly breast self-examination (American Cancer Society, 2011).

Nurses help older adults change the habits that place them at high risk for developing cancer. Following nutritional guidelines (as suggested earlier in this chapter), reducing stress, adopting a program of regular exercise, and stopping smoking and other use of tobacco products are a few of the approaches that nurses can advise to promote individual wellness. Periodic monitoring and screening in the form of regular visits with a primary health care provider or community screening can alert older adults to early signs and symptoms of cancers that occur during the later years.

Chemical Agents

Chemical agents can be both therapeutic and harmful depending on their use. The increased use of prescription and over-the-counter medications can result in increased adverse drug events. The use of alcohol and tobacco products can be especially harmful for older adults.

Drug Use

Normal changes of aging have a significant effect on the pharmacodynamics of drugs in older adults. The ways in which medications are absorbed, distributed, metabolized, and excreted from the body are affected by normal physiological changes and by illness. Even when medications are taken as prescribed, age-related changes and disease can increase the risk of undesirable side effects. According to the Food and Drug Administration (USDHHS, FDA, 2009), older adults are more likely to take multiple medications, resulting in increased risk for serious drug interactions. In addition to potential adverse effects caused by prescription drugs, older adults take many types of nonprescription substances including over-the-counter medications; vitamins, minerals, and supplements; herbal remedies; and foods and other traditional remedies used to resolve common ailments. Polypharmacy, or the use of multiple medications for the same or for different health problems, is a major concern for the elderly. The Food and Drug Administration (2009) estimates that the rate of polypharmacy in the elderly is between 9% and 39%, with 29% taking as many as five or more prescription drugs. Additionally, 42% of older adults take at least one over-the-counter drug, and 49% take at least one supplement. The Beers criteria (American Geriatric Society, 2012), developed from the Health Care Financing Administration Guidelines for Potentially Inappropriate Medications in the Elderly, presents medications known to place older adults at risk for adverse reactions.

Many older adults who reside at home take their medications independently. Although self-medication with prescription and nonprescription substances is an effective method of disease management, little is known about the process of taking medications after the person leaves the health care practice or facility. Although it is generally assumed that medications are taken as prescribed, sensory disturbances; lack of knowledge; and alternative drug, alcohol, and nutrition practices may present challenges to medication self-administration that interfere with medical management of health problems. Nurses must take a thorough medication history to assess for past drug reactions, and identify all currently prescribed and nonprescription substances taken. New medications should be started at their lowest effective dose and increased slowly as necessary.

One of the major barriers to drug adherence in the older adult is affordability. Medicare provides prescription drug coverage to everyone eligible for Medicare under Medicare Part D. One can get Medicare drug coverage in one of two ways: a Medicare Prescription Drug Plan (PDP) or a Medicare Advantage Drug Plan (PPO or HMO). For poor older adults, assistance for the purchase of prescription drugs is available in several ways: switching coverage to a less costly drug plan; or applying for assistance to pharmaceutical company assistance programs, state pharmaceutical assistance programs, national and community based charitable programs, and the Extra Help program through Medicare and Social Security (Medicare.gov, 2012).

Alcohol and Drug Abuse

Alcohol and drug abuse problems among older adults have been underestimated and hidden. According to the Centers for Disease Control and Prevention (CDC, 2011a), 3.8% of adults 65 years of age and older reported binge drinking in 2009 on at least one occasion within the previous 30 days. Alcohol and drug abuse in older adults is often unreported and unnoticed, because the symptoms can be similar to those of other common problems of aging, and health care providers often do not ask persons about alcohol use. The longer the problem remains undetected, the greater it becomes and the more potential harm related to other chronic health problems.

Older adults are more vulnerable to the effects of alcohol and illicit drugs, because their systems do not detoxify and excrete as efficiently as do those of younger people. Alcoholism and drug abuse predispose older adults to accidents and injury, cognitive decline, physical debility, nutritional deficiencies, disease, and decreased function. Additionally, alcohol use while taking medications can interfere with the desired effect of the medication. The National Prevention Council (NPC, 2011) recommends screening to identify alcohol and drug abuse early, to provide brief intervention, and to refer for treatment in appropriate facilities.

Tobacco Use

Tobacco use includes cigarette, cigar, and pipe smoking; and the use of chewing tobacco. Use of tobacco products is associated with cardiovascular disease, several types of cancer, and chronic lung disease (CDC, 2011h). Older men and women today may be the first generation to have smoked throughout their lives, starting in their teens or twenties when smoking seemed fashionable. The results of smoking occur slowly over time, and problems usually are not experienced until signs and symptoms of smoking-related health problems occur. Because smoking can initiate and promote disease processes, it is one of the most important negative predictors of longevity. Smoking is a particular problem for older adults because of the large number of medications they take and the potential for drug interactions. Nicotine-drug interactions can potentiate or interfere with a desired drug effect.

Older adults can experience the benefits of smoking cessation even after the age of 65. These people may be more motivated to quit smoking than when they were younger, because they are likely to see some of the damage that smoking has caused and anticipate that smoking cessation will restore or improve their health. Nurses can assist older adults in making the commitment to quit smoking through education and referral to smoking cessation programs.

DETERMINANTS OF HEALTH

Social Factors and Environment

The incidence of chronic and acute illnesses, the subsequent decline in functional status, changes in economic status, and changes in family structure frequently place older adults in situations for which they are admitted to acute-care facilities or must make a temporary or permanent move into a residential situation or a long-term care facility. When providing health-promotion services to older adults, nurses must take into account the type of setting in which the person lives.

When older adults leave their homes, they enter a continuum of care extending from the acute-care facility to the long-term care or community setting. Nurses who work in each of the settings on the continuum can promote health to this population in many ways. From the acute-care setting through each stage of the continuum until the person returns home, opportunities are available for nurses to introduce older adults and their families to community resources (Table 24-4). The acute care nurse

TABLE 24-4 LONG-TERM CARE HOUSING AND ASSESSMENT CONTINUUM

	INDEPENDENT LIVING	RETIREMENT COMMUNITY	ASSISTED LIVING	NURSING FACILITY
Description	Covers a broad range of housing options (residential houses, apartments, condominiums, townhouses, subsidized senior housing) for older persons who are functionally and socially independent	Provides a living arrangement that integrates shelter and services for older people who do not need 24-hour protective oversight	Provides a living arrangement that integrates shelter and services for frail older people who are functionally and/or socially impaired and require 24-hour protective oversight	Provides a living arrangement that integrates shelter with medical, nursing, psychosocial, and rehabilitation services for older people who require 24-hour nursing supervision
Primary services	-A- Environmental security Possibly coordination of resident services (transportation, activities, housekeeping) Or no services are available	-B- "A" plus: Meals (1 to 3 per day) Transportation Activities Housekeeping assistance Assistance with coordination of community-based services	-C- "A & B" plus: Assistance with activities of daily living Medication monitoring, 24-hour protective oversight	-D- "A, B, & C" plus: Medication administration, 24-hour nursing supervision

TABLE 24-4   LONG-TERM CARE HOUSING AND ASSESSMENT CONTINUUM—cont'd

	INDEPENDENT LIVING	RETIREMENT COMMUNITY	ASSISTED LIVING	NURSING FACILITY
Mobility	Capable of moving about independently OR ambulatory with cane or walker Independent with wheelchair, but needs help in an emergency	Capable of moving about independently Able to seek and follow directions Able to evacuate independently in emergency OR ambulatory with cane or walker Independent with wheelchair, but needs help in an emergency	Mobile, but may require escort or assistance resulting from confusion, poor vision, weakness, or poor motivation OR requires occasional assistance to move about, but is usually independent	May require assistance with transfers from bed, chair, toilet OR requires transfer and transport assistance Requires turning and positioning in bed and wheelchair
Nutrition	Able to prepare own meals; eats without assistance	Able to prepare own meals; eats without assistance. Generally a minimum of one meal a day is available	All meals and snacks are provided. May require assistance getting to dining room or requires minimal assistance (opening cartons or other packages, cutting food, or preparing trays)	May be unable or unwilling to go to dining room. May be dependent on staff for eating or feeding needs OR fully dependent on staff for nourishment (includes reminders to eat)
Hygiene	Independent in all care, including bathing	Independent in all care, including bathing and personal laundry	May require assistance with bathing or hygiene OR may require assistance, initiation, structure, or reminders. Resident may be able to complete tasks	May be dependent on staff for all personal hygiene
Housekeeping	Independent in performing housekeeping functions (includes making bed, vacuuming, cleaning, and laundry)	Independent in performing housekeeping functions (includes making bed, vacuuming, cleaning, and laundry) OR may need assistance with heavy housekeeping, vacuuming, laundry, and linens	Housekeeping and laundry services provided	Housekeeping and laundry services provided
Dressing	Independent and dresses appropriately	Independent and dresses appropriately	May require occasional assistance with shoelaces, zippers, or medical appliances or garments OR may require reminders, initiation, or motivation	May be dependent on staff for dressing
Toileting	Independent and continent	Independent and completely continent OR may have incontinence, colostomy, or catheter, but independent in caring for self through proper use of supplies	Same as "retirement community" OR may have occasional problem with incontinence, colostomy, or catheter and may require assistance in caring for self through proper use of supplies	May have problem with incontinence, colostomy, or catheter and requires assistance OR may be dependent and unable to communicate needs
Medications	Responsible for self-administration of all medications	Responsible for self-administration of all medications OR may arrange for family or home health agency to establish a medication administration system	Able to self-administer medications OR facility staff may remind or monitor the actual process OR facility staffed by RN or LPN who administers medications	Medications administered by staff personnel or self if assessed as capable
Mental status	Oriented to person, place, and time Memory intact, but has occasional forgetfulness AND able to reason, plan, and organize daily events. Mentally capable of identifying needs and meeting them	Oriented to person, place, and time AND memory is intact, but has occasional forgetfulness without consistent pattern of memory loss AND able to reason, plan, and organize daily events. Mentally capable of identifying environmental needs and meeting them	May require occasional direction or guidance in getting from place to place OR may have difficulty with occasional confusion that may result in anxiety, social withdrawal, or depression OR orientation to time or place or person may be impaired	Judgment can be poor and may attempt tasks that are not within capabilities OR may require strong orientation and reminder program. May need guidance in getting from place to place OR disoriented to time, place, and person OR memory is severely impaired
Behavioral status	Deals appropriately with emotions and uses available resources to cope with inner stress	Deals appropriately with emotions and uses available resources to cope with inner stress AND deals appropriately with other residents and staff OR may require periodic intervention from staff to resolve conflicts with others to cope with situational stress	May require periodic intervention from staff to facilitate expression of feelings to cope with inner stress OR may require periodic intervention from staff to resolve conflicts with others to cope with situational stress	May require regular intervention from staff to facilitate expression of feelings and to deal with periodic outbursts of anxiety or agitation OR maximal staff intervention is required to manage behavior

LPN, Licensed practical nurse; *RN,* registered nurse.

has the opportunity to present health-promotion strategies at a time during which individuals may perceive the greatest need to change their lifestyle behaviors so that they can return to an improved health state. In most cases an acute-care admission is an opportunity to introduce health-promotion teaching. However, the acute-care nurse may feel frustrated by the inability to see the results of this teaching and may therefore give it a low priority in the plan of care.

Some older adults will rapidly grasp material that they believe will prevent future hospital admissions and restore their health. Home health nursing appointments, transportation services, housekeeping services, adult day care, and assistance with grocery shopping or home-delivered meals will help older adults return to the home environment better prepared to recover from the illness. Helping older adults and their families locate adult day care programs, smoking-cessation programs, stress-management workshops, or weight-loss and exercise programs before leaving the hospital will encourage them to enter these programs immediately after discharge, while they are motivated.

Long-term care nurses are able to locate and plan community resources during the resident's stay. Some community services will enable an older person to return home to an environment in which health promotion can continue. Community resources that may help older adults who are discharged from long-term care facilities include adult day care programs, support groups and medical resources, telephone and Internet information, and referral services. In addition to their role in individual care planning, long-term care nurses can be more involved in institutional policy changes. Recommendations about smoking policies, healthy diets, and exercise programs may prompt interdisciplinary changes that will result in improved health for the entire institution.

The geriatric care manager who visits older adults in their homes or in other residential facilities may be charged with individual health-promotion planning. Home care nurses provide health care information and services to individuals and their families. The resources available to community health nurses frequently are rich and enable the nurses to draw on a variety of sources to assist in promoting the health of community-dwelling older adults. Transportation options, home-delivered meals, assistance with housekeeping, socialization activities, exercise programs, and self-help groups are only a few of the health-promotion resources available within the community. Nurses in all settings can consult a social worker or contact the community older adult services office for information on available resources.

It is important for the nurse to consider the health literacy level of the older adult and their family when providing information and health teaching. The U.S. Department of Health and Human Services (2012e) defines health literacy as "the degree to which individuals have the capacity to obtain, process, and understand basic health information needed to make appropriate health decisions and services needed to prevent or treat illness." Persons who are at risk for low health literacy are the elderly, minorities, persons of low socioeconomic level, and the medically underserved. Older adults with low health literacy

may have difficulty finding appropriate health care providers, seeking preventive health care, filling out health forms, managing chronic illness, following directions, understanding the relationship between risk behaviors and health problems, and following medication and treatment plans. It is important for nurses to identify older adults who have low health literacy and develop instructional materials that use simple language and short sentences, avoiding or defining technical terms. Nurses can provide assistance for older adults who have difficulty completing forms. For older adults who have limited English skills, written and oral instruction can be provided in their native language.

In recent years there has been a substantial increase by older adults in the use of palliative and hospice care. Palliative care is provided for persons with a serious illness who will continue to receive curative treatment and symptom relief. While palliative care is available to anyone with a serious illness, hospice care requires a terminal prognosis with an expected death within 6 months. Once the person is placed in hospice care, treatment to relieve pain and other symptoms is continued but the person and their physician have decided to end all curative treatment (National Hospice and Palliative Care Organization, n.d.). In 2010 there were 5150 hospice providers in the United States. Of approximately 2½ million deaths in the United States in 2010, slightly more than 1 million, or 42%, died under hospice care. The majority of hospice care provided in 2010 was in the person's home (41.1%), followed by a hospice inpatient facility (21.9%), nursing home (18%), and acute-care hospital (11.4%). The majority of hospice care recipients were female (56.1%), White (77.3%), and 65 years of age or older (82.7%). Hospice services provided include direct clinical care for persons and bereavement services for the person and their family (National Hospice and Palliative Care Organization, 2012).

Hospice persons are empowered to live with dignity, alert and free of pain. The goal of hospice care is to facilitate a "good death" for individuals. Families and loved ones are consistently engaged in caregiving for the dying and helping them maintain the highest possible quality of life. The hospice environment promotes quality of life within the context of differing cultural and spiritual values and beliefs. Nurses in all settings may identify and refer individuals for palliative or hospice care and facilitate usage of these services to promote wellness during serious or terminal illness.

The American Association of Retired Persons (AARP) provides many services to people over age 50, including excellent educational materials and community program packages. The topics reflect a broad range of concerns and generally are presented in a self-help manner. Among the topics covered are smoking, exercise, nutrition, and wellness. Each program serves as a guide to negotiate a system or learn more about a health problem. These topics are written in lay terms (in easily understood language) and are printed in large print to accommodate vision changes. This self-help method is especially important for those who feel uncomfortable addressing questions on finances or sexuality to nurses and physicians.

The National Institute for Aging (NIA) conducts research to examine many aspects of aging in order to improve the quantity and quality of life in older years. NIA (www.nia.nih.gov) provides free educational publications called *Age Pages* that can be given to older adults to help them adapt safely and successfully to the many changes and concerns encountered as a person ages. *Age Pages* are easily accessed on the Internet, and are written in large font and language easily understandable to the lay public.

Two additional environments of care emerged in the United States over the last half of the twentieth century: continuing care retirement communities (CCRCs) and assisted living facilities (ALFs). CCRCs are full-service communities offering long-term contracts that provide older adults with a continuum of care, extending from retirement services through assisted living to skilled nursing, all in one location. The mission behind CCRCs is "aging in place." CCRCs are expensive and require an entrance fee, and a monthly payment. Residence in a CCRC requires commitment to a long-term contract that specifies the housing, services, and nursing care provided. ALFs are defined as homelike settings that promote resident autonomy, privacy, independence, dignity, and respect while providing necessary support. The lower cost of ALFs in comparison with that of skilled nursing facilities and the greater emphasis on functional autonomy make these facilities appealing to older consumers and their families. Although ALF residents have many long-term health care needs, it is important to understand that the role and availability of nurses in these facilities vary greatly by state guidelines.

Diversity Awareness

The percentage of White older adults is expected to decrease from 1990 to 2030, while the percentages of Black, Asian, and Hispanic elders are expected to increase. These changes in the diversity of the nation bring unprecedented challenges to the U.S. health care delivery system. Challenges will continue to present in the way that each culture perceives the status of the older person within society, the way health is maintained or improved, the causes and meanings of disease throughout life, and the ways in which disease and injury are managed from the cultural perspective versus how they are managed according to the health care system.

Nurses must be aware of the cultural diversity of older adults for whom they care and the cultural beliefs that influence health care decisions of older adults. Cultural competence refers to the ability of nurses to understand and accept the cultural backgrounds of individuals and provide care that best meets the persons' needs—not the nurses' needs. In order to develop cultural competence the first step is to examine personal beliefs and the effect of these beliefs on professional behavior. This may best be accomplished by conducting personal cultural assessments. After identifying personal cultural biases that influence care, nurses must bracket these beliefs to make sure they do not affect delivery of care. After this step is accomplished, it is important to increase understanding about population-specific health-related cultural values, beliefs, and behaviors. It is important to remember that although an older person may be part of a cultural group, the individual may have become acculturated while living in the United States. A cultural history is therefore an essential first step in determining the person's health care beliefs and practices. When conducting cultural assessments, it is necessary to remember that some of the standardized assessment tools, such as the Geriatric Depression Scale and the MMSE, are available in languages other than English. Caution must be taken in interpreting a tool that has not been formally translated, because the meanings of many words and phrases may not have an appropriate translation. The nurse must also be cautious when using assessment tools that have not been tested and validated with people of different cultures and nationalities.

The final stage in attaining cultural competence is to develop skills for working with culturally diverse populations. This entails the development of knowledge in working with culturally diverse populations and consistently using those skills with older adults. Conducting cultural assessments, using translation services, and providing culturally competent care are integral components to developing culturally competent institutions and improving care.

Levels of Policy Making and Health

This chapter has attempted to emphasize the need for health-promotion services for older adults. Governmental efforts to improve health promotion and illness/injury prevention continue. The Affordable Care Act of 2010 (www.HealthCare.gov) strengthens Medicare by providing important new benefits including free or low-cost preventive services, free annual wellness visits, and a discount on prescription drugs for Medicare recipients in the "donut hole." Older adults continue to be able to choose their own physician. Preventive immunizations include influenza, pneumonia, and hepatitis B. Preventive screening exams include those for diabetes, cholesterol and other cardiovascular diseases, colorectal cancer, breast cancer, cervical cancer, and prostate cancer. Counseling services for smoking cessation and for medical nutrition therapy for those with diabetes or kidney disease are also provided.

Medicare and other federal expenditures for older adults (direct or indirect) constitute a large part of the federal budget. Most goes to old age and retirement programs, disability, and Medicaid. Because of the large percentage of the federal budget consumed by Medicare, this insurance program is undergoing much scrutiny. Legislation to more effectively manage or cut the Medicare budget is under review. Lawmakers anticipate that approximately $49 billion in savings could come from more effective use of health maintenance organizations and prospective payment systems instituted in the home. Regardless of the nature of funding cuts, illness and injury prevention contributes to financial stability of the older adult. Nurses continue to play a key role during the years of Medicare reform in promoting health not only to prevent illness and injury, but also to prevent older adults from losing all their savings and becoming impoverished.

Medigap policies have been promoted to pay for the health care coverage not afforded by Medicare. The various policies provide varying levels of coverage. Choices about whether to purchase coverage for durable health care supplies, prescription medications, and other medical charges must be made to select the most appropriate policy. The charge for the policy varies according to the level of coverage selected.

Nongovernmental organizations also influence policy decisions affecting older adults and health. Professional health care provider organizations such as the American Nurses Association, the National Gerontological Nurses Association, and the American Medical Association conduct research to determine best practices in elder care and to provide information to policymakers. The American Association of Retired Persons and the Gray Panthers are examples of two consumer organizations that gather information, fund research related to issues of older adults, and advocate for older adults in policy making organizations.

Health Services/Delivery Systems

Unfortunately, many people are not financially prepared for older adulthood. Although some individuals receive supplemental income from pensions or individual retirement accounts, many do not, and the amount of income from these sources is often very limited. Most older adults live on limited incomes. Several resources are available to help those with limited finances live quality lives. Medicaid, authorized by Title 19 of the Social Security Act, is designed to help older adults who are receiving public assistance pay for medical expenses. Both federal and state governments fund the Medicaid program. To qualify for Medicaid, an individual must have limited income and assets. The coverage afforded by Medicaid is more extensive than that of Medicare. For example, Medicaid covers stays in long-term care facilities, transportation for health care visits, and prescription drug services. Medicare covers these services in limited and medically acute situations. Frequently older adults and their caretakers desire the more extensive coverage provided by Medicaid. These individuals are required to "spend down" their assets to be eligible.

Other resources are available to help older adults live this last stage of life in a better manner. SNAP is available to those who meet certain economic criteria. SNAP can help older adults obtain nutritious food at participating markets without depleting their limited budgets.

Careful financial planning before the onset of illness is ideal to avoid the need to spend down assets and to help the older adult live at a desirable income level. This task can be accomplished through meeting with lawyers and financial planners as early in life as 30 years of age. Completing advance directives, including naming a conservator in advance of illness, assists caregivers, physicians, clergy, and the family in making difficult decisions at the end of life, when the affected person is no longer able to make them. The better prepared the older adult is, the easier it is to receive appropriate care and treatment during times of illness. Reverse annuity mortgages are one option for increased income during the later years. A reverse annuity mortgage is obtained when a bank or private business purchases the home of an older adult. The bank pays the person a set amount of money each month until the house is paid for in its entirety. The senior continues to live in the home. This approach provides the person with necessary funds and negates the need to move and sell the house if an illness arises. When the older adult (mortgagee) dies, the bank or mortgager then owns the property.

Long-term care insurance is an option for those planning for the possibility of long-term care. As with other insurance programs, younger adults can purchase a policy, now widely available from insurance agents. A premium is paid each month that entitles the beneficiary to receive long-term care benefits at home, in assisted living, in day care, or in a long-term care facility. Older individuals are cautioned to explore the many options available for this type of insurance. The benefits and coverage vary, and exclusions frequently are written into the contract to prevent care in certain situations. An important feature of these policies is the option to hire a personal caregiver if the need arises.

Because population shifts have created a large number of older adults in the United States, political movements toward protecting the rights of older adults are abundant and strong. Nowhere is there more political activity than among the groups responsible for social policy and aging. However, this has created problems of consistency, equity, and authority. Several large programs, including those directed by the Social Security Administration, the Health Care Financing Administration, and the Department of Veterans Affairs, have coordination problems because of their size and the large number of cases they handle.

The nurse who specializes in the care of older adults can do a great deal to promote their health and well-being through education, research, and practice. Educational curricula must be evaluated continually to ensure that content is appropriate and accurate with respect to aging. The quality of care depends on the clinician's knowledge base. Education for the older person is equally important and begins with an assessment of the individual's level of understanding of health-promotion activities.

Health-promotion and illness/injury-prevention research for this population is only beginning. Much more remains to be done in exploring the concepts of health promotion, relating these concepts, and developing and testing hypotheses. Research may best begin with an attempt to debunk commonly held beliefs, myths, and stereotypes about aging. Defining some of the concepts of health promotion, such as quality of life and functional ability, will yield immeasurable amounts of information that can be tested. Eventually, with the commitment of qualified nurses, health promotion will be respected for the integral role it plays in the quality of life of older adults.

NURSING APPLICATION

Nurses in a position of providing care to older adults focus on promoting quality of life, promoting the health of the population, maintaining self-care, and preventing disease and its complications. Nursing activities with the older adult often focus on the management of chronic conditions. While concentrating on healing, the nurse delivers care in a holistic manner that addresses the functional and psychosocial needs of the older adult.

Nurses assist older adults by engaging them in health-promotion activities. Some of the major areas of focus are healthy weight and diet, activity, fall prevention and home safety, and medical appointments for screening. Pneumococcal and seasonal influenza immunizations are extremely important for the older adult. Additionally, the older adult is educated about cancer screenings and other screenings aimed at detecting diabetes, late-onset heart disease, osteoporosis, and hypertension. An effective method of ensuring that older

adults participate in screenings is to coordinate health fairs in senior centers. The nurse is able to provide a common location where the senior can obtain vaccinations, necessary education, blood pressure checks, and fingerstick glucose monitoring. The nurse offers counseling as needed and refers the older adult to his or her primary care provider for follow-up.

CASE STUDY

Unsafe Driving: Larry Johnson

Larry Johnson, a healthy 75-year-old man, lives in his own apartment and is completely independent in ADLs and IADLs. Last Friday morning, Larry left his apartment complex at 8:00 AM to go to the store. While backing out of his driveway, he failed to see a school bus passing on the intersecting street, and his car struck the bus. Although no one was injured, this incident indicated the need for a sensory and neurological assessment. The assessment revealed both hearing and visual deficits.

Reflective Questions

1. What would the nurse do to help with the results of the assessment?
2. Should this person undergo further neuropsychological tests?
3. How best can the nurse support this person during this difficult time in his life?

ADLs, Activities of daily living; IADLs, instrumental activities of daily living.

CARE PLAN

Unsafe Driving: Larry Johnson

*NURSING DIAGNOSIS: Risk for Injury related to unsafe driving

Defining Characteristics
- Altered response time
- Change in vision or hearing

Related Factors
- Past accident
- Stressful life events
- Receipt of traffic tickets
- Witnessed poor driving

Expected Outcomes
- Person will have realistic expectations of ability to drive.
- Person and nurse will set appropriate limitations on driving.
- Person will take a driver refresher course.
- Person will have no further accidents.

Interventions
- Assist Larry in registering for a renewal driving program.
- Assist Larry in finding alternative modes of transportation until visual and hearing alterations are corrected and instead of driving in the evening.
- Schedule hearing and vision appointments for Larry and assist in transportation to appointments.

*NANDA Nursing Diagnoses—Definitions and Classification 2012-2014, Herdman T.H. (ED). Copyright © 2012, 1994-2012 NANDA International. Used by arrangement with John Wiley & Sons Limited. In order to make safe and effective judgments using the NANDA-I nursing diagnoses it is essential that nurses refer to the definitions and defining characteristics of the diagnoses listed in this work.

SUMMARY

Life expectancy is now beyond 75 years for both men and women, with the fastest-growing age group being those older than 85. This phenomenon is indeed wonderful. However, aging causes physiological changes in many body functions. Although some of these changes are benign, older adults have a higher frequency of illness than the younger population. The many physical, emotional, and role changes of aging are complicated by the increased diversity in cultural and spiritual backgrounds. Older adults who have immigrated to the United States have brought with them different languages, values and beliefs, spiritual patterns, eating habits, views toward modern medicine, and other customs foreign to U.S. culture. Culturally competent health-promotion services are integral to helping older adults lead high-quality lives throughout their extended life spans.

Many problems of old age are related to lifestyle. Changes in nutritional needs, sleep patterns, and activity level are required to adapt to normal and pathological processes. Psychological health depends on reassessing spirituality, self-concept, and role functions. Change and adaptation are possible. With the assistance of nurses and other health care professionals, older adults can be empowered to live their final years with integrity.

Some of the dysfunctional aspects of aging have extrinsic causes, such as environmental pollution. Older adults are as susceptible as any age group to society's problems, such as homelessness, mistreatment, and drug and alcohol abuse. In conjunction with physiological and pathological changes, multiple acute and chronic diseases can result. Internal and public policy changes will continue to help older adults live in a world in which old age can be the most rewarding stage of life.

REFERENCES

Agency for Healthcare Research and Quality. (1996). *Urinary incontinence in adults: Clinical practice guideline update*. Retrieved February 16, 2012, from www.ahrq.gov/clinic/uiovervw.htm.

Agency for Healthcare Research and Quality. (2005). *Manifestations and management of chronic insomnia in adults*. Retrieved February 16, 2012, from http://ahrq.gov/clinic/epcsums/insomnsum.htm.

Alexopoulos, G. S. (2005). Depression in the elderly. *Lancet, 365*, 1961–1970.

Alzheimer's Association. (2012). *Common types of dementia*. Retrieved February 17, 2012, from www.alz.org/alzheimers_disease_related_diseases.asp.

Alzheimer's Disease International. (2009). *World Alzheimer report 2009: Executive summary*. Retrieved February 17, 2012, from www.alz.org/national/documents/report_summary_2009worldalzheimerreport.pdf.

American Association of Retired Persons. (2008). *Fact Sheet: The food stamp program and older Americans*. Retrieved from http://assets.aarp.org/rgcenter/il/fs20r_food_stamps.pdf.

American Association of Retired Persons. (2010). *10 signs that it's time to limit or stop driving*. Retrieved February 14, 2012, from www.aarp.org/home-garden/transportation/info-05-2010/Warning_Signs_Stopping.html.

American Association of Retired Persons. (2012). *5 myths about sex and aging*. Retrieved May 20, 2012, from www.aarp.org/relationships/love-sex/info-05-2011/sex-myths.print.html.

American Cancer Society. (2010). *Cancer facts & figures 2010*. Atlanta: Author. Retrieved February 23, 2012, from www.cancer.org/acs/groups/content/@epidemiologysurveilance/documents/document/acspc-026238.pdf.

American Cancer Society. (2011). *Cancer prevention and early detection: Facts and figures 2011*. Atlanta: Author. Retrieved February 23, 2012, from www.cancer.org/acs/groups/content/@epidemiologysurveilance/documents/document/acspc-029459.pdf.

American Geriatric Society. (2010). *A pocket guide to the AGS Beers criteria*. New York: Author.

Beatty, G. (2006). Shedding light on Alzheimer's. *Nurse Practitioner, 31*(9), 32–45.

Bixby, M. B. (2011). Evidence-based transitional care for chronically ill older adults and their caregivers. *Journal of Geriatric Care Management, 21*(2), 20–24.

Butler, R., & Olshansky, S. J. (2002). Has anybody ever died of old age? *Gerontologist, 42*(Special Issue 1), 285–286.

Centers for Disease Control and Prevention. (2011a). *Enhancing use of clinical preventive services among older adults—Closing the gap*. Retrieved May 22, 2012, from www.cdc.gov/aging/pdf/Clinical_Preventive_Services_Closing_the_Gap_Report.pdf.

Centers for Disease Control and Prevention. (2011b). *How much physical activity do older adults need?* Retrieved from www.cdc.gov/physicalactivity/everyone/guidelines/olderadults.html.

Centers for Disease Control and Prevention. (2011c). *Dementia/Alzheimer's disease*. Retrieved from www.cdc.gov/mentalhealth/basics/mental-illness/dementia.htm.

Centers for Disease Control and Prevention. (2011d). *Depression statistics*. Retrieved February 20, 2012, from www.cdc.gov/mentalhealth/data_stats/depression.htm.

Centers for Disease Control and Prevention. (2011e). *Falls in older adults: An overview*. Retrieved February 26, 2012, from www.cdc.gov/HomeandRecreationalSafety/Falls/adultfalls.html.

Centers for Disease Control and Prevention. (2011f). *Older adult drivers*. Retrieved February 20, 2012, from www.cdc.gov/Motorvehiclesafety/Older_Adult_Drivers/data.html.

Centers for Disease Control and Prevention. (2011g). Update: Influenza activity—United States, 2010-11 season, and composition of the 2011-2012 influenza vaccine. *Morbidity and Mortality Weekly Report, 60*(21), 708–711. Retrieved from www.cdc.gov/mmwr/pdf/wk/mm6021.pdf.

Centers for Disease Control and Prevention. (2011h). *Smoking & tobacco use fact sheet*. Retrieved February 24, 2012, from www.cdc.gov/tobacco/data_statistics/fact_sheets/health_effects/effects_cig_smoking/index.htm.

Centers for Disease Control and Prevention. (2012a). *National Vital Statistics Reports: Deaths: Preliminary Data for 2010, 60*. Retrieved February 22, 2012, from www.cdc.gov/nchs/data/nvsr/nvsr60/nvsr60_04.pdf.

Centers for Disease Control and Prevention. (2012b). *Sexual health*. Retrieved from www.cdc.gov/sexualhealth/.

Centers for Disease Control and Prevention. (n.d.). *Suicide*. Retrieved from www.cdc.gov/violenceprevention.

Centers for Disease Control and Prevention, National Center for Health Statistics. (2010). *Summary health statistics for U.S. adults: National Health Interview Survey 2010*. Retrieved May 20, 2012, from www.cdc.gov/nchs/data/series/sr_10/sr10_252.pdf.

Centers for Disease Control and Prevention, National Center for Health Statistics. (2012a). *Data table: Percentage of adults aged 18 and over who met the 2008 federal physical activity guidelines for aerobic activity through leisure-time aerobic activity, by age group and sex: United States, January-September 2011*. Retrieved May 20, 2012, from www.cdc.gov/nchs/data/nhis/earlyrelease/201203_07.pdf.

Centers for Disease Control and Prevention, National Center for Health Statistics. (2012b). *Health data interactive*. Retrieved May 23, 2012, from www.cdc.gov/nchs/hdi.htm.

Erikson, E. H. (1982). *Life cycle completed: A review*. New York: W. W. Norton.

Erikson, E. H. (1997). *The life cycle completed*. New York: W.W. Norton.

Erikson, E. H., Erikson, J. H., & Kivnick, H. Q. (1986). *Vital involvement in old age: The experience of old age in our time*. New York: W.W. Norton.

Folstein, M. E., Folstein, S. E., & McHugh, P. (1975). "Mini-mental state." A practical method for grading the cognitive state of patients for the clinician. *Journal of Psychiatric Research, 12*, 189–198.

Gall, T. L., Charbonneau, C., Clarke, N. H., Grant, K., Joseph, A., & Shouldice, L. (2005). Understanding the nature and role of spirituality in relation to coping and health: A conceptual framework. *Canadian Psychology, 46*, 88–104.

Garnefski, N., & Kraaij, V. (2006). Relationships between cognitive emotion regulation strategies and depressive symptoms: A comparative study of five specific samples. *Personality and Individual Differences, 40*, 1659–1669.

Haight, B. K. (2005). Reminiscence. In J. Fitzpatrick & M. Wallace (Eds.), *Encyclopedia of nursing research*. New York: Springer.

Haight, B. K., Michel, Y., & Hendrix, S. (2000). The extended effects of the life review in nursing home residents. *International Journal of Aging & Human Development, 50*(2), 151–168.

Harvard Medical School. (2003). Forestalling frailty. *Harvard Women's Health Watch, 27*.

Hodge, D., Bonifas, R., & Chou, R. (2010). Spirituality and older adults: Ethical guidelines to enhance service provision. *Advances in Social Work, 11*, 1.

Hooyman, N., & Kiyak, H. (2011). *Social gerontology: A multidisciplinary perspective* (9th ed.). Boston: Allyn & Bacon.

Medicare.gov. (2012). *Medicare prescription drug coverage: Part D*. Retrieved February 26, 2012, from www.medicare.gov/navigation/medicare-basics/medicare-benefits/part-d.aspx?AspxAutoDetectCookieSupport=1.

National Center for Elder Abuse. (2012). *Why should I care about elder abuse?* Retrieved February 27, 2012, from www.ncea.aoa.gov/ncearoot/Main_Site/pdf/publication/NCEA_WhatIsAbuse-2010.pdf.

National Center for Statistics and Analysis. (2005). *Traffic safety facts: Older population.* Retrieved July 19, 2007, from www.nrd.nhtsa.dot.gov/pubs/810622.pdf.

National Highway Traffic Safety Administration (NHTSA). (2010). *Older driver program: Five year strategic plan 2012-2017.* Retrieved February 26, 2012, from www.nhtsa.gov/staticfiles/nti/pdf/811432.pdf.

National Hospice and Palliative Care Organization. (2012). *NHPCO facts and figures: Hospice care in America. 2011 Edition.* Alexandria, VA: Author. Retrieved February 26, 2012, from www.nhpco.org/files/public/Statistics_Research/2011_Facts_Figures.pdf.

National Hospice and Palliative Care Organization. (n.d.). *Some differences between palliative care and hospice.* Retrieved February 26, 2012, from www.nia.nih.gov/print/health/publication/end-life-helping-comfort-and-care/finding-care-end-life.

National Institute on Aging. (2011). *Biology of aging: Research today for a healthier tomorrow.* Retrieved May 22, 2012, from www.nia.nih.gov/sites/default/files/biology_of_aging.pdf.

National Institute of Mental Health. (2007). *Older adults: Depression and suicide facts (Fact sheet).* Retrieved February 20, 2012, from www.nimh.nih.gov/health/publications/older-adults-depression-and-suicide-facts-fact-sheet/index.shtml.

National Prevention Council. (2011). *National prevention strategy: America's plan for better health and wellness.* Retrieved May 25, 2012, from www.healthcare.gov/prevention/nphpphc/strategy/report.pdf.

National Resource Center on Nutrition, Physical Activity & Aging. (2012). *Malnutrition and older Americans.* Retrieved May 22, 2012, from http://nutritionandaging.fiu.edu/aging_network/malfact2.asp.

National Strategy for Suicide Prevention. (2007). *At a glance—suicide among the elderly.* Retrieved July 19, 2007, from http://mentalhealth.samhsa.gov/suicideprevention/elderly.asp.

National Survey on Drug Use and Health. (2005). *The NSDUH report: Substance use among older adults: 2002-2003.* Retrieved February 26, 2012, from http://oas.samhsa.gov/2k5/olderadults/olderadults.pdf.

Neikrug, A. B., & Ancoli-Israel, S. (2010). Sleep disorders in the older adult—A mini review. *Gerontology, 56*(2), 181–189.

Nies, M. A., & McEwan, M. (2011). *Community/public health nursing: Promoting the health of populations* (6th ed.). Philadelphia: Saunders.

Ogden, C. L., Carroll, M. D., Kitt, B. K., & Flegal, K. M. (2012). *Prevalence of obesity in the United States, 2009-2010.* NCHS Data Brief, No. 82, Retrieved May 22, 2012, from www.cdc.gov/nchs/data/databriefs/db82.htm.

Redline, S., Yenokyan, G., Gottlieb, D. J., et al. (2010). Obstructive sleep apnea hypopnea and incident stroke: The sleep heart health study. *American Journal of Respiratory Critical Care Medicine, 182*(2), 269–277.

Ross, M. E., & Aday, L. A. (2006). Stress and coping in African American grandparents who are raising their grandchildren. *Journal of Family Issues, 27,* 912–932.

Smyth, C. A. (2008). Evaluating sleep quality in older adults. *American Journal of Nursing, 108*(5), 42–50.

Social Security Administration. (2012). *Annual statistical supplement to the Social Security Bulletin, 2011.* Retrieved February 18, 2012, from www.ssa.gov/policy/docs/statcomps/supplement/2011/supplement11.pdf.

Touhy, T. (2012a). Communicating with older adults. In T. Touhy & K. Jett (Eds.), *Toward healthy aging: Human needs & nursing response* (8th ed.). St. Louis: Elsevier/Mosby.

Touhy, T. (2012b). Mental health. In T. Touhy & K. Jett (Eds.), *Toward healthy aging: Human needs & nursing response* (8th ed.). St. Louis: Elsevier/Mosby.

Touhy, T., & Jett, K. (2012). *Toward healthy aging: Human needs & nursing response* (8th ed.). St. Louis: Elsevier/Mosby.

Umlauf, M. G., Williams, L. L., & Chasens, E. R. (2008). Sleep: Nursing standard practice protocol: Excessive sleepiness. *Hartford Institute for Geriatric Nursing.* Retrieved from http://consultgerirn.org/topics/sleep/want_to_know_more.

U.S. Administration on Aging. (2011). *Older population as a percentage of the total population: 1900-2050.* Retrieved January 14, 2012, from www.aoa.gov/AoARoot/Aging_Statistics/future_growth/future_growth.aspx#age.

U.S. Census Bureau. (2010). *Deaths and death rates by selected causes: 2006-2007. Statistical Abstract of the United States: 2012.* Retrieved February 22, 2012, from www.census.gov/compendia/statab/2012/tables/12s0120.pdf.

U.S. Census Bureau. (2011a). *Current population survey: Annual social and economic supplement, 2010.* Retrieved January 14, 2011, from www.census.gov/population/www/socdemo/age/age_sex_2010.html.

U.S. Census Bureau. (2011b). *Living arrangements of children 2009.* Retrieved February 18, 2012, from www.census.gov/prod/2011pubs/p70-126.pdf.

U.S. Consumer Product Safety Commission. (n.d.). *National safety network: Older adults.* Retrieved February 26, 2012, from www.cpsc.gov/nsn/seniors.html.

U.S. Department of Agriculture (USDA). (2010). *Dietary Guidelines for Americans, 2010.* Retrieved February 17, 2012, from www.health.gov/dietaryguidelines/dga2010/DietaryGuidelines2010.pdf.

U.S. Department of Health and Human Services. (2007). *Healthy retirement study.* Retrieved July 17, 2007, from www.nia.nih.gov/NRI rdonlyreslD164FE6C-C6E0–4E78-B27F-7E8D8C0FFEE5l0IHRS_Text_WEB.pdf.

U.S. Department of Health and Human Services. (2012a). *Healthy People 2020: Topics & Objectives.* Retrieved February 17, 2012, from www.healthypeople.gov/2020/topicsobjectives2020/default.aspx.

U.S. Department of Health and Human Services. (2012b). *Healthy People 2020: Dementia, including Alzheimer's disease.* Retrieved February 17, 2012, from www.healthypeople.gov/2020/topicsobjectives2020/overview.aspx?topicid=7.

U.S. Department of Health and Human Services. (2012c). *Healthy People 2020: Oral health.* Retrieved February 18, 2012, from www.healthypeople.gov/2020/topicsobjectives2020/objectiveslist.aspx?topicId=32.

U.S. Department of Health and Human Services. (2012d). *Healthy People 2020: Injury and violence prevention.* Retrieved February 23, 2010, from http://healthypeople.gov/2020/topicsobjectives2020/objectiveslist.aspx?topicId=24.

U.S. Department of Health and Human Services. (2012e). *About health literacy.* Retrieved February 27, 2012, from www.hrsa.gov/publichealth/healthliteracy/healthlitabout.html.

U.S. Department of Health and Human Services, Food and Drug Administration. (2009). *FDA's safe use initiative: Collaborating to reduce preventable harm from medications.* Retrieved May 25, 2012, from www.fda.gov/downloads/Drugs/NewsEvents/UCM234184.pdf?utm_campaign=Google2&;utm_source=fdaSearch&utm_medium=website&utm_term=Adverse drug events in older adultsutm_content=10.

U.S. Department of Health and Human Services, Health Resources and Services Administration, Maternal and Child Health Bureau. (2010). *Women's health USA 2010.* Retrieved February 27, 2012, from http://mchb.hrsa.gov/whusa10/hstat/wa/pages/243ia.html.

Wagner, L. M., Scott, V., & Silver, M. (2011). Current approaches to fall risk assessment in nursing homes. *Geriatric Nursing, 32,* (4), 238–244.

Wallhagen, M., & Pettengill, E. (2008). Hearing impairment significant but underassessed in primary care settings. *Journal of Gerontological Nursing, 34,* 36.

Wellman, N., & Kamp, B. (2004, Fall). Federal food and nutrition assistance programs for older people. *Generations, 28*(3), 78–85.

Wood, D., & Roberts, B. W. (2006). The effect of age and role information on expectations for big five personality traits. *Personality Social Psychology Bulletin, 32*(11), 1482–1496.

Yesavage, J., Brink, T., Rose, T., Lum, O., Huang, V., Adey, M., et al. (1983). Development and validation of a geriatric depression screening scale: A preliminary report. *Journal of Psychiatric Research, 17,* 37–49.

Health Promotion for the Twenty-First Century: Throughout the Life Span and Throughout the World

Ratchneewan Ross and Jeffrey Ross

evolve WEBSITE

http://evolve.elsevier.com/Edelman/
- Study Questions
- Glossary

OBJECTIVES

After completing this chapter, the reader will be able to:
- Identify global trends and directions for health promotion and disease prevention.
- Discuss problems and implications related to community-associated methicillin-resistant *Staphylococcus aureus*.
- Describe problems and implications related to human immunodeficiency virus/acquired immunodeficiency syndrome.
- Discuss problems and implications related to violence.
- Discuss problems and implications related to bioterrorism and terrorism.

KEY TERMS

Anthrax (*Bacillus anthracis*)
Bioterrorism
Botulism
Centers for Disease Control and Prevention (CDC)
Community-associated methicillin-resistant *Staphylococcus aureus* (CA-MRSA)

Human immunodeficiency virus/acquired immunodeficiency syndrome (HIV/AIDS)
Malnutrition
Plague
Self-abuse
Smallpox (*Variola major*)
Suicide

Terrorism
Violence
World Health Organization (WHO)

? THINK ABOUT IT

HIV Infection and Cultural Practices

Adila lives in Kenya with her two children, ages 11 and 7 years old. Her husband died a week ago from AIDS. Adila learned 6 months earlier that she is HIV-positive, contacting the virus from her husband. Now Adila is being told by the village leader that she must undergo a traditional sexual cleansing. Also, the village leader told her that her husband's older brother is to inherit her as his second wife.

- What kind of problems would you anticipate that Adila will encounter if she does not follow the village leader's advice?
- What do you think could be done in this Kenyan village to prevent further HIV infections?
- Visit the World Health Organization website (www.who.org) to identify the incidence and prevalence of HIV and AIDS in Kenya.

In the new millennium the gap in life expectancies between people in developed and developing cultures has been widening. In many developed nations, such as Japan, France, and the United States, people have a life expectancy at birth ranging from 78 to 82 years (Central Intelligence Agency [CIA], 2012a), whereas residents of some countries in Africa, such as Angola and Swaziland, can have a life expectancy as low as 38 years, attributable primarily to high rates of human immunodeficiency virus (HIV) infections and poverty (CIA, 2012b; United Nations Programme on HIV and AIDS [UNAIDS], 2011a).

In 2002 there were 57 million deaths worldwide: More than 10 million deaths were among children younger than 5 years, and approximately 98% of these deaths occurred in developing countries (World Health Organization [WHO], 2011a). Based on WHO's 2008 statistics, lower respiratory tract infections (11.3%), diarrheal diseases (8.2%), and HIV/acquired immunodeficiency syndrome (AIDS) (7.8%) were the leading causes of deaths for people in low-income countries, whereas cardiovascular disorders (26.5%) and chronic obstructive pulmonary diseases were the leading causes of deaths in middle-income countries, and cardiovascular disorders (23.6%) and lower respiratory tract infections (6.1%) were the leading causes of deaths in high-income countries (WHO, 2011b) (Box 25-1: Quality and Safety Scenario). Approximately 13.1% of the world's population, or 925 million out of 7 billion, are undernourished and 5 million children die annually from starvation (World Hunger Education Service, 2012) (Figure 25-1). On the other end of the spectrum, obesity is a rising cause of health problems in both medium- and high-income countries. The number of the world population with obesity has more than doubled from 1980 to 2008, and almost 43 million children 5 years or younger were obese in 2008 (WHO, 2012a). While urgent interventions to combat hunger and infectious diseases (such as HIV infection and diarrheal diseases) are needed in many developing countries, behavioral interventions to fight cardiovascular disorders and obesity are crucial in medium-income and high-income countries.

Emerging infections (e.g., methicillin-resistant *Staphylococcus aureus* and tuberculosis), varied forms of intercultural and interpersonal violence, terrorism, and bioterrorism also pose great worries and risks to the world. This chapter presents information on malnutrition, emerging infections, HIV infection, violence, bioterrorism, and terrorism, followed by discussions on their important implications for the future.

MALNUTRITION

The World Health Organization (WHO, 2000) defines malnutrition as "bad nourishment" that can be associated with "either too much or too little food intake and [is] not limited to the wrong types of food." Malnutrition is characterized by "inadequate or excess intake of protein, energy, and micronutrients such as vitamins." In general, malnutrition can be classified into three categories: protein-energy malnutrition, micronutrient deficiencies, and obesity (WHO, 2000). This chapter will address only protein-energy malnutrition because it is the most serious among the three types (WHO, 2000).

FIGURE 25-1 Lunchtime for school children in a remote area of Thailand. The food was made possible through donations from health care providers.

Protein-Energy Malnutrition

Protein-energy malnutrition (PEM), a lack of calories and protein, is widespread in low-income countries and is the most lethal form of malnutrition/hunger (World Hunger Education Service, 2012). Humans convert food into energy, and the energy contained in food is measured by calories. Protein is necessary for key body functions including provision of essential amino acids and development and maintenance of muscles (WHO/United Nations Children's Fund [UNICEF], 2009). PEM can be severely harmful to the mental and physical development of individuals, especially children younger than age 5 (WHO, 2008). Children born to undernourished mothers have been reported to be at high risk for low birth weight, birth defects,

	No appetite · Medical complications		Appetite · No medical complications
Independent additional criteria			
Type of therapeutic feeding	Facility-based		Community-based
Intervention	F75 ► F100/RUTF And 24 hour medical care		RUTF, basic medical care
Discharge criteria (Transition criteria from facility to community-based care)	Reduced oedema Good appetite (with acceptable[a] intake of RUTF)		15 to 20% weight gain

[a]Child eats at least 75% of their calculated RUTF ration for the day

FIGURE 25-2 Severe acute malnutrition management. (Reprinted with permission from World Health Organization. [2011a]. *The WHO child growth standards.* Retrieved from www.who.int/childgrowth/standards/en/.)

low immunity levels and infection susceptibility, growth retardation, learning disabilities, mental retardation, blindness, and, most severely, premature death (WHO, 2008). Worldwide, one out of two deaths among children younger than 5 years old stems from protein-energy malnutrition (WHO, 2008). One out of four children is underweight and one out of three is stunted (WHO, 2000).

Severe Acute Malnutrition

Severe protein-energy malnutrition, or severe acute malnutrition (SAM), can be lethal. WHO defines SAM as the presence of serious wasting and/or edema (WHO/UNICEF, 2009). Severe wasting is defined as the weight of a child being less than 70% (or <3 standard deviations) of the median weight-for-height (WHO, 2011b) and/or having a mid-upper arm circumference (MUAC) below 115 mm—a new cut-off MUAC (WHO/UNICEF, 2009). Children with SAM require immediate treatment because they have a higher risk of death than children without SAM (WHO/UNICEF, 2009).

Severe wasting is caused by loss of subcutaneous fat and skeletal muscle and is highly noticeable because of underdeveloped buttocks, thighs, and upper arms. It is also characterized by sunken eyes, visible ribs, and protruding shoulder blades (WHO, 2004a). Children with severe wasting usually have a distended abdomen and general overall appearance in some way similar to an older adult. In general, these children are irritable, anxious, and cry easily; yet they will often have an absence of tears while crying because of lacrimal gland atrophy (WHO, 2004a).

Edema in children with undernutrition is caused by the leaking of potassium from cells, leading to an electrolyte imbalance and fluid retention in the feet, lower legs, arms, and face. The skin of children with edema is abnormally dark with peeling patches and is sensitive to the touch.

At present, treating children with SAM involves providing special therapeutic, milk-based foods called Ready-to-Use-Therapeutic Foods (RUTFs), which are soft, crushable, and tasty nutrient- and energy-rich foods that can be consumed by children 6 months or older (WHO/UNICEF, 2009). When a child has a good appetite with no medical conditions (e.g., hypoglycemia, hypothermia, dehydration, electrolyte imbalance, and/or infections), use of RUTFs under community-based care is appropriate. However, when a child does not have an appetite and/or medical conditions are present, the child needs to receive facility-based care (WHO/UNICEF, 2009). The child may be transferred from a facility-based care setting to a community-based setting when the following conditions are met: the child is absent of bilateral edema, regains a good appetite, and eats at least 75% of his/her calculated RUTF ration for the day (WHO/UNICEF, 2009). The child can be discharged from a community-based care setting when he or she has a weight gain of 15% since admission (WHO/UNICEF, 2009) (Figure 25-2).

Addressing Malnutrition at the Global Level

Different organizations, such as the Centers for Disease Control and Prevention (CDC), the World Health Organization (WHO), UNICEF, and the United Nations, have worked collaboratively to create several initiatives in order to address the malnutrition issue. These include the *Baby Friendly Hospital Initiative* programs to manage nutrition needs during emergencies, global nutrition data banks, a global network of collaborating centers in nutrition (UNICEF, 2012), and the *International Micronutrient Malnutrition Prevention and Control* (IMMPaCt) program (CDC, 2012a).

The *Baby Friendly Hospital Initiative,* launched in 1991 by UNICEF and WHO, has as its goal to promote exclusive breastfeeding during the first 4 months of life when it is most required by the infant (UNICEF, 2012). The program involves at least 170 countries and more than 16,000 hospitals (UNICEF, 2012). Through the initiative, a mother starts breastfeeding as soon as her child is born and continues to breastfeed her child exclusively, unless medically otherwise indicated or until the child is 4 months old. This includes avoiding supplemental food and drink until the older child is ready for such intake (UNICEF, 2012).

The *International Micronutrient Malnutrition Prevention and Control* (IMMPaCt) program, established in 2000 by the CDC, works with global partners such as WHO, UNICEF, and U.S. Agency for International Development (USAID) to provide its skills and resources toward working to eradicate vitamin and mineral deficiencies around the globe (CDC, 2012a). The IMMPaCt program's activities include conducting surveys; providing micronutrients to infants, young children, and women of childbearing age; and monitoring and evaluating intervention systems (CDC, 2012a). Since its establishment, the IMMPaCt program has provided assistance and/or training in more than 70 countries around the world.

EMERGING INFECTIONS

Methicillin-Resistant *Staphylococcus aureus* (MRSA)

Colonizing of *Staphylococcus aureus* in the nasal area is common and asymptomatic in one out of three healthy individuals (CDC, 2011a; Perencevich & Diekema, 2010). On the other hand, methicillin-resistant *Staphylococcus aureus* (MRSA), a form of staph bacteria that causes skin/soft tissue infections, is resistant to beta-lactams (e.g., methicillin, oxacillin, penicillin, and amoxicillin) (CDC, 2012b) and is estimated to be colonized in only 1% of healthy individuals (CDC, 2011a).

Health care–associated MRSA (HA-MRSA) may occur in hospitalized persons who receive medical or surgical procedures, such as administration of ventilation apparatus or introduction of a nasogastric tube or catheter (particularly in those with minimized immune functions), and can lead to life-threatening infections, such as pneumonia and bacteremia. However, a study that reviewed 82% of all MRSA cases in the United States from 2005 through 2008 showed that life-threatening HA-MRSA infections dropped 28% from 2005 to 2008 (Kallen et al., 2010). Yet, factors related to the decline were not reported.

In the community setting, community-associated methicillin-resistant *Staphylococcus aureus* (CA-MRSA) strains have emerged as serious threats in the past two decades and can cause dermatitis and soft tissue infections (CDC, 2010a, 2012b) with the ability also to cause fatal infections in the lungs (e.g., necrotizing pneumonia, purpura fulminans, and postviral toxic shock syndrome) (Schlievert et al., 2010). In general, CA-MRSA spreads more easily, has higher recurrence rates, and causes more skin problems and serious damage than the traditional HA-MRSA found in hospital settings (CDC, 2012b). More than three different *S. aureus* strains are found to cause CA-MRSA infections. In the United States, the most common strains are USA-300 and USA-400, and these strains are different from the USA-100 and USA-200 strains of HA-MRSA also found in health care settings (Fekete, 2007).

CA-MRSA cases have been reported by emergency departments, day care centers, schools, correctional facilities, sports facilities, dormitories, and military stations (CDC, 2011; Sedighi et al., 2011). Persons who are generally healthy can contact the bacteria through close skin-to-skin contact, cuts or abrasions in the skin, crowded conditions, shared utilities (e.g., clothing items and towels), and poor hygiene (CDC, 2011a; Kirkland & Adams, 2008). Also, those who are taking or have previously received antibiotic therapy have a greater risk of infections than those who do not have a history of previous antibiotic intake (Fekete, 2007).

Most CA-MRSA cases are mild and include a skin or soft tissue infection (i.e., a boil or abscess). Usually, the infected area resembles a red, swollen, and painful "spider bite" (CDC, 2010). Pus or other drainage may be present. If the infection is limited to the skin, it can be difficult to distinguish CA-MRSA from HA-MRSA (CDC, 2010a). Among severely CA-MRSA–infected people, complications may include serious necrotizing infection, septicemia, pneumonia, and death (CDC, 2010a). To diagnose CA-MRSA infections, a culture is taken by obtaining a specimen from the infection site (i.e., a small biopsy of skin or drainage and/or a sample of sputum, blood, or urine).

The most updated clinical guidelines for CA-MRSA management were published in 2006 by the CDC (2006). The guidelines suggest that CA-MRSA skin infections, such as boils or abscesses, may be treated by incision and drainage. Antibiotic regimens guided by sensitivity test results should be administered to infected individuals. Intravenous antibiotic treatment should be considered among hospitalized individuals who show signs of oral therapy nonadherence. Oral antibiotics may include sulfamethoxazole/trimethoprim, clindamycin, doxycycline, minocycline, and linezolid. To prevent MRSA cross-infection, meticulous hand washing has been found to be important and is recommended as a cost-effective everyday practice (see more details at www.cdc.gov/mrsa/pdf/MRSA-Strategies-ExpMtgSummary-2006.pdf).

In the United States, MRSA outbreaks are reportable in some states. Examples of reportable states include Connecticut (the first state to require such reports), Indiana, Kentucky, New Jersey, New York, Ohio, and Vermont. Whether or not CA-MRSA infections are reportable in a given area, having knowledge of this disease is essential to enable health care professionals to provide appropriate infection control initiations. Standard precautions—a combination and expansion of universal precautions and body substance isolation—are required among health care professionals to prevent cross-contamination (CDC, 2011a).

HIV/AIDS

Throughout the world, approximately 34 million people are living with human immunodeficiency virus/acquired immunodeficiency syndrome (HIV/AIDS), with 22.9 million in sub-Saharan Africa, 4 million in South/Southeast Asia, 1.5 million in Latin America, 1.5 million in Eastern Europe and Central Asia, 1.3 million in North America, 840,000 in Western/Central Europe, 790,000 in East Asia, 470,000 in the Middle

BOX 25-2 HOT TOPICS
Ethical Dilemmas

- Is it ethical in a clinical trial not to give HIV-positive persons in the control group the most recent antiretroviral drugs?
- Is it ethical to prosecute a local man who lives in Africa and wants to cure his HIV infection by having sex with a young virgin?

East/North Africa, 200,000 in the Caribbean, and 54,000 in Oceania (islands in the pacific and vicinity) (United Nations Programme on HIV/AIDS, 2011a). Sub-Saharan Africa—the region hardest hit by HIV—had 68% of the global HIV cases in 2010 (UNAIDS, 2011a), and life expectancy rates in this region had been reduced by 20 years because of HIV/AIDS. Swaziland, Botswana, Lesotho, and Zimbabwe—all in sub-Saharan Africa—are being particularly affected by the disease, despite the fact that antiretroviral medicines have been used to decrease mother-to-child transmission in these areas (UNAIDS, 2011a) (Box 25-2: Hot Topics).

In low-income countries, HIV prevalence rates in the adult population are much higher than those in high-income countries. For instance, the rate is approximately 0.6% in the United States and 0.1% in Japan. In Swaziland, the 2009 rate was 25.9% (CIA, 2012a) and 24.8% in Botswana (CIA, 2012b). Although economic level is found to be negatively associated with HIV rates, evidence also shows that cultural beliefs and practices are significant factors contributing to HIV infections; these include *wife inheritance, traditional sexual cleansing,* and *virgin cleansing* (Olugu et al., 2010; Robson, 2009).

Wife inheritance is a cultural practice among some Kenyans (Olugu et al., 2010). It is considered a heroic act of a male family member to assume the responsibility of being the new husband of a new widow. One male HIV prevention teacher states, "I don't see why I should not be allowed to look after my sister-in-law in all ways possible. The one inheriting the widow, a brother or cousin to the deceased, has to perform the duties of a husband, including providing and receiving conjugal rights" (Olugu et al., 2010, p. 374). If the new widow's husband has died of HIV/AIDS, the risk of further infection is compounded.

Traditional sexual cleansing, a cultural practice performed among particular tribes in sub-Saharan African countries, is usually undertaken after the spouse of a survivor has died. In this ritual, the widow or widower is required to have penetrative sex with a *cleanser* to avoid misfortune and to chase away the spirit of the dead from the self and the community (Olugu et al., 2010). The cleanser could be anyone, ranging from an in-law to a stranger, or commercial performer (Ayikukwei et al., 2007; Olugu et al., 2010). However, in Zambia, a study showed that 69% of widowers and widows are choosing to use combined alternative practices (i.e., sliding over a half-naked person, body-brushing, cow jumping, hair cutting, or mud throwing at the widow/widower) instead of traditional sexual cleansing (Malungo, 2001). Such alternative practices are helpful in that they do not pose any HIV infection risks for the survivors as does sexual cleansing.

In contrast to Zambia, the ritual of sexual cleansing persists widely in Kenya (Robson, 2009). Luo (a tribe in Kenya) members believe that this ritual will set the dead husband's spirit free and help the widow and her community avoid misfortune (Olugu et al., 2010; Robson, 2009). The female widow needs to be cleansed by having sex after the period of mourning over her husband's death is over. The mourning period can last from 1 to 12 months (Ayikukwei et al., 2007). Although there have been some movements to modify the cleansing procedures (e.g., dress code, mourning period), having sex with a cleanser is still a requirement for Luo members (Olugu et al., 2010; Robson, 2009).

In terms of gender, women with HIV in African countries are overall more vulnerable to progression to AIDS than their male counterparts because of their unequal socioeconomic status. Furthermore, African females in general are the caretakers for the sick in their families and they can lose their property when they become widows. In Kenya, a widow in Luo clans is ostracized by her community members and not allowed to join any social functions immediately upon her husband's death. To be accepted back to the community, the Kenyan widow needs to undergo traditional sexual cleansing (Olugu et al., 2010).

Concerning *virgin cleansing* in sub-Saharan countries, literature reveals that male HIV-positive individuals in Kenya and Tanzania are advised by traditional healers that their infection is caused by a curse and can only be cured by having sex with a virgin female child younger than 12 years of age (Murry & Burnham, 2009; Olugu et al., 2010). Some argue that this is not the case in Malawi and South Africa (Epstein & Jewkes, 2009; Mtibo et al., 2011). Clearly, however, the rituals of widow inheritance, traditional sexual cleansing, and virgin cleansing contribute to the spread of HIV in some sub-Saharan communities. Other cultural practices in regions as diverse as Russia, sub-Saharan Africa, and Thailand have been found to contribute to HIV transmission, including promiscuity among heterosexual individuals (Amirkhanian et al., 2010; Olugu et al., 2010; Ross et al., 2009a; Ross et al., 2011).

Even though HIV prevention education efforts have been undertaken, these efforts can be complicated in places by the existence of certain unique cultural practices. A study in Kenya and Tanzania reveals how *mila potofu* (deceptive cultural practices) hinders the effectiveness of HIV prevention education there (Olugu et al., 2010). *Mila potofu,* as identified by HIV teacher trainees and their mentors in this study, include *the taboo of talking about sex, wife inheritance,* and *sexual cleansing.* Teacher trainees in the study conducted by Olugu and colleagues reported that it is not acceptable to talk about sex with female children and adolescents in Kenya and Tanzania because any female child who listens to a sex talk is considered immoral. Also, the beliefs and practices of *wife inheritance* and *sexual cleansing* (*traditional cleansing* and *virgin cleansing*) still exist in some communities (Olugu et al., 2010).

Clearly, the challenges of reducing HIV/AIDS rates are complex and the solutions require multidisciplinary and multidimensional approaches. Ordinary people, community leaders, health care professionals, and organizations at all levels must work collaboratively. Together, we can consider gender/social inequalities and cultural/religious beliefs and practices as we work to identify barriers to understanding and facilitate the reduction of HIV infections. Support from all parties will enable us to set priorities and fight HIV/AIDS more effectively. Including indigenous people from the community in educational efforts and taking advantage of alternative cultural beliefs, such as modified sexual cleansing, for example, could be helpful in some sub-Saharan countries.

To fight against HIV/AIDS at the global level, UNAIDS (2011b) is working collaboratively with its partner organizations, such as UNICEF, UNESCO, WHO, and the World Bank. The ambitious visions of UNAIDS include zero new HIV infections, zero AIDS-related deaths, and zero discrimination; the commitment is that everyone globally should have universal access to HIV prevention, treatment, care, and support (UNAIDS, 2011b). To reach these optimal goals, UNAIDS has outlined three strategic directions: *revolutionizing HIV prevention; catalyzing the next generation for treatment, care, and support;* and *advancing human rights and gender equality in responses to HIV* (UNAIDS, 2011b).

Revolutionizing HIV prevention means that the focus is shifted from HIV rates of "prevalence" to "incidence" (UNAIDS, 2011b). "Incidence" deals with the number of new HIV infections in a particular population during a certain period of time, whereas HIV "prevalence" is the percentage of all cases (new and old) of HIV infections at a certain time point (AVERT, 2012). In this focus, hot spot transmissions need to be identified, and empowerment (especially among young people) needs to be encouraged so that all involved people will adopt more proactive behaviors to decrease the number of new HIV infections. UNAIDS (2011b) has announced its support of political change in terms of HIV, new approaches to technology, the reduction of stigma and discrimination associated with HIV, and comprehensive sexuality education for HIV-positive individuals, networks, and related key populations.

Catalyzing the next generation of treatment, care, and support involves universal antiretroviral (ARV) treatment access for all HIV-positive individuals who need medication (Box 25-3: Research for Evidence-Based Practice). UNAIDS (2011b) expects that all HIV-positive individuals and their families will have access to essential care and support. UNAIDS (2011b) will act with each nation to make it possible that simpler, more effective, and more affordable therapy will be universally accessible so that HIV deaths related to tuberculosis (TB) infection will be minimized.

Advancing human rights and gender equality for the HIV response means working toward the day that gender inequality, violence against women and girls, and stigmatization and discrimination related to HIV will be eradicated (UNAIDS, 2011b). Punitive laws and practices against HIV-positive individuals need to be eliminated. UNAIDS (2011b) will work with each government to reinforce the rights of HIV-positive individuals and to better educate infected individuals about their rights. UNAIDS proposes to accelerate the full implementation of these goals within countries by building synergies with communities and other organizations.

BOX 25-3   RESEARCH FOR EVIDENCE-BASED PRACTICE

Abstract

Atazanavir (ATV/r) has been found to be an effective ARV medication for HIV-positive adults. However, because atazanavir is not always affordable, a prospective study was conducted among 84 Thai adults to examine if the effectiveness of atazanavir would be maintained when lowering the dosage from 300/100 mg to 200/100 mg once daily. After following participants for more than 60 weeks, results showed that adequate atazanavir plasma concentrations were found. Moreover, CD4 counts increased over time with no change for cholesterol, triglyceride, LDL, or HDL levels, whereas bilirubin levels decreased over time. These results suggest that a lower dose of atazanavir is still effective, safe, and economical. A future larger study using a randomized controlled trial will be helpful.

Data from Avihingsanon, A., Apornpong, R., Kerr, S. J., Ananworanich, J., & Ruxrungtham, K. (2010). Long-term efficacy and safety of low-dose ritonavir-boosted atazanavir (ATV/r) 200/100 mg in HIV-infected Thai patients. *Journal of International AIDS Society, 13*(Suppl/4), 60.

VIOLENCE

Violence can happen to individuals anywhere, regardless of gender, age, or nationality, and is among the leading causes of physical, sexual, reproductive, and mental health problems worldwide. Each year, violence has been estimated to cause the loss of 1.6 million lives globally. In addition, violence costs nations immeasurable amounts of money in terms of health care, law enforcement, and loss of productivity (WHO, 2011c). Many of these costs and harms are "hidden" and underestimated (WHO, 2010).

Definition of Violence

Violence is defined differently in different parts of the world, depending on people's beliefs and cultures. The definition proposed by WHO is used in this chapter. According to WHO (2012b), violence is defined as:

> *intentional use of physical force or power, threatened or actual, against oneself, another person, or against a group or community, that either results in or has a high likelihood of resulting in injury, death, psychological harm, maldevelopment or deprivation.*

In response to violence, WHO has proposed the four-step public health approach that includes the following steps: defining the problem; identifying risks and protective factors; devising and testing means of dealing with violence; and applying successful means on a large scale (CDC, 2012c). Successful response prevention of violence should be based on rigorous research and collaboration among health care professionals and other experts in areas such as epidemiology, criminology, education, and economics.

The CDC is an example of an organization in the United States that is applying the preceding four-step public health model. Activities, projects, and funding supported by the CDC are outlined below as an exemplar.

Defining the Problem

To understand the magnitude of violence in the United States, different data sources are needed. Such sources may include police reports, medical examiner files, vital records, medical charts, population-based surveys, and research results. Extrapolations of the data from these sources can help us to learn about violence frequencies, places, trends, and perpetrators. The CDC has provided funding to studies deemed to be helpful in defining violence problems. The National Violent Death Reporting System (NVDRS) is an example of a project funded by the CDC to ensure that timely, complete, and accurate data are collected about violent deaths for different states in the United States. It is hoped that the data will enable each state to gain a clearer picture of violence in order to respond more effectively (CDC, 2012c).

Identifying Risk and Protective Factors

A "risk factor" is defined as "a characteristic that increases the likelihood of a person becoming a victim or perpetrator of violence," and a "protective factor" as "a characteristic that decreases the likelihood of a person becoming a victim or perpetrator of violence" (CDC, 2012c). Knowing risk and protective factors can help responsible organizations and personnel to estimate violence magnitudes and devise appropriate prevention measures. It is important to note that the identification of risk factors should not be used to blame victims of violence, but rather as a focus for intervention.

Devising and Testing Means for Dealing with Violence

In this step, data on violence from all available sources are extrapolated and assessed. Based on the evidence, programs and interventions are planned. Such programs and interventions are then implemented, tested, and rigorously evaluated to determine their effectiveness. An example of step 3 activities is the *Choose Respect* project—a communication initiative for sixth- to eighth-grade students to guide adolescents in forming healthy relationships in order to prevent dating violence (CDC, 2012c).

Applying Successful Means on a Large Scale

After a program has been tested successfully for its effectiveness, large-scale dissemination should be provided. At this stage, communities are encouraged to adopt a program tailored to their own problems and needs. An evaluation of the program should be performed in each community. Training, networking, technical assistance, and process evaluations are to be supported by all involved parties. An example of step 4 activities initiated by the CDC is the National Youth Violence Prevention Resource Center with its goal to prevent youth violence and suicide. In this project, a website, toll-free hotline, and fax-on-demand service were created as helpful resources for youth. Any interested community can request more information from the CDC.

Forms and Context of Violence

WHO (2012c) classifies violence into three major categories: interpersonal, self-directed, and collective.

Interpersonal Violence (IPV)

Interpersonal violence is violence committed by an individual or a small group of people in a wide range of acts and behaviors (emotional, physical, sexual, and psychological). The violence could happen to people of any age (adolescents, children, and older adults). It could also occur anywhere, including the home, workplace, neighborhood, and unfamiliar places.

Whereas violence in the community (e.g., youth violence or crimes) is highly visible, violence in the home is usually hidden. The impact of such hidden violence is complicated by the fact that authorities or health personnel are less willing or prepared to deal with it (WHO, 2010).

Risk factors for IPV may include a victim's low self-esteem, low self-control, and personality/conduct disorders (Fowler & Westen, 2011; Peralta et al., 2010). Other risk factors are reported to be lack of social support, dysfunctional family structure, family history of violence, and drug and alcohol abuse (Clements & Schumacher, 2010; Fowler & Westen, 2011; Ross, 2012). Alcohol intoxication may increase violent actions by impairing the drinker's cognitive functions and processes through alterations of social cue perceptions and inhibitions (Clements & Schumacher, 2010). Also, three subtypes of male perpetrators are reported as psychopathic, hostile/controlling, and borderline/dependent (Fowler & Westen, 2011). Psychopathic male perpetrators are likely to have a history of violent behavior in all types of relationships, starting in childhood. Hostile/controlling male perpetrators tend to anger easily and are hypersensitive to criticism, blame others, and hold grudges. Borderline/dependent male perpetrators tend to be depressed, need emotional support from their partners, and become out of control when stress builds beyond a given point (Fowler & Westen, 2011).

Mothers who are victims of violence along with their children who witness such violence are at risk for physical, emotional, psychological, and developmental damage (Meyer, 2010). A study in Finland revealed that female victims of violence tended to seek treatment at the emergency department at least once a month (Leppäkoski et al., 2010). In Australia, help-seeking action is increased among abused women whose children witnessed the abuse in order to protect their children from further harm (Meyer, 2010).

Culture and gender inequality are also significant factors of IPV. Evidence shows that women in countries where gender equality is emphasized experience violence less than those in countries with gender inequality (Kaya & Cook, 2010). Kaya and Cook reported that the highest rates of physical violence among women were found in Zambia (27%) and Kenya (24%), whereas the rate of 1% was reported in Denmark, Hong Kong, Switzerland, and the United States (Kaya & Cook, 2010).

Gender equality in Ghana, as shown by equal household contributions to decision-making, is related to a low acceptance of abuse toward women (Mann & Takyi, 2009). A study among 245 obstetric/gynecological (OB/GYN) patients in Thailand revealed that the rate for emotional abuse was at 88.2%, physical abuse at 59.2%, and sexual abuse at 23.9% (Ross, 2012). Predictors of emotional abuse included partner's drug use and gambling behavior. The predictor of physical abuse was drug abuse. No predictor was found for sexual abuse. Violence in this study was found to be associated with depression and physical problems (Ross, 2012). This result aligns with a study of more than 6000 women in Canada, which revealed that women who were abused reported higher rates of postpartum depression than those who did not experience abuse (Beydoun et al., 2010). Social support was found to mediate the effects of IPV on depression and physical health in the Thai study (Ross, 2012).

It is important for health care providers to understand the seriously negative impact that interpersonal violence can have on individuals. They should be able to identify such violence and be aware of helpful resources for persons affected by violence as well as their children. Local domestic violence crisis contact information (i.e., numbers and counseling services) should be readily provided to these persons. A sexual violence assessment and care guide as proposed by Ross and colleagues (2009b) is a helpful resource for health care professionals who work with care recipients of OB/GYN services, especially for those who feel uncomfortable mentioning the subject (Ross et al., 2010).

Self-Directed Violence

Self-directed violence is defined by WHO (2012c) as "violence in which the perpetrator and the victim are the same individual and is subdivided into self-abuse and suicide." It is estimated that almost 1 million individuals die from suicide (a person commits suicide every 40 seconds) (WHO, 2012d). Previously, suicide rates had been highest among the male older adult. However, rates among young people ages 15 to 24 have been increasing to such an extent that suicide is the second leading cause of death in this age group in some developed and developing countries (WHO, 2012d). Although major factors contributing to suicide in Europe and North America include mental disorders, especially depression, and alcohol use disorders, impulsiveness is found to be a major factor in Asian countries (WHO, 2012e).

WHO (2012f) recommends that effective suicide prevention interventions should include restriction of access to common methods of suicide where possible or when prudent, along with effective prevention and treatment of depression and alcohol and substance abuse. However, there are clearly challenges to such interventions. In many countries, for example, a lack of awareness about suicide and the taboo to discuss suicide openly exist. Many countries will need to initiate training for prevention of suicide, including appropriate certification for health care personnel, and to seek the involvement of individuals from sectors other than health care, including education, labor, law, politics, police, justice, religion, and the media.

Collective Violence

Collective violence is defined as the instrumental use of violence by a particular group of people for specific political, economic, or social objectives. Such violence may include armed conflicts within or between states or nations, genocide, terrorism, repression, and other abuses of human rights (WHO, 2012d) (Figure 25-3).

In the twentieth century, it is estimated that 191 million people lost their lives as a result of armed conflict. More than half of these people were civilians. In the year 2000, more than 300,000 people died because of collective violence. The majority of victims lived in the poorer regions of the world (WHO, 2012d). Besides death, the aftermath of collective violence includes physical and

FIGURE 25-3 Armed conflicts can be within or between states and nations.

FIGURE 25-4 The need to be able to respond to terrorism poses important challenges to all.

psychological disabilities that exert burdens on families, communities, and nations. Young children and refugees are usually among the most vulnerable to the aftermaths of disease and posttraumatic stress disorders related to violence (WHO, 2012c).

WHO (2012c) is committed to working with its partners at the regional, national, and international levels to prevent collective violence. Its goal is to identify and implement preventive strategies. Data collection systems are used to support and evaluate the success of their strategies. In this effort, political commitment and momentum are required from a wide variety of concerned parties to strengthen and increase violence prevention endeavors in the next 5 years (WHO, 2012c).

TERRORISM

The threat of terrorism—whether homegrown or international— creates a unique brand of fear among individuals and communities within our increasingly interconnected global cultures (Napoleoni, 2010). Moreover, the need to be able to respond to terrorism—potential or actual— poses important challenges to health care professionals and community planners at all levels of our society (Figure 25-4). The International Council for Nurses

(ICN) describes its position on the role of nursing concerning disaster preparedness to include risk assessment as well as management strategies bridging multiple disciplines and system levels.

Nursing plays a key role in responding to short-, medium-, and long-term requirements of populations stricken by disaster. To coordinate health sector preparedness, regulatory meetings and frameworks across cultures will help nurses plan for and streamline health care responses to such mass events internationally (Welner, 2011). Much work in laying the foundations for such a broader, more global preparedness has already been started.

Research on the surgical responses to the 2008 terrorist attacks in Mumbai, India, reveals the importance of an initial disaster management plan to treat casualties. The earliest victims of firearm and blast trauma were received in a primary triage zone and then sent to different stations for further treatment. The study concluded that onsite triage—established as soon as a site is found to be safe—optimizes the treatment of bullet and blast injuries (Bhandarwar et al., 2011). Another study examined the effectiveness of including a pediatric trauma center (PTC) in responding to victims of a disaster surge. This study added a hypothetical PTC to the response of the Israeli Defense Forces field hospital to the Haiti earthquake in 2010 and measured its effectiveness mathematically, concluding that "aggressive inclusion of PTCs in planning for disasters by public health agencies" (Barthel et al., 2011, p. 1) can significantly increase overall rates of admission and greatly reduce treatment times (Barthel et al., 2011). Regarding the responses of health care providers to the repercussions of mass disasters, results from the literature are sometimes conflicting. In the United Sates, studies among victims of the World Trade Center disaster (WTCD) in terms of post-traumatic stress disorder (PTSD) suggest that early and brief interventions at the worksite were most effective in responding to PTSD, and that informal support from family, friends, and spiritual communities was also beneficial. Conversely, more extensive post-disaster psychotherapy was not found to be beneficial and sometimes led to worse outcomes (Boscarino & Adams, 2008). Mental resilience following the WTCD tended to be linked with victims who had higher self-esteem and more social support, while victims who experienced "delayed" PTSD following the attacks tended to be "non-native born, or to have recently experienced lower self-esteem and/or negative life events" (Boscarino, 2011). In Thailand, cognitive-behavioral therapy (CBT) as a means to treat PTSD was studied in a randomized controlled effectiveness trial. The researchers found that CBT can successfully treat PTSD, even "in settings where very regular [terrorist] attacks are made upon communities in which the patient lives" (Bryant et al., 2011).

Among its overarching influences, one must also weigh terrorism's negative consequences for economies around the world. These include changes in "variables such as Gross Domestic Product (GDP), unemployment, foreign direct investment (FDI), and the tourism industry" (Waxman, 2011). Such economic changes affect the lives of everyday people and, in turn, their health. The threat of terrorism is thus real, and its actual and potential negative effects are pervasive and far reaching, spanning cultures and ranging from the concrete and immediate to the psychosocial and lasting. Nurses and health care professionals must be among the front lines of response.

Bioterrorism

A bioterrorism attack is the deliberate release of viruses, bacteria, or other germs (agents) used to cause illness or death in people, animals, or plants. These agents are typically found in nature, but it is possible that they could be changed to increase their ability to cause disease, make them resistant to current medicines, or to increase their ability to be spread into the environment. Biological agents can be spread through the air, through water, or in food. Terrorists may use biological agents because they can be extremely difficult to detect and do not cause illness for several hours to several days. Some bioterrorism agents, like the smallpox virus, can be spread from person to person and some, like anthrax, cannot.

(CDC, 2012d)

The preceding definition reflects what many people in different nations may feel or know about bioterrorism. As health care professionals, we are required to be knowledgeable about possible diseases/agents that could be used for bioterrorism and the proper responses we should take to an act of bioterrorism.

Bioterrorism is classified by the CDC (2012d) into three different categories: A, B, and C. These categories are based on the ease with which the disease or agent might be spread; the potential negative impact it could have on public health; the extent to which it could cause public panic or social disruption; and the degree to which it would require the public to prepare for an attack.

Category A Diseases/Agents

Category A diseases/agents include various biological agents and pathogens that are not usually seen in the United States and pose the highest risks and priority. They include anthrax, botulism, plague, smallpox, tularemia, and viral hemorrhagic fevers.

Anthrax (Bacillus anthracis). Since the anthrax (*Bacillus anthracis*) mailing attacks to a few recipients in the United States in 2001, no other attacks have been reported (CDC, 2012e). These unfortunate mail recipients contracted the bacillus either cutaneously or inhalationally. Cutaneous anthrax contractors developed erythema (red, inflamed area similar to cellulitis) on exposed areas of the hands, arms, or face that later transformed into painful vesicles and then necrotic painless, depressed, black eschar. Inhalation contractors had fever, dyspnea, cough, and chest discomfort (CDC, 2012e). Usually, respiratory failure and hemodynamic collapse will follow. Other symptoms may include lymphangitis and painful lymphadenopathy. It is recommended that persons receive a complete treatment of ciprofloxacin, levofloxacin, doxycycline, or penicillin for 60 days (CDC, 2012e). Vaccines against anthrax have been developed and evidence shows that they can be effective in preventing the disease (Chitlaru et al., 2011). The CDC (2012f) and its partners are working collaboratively to develop more effective anthrax vaccines. Questions and answers about anthrax vaccines can be found at www.bt.cdc.gov/agent/anthrax/faq/vaccination.asp.

Smallpox *(Variola major).* It is believed that smallpox *(Variola major)* was eradicated in 1977. However, there are fears that a strain kept in a laboratory could be used as a bioweapon. According to the CDC (2012g), however, the United States has enough vaccines for everyone if needed. Side effects from smallpox vaccination mostly involve a low fever, soreness in the injection area, and enlarged glands in the armpit (CDC, 2012h). In rare circumstances, severe side effects may occur and need medical attention. Follow this link to learn more about potentially serious and life-threatening side effects: www.bt.cdc.gov/agent/smallpox/vaccination/reactions-vacc-public.asp.

Smallpox symptoms usually resemble influenza symptoms, which include fever and myalgias, followed by a rash. Rashes in smallpox can be differentiated from those of chickenpox (varicella). A rash from smallpox is most prominent on the face and extremities with the same stage of lesion development. A rash of chickenpox is more prominent on the trunk, with different stages of lesion development and resolution. The CDC (2012i) provides an acute, generalized vesicular or pustular rash illness testing protocol in the United States: www.bt.cdc.gov/agent/smallpox/diagnosis/pdf/poxalgorithm1-5-12.pdf. The CDC also provides an online assessment of a rash as a way to identify whether or not the rash is an indicator of a smallpox infection: www.bt.cdc.gov/agent/smallpox/diagnosis/riskalgorithm/.

Category B Diseases/Agents

Category B diseases/agents are those that pose the second highest risks for world and national security. They include brucellosis; food safety threats (e.g., *Salmonella* sp., *Escherichia coli* O157:H7, *Shigella*); glanders; melioidosis; psittacosis; Q fever; ricin toxin; staphylococcal enterotoxin B; typhus fever; viral encephalitis; and water safety threats (e.g., *Vibrio cholerae*, *Cryptosporidium parvum*).

Category C Diseases/Agents

Category C diseases/agents are emerging pathogens that could be reproduced for mass dissemination. They include emerging infectious diseases such as Nipah virus and hantavirus.

Epidemic and Pandemic Alert and Response (EPR)

The CDC created a public health emergency response guide to help public health professionals at the state, local, and tribal levels respond to an emergency in the first 24 hours. Health care providers should be alerted to any unusual symptoms indicative of infectious outbreak related to bioterrorism. In turn, if a bioterrorist action is suspected, health care providers should report it to their local or state health department. According to the CDC (2011b), indications of bioterrorism include "an unusual temporal or geographic clustering of illness (e.g., persons who attended the same public event or gathering) or individuals presenting with clinical signs and symptoms that suggest an infectious disease outbreak (e.g., more than two persons presenting with an unexplained febrile illness associated with sepsis, pneumonia, respiratory failure, or rash or a botulism-like syndrome with flaccid muscle paralysis, especially if

occurring in otherwise healthy persons); an unusual age distribution for common diseases (e.g., an increase in what appears to be a chickenpox-like illness among adult persons, but which might be smallpox); and a large number of cases of acute flaccid paralysis with prominent bulbar palsies, suggestive of a release of *botulinum* toxin." To learn more about clinical diagnosis, management, and responses to bioterrorism, refer to the CDC website available at www.bt.cdc.gov and www.cdc.gov/mmwr/preview/mmwrhtml/mm5041a2.htm.

At the international level, responses to bioterrorism also have been prepared. WHO is a core organization responding to needs for such preparation at this level. WHO works collaboratively with agencies in many countries to gather reports of suspected outbreaks and rumors regarding bioterrorism through advanced technologies from all sources available, both formally and informally.

The Global Public Health Intelligence Network (GPHIN), a significant source of informal information related to outbreaks, was also collaboratively established by Health Canada and WHO. Its multilingual capabilities are Internet-based, constantly searching data worldwide to identify information regarding disease outbreaks that can place international public health sectors at risk (WHO, 2012g).

The 2005 *International Health Regulations* (IHR)—legally-binding regulations across countries led by WHO—are embraced by most nations throughout the world. IHR's mission is to provide legal frameworks to ensure health security among nations without unnecessary international traffic and trade interference (WHO, 2012h). To learn more about *International Health Regulations*, go to www.who.int/features/qa/39/en/index.html.

NATURAL DISASTERS

Natural disasters have existed since the earth was formed. They are phenomena that occur through natural forces involving land, air, or water, and they often have large-scale negative impacts on humans who live in the affected areas. Examples of natural disasters include tsunamis, earthquakes, floods, landslides, mudslides, tornadoes, hurricanes, cyclones, typhoons, wildfires, volcano eruptions, extreme heat, winter weather, and others (CDC, 2012j). Natural disasters in recent decades have been reported to cause more harm in developing countries than developed countries, attributable in part to deforestation and inadequate warning and emergency management systems (Kar, 2009). Health care professionals should be aware of recent large-scale natural disasters and familiar with their negative impact on human well-being. Critically, lessons learned from the successful or unsuccessful management of these disasters should be shared among health care professionals in order to appropriately address and minimize the effects of future disasters.

Effects of Natural Disasters on Human Well-Being

All humans are affected by natural disasters economically, physically, and psychologically. In 2011, a record $366 billion in economic losses included $210 billion resulting from the earthquake/tsunami in Japan and $40 billion attributable to flooding in Thailand. Overall in 2011, approximately 200 million people suffered the effects of at least 300 human-impact disasters. These included approximately 105 million people who endured the effects of flooding. Additionally, more than 60 million humans were affected by drought conditions and more than 30 million suffered tropical storms. More than 29,000 deaths resulted from 302 major disaster events in 2011, including almost 20,000 deaths from Japan's earthquake/tsunami in March of that year (United Nation International Strategy for Disaster Reduction [UNISDR], 2011).

Concerning the physical effects of natural disasters, victims tend to have limited access to essential infrastructures for survival related to food, water, shelter, and sanitation. These deficiencies can lead to infections and undernutrition (Bae et al., 2009; Burkle et al., 2011; Gribble & Berry, 2011; Kouadio et al., 2012; Sri-Aroon et al., 2010). Undernutrition, in turn, can lead to malnutrition and starvation—especially among infants and children in low-resource countries (Burkle et al., 2011). Infection outbreaks commonly diagnosed after natural disasters during the period 2000 to 2011 include, for example, diarrhea, acute respiratory tract infections, viral hepatitis, and snail and trematode infections (Kouadio et al., 2012; Sri-Aroon et al., 2010).

In terms of the psychological impact of natural disasters, post-traumatic stress disorder (PTSD) is a classic negative effect that occurs among victims of all ages. For instance, a survey of 1615 Thai students who experienced the 2004 tsunami showed that 6 weeks after the event 57.3% of these students reported symptoms for PTSD, and more than 2% of the students continued to have PTSD symptoms at the end of the fifth year after the event (Piyasil et al., 2011). A case-control study reported that 1463 Swedes who experienced a tsunami reported more psychological distress than those who had no such experience (Wahlstrom et al., 2009). Research results among 63 Norwegians who experienced the 2004 tsunami while visiting Thailand showed that 30.2% of the participants reported specific phobia, 17.5% agoraphobia, and 11.1% each for social anxiety disorder, PTSD, and major depressive disorder (Hussain et al., 2011). In conclusion, psychological trauma has been reported as a result of natural disasters regardless of age or country of residence.

Natural Disaster Responses and Preparedness

In general, emergency care for victims of natural disasters, especially for children and women, is reported to be inadequate regardless of the country type (Burkle et al., 2011; Rose et al., 2011). However, the inadequacy of emergency care is heightened in developing nations (Burkle et al., 2011). For example, with the 2010 earthquake in Haiti, more than 200,000 people lost their lives with 1.5 million people losing shelter (Rose et al., 2011). As the poorest country in the Western world, Haiti already had limited resources before the earthquake. As many as 40% of rural Haitians did not have access to primary health care before the disaster, and 70% of health provisions in Haiti overall before the disaster were offered by nongovernmental organizations (Rose et al., 2011). While psychiatric mental health needs surged after the earthquake, existing mental health services in Haiti were damaged by the two crumpled understaffed psychiatric hospitals as a consequence of the earthquake. The psychiatrist to person ratio was 0.2 to 100,000 before the earthquake, and this ratio only became worse when some health care workers were among the injured (Rose et al., 2011). *Vodou*, a common belief about magic and illness in Haiti, is deemed by some to function as the main Haitian health care system (Vonarx, 2011). *Vodou* beliefs might be considered by some professionals as a hindrance to modern mental health acquisition. Yet, evidence shows that if a strong collaboration is established between traditional healers and health care providers, mental health services can be enhanced in the process (Khoury et al., 2012).

International Standard Guidelines for Emergency Mental Health Response

Before 2007, there was a lack of consensual international guidelines for emergency mental health response (Burkle et al., 2011). However, after the Asian tsunami in 2004, a taskforce was established composed of both governmental and nongovernmental experts from more than 100 various organizations and 27 different countries (Burkle et al., 2011). This taskforce, Inter-Agency Standing Committee (IASC), developed the 2007 *IASC Guidelines on Mental Health and Psychosocial Support in Emergency Settings,* reflecting standards for appropriate emergency mental health care for victims around the world (Burkle et al., 2011). The *IASC Guidelines* are consistent with the WHO's recommendations for emergency among developing nations in that all victims and affected families should have access to emergency assistance with equality and dignity, and that helping people to remain resilient after a disaster is important. Besides these general principles, the minimum response for primary care clinics to help victims with severe psychological needs is outlined by the IASC and includes 10 major tenets (Burkle et al., 2011):

- Each victim is assessed holistically.
- Each victim will have access to essential psychiatric drugs.
- At least one emergency primary health care (PHC) professional is available to tend to victims' mental health in the affected area.
- The care provided by the PHC professional is adequately supervised.
- PHC professionals will be assigned to specific trainings and not be overwhelmed by unnecessary training sessions.
- Additional mental health service points will be established for victims' accessibility.
- Unnecessary duplicating services should be avoided.
- All people affected by a disaster are informed about available mental health services.
- Primary care clinics should work collaboratively with local community agencies to discover, visit, and help the target population.
- Primary care clinics should have a major role in collaboration with other mental health agencies.

To learn more about the IASC's guidelines and related work, the reader can log onto www.humanitarianinfo.org/iasc/pageloader.aspx?page=content-subsidi-tf_mhps-default.

Emergency Management for Infants in Developed Countries

Most infants in developing countries are breastfed. Thus, when natural disasters occur they tend to do better than infants in developed countries because their mothers have mobile fresh milk supplies for them as long as they are with their mothers during the disaster (Gribble & Berry, 2011). Likewise, infants in developed countries whose primary food is based on formula feeding can be vulnerable because of a lack of supplies during a disaster (Gribble & Berry, 2011). Therefore, emergency preparedness for these infants should be in place. In general, it is recommended that a week's supply of necessary items is available for infants. For exclusively breastfed infants, 100 diapers and 200 wipes are the only needed items. For bottle-fed infants, more items are recommended for their survival (Gribble & Berry, 2011). Mothers of infants with ready-to-use formula will need the following items: 56 single serves of the formula, 84 liters of drinking water, 56 feeding bottles or cups, 56 zip-lock plastic bags, a large storage container, a small bowl, a metal knife, 120 antiseptic wipes, detergent, 200 sheets of paper towels, 100 diapers, and 200 wipes (Gribble & Berry, 2011). Mothers of infants with powdered infant formula will need the following items: 2 cans of infant formula, 170 liters of drinking water, a feeding cup, a large storage container, a measuring cup, a large cooking pot with a lid, a kettle, a gas stove, a box of matches/lighters, 14 kilograms of liquid cooking gas, a metal knife, a pair of metal tongs, 120 antiseptic wipes, detergent, 300 sheets of paper towels, 100 diapers, and 200 wipes (Gribble & Berry, 2011). Health care professionals who care for mothers with their infants should be trained to provide appropriate information to the mothers based on their feeding strategy. To learn more about the information provided by Gribble and Berry (2011), the reader can log onto www.internationalbreastfeedingjournal.com/content/pdf/1746-4358-6-16.pdf.

The Office of Public Health Preparedness and Response (OPHPR) also provides very helpful information about steps and types of emergency responses on a CDC (2012j) website. To learn more, interested readers should log onto www.bt.cdc.gov/hazards-all.asp.

IMPLICATIONS

The health-promotion and disease-prevention priorities that have been outlined in this chapter present challenges and opportunities for health care providers—as individuals and as a collective profession—to play key roles in emerging systems emphasizing health promotion and disease prevention. Goals for optimal health of individuals include greater longevity and quality of life, while decreasing gender, racial, and ethnic disparities (Purnell, 2008). The principles of primary prevention, health care policies, cultural diversity, cultural competency, and multidisciplinary teamwork in health promotion are critical to a new era that strives to achieve dramatic changes in health care delivery (Purnell, 2008). Through a perspective on the development of community-based, health-promotion programs, health

care professionals can bring a balance to decisions that will be made about the appropriate use of traditional and newer health care resources (Box 25-4: *Healthy People 2020*).

Ten **essential public health services** as proposed by the CDC (2010b) were developed in 1994 by the Core Public Health Functions Steering Committee, comprising representatives from various U.S. Public Health Service agencies and other key public health organizations. This framework can be instrumental for health care professionals in various fields and be applied at all levels, ranging from local to international. The 10 essentials include:

- Monitoring the health status of individuals and communities in order to address identified health problems
- Diagnosing and investigating health problems and health hazards among individuals in the community
- Informing, educating, and empowering people about health problems and various ways to address problems, including applying strengths found in the community
- Mobilizing community partnerships and community actions so that health problems can be identified and addressed
- Developing policies and plans that will assist individuals and their communities to address identified problems
- Enforcing laws and regulations to provide and protect the safety and health of individuals and communities
- Linking people to appropriate health services to ensure accessible health care
- Ensuring proficient personal and public health care workforces
- Evaluating the accessibility, effectiveness, and quality of health services
- Searching for innovative ideas and solutions to identified health problems

For more information about the 10 essentials, go to www.cdc.gov/nphpsp/essentialservices.html. These 10 essentials—along with an awareness of human rights, empowerment, cultural diversity, and cultural competence (Box 25-5: Diversity Awareness)—can help health care professionals effectively deliver care to individuals and communities. It is important, moreover, to help individuals, families, and communities become active participants in defining their own health needs, in making informed decisions to meet those needs, and, ultimately, in bringing about real improvements in their own health status and quality of life.

An increasing demand for primary health care providers will continue to spur the need for more advanced practice nurses, including nurses with degrees of Doctor of Nursing Practice and Doctor of Philosophy. This demand can be met if undergraduate students are introduced early to concepts of health promotion and disease prevention with an emphasis on evidence-based practice, human rights, cultural diversity, and cultural competency, and with a global perspective (Purnell, 2008). In this way, health promotion, quality of life, and socioeconomic justice might become increasingly valued in cultures throughout the world.

Also, health care educational programs in culturally diverse global frameworks that teach about malnutrition,

BOX 25-4 HEALTHY PEOPLE 2020

Topic Area: Genomics
- To increase the proportion of women with a family history of breast and/or ovarian cancer who receive genetic counseling. (In 2005, 23.3% of U.S. females with such a history obtained genetic counseling. The target for 2020 is 25.6%.)
- To increase the proportion of individuals with newly diagnosed colorectal cancer who receive genetic testing to identify Lynch syndrome (or familial colorectal cancer syndromes).

Topic Area: Global Health
- To reduce the number of cases of malaria reported in the United States. (In 2008, 1298 new cases of malaria were reported in the United States. The target for 2020 is 999 new cases.)
- To decrease the tuberculosis (TB) case rate for foreign-born individuals living in the United States. (In 2008, 20.2 cases of TB per 100,000 population were reported for foreign-born individuals living in the United States. The target for 2020 is 14.0 cases per 100,000 population.)
- To increase the number of Global Disease Detection Regional Centers (GDDRCs) worldwide to detect and contain emerging health threats. (In 2009, 7 GDDRCS were active. The target for 2020 is to have 13 active GDDRCs.)
- To increase the number of public health professionals (PHPs) trained by Global Disease Detection (GDD) programs worldwide. (In 2009, 37,132 PHPs were trained by GDD programs. The target is to have 144,132 trained by GDD programs.)
- To increase diagnostic testing capacity in host countries and regionally through the GDDRCs. (In 2009, 154 tests were established or substantially improved by GDD programs. The target for 2009 is 264 established/substantially improved tests.)

Topic Area: Health Care–Associated Infections
- To reduce central line–associated bloodstream infections (CLABSIs). (In 2006-2008, a Standardized Infection Ratio (SIR) of 1.00 was reported. The target for 2020 is 0.25 SIR or a 75% reduction.)
- To reduce invasive health care–associated methicillin-resistant *Staphylococcus aureus* (MRSA) infections. (In 2007-2008, 26.24 infections per 100,000 persons were reported. The target for 2020 is 6.56 infections per 100,000 persons or a 75% reduction. The target for 2020 is 27.5% after-action reports and improvement plans following responses to public health emergencies and exercises.) In 2009, 46 days were required for state public health agencies to establish such reports and plans. (The target for 2020 is 41 days.)

Topic Area: (Selected) Health Communication and Health IT
- To increase the proportion of individuals who report that their health care professional (HCP) always listened carefully to them. (In 2007, 59% of individuals reported that their HCP always listened carefully to them. The target for 2020 is 65%.)
- To increase the proportion of individuals who report that their HCP always explained things so they could understand them. (In 2007, 60% of individuals reported that their HCP always explained things so they could understand them. The target is 66%.)

- To increase the proportion of individuals who report that their health care professionals always involved them in decisions about their health care as much as they wanted. (In 2007, 51.6% of individuals reported that their health care professionals always involved them in decisions about their health care as much as they wanted. The target for 2020 is 56.8%.)
- To increase the proportion of individuals who use the Internet to keep track of personal health information, such as care received, test results, or upcoming medical appointments. (In 2007, 14.3% of persons reported using the Internet to keep track of personal health information, such as care received, test results, or upcoming medical appointments.)
- To increase the proportion of individuals who use the Internet to communicate with their provider. (In 2007, 13.6% of persons reported using the Internet to communicate with their provider. The target for 2020 is 15.0%.)
- To increase the proportion of individuals with access to the Internet. (In 2007, 68.5% of individuals reported having access to the Internet. The target for 2020 is 75.4%.)
- To increase the proportion of individuals with broadband access to the Internet. (In 2007, 75.6% of individuals reported having broadband access to the Internet. The target for 2020 is 83.2%.)
- To increase the proportion of individuals who use mobile devices. (In 2007, 6.7% of individuals reported using mobile devices. The target for 2020 is 7.7%.)
- To increase the proportion of adults who report having friends or family members whom they talk with about their health. (In 2007, 79.5% of adults reported having friends or family members that they talk to about their health. The target for 2020 is 87.5%.)
- To increase the proportion of online health information seekers who report easily accessing health information. (In 2007, 37.3% of online health information seekers reported easily accessing health information. The target for 2020 is 41.0%.)
- To increase the proportion of medical practices that use electronic health records. (In 2007, 25.0% of medical practices reported using electronic health records. The target for 2020 is 27.5%.)

Topic Area: Selected Preparedness
- To reduce the time necessary to activate designated personnel in response to a public health emergency. (In 2009, 66 minutes were needed for designated personnel to report for immediate duty with no advance notice. The target for 2020 is 60 minutes.)
- To increase the proportion of Laboratory Response Network (LRN) biological laboratories that meet proficiency standards for Category A and B threat agents.
- To increase the proportion of LRN chemical laboratories that meet proficiency standards for chemical threat agents. (In 2008, 92% of LRN chemical laboratories met proficiency standards for chemical threat agents. The target for 2020 is 95%.)
- To reduce the time for state public health agencies to establish after-action reports and improvement plans following responses to public health emergencies and exercises. (In 2009, 46 days were required for state public health agencies to establish such reports and plans. The target for 2020 is 41 days.)

From U.S. Department of Health and Human Services. (2010). *Healthy People 2020.* Washington, DC: U.S. Government Printing Office.

emerging diseases, HIV/AIDS, bioterrorism, violence, and other contemporary challenges will help nurses and other professionals play innovative roles in health care and maximize the quality of life around the world. Faculty and students will ideally increase their work together in interdisciplinary teams, using an expanding variety of health-promotion services and guided by national and international standards. Given the increasing focus on cultural diversity and self-care in disease prevention and health promotion, nurses can respond directly to the health needs of individuals, families, communities, and groups by focusing on health promotion and disease prevention tailored to particular cultures and spiritual beliefs and by supporting new ways to work and live.

In the area of research, understanding health care practices and the impact of culture on people from different nations will enable health care professionals to create appropriate health-promotion and disease-prevention interventions. Thus, international collaborative research is important. Gender Age Disaggregated Data (GADD) quantitative and qualitative analysis needs to be used more widely in research so that data can be categorized by gender and age/age group, which will allow for examination and identification of needs that are specific to each gender and age group (Mazurana et al., 2011). GADD could be especially beneficial in the assessment of crisis situations such as bioterrorism and terrorism because it helps to identify the immediate needs of particular groups, the reasons they need immediate help, and the resources that can be most helpful (Inter-Agency Standing Committee Gender Sub-Working Group, 2009).

To be advocates for newly emerging priorities for disease prevention and health promotion, nurses in the twenty-first century need to engage in the following:

- Participate in policy development for health promotion as the health care of individuals in acute settings shifts from hospitals to home and community settings. Thus the attention to health-promoting behaviors in home and community environments provides an entry point for the development of models of primary care that emphasize both health promotion and disease prevention in communities.
- Influence public expectations about health promotion. Presentations and other forms of public dialogue and

---

BOX 25-5 DIVERSITY AWARENESS

Health and Health Promotion in a Native American Tribe: The Navajo

The Navajo people of the *Dine' Bike'yah* live on a vast land in which the four states of Arizona, Utah, New Mexico, and Colorado intersect. The *Dine'* hold this land as sacred and as an integral part of their lives. The Navajo believe that health is a part of the *Hozho'*, which is a personal sense of well-being and rightness with the world and is all-inclusive. For the Navajo, health is not separate from the overall state of balance among the body, mind, spirit, and the surrounding environment. When one of these is out of balance, *Hozho'* is not achieved. *Hozho'* is everything that a Navajo thinks of as being good, in terms of good and evil or favorable and unfavorable. The Navajo strive to maintain *Hozho'* and to live in harmony with all things that surround them. The goal of Navajo life in this world is to live to attain maturity with *Hozho'* and to die of old age, the result of which incorporates beauty, harmony, and happiness or *sa'ah naagh"ii bik'eh*

hozho'. When the body, spirit, or mind fall out of *Hozho'*, a traditional healer or medicine man is sought. In many instances, the medicine man recommends that the individual seek both Western medicine and the traditional ways to cure the problem.

Since 1955, trends in Navajo health have demonstrated a progressive improvement, particularly in the areas of maternal and infant mortality. However, on the increase are lifestyle-related diseases and premature deaths for which health-promotion activities can have an effect. Among these lifestyle-related diseases are adult-onset diabetes, AIDS, and alcohol and substance abuse. Health care providers who work with the Navajo must address all health-promotion and disease-prevention activities in terms of an appreciation for the cultural and economic realities and the needs of this community.

Compiled from Anonymous. (n.d.). *Navajo land.* Retrieved June 4, 2008, from www.discovernavap.comlculture.html; The Official Navajo Nation Visitor Guide. (2002). *Navajo cultural history and legends.*

BOX 25-6 INNOVATIVE PRACTICE

Haitian Health Foundation: A Charitable Outreach to Neighbors in Need

A volunteer effort of health professionals initiated in Haiti in 1982 by Dr. Jeremiah Lowney and his wife, Virginia, has grown into an outpatient health care facility supported by a nondenominational foundation called the Haitian Health Foundation, Inc. (HHF). In 1985, after working for 4 years in Port au Prince, HHF moved its outreach to Jeremie, Haiti, at the suggestion of Mother Teresa of Calcutta, to bring health care, hope, and opportunity to this especially poor and remote area. The clinic at Jeremie employs 105 people, including 2 full-time physicians, 1 full-time dentist, 10 registered nurses, 2 licensed professional nurses, a medical technician, a dental assistant, and 70 to 80 auxiliary personnel (all Haitians). The clinic provides health care to 350 to 400 Haitians daily.

The Haitian Agents de Sante program currently employs villagers in 936 villages surrounding Jeremie. This program was initiated by a nurse who enlisted an individual who had a seventh-grade education in each village. After being educated in health promotion, the person became the Health Agent of that village. These Health Agents are trained by HHF to provide preventive and basic health care and education. Many villages have also begun mothers' groups, by which women can share experiences and knowledge relating to nutrition, health care, and other topics that have an effect on their quality of life. Breastfeeding classes and immunization programs are available.

Another program was begun by building a food distribution pavilion. This building will be used to store and distribute food to more than 1000 children and pregnant women 3 times a week. The pavilion will also be used to educate participants in nutrition and preventive health care. Much of the education in these programs is accomplished through song, primarily because this approach appears to enable the Haitians to remember what is being taught.

For more than 8 years, another education program has provided access to schools for poor children in a country in which education is neither free nor mandatory. As of 2004, 1250 students were attending school through this program. Tuition, uniforms, books, and shoes are provided by HHF funds or through the Save-a-Family Program.

The HHF relies heavily on the generosity of donors and the many volunteers who donate their time and talents to supplement the staff in Haiti. Volunteers travel to Jeremie at their own expense from America, Canada, and Europe to share their skills and resources with the poor. These volunteers include health care providers, electricians, plumbers, teachers, clergy, and students.

These programs are only a few examples of the health-promotion programs sponsored by the HHF. These efforts show how dedicated professionals can make a difference, even in third-world countries in which health care resources are rare.

Courtesy Jeremiah Lowney, MD, MPH.

education will help raise awareness of the value of individual and community health promotion. Nurses have the collective capacity to change the philosophy of the system from selling health care in the marketplace to creating a milieu for changing health behaviors. Encouraging meaningful community participation in addressing health issues provides a significant opportunity to narrow the gap between what is possible in terms of health promotion in each country and what is reality. As mentioned earlier, violence and emerging diseases are among the challenges today that require heightened public awareness.

- Promote equitable access to preventive health care. Given the higher rates of preventable conditions among populations in resource-poor countries, a need to promote the justified distribution and utilization of preventive health services is apparent. Community-based efforts that combine public and private resources should be targeted to those most in need of health care. Delivery models that focus on integrating preventive and primary care should be expanded.

Preventive health care delivery should be based on broad research agendas that encompass multiple health and social science perspectives. Health care providers should participate in areas of research that will cost-effectively influence both personal and community health. Service delivery can also benefit from expanded health service research agendas that foster collaboration among disciplines and countries. Most important, preventive health care should be adapted to the health and social problems of specific groups and cultures. Alternate approaches to health-promotion and preventive service delivery should be used where most effective to meet new international health challenges, including mobile vans, school and worksite clinics, and other community-based, collaborative actions (Box 25-6: Innovative Practice).

CASE STUDY

Nutrition: Don

Don is a 4-year-old boy who is brought to a rural health department clinic by his grandmother. Don and his family are recent immigrants from Laos and have lived in this area for less than a year. This is Don's first visit to the clinic. Don looks weak with sunken eyes and dry mouth. His weight is less than 70% (or <3 standard deviations) of the median weight-for-height with underdeveloped buttocks, thighs, and upper arms. Through a translator, Don's grandmother tells the community health nurse that Don has had diarrhea for more than 2 days and that the family can barely "make ends meet." Don's parents are seasonal farm workers and are at work today.

Reflective Questions

1. Don's grandmother is his caretaker during the day.
2. How can the nurse help Don's family learn about the resources available in their community?
3. Where does the nurse direct Don's family for immediate help?
4. How would the nurse follow-up with the family to prevent further problems with this child?

CARE PLAN

Nutrition: Don

***NURSING DIAGNOSIS: Imbalanced Nutrition—Less than body requirement related to inadequate food intake and diarrhea as evidenced by the weight of less than 70% (or <3 standard deviations) of the median weight-for-height; underdeveloped buttocks, thighs, and upper arms; and sunken eyes and dry mouth**

Defining Characteristics
- A weight of less than 70% (or <3 standard deviations) of the median weight-for-height
- Underdeveloped buttocks, thighs, and upper arms
- Sunken eyes, dry mouth, and a history of diarrhea

Related Factors
- Poverty, lack of knowledge about available resources

Short-Term Expected Outcomes
Grandmother will:
- Increase health-promotion and health-maintenance knowledge regarding Don's nutrition
- Increase health-promotion and health-maintenance practices regarding Don's nutrition

- Gain access to available resources, such as Food Stamps and the Women, Infants, and Children Program

Long-Term Expected Outcome
- Don will show no sign of malnutrition.

Interventions
- Give Don fluids/food per protocol.
- Observe Don's fluids/food intake and monitor his signs and symptoms.
- If necessary, refer Don to an appropriate health setting.
- Assess grandmother's knowledge and practices about Don's nutrition.
- Educate grandmother about negative effects of malnutrition on Don's growth and development.
- Educate grandmother about appropriate food choices for Don.
- Assist family to access and connect with available nutrition community resources.
- Assist Don's parents to access community career center.
- Provide for follow-ups to monitor Don's physical progress (body weight for age and height) and family's access to available resources.

*NANDA Nursing Diagnoses—Definitions and Classification 2012-2014, Herdman T.H. (ED). Copyright © 2012, 1994-2012 NANDA International. Used by arrangement with John Wiley & Sons Limited. In order to make safe and effective judgments using the NANDA-I nursing diagnoses it is essential that nurses refer to the definitions and defining characteristics of the diagnoses listed in this work.

SUMMARY

This chapter has presented priority issues and future directions for health professions in the areas of health promotion and disease prevention from a world perspective. Current emerging health care reform efforts pose significant challenges and opportunities for health care providers, educators, and researchers with the emphasis on human rights, cultural diversity, and cultural sensitivity; health promotion and disease prevention; evidence-based practice and advanced technology; and global perspectives. Nurses in the new millennium are required to have sufficient vision, expertise, and the ability to truly make a difference in the health of the persons for whom they care at the individual, local community, national, and international levels. Through leadership, creativity, and determination, nurses and other health care providers can establish a healthier future for people around the globe with a respect for human needs, cultural diversity, and human rights.

REFERENCES

Amirkhanian, Y. A., et al. (2010). Male labor migrants in Russia: HIV risk behavior levels, contextual factors, and prevention needs. *Journal of Immigrant Minority Health, 13*, 918–928.

AVERT. (2012). *Understanding HIV and AIDS statistics.* Retrieved from www.avert.org/statistics.htm.

Avihingsanon, A., Apornpong, R., Kerr, S. J., Ananworanich, J., & Ruxrungtham, K. (2010). Long-term efficacy and safety of low-dose ritonavir-boosted atazanavir (ATV/r) 200/100 mg in HIV-infected Thai patients. *Journal of International AIDS Society, 13* (Suppl/4), 60.

Ayikukwei, R. M., Ngare, D., Sidle, J. E., Ayuku, D. O., Baliddawa, J., & Greene, J. Y. (2007). Social and cultural significance of the sexual cleansing ritual and its impact on HIV prevention strategies in Western Kenya. *Sexuality & Culture, 11*(3), 23–50.

Bae, J., Kim, K. -Y., Panuncio, R. L., Choi, N., & Im, S. -B. (2009). Inauguration of the first psychological support center for disaster victims in Korea. *Nursing and Health Sciences, 11*, 351–356.

Barthel, E. R., Pierce, J. R., Goodhue, C. J., Ford, H. R., Grikscheit, T. C., & Upperman, J. S. (2011). Availability of a pediatric trauma center in a disaster surge decreases triage time of the pediatric surge population: A population kinetics model. *Theoretical Biology and Medical Modeling, 8*(38), 1–32.

Beydoun, H. A., al-Sahab, B., Beydoun, M. A., & Tamim, H. (2010). Intimate partner violence as a risk factor for postpartum depression among Canadian women in the maternity experience survey. *Annals of Epidemiology, 20*, 575–583.

Bhandarwar, A. H., Bakhshi, G. D., Tayade, M. B., Borisa, A. D., Thadeshwar, N. R., & Gandhi, S. S. (2011). *British Journal of Surgery.* [Epub ahead of print].

Boscarino, J. A. (2011). Introduction to special issue commemorating the 10th anniversary of September 11, 2001. *International Journal of Emergency Mental Health, 13*(2), 65–67.

Boscarino, J. A., & Adams, R. E. (2008). Overview of findings from the World Trade Center disaster outcome study: Recommendations for future research after exposure to psychological trauma. *International Journal of Emergency Mental Health, 10*(4), 275–290.

Bryant, R. A., Ekasawin, S., Chakrabhand, S., Suwanmitri, S., Duangchun, O., & Chantaluckwong, T. (2011). A randomized controlled effectiveness trial of cognitive behavior therapy for post-traumatic stress disorder in terrorist-affected people in Thailand. *World Psychiatry, 10*, 205–209.

Burkle, F. M., Argent, A. C., & Kisson, N. (2011). The reality of pediatric emergency mass critical care in the developing world. *Pediatric Critical Care Medicine, 12*(6-Suppl), S169–S179.

Centers for Disease Control and Prevention. (2006). *Strategies for clinical management of MRSA in the community: Summary of an experts' meeting convened by the Centers for Disease Control and Prevention.* Retrieved from www.cdc.gov/mrsa/pdf/MRSA-Strategies-ExpMtgSummary-2006.pdf.

Centers for Disease Control and Prevention. (2010a). *Diagnosis and testing of MRSA infections.* Retrieved from www.cdc.gov/mrsa/diagnosis/index.html#reporting.

Centers for Disease Control and Prevention. (2010b). *10 essentials of public health services.* Retrieved from www.cdc.gov/nphpsp/essentialservices.html.

Centers for Disease Control and Prevention. (2011a). *MRSA and the workplace.* Retrieved from www.cdc.gov/niosh/topics/mrsa/.

Centers for Disease Control and Prevention. (2011b). *Bioterrorism rapid response information.* Retrieved from http://beprepared california.ca.gov/EPO/Partners/HealthcareProviders/ForHealthcare Providers/PracticeGuidelinesFactSheets/BioterrorismPreparedness/BioterrorismRapidResponseInformation.htm.

Centers for Disease Control and Prevention. (2012a). *Global health programs: International Micronutrient Malnutrition Prevention and Control Program (IMMPaCT).* Retrieved from www.cdc.gov/global health/programs/IMMPaCT.htm.

Centers for Disease Control and Prevention. (2012b). *Protect yourself from MRSA.* Retrieved from www.cdc.gov/Features/MRSAin Healthcare/.

Centers for Disease Control and Prevention. (2012c). *Violence prevention.* Retrieved from www.cdc.gov/violenceprevention/.

Centers for Disease Control and Prevention. (2012d). *Bioterrorism overview.* Retrieved from www.bt.cdc.gov/bioterrorism/overview.asp.

Centers for Disease Control and Prevention. (2012e). *Anthrax: What you need to know.* Retrieved from www.bt.cdc.gov/agent/anthrax/needtoknow.asp.

Centers for Disease Control and Prevention. (2012f). *Anthrax Q & A: Vaccination.* Retrieved from www.bt.cdc.gov/agent/anthrax/faq/vaccination.asp.

Centers for Disease Control and Prevention. (2012g). *Smallpox vaccines.* Retrieved from www.bt.cdc.gov/agent/smallpox/vaccination/vaccine.asp.

Centers for Disease Control and Prevention. (2012h). *Side effects of smallpox vaccination.* Retrieved from www.bt.cdc.gov/agent/small pox/vaccination/reactions-vacc-public.asp.

Centers for Disease Control and Prevention. (2012i). *Small pox diagnosis.* Retrieved from www.bt.cdc.gov/agent/smallpox/diagnosis/pdf/poxalgorithm1-5-12.pdf.

Centers for Disease Control and Prevention. (2012j). *Emergency preparedness and response.* Retrieved from www.bt.cdc.gov/disasters/.

Central Intelligence Agency. (2012a). *Country comparisons: Life expectancy at birth.* Retrieved from www.cia.gov/library/publications/the-world-factbook//rankorder/2102rank.html.

Central Intelligence Agency. (2012b). *Country comparison: HIV/AIDS—adult prevalence rate.* Retrieved from www.cia.gov/library/publications/the-world-factbook/rankorder/2155rank.html.

Chitlaru, T., Altboum, Z., Reuveny, S., & Shafferman, A. (2011). Progress and novel strategies in vaccine development and treatment of anthrax. *Immunological Reviews, 239*(1), 221–236. doi:10.1111/j.1600-065X.2010.00969.x.

Clements, K., & Schumacher, J. A. (2010). Perceptual biases in social cognition as potential moderators of the relationship between alcohol and intimate partner violence: A review. *Aggression and Violent Behavior, 15*, 357–368.

Epstein, H., & Jewkes, R. (2009). The myth of the virgin rape myth. *Lancet, 374*(9699), 1419.

Fekete, T. (2007). Emerging infections: What you need to know, Part 1. *Consultant, 47*(12), 1013–1016.

Fowler, K. A., & Westen, D. (2011). Subtyping male perpetrators of intimate partner violence. *Journal of Interpersonal Violence, 26*(4), 607–639.

Gribble, K. D., & Berry, N. (2011). Emergency preparedness for those who care for infants in developed country contexts. *International Breastfeeding Journal, 6*(16). Retrieved from www.international breastfeedingjournal.com/content/pdf/1746-4358-6-16.pdf.

Hussain, A., Weisaeth, L., & Heir, T. (2011). Psychiatric disorders and functional impairment among disaster victims after exposure to a natural disaster: A population based study. *Journal of Affective Disorders, 128*(1-2), 135–141.

Inter-Agency Standing Committee Gender Sub-Working Group (2009). *Sex and age disaggregated data in humanitarian action: SADD project.* New York: Author.

Kallen, A. J., Yi, M., Bulens, S., Reingold, A., Petit, S., Gershman, K., et al. (2010). Health care-associated invasive MRSA infections, 2005-2008. *Journal of the American Medical Association, 304*(6), 641–648. doi:10.1001/jama.2010.1115.

Kar, N. (2009). Natural disasters in developing countries: Mental health issues. *Indian Journal of Medical Science, 63*(8), 327–329.

Kaya, Y., & Cook, K. J. (2010). A cross-national analysis of physical intimate partner violence against women. *International Journal of Comparative Sociology, 51*(6), 423–444. doi:10.1177/0020715210386155.

Khoury, N. M., Kaiser, B. N., Keys, H. M., Brewster, A. R., & Kohrt, B. A. (2012). Explanatory models and mental health treatment: Is vodou an obstacle to psychiatric treatment in rural Haiti? *Culture, Medicine, and Psychiatry.* Apr 28. [Epub ahead of print]. Retrieved from www.ncbi.nlm.nih.gov/pubmed?term=Khoury%20NM%5B Author%5D&;cauthor=true&cauthor_uid=22544545.

Kirkland, E. B., & Adams, B. B. (2008). Methicillin-resistant *Staphylococcus aureus* and athletes. *Journal of the American Academy of Dermatology, 59*(3), 494–502.

Kouadio, I. K., Aljunid, S., Kamigaki, T., Hammad, K., & Oshitani, H. (2012). *Expert Review of Anti-infective Therapy, 10*(1), 95–104.

Leppäkoski, T., Astedt-Kurki, P., & Paavilainen, E. (2010). Identification of women exposed to acute physical intimate partner violence in an emergency department setting in Finland. *Scandinavian Journal of Caring Sciences, 24*, 638–647.

Malungo, J. R. S. (2001). Sexual cleansing (Kusalazya) and levirate marriage (Kunjilila mung'anda) in the era of AIDS: Changes in perceptions and practices in Zambia. *Social Science & Medicine, 53*(3), 371–382.

Mann, J. R., & Takyi, B. K. (2009). Autonomy, dependence or culture: Examining the impact of resources and socio-cultural processes on attitudes towards intimate partner violence in Ghana, Africa. *Journal of Family Violence, 24*, 323–335. doi:10.1007/s10896-009-9232-9.

Mazurana, D., Benelli, P., Gupta, H., & Walker, P. (2011). *Sex and age matter: Improving humanitarian response in emergencies.* Medford, MA: Feinstein International Center, Tufts University.

Meyer, S. (2010). Seeking help to protect the children? The influence of children on women's decisions to seek help when experiencing intimate partner violence. *Journal of Family Violence, 25*, 713–725. doi:10.1007/s10896-010-9329-1.

Mtibo, C., Kennedy, N., & Umar, E. (2011). Explanations for child sexual abuse given by convicted offenders in Malawi: No evidence for "HIV cleansing." *Child Abuse & Neglect, 35*(2), 142–146.

Murray, L., & Burnham, G. (2009). Understanding childhood sexual abuse in Africa. *Lancet, 373*(9679), 1924–1926.

Napoleoni, L. (2010). *Terrorism and the economy: How the war on terror is bankrupting the world.* New York: Seven Stories Press.

Oluga, M., Kiragu, S., Mohamed, M., & Walli, S. (2010). 'Deceptive' cultural practices that sabotage HIV/AIDS education in Tanzania and Kenya. *Journal of Moral Education, 39*(3), 365–380.

Peralta, R. L., Tuttle, L., & Steele, J. L. (2010). At the intersection of interpersonal violence, masculinity, and alcohol use: The experiences of heterosexual male perpetrators of intimate partner violence. *Violence Against Women, 16*(4), 387–409.

Perencevich, E. N., & Diekema, D. J. (2010). Decline in invasive MRSA infection: Where to go from here? *Journal of the American Medical Association, 304*(6), 687–689. doi:10.1001/jama.2010.1125.

Piyasil, V., Ketumarn, P., Prubrukarn, R., Ularntinon, S., Sitdhiraksa, N., Pithayaratsathien, N., et al. (2011). Post-traumatic stress disorder in children after the tsunami disaster in Thailand: A 5-year follow-up. *Journal of Medical Association of Thailand* (Suppl. 3), S138–S144.

Purnell, L. D. (2008). Transcultural diversity and health care. In L. D. Purnell & B. J. Paulanka (Eds.), *Transcultural health care: A culturally competent approach* (pp. 1–18). Philadelphia: F.A. Davis.

Robson, A. (2009, April). Male cleansers for hire. *New Internationalist Magazine, 421.* Retrieved from www.newint.org/columns/currents/2009/04/01/kenya/.

Rose, N., Hughes, Ali S., & Jones, L. (2011). Interrating mental health into primary health care settings after an emergency: Lessons for Haiti. *Intervention, 9*(3), 211–224.

Ross, R. (2012, April). *Social support as a mediator of the effects of intimate partner violence (IPV) on depression and physical health among OB/GYN patients in Thailand.* Dearborn, MI: A paper presented at the 36th Annual MNRS Research Conference.

Ross, R., Sawatphanit, W., & Zeller, R. (2009a). Depressive symptoms among HIV-positive pregnant women in Thailand. *Journal of Nursing Scholarship, 41*(4), 344–350.

Ross, R., Roller, C. G., Rusk, T., Martsolf, D. S., & Draucker, C. B. (2009b). The Satellite sexual violence assessment and care guide. *Women's Health Care, 8*(11), 25–31.

Ross, R., Draucker, C. B., Martsolf, D. S., Adamle, K., Chiang-Hanisko, L., & Lewandowski, W. (2010). The bridge: Providing nursing care for survivors of sexual violence. *Journal of the American Academy of Nurse Practitioner, 22*, 1–8.

Ross, R., Sawatphanit, W., Mizuno, M., & Takeo, K. (2011). Depressive symptoms among HIV-positive postpartum women in Thailand. *Archives of Psychiatric Nursing, 25*(1), 36–42.

Ross, R., Sawatphanit, W., Suwansujarid, T., Stidham, A. W., & Drew, D. (in press). The effect of telephone support on depressive symptoms among HIV-positive pregnant women in Thailand: A mixed-methods study. *Journal of Association of Nurses in AIDS Care.*

Schlievert, P. M., Nemeth, K. A., Davis, C. C., Peterson, M. L., & Jones, B. E. (2010). *Staphylococcus aureus* exotoxins are present in vivo in tampons. *Clinical Vaccine Immunology, 17*(5), 722–727. doi:10.1128/CVI.00483-09.

Sedighi, I., Moez, H. J., & Alikhani, M. Y. (2011). Nasal carriage of methicillin resistant Staphylococcus aureus and their antibiotic susceptibility patterns in children attending day-care centers. *Acta Microbiologica et Immunologica Hungarica, 58*(3), 227–234.

Sri-Aroon, P., Chusongsang, P., Chusongsang, Y., Pornpimol, S., Butraporn, P., & Lohachit, C. (2010). Snails and trematode infection after Indian Ocean tsunami in Phang_nga proice, southern Thailand. *Southest Asian Journal of Tropical Medicine and Public Health, 41*(1), 48–60.

United Nations Children's Fund. (2012). *The Baby-Friendly Hospital Initiative.* Retrieved from www.unicef.org/programme/breast feeding/baby.htm.

United Nations International Strategy for Disaster Reduction. (2012). 2011: Record year for economic losses. *Evidence, 4,* 1.

United Nations Programme on HIV and AIDS. (2011a). *World AIDS Day report.* Retrieved from www.unaids.org/en/media/unaids/contentassets/documents/. unaidspublication/2011/JC2216_WorldAIDSday_report_2011_en.pdf.

United Nations Programme on HIV and AIDS. (2011b). *Getting to zero: UNAIDS strategies2011–2015.* Retrieved from www.unaids.org/en/media/unaids/contentassets/.documents/unaidspublication/2010/JC2034_UNAIDS_Strategy_en.pdf.

Vonarx, N. (2011). Haitian vodou as a health care system: Between magic, religion, and medicine. *Alternative Therapies in Health and Medicine, 17*(5), 44–51.

Wahlstrom, L., Michelsen, H., Schulman, A., & Backheden, M. (2009). Psychological distress and sick leave in Swedish survivors of the 2004 tsunami: A comparison with a population sample. *Journal of Nervous and Mental Disease, 197*(12), 918–922.

Waxman, D. (2011). Living with terror, not living in terror: The impact of chronic terrorism on Israeli society. *Perspectives on Terrorism, 5*(5-6), 4–26.

Welner, E. (2011). Research issues for nursing and midwifery contributions in emergencies. *Prehospital & Disaster Medicine, 26*(2), 109–113.

World Health Organization. (2000). *Turning the tide of malnutrition: Responding to the challenge of the 21st century.* Geneva, Switzerland: WHO. 2000 (WHO/NHD/00.7).

World Health Organization (2004). Serious childhood problems in countries with limited resources: Background book on management of the child with a serious infection or severe malnutrition. Geneva.

World Health Organization. (2008). *Challenges.* Retrieved from www.who.int/nutrition/en/print.html.

World Health Organization. (2010). *Preventing intimate partner and sexual violence against women: Taking action and generating evidence.* Retrieved from www.who.int/violence_injury_prevention/publications/violence/9789241564007_eng.pdf.

World Health Organization. (2011a). *Global status report on noncommunicable diseases 2010.* Retrieved from www.who.int/nmh/publications/ncd_report_full_en.pdf.

World Health Organization. (2011b). *The WHO child growth standards.* Retrieved from www.who.int/childgrowth/standards/en/.

World Health Organization. (2011c). *Violence and injury prevention and disability (VIP).* Retrieved from www.who.int/violence_injury_prevention/violence/en/.

World Health Organization. (2012a). *Obesity and overweight.* Retrieved from www.who.int/mediacentre/factsheets/fs311/en/.

World Health Organization. (2012b). *Violence.* Retrieved from www.who.int/topics/violence/en/.

World Health Organization. (2012c). *Definition and typology of violence.* Retrieved from www.who.int/violenceprevention/approach/definition/en/index.html.

World Health Organization. (2012d). *Suicide prevention (SUPRE).* Retrieved from www.who.int/mental_health/prevention/suicide/suicideprevent/en/.

World Health Organization. (2012e). *Mental health.* Retrieved from www.who.int/mental_health/prevention/suicide_rates/en/index.html#.

World Health Organization. (2012f). *Suicide prevention (SUPRE).* Retrieved from www.who.int/mental_health/prevention/suicide/suicideprevent/en/.

World Health Organization. (2012g). *Epidemic intelligence—systematic event detection.* Retrieved from www.who.int/csr/alertresponse/epidemicintelligence/en/index.html.

World Health Organization. (2012h). *What are the international health regulations?* Retrieved from www.who.int/features/qa/39/en/index.html.

World Health Organization/United Nations Children's Fund. (2009). *Child growth standards and the identification of severe acute malnutrition in infants and children.* Retrieved from www.who.int/nutrition/publications/severemalnutrition/9789241598163_eng.pdf.

World Hunger Education Service. (2012). *2011 World hunger and poverty facts and statistics.* Retrieved from www.worldhunger.org/articles/Learn/world%20hunger%20facts%202002.htm.

Page numbers followed by *f* indicates figures; *t*, indicates tables; *b*, indicates boxes.

Community *(Continued)*
  infant development affected by, 418
  interaction of, 183
  nurse's role in health of, 179–181
  nursing process and, 178–179
  nursing process evaluation with, 191–193
  nursing process implementation for, 191
  nutritional-metabolic pattern of, 184
  planning with, 189–191
  risk factors for, 183–184
  roles-relationship pattern and, 140, 186
  self-perception–self-concept pattern of, 185–186
  sexuality-reproductive pattern of, 186
  sleep-rest pattern of, 185
  sources of information about, 182
  strengths of, 188, 188t
  structure of, 182–183
  support of, for pregnant female, 380
  systems theory for framework on, 182–183
  values-belief pattern of, 186
  young adult development affected by, 557
Community-associated methicillin-resistant *Staphylococcus aureus*, 624
Community-based care, 15
Community guide, screening and, 210–212
Community health nurse, 584
Community outcomes, 189
Community preventive services, 196
Community resources, screening and, 200–202
Competency, proxy decision-making and, 115
Complementary and alternative medicine (CAM), 2b. *See also* Complementary and alternative strategies
  Affordable Care Act and, 323–324
  clinical practice guidelines for, 321, 323b
  definition of, 320–321
  effectiveness of, 330–332
  evaluation of, 322b
  safety of, 330–332
  traditional medicine *versus*, 323b
  website information for, 331b
Complementary and alternative strategies, 319–334
  effectiveness of, 330–332
  nursing interventions for, 324–330
  safety of, 330–332
  website information for, 331b
Complementary and alternative therapy
  ethnic minority populations and, 30b
  stress management with, 306–307
Complementary therapy, definition of, 320–321
Compliance, exercise program and, 286–288
Computer games, school-age child development and, 504–505
Computer learning, health teaching by, 224–225
Computer use, limits on, for toddler, 435
Conception, 352
Concierge care, 57
Concierge practice, 57–58
Concrete operation, school-age child development and, 489
Concrete thinking, preschool child development and, 458
Conditioned-play audiometry, toddler's hearing screened with, 437
Condom, sexually transmitted disease prevention and, 552–553

Confidentiality, 116–117
Confrontation, constructive, effective communication and, 95–96
Congenital defect, 353, 554
Congenital rubella syndrome, 543
Congregate Nutrition Services Program, 247
Consequentialism, 105–106
Conservation, school-age child development and, 489
Constipation
  in middle-age adult, 563–564, 571
  nutrition deficiency as cause of, 231t
  in older adult, 597
Consultant, nurse as, 16
Continuing care retirement community, 615
Contraception
  counseling for, 550
  emergency, 550–551
  overview of methods of, 551t
  USPSTF recommended services for, 208b
  young adult use of, 550
Control, sense of, school-age child development and, 493
Cool-down period, exercise and, 282
Copayment, definition of, 56b
Coping
  adolescent stress and, 525b
  effective, 314–316
    care plan for, 315b–316b
    case study of, 315b
  function of, 141
  ineffective, care plan for, 475b
  older adult and, 606
  preschool child development and, 465–466
  primary appraisal of, 303
  secondary appraisal of, 303
  strategy for, 141–142
    school-age child's use of, 496, 496t
  stress management with, 298, 310
Coping-stress tolerance pattern, 141–142
  adolescent development and, 525–526
  community assessment and, 186
  description of, 130t
  family assessment and, 164
  infant development and, 408
  middle-age adult health and, 579–580
  older adult health and, 606–607
  pregnancy assessment and, 362b, 372
  preschool child development and, 465–466
  school-age child development and, 495–497
  toddler development and, 441
  young adult development and, 553–554
Coronary artery disease
  in Arab Americans, 27
  in female, 144b
  in young adult, 538–540
Coronary heart disease (CHD), 248
  diet and, 231
  exercise following, 284–286
  nutrition guidelines and, 238
  risk factors for, 268–271
Corticosteroids, stress response and, 300–301
Cost-benefit ratio, screening and, 203–204
Cost-effectiveness, screening and, 204
Cost-efficiency, screening and, 204
Cost sharing, definition of, 56b
Counseling. *See* Health counseling

Countertransference, communication barriers caused by, 96–97
Course of action, determination of, 122
CRAFFT, adolescent substance abuse screening with, 530b
Crib, safety standards for, 410
Crime rate, community self-perception and, 185–186
Critical thinking, health education and, 214b–215b
Cross-training, 279
CRS. *See* Congenital rubella syndrome
Cultural competence, 25–26
  care of pregnant woman and, 380–381
  family nursing diagnosis and, 170
  health care delivery and, 7b
  older adult health care and, 615
Culturally competent care, 38
  functional health pattern assessment and, 131
  nursing roles in, 381b
Culture, 24–25
  adolescent development affected by, 531
  communication and, 97b
  definition of, 24
  development affected by, 345
  fetal health and, 360
  food and, 239b
  functional health pattern assessment affected by, 132
  health teaching affected by, 222b
  human immunodeficiency virus education and prevention affected by, 625
  infant development affected by, 419
  middle-age adult health affected by, 582
  pregnancy affected by, 380–381
  preschool child development and, 473
  school-age child development and, 504
  school-age child health beliefs and, 482–483
  toddler development affected by, 445
  veracity of health information and, 118
  young adult development and, 554–555
Culture Care Diversity and Universality theory, 38
Cupping, description of, 440b
Curandero, 31, 328
CVD. *See* Cardiovascular disease (CVD)
Cyberbullying, 527
Cycling, benefits of, 281–282
Cystic fibrosis, in preschool child, 453
Cytomegalovirus, 373t
  fetus affected by, 374
  in young adult, 551–552

D

DALY. *See* Disability Adjusted Life Year (DALY)
Dance therapy, 327
DASH program, 236–238, 250–251
Data
  analysis of, 187–188
  collection and analysis of, 143–145
  community health and, 178
  demographic, 182–183
  environmental, 182
  family, analysis of, 166–170
  guidelines for analysis of, 187–188
  measurement, 182
  organization of, 186–187
Data collection, methods of, 181–182

National Heart, Lung and Blood Institute, 250–251
National Institute on Aging, 614–615
National Institute for Occupational Health and Safety, 585
National Institute of Nursing Research, 16
National Institute on Minority Health and Health Disparities, 37
National Institutes of Health (NIH), 37, 60b, 63, 240
National League for Nursing, response to emerging populations by, 38
National Occupational Research Agenda, 585
National Partnership for Action to End Health Disparities, 37–38
National Prevention, Health Promotion, and Public Health Council, 52
National Prevention Council, 207
National Prevention Strategy, 206–209, 210f, 323–324
National School Breakfast Program (NSBP), 244–246
National School Lunch Program (NSLP), 244–246
National Survey of Children's Health, 153–155
Native American, 33–34. *See also* American Indian/Alaska Native
  health care access for, 34
  health issues of, 33–34
  health promotion for, example of, 634b
  as minority population, 23
  obesity in, 34
  pregnancy and childbirth values of, 356t
Native Hawaiians, as percentage of Asian American population, 28
Natural disaster, 630–632
  preparedness for, 631
  response to, 631
Natural products, complementary and alternative strategies and, 325
Naturopathy, 324–325
Navajo, health promotion for, example of, 634b
NCCAM. *See* National Center for Complementary and Alternative Medicine (NCCAM)
NCEP. *See* National Cholesterol Education Program (NCEP)
Nearsightedness, in school-age child, 490
Neighborhood, family health affected by, 165
Neonatal care, in Black/African American population, 32
Neonate, siblings of, 371b
Nervous system
  growth and development of, through life cycle, 337t–342t
  preschool child development and, 451
  relaxation effect on, 305–306
  stress response and, 300–301
Netherlands
  health care cost per capita in, 59f
  health care total expenditures in, 66f
Neural tube defect (NTD), 364
Neuroblastoma, 417, 472
Neuroendocrine system, effect of exercise on, 277–278
Neurolinguistic programming, 326–327
Neuromuscular therapy, 326

Newborn. *See also* Infant
  reflexes in, 392–393
  transition of fetus to, 359–360
NHANES. *See* National Health and Nutrition Examination Survey (NHANES)
NIA. *See* National Institute on Aging
Niacin, toxicity of, 241
Nicotine
  effects of, 582
  pregnancy affected by, 378
Nicotine replacement therapy, pregnancy and, 379b
Night terrors, 436, 457
Nightingale, Florence, 50
Nightmares, preschool child and, 457
NIH. *See* National Institutes of Health (NIH)
NINR. *See* National Institute of Nursing Research
Nitrogen dioxide, health effects of, 416t
NLN. *See* National League for Nursing
No Child Left Behind Act, 506
Nocturnal emissions, adolescent development and, 518
Noise pollution, 555, 581
Noncompliance, health behavior and, 220
Nondiet movement, 257b
Nonmaleficence, 118
Norepinephrine, stress response and, 300
North American Nursing Diagnosis Association International (NANDA-I)
  nursing diagnosis and, 144b
  nursing diagnosis definition from, 129
  taxonomy of, 129, 143
Norway
  health care cost per capita in, 59f
  health care total expenditures in, 66f
Noun, effective communication and use of, 96
NP. *See* Nurse practitioner
NPS. *See* National Prevention Strategy
NTD. *See* Neural tube defect (NTD)
Nurse
  acute care, 612–614
  advanced practice. *See* Advanced practice nurse
  advocate role of, 15, 110, 180, 634
  assessment by, 129t
  care manager role of, 15–16
  code of ethics for, 105b
  communication barriers for, 96
  communication strategies for, 87b
  community, 191
    homelessness and, 37
    role of, 179–181
  community health, 179–181, 584
  consultant role of, 16, 16
  core role of, 16
  cultural competency for, 26b
  as deliverer of services, 16
  as educator, 16
  emotional and spiritual reconnecting for, 331b
  family assessment by, 150–151
  as genetic counselor, 107b
  healer role of, 16
  as health counselor, 215
  health education responsibility of, 215–221
  health literacy and, 217
  health policy influenced by, 180–181
  health promotion role of, 15–17, 50

Nurse *(Continued)*
  home care, 614
  long-term care, 614
  occupational health, 584
  political involvement of, 180
  pregnancy education from, 355
  prejudice in, 381
  presence of, 330
  role of
    in combating homelessness, 408
    in community screening, 209–210
    in family assessment, 151
    in family health promotion, 173t
    in health care change, 62
    in health care policy, 421
    in infant health care promotion, 422–425
    during labor, 359
  school (*See* School nurse)
  self-disclosure by, 84–85
  statistics on, 70
  stereotyping by, 381
  stress management strategy for, 306b
  teaching and organizing skills for, 226
  unintentional harm by, 118
  values of, client values and, 82, 82b
Nurse anesthetist, statistics on, 70
Nurse midwife, statistics on, 70
Nurse practitioner
  health care delivery by, 54–55
  history of, 54–55
  statistics on, 70
Nurse Professional Advisory Committee, 63
Nurses Strategic Action Team (N-STAT), 180
Nursing
  assessment in, 129t
  "being there" and "being with" in, 330, 330t
  code of ethics for, 104
  communication in, 87
  community, system theory and, 178–179
  concept of care in, 108
  cross-cultural, 420b
  cultural competency in, 26b, 381b, 420b
  definition of, 128
  future of, 63b
  health education and, 215–221
  health promotion in, 14
  holistic, 320, 324
  presence in, 330
  response to emerging populations by, 38–41
  responsibility in, 109–111
  role of, in health care change, 62
  transcultural, 38
Nursing: Scope and Standards of Practice, 215
Nursing center, health care delivery through, 54–55
Nursing diagnosis
  classification systems for, 144b
  community, 188–189
  definition of, 129
  family, 170
  family analysis and, 166–170
  format of, 143
  variables in, 144–145
Nursing home
  assessment of, 612t–613t
  risk of falls in, 608b